CONTEMPORARY NURSING KNOWLEDGE

Analysis and Evaluation of Nursing Models and Theories

CONTEMPORARY NURSING KNOWLEDGE

Analysis and Evaluation of Nursing Models and Theories

SECOND EDITION

JACQUELINE FAWCETT, PhD, FAAN

F.A. Davis Company • Philadelphia

F. A. Davis Company
1915 Arch Street
Philadelphia, PA 19103
www.fadavis.com

Printed in the United States of America

Last digit indicates print number: 10 9 8 7 6 5 4 3 2

Acquisitions Editor: Joanne P. DaCunha, RN, MSN
Developmental Editor: Kristin L. Kern
Production Editor: Jessica Howie Martin
Design Manager: Joan Wendt

As new scientific information becomes available through basic and clinical research, recommended treatments and drug therapies undergo changes. The author and publisher have done everything possible to make this book accurate, up to date, and in accord with accepted standards at the time of publication. The author, editors, and publisher are not responsible for errors or omissions or for consequences from application of the book, and make no warranty, expressed or implied, in regard to the contents of the book. Any practice described in this book should be applied by the reader in accordance with professional standards of care used in regard to the unique circumstances that may apply in each situation. The reader is advised always to check product information (package inserts) for changes and new information regarding dose and contraindications before administering any drug. Caution is especially urged when using new or infrequently ordered drugs.

Library of Congress Cataloging-in-Publication Data

Fawcett, Jacqueline.
  Contemporary nursing knowledge : analysis and evaluation of nursing models
and theories / Jacqueline Fawcett. — 2nd ed.
    p. cm.
  Combines the content from the author's previous books titled: Analysis and
evaluation of conceptual models of nursing.
  Includes bibliographical references and index.
  ISBN 10: 0-8036-1194-3   ISBN 13: 978-0-8036-1194-8
  1. Nursing models. 2. Nursing models—Evaluation. I. Fawcett, Jacqueline.
Analysis and evaluation of conceptual models of nursing. II. Title.
  [DNLM: 1. Models, Nursing. 2. Nursing Theory. WY 100 F278c 2005]
RT84.5.F393 2005
610.73—dc22

2004017695

Preface

As we continue to be challenged by the organization and financing of the contemporary health care system, as well as a worldwide nursing shortage, the need to articulate what nursing is and can be has never been more critical. Conceptual models of nursing and nursing theories provide clear answers to questions about what nursing is, what nursing can be, and how what nursing is and can be influences what nurses do—or should do. Conceptual models of nursing and nursing theories also provide:

- Answers for nurse educators, who continue to seek better ways to prepare students for current and future trends in health services.
- Answers for nurse researchers, who continue to seek ways to identify the phenomena of central interest to nursing and to design studies that reflect nursing's distinctive perspective of people in matters of health.
- Answers for nurse administrators, who continue to seek ways to organize the delivery of nursing services in an efficient and effective manner and to document the quality of nursing practice.
- Answers for practicing nurses, who continue to seek ways to improve the quality of people's lives.

This edition of the book is the culmination of years of thinking, talking, and writing about the structure and nature of contemporary nursing knowledge. It was written for all nurses and nursing students who are interested in the development of nursing knowledge and the use of that knowledge to guide nursing research, education, administration, and practice. Although some reviewers have indicated that the book is most appropriate for graduate students, others, with whom I agree, insist that the book also is a valuable resource for undergraduates.

As with my previous books, this edition represents an ongoing attempt to clarify the confusion between conceptual models and theories that remains in the nursing literature. To that end, the book includes the abstract and general formulations of nursing knowledge that are called conceptual models of nursing, the somewhat less abstract and general formulations that are called grand nursing theories, and the relatively concrete and specific formulations that are called middle-range nursing theories. The book continues the tradition of my previous books by presenting the most up-to-date information available about the major conceptual models of nursing and nursing theories.

The book is divided into four parts. Part One introduces the reader to the world of contemporary nursing knowledge, as formalized in conceptual models of nursing and nursing theories. Chapter 1 acquaints the reader with what I regard as the components of contemporary nursing knowledge, including the metaparadigm, philosophies, conceptual models, theories, and empirical indicators. That chapter contains my latest thinking about the nature and structure of contemporary nursing knowledge, with attention to the current dialogue about nursing knowledge and others' critique of my work in this area. That chapter also contains discussion about my understanding of the relations among the metaparadigm of nursing, philosophies of nursing, conceptual models of nursing, nursing theories, and empirical indicators. Chapter 2 acquaints the reader with strategies used to implement conceptual models of nursing and nursing theories in the real world of nursing practice.

Part Two introduces the reader to conceptual models of nursing. Chapter 3 presents a distinctive framework for the analysis and evaluation of nursing models. Chapters 4, 5, 6, 7, 8, 9, and 10 illustrate the application of the analysis and evaluation framework, and acquaint the reader with the most widely recognized and most frequently cited nursing models. In these chapters, the reader enters the world of nursing as conceptualized by Dorothy Johnson in her Behavioral System Model, Imogene King in her Conceptual System, Myra Levine in her Conservation Model, Betty Neuman in her Systems Model, Dorothea Orem in her Self-Care Framework, Martha Rogers in her Science of Unitary Human Beings, and Sister Callista Roy in her Adaptation Model.

Part Three introduces the reader to nursing theories. Chapter 11 presents a distinctive framework for the analysis and evaluation of nursing theories. Chapters 12, 13, 14, 15, and, 16 illustrate the application of the analysis and evaluation framework. These chapters acquaint the reader with the most widely recognized and most frequently cited nursing theories. In Chapters 12 and 13, the reader learns about two grand theories—Margaret Newman's Theory of Health as Expanding Consciousness and Rosemarie Parse's Theory of Human Becoming. In Chapters 14, 15, and 16, the reader learns about three middle-range theories—Ida Jean Orlando's Theory of the Deliberative Nursing Process, Hildegard Peplau's Theory of Interpersonal Relations, and Jean Watson's Theory of Human Caring.

Part Four introduces the reader to the possibilities of nursing knowledge now and in the future. Chapter 17, the last chapter in this book, offers the reader an opportunity to consider a strategy to promote the integration of nursing knowledge with nursing research and nursing practice and to explore what the discipline of nursing could become.

The Appendix includes such resources as societies devoted to the advancement of particular conceptual models of nursing and nursing theories, internet home pages, audio and video productions, CD-ROMs, and strategies for computer-based literature searches.

Chapters 1 and 2 should be read before the remainder of the book. Those first two chapters provide the background that facilitates understanding of the place of conceptual models of nursing and nursing theories in the structural hierarchy of contemporary nursing knowledge and the use of nursing models and theories in nursing practice. Chapter 17 may be read at any time. That chapter should be of special interest to nurses who are committed to fostering the survival and advancement of the discipline of nursing. Chapter 3 should be read before the subsequent chapters dealing with various conceptual models of nursing. Similarly, Chapter 11 should be read before the chapters dealing with various nursing grand theories and middle-range theories.

I have continued to draw from my extensive personal conversations and correspondence with the authors of the conceptual models and theories, as well as from the vast literature about the conceptual models and theories, with emphasis on the latest primary source materials. The book includes comprehensive reviews of virtually all of the published literature dealing with the use of conceptual models of nursing and nursing theories as guides for nursing practice, nursing administration, nursing education, and nursing research. In an attempt to make the primary source material and other literature in each chapter more immediately accessible to readers, tables are used to present practice and research methodologies for each conceptual model and theory, as well as lists of uses of each conceptual model and theory as a guide for nursing research, nursing education, nursing administration, and nursing practice.
Special features of this edition include:

- An overview and list of key terms for each chapter
- A nursing process format, that is, a nursing practice methodology, for each conceptual model and theory
- Rules or guidelines for nursing research, education, administration, and practice for each conceptual model
- A research methodology for each nursing theory
- Strategies for the implementation of each conceptual model and theory in nursing practice
- A bibliography for each chapter on a searchable compact disk (CD)

Readers are encouraged to use this book in combination with the primary source materials that are cited in the chapter references and bibliographies. The references at the end of each chapter are supplemented by the CD, which comes with the book. The CD includes comprehensive bibliographies of all relevant literature that could be located through hand and computer-assisted searches of an extensive list of nursing books and journals. The bibliographies include citations to the full range of debate and dialogue about contemporary nursing knowledge and each conceptual model and theory. The bibliographies for each of the conceptual model and theory chapters are divided into several sections: Primary Sources; Commentary: General; Commentary: Research; Commentary: Education; Commentary: Administration; Commentary: Practice; Research; Doctoral Dissertations; Master's Theses; Research Instruments and Nursing Practice Tools; Education; Administration; and Practice. I continue to be grateful to the authors of the conceptual models and theories and to my students and colleagues for the many citations of relevant publications they have shared with me. I also continue to be grateful to the staff of the Cumulative Index of Nursing and Allied Health Literature (CINAHL) for their technical support, which has greatly facilitated my searches of the literature over the years.

I believe that a hallmark of this book, as with my other books about nursing conceptual models and theories, is the care that I take to present an accurate account of each conceptual model and theory as it was developed by its author rather then to draw from secondary analyses and other interpretations of the author's work. Each of those chapters includes many direct quotes from the author's original works. The quotations reflect the author's writing style and the language customs at the time of publication of the particular book or journal article. Despite some criticism from colleagues, I have decided to continue to not alter pronouns to reflect current gender-neutral language. However, in this edition I have endeavored to replace the word "clinical" with "practice" or "nursing practice," in response to contemporary dialogue about "clinical" referring solely to bedside nursing. A chapter about Leininger's Theory of Culture Care Diversity and Universality has not been included in this edition of the book because I was unable to obtain permission for the quotations needed for the analysis of the theory. Readers interested in that grand theory are referred to the many books, book chapters, and journal articles by Madeleine Leininger and those who use her theory to guide their research and practice.

The success of the previous editions of my books, as well as the successive editions of other texts dealing with conceptual models of nursing and nursing theories, indicates continued interest of nurses in *nursing* knowledge, rather than in the knowledge of other disciplines. Nurses are especially fortunate to be able to select as a guide for their work any one of many conceptual models and theories that already have been used widely. Thus, novice users can draw from the experiences of those who forged the way. And, experienced users can expand their work by examining what other users have done.

The works included in the book continue, in my opinion, to be the major representatives of conceptual models and nursing theories in the contemporary nursing literature. Readers who are interested in understanding the content of other nursing conceptual models and theories are encouraged to use the frameworks for analysis and evaluation of conceptual models of nursing and nursing theories that are given in Chapters 3 and 11. My sincere hope is that this book will stimulate readers to continue their study of conceptual models and nursing theories and to adopt explicit conceptual-theoretical-empirical structures for their nursing activities.

The writing of this edition of the book was, as always, a consuming, stimulating, and growth-enhancing experience. Thanks for its preparation is owed to many people. First, I continue to be indebted to Dorothy Johnson, Imogene King, Myra Levine, Betty Neuman, Dorothea Orem, Martha Rogers, Callista Roy, Margaret Newman, Ida Jean Orlando, Rosemarie Parse, Hildegard Peplau, and Jean Watson, whose efforts to continuously refine the knowledge base for the discipline of nursing made this book possible. My conversations and written communications with those nursing pioneers have greatly enhanced my understanding and appreciation of all the obstacles they have overcome to share their visions of nursing with us. I am greatly saddened by the deaths of Martha Rogers, Myra Levine, Hildegard Peplau, and Dorothy Johnson, but am heartened by the works of other nurses who have had the courage to advance Martha's, Myra's, Hildegard's, and Dorothy's ideas about nursing. I also am indebted to those courageous researchers, educators, administrators, and clinicians who stand for *nursing* by using explicit conceptual models of nursing and nursing theories to guide their work.

Moreover, I am indebted to my students and colleagues at the universities where I have been privileged to teach, serve as a visiting faculty member, or to present a paper, for their support, intellectual challenges, and constructive criticism. In addition, I am indebted to Joanne DaCunha of F.A. Davis Company for her encouragement and the time spent discussing the content and design of this edition of the book. Finally, I continue to be indebted to Robert G. Martone of F.A. Davis Company for his steadfast support of my work.

My gratitude to my husband, John S. Fawcett, for his unconditional love and support throughout our 40 years of marriage and his understanding of the demands of my nursing career, continues to extend to the infinite universe.

Jacqueline Fawcett
Waldoboro, Maine

Credits

Quotations and Figure 2–2 from Rogers, M.E. (1992). *Transformative learning: Understanding and facilitating nurses' learning of nursing conceptual frameworks.* Unpublished manuscript, were reprinted with permission of M.E. Rogers. Copyright 1991.

Quotations from King, I.M. (1971). *Toward a theory for nursing* were reprinted with permission of Imogene M. King.

Quotations and Figures 5–1 and 5–2 from King, I.M. (1981). *A theory for nursing* were reprinted with permission of Imogene M. King.

Quotations from Levine, M.E. (1973). *Introduction to clinical nursing* (2nd ed.) were reprinted with permission of F.A. Davis Company, Publishers. Copyright 1973.

Quotations from Schaefer, K.M., & Pond, J.B. (Eds.). (1991). *Levine's conservation model* were reprinted with permission of F.A. Davis Company, Publishers. Copyright 1991.

Quotations and Figure 7–1 from Neuman, B., & Fawcett, J. (Eds.) (2002). *The Neuman systems model* (4th ed.) were reprinted with permission of Prentice-Hall, Inc., Upper Saddle River, N.J. Copyright 1995.

Quotations from Newman, M.A. (1994). *Health as expanding consciousness* were reprinted by permission of Margaret A. Newman.

Quotations from Orem, D.E. (2001). *Nursing: Concepts of practice* (6th ed.) were reprinted with permission of Elsevier. Copyright 2001.

A portion of Table 14–1 was adapted from Orlando, I.J. (1972). *The discipline and teaching of nursing process (An evaluation study)* (pp. 60–61, 63) with permission of Ida Jean Orlando Pelletier.

Quotations from Orlando, I.J. (1972). *The discipline and teaching of nursing process (An evaluation study)* were reprinted with permission of the Ida Jean Orlando Pelletier.

Quotations from Parker, M.E. (2001). *Nursing theories and nursing practice* were reprinted with permission of F.A. Davis Company, Publishers. Copyright 2001.

Quotations from Parse, R.R. (1998). *The human becoming school of thought: A perspective for nurses and other health professionals.* Copyright 1998 by Sage Publications. Reprinted by permission of Sage Publications, Inc.

Quotations from Parse, R.R. (2003). *Community: A human becoming perspective* were reprinted with permission from Jones and Bartlett Publishers, Sudbury, MA. *www.jbpub.com.*

Quotations from Rogers, M.E. (1970). *An introduction to the theoretical basis of nursing* were reprinted with permission of F.A. Davis Company, Publishers. Copyright 1970.

Table 9–1 was adapted from Rogers, M.E. (1990). Nursing: Science of unitary, irreducible, human beings: Update 1990. In E.A.M. Barrett (Ed.), *Visions of Rogers' science-based nursing* (p. 9) with permission of the National League for Nursing. Copyright 1990 by the

Contents

Part four
NURSING KNOWLEDGE IN THE 21ST CENTURY   587

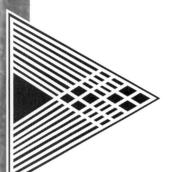

Part One

STRUCTURE AND USE OF NURSING KNOWLEDGE

Part One introduces the reader to the world of contemporary nursing knowledge, as formalized in conceptual models of nursing and nursing theories.

Chapter 1 introduces the reader to the components of contemporary nursing knowledge, including the metaparadigm, philosophies, conceptual models, theories, and empirical indicators.

Chapter 2 introduces the reader to the strategies used to implement conceptual models of nursing and nursing theories in the real world of nursing practice.

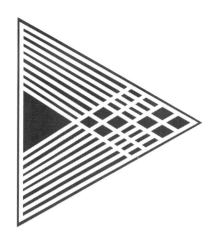

Chapter **1**

The Structure of Contemporary Nursing Knowledge

This book celebrates nursing as a distinct discipline, and this chapter lays the groundwork for the remainder of the book. Here, a structural holarchy of contemporary nursing knowledge is identified and described. Each component of the structure—metaparadigm, philosophies, conceptual models, theories, and empirical indicators—is defined and its functions are delineated. Then the distinctions between the components are discussed, with special emphasis on the differences between conceptual models and theories and the need to view and use these two knowledge components in different ways.

Overview

The structural holarchy differentiates the various components of contemporary nursing knowledge according to their level of abstraction. Drawing from Wilber (1998), the term holarchy, rather than hierarchy, is used to denote components that are whole within themselves but also part of a larger whole. In this case, the larger whole is contemporary nursing knowledge. Thus, each component of contemporary nursing knowledge is a complete whole but also part of a larger whole. The components of the structural holarchy of contemporary nursing knowledge are listed here. Each component is defined and described in detail in this chapter.

Key Terms

STRUCTURAL HOLARCHY OF CONTEMPORARY
  NURSING KNOWLEDGE

CONCEPTS
PROPOSITIONS
    Nonrelational Proposition
    Relational Proposition
METAPARADIGM
    Requirements for a Metaparadigm
    Metaparadigm of Nursing
PHILOSOPHIES
    Philosophies of Nursing
    Reaction World View
    Reciprocal Interaction World View
    Simultaneous Action World View
    Categories of Nursing Knowledge
CONCEPTUAL MODELS
    Conceptual Models of Nursing
THEORIES
    Grand Theory
    Middle-Range Theory
    Nursing Theories
EMPIRICAL INDICATORS

STRUCTURAL HOLARCHY OF CONTEMPORARY NURSING KNOWLEDGE

An analysis of the terminology used to describe contemporary nursing knowledge led to the identification of five components: metaparadigm, philosophies, conceptual models, theories, and empirical indicators (Fawcett, 1993a; King & Fawcett, 1997a). These components comprise the unique disciplinary knowledge of nursing, the knowledge that separates nursing from other disciplines (Parse, 2001b).

The **STRUCTURAL HOLARCHY OF CONTEMPORARY NURSING KNOWLEDGE** is *a heuristic device that places the five components of contemporary nursing knowledge into a holarchy based on level of abstraction.* Similar structures have long been proposed by scholars in other disciplines, including Feigl (1970), Gibbs (1972), and Margenau (1972). The holarchy is depicted in Figure 1–1.

CONCEPTS AND PROPOSITIONS

With the exception of empirical indicators, the components of the structural holarchy are composed of concepts and propositions. Empirical indicators measure concepts. A **CONCEPT** is *a word or phrase that summarizes ideas, observations, and experiences.* Concepts are tools that provide mental images that can facilitate communication about and understanding of phenomena; they are not real entities (Babbie, 1998). A **PROPOSITION** is *a statement* about a concept or a statement of the relation between two or more concepts. A **nonrelational proposition** is a description or definition of a concept. A nonrelational proposition that states the meaning of a concept is called a constitutive definition. A nonrelational proposition that states how a concept is observed or measured is called an operational definition. A **relational proposition** asserts the relation, or linkage, between two or more concepts.

METAPARADIGM

The first component of the structural holarchy of contemporary nursing knowledge is the **METAPARADIGM** (see Fig. 1–1). A metaparadigm is defined as *the global concepts that identify the phenomena of central interest to a discipline, the global propositions that describe the concepts, and the global propositions that state the relations between or among the concepts.* That definition of a metaparadigm indicates that concepts alone are not sufficient to identify the subject matter of a discipline or to delineate the boundary for the subject matter of interest to a discipline (Kim, 2000b). Rather, both concepts and propositions about those concepts are required to specify the subject matter.

The metaparadigm is the most abstract component of the structural holarchy of contemporary nursing knowledge, and acts as "an encapsulating unit, or framework, within which the more restricted … structures develop" (Eckberg & Hill, 1979, p. 927). The concepts and propositions of a metaparadigm are admittedly extremely global and provide no definitive direction for activities such as research and practice. That is to be expected because the metaparadigm "is the broadest consensus within a discipline. It provides the general parameters of the field and gives scientists a broad orientation from which to work" (Hardy, 1978, p. 38). In other words, a metaparadigm "is concerned with general issues of the subject matter of a discipline … [that is,] what a discipline is concerned with" (Kim, 2000b, p. 28).

The idea for a component of knowledge called the metaparadigm arose in discussion of the multiple meanings Kuhn (1962) had given to the term, paradigm. Masterman (1970) pointed out that one meaning reflected a metaphysical rather than scientific notion or entity and labeled that meaning as the metaparadigm.

FUNCTIONS OF A METAPARADIGM

Articulation of the metaparadigm brings a certain unity to a discipline. In particular, specification of the concepts and propositions that represent the subject matter of a disci-

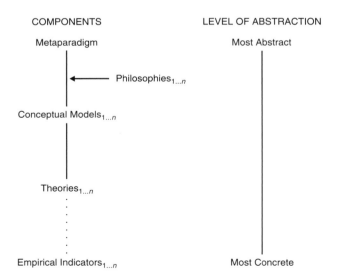

COMPONENTS   LEVEL OF ABSTRACTION

Metaparadigm — Most Abstract

Philosophies$_{1…n}$

Conceptual Models$_{1…n}$

Theories$_{1…n}$

Empirical Indicators$_{1…n}$ — Most Concrete

FIG. 1–1. The structural holarchy of contemporary nursing knowledge: components and levels of abstraction.

pline permits the members of that discipline to communicate to members of other disciplines and to the general public what is of special interest to that discipline. In other words, the members of the discipline can say, "This is who we are and what our work is all about." Similarly, specification of the metaparadigm concepts and propositions facilitates communication of what the discipline is *not* about. Thus, members of the discipline can also say, "This is what we are not about." In addition, the boundary imposed by the metaparadigm concepts and propositions helps the members of the discipline identify the focus of their knowledge development activities and to have confidence that what they are doing is, indeed, consistent with the subject matter of the discipline. Members of the discipline then can say, "This is *why* I am doing what I am doing."

The functions of a metaparadigm, then, are to summarize the intellectual and social missions of a discipline and place a boundary on the subject matter of that discipline (Kim, 1989, 2000b). Those functions are reflected in four **requirements for a metaparadigm** (Fawcett, 1992, 1996.). The four requirements, which pertain to the metaparadigm of any discipline, are:

1. The metaparadigm must *identify a domain that is distinctive from the domains of other disciplines*. That requirement is fulfilled only when the concepts and propositions represent a unique perspective for inquiry and practice.
2. The metaparadigm must *encompass all phenomena of interest to the discipline in a parsimonious manner*. That requirement is fulfilled only if the concepts and propositions are global and if there are no redundancies in concepts or propositions.
3. The metaparadigm must *be perspective neutral*. That requirement is fulfilled only if the concepts and propositions do *not* represent a specific perspective, that is, a specific paradigm or conceptual model, or a combination of perspectives.
4. The metaparadigm must *be international in scope and substance*. That requirement, which is a corollary of the third requirement, is fulfilled only if the concepts and propositions do not reflect particular national, cultural, or ethnic beliefs and values.

The requirements indicate that the metaparadigm of any discipline must be highly abstract and general; concise and free of redundant terms; not aligned with a particular disciplinary frame of reference; and free of particular national, cultural, or ethnic group orientations. Conflicting opinions have been voiced about the third requirement, which calls for perspective neutrality. That means that the metaparadigm should not embrace a particular philosophic stance or conceptual model within a discipline that encompasses diverse philosophies and conceptual models. Thorne and colleagues' (1998) comments reflect support for the third requirement. They stated, "We believe that our central concepts ought to be characterized by paradigmatic neutrality" (p. 1265). In contrast, Cody (1996) and Malinski (1996) maintained that the third requirement is not appropriate or even possible. Cody asserted that the requirement is "an impossibility recognized throughout post-positivist philosophy of science and the human science perspectives of hermeneutics and critical theory" (p. 98). Malinski (1996) pointed out that the metaparadigm of nursing, at least the proposal put forth by Fawcett (1996), "is reflective of the dominant view in nursing," which she labeled as the totality paradigm (p. 101). The differences of opinion about the requirement of perspective neutrality indicate that consensus about the appropriate requirements for the metaparadigm of any discipline does not yet exist within nursing.

METAPARADIGM OF NURSING

Origins of the Metaparadigm of Nursing

The notion of a metaparadigm was introduced in the nursing literature in the late 1970s, when nursing, as Rawnsley (1996) pointed out, "was struggling to defend its self-nominated status as a science" (p. 102). In 1978, Hardy defined a metaparadigm as "a gestalt … within a discipline" (p. 38). Hardy went on to explain that a metaparadigm "provides a map which guides the scientist thought the vast, generally incomprehensible world. It gives focus to scientific endeavor which would not be present if scientists were to explore randomly" (p. 38). Hardy likened the metaparadigm to the "prevailing paradigm in a discipline [that] presents a general orientation … that holds the commitment and consensus of the scientists in a particular discipline" (p. 39). In 1979, Smith used the term metaparadigm to refer to a way of organizing and structuring nursing phenomena. Later, Fawcett (1984b) defined the metaparadigm of any discipline as "a statement or group of statements identifying its relevant phenomena" (p. 84). She claimed that a review of the literature of the time revealed "evidence supporting the existence of a metaparadigm of nursing" (p. 84).

Proposals for the Nursing Metaparadigm

Fawcett (1978) initially identified what she called the central units of nursing as person, environment, health, and nursing. She then formalized those units as the concepts of the metaparadigm of nursing in her article, "The

Metaparadigm of Nursing: Present Status and Future Refinements" (Fawcett, 1984b). In her response to Fawcett's paper, Brodie (1984) pointed out, "Fawcett's metaparadigm can be viewed as an evolution of a nursing metaparadigm and an organization of the growth of nursing knowledge rather than as a completed and finalized product" (p. 87). Indeed, several proposals for different versions of the nursing metaparadigm have emerged since that time. Some of those proposals were in direct response to Fawcett's proposal, whereas others were offered without reference to Fawcett's work.

The Fawcett Proposal. The metaparadigm of nursing is made up of four concepts, four nonrelational propositions, and four relational propositions. The four concepts are:

- Human beings
- Environment
- Health
- Nursing

The nonrelational propositions of the metaparadigm of nursing, which are constitutive definitions of the metaparadigm concepts, are:

- The metaparadigm concept of human beings refers to the individuals, if individuals are recognized in a culture, as well as to the families, communities, and other groups or aggregates who are participants in nursing.
- The metaparadigm concept of environment refers to human beings' significant others and physical surroundings, as well as to the settings in which nursing occurs, which range from private homes to health-care facilities to society as a whole. The metaparadigm concept of environment also refers to all local, regional, national, and worldwide cultural, social, political, and economic conditions that are associated with human beings' health.
- The metaparadigm concept of health refers to human processes of living and dying.
- The metaparadigm concept of nursing refers to the definition of nursing, the actions taken by nurses on behalf of or in conjunction with human beings, and the goals or outcomes of nursing actions. Nursing actions are viewed as a mutual process between the participants in nursing and nurses. The process encompasses activities that are frequently referred to as assessment, labeling, planning, intervention, and evaluation.

The relational propositions of the metaparadigm of nursing, which were drawn from work by Donaldson and Crowley (1978) and Gortner (1980), assert the linkages between metaparadigm concepts. Relational proposition 1 links the concepts human beings and health. Relational proposition 2 links the concepts human beings and environment. Relational proposition 3 links the concepts health and nursing. Relational proposition 4 links the concepts human beings, environment, and health. The relational propositions are:

1. The discipline of nursing is concerned with the principles and laws that govern human processes of living and dying.
2. The discipline of nursing is concerned with the patterning of human health experiences within the context of the environment.
3. The discipline of nursing is concerned with the nursing actions or processes that are beneficial to human beings.
4. The discipline of nursing is concerned with the human processes of living and dying, recognizing that human beings are in a continuous relationship with their environments.

This version of Fawcett's proposal for the metaparadigm of nursing represents refinement of earlier versions (Fawcett, 1984b, 2000). One refinement is the modification in the labels for the four metaparadigm concepts. The frequently cited metaparadigm concepts of person, environment, health, and nursing were a modification of labels for four concepts induced from the conceptual frameworks of baccalaureate programs accredited by the National League for Nursing. The original concepts were labeled man, society, health, and nursing (Yura & Torres, 1975). "Man" was changed to "person" to avoid gender-specific language, and "society" was changed to "environment" to more fully encompass phenomena relevant to the person (Fawcett, 1978). In the current version of the metaparadigm, "person" has been changed to "human beings." That change was made in response to Leininger's (1991a) argument that the concept of person is not a globally understood term. She stated, "From an anthropological and nursing perspective, the use of the term person has serious problems when used transculturally, as many non-Western cultures do not focus on or believe in the concept person, and often there is no linguistic term for person in a culture, family and institutions being more prominent" (pp. 39–40). Furthermore, the change may address Jacobs' (2001) charge that "The concept of 'person' … is … insufficient to represent all of nursing's phenomena, thereby indicating a continued need for clarification and validation" (pp. 19–20).

Another refinement is the inclusion of a constitutive definition for each metaparadigm concept. Continued refinement of the constitutive definitions of the metaparadigm concepts has resulted in the current reference to the human being as a participant in nursing, rather than a recipient of nursing. In keeping with Thorne and colleagues' (1998) belief that the central concepts of nursing should be characterized by "common currency" (p. 1265), that change was made to better reflect the contemporary emphasis on human beings as active participants in the process of nursing, rather than passive recipients of pronouncements by and ministrations from nurses. Continued refinement also has resulted in an expansion of the constitutive definition for the metaparadigm concept environment. That refinement was made to better reflect the multitude of environmental conditions that are relevant in nursing (Kleffel, 1991). In addition, refinement of the constitutive definitions has resulted in a change in the definition of health from states of wellness and illness to human processes of living and dying. That change was made in response to Cody's (1996) point that Fawcett's "view of health as a 'state' that can be characterized on a continuum from 'high-level wellness to terminal illness' ... [implies that] everyone's health ultimately and unavoidably reaches abysmal levels in the natural dying process" (p. 98). Other refinements include the formalization of metaparadigm themes into relational propositions and the addition of the fourth relational proposition.

The current version of the metaparadigm meets the four requirements for a metaparadigm given earlier in this chapter. In particular, the four metaparadigm concepts—human beings, environment, health, nursing—generally are regarded as the central or domain concepts of nursing (Flaskerud & Halloran, 1980; Jennings, 1987; Thorne et al., 1998; Wagner, 1986). Additional support for the centrality of the four metaparadigm concepts comes from the successful use of those concepts as a schema for analysis of the content of conceptual models of nursing and nursing theories (Fitzpatrick & Whall, 1996; George, 2002; Marriner-Tomey & Alligood, 2002; Parker, 2001). The utility of the four metaparadigm concepts is underscored by their adoption, with appropriate modifications, as the concepts of the metaparadigm of dental hygiene. More specifically, Darby and Walsh (1994) identified the concepts of the dental hygiene metaparadigm as client, environment, health/oral health, and dental hygiene actions.

The relational propositions of the metaparadigm provide a unique perspective of the metaparadigm concepts that helps to distinguish nursing from other disciplines. Relational propositions 1, 2, and 3 represent recurrent themes identified in the writings of Florence Nightingale and many other nursing scholars and practitioners of the 19th and 20th centuries. Donaldson and Crowley (1978) commented, "These themes suggest boundaries of an area for systematic [i]nquiry and theory development with potential for making the nature of the discipline of nursing more explicit than it is at present" (p. 113). Relational proposition 4, according to Donaldson and Crowley (1978), "evolve[d] from the practical aim of optimizing of human environments for health" (p. 119).

Taken together, the four concepts, the four nonrelational propositions, and the four relational propositions identify the unique focus of the discipline of nursing and encompass all relevant phenomena in a parsimonious manner. The concepts and propositions are perspective-neutral because they do not reflect a specific philosophic perspective, a specific paradigm, or a specific conceptual model. Furthermore, the metaparadigm concepts and propositions do not reflect the beliefs and values of nurses from any one country or culture and, therefore, are international in scope and substance.

There is, however, some debate about whether the Fawcett proposal does, indeed, meet the four requirements for a metaparadigm. Cody (1996) explicitly rejected the claim that the Fawcett proposal meets the four requirements for a metaparadigm. He maintained that it is unreasonable to believe that "four common, global, disparate concepts, all studied by many disciplines, [could] reflect the unique focus of nursing at all, much less 'parsimoniously'" (p. 97). Continuing, Cody maintained that Fawcett's claim that the four metaparadigm concepts meet the requirement of encompassing all phenomena of interest to nursing is "manifestly unfounded in light of the many prevalent concepts in nursing that are excluded" (pp. 97–98). In addition, Cody maintained that it is impossible to present a perspective-neutral statement of disciplinary phenomena. Inasmuch as Cody most likely does not recognize a need for a disciplinary metaparadigm, it is not surprising that he did not offer an alternative to Fawcett's proposal.

Morse (1996) maintained that the four metaparadigm concepts in the Fawcett proposal "were—and remain—inappropriate and restrictive" (p. 78). She did not, however, explain in what way the concepts were inappropriate and restrictive, nor did she offer a different set of concepts.

Leininger (1991a) questioned the inclusion of environment as a metaparadigm concept. She commented, "While environment is very important to nursing, I would contend it is certainly not unique to nursing, and there are very few nurses who have advanced formal study and are prepared to study a large number of different types of environments or ecological niches worldwide" (p. 40). Cody (1996) also noted that environment is not unique to nursing, because it is studied by other disciplines. Leininger and Cody have failed to acknowledge that the point of the inclusion of the concept environment in Fawcett's proposal for the metaparadigm was to provide a context for human beings, to indicate that participants in nursing actions are surrounded by and interact or engage in mutual process with other people and the social structure.

Although Leininger (1991a) did not reject the inclusion of health as a metaparadigm concept, she did point out that the concept is not unique to nursing, because many disciplines study health. Cody (1996) also pointed out that health is studied by many other disciplines. Several scholars have addressed the metaparadigm concept of nursing. Their comments indicate that the inclusion of this concept does not meet the requirement of a metaparadigm for parsimony. Conway (1985, 1989) responded directly to Fawcett's (1984) initial presentation of the metaparadigm of nursing. She claimed that the term "nursing" represents the discipline or the profession and is not an appropriate metaparadigm concept because it creates a tautology. Rawnsley (1996), who agreed with Conway's position, explained, "The rationale, or perhaps the rationalization, that [the] inclusion [of nursing] within the metaparadigm refers primarily to nursing actions and activities rather than to a holistic worldview is simply unacceptable. Such a myopic view of our discipline only reinforces reductionist themes that have too long stymied creative scientific breakthroughs" (p. 104).

Leininger (1988) also rejected the metaparadigm concept of nursing in Fawcett's proposal. She commented, "[I] reject the idea that nursing … explain[s] nursing, for one cannot explain nor predict the same phenomenon one is studying. Nursing is the phenomenon to be explained" (p. 154). Adding to her position in a later publication, Leininger (1991b) noted, "Nursing cannot be logically used to explain and predict nursing. The [concept] is a redundancy and a contradiction to explain the same phenomenon being studied by the same concept" (p. 152).

Cody (1996) and Meleis (1997) also regarded the inclusion of nursing in the metaparadigm of nursing as a tautology. Meleis commented, "It would be an instance of tautological conceptualizing to define nursing by all the concepts and then include nursing as one of the concepts" (p. 106). Cody (1996) asserted, "One could hardly ask for a better textbook example of a tautology" (p. 98).

Kolcaba and Kolcaba (1991) rejected the charge of a tautology. They noted that, inasmuch as the metaparadigm concept of nursing stands for nursing activities or actions, a tautology is not created. Furthermore, other scholars view nursing as a distinct phenomenon of interest to the discipline. Kim (1987) identified nursing as a component of two domains of nursing knowledge. She regarded nursing as the central feature of the practice domain and as an essential component of the client-nurse domain. In addition, Barnum (1998) identified nursing acts as a commonplace, that is, a topic addressed by most nursing theories; Newman (1983) included nursing as an action in her list of nursing metaparadigm concepts; and King (1984) found that nursing was a central concept in the philosophies of nursing education of several nursing education programs. That finding suggests that the concept nursing is an important concept that should be included in the metaparadigm. Furthermore, Thorne and her colleagues (1998)

maintained that nursing should remain a part of the metaparadigm. They stated, "We contend that the term 'nursing' ought to remain prominent in our lexicon, whatever additional terms we use to qualify it, and that its essence retain the notion of an expert service that we can offer to individuals and society" (p. 1265).

The Newman Proposal. Newman (1983) proposed that the term "client" be one of four concepts that make up the domain of nursing, or what she called the nursing paradigm. Elaborating, she stated, "The phenomena of our concern—the major components of the nursing paradigm—are nursing (as an action), client (human being), environment (of the client and of the nurse-client), and health" (p. 388). Newman also offered what can be considered a relational proposition for her version of the nursing metaparadigm: "The nurse interacts with the client and the environment for the purpose of facilitating the health of the client" (p. 388). Despite its merits, Newman's proposal is not completely perspective-neutral, in that the concept of client reflects a particular view of human beings. Indeed, Levine (1996) maintained that "client" means "follower," which is not an appropriate perspective for participants in nursing processes.

The King Proposal. King's (1984) review of the philosophies of a representative sample of National League for Nursing accredited nursing education programs in the United States revealed nine concepts: man, health, environment, social systems, role, perceptions, interpersonal relations, nursing, and God. King found that not all nine concepts were evident in the philosophies of all schools included in the sample. She recommended that the most frequently cited concepts could represent the domain of nursing. Those concepts are man, health, role, and social systems.

King's proposal falls short of meeting all requirements for a metaparadigm. First, the inclusion of role and social systems reflects a sociologic orientation to nursing. Second, the elimination of environment and nursing results in a narrow view of the domain, and leaves a list of concepts more closely aligned with the discipline of social work (Ben-Sira, 1987) than with nursing.

The Kim Proposal. Kim (1987, 1997, 2000b) identified four domains of nursing knowledge. The client domain is concerned with the client's essential characteristics, pathologic or abnormal deviations from normal patterns of healthy living, and experiences in the health-care system. Kim (2000a) has proposed that the client domain be viewed as human living, which she conceptualized within three dimensions: living of oneself, living with others, and living in situations. She explained, "By orienting its mission to clients' living rather than limiting its focus to clients' states, nursing can clarify its distinctive role within the community of healthcare providers, formulate client-centered outcomes that are uniquely related to its knowledge-based practice, and ensure public recognition of its distinctive professional contribution in healthcare" (Kim, 2000a, p. 38).

The client-nurse domain focuses on direct contacts, communication, and interactions between the client and the nurse. The practice domain emphasizes the cognitive, behavioral, social, and ethical aspects of professional nursing actions and activities performed in relation to patient care. The environment domain focuses on the physical, social, and symbolic boundaries of the client's environment.

Hinshaw (1987) pointed out that Kim's (1987) proposal work did not include the concept of health, and asked: "Is health a strand that permeates each of the ... domains ... rather than a major separate domain?" (p. 112). Kim (personal communication, October 31, 1986) indicated that the client domain could encompass health. In the most recent version of her proposal, Kim (2000b) has explicitly identified health within the client domain. She explained, "In a holistic posture, phenomena in the domain of client are conceptualized as systems of interlinked elements, either with respect to the nature of human beings or to that of health" (p. 61). Kim's proposal may be regarded as an informative explication of the discipline of nursing. However, her use of the term client for a domain of the discipline introduces a particular perspective, as noted earlier in the discussion of the Newman proposal. Her recent focus on human living may reflect her recognition of that problem and represent an attempt at perspective-neutrality. Rawnsley (2000), however, pointed out that Kim's descriptions of the processes within each of the dimensions of human living reflect a particular perspective.

The Newman, Sime, and Corcoran-Perry Proposal. Newman, Sime, and Corcoran-Perry (1991) claimed that the focus of the discipline of nursing is summarized in the following statement: "Nursing is the study of caring in the human health experience" (p. 3). In a later publication, they asserted, "The theme of caring is sufficiently dominant, when combined with the theme of the human health experience, to be considered as the focus of the discipline" (Newman, Sime, & Corcoran-Perry, 1992, p. vii).

Despite Newman and colleagues' (1992) claims to the contrary, their proposition represents just one frame of reference for nursing and for health. In fact, Newman and her colleagues (1991) ended their initial treatise by maintaining that caring in the human health experience can be most fully elaborated only through a unitary-transformative perspective. Moreover, although Newman et al. (1991) offered their proposition as a single statement that integrates "concepts commonly identified with nursing at the metaparadigm level" (p. 3), and they identified the metaparadigm concepts as person, environment, health, and nursing, their proposition does not include environment. In an attempt to clarify their position, Newman, Sime, and Corcoran-Perry (1992) later stated, "We view the concept of environment as inherent in and inseparable from the integrated focus of caring in the human health experience" (p. vii). Despite that clarification, their proposal is neither sufficiently comprehensive nor perspective-neutral.

The Malloch, Martinez, Nelson, Predeger, Speakman, Steinbinder, and Tracy Proposal. Malloch, Martinez, Nelson, Predeger, Speakman, Steinbinder, and Tracy (1992) suggested a revision of the Newman, Sime, and Corcoran-Perry (1991) statement. Their focus statement is: "Nursing is the study and practice of caring within contexts of the human health experience" (p. vi). Malloch and her colleagues (1992) maintained that their statement extends the focus of the discipline to nursing practice and incorporates the environment by the use of the term contexts. They noted that environment "includes, but is not limited to, culture, community, and ecology" (p. vi). Moreover, they claimed that the use of the term caring brings unity to the metaparadigm concepts of person, environment, health, and nursing. Apparently, they do not regard caring as a particular perspective of nursing. Thus, although the Malloch et al. proposal is sufficiently comprehensive, it is not perspective neutral.

The Leininger, Watson, and Lewis Proposals. Leininger (1995) asserted, "With transcultural nurse knowledge and consumer demands, many nurses are recognizing that human care, health, and environmental cultural context must become the central focus, essence, and dominant domains of nursing knowledge to replace the 'Eastern' four concept metaparadigm" (p. 97). In setting the stage for her proposal, Leininger charged that "a small group of 'Eastern' USA nurse researchers ... declared in nursing publications that nursing's major foci or 'metaparadigm' for the discipline ... would be health, nursing, person, and environment. It was quite clear to me that these nurses blatantly failed to recognize [that] human care, caring, and cultural factors were important phenomena of nursing. It appeared to me and other care scholars that this small elite group was lobbying against the rapidly growing interest in care and transcultural nursing" (p. 96). Leininger's charge regarding lobbying against her ideas by a small, elite group of "Eastern" nurses has no basis—none of the discussions of the metaparadigm concepts have included negative comments about caring or transcultural nursing.

In another publication, Leininger (1990) claimed that "human care/caring [is] the central phenomenon and essence of nursing" (p. 19) and Watson (1990) maintained that "human caring needs to be explicitly incorporated into nursing's metaparadigm" (p. 21). Even more to the point, Leininger (1991a) maintained: "Care is the essence of nursing and the central, dominant, and unifying focus of nursing" (p. 35). She also has claimed that "human care and caring [are] the central, distinct, and dominant foci to explain, interpret, and predict nursing as a discipline and profession" (Leininger, 2002, p. 47). Lewis (2003) asserted, "I believe that caring and healing are core processes of nursing" (p. 37). She went on to explain that she regards caring as "being with others" (p. 37).

Both Leininger and Watson failed to acknowledge that although the term caring is included in several conceptualizations of the discipline of nursing (Morse, Solberg, Neander, Bottorff, & Johnson, 1990), it is not a dominant theme in every conceptualization and, therefore, does not represent a discipline-wide viewpoint (Wilson, 1994). Indeed, caring reflects a particular view of nursing and a particular kind of nursing (Eriksson, 1989). Lewis (2003) acknowledged that point by explaining, "The frame of reference that guides my thinking is aligned with the unitary-transformative perspective (Newman, Sime, & Corcoran-Perry, 1991)" (p. 37). Furthermore, as Swanson (1991) pointed out, although there may be "characteristic behavior patterns that are universal expressions of nurse caring … caring is not uniquely a nursing phenomenon" (p. 165). Lewis (2003) has attempted to identify the unique features or characteristics of caring as being in nursing. She identified four pathways—honoring one another through artistic endeavors, moving beyond ourselves through caring relationships and spirituality, being grounded in our healing environment, and soulful caring consciousness—as the "ubiquitous or unique nature of caring as *being*" (p 38).

Caring behaviors, moreover, may not be generalizable across national and cultural boundaries (Mandelbaum, 1991). And, as Rogers (1992) asserted, "As such, caring does not identify nurses any more than it identifies workers from another field. Everyone needs to care" (p. 33). Rogers (1994b) went on to say, "I don't think nurses care any more than anybody else, or that it's a characteristic any more peculiar to nursing than to any other field. [But caring] does differ among different groups … It is the body of knowledge about the phenomenon of concern that determines the nature of the caring that one is going to demonstrate" (p. 34). Elaborating, Rogers (1994a) added, "Caring is doing, it is practice. Caring is a way of using knowledge" (p. 7). Viewed from a different vantage point, Roper (1994) commented, "I consider that 'care' is implicit in 'nursing' and therefore 'nursing care' is a tautology" (p. 460).

The Meleis Proposal. Meleis (1997) proposed that the central concepts of nursing are nursing client, transitions, interaction, nursing process, environment, nursing therapeutics, and health. She explained, "The nurse interacts (interaction) with a human being in a health/illness situation (nursing client) who is in an integral part of his sociocultural context (environment) and who is in some sort of transition or is anticipating a transition (transition); the nurse/patient interactions are organized around some purpose (nursing process, problem solving, holistic assessment, or caring actions) and the nurse uses some actions (nursing therapeutics) to enhance, bring about, or facilitate health (health)" (p. 106). Meleis and Trangenstein (1994) and Schumacher and Meleis (1994) highlighted the importance and centrality of the concept transitions. In particular, Meleis and Trangenstein (1994) maintained that "the transition experience of clients, families, communities, nurses, and organizations, with health and well-being as a goal and an outcome, meets … the criteria … of an organizing concept that allows for a variety of viewpoints and theories within the discipline of nursing, … [is] not culture bound, and … should help in identifying the focus of the discipline" (p. 255).

Although Meleis' proposal is meritorious, the inclusion of nursing process, nursing therapeutics, and interactions represents a redundancy that can be avoided by use of the single concept, nursing. The inclusion of transitions reflects a particular perspective of human life. Indeed, Meleis and Trangenstein (1994) referred to their discussion of transitions as a "conceptual framework" (p. 258).

The Parse Proposal. Parse (1997) asserted, "The core focus of nursing, the metaparadigm, is the human-universe-health process" (p. 74). She went on to explain that the "hyphens between the words create a … construct incarnating the notion that the study of nursing is the science of the human-universe-health process. Consequently, all nursing knowledge is in some way concerned with this phenomenon" (p. 74).

Parse's proposal has merit in that her use of the term universe extends the environment far beyond the immediate surroundings of human beings and the settings in which nursing occurs. However, her proposal does not explicitly name nursing as a concept of the metaparadigm. That omission is a problem in that many disciplines could be interested in humans, the universe, and health. Furthermore, the meaning Parse ascribed to the hyphens used reflects a particular perspective of the named phenomenon. That is, humans, the universe, and health must be viewed as unitary.

The Thorne, Canam, Dahinten, Hall, Henderson, and Kirkham Proposal. Thorne, Canam, Dahinten, Hall,

Henderson, and Kirkham (1998) presented a proposal for the metaparadigm of nursing that encompasses the four metaparadigm concepts of human beings, environment, health, and nursing but describes those concepts differently. Their proposal states: "Nursing is the study of human health and illness processes. Nursing practice is facilitating, supporting and assisting individuals, families, communities, and/or societies to enhance, maintain and recover health, and to reduce and ameliorate the effects of illness. Nursing's relational practice and science are directed toward the explicit outcome of health related quality of life within the immediate and larger environmental contexts" (p. 12 of on-line full text version of manuscript).

Thorne, Canam, Dahinten, Hall, Henderson, and Kirkham regard their statement as a perspective-neutral proposal that represents a "common core of purpose" (p. 12 of on-line full text version of manuscript). Certainly their proposal has merit, although it does not overcome objections to an inclusion of individuals and also raises questions about whether the inclusion of the terms, health and illness, reflect a particular perspective of health, such as health as dichotomous with illness.

The Jacobs Proposal. Jacobs (2001) proposed that "the central phenomenon of nursing is not health or some sort of restoration of holistic balance and harmony but respect of human dignity" (p. 26). Elaborating, she stated, "The central phenomenon [of nursing] is the respect for or the restoration of human dignity, our being in community, our sea, our moral imperative" (p. 33). One could argue that respect for human dignity is perspective-neutral and international in scope and substance, but it is not necessarily unique to nursing nor does this single idea encompasses all phenomena of interest to the nursing discipline.

The merits of the various proposals for the nursing metaparadigm deserve attention from all nurses, and they should not be regarded as premature closure on an explanation of phenomena of interest to the discipline of nursing. It is anticipated that modifications in the metaparadigm concepts and propositions will continue to be offered as the discipline of nursing evolves. All nurses are urged to offer their proposals so that members of the discipline and the public will better understand what the field of nursing encompasses and how what is studied guides practice. Modifications must, however, fulfill the four requirements for a metaparadigm.

Contemporary Issues Related to the Metaparadigm of Nursing

Many years ago, Brodie (1984) asked, "To whom in the discipline of nursing will the metaparadigm make a valued

and substantial contribution?" (p. 89). Her question has never been explicitly answered. Apparently, nurses have assumed that Donaldson and Crowley's (1978) claim that nursing is a professional discipline was enhanced by the claim of a formal metaparadigm.

Contemporary scholars are, however, raising questions with regard to the need for a metaparadigm of nursing. Rawnsley (1996) acknowledged that although "the word metaparadigm will not easily disappear from nursing's lexicon," nurses should demythologize the power of the metaparadigm over nursing science (p. 105). Cody (1996) implied that there is no need for a metaparadigm of nursing. He claimed, "There is no way to circumscribe all of nursing without leaving some nurses out" (p. 99). Instead, he urged each nurse to be responsible for "identifying the nature and parameters of his or her own view" (p. 99). It is unclear how such an essentially anarchistic view would serve the discipline as a whole. Malinski (1996) also advocated for elimination of the basic idea of a nursing metaparadigm. She asserted, "Perhaps it is time to drop the metaparadigm entirely. The desire to identify some grand, unifying schema for all of nursing is no longer warranted" (p. 100). Malinski went on to point out that given the diversity of contemporary views of nursing, a nursing metaparadigm would have to be "so broad and general as to be relatively meaningless in terms of defining the scope of nursing and providing direction for all of its members" (p. 100). Cody's and Malinski's comments suggest that they may have failed to fully appreciate the global nature of a metaparadigm and the necessity of some means of distinguishing one discipline from another, if for no other reason than to create manageable units with institutions of higher learning, and organize funding agencies and scholarly societies.

Kim (2000b) has offered a stronger rationale for a metaparadigm of nursing than manageable units and organization of agencies and societies. She pointed out that the metaparadigm of nursing is the way in which the professional discipline of nursing delineates and makes public its particular nature and distinguishes itself from the natural, social, and human sciences. Kim also pointed out that public articulation of the metaparadigm of nursing is necessary because the metaparadigm serves as the primary guide for the development of nursing knowledge.

 ## PHILOSOPHIES

The second component of the structural holarchy of contemporary nursing knowledge is the **PHILOSOPHY** (see Fig. 1–1). A philosophy may be defined as *a statement encompassing ontological claims about the phenomena of central interest to a discipline, epistemic claims about how those*

phenomena come to be known, and ethical claims about what the members of a discipline value.

FUNCTION OF A PHILOSOPHY

Philosophies are directed at discovery of knowledge and truth, as well as the identification of what is valuable and important to members of a discipline; philosophic problems focus on the nature of existence, knowledge, morality, reason, and human purpose (McEwen, 2002). The function of a philosophy, then, is to communicate what the members of a discipline believe to be true in relation to the phenomena of interest to that discipline, what they believe about the development of knowledge about those phenomena, and what they value with regard to their actions and practices (Kim, 1989; Salsberry, 1994; Seaver & Cartwright, 1977). In other words, the function of each philosophy is to inform the members of disciplines and the public about the beliefs and values of a particular discipline.

PHILOSOPHIES OF NURSING

Grace (2002) pointed out that philosophies of nursing "attempt to answer the question, 'What is nursing?' as well as a related significant question—'Why is nursing important to human beings?'" (p. 64). In particular, philosophies of nursing encompass ontological and epistemic claims about the phenomena of interest to the discipline of nursing and ethical claims about nursing actions, nursing practices, and the character of individuals who choose to practice nursing (Salsberry, 1994). Ontological claims address "the totality of assumptions about the nature of the world or the portion of reality in question ... [that is,] the nature of being" (Young, Taylor, & McLaughlin-Renpenning, 2001, p. 9). The ontological claims in philosophies of nursing state what is believed about the nature of human beings, the environment, health, and nursing. Epistemic claims address "knowledge itself: what is it, what its properties are, and why it has these properties. [These claims focus on] answers about the properties of truth and falsity, the nature of evidence, and the certainty that evidence produces in scientific knowledge" (Young et al., 2001, p. 10). Epistemic claims in philosophies of nursing provide "some information on how one may come to learn about the world [and] about how the basic phenomena can be known" (Salsberry, 1994, p. 13). Epistemic claims in nursing extend the ontological claims by directing how knowledge about human beings, the environment, health, and nursing is developed.

Ontological and epistemic claims in philosophies of nursing reflect one or more of three contrasting world views: the reaction world view, the reciprocal interaction world view, and the simultaneous action world View (Fawcett, 1993b.). Those three world views emerged from an analysis of five other sets of world views: mechanism and organicism (Ackoff, 1974; Reese & Overton, 1970); change and persistence (Hall, 1981, 1983; Thomae, 1979; Wells & Stryker, 1988); totality and simultaneity (Parse, 1987); particulate-deterministic, interactive-integrative, and unitary-transformative (Newman, 1992); and heuristic and complementarity (Rawnsley, 2003). The different world views lead to different conceptualizations of the metaparadigm concepts, different statements about the nature of the relations between those metaparadigm concepts (Altman & Rogoff, 1987), and different ways to generate and test knowledge about the concepts and their connections.

Reaction World View

This world view, which contains elements of the mechanistic, persistence, totality, and particulate-deterministic world views, has these features:

- *Humans are bio-psycho-social-spiritual beings.* The metaphor is the compartmentalized human being, who is viewed as the sum of discrete biological, psychological, sociological, and spiritual parts.
- *Human beings react to external environmental stimuli in a linear, causal manner.* Human beings are regarded as inherently at rest, responding in a reactive manner to external environmental stimuli. Behavior is considered a linear chain of causes and effects, or stimuli and reactions.
- *Change occurs only for survival and as a consequence of predictable and controllable antecedent conditions.* Change occurs only when human beings must modify behaviors to survive. Consequently, stability is valued. Threats to stability are, however, predictable and controllable if enough is known about the stimuli that would force a change.
- *Only objective phenomena that can be isolated, observed, defined, and measured are studied.* Knowledge is developed only about objective, quantifiable phenomena that can be isolated and observed, defined in a concrete manner, and measured by objective instruments.

Reciprocal Interaction World View

This world view, which is a synthesis of elements from the organismic, simultaneity, totality, change, persistence, and interactive-integrative world views, has these features:

- *Human beings are holistic; parts are viewed only in the context of the whole.* The metaphor is the holistic, interacting human being, who is viewed as an integrated, organized entity not reducible to discrete parts. Although parts are acknowledged, they have meaning only within the context of the whole human being.
- *Human beings are active, and interactions between human beings and their environments are reciprocal.* Human beings are regarded as inherently and spontaneously active. Human beings and the environment interact in a reciprocal manner.
- *Change is a function of multiple antecedent factors, is probabilistic, and may be continuous or may be only for survival.* Changes in behavior occur throughout life as the result of multiple factors within the individual and within the environment. At times, changes are continuous. At other times, persistence or stability reigns and change occurs only to foster survival. The probability of change at any given time can only be estimated.
- *Reality is multidimensional, context dependent, and relative.* Both objective and subjective phenomena are studied through quantitative and qualitative methods of inquiry; emphasis is placed on empirical observations, methodological controls, and inferential data analytic techniques. Knowledge development focuses on both objective phenomena and subjective experiences and is accomplished by means of both quantitative and qualitative methodologies. Multiple dimensions of experience are taken into account, the context of the human being-environment interaction is considered, and the product of knowledge development efforts is regarded as relative to historical time and place. Emphasis always is placed on empirical observations within methodologically controlled situations, and quantitative data typically are analyzed objectively by means of descriptive and inferential statistics.

Simultaneous Action World View

This world view, which combines elements of the organismic, simultaneity, change, and unitary-transformative world views, has these features:

- *Unitary human beings are identified by pattern.* The metaphor is the unitary human being, who is regarded as a holistic, self-organized field. The human being is more than and different from the sum of parts and is recognized through patterns of behavior.
- *Human beings are in mutual rhythmical interchange with their environments.* The human being-environment interchange is a mutual, rhythmical process.
- *Human beings change continuously, unpredictably, and in the direction of more complex self-organization.* Changes

in patterns of behavior occur continuously, unidirectionally, and unpredictably as the human being evolves. Although the patterns are sometimes organized and sometimes disorganized, change ultimately is in the direction of increasing organization of behavioral patterns.

- *The phenomena of interest are personal knowledge and pattern recognition.* Knowledge development emphasizes personal becoming through recognition of patterns. The phenomena of interest are, therefore, human beings' inner experiences, feelings, values, thoughts, and choices.

Newman (2002) regards the diverse world views not as separate realms of knowledge or as competitive bodies of knowledge but rather as ever inclusive. She explained, "Just as relatively theory includes mechanistic theory as special cases, the unitary perspective includes the more particulate view" (p. 3). If Newman's position is accepted, the simultaneous action world view would be the most inclusive, the reaction world view would be a special case of the reciprocal interaction world view, and the reciprocal interaction world view would be a special case of the simultaneous action world view.

Categories of Knowledge

Ontological claims in philosophies of nursing also reflect one or more broad categories of knowledge found in adjunctive disciplines and in nursing. Categories of knowledge from adjunctive disciplines are developmental, systems, and interaction (Johnson, 1974; Reilly, 1975; Riehl & Roy, 1980). Bunkers (Pilkington, Bunkers, Clarke, & Frederickson, 2002) wondered whether there is a category of knowledge that is unique to nursing. Inasmuch as nurse theorists have drawn liberally from other disciplines to create distinctive or unique nursing conceptual models and theories, evidence of a unique category into which nursing knowledge might fit is not evident. Categories of knowledge that have been mentioned in the nursing literature are needs and outcomes (Meleis, 1997); client-focused, person-environment focused, and nursing therapeutics focused (Meleis, 1997); energy fields (Hickman, 1995; Marriner-Tomey, 1989); and intervention, substitution, conservation, sustenance/support, and enhancement (Barnum, 1998). None of these seems particularly unique to nursing. Clearly, Bunkers' question deserves more thought and study.

The various categories of knowledge are "different classes of approaches to understanding the person who is a patient, [so that they] not only call for differing forms of practice toward different objectives, but also point to different kinds of phenomena, suggest different kinds of questions, and lead eventually to dissimilar bodies of knowledge" (Johnson, 1974, p. 376). Each category, then, emphasizes different phenomena and leads to different questions about nursing situations. Consequently, each category fosters development of a different body of knowledge about human beings, the environment, health, and nursing. The characteristics of each category of knowledge are summarized in the following paragraphs.

Developmental Category of Knowledge. The origin of this category of knowledge is the discipline of psychology. In this category:

- Identification of actual and potential developmental problems and delineation of intervention strategies that foster maximum growth and development of people and their environments are emphasized.
- Processes of growth, development, and maturation also are emphasized.
- Change is the major focus, with the assumption made "that there are noticeable differences between the states of a system at different times, that the succession of these states implies the system is heading somewhere, and that there are orderly processes that explain how the system gets from its present state to wherever it is going" (Chin, 1980, p. 30).
- Changes are regarded as directional—the individuals, groups, situations, and events of interest are headed in some direction. The direction of change is: "(a) some goal or end state (developed, mature), (b) the process of becoming (developing, maturing), or (c) the degree of achievement toward some goal or end state (increased development, increase in maturity)" (Chin, 1980, p. 31).
- Different states of human beings are examined over time. Those states frequently are termed stages, levels, phases, or periods of development; they may be quantitatively or qualitatively differentiated from one another. Shifts in state may be either small, nondiscernible steps that eventually are recognized as change, or sudden, cataclysmic changes (Chin, 1980).
- Developmental change is thought to be possible through four different forms of progression: (1) unidirectional development may be postulated, such that "once a stage is worked through, the client system shows continued progression and normally never turns back;" (2) developmental change may take the form of a spiral, so that although return to a previous problem may occur, the problem is dealt with at a higher level; (3) development may be seen as "phases which occur and recur ... where no chronological priority is assigned to each state; there are cycles;" or (4) development may take the form of "a branching out into differentiated forms and processes, each part increasing in its specialization and at the same time acquiring its own autonomy and significance" (Chin, 1980, pp. 31–32).
- Forces are regarded as "causal factors producing devel-

opment and growth" (Chin, 1980, p. 32), and may be viewed as (a) a natural component of human beings undergoing change, (b) a coping response to new situations and environmental factors that leads to growth and development, or (c) internal tensions within a human being that at some time reach a peak and cause a disruption that leads to further growth and development.
- Human beings are assumed to have the inherent potential for change; potentiality may be overt or latent, triggered by internal states or certain environmental conditions.

Systems Category of Knowledge. The origins of this category of knowledge are the disciplines of biology and physics. In this category:

- Identification of actual and potential problems in the function of systems and delineation of intervention strategies that maximize efficient and effective system operation is emphasized; change is of secondary importance.
- A system is defined as "a set of objects together with relationships between the objects and between their attributes" (Hall & Fagen, 1968, p. 83).
- Phenomena are treated "as if there existed organization, interaction, interdependency, and integration of parts and elements" (Chin, 1980, p. 24).
- Systems are viewed as open or closed. An open system "maintains itself in a continuous inflow and outflow, a building up and breaking down of components," [whereas a closed system is] "considered to be isolated from [its] environment" (von Bertalanffy, 1968, p. 39). Open systems continuously import energy in a process called negative entropy or negentropy, so that the system may become more differentiated, more complex, and more ordered. Conversely, closed systems exhibit entropy, such that they move toward increasing disorder. All living organisms are open systems (von Bertalanffy, 1968). Although closed systems therefore do not exist in nature, it sometimes is convenient to view a system as if it did not interact with its environment (Chin, 1980). The artificiality of that view, however, must be taken into account.
- Environment is defined as "The set of all objects a change in whose attributes affects the system and also those objects whose attributes are changed by the behavior of the system" (Hall & Fagen, 1968, p. 83).
- The boundary is the line of demarcation between a system and its environment, "the line forming a closed circle around selected variables, where there is less interchange of energy ... across the line of the circle than within the delimiting circle" (Chin, 1980, p. 24). The placement of the boundary must take all relevant system parts into account. Boundaries may be thought of as

more or less permeable. The greater the boundary permeability, the greater the interchange of energy between the system and its environment.

- Tension, stress, strain, and conflict are the forces that alter system structure. The differences in system parts, as well as the need to adjust to outside disturbances, lead to different amounts of tension within the system (Chin, 1980). Internal tensions arising from the system's structural arrangements are called the stresses and strains of the system (Chin, 1980). Conflict occurs when tensions accumulate and become opposed along the lines of two or more components of the system. Change then occurs to resolve the conflict.

- Systems are assumed to tend to move toward a balance between internal and external forces. "When the balance is thought of as a fixed point or level, it is called 'equilibrium.' 'Steady state,' on the other hand, is the term … used to describe the balanced relationship of parts that is not dependent upon any fixed equilibrium point or level" (Chin, 1980, p. 25). Steady state, which also is referred to as a dynamic equilibrium, is characteristic of living open systems and is maintained by a continuous flow of energy within the system and between the system and its environment (von Bertalanffy, 1968).

- Feedback is the flow of energy between a system and its environment. Systems "are affected by and in turn affect the environment. While affecting the environment, a process we call output, systems gather information about how they are doing. Such information is then fed back into the system as input to guide and steer its operations" (Chin, 1980, p. 27). The feedback process works so that, as open systems interact with their environments, any change in the system is associated with a change in the environment, and vice versa.

Interaction Category of Knowledge. The origin of this category of knowledge is symbolic interactionism, from the discipline of sociology. Symbolic interactionism views human beings "as creatures who define and classify situations, including themselves, and who choose ways of acting toward and within them" (Benoliel, 1977, p. 110), and "postulates that the importance of social life lies in providing [human beings] with language, self-concept, role-taking ability, and other skills" (Heiss, 1976, p. 467). In this category:

- Identification of actual and potential problems in interpersonal relationships and delineation of intervention strategies that promote optimal socialization are emphasized.
- Social acts and relationships between human beings are also emphasized.
- The human being's perceptions of other people, the environment, situations, and events—that is, the awareness

and experience of phenomena—depend on meanings attached to those phenomena. The meanings, or definitions of the situation, determine how human beings behave in a given situation. Human beings actively set goals based on their perceptions of the relevant factors in a given situation, which are derived from social interactions with others.

- Communication is through language, "a system of significant symbols" (Heiss, 1981, p. 5). Communication, therefore, involves the transfer of arbitrary meanings of things from one human being to another. Human beings are thought to actively evaluate communication from others, rather than passively accept their ideas.

- Roles are "prescriptions for behavior which are associated with particular actor-other combinations … the ways we think people of a particular kind ought to act toward various categories of others" (Heiss, 1981, p. 65). Each human being has many different roles, each one providing a behavioral repertoire. Human beings adopt the behaviors associated with a given role, when, through communication, they determine that a given role is called for in a particular situation.

- Self-concept is defined as "the individual's thoughts and feelings about him[her]self" (Heiss, 1981, p. 83). An important aspect of self-concept is self-evaluation, which refers to "our view of how good we are at what we think we are" (Heiss, 1981, p. 83).

Needs Category of Knowledge. This category:

- Focuses on nurses' functions and consideration of the patient in terms of a hierarchy of needs. When patients cannot fulfill their own needs, nursing is required. The function of the nurse is to provide the necessary action to help patients meet their needs. The human being is reduced to a set of needs, and nursing is reduced to a set of functions. Nurses are portrayed as the final decision makers for nursing practice (Meleis, 1997).

Outcomes Category of Knowledge. In this category:

- Emphasis is placed on the outcomes of nursing practice and comprehensive descriptions of the recipient of that practice (Meleis, 1997).

Client-Focused Category of Knowledge. This category:

- Refers to a comprehensive focus on the client as viewed from a nursing perspective (Meleis, 1997).

Person-Environment-Focused Category of Knowledge. In this category:

- Emphasis is placed on the relationships between clients and their environments (Meleis, 1997).

Nursing Therapeutics Category of Knowledge. In this category:

- Emphasis is placed on what nurses should do and under what circumstances they should act (Meleis, 1997).

Energy Fields Category of Knowledge. This category:

- Incorporates the concept of energy (Marriner-Tomey, 1989), and focuses on human beings as energy fields in constant interaction with their environment or the universe (Hickman, 1995).

Intervention Category of Knowledge. This category:

- Emphasizes the nurse's professional actions and decisions and regards the patient as an object of nursing rather than a participant in nursing. Agency, or action, rests with the nurse, who makes the practice decisions and manipulates selected patient or environmental variables to bring about change (Barnum, 1998).

Conservation Category of Knowledge. This category:

- Emphasizes preservation of beneficial aspects of the patient's situation that are threatened by illness or actual or potential problems. Agency rests with the nurse, but he or she acts to conserve the existing capabilities of the patient (Barnum, 1998).

Substitution Category of Knowledge. This category:

- Focuses on provision of substitutes for patient capabilities that cannot be enacted or have been lost. Agency rests with the patient, in that the patient exercises his or her will and physical control to the greatest possible extent. Nursing acts as a substitute for the patient's will or intent when the patient is incapacitated (Barnum, 1998).

Sustenance/Support Category of Knowledge. This category:

- Focuses on helping the patient endure insults to health and supporting the patient while building psychological and physiological coping mechanisms. Required nursing is determined by the extent to which the patient can or cannot cope without assistance in a particular situation (Barnum, 1998).

Enhancement Category of Knowledge. In this category:

- Nursing is regarded as a way to improve the quality of the patient's existence following a health insult. Nursing enables the patient to emerge from a health insult somehow stronger, better, or improved because he or she experienced or overcame the health insult (Barnum, 1998).

The ethical claims in philosophies of nursing address the values "that guide the nurse's relationship with patients/clients, … the character of the persons entering and remaining in the field of nursing … [and] the values that regulate nursing practice" (Salsberry, 1994, p. 18). Ethical claims in nursing are summarized in the dominant collective philosophy of humanism (Gortner, 1990), which emphasizes "humanistic (moral) values of caring and the promotion of individual welfare and rights" (Fry, 1981, p. 5). Ethical claims in nursing also articulate values about "the treatment of others," including the respect that should be accorded human beings "simply for what they are," values about consideration of human dignity when engaging in nursing practice, values about caring, values about autonomy, values about the rights of people to health care, and values about beneficence (Salsberry, 1994, pp. 13–14).

 CONCEPTUAL MODELS

The third component of the structural holarchy of contemporary nursing knowledge is the **CONCEPTUAL MODEL** (see Fig. 1–1). A conceptual model is defined as *a set of relatively abstract and general concepts that address the phenomena of central interest to a discipline, the propositions that broadly describe those concepts, and the propositions that state relatively abstract and general relations between two or more of the concepts.*

The term conceptual model is synonymous with the terms conceptual framework, conceptual system, paradigm, and disciplinary matrix. Conceptual models have existed since people began to think about themselves and their surroundings. They now exist in all areas of life and in all disciplines. Indeed, everything that human beings see, hear, read, and experience is filtered through the cognitive lens of some conceptual frame of reference (Kalideen, 1993; Lachman, 1993).

The concepts of a conceptual model are so abstract and general that they are not directly observed in the real world, nor are they limited to any particular individual, group, situation, or event. Human adaptive system is an example of a conceptual model concept (Roy & Andrews, 1999). It can refer to several types of human systems, including individuals, families, groups, communities, and entire societies.

The propositions of a conceptual model also are so abstract and general that they are not amenable to direct empirical observation or test. Nonrelational propositions found in conceptual models are general descriptions or constitutive definitions of the conceptual model concepts. Because conceptual model concepts are so abstract, their constitutive definitions typically are broad. Adaptation level, for example, is defined as "a changing point influenced by the demands of the situation and the internal resources [of the human adaptive system, including] capabilities, hopes, dreams, aspirations, motivations, and all that makes humans constantly move toward mastery" (Roy & Andrews, 1999, p. 33). Moreover, because the concepts are so abstract, nonrelational propositions that are operational definitions, that is, propositions that state how the concepts are empirically observed or measured, are not found in conceptual models, nor should they be expected.

The relational propositions of a conceptual model state the relations between conceptual model concepts in a relatively abstract and general manner. They are exemplified by the following statement: "Adaptation level affects the human [adaptive] system's ability to respond positively in a situation" (Roy & Andrews, 1999, p. 36).

Conceptual models evolve from the empirical observations and intuitive insights of scholars or from deductions that creatively combine ideas from several fields of inquiry. A conceptual model is inductively developed when generalizations about specific observations are formulated and is deductively developed when specific situations are seen as examples of other more general events. For example, much of the content of the self-care framework was induced from Orem's observations of "the constant elements and relationships of nursing practice situations" (Orem & Taylor, 1986, p. 38). In contrast, Levine (1969) indicated that she deduced the conservation model from "ideas from all areas of knowledge that contribute to the development of the nursing process" (p. viii).

FUNCTIONS OF A CONCEPTUAL MODEL

A conceptual model provides a distinctive frame of reference—"a horizon of expectations" (Popper, 1965, p. 47)—and "a coherent, internally unified way of thinking about ... events and processes" (Frank, 1968, p. 45) for its adherents that tells them how to observe and interpret the phenomena of interest to the discipline. Each conceptual model, then, presents a unique focus that has a profound influence on individuals' perceptions. The unique focus of each conceptual model is a characterization of a possible reality. Each conceptual model includes concepts and propositions that the model author considers relevant and as aids to understanding (Lippitt, 1973; Reilly, 1975). Thus, although conceptual models address all of the concepts representing the subject matter of the discipline, as identified in the metaparadigm, each metaparadigm concept is defined and described in a different way in different conceptual model.

Conceptual models, then, provide alternative ways to view the subject matter of the discipline; there is no "best" way. More specifically, certain aspects of the phenomena of interest to a discipline are regarded as particularly relevant,

and other aspects are ignored. For example, Neuman's Systems Model (Neuman & Fawcett, 2002) focuses on preventing a deleterious reaction to stressors, whereas Orem's (2001) self-care framework emphasizes enhancing each human being's self-care capabilities and actions. Note that Neuman's conceptual model does not deal with self care, and Orem's does not focus on reactions to stressors. Furthermore, different conceptual models place varying emphasis on the metaparadigm concepts. For example, King's (1995) General Systems Framework does not ignore but does not emphasize the nursing metaparadigm concept of environment, whereas Rogers' (1994b) Science of Unitary Human Beings places equal emphasis on the nursing metaparadigm concepts of human beings and environment.

Each conceptual model also provides a structure and a rationale for the scholarly and practical activities of its adherents, who comprise a subculture or community of scholars within a discipline (Eckberg & Hill, 1979). More specifically, each conceptual model gives direction to the search for relevant questions about the phenomena of central interest to a discipline and suggests solutions to practical problems. Each one also provides general criteria for knowing when a problem has been solved. Those features of a conceptual model are illustrated in the following example. The Roy Adaptation Model focuses on adaptation of human beings to environmental stimuli and proposes that management of the most relevant stimuli leads to adaptation (Roy & Andrews, 1999). Here, a relevant question might be, "What are the most relevant stimuli in a given situation?" Anyone interested in solutions to adaptation problems would focus on the various ways of managing stimuli, and one would be led to look for manifestations of adaptation when seeking to determine if the problem has been solved.

Kaplan (1964) pointed out that advances in knowledge occur "when scientists understand one another with as little uncertainty as possible" (p. 269). In addition, he noted that uncertainty is reduced when the scientist "make[s] clear to others just what he [or she] had in mind" by explicating the conceptual model that is being used to guide the work (p. 269).

CONCEPTUAL MODELS OF NURSING

Conceptual models are not new to nursing; they have existed since Nightingale (1859/1946) first advanced her ideas about nursing. Most early conceptualizations of nursing, however, were not presented in the formal manner of models. It remained for the Nursing Development Conference Group (1973, 1979), Johnson (1974), Riehl and Roy (1974, 1980), and Reilly (1975) to explicitly label various perspectives of nursing as conceptual models.

Peterson (1977) and Hall (1979) linked the proliferation of formal conceptual models of nursing with interest in conceptualizing nursing as a distinct discipline and the concomitant introduction of ideas about nursing theory. Meleis (1997) reached the same conclusion in her historiography of nursing knowledge development. Readers who are especially interested in the progression of nursing knowledge are referred to Meleis' (1997) excellent work, because a comprehensive historic review is beyond the scope of this book.

The works of several nurse scholars currently are recognized as conceptual models. Among the best known are Johnson's Behavioral System Model, King's General Systems Framework, Levine's Conservation Model, Neuman's Systems Model, Orem's Self-Care Framework, Rogers' Science of Unitary Human Beings, and Roy's Adaptation Model (Johnson, 1980, 1990; King, 1971, 1981, 1990; Levine, 1969, 1991; Neuman & Fawcett, 2002; Neuman & Young, 1972; Orem, 1971, 2001; Rogers, 1970, 1990; Roy, 1976; Roy & Andrews, 1999). Those conceptual models of nursing are discussed in Chapters 4 through 10 of this book.

The development of conceptual models of nursing and the labeling of them as such was an important advance for the discipline. Reilly's (1975) comments help underscore this point:

> We all have a private image (concept) of nursing practice. In turn, this private image influences our interpretation of data, our decisions, and our actions. But can a discipline continue to develop when its members hold so many differing private images? The proponents of conceptual models of practice are seeking to make us aware of these private images, so that we can begin to identify commonalities in our perceptions of the nature of practice and move toward the evolution of a well-ordered concept (p. 567).

Johnson (1987) also pointed out that nurses always use some frame of reference for their activities and explained the drawbacks of implicit frameworks:

> It is important to note that some kind of implicit framework is used by every practicing nurse, for we cannot observe, see, or describe, nor can we prescribe anything for which we do not already have some kind of mental image or concept. Unfortunately, the mental images used by nurses in their practice, images developed through education and experience and continuously governed by the multitude of factors in the practice setting, have tended to be disconnected, diffused, incomplete and frequently heavily weighted by concepts drawn from the conceptual schema used by medicine to achieve its own social mission (p. 195).

In a similar vein, Bradshaw (1995) stated:

> Both the modern academic nursing approach and the old-fashioned practical training nursing approach presume some kind of [conceptual model] about the needs of patients and clients and how nurses can best provide for these needs. The difference may be that for modern nursing such [a conceptual model] is self-consciously explicit, while for nurses trained in the traditional manner [the conceptual model] was implicit; it was the hidden mutually accepted but taken for granted understanding that underpinned the fabric of care (p. 82).

Elaborating, Kalideen (1993) stated:

> Whatever you may think, we all use models to guide our actions, be it the way we conduct our personal lives or the way we nurse. These are based on the beliefs and values of family, friends, peers, and those we respect or those who have influenced us greatly. One of the problems of each of us using an individual model of practice is that it is difficult for others to understand how we think, and why we do what we do. Since none of us care for patients in isolation, it is important that others (our peers, ward colleagues, medical staff) can understand us (p. 4).

Conceptual models of nursing, then, are the explicit and formal presentations of some nurses' implicit, private images of nursing. Explicit conceptual models of nursing "provide [explicit] philosophical and pragmatic orientations to the service nurses provide patients—a service which only nurses can provide—a service which provides a dimension to total care different from that provided by any other health professional" (Johnson, 1987, p. 195). Explicit conceptual models of nursing provide explicit orientations not only for nurses but also for other health professionals and the public. They identify the purpose and scope of nursing and provide frameworks for objective records of the effects of nursing. Johnson (1987) explained that explicit conceptual models "specify for nurses and society the mission and boundaries of the profession. They clarify the realm of nursing responsibility and accountability, and they allow the practitioner and/or the profession to document services and outcomes" (pp. 196–197). Moreover, use of an explicit conceptual model helps achieve consistency in nursing practice by facilitating communication among nurses, reduces conflict among nurses who might have different implicit goals for practice, and provides a systematic approach to nursing research, education, administration, and practice.

THEORIES

The fourth component of the structural holarchy of contemporary nursing knowledge is the **THEORY** (see Fig. 1–1). A theory is defined as *one or more relatively concrete and specific concepts that are derived from a conceptual model, the propositions that narrowly describe those concepts, and the propositions that state relatively concrete and specific relations between two or more of the concepts.*

Scholars have used many different terms to refer to theory, as defined in this chapter. Among those terms are atomistic theory, grand theory, macro theory, micro theory, middle-range theory, mid-range theory, practice theory, praxis theory, and theoretical framework (King & Fawcett, 1997b). This book focuses on grand theories and middle-range theories.

GRAND THEORY AND MIDDLE-RANGE THEORY

Theories vary in their level of abstraction and scope. The more abstract and broader type of theory is referred to as a **grand theory**. The more concrete and narrower type of theory is referred to as a **middle-range theory**.

Grand theories are broad in scope. They are composed of concepts and propositions that are less abstract and general than the concepts and propositions of a conceptual model but are not as concrete and specific as the concepts and propositions of a middle-range theory. Consciousness is an example of a grand theory concept (Newman, 1994). An example of a grand theory nonrelational proposition is as follows: Consciousness is the informational capacity of the human system and encompasses interconnected cognitive (thinking) and affective (feeling) awareness, physiochemical maintenance including the nervous and endocrine systems, growth processes, the immune system, and the genetic code (Newman, 1994). An example of a grand theory relational proposition, which links the concepts consciousness and pattern, is as follows: "The evolving pattern of person-environment can be viewed as a process of expanding consciousness" (Newman, 1994, p. 33).

Middle-range theories are narrower in scope than grand theories. They are composed of a limited number of concepts and propositions that are written at a relatively concrete and specific level. Nurse's activity is an example of a middle-range theory concept (Orlando, 1961). An example of a middle-range theory nonrelational proposition is as follows: Nurse's activity is "only what [the nurse] says or does with or for the benefit of the patient," such as instructions, suggestions, directions, explanations, information, requests, and questions directed toward the patient; making decisions for the patient; handling the patient's body; administering medications or treatments; and changing the patient's immediate environment (Orlando, 1961, p. 60). An example of a middle-range theory relational proposition, which links the concepts nurse's reaction and nurse's activity, is as follows: "What a nurse says or does is necessarily an outcome of her reaction to something in the situation" (Orlando, 1961, p. 61).

Each middle-range theory addresses a more or less relatively concrete and specific phenomenon by describing what the phenomenon is, explaining why it occurs, or predicting how it occurs. Middle-range descriptive theories are the most basic type of middle-range theory. They describe or classify a phenomenon and, therefore, may encompass just one concept. When a middle-range descriptive theory describes a phenomenon, it simply names the commonalities found in discrete observations of individuals, groups, situations, or events. When a middle-range descriptive theory classifies a phenomenon, it categorizes the described commonalities into mutually exclusive, overlapping, hierarchical, or sequential dimensions. A middle-range classification theory may be referred to as a typology or a taxonomy.

Middle-range explanatory theories specify relations between two or more concepts. They explain why and the extent to which one concept is related to another concept. Middle-range predictive theories move beyond explanation to the prediction of precise relations between concepts or the effects of one or more concepts on one or more other concepts. This type of middle-range theory addresses how changes in a phenomenon occur.

The definition of a theory used in this book indicates that a conceptual model is always the precursor to a grand theory or a middle-range theory. Indeed, Popper (1970) maintained that inasmuch as "we approach everything in the light of a preconceived theory (p. 52), the belief held by some that theory development proceeds outside the context of a conceptual frame of reference is "absurd" (Popper 1965, p. 46). As Slife and Williams (1995) explained, "All theories have implied understandings about the world that are crucial to their formulation and use... [In other words,] all theories have assumptions and implications embedded in them [and] stem from cultural and historic contexts that lend them meaning and influence how they are understood and implemented" (pp. 2, 9).

Moreover, inasmuch as each grand theory and each middle-range theory deals only with a limited aspect of reality, many theories are needed to deal with all of the phenomena encompassed by a conceptual model. Each conceptual model, then, is more fully specified by several grand or middle-range theories, as indicated in Figure 1–1 by the subscript notation 1 ... n.

Grand theories are derived directly from conceptual models (Fig. 1–2). For example, Rogers (1986) derived three grand theories from her conceptual model, the Science of Unitary Human Beings: the Theory of Accelerating Evolution, the Theory of Rhythmical Correlates of Change, and the Theory of Paranormal Phenomena.

The grand theories derived from conceptual models can serve as the starting points for middle-range theory development (see Fig. 1–2). Alligood (1991), for example, derived a middle-range theory of creativity, actualization, and empathy from Rogers' (1986) grand theory of accelerating evolution.

Alternatively, middle-range theories can be derived

directly from the conceptual model (see Fig. 1–2). For example, King (1981) derived the middle-range theory of goal attainment from her Conceptual System.

FUNCTIONS OF A THEORY

One function of a theory is to narrow and more fully specify the phenomena contained in a conceptual model. Another function is to provide a relatively concrete and specific structure for the interpretation of initially puzzling behaviors, situations, and events.

NURSING THEORIES

A few nurses have presented their ideas about nursing in the form of explicit grand theories. For example, Newman (1986, 1994) has presented her Theory of Health as Expanding Consciousness and Parse (1981, 1998) has presented her Theory of Human Becoming. These grand theories are discussed in Chapters 12 and 13 of this book.

A few other nurses have presented their ideas about nursing in the form of explicit middle-range theories. Orlando (1961) presented her Theory of the Deliberative Nursing Process, Peplau (1952, 1992) presented her Theory of Interpersonal Relations, and Watson (1985, 1997) presented her Theory of Human Caring. Peplau's work is a middle-range descriptive classification theory, Watson's

work is a middle-range explanatory theory, and Orlando's work is a middle-range predictive theory. These theories are discussed in Chapters 14 through 16 of this book.

It is likely that many other middle-range nursing theories exist (Smith & Liehr, 2003), but they are not always recognizable as such. The paucity of recognizable middle-range nursing theories is a result of nurse researchers' failure to be explicit about the theoretical components of their studies and to label their work as theories and to practicing nurses' failure to be explicit about the theoretical elements in their discussions of nursing practice. Therefore, the ideas presented by nurses in books, monographs, and journal articles should be closely examined for evidence of the concepts and propositions that compose middle-range theories. Identification of the components of a theory is accomplished by the technique of theory formalization, also called theoretical substruction. Discussion of that technique is beyond the scope of this book. Readers who are interested in theory formalization are referred to Hinshaw's (1979) pioneering work and Fawcett's (1999) more recent work.

Unique, Borrowed, and Shared Nursing Theories

Some theories used by nurses are unique to nursing, and others are borrowed from adjunctive disciplines (Smith & Liehr, 2003). The theories developed by Newman,

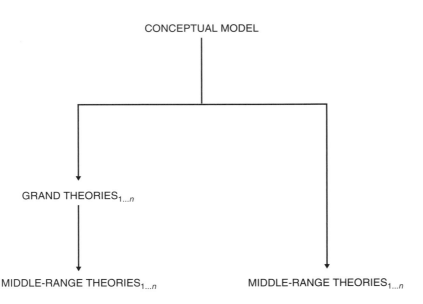

FIG. 1–2. Derivation of grand theories and middle-range theories from a conceptual model.

Orlando, Parse, Peplau, and Watson are unique nursing theories. Many other theories used by nurses have been borrowed from other disciplines. Theories of stress, coping, locus of control, reasoned action, planned behavior, and self-efficacy are just a few examples of borrowed theories. Unfortunately, few nurses have attempted to present a rationale for the use of such theories as guides for nursing research or practice by linking the theory with a nursing conceptual model. One exception is the linkage of the theory of planned behavior with Neuman's Systems Model and Orem's Self-Care Framework (Villarruel, Bishop, Simpson, Jemmott, & Fawcett; 2001).

Also unfortunately, these theories sometimes are used with no consideration given to their empirical adequacy in nursing situations. There is, however, increasing awareness of the need to test borrowed theories to determine if they are empirically adequate in nursing situations. The theory testing work by Lowery and associates (1987) is an especially informative example of what can happen when a theory, borrowed in this case from the discipline of psychology, is tested in the real world of acute and chronic illness. The investigators determined that a basic proposition of attribution theory, stating that people search for causes to make sense of their lives, was not fully supported in their research with patients with arthritis, diabetes mellitus, hypertension, or myocardial infarction. Further research should determine whether a modification of attribution theory is empirically adequate in nursing situations or if an entirely new theory is required. The available results, however, mean that attribution theory cannot be considered a shared theory, that is, a theory that is borrowed from another discipline and found to be empirically adequate in nursing situations (Barnum, 1990).

In contrast, the theory of self-efficacy is a borrowed theory that appears to be developing into a shared theory. This theory was developed initially in the discipline of social psychology and has received empirical support in some nursing situations (e.g., Burns, Camaione, Froman, & Clark, 1998; Froman & Owen, 1990; Hickey, Owen, & Froman, 1992; Lev & Owen, 2002).

 EMPIRICAL INDICATORS

The fifth and final component of the structural holarchy of contemporary nursing knowledge is the **EMPIRICAL INDICATOR** (see Fig. 1–1). An empirical indicator is defined as *a very concrete and specific real world proxy for a middle-range theory concept; an actual instrument, experimental condition, or procedure that is used to observe or measure a middle-range theory concept.* The information obtained from empirical indicators is typically called data.

Empirical indicators are one aspect of the empirical research methods or methods of inquiry that are used to gather evidence about the empirical adequacy of a middle-range theory. The other aspects include the participants from whom the data are collected and the procedures used to collect and analyze the data.

FUNCTION OF AN EMPIRICAL INDICATOR

The function of empirical indicators is to provide the means by which middle-range theories are generated or tested. Empirical indicators that are instruments yield data that can be sorted into qualitative categories or calculated as quantitative scores. For example, responses to an interview schedule composed of open-ended questions can be analyzed to yield categories or themes, and responses to questionnaires composed of fixed-choice items can be subjected to mathematical calculations that yield a number or score.

Empirical indicators that are experimental conditions or procedures tell the researcher or practitioner exactly what to do. They are, in effect, protocols or scripts that direct actions in a precise manner.

NURSING EMPIRICAL INDICATORS

Nurses have developed a plethora of empirical indicators in the form of research instruments and nursing practice tools. Those that measure concepts associated with the conceptual models of nursing and nursing theories discussed in this book are listed and described in tables in Chapters 4 through 10 and 12 through 17.

 DISTINCTIONS BETWEEN THE COMPONENTS OF THE STRUCTURAL HOLARCHY OF CONTEMPORARY NURSING KNOWLEDGE

The distinctions between the various components of the structural holarchy of contemporary nursing knowledge require some discussion. The discussion that follows should be kept in mind when reading the remainder of this book.

THE METAPARADIGM, PHILOSOPHIES, CONCEPTUAL MODELS, THEORIES, AND EMPIRICAL INDICATORS

Empirical indicators are directly connected to theories by means of the operational definition for each middle-range theory concept. As can be seen in Figure 1–1, there is no direct connection between empirical indicators and conceptual models, philosophies, or the metaparadigm. Consequently, those components of the structural holarchy of contemporary nursing knowledge cannot be subjected to empirical testing. Rather, the credibility of a conceptual model is determined indirectly through empirical testing of middle-range theories that are derived from or linked with the model. Furthermore, philosophies cannot be empirically tested either directly or indirectly because they are statements of beliefs and values. Philosophies should, however, be defendable based on logic or through dialogue. More specifically, philosophies can and should be "reconsidered, rejected, or modified through a process of considered reflection spurred on by debate and discussion with one's peers" (Salsberry, 1994, p. 18). Similarly, the metaparadigm cannot be empirically tested, but should be defendable based on dialogue and debate about the phenomena of interest to the discipline as a whole.

THE METAPARADIGM, PHILOSOPHIES, CONCEPTUAL MODELS, AND THEORIES

When viewed from the perspective of the structural holarchy of contemporary nursing knowledge (see Fig. 1–1), it is clear that the metaparadigm, philosophies, conceptual models, and theories are distinct formulations. Yet Kikuchi (1997) argued that certain aspects of the structural holarchy of contemporary nursing knowledge are "problematic in that they contain seeds of confusion regarding the nature of conceptions about nursing—seeds sown, it would seem, by virtue of the failure to see that the conceptions are philosophical, rather than scientific in nature and the eclectic amalgamation of ideas" (p. 102). She went on to argue that, with the exception of empirical indicators, all other components of the structural holarchy are better thought of as philosophies of nursing, "having the form of a philosophic nursing theory" (p. 107).

Moreover, Salsberry (1994) implied that what are called conceptual models in this book actually are philosophies. She noted, "Much of what has been referred to a conceptual model is, in fact, a philosophy—that is, a set of beliefs about what the basic entities of nursing are, how these entities are known, and what values should guide the discipline. The model development arises when these philosophical claims are arranged into a particular structure" (p. 18).

Support for the structural holarchy as presented in this book is especially evident in the content of Chapters 4 through 10, where clear distinctions are made between philosophical claims and the concepts and propositions that comprise conceptual models of nursing and reflect underlying philosophical claims. Further support is evident in the content of Chapters 12 through 17, where clear distinctions are made between philosophical claims and propositions that compose grand theories or middle-range theories and reflect underlying philosophical claims. More specifically, each of these chapters explicitly identifies statements that are beliefs and values, that is, philosophical claims, and then identifies the concepts and propositions of the conceptual model, grand theory, or middle-range theory that clearly reflect—but do not duplicate—those philosophical claims.

THE METAPARADIGM, PHILOSOPHIES, AND CONCEPTUAL MODELS

Philosophies do not follow directly in line from the metaparadigm of the discipline, nor do they directly precede conceptual models (see Fig. 1–1). Rather, the metaparadigm of a discipline identifies the phenomena about which ontological, epistemic, and ethical claims are made. The unique focus and content of each conceptual model then reflect certain philosophical claims. The philosophies therefore are the foundation for other formulations, including conceptual models, grand theories, and middle-range theories. Salsberry (1994) explained, "A philosophy consists of the basic assumptions and beliefs that are built upon in theorizing" (p. 18).

For example, a metaparadigm might identify people as a central concept. A philosophy then might make the claim that all people are equal. That philosophical claim then would be reflected in a conceptual model that depicts the nurse and the patient as equal partners in the process of nursing.

THE METAPARADIGM AND CONCEPTUAL MODELS

Most disciplines have a single metaparadigm but multiple conceptual models, as indicated by the subscript notation $1 \ldots n$ in Figure 1–1. For example, this book identifies seven different conceptual models that address the concepts of the metaparadigm of nursing, and Darby and Walsh (1994) identified eight different conceptual models that address the concepts of the metaparadigm of dental hygiene. Moreover, Waters (1994) identified five different general conceptual models, and Nye and Berardo (1981) identified 16 different conceptual models of the family that address the concepts of the discipline of sociology.

Multiple conceptual models allow the members of a discipline to think about the phenomena of central interest in different ways. They speak to the view that "there is no one reality of [a discipline]. There is no clear and universal [conceptual model] of what should underpin practice precisely because there is no such thing as universal knowledge" (Bradshaw, 1995, p. 83).

Conceptual models address the phenomena identified by a metaparadigm and, therefore, incorporate the most global concepts and propositions in a more restrictive yet still abstract manner. Each conceptual model, then, provides a different view of the metaparadigm concepts. As Kuhn (1970) explained, although adherents of different conceptual models are looking at the same phenomena, "in some areas they see different things, and they see them in different relations to one another" (p. 150). The acceptance of multiple conceptual models is an outgrowth of the recognition of the advantages of diverse perspectives for a discipline (Moore, 1990; Nagle & Mitchell, 1991).

As in other disciplines, the conceptual models of nursing represent various paradigms that address the phenomena identified by the metaparadigm of the discipline of nursing. Thus, it is not surprising that each defines the four metaparadigm concepts differently and links those concepts in diverse ways (see Chapters 4 through 10).

Examination of conceptual models of nursing reveals that human beings usually are identified as integrated bio-psycho-social beings, but are defined in diverse ways, such as adaptive systems (Roy & Andrews, 1999), behavioral systems (Johnson, 1990), self-care agents (Orem, 2001), or energy fields (Rogers, 1990). Environment frequently is identified as internal structures and external influences, including family members, the community, and society, as well as human beings' physical surroundings. The environment is seen as a source of stressors in some models (Neuman & Fawcett, 2002), but a source of resources in others (Rogers, 1990). Health is presented in various ways, such as a continuum of client system wellness or stability (Neuman & Fawcett, 2002), a dichotomy of behavioral stability or instability (Johnson, 1990), or a value identified by each cultural group (Rogers, 1990).

The conceptual models also present descriptions of the concept of nursing, usually by defining nursing and then specifying goals of nursing actions and a nursing process. The goals of nursing action frequently are derived directly from the definition of health given by the model. For example, a nursing goal might be to assist people to attain, maintain, or regain client system stability (Neuman & Fawcett, 2002). The nursing process, or practice methodology, described in each conceptual model emphasizes assessing and labeling human beings' health conditions, setting goals for nursing action, implementing nursing actions, and evaluating health conditions after nursing intervention. The labels for and content of the steps or components of the process, however, frequently differ from one conceptual model to another.

CONCEPTUAL MODELS AND THEORIES

A central thesis of this book is that a conceptual model is not a theory, nor is a theory a conceptual model. This thesis requires further discussion because considerable confusion about those two components of the structural holarchy of contemporary nursing knowledge still exists in the minds of some students and scholars. The distinctions between conceptual models and theories described here and the meaning ascribed to conceptual models are in keeping with earlier works by Rogers (1970), Johnson (1974), and Reilly (1975) in nursing; Hempel (1970) in philosophy; Reese and Overton (1970) in developmental psychology; and Nye and Berardo (1966) in sociology; and more recent work by Darby and Walsh (1994) in dental hygiene. Although some writers consider distinctions between conceptual models and theories a semantic point (e.g., Flaskerud & Halloran, 1980; Meleis, 1997), the issue should not be dismissed so easily. Indeed, King (1997) called for "a consensus on a definition of the term 'theory' to clearly differentiate it from 'conceptual system'" (p. 16), which is the term she prefers over conceptual model, conceptual framework, or paradigm.

The distinction between a conceptual model and a theory should be made because of the differences in the way that each is used—if one is to know what to do next, one must know whether the starting point is a conceptual model or a theory. As can be seen in Figure 1–1, conceptual models and theories differ in their level of abstraction. A conceptual model is composed of several abstract and general concepts and propositions. A grand theory or a middle-range theory, in contrast, deals with one or more relatively concrete and specific concepts and propositions.

Distinguishing between conceptual models, grand theories, and middle-range theories on the basis of level of abstraction raises the question of how abstract is abstract enough for a work to be considered a conceptual model. Although the decision in a few cases may be somewhat arbitrary, the following rule serves as one guideline for distinguishing between conceptual models and theories. The rule requires determination of the purpose of the work.

If the purpose of the work is to articulate a body of distinctive knowledge for the whole of the discipline of nursing, the work most likely is a conceptual model. Given that this was the explicitly stated purpose of authors such as Johnson (1980), King (1971), Levine (1969), Neuman (Neuman & Young, 1972), Orem (1971), Rogers (1970), and Roy (1976), their works are classified as conceptual models.

If the purpose of the work is to further develop one aspect of a conceptual model, the work most likely is a grand theory. For example, both Newman (1986) and Parse (1981) explained that they elected to further develop the concept of health from the perspective of Rogers' (1970) conceptual model. As can be discerned from these examples, nurse scholars who consider conceptual models and grand theories to be synonymous (e.g., Barnum, 1998; Kim, 1983; Marriner-Tomey & Alligood, 2002) mislead their readers.

If the purpose of the work is to describe, explain, or predict concrete and specific phenomena, the work most likely is a middle-range theory. For example, Peplau's (1952) theory of interpersonal relations is a classification of the stages of the nurse-patient relationship. Peplau did not, nor did she intend to, address the entire domain of nursing. Consequently, her theory is classified as a middle-range theory. In summary, if a given work is an abstract and general frame of reference addressing all four concepts of the metaparadigm of nursing, it is a conceptual model. If the work is more concrete, specific, and restricted to a more limited range of phenomena than that identified by the conceptual model, it is a grand theory or middle-range theory.

Another rule for distinguishing between conceptual models and theories requires determination of how many levels of knowledge are needed before the work may be applied in particular nursing situations. If, for example, the work identifies physiologic needs as an assessment parameter, but does not explain the differences between normal and pathologic functions of body systems in concrete terms, it most likely is a conceptual model. As such, the work is not directly applicable in practice. A theory of normal and pathologic functions must be linked with the conceptual model so that judgments about the physiological functions of body systems may be made. Conversely, if the work includes a detailed description of particular people's behavior, or an explanation of how particular factors influence particular behaviors, it most likely is a middle-range theory. In that case, the work may be directly applied in practice. The rule also is exemplified by the number of steps required before empirical testing can occur (Reilly, 1975). A conceptual model cannot be tested directly, because its concepts and propositions are not empirically measurable. More concrete and specific concepts and propositions have to be derived from the conceptual model; that is, a middle-range theory must be formulated. Those more concrete concepts then must be operationally defined and empirically testable hypotheses must be derived from the propositions of the theory. Four steps are required before a conceptual model can be tested, albeit indirectly. First, the conceptual model must be formulated; second, a middle-range theory must be derived from the conceptual model; third, empirical indicators must be identified; and fourth, empirically testable hypotheses must be specified. In contrast, only three steps are required

for empirical testing of a middle-range theory. First, the theory must be stated; second, empirical indicators must be identified; and third, empirically testable hypotheses must be specified.

Failure to distinguish between a conceptual model and a theory leads to considerable misunderstanding and inappropriate expectations about the work. When a conceptual model is labeled a grand theory or, especially, a middle-range theory, expectations regarding empirical testing and applicability in practice immediately arise. When such expectations cannot be met, the work is frequently regarded as inadequate. Similarly, when a grand theory or a middle-range theory is labeled a conceptual model, expectations regarding comprehensiveness arise. When those expectations cannot be met, that work also may be regarded as inadequate.

 ## NOTES ON LANGUAGE

The meaning given to conceptual models in this book should not be confused with the meaning of model found in the philosophy of science literature and some nursing literature. The latter refers to representations of testable theories. Rudner (1966), for example, defined a model for a middle-range theory as "an alternative interpretation of the same calculus of which the theory itself is an interpretation" (p. 24). That kind of a model is composed of ideas or diagrams that are more familiar to the novice than are the concepts and propositions of the theory. Thus, the model is a heuristic device that facilitates understanding of the theory. Rudner illustrated this by the analogy of the flow of water through pipes as a model for a middle-range theory of electric current wires. So-called models that actually are diagrams of theories are found with increasing frequency in reports of nursing research. For example, Hamner (1996) labeled her diagrams of the relations between the concepts of a middle-range theory of factors associated with patient length of stay in an intensive care unit as a model.

The concepts and propositions of each conceptual model and each theory often are stated in a distinctive vocabulary. One conceptual model, for example, uses the term conservation (Levine, 1996), another uses the terms stimuli and adaptation level (Roy & Andrews, 1999), and still another uses the terms resonancy, helicy, and integrality (Rogers, 1990). Furthermore, the meaning of each term is usually connected to the unique focus of the conceptual model or theory. Thus, the same or similar terms may have different meanings in different conceptual models and theories. For example, adaptation is defined in one conceptual model as "the process and outcome whereby thinking and feeling persons, as individuals or in groups, use conscious awareness and choice to create human and environmental integration" (Roy & Andrews, 1999, p. 30), and in another conceptual model as "the process by which individuals 'fit' the environments in which they live" (Levine, 1996, p. 38).

The vocabulary of each conceptual model and each theory should not be considered unnecessary jargon. Rather, the terminology used by the author of each conceptual model and each theory is the result of considerable thought about how to precisely convey the meaning of that particular perspective to others (Biley, 1990). Nurses have long understood the need for a distinctive vocabulary that differentiates nursing from other sciences and especially from medicine (Watson, 1996). "Language," Batey and Eyres (1979) explained, "is fundamental to the evolution of all disciplines [and] [w]ithin any discipline, selected terminology evolves to become the concepts that denote the specific knowledge domains and methodologies of that discipline" (p. 139). Akinsanya (1989) added, "Every science has its own peculiar terms, concepts and principles which are essential for the development of its knowledge base. In nursing, as in other sciences, an understanding of these is a prerequisite to a critical examination of their contribution to the development of knowledge and its application to practice" (p. ii). Finally, Barrett (2003) commented, "How would one understand anatomy and physiology, microbiology, pharmacology, … without the precise use of language reflecting those domains of knowledge? … various professional groups and consumers may be able to grasp the meaning precisely due to the specificity of description. How else is substantive knowledge to be communicated without saying it is what it is that it is!" (p. 280).

Although decried by some readers as unnecessary and distracting (e.g., Bowie, 2003), some jargon is to be expected in any conceptual model or theory. The amount of jargon can be calculated using a formula given by Crovitz (1970): Jargon is the ratio of x words to y words, where x is the number of words in a conceptual model or theory that are specific to that conceptual model or theory, and y is the number of words that might appear in any conceptual model or theory.

Knowing the unique language of a discipline, then, is required to understand the knowledge that comprises that discipline (Parse, 2001a). Watson (1997) pointed out, "The attention to language is especially critical to an evolving discipline, in that during this postmodern era, one's survival depends upon having language; writers in this area remind us 'if you do not have your own language you don't exist'" (p. 50). Mitchell (2002) added that a unique language is required for a discipline to be visible.

 ## CONCLUSION

This chapter presented the definition and function of each component of the structural holarchy of contemporary nursing knowledge. It is important to point out that metaparadigms, philosophies, conceptual models, and theories are not real or tangible entities. Rather, they are tentative formulations that represent scholars' best efforts to understand phenomena (Payton, 1994; Polit & Beck, 2004). Their tentative nature means that the knowledge contained in metaparadigms, philosophies, conceptual models, and theories carries with it a degree of uncertainty. Thus metaparadigms, philosophies, conceptual models, and theories are not unchangeable ideologies but rather ideas that are subject to continual revision or even rejection in response to ongoing dialogue, debate, and systematic inquiry.

This chapter also presented a discussion of the distinctions between the various components of the structural holarchy of contemporary nursing knowledge, with emphasis on the distinctions between conceptual models and theories. The distinctions between conceptual models and theories mandate separate analysis and evaluation schemata. Chapter 3 presents a framework expressly designed for the analysis and evaluation of conceptual models of nursing. The framework expressly designed for the analysis and evaluation of nursing theories is presented in Chapter 11.

 ## REFERENCES

Ackoff, R.L. (1974). Redesigning the future: A systems approach to societal problems. New York: Wiley.

Akinsanya, J.A. (1989). Introduction. Recent Advances in Nursing, 24, i–ii.

Alligood, M.R. (1991). Testing Rogers' theory of accelerating change: The relationships among creativity, actualization, and empathy in persons 18 to 92 years of age. Western Journal of Nursing Research, 13, 84–96.

Altman, I., & Rogoff, B. (1987). World views in psychology: Trait, interactional, organismic, and transactional perspectives. In D. Stokols & I. Altman (Eds.), Handbook of environmental psychology (pp. 7–40). New York: Wiley.

Babbie, E. (1998). The practice of social research (8th ed.). Belmont, CA: Wadsworth.

Barnum, B.J.S. (1990). Nursing theory: Analysis, application, evaluation (3rd ed.). Glenview, IL: Scott, Foresman/Little Brown Higher Education.

Barnum, B.J.S. (1998). Nursing theory: Analysis, application, evaluation (5th ed.). Philadelphia: Lippincott.

Barrett. E.A.M. (2003). Response to Letter to the Editor. Nursing Science Quarterly, 16, 27–280.

Batey, M.V., & Eyres, S.J. (1979). Interdisciplinary semantics: Implications for research. Western Journal of Nursing Research, 1, 139–141.

Benoliel, J.Q. (1977). The interaction between theory and research. Nursing Outlook, 25, 108–113.

Ben-Sira, Z. (1987). Social work in health care: Needs, challenges and implications for structuring practice. Social Work in Health Care, 13, 79–100.

Biley, F. (1990). Wordly wise. Nursing (London), 4(24), 37.

Bowie, B.H. (2003). Letter to the Editor re: "What is nursing science?" Nursing Science Quarterly, 16, 279.

Bradshaw, A. (1995). What are nurses doing to patients? A review of theories of nursing past and present. Journal of Clinical Nursing, 4, 81–92.

Brodie, J.N. (1984). A response to Dr. J. Fawcett's paper: "The metaparadigm of nursing. Current status and future refinements." Image. The Journal of Nursing Scholarship, 16, 87–89.

Burns, K.J., Camaione, D.N., Froman, R.D., & Clark, B.A. III. (1998). Predictors of referral to cardiac rehabilitation and cardiac exercise self-efficacy. Clinical Nursing Research, 7, 147–163.

Chin, R. (1980). The utility of systems models and developmental models for practitioners. In J.P. Riehl and C. Roy (Eds.), Conceptual models for nursing practice (2nd ed., pp. 21–37). New York: Appleton-Century-Crofts.

Cody, W. K. (1996). Response to: "On the requirements for a metaparadigm: An invitation to dialogue." Nursing Science Quarterly, 9, 97–99.

Conway, M.E. (1985). Toward greater specificity in defining nursing's metaparadigm. Advances in Nursing Science, 7(4), 73–81.

Conway, M.E. (1989, April). Nursing's metaparadigm: Current perspectives. Paper presented at the Spring Doctoral Forum, Medical College of Georgia School of Nursing, Augusta.

Crovitz, H.F. (1970). Galton's walk. New York: Harper.

Darby, M.L., & Walsh, M.M. (1994). Dental hygiene theory and practice. Philadelphia: Saunders.

Donaldson, S.K., & Crowley, D.M. (1978). The discipline of nursing. Nursing Outlook, 26, 113–120.

Eckberg, D.L., & Hill, L., Jr. (1979). The paradigm concept and sociology: A critical review. American Sociological Review, 44, 925–937.

Eriksson, K. (1989). Caring paradigms: A study of the origins and the development of caring paradigms among nursing students. Scandinavian Journal of Caring Sciences, 3, 169–176.

Fawcett, J. (1978). The "what" of theory development. In Theory development: What, why, how? (pp. 17–33). New York: National League for Nursing.

Fawcett, J. (1984). The metaparadigm of nursing: Current status and future refinements. Image: Journal of Nursing Scholarship, 16, 84–87.

Fawcett, J. (1992). The metaparadigm of nursing: International in scope and substance. In K. Krause & P. Astedt-Kurki (Eds.), International perspectives on nursing. A joint effort to explore nursing internationally (Series A 3/92, pp. 13–21). Tampere, Finland: Tampere University Department of Nursing.

Fawcett, J. (1993a). Analysis and evaluation of nursing theories. Philadelphia: F.A. Davis.

Fawcett, J. (1993b). From a plethora of paradigms to parsimony in world views. Nursing Science Quarterly, 6, 56–58.

Fawcett, J. (1996). On the requirements for a metaparadigm: An invitation to dialogue. Nursing Science Quarterly, 9, 94–97.

Fawcett, J. (1999). The relationship of theory and research (3rd ed). Philadelphia: F.A. Davis.

Fawcett, J. (2000). Analysis and evaluation of contemporary nursing knowledge: Nursing models and theories. Philadelphia: F.A. Davis.

Feigl, H. (1970). The "orthodox" view of theories: Remarks in defense as well as critique. In M. Radner & S. Winokuk (Eds.), Minnesota studies in the philosophy of science. Volume IV: Analyses of theories and methods of physics and psychology (pp. 3–16). Minneapolis: University of Minnesota Press.

Fitzpatrick, J.J., & Whall, A.L. (1996). Conceptual models of nursing: Analysis and application (3rd ed.). Stamford, CT: Appleton and Lange.

Flaskerud, J.H., & Halloran, E.J. (1980). Areas of agreement in nursing theory development. Advances in Nursing Science, 3(1), 1–7.

Frank, L.K. (1968). Science as a communication process. Main Currents in Modern Thought, 25, 45–50.

Froman, R.D., & Owen, S.V. (1990). Mothers' and nurses' perceptions of infant care skills. Research in Nursing and Health, 13, 247–253.

Fry, S. (1981). Accountability in research: The relationship of scientific and humanistic values. Advances in Nursing Science, 4(1), 1–13.

George, J.B. (2002). Nursing theories: The base for professional nursing practice (5th ed.). Upper Saddle River, NJ: Prentice Hall.

Gibbs, J. (1972). Sociological theory construction. Hinsdale, IL: Dryden Press.

Gortner, S.R. (1980). Nursing science in transition. Nursing Research, 29, 180–183.

Gortner, S. R. (1990). Nursing values and science: Toward a science philosophy. Image: Journal of Nursing Scholarship, 22, 101–105.

Grace, P.J. (2002). Philosophies, models, and theories: Moral obligations. In M.R. Alligood & A. Marriner Tomey (Eds.), Nursing theory: Utilization and application (2nd ed., pp. 63–79.). St. Louis: Mosby.

Hall, A.D., & Fagen, R.E. (1968). Definition of system. In W. Buckley (Ed.), Modern systems research for the behavioral scientist (pp. 81–92). Chicago: Aldine.

Hall, B.A. (1981). The change paradigm in nursing: Growth versus persistence. Advances in Nursing Science, 3(4), 1–6.

Hall, B.A. (1983). Toward an understanding of stability in nursing phenomena. Advances in Nursing Science, 5(3), 15–20.

Hall, K.V. (1979). Current trends in the use of conceptual frameworks in nursing education. Journal of Nursing Education, 18(4), 26–29.

Hamner, J.B. (1996). Preliminary testing of a proposition from the Roy adaptation model. Image: Journal of Nursing Scholarship, 28, 215–220.

Hardy, M.E. (1978). Perspectives on nursing theory. Advances in Nursing Science, 1(1): 37–48.

Heiss, J. (1976). Family roles and interaction (2nd ed.). Chicago: Rand McNally.

Heiss, J. (1981). The social psychology of interaction. Englewood Cliffs, NJ: Prentice-Hall.

Hempel, C.G. (1970). On the "standard conception" of scientific theories. In M. Radner & S. Winokuk (Eds.), Minnesota studies in the philosophy of science. Volume IV: Analyses of theories and methods of physics and psychology (pp. 142–163). Minneapolis: University of Minnesota Press.

Hickey, M.L., Owen, S.V., & Froman, R.D. (1992). Instrument development: Cardiac diet and exercise self-efficacy. Nursing Research, 41, 347–351.

Hickman, J.S. (1995). An introduction to nursing theory. In J.B. George (Ed.), Nursing theories: The base for professional nursing practice (4th ed., pp. 1–14). Norwalk, CT: Appleton & Lange.

Hinshaw, A.S. (1979). Theoretical substruction: An assessment process. Western Journal of Nursing Research, 1, 319–324.

Hinshaw, A.S. (1987). Response to "Structuring the nursing knowledge system: A typology of four domains." Scholarly Inquiry for Nursing Practice, 1, 111–114.

Jacobs, B.B. (2001). Respect for human dignity: A central phenomenon to philosophically unite nursing theory and practice through consilience of knowledge. Advances in Nursing Science, 24(1), 17–35.

Jennings, B.M. (1987). Nursing theory development: Successes and challenges. Journal of Advanced Nursing, 12, 63–69.

Johnson, D.E. (1974). Development of theory: A requisite for nursing as a primary health profession. Nursing Research, 23, 372–377.

Johnson, D.E. (1980). The behavioral system model for nursing. In J.P. Riehl & C. Roy (Eds.), Conceptual models for nursing practice (2nd ed., pp. 207–216). New York: Appleton-Century-Crofts.

Johnson, D.E. (1987). Guest editorial: Evaluating conceptual models for use in critical care nursing practice. Dimensions of Critical Care Nursing, 6, 195–197.

Johnson, D.E. (1990). The behavioral system model for nursing. In M.E. Parker (Ed.), Nursing theories in practice (pp. 23–32). New York: National League for Nursing.

Kalideen, D. (1993). Is there a place for nursing models in theatre nursing? British Journal of Theatre Nursing, 3(5), 4–6.

Kaplan, A. (1964). The conduct of inquiry: Methodology for behavioral science. San Francisco: Chandler.

Kikuchi, J.F. (1997). Clarifying the nature of conceptualizations about nursing. Canadian Journal of Nursing Research, 29, 97–110.

Kim, H.S. (1983). The nature of theoretical thinking in nursing. Norwalk, CT: Appleton-Century-Crofts.

Kim, H.S. (1987). Structuring the nursing knowledge system: A typology of four domains. Scholarly Inquiry for Nursing Practice, 1, 99–110.

Kim, H.S. (1989). Theoretical thinking in nursing: Problems and prospects. Recent Advances in Nursing, 24, 106–122.

Kim, H.S. (1997). Terminology in structuring and developing nursing knowledge. In I.M. King & J. Fawcett (Eds.), The language of nursing theory and metatheory (pp. 27–36). Indianapolis: Sigma Theta Tau International Center Nursing Press.

Kim, H.S. (2000a). An integrative framework for conceptualizing clients: A proposal for a nursing perspective in the new century. Nursing Science Quarterly, 13, 37–40.

Kim, H.S. (2000b). The nature of theoretical thinking in nursing (2nd ed.). New York: Springer.

King, I.M. (1971). Toward a theory for nursing: General concepts of human behavior. New York: Wiley.

King, I.M. (1981). A theory for nursing. Systems, concepts, process. New York: Wiley.

King, I.M. (1984). Philosophy of nursing education: A national survey. Western Journal of Nursing Research, 6, 387–406.

King, I.M. (1990). King's conceptual framework and theory of goal attainment. In M.E. Parker (Ed.), Nursing theories in practice (pp. 73–84). New York: National League for Nursing.

King, I.M. (1995). A systems framework for nursing. In M.A. Frey & C.L. Sieloff (Eds.), Advancing King's systems framework and theory of nursing (pp. 14–22). Thousand Oaks, CA: Sage.

King, I.M. (1997). Reflections on the past and a vision for the future. Nursing Science Quarterly, 10, 15–17.

King, I.M., & Fawcett, J. (1997a). Epilogue. In I.M. King & J. Fawcett (Eds.), The language of nursing theory and metatheory (pp. 89–91). Indianapolis: Sigma Theta Tau International Center Nursing Press.

King, I. M., & Fawcett, J. (Eds.) (1997b). The language of nursing theory and metatheory. Indianapolis: Sigma Theta Tau International Center Nursing Press.

Kleffel, D. (1991). Rethinking the environment as a domain of nursing knowledge. Advances in Nursing Science, 14(1), 40–51.

Kolcaba, K.Y., & Kolcaba, R.J. (1991). In defense of the metaparadigm for nursing. Unpublished manuscript.

Kuhn, T.S. (1962). The structure of scientific revolutions. Chicago: University of Chicago Press.

Kuhn, T.S. (1970). The structure of scientific revolutions (2nd ed.). Chicago: University of Chicago Press.

Lachman, V.D. (1993, June). Communication skills for effective interpersonal relations. Concurrent session presented at the American Nephrology Nurses Association 24th National Symposium, Orlando, FL.

Leininger, M.M. (1988). Leininger's theory of nursing: Cultural care diversity and universality. Nursing Science Quarterly, 1, 152–160.

Leininger, M.M. (1990). Historic and epistemologic dimensions of care and caring with future directions. In J.S. Stevenson & T. Tripp-Reimer (Eds.), Knowledge about care and caring: State of the art and future developments (pp. 19–31). Kansas City, MO: American Academy of Nursing.

Leininger, M.M. (1991a). The theory of culture care diversity and universality. In M.M. Leininger (Ed.), Culture care diversity and universality: A theory of nursing (pp. 5–65). New York: National League for Nursing.

Leininger, M.M. (1991b). Looking to the future of nursing and the relevancy of culture care theory. In M.M. Leininger (Ed.), Culture care diversity and universality: A theory of nursing (pp. 391–418). New York: National League for Nursing.

Leininger, M.M. (1995). Transcultural nursing: Concepts, theories, research and practices. New York: McGraw-Hill.

Leininger, M. (2002). Essential transcultural nursing care concepts, principles, examples, and policy statements. In M. Leininger & M.R. McFarland, Transcultural nursing: Concepts, theories, research, and practice (3rd ed., pp. 45–69). New York: McGraw-Hill.

Lev, E.L., & Owen, S.V. (2002). Association of cancer patients' quality of life, symptoms, moods, and self-care self-efficacy with family care givers' depression, reaction and health. Self-Care, Dependent Care, and Nursing, 10(2), 3–12.

Levine, M.E. (1969). Introduction to clinical nursing. Philadelphia: F.A. Davis.

Levine, M.E. (1991). The conservation principles: A model for health. In K.M. Schaefer & J.B. Pond (Eds.), Levine's conservation model: A framework for nursing practice (pp. 1–11). Philadelphia: F.A. Davis.

Levine, M.E. (1996). The conservation principles: A retrospective. Nursing Science Quarterly, 9, 38–41.

Lewis, S.M. (2003). Caring as being in nursing: Unique or ubiquitous. Nursing Science Quarterly, 16, 37–43.

Lippitt, G.L. (1973). Visualizing change. Model building and the change process. Fairfax, VA: NTL Learning Resources.

Lowery, B.J., Jacobsen, B.S., & McCauley, K. (1987). On the prevalence of causal search in illness situations. Nursing Research, 36, 88–93.

Malinski, V.M. (1996). Response to: "On the requirements for a metaparadigm: An invitation to dialogue." Nursing Science Quarterly, 9, 100–102.

Malloch, K., Martinez, R., Nelson, L., Predeger, B., Speakman, L., Steinbinder, A., & Tracy, J. (1992). To the editor [Letter]. Advances in Nursing Science, 15(2), vi–vii.

Mandelbaum, J. (1991). Why there cannot be an international theory of nursing. International Nursing Review, 38; 48, 53–55.

Margenau, H. (1972). The method of science and the meaning of reality. In H. Margenau (Ed.), Integrative principles of modern thought (pp. 3–43). New York: Gordon and Breach.

Marriner-Tomey, A. (1989). Nursing theorists and their work (2nd ed.). St. Louis: Mosby.

Marriner-Tomey, A., & Alligood, M.R. (2002). Nursing theorists and their work (5th ed.). St. Louis: Mosby.

Masterman, M. (1970). The nature of paradigm. In I. Lakatos & A. Musgrave (Eds.), Criticism and the growth of knowledge (pp. 59–89). Cambridge, England: Cambridge University Press.

McEwen, M. (2002). Philosophy, science, and nursing. In M. McEwen & E. Wills, Theoretical basis for nursing (pp.3–22). Philadelphia: Lippincott Williams & Wilkins.

Meleis, A.I. (1997). Theoretical nursing: Development and progress (3rd ed.). Philadelphia: Lippincott.

Meleis, A.I., & Trangenstein, P.A. (1994). Facilitating transitions: Redefinition of the nursing mission. Nursing Outlook, 42, 255–259.

Mitchell, G.J. (2002). Learning to practice the discipline of nursing. Nursing Science Quarterly, 15, 209–213.

Moore, S. (1990). Thoughts on the discipline of nursing as we approach the year 2000. Journal of Advanced Nursing, 15, 825–828.

Morse, J.M (1996). Nursing scholarship: Sense and sensibility. Nursing Inquiry, 3, 74–82.

Morse, J.M., Solberg, S.M., Neander, W.L., Bottorff, J.L., & Johnson, J.L. (1990). Concepts of caring and caring as a concept. Advances in Nursing Science, 13(1), 1–14.

Nagle, L.M., & Mitchell, G.J. (1991). Theoretic diversity: Evolving paradigmatic issues in research and practice. Advances in Nursing Science, 14(1), 17–25.

Neuman, B., & Fawcett, J. (Eds.). (2002). The Neuman systems model (4th ed.). Upper Saddle River, NJ: Prentice Hall.

Neuman, B., & Young, R.J. (1972). A model for teaching total person approach to patient problems. Nursing Research, 21, 264–269.

Newman, M.A. (1983). The continuing revolution: A history of nursing science. In N.L. Chaska (Ed.), The nursing profession: A time to speak (pp. 385–393). New York: McGraw-Hill.

Newman, M.A. (1986). Health as expanding consciousness. St. Louis: Mosby.

Newman, M.A. (1992). Prevailing paradigms in nursing. Nursing Outlook, 40; 10–13, 32.

Newman, M.A. (1994). Health as expanding consciousness (2nd ed). New York: National League for Nursing Press.

Newman, M.A. (2002). The pattern that connects. Advances in Nursing Science, 24(3), 1–7.

Newman, M.A., Sime, A.M., & Corcoran-Perry, S.A. (1991). The focus of the discipline of nursing. Advances in Nursing Science, 14(1), 1–6.

Newman, M.A., Sime, A.M., & Corcoran-Perry, S.A. (1992). Authors' reply [Letter to the editor]. Advances in Nursing Science, 14(3), vi–vii.

Nightingale, F. (1859). Notes on nursing: What it is, and what it is not. London: Harrison. [Reprinted 1946. Philadelphia: Lippincott.]

Nursing Development Conference Group. (1973). Concept formalization in nursing. Process and product. Boston: Little, Brown.

Nursing Development Conference Group. (1979). Concept formalization in nursing. Process and product (2nd ed.). Boston: Little, Brown.

Nye, F.I., & Berardo, F.N. (Eds.). (1966). Emerging conceptual frameworks in family analysis. New York: Macmillan.

Nye, F.I., & Berardo, F.N. (Eds.). (1981). Emerging conceptual frameworks in family analysis. New York: Praeger.

Orem, D.E. (1971). Nursing: Concepts of practice. New York: McGraw-Hill.

Orem, D.E. (2001). Nursing: Concepts of practice (6th ed.). St. Louis: Mosby.

Orem, D.E., & Taylor, S.G. (1986). Orem's general theory of nursing. In P. Winstead-Fry (Ed.), Case studies in nursing theory (pp. 37–71). New York: National League for Nursing.

Orlando, I.J. (1961). The dynamic nurse-patient relationship. New York: G.P. Putnam's Sons.

Parker, M. (2001). Nursing theories and nursing practice. Philadelphia: F.A. Davis.

Parse, R.R. (1981). Man-living-health: A theory of nursing. New York: Wiley.

Parse, R.R. (1987). Nursing science: Major paradigms, theories, and critiques. Philadelphia: Saunders.

Parse, R.R. (1997). The language of nursing knowledge: Saying what we mean. In I.M. King & J. Fawcett (Eds.), The language of nursing theory and metatheory (pp. 73–77). Indianapolis: Sigma Theta Tau International Center Nursing Press.

Parse, R.R. (1998). The human becoming school of thought: A perspective for nurses and other health professionals. Thousand Oaks, CA: Sage.

Parse, R.R. (2001a). Language and the sow-reap rhythm. Nursing Science Quarterly, 14, 273.

Parse, R.R. (2001b). Nursing: Still in the shadow of medicine. Nursing Science Quarterly, 14, 181.

Payton, O.D. (1994). Research: The validation of clinical practice (3rd ed.). Philadelphia: F.A. Davis.

Peplau, H.E. (1952). Interpersonal relations in nursing. New York: G.P. Putnam's Sons.

Peplau, H.E. (1992). Interpersonal relations: A theoretical framework for application in nursing practice. Nursing Science Quarterly, 5, 13–18.

Peterson, C.J. (1977). Questions frequently asked about the development of a conceptual framework. Journal of Nursing Education, 16(4), 22–32.

Pilkington, F.B., Bunkers, S.S., Clarke, P.N., & Frederickson, K. (2002). Critiquing contemporary nursing knowledge. Nursing Science Quarterly, 15, 171–177.

Polit, D.F., & Beck, C.T. (2004). Nursing research: Principles and methods (7th ed.). Philadelphia: Lippincott, Williams, and Wilkins.

Popper, K.R. (1965). Conjectures and refutations: The growth of scientific knowledge. New York: Harper and Row.

Popper, K.R. (1970). Normal science and its dangers. In I. Lakatos & A. Musgrave (Eds.), Criticism and the growth of knowledge (pp. 51–58). London: Cambridge University Press.

Rawnsley, .M. (1996). Response to: "On the requirements for a metaparadigm: An invitation to dialogue." Nursing Science Quarterly, 9, 102–106.

Rawnsley, M.M. (2000). Response to Kim's human living concept as a unifying perspective for nursing. Nursing Science Quarterly, 13, 41–44.

Rawnsley, M.M. (2003). Dimensions of scholarship and the advancement of nursing science: Articulating a vision. Nursing Science Quarterly, 16, 6–13.

Reese, H.W., & Overton, W.F. (1970). Models of development and theories of development. In L.R. Goulet & P.B. Baltes (Eds.), Life span developmental psychology: Research and theory (pp. 115–145). New York: Academic Press.

Reilly, D.E. (1975). Why a conceptual framework? Nursing Outlook, 23, 566–569.

Riehl, J.P., & Roy, C. (1974). Conceptual models for nursing practice. New York: Appleton-Century-Crofts.

Riehl, J.P., & Roy, C. (1980). Conceptual models for nursing practice (2nd ed.). New York: Appleton-Century-Crofts.

Rogers, M.E. (1970). An introduction to the theoretical basis of nursing. Philadelphia: F.A. Davis.

Rogers, M.E. (1986). Science of unitary human beings. In V.M. Malinski (Ed.), Explorations on Martha Rogers' science of unitary human beings (pp. 3–8). Norwalk, CT: Appleton-Century-Crofts.

Rogers, M.E. (1990). Nursing: Science of unitary, irreducible, human beings: Update 1990. In E.A.M. Barrett (Ed.), Visions of Rogers' science-based nursing (pp. 5–11). New York: National League for Nursing.

Rogers, M.E. (1992). Nursing science and the space age. Nursing Science Quarterly, 5, 27–34.

Rogers, M.E. (1994a). Nursing science evolves. In M. Madrid & E.A.M. Barrett (Eds.), Rogers' scientific art of nursing practice (pp. 3–9). New York: National League for Nursing Press.

Rogers, M.E. (1994b). The science of unitary human beings: Current perspectives. Nursing Science Quarterly, 7, 33–35.

Roper, N. (1994). Definition of nursing: 2. British Journal of Nursing, 3, 460–462.

Roy, C. (1976). Introduction to nursing: An adaptation model. Englewood Cliffs, NJ: Prentice-Hall.

Roy, C., & Andrews, H.A. (1999). The Roy adaptation model (2nd ed.). Stamford, CT: Appleton & Lange.

Rudner, R.S. (1966). Philosophy of social science. Englewood Cliffs, NJ: Prentice-Hall.

Salsberry, P. (1994). A philosophy of nursing: What is it? What is it not? In J.F. Kikuchi & H. Simmons (Eds.), Developing a philosophy of nursing (pp. 11–19). Thousand Oaks, CA: Sage.

Schumacher, K.L., & Meleis, A.I. (1994). Transitions: A central concept in nursing. Image: Journal of Nursing Scholarship, 26, 119–127.

Seaver, J.W., & Cartwright, C.A. (1977). A pluralistic foundation for training early childhood professionals. Curriculum Inquiry, 7, 305–329.

Slife, B.D., & Williams, R.N. (1995). What's behind the research? Discovering hidden assumptions in the behavioral sciences. Thousand Oaks, CA: Sage.

Smith, M.C. (1979). Proposed metaparadigm for nursing research and theory development. Image, 11, 75–79.

Smith, M.J., & Liehr, P.R. (Eds.) (2003). Middle range theory for nursing. New York: Springer.

Swanson, K.M. (1991). Empirical development of a middle range theory of caring. Nursing Research, 40, 161–165.

Thomae, H. (1979). The concept of development and life-span developmental psychology. In P.B. Baltes & O.G. Brim, Jr. (Eds.), Life-span development and behavior (Vol. 2, pp. 281–312). New York: Academic Press.

Thorne, S., Canam, C., Dahinten, S., Hall, W., Henderson, A., & Kirkham, S. (1998). Nursing's metaparadigm concepts:

Disimpacting the debates. Journal of Advanced Nursing, 27, 1257–1268.

Villarruel, A.M., Bishop, T.L., Simpson, E.M., Jemmott, L.S., & Fawcett, J. (2001). Borrowed theories, shared theories, and the advancement of nursing knowledge. Nursing Science Quarterly, 14, 158–163.

von Bertalanffy, L. (1968). General system theory. New York: George Braziller.

Wagner, J.D. (1986). Nurse scholars' perceptions of nursing's metaparadigm. Dissertation Abstracts International, 47, 1932B.

Waters, M. (1994). Modern sociological theory. Thousand Oaks, CA: Sage.

Watson, J. (1985). Nursing: Human science and human care: A theory of nursing. Norwalk, CT: Appleton-Century-Crofts.

Watson, J. (1990). Caring knowledge and informed moral passion. Advances in Nursing Science, 13(1), 15–24.

Watson, J. (1996). Watson's theory of transpersonal caring. In P. Hinton Walker & B. Neuman (Eds.), Blueprint for use of nursing models: Education, research, practice, and administration (pp. 141–184). New York: NLN Press.

Watson, J. (1997). The theory of human caring: Retrospective and prospective. Nursing Science Quarterly, 10, 49–52.

Wells, L.E., & Stryker, S. (1988). Stability and change in self over the life course. In P.B. Baltes, D.L. Featherman, & R.M. Lerner (Eds.), Life-span development and behavior (pp. 191–229). Hillsdale, NJ: Lawrence Erlbaum Associates.

Wilber, K. (1998). The marriage of sense and soul. New York: Random House.

Wilson, C. (1994). Care: Superior ideal for nursing? Nursing Praxis in New Zealand, 9(3), 4–11.

Young, A., Taylor, S.G., & McLaughlin-Renpenning, K. (2001). Connections: Nursing research, theory, and practice. St. Louis: Mosby.

Yura, H., & Torres, G. (1975). Today's conceptual framework within baccalaureate nursing programs. In Faculty-curriculum development. Part III: Conceptual framework—Its meaning and function (pp. 17–25). New York: National League for Nursing.

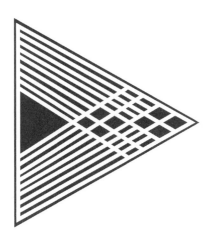

Chapter **2**

Implementing Nursing Models and Theories in Practice

The application of a conceptual model of nursing or a nursing theory in the real world of research, education, administration, or practice occurs when a conceptual model, one or more theories, and one or more empirical indicators are linked to create a conceptual-theoretical-empirical system of nursing knowledge. Consequently, conceptual model-based or theory-guided scientific and practical activities actually involve implementation of a full conceptual-theoretical-empirical system of nursing knowledge. Typically, however, when discussion centers on conceptual model-based nursing practice, theories and empirical indicators are not mentioned. Similarly, when discussion centers on theory-guided nursing practice, conceptual models and empirical indicators are not mentioned. This chapter extends discussions of conceptual model-based and theory-guided nursing practice, including those in Chapters 4 through 10 and 12 through 17 of this book, by focusing on full conceptual-theoretical-empirical systems of nursing knowledge.

More specifically, this chapter presents a discussion of the substantive and process elements of the implementation of conceptual-theoretical-empirical systems of nursing knowledge (C-T-E systems) in the real world of nursing practice. The chapter begins with a definition and discussion of C-T-E system-based nursing practice. The chapter continues with an explanation of the substantive elements of implementing C-T-E systems that emphasizes the translation of the components of the structural holarchy of contemporary nursing knowledge into C-T-E systems for nursing practice. Included in the section on substantive elements is discussion of the guidelines for use of conceptual models as guides for nursing practice, nursing research, nursing education, and nursing administration. Next, the process elements of implementing C-T-E systems are discussed, including identification of 10 phases of implementation. The chapter concludes with a description of the perspective transformation that nurses experience when they adopt an explicit C-T-E system as a guide for nursing practice.

Although the discussion in this chapter emphasizes implementation of C-T-E systems in nursing departments within larger health care institutions, the substantive and process elements are equally applicable to the individual practitioner who works in a health-care institution or has a private practice (Fawcett, 1997), and to practitioners who work together in group practices or free-standing nursing organizations. The substantive and process elements are also applicable in nursing education, where the emphasis is on using C-T-E systems to guide curriculum construction and teaching students to base nursing practice on explicit C-T-E systems (Lowry, 1998).

Overview

The implementation of conceptual-theoretical-empirical systems of nursing knowledge (C-T-E systems) requires attention to elements of both substance and process, as well as considerable thought, careful planning, and commitment to a long-term project that typically involves much change in the form and scope of nursing practice. Recommendations regarding the substantive elements and the process elements of implementation are presented in this chapter. These recommendations are based on an integration of published descriptions of successful projects that were designed to implement specific conceptual models of nursing and nursing theories in nursing practice settings, and extend typical discussions of factors involved in change. The substantive and process elements associated with implementation of C-T-E systems, as well as the phases of the transformation nurses experience when they adopt an explicit C-T-E system, are listed here. Each element and phase is defined and described in detail in this chapter.

Key Terms

CONCEPTUAL-THEORETICAL-EMPIRICAL SYSTEM-BASED NURSING PRACTICE

CONCEPTUAL-THEORETICAL-EMPIRICAL (C-T-E) SYSTEM-BASED NURSING PRACTICE is defined as *service to society guided by knowledge that is specific to the discipline of nursing, as articulated in conceptual models of nursing and nursing theories.*

Kenney (1995) explained that nurses apply C-T-E systems in practice "through critical thinking, psychomotor skills, and interpersonal actions to assist [nursing participants] to achieve their optimum health potential" (p. 6). Elaborating, she noted that "The art of nursing is the interpersonal relationship and interaction process between the person and the nurse within a social environment during delivery of nursing. … The science and art of nursing are creatively applied within the nursing process [or practice methodology of each conceptual model and theory] by critical thinking" (p. 6).

When nurses engage in C-T-E system–based nursing practice, "they are able to systematically identify, label, aggregate and synthesize phenomena. Nurses need a [C-T-E system] to help them understand which data are important, how these data relate, what can be predicted by these relationships, and what interventions are needed to deal with specific relationships. ... Without this understanding, data are often collected and left uninterpreted or never collected at all" (Raudonis & Acton, 1997, pp. 138–139). Furthermore, C-T-E system-based nursing practice provides an "anchor in the sea of issues and problems" and constant change that characterize contemporary health care throughout the world (Parker, 1990, p. 4).

FUNCTIONS OF CONCEPTUAL-THEORETICAL-EMPIRICAL SYSTEM-BASED NURSING PRACTICE

One function of C-T-E system-based nursing practice is to provide an intellectual lens for viewing the human beings who participate in nursing, their environments, and their health. Another function is to provide a purposeful and systematic process for practice, that is, a practice methodology. "When nurses practice purposefully and systematically, they are more efficient, have better control over outcomes of their [practice], and are better able to communicate with others" (Raudonis & Acton, 1997, p. 139).

SUBSTANTIVE ELEMENTS OF IMPLEMENTING A CONCEPTUAL-THEORETICAL-EMPIRICAL SYSTEM OF NURSING KNOWLEDGE

The **SUBSTANTIVE ELEMENTS OF IMPLEMENTING A CONCEPTUAL-THEORETICAL-EMPIRICAL SYSTEM OF NURSING KNOWLEDGE** in nursing practice involve the translation of the components of the structural holarchy of contemporary nursing knowledge for the real world of nursing practice (Fig. 2–1). The components of the structural holarchy of contemporary nursing knowledge—the metaparadigm, philosophies, conceptual models, theories, and empirical indicators—were described in detail in Chapter 1 of this book. Successful implementation of C-T-E systems in nursing practice requires consideration of each component of the structural holarchy as it relates to the particular nursing department and health care institution.

TRANSLATING THE METAPARADIGM CONCEPTS FOR NURSING PRACTICE

The first substantive element of implementing C-T-E system-based nursing practice is the **translation of the metaparadigm of nursing**. The concepts of the metaparadigm of nursing identify the phenomena of interest to the discipline of nursing as human beings, environment, health, and nursing (see Chapter 1). When translated for practice, the metaparadigm concepts become the nursing participant, who may be an individual, a family, or a community requiring nursing; the environment of the nursing participant, including significant others, physical surroundings, and the nursing practice setting; the health condition of the nursing participant; and the nursing process, or practice methodology, used.

The mission statement of each health care institution identifies the particular characteristics and health conditions of the population of nursing participants served by that institution. For example, a children's hospital provides services for children with various health conditions, whereas a children's rehabilitation hospital provides services only to children with health conditions requiring intensive inpatient or outpatient rehabilitation. Similarly, a large inner city tertiary medical center serves all residents of the city and people referred from other locations, whereas a small community hospital typically serves only the members of the immediate community.

The limitations imposed by the mission of the health care institution on the population of nursing participants served and types of health conditions considered, as well as the structural design of the institution, have an influence on the relevant environments of nursing participants and the scope of the nursing practice methodology. For example, the physical structure of units may require nursing to be provided in large open wards or in private rooms. Moreover, direct assessment of nursing participants' home resources and frequent face-to-face contact with family members may be difficult or impossible if the nursing participants have been referred from distant communities. In addition, nursing activities that emphasize primary prevention and health promotion may be more limited in an institution whose mission is trauma care than in an institution whose mission is ambulatory care.

TRANSLATING THE PHILOSOPHY FOR NURSING PRACTICE

The second substantive element is the **translation of philosophies** for nursing practice. When translated for nursing practice, the philosophy refers to statements that reflect beliefs and values about nursing as a discipline and

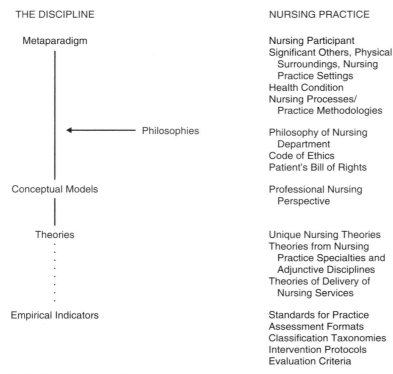

THE DISCIPLINE		NURSING PRACTICE
Metaparadigm		Nursing Participant
		Significant Others, Physical
		Surroundings, Nursing
		Practice Settings
		Health Condition
		Nursing Processes/
		Practice Methodologies
	←——— Philosophies	Philosophy of Nursing
		Department
		Code of Ethics
		Patient's Bill of Rights
Conceptual Models		Professional Nursing
		Perspective
Theories		Unique Nursing Theories
		Theories from Nursing
		Practice Specialties and
		Adjunctive Disciplines
		Theories of Delivery of
		Nursing Services
Empirical Indicators		Standards for Practice
		Assessment Formats
		Classification Taxonomies
		Intervention Protocols
		Evaluation Criteria

FIG. 2–1. The structural holarchy of contemporary nursing knowledge translated for nursing practice.

a profession, the beliefs and values held by a particular health care institution about the nursing participant and health care, and the beliefs and values of the nurses who work in the institution about nursing participants, the environment, health, and methodologies for nursing practice. Philosophical statements about the discipline and the profession of nursing appear in documents such as the American Nurses' Association Code of Ethics, and philosophical statements about human beings and health care appear in the Patient's Bill of Rights. The philosophy of the nursing department of each health care institution typically incorporates relevant notions from a code of ethics and a patient's bill of rights and further articulates the nurses' particular beliefs and values.

TRANSLATING THE CONCEPTUAL MODEL, THEORIES, AND EMPIRICAL INDICATORS INTO A PROFESSIONAL PRACTICE MODEL

The third substantive element of implementing C-T-E system–based nursing practice is **translation of the con-**

ceptual model, theories, and empirical indicators into a formal nursing knowledge system. Creation of a C-T-E system of nursing knowledge requires the linkage of a conceptual model of nursing, one or more theories, and one or more empirical indicators. The starting point may be a conceptual model of nursing (Chapters 4 through 10), a nursing grand theory (Chapters 12 through 14), or a nursing middle-range theory (Chapters 15 through 17). Regardless of the starting point, a full C-T-E system—not just a conceptual model or a theory—actually is used to guide nursing practice.

C-T-E systems are comprehensive professional practice models that extend the statement of values, professional and structural relationships, communication channels, management approach, governance structure, and compensation and rewards packages that compose the so-called professional practice models described in the nursing literature (e.g., Hoffart & Woods, 1996; Stenglein et al., 1993; Zelauskas & Howes, 1992). Here, the meaning of a professional practice model is extended to also include the conceptual models and theories that always guide scientific and practical nursing activities (Brooks & Rosenberg, 1995).

The process of selecting the conceptual model of nursing or nursing theory that is the starting point for the creation of a C-T-E system is discussed later in this chapter. Suffice it to say that the conceptual model of nursing or nursing theory that is selected must be appropriate for the population of nursing participants served by the healthcare institution and congruent with the philosophy of the nursing department. If the starting point is a nursing theory, the conceptual model from which the theory was derived has to be identified, as do appropriate empirical indicators. If the starting point is a conceptual model, unique nursing theories and theories from adjunctive disciplines that address the specific knowledge required for practice with the population of nursing participants served by the health care institution have to be identified. These theories represent practice knowledge that is in the form of relatively concrete and specific descriptions, explanations, and predictions about elements of nursing practice that come from the results of nursing research and research in such adjunctive disciplines as physiology, biochemistry, nutrition, pharmacology, sociology, psychology, and education. The reports of relevant research can be found in textbooks, practice specialty journals, and research journals.

In addition, a theory of delivery of nursing services must be included in the C-T-E system. Such theories address methods used to deliver nursing services, including team nursing, primary nursing, case management, and managed care (Hood & Leddy, 2003; Manthey, 1990; Rafferty, 1992; Zander, 1990). Inasmuch as C-T-E system-based nursing practice virtually mandates individualized practice for each nursing participant, the service delivery theory should facilitate that type of practice. Primary nursing has been recommended as a particularly appropriate theory for C-T-E system-based nursing practice (Shea et al., 1989; Walsh, 1989). Another appropriate theory is nursing case management (Ethridge, 1991).

The theories of delivery of nursing services address only the way in which nursing services are organized and delivered to the nursing participant; they do not provide the substance of those nursing services (Brazen, 1992). The substance comes from the conceptual model and theories.

The recognition of the need to link theories with conceptual models reflects an understanding of the different functions of conceptual models and theories. As Aggleton and Chalmers (1990) explained,

> While it is reasonable to expect a model of nursing to provide general guidelines for intervention, it is unlikely that [the model] will give detailed guidance on the precise ways in which nurses can act. It is crucial for the model to have this kind of emphasis, since it alerts nurses to the need to look elsewhere to find out more about a particular issue. Indeed, it is probably undesirable for a model to go beyond advocating

certain broad principles of intervention. This way, nurses will be encouraged to make use of up-to-date studies to inform practice (p. 42).

The results of studies inform practice in a very formal manner when those results are regarded as the theories that further specify the general parameters of assessment, labeling, planning, intervention, and evaluation that are provided by the conceptual model. Thus, research results become one way to specify the theory part of a C-T-E system of nursing knowledge.

The conceptual model and theories selected for inclusion in a C-T-E system must be logically congruent. Whall (1980) presented the first substantial discussion in the nursing literature of elements to consider when assessing logical congruence between conceptual models of nursing and theories. She proposed that conceptual models and theories must be examined for their stands on holism and linearity. Holism is a major characteristic of both the reciprocal interaction and simultaneous action world views, whereas linearity is a central characteristic of the reaction world view (Fawcett, 1993) (see Chapter 1). Whall's (1980) discussion suggested that if the world views of the conceptual model and the theory are not congruent, the theory should be discarded and another more congruent one chosen; otherwise, the theory should be reformulated so that it is congruent with the model. Inasmuch as the conceptual model is the more abstract starting point, the theory—not the model—is reformulated to ensure congruence. Examples of linkage of logically congruent conceptual models and theories, using reformulated theories from adjunctive disciplines, are given in Fitzpatrick and colleagues (1982), McFarlane (1988), and Whall (1986). An example of the linkage of two conceptual models of nursing—Neuman's Systems Model and Orem's Self-Care Framework—with the logically congruent theory of planned behavior from the discipline of psychology, is given in Villarruel, Bishop, Simpson, Jemmott, and Fawcett (2001).

Empirical indicators are selected after the conceptual model and relevant theories have been selected. When translated for nursing practice, empirical indicators refer to the documents and technology—the practice tools—used to guide and direct nursing practice, to record observations and results of interventions, and to describe and evaluate nursing job performance. In other words, the empirical indicators encompass the standards for nursing practice, department and unit objectives, nursing care plans, patient database and classification tools, flow sheets, Kardex forms, computer information systems, quality assurance tools, nursing job descriptions and performance appraisal tools, and other relevant documents and technologies (Fawcett, 1992; Fitch et al., 1991; Laurie-Shaw & Ives, 1988). Each practice tool selected for inclusion in a C-T-E system must be logically congruent with the conceptual model and must be a reliable and valid indicator of the theory concept it is to measure.

General Guidelines for Nursing

Each conceptual model is a distinctive professional nursing perspective (see Fig. 2–1) that stipulates rules, or guidelines, for nursing activities. Guidelines that are inherent in each conceptual model of nursing provide broad guidelines for nursing practice, as well as for nursing research, education, and administration. Inasmuch as nursing practice should be based on the findings of nursing research, is learned through nursing education, and is organized through nursing administration, guidelines for research, education, and administration are specified here, along with those for practice. The general guidelines for nursing practice are listed in the following paragraphs, followed by those for nursing research, nursing education, and nursing administration. The particular guidelines for each conceptual model included in this book are given in Chapters 4 through 10. The guidelines encompass a set of statements about a domain of interest and epistemic and methodological norms about how that domain can be applied in real world situations (Laudan, 1981), and are followed when conceptual models are linked with theories and empirical indicators to form C-T-E systems.

General Guidelines for Nursing Practice. Conceptual models of nursing provide general guidelines for nursing practice. A fully developed conceptual model represents a particular view of and approach to nursing practice. When a conceptual model is used to guide nursing practice, the metaparadigm concept of human beings refers to the nursing participant, who may be an individual, a family, or a community requiring nursing. Environment refers to the nursing participant's significant others and physical surroundings, as well as to the nursing practice setting. Health refers to the health-related condition of the nursing participant. Nursing refers to the nursing process, or practice methodology, used. The domain of nursing practice and nursing processes are specified in six guidelines that are inherent in each conceptual model:

- The first guideline identifies the purposes to be fulfilled by nursing practice.
- The second guideline identifies the general nature of the practice problems to be considered.
- The third guideline identifies the settings in which nursing practice occurs.

- The fourth guideline identifies the characteristics of legitimate participants in nursing practice.
- The fifth guideline identifies the nursing process to be employed and the technologies to be used, including parameters for assessment, labels for practice, a strategy for planning, a typology of interventions, and criteria for evaluation of outcomes.
- The sixth guideline identifies the nature of contributions that nursing practice makes to the well-being of nursing participants.

A conceptual model guides all aspects of practice and all aspects of the nursing practice methodology. The specifics of nursing assessment, labeling, planning, intervention, and evaluation must, however, come from theories. Although the conceptual model may, for example, direct the practitioner to look for certain categories of problems in adaptation, theories of adaptation are needed to describe, explain, and predict manifestations of actual or potential patient problems in particular situations. Similarly, theories are needed to direct the particular nursing interventions required in such situations (Lipsey, 1993; Sidani & Braden, 1998). The C-T-E structure is completed when relevant empirical indicators, such as standards for nursing practice, an assessment format, a classification system, intervention protocols, a quality assurance program, and an information system, are identified.

General Guidelines for Nursing Research. The function of nursing research is to generate or test nursing theories. Every theory development effort is guided by a conceptual model, which acts as a research tradition. Laudan (1981) explained the relations between conceptual models (which he called research traditions), theories, and empirical testing. He stated,

> Research traditions are not directly testable, both because their ontologies are too general to yield specific predictions and because their methodological components, being guidelines or norms, are not straightforwardly testable assertions about matters of fact. Associated with any active research tradition is a family of theories. … The theories … share the ontology of the parent research tradition and can be tested and evaluated using its methodological norms (p. 151).

When a conceptual model is used to guide nursing research, the metaparadigm concept of human beings becomes the study participant. Environment becomes the relevant surroundings of the study participant, as well as the research infrastructure available to the investigator. Health refers to the study participant's health-related condition, and nursing refers to the research methods.

A fully developed conceptual model reflects a particular

research tradition that includes seven guidelines that guide theory generation and testing through all phases of a study (Laudan, 1981; Schlotfeldt, 1975):

- The first guideline identifies the purposes to be fulfilled by the research.
- The second guideline identifies the phenomena that are to be studied.
- The third guideline identifies the nature of the problems to be studied.
- The fourth guideline identifies the source of the data (individuals, groups, animals, documents) and the settings in which data are to be gathered.
- The fifth guideline identifies the research designs, instruments, and procedures that are to be employed.
- The sixth guideline identifies the methods to be employed in reducing and analyzing the data.
- The seventh guideline identifies the nature of contributions that the research will make to the advancement of knowledge.

A conceptual model contains the concepts from which specific variables are derived for the research and the general propositions from which testable hypotheses are eventually derived. In addition, the conceptual model guides the selection of appropriate empirical indicators. The subject matter of the study might be one concept or the relation between two or more concepts. A study may involve generation or testing of a unique nursing theory, or theories borrowed from other disciplines may be linked with the conceptual model to test the empirical adequacy of the theory in nursing situations. Care must be taken, however, to ensure that the conceptual model and the theory are logically congruent; that is, the model and the theory must reflect compatible world views about the nature of the phenomena to be studied (Fawcett, 1993; Whall, 1980).

The findings of research based on explicit C-T-E systems of nursing knowledge are, of course, used to evaluate the empirical adequacy of the theory. Those findings also constitute indirect evidence regarding the conceptual model and are used to evaluate its credibility. Thus, the credibility of the conceptual model should be considered in addition to the empirical adequacy of the theory whenever research is conducted.

General Guidelines for Nursing Education. In nursing education, the conceptual model, or conceptual framework as it usually is called, provides the general outline for curriculum content and teaching-learning activities. A fully developed conceptual model represents a particular view of and approach to nursing education. When a conceptual model is used to guide nursing education, the metaparadigm concept human beings becomes the student, and environment

becomes the educational setting. Health refers to the student's health-related condition, and nursing refers to the educational goals, outcomes, and processes.

The curricular structure and educational processes are specified in five guidelines that are inherent in each conceptual model:

- The first guideline identifies the distinctive focus of the curriculum and the purposes to be fulfilled by nursing education.
- The second guideline identifies the general nature and sequence of the content to be presented.
- The third guideline identifies the settings in which nursing education occurs.
- The fourth guideline identifies the characteristics of legitimate students.
- The fifth guideline identifies the teaching-learning strategies to be used.

When a conceptual model is used for curriculum construction, it must be linked with theories about education and the teaching-learning process, as well as with substantive theoretical content from nursing and adjunctive disciplines (Fawcett, 1985). In addition, appropriate empirical indicators, in the form of the actual classroom content, practicum experiences, and student assignments, must be identified. The resulting C-T-E system then applies to the nursing participant, the student, and the educator.

General Guidelines for Nursing Administration. When a conceptual model is used in nursing administration, it provides a systematic structure for thinking about administrative structures, for observations of the administrative situation, and for interpreting what is seen in administrative settings (Fawcett et al., 1989). Each fully developed conceptual model represents a particular view of and approach to administration of nursing services. When a conceptual model is used to guide nursing administration, the metaparadigm concept of human beings may refer to the staff of a health-care institution, the department of nursing as a whole, or even the entire institution. Environment becomes the relevant practice milieu for the staff and the surroundings of the department of nursing and the health-care institution. Health refers to the health-related conditions of the staff or the functional condition of the department or institution. Nursing encompasses the management strategies and administrative policies used by the nurse administrator on behalf of or in conjunction with the staff, the department of nursing, and the institution.

The administrative structure and management practices are specified in five guidelines that are inherent in each conceptual model:

- The first guideline identifies the distinctive focus of nursing in the health care institution.
- The second guideline identifies the purpose to be fulfilled by nursing services.
- The third guideline identifies the characteristics of legitimate nursing personnel.
- The fourth guideline identifies the settings in which nursing services are delivered.
- The fifth guideline identifies the management strategies and administrative policies to be used.

When a conceptual model is used to guide administrative practices, it must be linked with theories of organizations and management developed in nursing and adjunctive disciplines. Moreover, empirical indicators in the form of specific management strategies must be identified, and administrative policies must be formulated. The resulting C-T-E structure is then applicable to the nursing participant, the nursing staff, and the nurse administrator.

 ## PROCESS ELEMENTS OF IMPLEMENTING A CONCEPTUAL-THEORETICAL-EMPIRICAL SYSTEM OF NURSING KNOWLEDGE

The **PROCESS ELEMENTS OF IMPLEMENTING A CONCEPTUAL-THEORETICAL-EMPIRICAL SYSTEM OF NURSING KNOWLEDGE** encompass 10 phases. These 10 phases of an implementation project require at least 27 to 36 months. The first 5 phases take approximately 9 to 12 months. The sixth phase takes at least another 6 months. The 7th through 10th phases require at least an additional 12 to 18 months. Consequently, the decision to implement C-T-E system-based nursing practice in a health-care institution involves not only the willingness to do so but also the motivation and resources to continue a long-term project.

FIRST PHASE: IDEA OR VISION

The **First Phase: Idea or Vision** of the implementation of an explicit C-T-E system focuses on envisioning what nursing practice should be and can be, rather than what it currently is. The idea may be put forth by one or more staff nurses, clinical specialists, or nurse managers, or by the nurse executive. Regardless of who initiates the idea, it is crucial that both administrators and staff are willing to at least consider a new approach to the practice of nursing in the health-care institution. Moreover, a spirit of adventure and risk taking on the part of administrators and staff, as well as a high tolerance for ambiguity and resistance to change, will greatly facilitate the continuation of the implementation project.

SECOND PHASE: FORMATION OF A TASK FORCE FOR FEASIBILITY STUDY

The **Second Phase: Formation of a Task Force for Feasibility Study** deals with determining the feasibility of implementing C-T-E system-based nursing practice. Much time can be saved and much frustration can be avoided if the originators of the idea of practicing using an explicit C-T-E system conduct a feasibility study in the form of an initial assessment of the practice climate to determine if it is conducive to using an explicit C-T-E system (Capers, 1986; Gray, 1991). The task force should include key nursing personnel, including the nurse executive or designee and a representative from each category of nursing personnel who work in the health-care institution. The feasibility study questionnaire, which should be sent to all nursing personnel, should focus on the physical, psychological, and organizational climate for change to a new way of practicing nursing (Gray, 1991).

THIRD PHASE: PLANNING COMMITTEE AND LONG-RANGE PLAN

Implementation proceeds to the **Third Phase: Planning Committee and Long-Range Plan.** if the results of the feasibility study reveal a favorable climate for C-T-E system-based nursing practice. The third phase encompasses formation of a planning committee and the development of a long-range plan, a formal action plan, or a strategic plan (Craig & Beynon, 1996). A business plan also should be developed, so that costs can be tracked.

The planning committee may include the original task force members or other interested nurses. The committee also should include representatives from other organizational units of the health-care institution, such as the institution administrator or designee and representatives from medicine, social work, dietetics, physical therapy, occupational therapy, respiratory therapy, and other relevant departments. Although such a broad membership may seem cumbersome, it is important that all individuals who will be affected by the change in nursing practice be directly involved in that change. Indeed, the "key to success of [C-T-E system-based nursing practice is] the commitment and ability of nurses [and others] to become more active in their selection, implementation, and evaluation" (Barr, 1997, p. 689). Subcommittees can be formed to carry out various tasks involved in planning and implementing C-T-E system-based nursing practice. In addition, the planning committee should include an on-site consultant who is an expert in the content of conceptual models of nursing and nursing theories and the process of implementing C-T-E system-based nursing practice (Northrup & Cody, 1998). Although one or more nurses within the health-care institution may have such expertise, a nurse consultant who has no formal tie to the institution frequently is more effective in moving the implementation project forward. A major function of the consultant is to help all personnel to understand that conceptual models of nursing and nursing theories provide a scientific base for nursing practice, which, in turn, helps the nurse to "understand people, the causes of illness and its treatment, and the organizational settings within which nursing is practiced" (Anderson, 1997, p. 249).

The long-range and business plans should contain a specific timeline for actions and the human and material resources required. More specifically, the plan should address: (a) the outcomes that are anticipated from use of the C-T-E system; (b) the nursing personnel who will use the C-T-E system; (c) the identification of subsequent phases of implementation and the time required for each phase; and (d) the financial resources that are needed and those that are available.

The decision to implement C-T-E system-based nursing practice is typically undertaken in response to the quest for a way to articulate the substance and scope of professional nursing practice to members of other health care disciplines and the public and to improve the conditions and outcomes of nursing practice. Consequently, one anticipated outcome of C-T-E system-based nursing practice is enhanced understanding of the role of nursing in health care by administrators, physicians, social workers, dietitians, physical therapists, occupational therapists, respiratory therapists, and other health-care team members, as well as by the population of nursing participants served by the health-care institution. Another anticipated outcome is increased nursing staff satisfaction with the conditions and outcomes of nursing practice through an explicit focus on and identification of nursing problems and actions, as well as through enhanced communication and documentation (Fitch et al., 1991). Still another anticipated outcome is increased satisfaction of nursing participants and their families with the nursing received. Other more specific outcomes that are relevant to a particular health-care institution may be formulated as the long-range plan is developed. For example, a computerized documentation system or a patient classification system based on the C-T-E system may be a desired outcome. Indeed, such an outcome may be the catalyst for the implementation of C-T-E system–based nursing practice. Still other outcomes are tied to the particular C-T-E system selected. Anticipated and actual outcomes of the use of various conceptual models of nursing and nursing theories are identified in Chapters 4 through 10 and 12 through 17.

C-T-E system–based nursing practice is most effective when all categories of nursing personnel, from aides through the nurse executive, use the designated C-T-E system to guide their nursing activities. The C-T-E system can be adapted to the particular focus of each person's activities. For example, nurse managers and the nurse executive may use a version of the C-T-E system that is adapted for administration, whereas the nurse aides, practical nurses, registered nurses, clinical specialists, and nurse practitioners use the version that directly addresses nursing practice. The depth of use and the scope of phenomena addressed within the context of the particular C-T-E will vary according to the educational level and concomitant knowledge of each category of nursing personnel (Cox, 1991).

As the long-range plan develops, additional phases of planning and implementing C-T-E system-based nursing practice need to be identified, along with the estimated time for each phase. The typical implementation project proceeds through seven more phases: the fourth through the tenth.

The business plan should focus on expenditures. The actual cost of implementing C-T-E system-based nursing practice has not yet been fully addressed in the nursing or health-care literature. Costs most likely vary from institution to institution depending on the staff's current knowledge of conceptual models and theories, existing staff development resources, extent of change in documentation, and the like. Categories of costs include, but are not limited to, consultation fees, printing of all documents, staff orientation and development, and data analysis. Some cost categories represent existing budget items, but others represent new items. For example, most health-care institutions already allocate funds for staff orientation and development, but few regularly allocate funds for consultation from nurse experts. Consequently, the nurse executive must be prepared to negotiate with the finance officer and the institution administrator for the supplemental funds that will be needed to sustain the implementation project. In addition, the nurse executive may apply to federal agencies, foundations, or other extramural sources for funding (Capers et al., 1985).

FOURTH PHASE: REVIEW OF DOCUMENTS

The **Fourth Phase: Review of Documents** focuses on reviewing all documents that serve as a base for nursing practice. In particular, the mission statement of the health care institution and the philosophy of the nursing department should be reviewed at this point in the implementation project. The written mission statement of the health-care institution should be examined to determine its congruence with the actual situation. As the statement is examined, the opportunity for all members of the health-care team to reaffirm their commitment to a particular population of nursing participants is provided. The opportunity to discuss changes in the population of nursing participants served is, of course, also provided.

Next, the philosophy of the nursing department should be reviewed to determine if it reflects current beliefs about nursing held by the members of the discipline at large, as well as by the nurses at the health-care institution where the implementation project is taking place. The implementation project, then, may act as a catalyst for reaffirmation or revision of the nursing department's current philosophy of nursing.

A comprehensive review of the current philosophy could take the form of a survey of all nursing personnel that seeks to elicit each nurse's beliefs and values about nursing participants, their environments and health, and nursing processes. Or the review could be in the form of a request that all nursing personnel comment on the current philosophy and engage in "reflective deliberation" to reaffirm or develop a shared understanding of the beliefs and values undergirding nursing practice at the health care institution (Cheek, Gibson, & Heartfield, 1993, p. 69). Regardless of the approach taken, the result should be a document that articulates a philosophy representing the beliefs and values of those nurses who are responsible for the nursing of the population of nursing participants served by the health care institution.

Moreover, as Johns (1989) noted, the philosophy of the nursing department "must be relevant to the context of where [nursing] is carried out … [as well as] to how nursing organizes the delivery of [services] on the unit and the relationship nursing has with medicine and the organization in general" (p. 3). He pointed out that the document may go through successive drafts until both the philosophic content and the language in which it is expressed are clearly understood and accepted by all nursing personnel (Johns, 1990).

FIFTH PHASE: SELECTION AND DEVELOPMENT OF A CONCEPTUAL-THEORETICAL-EMPIRICAL SYSTEM OF NURSING KNOWLEDGE

The **Fifth Phase: Selection and Development of a Conceptual-Theoretical-Empirical System of Nursing Knowledge** involves the selection of a conceptual model or nursing theory as the starting point for development of a formal C-T-E system of nursing knowledge. The process of selecting a conceptual model of nursing or a nursing the-

ory as the starting point should proceed through the following four steps:

1. Thoroughly analyze and evaluate several conceptual models of nursing and nursing theories.
2. Compare the content of each conceptual model and theory with the mission statement of the health-care institution to determine if the model or theory is appropriate for use with the population of nursing participants served.
3. Determine if the philosophic claims undergirding each conceptual model or theory are congruent with the philosophy of the nursing department.
4. Select the conceptual model or theory that most closely matches the mission of the health care institution and the philosophy of the nursing department.

Chapters 4 through 10 and 12 through 16 of this book contain thorough analyses and evaluations of Johnson's Behavioral System Model, King's General Systems Framework, Levine's Conservation Model, Neuman's Systems Model, Orem's Self-Care Framework, Rogers' Science of Unitary Human Beings, Roy's Adaptation Model, Newman's Theory of Health as Expanding Consciousness, Parse's Theory of Human Becoming, Orlando's Theory of the Deliberative Nursing Process, Peplau's Theory of Interpersonal Relations, and Watson's Theory of Human Caring. Reading these chapters, along with the primary source material for each conceptual model or theory, provides the foundation for the selection of the conceptual model or theory.

The next step is the comparison of the content of various conceptual models and theories with the mission statement of the health care institution, with particular attention given to whether that content will lead to nursing actions that are appropriate for the population of nursing participants served by that institution. Next, the fit of the underlying philosophic claims of each conceptual model and theory with the philosophy of the nursing department should be determined.

The literature associated with the conceptual models of nursing and nursing theories included in this book suggests that each is appropriate in a wide range of nursing situations and for many different populations of nursing participants. Aggleton and Chalmers (1985) noted that such literature "might encourage some nurses to feel that it does not really matter which model [or theory] of nursing is chosen to inform nursing practice within a particular care setting" (p. 39). They also noted that the literature might "encourage the view that choosing between models [or theories] is something one does intuitively, as an act of personal preference. Even worse, it might encourage some nurses to feel that all their everyday problems might be eliminated were they to make the 'right choice' in selecting a particular model [or theory] for use across a care setting" (p. 39).

Nurses have not yet addressed the extent to which the fit of a conceptual model or theory to particular populations of nursing participants might have been forced. Furthermore, little attention has been given to the extent to which a particular conceptual model or theory is modified by an individual or group to fit a given situation or culture (C.P. Germain, personal communication, October 21, 1987; Fawcett, 2003). Although modifications certainly are acceptable, they should be acknowledged and serious consideration should be given to renaming the conceptual model or theory to indicate that modifications have been made. Clearly, systematic exploration of the nursing specialty practice implications of various conceptual models and theories, coupled with more practical experience with each model and each theory in a variety of settings and cultures, is required.

Although pluralism in conceptual models and theories has been advocated (Barr, 1997; Kristjanson, Tamblyn, & Kuypers, 1987; Nagle & Mitchell, 1991; Story & Ross, 1986), it is recommended that just one conceptual model or theory be selected for initial use on all nursing units of a health-care institution. Health-care institutions that serve just one particular population of nursing participants or encompass just one practice specialty area should not have difficulty using one conceptual model or one theory to guide all nursing practice activities. General-purpose health-care institutions, however, may encounter difficulties if the conceptual model or theory selected does not readily guide practice for all nursing specialty areas and all populations of nursing participants served. However, use of more than one conceptual model or theory within an institution may pose problems for a nurse who works on different units, as well as for nursing participants who are moved from unit to unit as their health condition changes. In addition, use of more than one conceptual model or theory in a health care institution could have a negative impact on continuity of nursing and could dramatically increase the cost of implementing C-T-E system-based nursing practice because different forms, teaching materials, and procedures would have to be developed (Dee, 1990).

Schmieding (1984) claimed that adopting a single conceptual model or theory as the starting point for C-T-E system-based nursing practice in a health care institution "can help nurses work together for [high] quality nursing care" (p. 759). Furthermore, "without commitment to one [conceptual model or theory] the confusion remains; attitudes, values, and beliefs about nursing vary from one nurse to another and the delivery of care is left to the whim of the moment, one day demanding patient self-care and

the next placing the patient back in a dependent and passive role" (Mascord, 1988/1989, p. 15). Moreover, all of the successful implementation projects that have been reported in the literature focused on just one conceptual model of nursing or nursing theory (see Chapters 4 through 10 and 12 through 17).

Once a conceptual model or theory has been selected, work can proceed to development of an explicit C-T-E system. The issues involved in the creation of an explicit C-T-E system were discussed earlier in this chapter, in the section on substantive elements. In short, care must be taken to link a conceptual model, one or more theories, and one or more empirical indicators that are logically congruent. Special attention should be given to reviewing each existing document and all current technology for congruence with the conceptual model and theories. Although revision in or replacement of existing documents and technologies is frequently required, and although the work may seem overwhelming at the outset, the importance of having documents and technologies that are congruent with the conceptual and theoretical components of the C-T-E system cannot be overemphasized. Indeed, congruence may be regarded as the *sine qua non* of C-T-E system-based nursing practice.

The need seems obvious for revisions in or development of new documents and technology that have a direct influence on nursing practice, such as standards of practice, nursing care plans, and patient classification systems, so that they are congruent with the conceptual and theoretical components of the C-T-E system. The need to revise job descriptions and performance appraisal tools so that they, too, are congruent with the conceptual and theoretical components may not be as obvious. Yet, as Laurie-Shaw and Ives (1988) pointed out, these documents should acknowledge the use of the C-T-E system and "reinforce the importance of operationalizing the nursing standards of the department" (p. 18).

SIXTH PHASE: EDUCATION OF THE NURSING STAFF

The **Sixth Phase: Education of the Nursing Staff** focuses on the education of the nursing staff for C-T-E system-based practice. Education may occur through participation in staff development or continuing education seminars, workshops, retreats, discussion groups, unit conferences, and nursing grand rounds; formal courses offered by local colleges or through distance learning programs; and independent study. Ongoing educational activities should be made available to the current nursing staff and other members of the health care team, as well as to individuals who join the health care institution as the implementation project proceeds. Educational programs should contain information about the content of the C-T-E system and realistic examples of its use in nursing practice. Initially, the consultant and other nurses who have experience with C-T-E system-based nursing practice may act as preceptors to the staff. As the staff members become proficient, they can take over the preceptor role during the orientation of new employees.

SEVENTH PHASE: DEMONSTRATION SITES

The **Seventh Phase: Demonstration Sites** encompasses the designation of certain nursing units to serve as demonstration sites and the implementation of C-T-E system-based practice on those units. Participants in many implementation projects credit their success to careful phasing in of C-T-E system-based practice through demonstration projects on pilot units before implementing the C-T-E system on all of the nursing units. Implementation of C-T-E system-based nursing practice appears to be most successful when the procedures are "tailored to the particular style and variables of each nursing unit" (Laurie-Shaw & Ives, 1988, p. 19). The seventh phase also includes evaluation of the results of C-T-E system–based nursing practice on the pilot units, with emphasis on refinement of nursing documents and procedures for implementation.

EIGHTH PHASE: INSTITUTION-WIDE IMPLEMENTATION

The **Eighth Phase: Institution-Wide Implementation** focuses on implementation of the C-T-E system on all nursing units throughout the health care institution. This phase requires continuing attention to the education of current staff and the orientation of new staff with regard to C-T-E system-based nursing practice, as well as ongoing monitoring of and refinements in the implementation procedures. Again, procedures for implementation should take the characteristics of each unit into account (Laurie-Shaw & Ives, 1988).

NINTH PHASE: EVALUATION OF OUTCOMES

The **Ninth Phase: Evaluation of Outcomes** focuses on evaluation of administrative, nurse, and nursing participant outcomes of the implementation of C-T-E system-based nursing practice. Although the evaluation phase actually overlaps with other phases, its importance to the entire implementation project mandates that it be highlighted as a separate phase (K.M.Tong, personal communication, January 29, 1995).

Evaluation should be done periodically throughout the entire implementation project, and especially during the eighth phase, "to capture the flow and timing of the change [in outcomes]" (Fitch et al., 1991, p. 25). The evaluation should be carefully and systematically designed, in the form of an experimental or a quasi-experimental study (McKenna, 1993).

Outcomes in terms of the quality of nursing practice should be emphasized and should encompass the interpersonal and technical competence of the nurses, the physical and technical conditions of the health-care institution, and the sociocultural atmosphere of the institution (Wilde et al., 1993). The evaluation also should include documentation of environmental factors that might influence nurse and nursing participant outcomes, such as a major organizational change or changes in leadership within nursing or the larger institution (Fitch et al., 1991). Other environmental factors to consider include changes in institution accreditation criteria and changes in standards developed by national and international nursing organizations. Conclusions drawn from the evaluation of administrative, nurse, and nursing participant outcomes should be in the form of statements documenting the merit of the C-T-E system, including strengths and limitations.

TENTH PHASE: DISSEMINATION OF IMPLEMENTATION PROJECT PROCEDURES AND OUTCOMES

The **Tenth Phase: Dissemination of Implementation Project Procedures and Outcomes** involves presentations and publications that disseminate the implementation project procedures and outcomes (K.M. Tong, personal communication, January 29, 1995). No implementation project should be considered complete until presentations are given and manuscripts are published. Indeed, sharing what was done to implement C-T-E system-based nursing practice and what happened as a result is a crucial aspect of any implementation project. Posters and oral presentations should be prepared for the administrators and staff of the health-care institution, the public served by the health-care institution, and nursing peers at local, regional, national, and international conferences. Manuscripts should be prepared for publication as books, book chapters, and journal articles.

 ## PERSPECTIVE TRANSFORMATION

The successful implementation of C-T-E system-based nursing practice requires recognition of the time needed by each nurse and the health-care institution as a whole to evolve from use of individual, implicit frames of reference for nursing practice to an explicit C-T-E system. Given the paucity of attention given to the teaching of the content of nursing conceptual models and theories in many nursing programs (Mitchell, 2002), it is likely that many nurses are using their own implicit frame of reference for their practice. This situation underscores the importance of the process that occurs during the period of evolution, which is referred to as **PERSPECTIVE TRANSFORMATION.** Drawing from Mezirow's (1975, 1978) early work in the development of adult learning theory, Rogers (1989) explained that perspective transformation is based on the assumption that "individuals have a personal paradigm or meaning perspective that structures the way in which they existentially experience, interpret, and understand their world" (p. 112). She went on to define and describe perspective transformation as the process "whereby the assumptions, values, and beliefs that constitute a given meaning perspective come to consciousness, are reflected upon, and are critically analyzed. The process involves gradually taking on a new perspective along with the corresponding assumptions, values, and beliefs. The new perspective gives rise to fundamental structural changes in the way individuals see themselves and their relationships with others, leading to a reinterpretation of their personal, social, or occupational worlds" (p. 112).

Thus, the process of perspective transformation when C-T-E system-based nursing practice is implemented in a health-care institution involves the shift from one meaning perspective about nursing and nursing practice to another, from one way "of viewing and being with human beings" to another (Nagle & Mitchell, 1991, p. 22). Inasmuch as practice that is not based on an explicit C-T-E system is based on an implicit, private image of nursing (Reilly, 1975), the shift in meaning perspective is from a private image of nursing to a public image, that is, to an explicit "professional meaning perspective" (Rogers, 1989, p. 113).

Rogers, a Canadian nurse who is not related to the author of the Science of Unitary Human Beings, commented that her work as a consultant to nurses who were implementing C-T-E system-based nursing practice in health-care institutions revealed that the cognitive and emotional aspects of perspective transformation represent "dramatic individual change for every nurse" (Rogers, 1989, p. 112). Moreover, she underscored the importance of recognizing, appreciating, and acknowledging that during the process of perspective transformation, each nurse evolves from feeling "a [profound] sense of loss followed by an ultimate sense of liberation and empowerment" (Rogers, 1992, p. 23). Clearly, as Nagle and Mitchell (1991) pointed out, perspective transformation requires considerable effort and a strong commitment to change.

Perspective transformation encompasses the nine phases depicted in Figure 2–2: **stability, dissonance, con-** **fusion, dwelling with uncertainty, saturation, synthesis, resolution, reconceptualization,** and **return to stability** (Rogers, 1992). The prevailing period of **stability** is disrupted when the idea of implementing C-T-E system-based nursing practice is introduced. **Dissonance** occurs as the nurses begin to examine their private images or meaning perspectives in light of the challenge to adopt a public, professional one. As the nurses begin to learn the content of the conceptual model or theory that is the starting point for an explicit C-T-E system, they see the discrepancies between the current way of practice and what nursing practice could be. A phase of **confusion** follows. As the nurses struggle to learn more about the conceptual model or theory and its implications for practice, they find themselves "lying in limbo between [meaning] perspectives" (Rogers, 1992, p. 22). Throughout the phases of **dissonance** and **confusion**, the nurses frequently feel anxious, angry, and unable to think. Rogers (1992) explained that those distressing emotions "seem to arise out of the grieving of a loss of an intimate part of the self. The existing meaning perspective no longer makes sense, yet the new perspective is not sufficiently internalized to provide resolution" (p. 22). Kappeli (1987) added that "confrontation with a model [or theory] can be threatening and produce hostility as it implies the requirement of change" (p. 38).

The phase of **confusion** is following by the phase of **dwelling with uncertainty**. At this point, each nurse acknowledges that his or her confusion "is not a result of some personal inadequacy" (Rogers, 1992, p. 22). As a consequence, anxiety is replaced by a "feeling of freedom to critically examine old ways and explore the new [meaning] perspective" (Rogers, 1992, p. 22). The phase of **dwelling with uncertainty** is spent immersed in information that frequently seems obscure and irrelevant. It is a time of "wallowing in the obscure while waiting for moments of coherence that lead to unity of thought" (Smith, 1988, p. 3).

The phase of **saturation** occurs when the nurses "feel that they cannot think about or learn anything more about the nursing conceptual [model or theory]" (Rogers, 1992, p. 22). That phase does not represent resistance but rather "the need to separate from the difficult process of transformation, [which] is part of the natural ebb and flow of the learning experience" (Rogers, 1992, p. 22).

The phase of **synthesis** occurs as insights render the content of the conceptual model or theory coherent and meaningful. The formerly obscure C-T-E system-based nursing practice becomes clear and worthy of the implementation effort. Increasing tension is followed by exhilaration as insights illuminate the connections between the content of the conceptual model or theory and its use in nursing practice (Rogers, 1992; Smith, 1988). "These insights," Smith (1988) explained, "are moments of coherence, flashes of unity, as though suddenly the fog lifts and

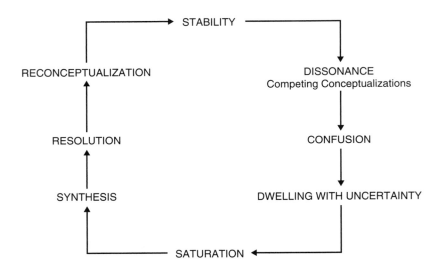

FIG. 2–2. Learning a conceptual model of nursing or a nursing theory: phases of the transformation process. (Source: Rogers, M.E. (1992, February–April). Transformative learning: Understanding and facilitating nurses' learning of nursing conceptual frameworks. Paper presented at Sigma Theta Tau Conferences, "Improving Practice and Education Through Theory." Chicago, IL; Pittsburgh, PA; Wilkes-Barre, PA. ©1991 Martha Rogers, with permission.)

clarity prevails. These moments of coherence push one beyond to deepened levels of understanding" (p. 3).

The phase of **resolution** is characterized by "a feeling of comfort with the new nursing conceptual [model or theory]. The feelings of dissonance and discontent … are resolved and the anxiety is dissipated" (Rogers, 1992, p. 23). During that phase, "nurses describe themselves as changed, as seeing the world differently and feeling a distinct sense of empowerment" (Rogers, 1992, p. 23).

The phase of **reconceptualization** occurs as the nurses consciously reconceptualize nursing practice using the new meaning perspective, that is, the C-T-E system (Rogers, 1992). During that phase, the nurses compare the activities of practice, from patient assessment through shift reports, according to the old and new meaning perspectives, and change those activities so that they are in keeping with the new perspective. The final phase, **return to stability**, occurs when the new meaning perspective prevails, that is, when nursing practice is based on an explicit C-T-E system.

Rogers' presentation of the phases of perspective transformation as a linear process (see Fig. 2–2) is based on Mezirow's (1975, 1978) empirical work. Bunkers proposed that nonlinear accounts of descriptions of nurses' participation in the process of learning new nursing models and theories be included (Pilkington, Bunkers, Clarke, & Frederickson, 2002). Although one may be philosophically inclined toward a nonlinear view of human processes, any adaptation of Rogers' and Mezirow's works requires further empirical study of the process nurses use to learn and adopt an explicit conceptual model of nursing as a guide for their activities.

The nine phases of perspective transformation described by Rogers (1992) are strikingly similar to three stages or phases of perspective transformation that occur when faculty members adopt an explicit conceptual model of nursing as a guide for curriculum construction. Heinrich (1989) identified three stages—upheaval, evolution, and integration—that were experienced by both faculty and students when the Roy Adaptation Model was adopted as a curriculum guide at the University of Hartford in Hartford, Connecticut. The stage of upheaval was characterized by a "right-wrong struggle;" the stage of evolution, by "facing the conflict;" and the stage of integration, by "humor, creativity, and cooperative learning" (p. 4).

Mengel and colleagues (1989) identified three periods of faculty evolution—excitement, reorganization, and acceptance—that occurred when the Roy Adaptation Model was adopted at the Community College of

Philadelphia, Pennsylvania. They explained, "In the period of excitement, we were naïvely overconfident that the revised curriculum would work. 'Why doesn't it work?' was the theme of the reorganization period. During reorganization we began to make changes to meet our needs. Finally, in the period of acceptance, we discovered that with further adaptations, a curriculum based on the Roy model does meet our needs" (p. 125).

The phases of perspective transformation experienced by adult learners and nurses is similar to the phases of transformative change experienced by members of business organizations as they create a new way of doing business (Nevis, Lancourt, & Vassallo, 1996). When undergoing transformative change, organization members progress from the status quo, or traditional phase, through exploration and generation to internalization. Like perspective transformation, transformative change requires each individual to significantly alter his or her understanding of the fundamental customs, values, and basic assumptions that guide the functions of the organization. Resistance to change occurs when people do not view the organization in the same way. The challenge is to facilitate evolution of a new shared reality that will, after a time, automatically guide the organization's functions.

STRATEGIES TO FACILITATE PERSPECTIVE TRANSFORMATION

Rogers (1989) identified several strategies that can be used to facilitate perspective transformation as C-T-E system-based nursing practice is being implemented in a health-care institution. Those strategies are especially effective during the early phases of perspective transformation, when the nurses are experiencing a move from their implicit, private images of nursing to a shared perspective in the form of an explicit C-T-E system.

One strategy is to use analogies to facilitate understanding of the term conceptual model. Such analogies as a chair or book can be used for conceptual, and the analogy of a model home or model airplane can be used for model. Rogers (1989) noted that the act of conceptualizing can be demystified "by stating that it is not a process reserved for intellectuals, but rather a cognitive process of all humans that begins in infancy as a baby puts together all the pieces to form the concept of mother" (p. 114).

Two other strategies are directed toward identification of the nurses' existing private images of nursing practice. One of those strategies is to ask each nurse to list words that reflect his or her view of nursing practice. Similarly, each nurse could be asked to depict his or her view of nursing practice in drawings or collages of photographs. Another strategy is to ask each nurse to present a detailed description of a recent interaction with a nursing participant. Regardless of the strategy selected, group discussion then is used to extract each nurse's underlying perspective of nursing practice from the words, pictures, or descriptions of interactions.

Once the nurses have gained a clear understanding of their private images, they should be helped to explore the difference between nursing practice as it is now and as it should be, between real and ideal nursing practice. This can be accomplished through the use of provocative strategies. One provocative strategy is to raise questions about how situations such as childbirth and death are actually managed and how they ought to be managed. Another strategy is to ask the nurses to describe what is unique about nursing practice or what they would do if they did not have to carry out physicians' orders for medications and treatments.

Rogers (1989) pointed out that as the nurses become aware of the differences between the real and the ideal, they experience a cognitive dissonance or discomfort that comes from "the awareness of the 'what is' versus 'what should be'" (p. 115). She went on to point out that

> Most nurses hold in the back of their minds a clear image of the ideal nurse and ideal practice. Much of the ideal image was learned in their educational programs and sustained, if at all, by collegial interaction with other nurses or mentors who shared the same image. It also appears that while many nurses have a clear sense of the ideal, they have had to sublimate that image to accommodate a system which does not share the same image. Many nurses can describe their feelings of loss as they let go of the ideal and came to accept the real. [Consequently,] nurses need to rekindle an image of the ideal, the what could be or should be [that is represented by the C-T-E system]. More importantly, nurses need to experience a sense of powerfulness to realize the ideal vision. Empowerment of nurses through discussion of the value and importance of nursing knowledge, acts, and processes is essential (pp. 115–116).

Rogers (1989) concluded by noting that when cognitive dissonance "has been experienced by nurses both individually or collectively, then perspective transformation can occur and a climate for the implementation of a nursing conceptual [model] will have been created" (p. 116).

Subsequent stages of perspective transformation and the implementation of C-T-E system-based nursing practice are facilitated by constant reinforcement. Accordingly, all nursing activities at the health-care institution should be tied to the C-T-E system in a systematic manner. The novice user of a C-T-E system should not become discouraged if initial experiences with that system seem forced or awkward. Adoption of an explicit C-T-E system does require restructuring the nurse's way of thinking about nursing situations and use of a new vocabulary. However, repeated use of the C-T-E system should lead to more systematic and organized endeavors. As Broncatello (1980) commented, "The nurse's consistent use of any [C-T-E system] for the interpretation of observable client data is most definitely not an easy task. Much like the development of any habitual behavior, it initially requires thought, discipline and the gradual evolvement of a mind set of what is important to observe within the guidelines of the [C-T-E system]. As is true of most habits, however, it makes decision making less complicated" (p. 23).

LEVELS OF INTEGRATION OF CONCEPTUAL-THEORETICAL-EMPIRICAL SYSTEM–BASED NURSING PRACTICE

Finally, it is helpful to realize that not all nurses in the health care institution will integrate the C-T-E system into their practice to the same degree and in the same amount of time. Weiss and her colleagues (1994) identified four **levels of integration**, based on their experience with the Roy Adaptation Model as the starting point for C-T-E system-based nursing practice at Sharp Memorial Hospital in San Diego, California.

- *Lack of integration* is evident when the nurse has limited knowledge of the C-T-E system but recognizes the relationship between the C-T-E system and the C-T-E system–based documentation and care planning systems. At that level, the nurse uses relevant concepts to guide practice but does not use the distinctive language of the C-T-E system.
- *Directed integration* is evident when the C-T-E system-based documentation and care planning systems are the impetus for using the model. At that level, the content required in the documentation forms provides the direction for the nurse's assessment of nursing participants and the creation of the nursing care plan.
- *Unconscious integration* is evident when the nurse uses concepts of the C-T-E system to guide practice but does not specifically relate those concepts to the C-T-E system. At that level, the basic concepts of the C-T-E system are integrated into the nurse's practice, but are not explicitly identified as such.
- *Conscious integration* is evident when the nurse specifically identifies the C-T-E system as his or her personal framework for nursing practice. At that level, the nursing process used by the nurse includes easily identifiable components of the C-T-E system.

Weiss and colleagues (1994) reported that the level of integration demonstrated by nurses was related to "prior learning about models in nursing education programs, participation in the hospital-based career advancement program, and participation in shared governance councils which actively promoted development of [C-T-E system]-based practice" (p. 83). Their findings clearly support the inclusion of courses addressing the content and application of C-T-E systems in nursing education programs, the linkage of practice career advancement programs to the use of an explicit C-T-E system, and the institution of shared governance councils that actively promote and support C-T-E system-based nursing practice.

 ## CONCLUSION

The major substantive and process elements involved in the implementation of C-T-E system-based nursing practice were identified in this chapter. Chapters 4 through 10 and 12 through 17 provide specific examples of the implementation of C-T-E systems within the context of particular conceptual models of nursing and nursing theories. Noteworthy is the ongoing work toward adoption of the notion of C-T-E system-based practice by pharmacy. More specifically, as the scope of pharmacy practice expands to encompass pharmaceutical clinical technology, the idea of C-T-E systems of knowledge as presented in this chapter is being adopted as a structure for pharmacy practice. (A. Heller, personal communications, January to July, 2003).

 ## REFERENCES

Aggleton, P., & Chalmers, H. (1985). Critical examination. Nursing Times, 81(14), 38–39.

Aggleton, P., & Chalmers, H. (1990). Model future. Nursing Times, 86(3), 41–43.

Anderson, C.A. (1997). What is nursing anyhow? Nursing Outlook, 45, 249–250.

Barr, O. (1997). The value of nursing models. Professional Nurse, 12, 689.

Brazen, L. (1992). Project 2000: The difference between conceptual models, practice models. Association of Operating Room Nurses Journal, 56; 840–842, 844.

Broncatello, K.F. (1980). Auger in action: Application of the model. Advances in Nursing Science, 2(2), 13–23.

Brooks, B.A., & Rosenberg, S. (1995). Incorporating nursing theory into a nursing department strategic plan. Nursing Administration Quarterly, 20(1), 81–86.

Capers, C.F. (1986). Some basic facts about models, nursing conceptualizations, and nursing theories. Journal of Continuing Education, 16, 149–154.

Capers, C.F., O'Brien, C., Quinn, R., Kelly, R., & Fenerty, A.

(1985). The Neuman systems model in practice. Planning phase. Journal of Nursing Administration, 15(5), 29–39.

Cheek, J., Gibson, T., & Heartfield, M. (1993). Holism, care and nursing: Points of reflection during the evolution of a philosophy of nursing statement. Contemporary Nurse, 2(2), 68–72.

Cox, Sr. R.A. (1991). A tradition of caring: Use of Levine's model in long-term care. In K.M. Schaefer & J.B. Pond (Eds.), Levine's conservation model: A framework for nursing practice (pp. 179–197). Philadelphia: F.A. Davis.

Craig, D., & Beynon, C. (1996). Nursing administration and the Neuman systems model. In P. Hinton Walker & B. Neuman (Eds.), Blueprint for use of nursing models (pp. 251–274). New York: NLN Press.

Dee, V. (1990). Implementation of the Johnson model: One hospital's experience. In M.E. Parker (Ed.), Nursing theories in practice (pp. 33–44). New York: National League for Nursing.

Ethridge, P. (1991). A nursing HMO: Carondelet St. Mary's experience. Nursing Management, 22(7), 22–27.

Fawcett, J. (1985). Theory: Basis for the study and practice of nursing education. Journal of Nursing Education, 24, 226–229.

Fawcett, J. (1992). Conceptual models and nursing practice: The reciprocal relationship. Journal of Advanced Nursing, 17, 224–228.

Fawcett, J. (1993). From a plethora of paradigms to parsimony in world views. Nursing Science Quarterly, 6, 56–58.

Fawcett, J. (1997). Conceptual models of nursing, nursing theories, and nursing practice: Focus on the future. In M.R. Alligood & A. Marriner-Tomey (Eds.), Nursing theory: Utilization and application (pp. 211–221). St. Louis: Mosby.

Fawcett, J. (2003). Conceptual models of nursing: International in scope and substance? The case of the Roy adaptation model. Nursing Science Quarterly, 16, 315–318.

Fawcett, J., Botter, M.L., Burritt, J., Crossley, J.D., & Frink, B.B. (1989). Conceptual models of nursing and organization theories. In B. Henry, C. Arndt, M. DiVincenti, & A. Marriner-Tomey (Eds.), Dimensions of nursing administration: Theory, research, education, practice (pp. 143–154). Boston: Blackwell Scientific.

Fitch, M., Rogers, M., Ross, E., Shea, H., Smith, I., & Tucker, D. (1991). Developing a plan to evaluate the use of nursing conceptual frameworks. Canadian Journal of Nursing Administration, 4(1), 22–28.

Fitzpatrick, J.J., Whall, A.L., Johnston, R.L., & Floyd, J.A. (1982). Nursing models and their psychiatric mental health applications. Bowie, MD: Brady.

Gray, J. (1991). The Roy adaptation model in nursing practice. In C. Roy & H.A. Andrews (Eds.), The Roy adaptation model: The definitive statement (pp. 429–443). Norwalk, CT: Appleton & Lange.

Heinrich, K. (1989). Growing pains: Faculty stages in adopting a nursing model. Nurse Educator, 14(1); 3–4, 29.

Hoffert, N., & Woods, C.Q. (1996). Elements of a nursing professional practice model. Journal of Professional Nursing, 12, 354–364.

Hood, L.J., & Leddy, S.K. (2003). Leddy and Pepper's conceptual bases of professional nursing (5th ed.). Philadelphia: Lippincott Williams & Wilkins.

Johns, C. (1989). Developing a philosophy. Nursing Practice, 3(1), 2–4.

Johns, C. (1990). Developing a philosophy [Part 2]. Nursing Practice, 3(2), 2–6.

Kappeli, S. (1987). The influence of nursing models on clinical decision making I. In K.J. Hannah, M. Reimer, W.C. Mills, & S. Letourneau (Eds.), Clinical judgment and decision making: The future with nursing diagnosis (pp. 33–41). New York: Wiley.

Kenney, J.W. (1995). Relevance of theory-based nursing practice. In P.J. Christensen & J.W. Kenney (Eds.), Nursing process: Application of conceptual models (4th ed., pp. 1–23). St. Louis: Mosby.

Kristjanson, L.J., Tamblyn, R., & Kuypers, J.A. (1987). A model to guide development and application of multiple nursing theories. Journal of Advanced Nursing, 12, 523–529.

Laudan, L. (1981). A problem-solving approach to scientific progress. In I. Hacking (Ed.), Scientific revolutions (pp. 144–155). Fairlawn, NJ: Oxford University Press.

Laurie-Shaw, B., & Ives, S.M. (1988). Implementing Orem's self-care deficit theory: Part II—Adopting a conceptual framework of nursing. Canadian Journal of Nursing Administration, 1(2), 16–19.

Lipsey, M.W. (1993). Theory as method: Small theories of treatment. In L.B. Sechrest & A.G. Scott (Eds.), New directions for program evaluation (No. 57: Understanding causes and generalizing about them, pp. 5–38). San Francisco: Jossey-Bass.

Lowry, L. (Ed.). (1998). The Neuman systems model and nursing education: Teaching strategies and outcomes. Indianapolis: Sigma Theta Tau International Center Nursing Press.

Manthey, M. (1990). Definitions and basic elements of a patient care delivery system with an emphasis on primary nursing. In G.G. Mayer, M.J. Madden, & E. Lawrenz (Eds.), Patient care delivery models (pp. 201–211). Rockville, MD: Aspen.

Mascord, P. (1988/1989). Five days: Five nursing theories. Australian Journal of Advanced Nursing, 6(2), 13–15.

McFarlane, A.J. (1988). A nursing reformulation of Bowen's family systems theory. Archives of Psychiatric Nursing, 2, 319–324.

McKenna, H. (1993). The effects of nursing models on quality of care. Nursing Times, 89(33), 43–46.

Mengel, A., Sherman, S., Nahigian, E., & Coleman, I. (1989). Adaptation of the Roy model in an educational setting. In J.P. Riehl-Sisca (Ed.), Conceptual models for nursing practice (3rd ed., pp. 125–131). Norwalk, CT: Appleton & Lange.

Mezirow, J. (1975). Education for perspective transformation: Women's re-entry programs in community colleges. New York: Center for Adult Education, Teachers College, Columbia University.

Mezirow, J. (1978). Perspective transformation. Adult Education, 28, 100–110.

Mitchell, G.J. (2002). Learning to practice the discipline of nursing. Nursing Science Quarterly, 15, 209–213.

Nagle, L.M., & Mitchell, G.J. (1991). Theoretic diversity: Evolving paradigmatic issues in research and practice. Advances in Nursing Science, 14(1), 17–25.

Nevis, E.C., Lancourt, J., & Vassallo, H.G. (1996). Intentional revolutions: A seven point strategy for transforming organizations. San Francisco: Jossey-Bass.

Northrup, D.T., & Cody, W.K. (1998). Evaluation of the human becoming theory in practice in an acute care psychiatric setting. Nursing Science Quarterly, 11, 23–30.

Parker, M.E. (1990). Developing perspectives on nursing theory in practice. In M.E. Parker (Ed.), Nursing theories in practice (pp. 3–6). New York: National League for Nursing.

Pilkington, F.B., Bunkers, S.S., Clarke, P.N., & Frederickson, K. (2002). Critiquing contemporary nursing knowledge. Nursing Science Quarterly, 15, 171–177.

Rafferty, D. (1992). Team and primary nursing. Senior Nurse, 12(1), 31–34, 39.

Raudonis, B.M., & Acton, G.J. (1997). Theory-based nursing practice. Journal of Advanced Nursing, 26, 138–145.

Reilly, D.E. (1975). Why a conceptual framework? Nursing Outlook, 23, 566–569.

Rogers, M.E. (1989). Creating a climate for the implementation of a nursing conceptual framework. Journal of Continuing Education in Nursing, 20, 112–116.

Rogers, M.E. (1992, February–April). Transformative learning: Understanding and facilitating nurses' learning of nursing conceptual frameworks. Paper presented at Sigma Theta Tau Conferences, "Improving Practice and Education Through Theory." Chicago, IL; Pittsburgh, PA; Wilkes-Barre, PA.

Schlotfeldt, R.M. (1975). The need for a conceptual framework. In P.J. Verhonick (Ed.), Nursing research I (pp. 3–24). Boston: Little, Brown.

Schmieding, N.J. (1984). Putting Orlando's theory into practice. American Journal of Nursing, 84, 759–761.

Shea, H., Rogers, M., Ross, E., Tucker, D., Fitch, M., & Smith, I. (1989). Implementation of nursing conceptual models:

Observations of a multi-site research team. Canadian Journal of Nursing Administration, 2(1), 15–20.

Sidani, S., & Braden, C.J. (1998). Evaluating nursing interventions: A theory-driven approach. Thousand Oaks, CA: Sage.

Smith, M.J. (1988). Wallowing while waiting. Nursing Science Quarterly, 1, 3.

Stenglein, E., Doepke, C., Hall, J., Lochner, L., Piersol, L., Szalapski, J., Vanderbilt, D., & Winston, P.B. (1993). Transforming beliefs into action: A professional practice model. Aspen's Advisor for Nurse Executives, 8(6); 1, 4–5, 8.

Story, E.L., & Ross, M.M. (1986). Family centered community health nursing and the Betty Neuman Systems Model. Nursing Papers, 18(2), 77–88.

Villarruel, A.M., Bishop, T.L., Simpson, E.M., Jemmott, L.S., & Fawcett, J. (2001). Borrowed theories, shared theories, and the advancement of nursing knowledge. Nursing Science Quarterly, 14, 158–163.

Walsh, M. (1989). Nursing models: Model example. Nursing Standard, 3(22), 22–24.

Weiss, M.E., Hastings, W.J., Holly, D.C., & Craig, D.I. (1994). Using Roy's adaptation model in practice: Nurses' perspectives. Nursing Science Quarterly, 7, 80–86.

Whall, A.L. (1980). Congruence between existing theories of family functioning and nursing theories. Advances in Nursing Science, 3(1), 59–67.

Whall, A.L. (1986). Family therapy theory for nursing: Four approaches. Norwalk, CT: Appleton-Century-Crofts.

Wilde, B., Starrin, B., Larsson, G., & Larsson, M. (1993). Quality of care from a patient perspective: A grounded theory study. Scandinavian Journal of Caring Sciences, 7, 113–120.

Zander, K. (1990). Managed care and nursing case management. In G.G. Mayer, M.J. Madden, & E. Lawrenz (Eds.), Patient care delivery models (pp. 37–61). Rockville, MD: Aspen.

Zelauskas, B., & Howes, D.G. (1992). The effects of implementing a professional practice model. Journal of Nursing Administration, 22(7/8), 18–23.

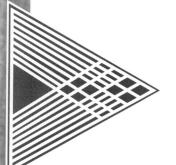

Part Two

ANALYSIS AND EVALUATION OF CONCEPTUAL MODELS OF NURSING

Part Two introduces the reader to conceptual models of nursing.

Chapter 3 presents a distinctive framework for the analysis and evaluation of nursing models.

Chapters 4 through 10 acquaint the reader with the most widely recognized and oft—cited nursing models. In these chapters, the reader enters the world of nursing as conceptualized by Dorothy Johnson in her Behavioral System Model, Imogene King in her Conceptual System, Myra Levine in her Conservation Model, Betty Neuman in her Systems Model, Dorothea Orem in her Self—Care Framework, Martha Rogers in her Science of Unitary Human Beings, and Callista Roy in her Adaptation Model.

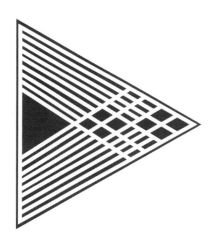

Chapter **3**

Framework for Analysis and Evaluation of Nursing Models

This chapter presents a framework for analysis and evaluation of conceptual models of nursing that highlights their most important features and is appropriate to their level of abstraction. This framework, like the framework for analysis and evaluation of nursing theories presented in Chapter 11, reflects critical reasoning and, therefore, "highlights strengths and exposes problems inherent in a line of reasoning" (Silva & Sorrell, 1992, p. 17). Application of the framework yields a descriptive, analytical, and critical commentary that enhances understanding of a conceptual model and can lead to refinements in the concepts and propositions of that model (Meleis, 1997).

   The framework was first published many years ago (Fawcett, 1980) and has undergone repeated refinement since that time. The initial development and continued refinement of the framework was motivated by dissatisfaction with other frameworks, primarily because of their continuing failure to distinguish among conceptual models, grand theories, and middle-range theories (e.g., Barnum, 1998; Fitzpatrick & Whall, 1996; George, 2002; Marriner-Tomey & Alligood, 2002; Meleis, 1997). The current version of the framework reflects increased understanding of the relation of conceptual models of nursing to the other components of the structural holarchy of contemporary nursing knowledge, that is, the metaparadigm, philosophies, theories, and empirical indicators. This version also reflects attention to language that encompasses all nursing practice situations and settings, not just those situations and settings that connote nursing at the bedside of the sick, or clinical nursing (Parse, 2002). In the interest of readability, conceptual models of nursing henceforth will be referred to as nursing models in this chapter.

Overview

The framework for analysis and evaluation of nursing models separates questions dealing with analysis from those more appropriate to evaluation. The analysis is an objective and nonjudgmental description of a nursing model. Evaluation, in contrast, requires judgments to be made about the extent to which a nursing model satisfies certain criteria. The steps of the framework are listed here. Each step is discussed in detail in this chapter.

Key Terms

ANALYSIS

 ANALYSIS OF NURSING MODELS

Analysis of a nursing model, using the framework presented in this chapter, requires a systematic, detailed review of all available primary sources, including publications and presentations by the author of the model, to determine exactly what has been said, rather than relying on inferences about what might have been meant or by referring to other authors' interpretations of the nursing model (Levine, 1994). When the author of the nursing model has not been clear about a point or has not presented certain information, it may be necessary to make inferences or to turn to other reviews of the model. That, however, must be noted explicitly, so that the distinction between the words of the nursing model author and those of others is clear (Levine, 1994). The analysis targets the **origins of the nursing model** as well as its **unique focus** and **content**.

ANALYSIS STEP 1: ORIGINS OF THE NURSING MODEL

The first step in the analysis of a nursing model is examination of four aspects of its **origins**. First, the historical evolution of the nursing model is described, and the author's motivation for developing the nursing model is explicated. Second, the author's philosophic claims about nursing and the knowledge development strategies used to formulate the nursing model are examined. Third, the influences on the author's thinking from nurse scholars and scholars of adjunctive disciplines are identified. Fourth, the world view reflected by the nursing model is specified.

A nursing model is derived from an author's philosophic claims about the phenomena of interest to nursing and the development of knowledge. The development of a nursing model is more an intellectual than an empirical endeavor, although empirical observations certainly may influence the work. The content of the nursing model frequently evolves as the author engages in an iterative process of inductive and deductive reasoning. Because it is not unusual to find that the content of a nursing model has undergone revisions as the author refines concepts and propositions and formulates new ideas about nursing, it is important to trace the evolution of the model from its initial version to the present one. An extensive review of the model author's publications and publicly available presentations will provide clues or explicit descriptions of the underlying beliefs and values and the factors that motivated model development, as well as the inductive and deductive strategies used to transform an implicit private image of nursing into an explicit nursing model.

The author's use of inductive reasoning, deductive reasoning, or both reflects a certain philosophical orientation to the development of knowledge and to the relationship between human beings and the environment. This orientation often can be traced to the author's educational experiences, as well as to exposure to the thinking of other nursing scholars and scholars of adjunctive disciplines. Accordingly, analysis of the origins of the nursing model should include identification of the author's references to the works of earlier scholars in nursing and other disciplines. In addition, the analysis of origins should include identification of the world view reflected by the nursing model. The reaction, reciprocal interaction, and simultaneous action world views, discussed in Chapter 1, are appropriate here. The questions that should be asked when analyzing the origins of the nursing model are:

- What is the historical evolution of the nursing model?
- What motivated development of the nursing model?
- On what philosophical beliefs and values about nursing is the nursing model based?
- What strategies for knowledge development were used to formulate the nursing model?
- What scholars influenced the model author's thinking?
- What world view is reflected in the nursing model?

ANALYSIS STEP 2: UNIQUE FOCUS OF THE NURSING MODEL

The second step in the analysis of a nursing model is examination of its **unique focus**. The need to identify the unique focus of the nursing model stems from the understanding that although most authors start with the same view of the general purpose of nursing, in final form the nursing models present distinctive views of the metaparadigm concepts (Johnson, 1974). Indeed, different models are concerned with different problems in nursing situations or different problems in interactions between human beings and their environments (Christensen & Kenney, 1995; Duffey & Muhlenkamp, 1974). They also are concerned with different actual and potential deviations from desired health conditions and with different modes of nursing intervention (Johnson, 1987).

The factors thought to influence the development of problems or deviations and to direct types of nursing interventions also vary from model to model. The unique focus of a nursing model is specified by its classification regarding one or more categories of nursing knowledge. As explained in Chapter 1, the relevant categories are developmental, systems, interaction, needs, outcomes, client focused, person-environment interaction focused, nursing therapeutics, energy fields, intervention, conservation, substitution, sustenance/support, and enhancement. The question is:

- What is the unique focus of the nursing model?

ANALYSIS STEP 3: CONTENT OF THE NURSING MODEL

The third step in the analysis of a nursing model is examination of its **content**. The content of a nursing model is presented in the form of abstract and general concepts and propositions. Most authors of nursing models have not

presented their ideas in the form of explicit statements about each of the metaparadigm concepts. Therefore this part of the analysis is most readily accomplished first by categorizing the content of the model into the concepts that represent human beings, the environment, health, and nursing. Next, the nonrelational propositions that define and describe those concepts are identified. Finally, the relational propositions that link the concepts are extracted and categorized according to linkages among the four metaparadigm concepts. The questions about the content of the nursing model are:

- How are human beings defined and described?
- How is environment defined and described?
- How is health defined? How are wellness and illness differentiated?
- How is nursing defined?
- What is the goal of nursing?
- How is nursing practice described?
- What statements are made about the relations among the four metaparadigm concepts?

 ## EVALUATION OF THE NURSING MODEL

Evaluation of a nursing model is accomplished by comparing its content with certain criteria. Those criteria address **explication of origins, comprehensiveness of content, logical congruence, generation of theory, credibility**, and **contributions to the discipline of nursing**. The evaluation is based on the results of the analysis, as well as on a review of previously published critiques, research reports, and reports of the application of the nursing model in nursing education, administration, and practice.

EVALUATION STEP 1: EXPLICATION OF ORIGINS

The first step of evaluation concerns **explication of origins** of the nursing model. Identification of the author's beliefs and values yields information about the philosophical foundations of the model and helps identify special points of emphasis in the view of nursing put forth by the nursing model.

The expectation is that philosophical claims have been made explicit by the author. Indeed, "a statement of one's value system is an essential accompaniment to a model" (Johnson, 1987, p. 197). Furthermore, because the content of most nursing models draws from existing knowledge in nursing and adjunctive disciplines (Levine, 1988, 1995), it is expected that the works of other scholars have been cited. The questions that should be asked when evaluating the origins of the nursing model are:

• Are the philosophical claims on which the nursing model is based explicit?
• Are the scholars who influenced the model author's thinking acknowledged and are bibliographical citations given?

EVALUATION STEP 2: COMPREHENSIVENESS OF CONTENT

The second step of evaluation deals with the **comprehensiveness of content** of the model. Emphasis is placed on the depth and breadth of content.

No well-established criterion for the depth of the content of a nursing model has been established. It seems reasonable to expect, however, that the content should encompass the four metaparadigm concepts and that the content is relatively unambiguous. Consequently, the expectation is that the nursing model includes concepts and nonrelational propositions that represent a description of human beings, an identification of the relevant environment, a description of the author's meaning of health, a definition of nursing, a statement of nursing goals or outcomes, and a description of nursing practice, which may be in the form of a nursing process or a methodology for nursing practice. In addition, the nursing process or practice methodology should be grounded in a base of scientific knowledge, permit dynamic movement between each component, and be compatible with ethical standards for nursing practice (Walker & Nicholson, 1980).

It also seems reasonable to expect the relational propositions of the nursing model to link all four metaparadigm concepts. This may be done in a series of propositions that reflect linkage of two or more metaparadigm concepts, or it may be accomplished by one summary statement encompassing all four metaparadigm concepts. These propositions will, of course, be stated in the vocabulary of the particular nursing model. The questions that should be asked when evaluating the depth of the content of a nursing model are:

• Does the nursing model provide adequate descriptions of all four concepts of nursing's metaparadigm?
• Do the relational propositions of the nursing model completely link the four metaparadigm concepts?

The criterion for the breadth of the content of a nursing model requires that it be sufficiently broad to provide guidance in practice situations of normalcy, risk, crisis, and morbidity (Magee, 1994) and to also serve as a basis for research, education, and administration. Although the ex-

pectation is that the nursing model is a useful frame of reference for many nursing activities, it is recognized that any one nursing model may not be appropriate for all practice situations in all cultures. Indeed, it is entirely possible that the content of the model precludes consideration of or application to certain situations or cultures (Fawcett, 2003a, 2003b). In such a case, potential users of the model must decide if the limitations are sufficient to warrant its elimination as a viable one for nursing. The questions to ask when evaluating the breadth of the content of the nursing model are based on suggestions from Johnson (1987) and reflect the guidelines for nursing research, education, administration, and practice that were described in Chapter 2. The questions are:

• Is the researcher given sufficient direction about what questions to ask and what methodology to use?
• Does the educator have sufficient guidelines to construct a curriculum?
• Does the administrator have sufficient guidelines to organize and deliver nursing services?
• Is the practitioner given sufficient direction to be able to make pertinent observations, decide that an actual or potential need for nursing exists, and prescribe and execute a course of action that achieves the goal specified in a variety of practice situations?

EVALUATION STEP 3: LOGICAL CONGRUENCE

The third step of evaluation of a nursing model considers the logic of its internal structure. **Logical congruence** is evaluated through an intellectual process that involves judging the congruence of the model author's espoused philosophical claims with the content of the model. In addition, the process requires judgments regarding congruence of the world view(s) and category(ies) of nursing knowledge reflected by the model. Evaluation of logical congruence is especially important if the nursing model incorporates more than one world view or category of nursing knowledge, because different schools of thought cannot be combined easily, if at all. However, viewpoints sometimes may be merged or translated by redefining all concepts in a consistent manner. More specifically, nursing models that strive to combine concepts and propositions derived from different world views or different categories of nursing knowledge must first reformulate or translate the concepts and propositions to ensure just one congruent frame of reference.

Reformulation or translation is accomplished by redefining concepts and restating propositions that do not reflect the preferred world view or category of nursing knowledge, so that all ideas presented in the nursing model are consistent (Reese & Overton, 1970; Whall, 1980) (see

Chapter 2). The expectation is that all elements of the nursing model are logically congruent. The questions that should be asked when evaluating logical congruence are:

- Does the model reflect more than one world view?
- Does the model reflect characteristics of more than one category of nursing knowledge?
- Do the components of the model reflect logical translation or reformulation of diverse perspectives?

EVALUATION STEP 4: GENERATION OF THEORY

The fourth step of the evaluation of a nursing model reflects the relationship between a more abstract and general conceptual model and a more concrete and specific theory. As explained in Chapter 1, grand theories and middle-range theories are derived from nursing models (see Fig. 1–2). Thus, the extent to which the nursing model leads to **generation of theory** should be judged.

The need for logically congruent conceptual-theoretical-empirical systems of nursing knowledge for nursing activities mandates that at least some theories be derived from each nursing model. The expectation, therefore, is that the abstract concepts and propositions of the model be sufficiently clear so that the more concrete concepts and propositions of grand theories and middle-range theories can be deduced and testable hypotheses can be formulated. The question is:

- What theories have been generated from the nursing model?

EVALUATION STEP 5: CREDIBILITY OF THE NURSING MODEL

The fifth step of evaluation focuses attention on the **credibility of the nursing model**. Credibility determination is necessary to avoid the danger of uncritical acceptance and adoption of nursing models, which could easily lead to their use as ideologies. Critical reviews of the evidence regarding the credibility of each nursing model must be encouraged and acceptance of work that is "fashionable, well-trodden or simply available in the nursing library" (Grinnell, 1992, p. 57) must be avoided.

The ultimate aim of credibility determination is to ascertain which nursing models are appropriate for use in which practice situations and with which populations. It is likely that determination of credibility will either support or refute the impression that any nursing model "can explain or guide any nursing intervention in any setting, and that all [models] are equally relevant for guiding the prac-tice of nursing" (See, 1986, p. 355). Acceptance or rejection of that impression by means of a thorough evaluation of the credibility of each nursing model is crucial if nursing is to continue to advance as a respected discipline characterized by excellent scholarship.

The credibility of a nursing model cannot be determined directly. Rather, the abstract and general concepts and propositions of the nursing model must be linked with the more concrete and specific concepts and propositions of a middle-range theory and appropriate empirical indicators to determine credibility. The resulting conceptual-theoretical-empirical system of nursing knowledge then is used to guide nursing activities, and the results of use are examined. Thus credibility of nursing models is determined through tests of conceptual-theoretical-empirical systems of nursing knowledge. In particular, credibility is examined by means of the criteria of *social utility, social congruence*, and *social significance*. Judgments regarding the extent to which the nursing model meets those criteria require a review of all available publications and presentations by the author of the nursing model, as well as those by other nurses who have used the model.

Social Utility

Social utility addresses the special education required to apply the nursing model; the feasibility of implementing the nursing model in nursing practice; and the extent to which the nursing model actually is used to guide nursing research, education, administration, and practice. Although model authors should strive to write and discuss their work clearly and concisely (Cormack & Reynolds, 1992), the abstract and general nature of nursing models and the special vocabulary of each one typically require collegiate or continuing education for mastery. In addition, special training in interpersonal and psychomotor skills may be necessary to apply the model in practice situations (Magee, 1994). The expectation is that the nurse has a full understanding of content of the nursing model, as well as the interpersonal and psychomotor skills necessary to apply it. Thus, the first question to be asked when evaluating the social utility of a nursing model is:

- Are education and special skill training required before applying the nursing model in nursing practice?

The evaluation of social utility also considers the feasibility of implementing practice protocols derived from the nursing model and related theories in nursing practice. The expectation is, of course, that the implementation of such protocols is feasible. Feasibility is determined by evaluating the human and material resources needed to establish the model-based nursing actions as customary practice (Magee, 1994). Requisite resources include the time required to learn and implement the protocols; the number, type, and expertise of personnel required for their application; and the funds for continuing education, salaries, equipment, and protocol-testing procedures. The question is:

- Is it feasible to implement practice protocols derived from the nursing model and related theories?

In addition, evaluation of social utility requires consideration of the extent to which the nursing model actually is used to guide nursing research, education, administration, and practice. The expectation is that the nursing model has been applied in some situations. Although a completely accurate appraisal of actual use is impossible, a continually growing body of literature documents the application of nursing models to the design of nursing studies, the construction of educational programs and administrative structures, and the care of people who require nursing. The question is:

- To what extent is the nursing model actually used to guide nursing research, education, administration, and practice?

Social Congruence

Social congruence refers to the compatibility of nursing model-based nursing activities with the expectations for nursing practice of the human beings who require nursing, the community, and the health-care system (Magee, 1994). In particular, the culturally determined expectations of people who require nursing and the community, as well as various discipline-oriented expectations of health care team members, with regard to appropriate areas of assessment, relevant goals, appropriate nursing interventions, and relevant outcomes must be taken into account (Aggleton & Chalmers, 1985; Jones, 1989; McLane, 1983). Furthermore, expectations based on the system of health care delivery in various countries should be considered (Cormack & Reynolds, 1992). If others' expectations for nursing are not congruent with the practice that is derived from the nursing model, they must be helped to expect a different kind of nursing. This is especially important, because without the expected affirmative answer to the question of social congruence, "nursing will not continue to be sanctioned as a profession or an occupation, and in a nursing shortage situation [or in any era of health care reform], … the nurse may be replaced with other health professionals" (Johnson, 1987, p. 197). The question is:

- Does the nursing model lead to nursing activities that meet the expectations of the public and health profes-

sionals of various cultures and in diverse geographic regions?

Social Significance

The criterion of *social significance* requires a judgment to be made with regard to the social value of a nursing model, with emphasis placed on the effect of use of a nursing model on the health conditions of people (Magee, 1994). "This criterion," according to Johnson (1974), "recognizes that a professional service is a highly valued one because it is critical to people in some way" (p. 376). The social significance of a nursing model is determined by analysis of data from practice projects and formal studies.

The practice project method of determining social significance is accomplished by examining the conclusions drawn by nurses who have applied the nursing model-based system of knowledge in the real world of nursing practice. The conceptual-theoretical-empirical system of knowledge is considered credible if practice outcomes are in accordance with expectations. If, however, outcomes are not in accordance with expectations, the credibility of the knowledge system, and hence the nursing model, must be questioned.

The formal study method of determining social significance is accomplished by examining the findings of research guided by conceptual-theoretical-empirical systems of nursing knowledge. More specifically, determination of credibility is accomplished by comparing the research findings with the propositions of the conceptual-theoretical-empirical system of nursing knowledge that was used to guide the research. If the research findings support the empirical adequacy of the theory, it is likely that the nursing model is credible. If, however, the research findings do not support hypothesized expectations, both the empirical adequacy of the theory and the credibility of the nursing model must be questioned.

The expectation for the criterion of social significance is that the use of the nursing model has a significant, positive impact on the well-being of the public. The question is:

- Does application of the nursing model, when linked with relevant theories and appropriate empirical indicators, make important and positive differences in the health conditions of the public?

EVALUATION STEP 6: CONTRIBUTIONS TO THE DISCIPLINE OF NURSING

The sixth and final step of evaluation of nursing models, which is as general as the conceptual models themselves, requires a judgment to be made with regard to the **contri-**

butions of the model to the discipline of nursing. The judgment is made following a thorough review of all the available literature dealing with the nursing model. Judgments should not be made on the basis of the comparison of one nursing model with another. Rather, each nursing model should be judged on its own merits and in accord with its own philosophical claims. One should not criticize a nursing model for failing to consider, for example, problems in self-care abilities when the model emphasizes the nurse's management of stimuli to promote adaptation. The expectation is that the nursing model enhances understanding of the phenomena of interest to nursing. The question is:

- What is the overall contribution of the nursing model to the discipline of nursing?

 ## CONCLUSION

In this chapter, a framework for analysis and evaluation of nursing models was presented. The framework, which is summarized in Table 3–1, will be applied in the next seven chapters. Each of those chapters will present a comprehensive examination of one nursing model. The framework for analysis and evaluation of nursing models presented in this chapter is not appropriate for examination of grand and middle-range nursing theories. The framework for analysis and evaluation of nursing theories is presented in Chapter 11.

TABLE 3–1
A FRAMEWORK FOR ANALYSIS AND EVALUATION OF NURSING MODELS

QUESTIONS FOR ANALYSIS

STEP 1: ORIGINS OF THE NURSING MODEL

- What is the historical evolution of the nursing model?
- What motivated development of the nursing model?
- On what philosophical beliefs and values about nursing is the nursing model based?
- What strategies for knowledge development were used to formulate the nursing model?
- What scholars influenced the model author's thinking?
- What world view is reflected in the nursing model?

STEP 2: UNIQUE FOCUS OF THE NURSING MODEL

- What is the unique focus of the nursing model?

STEP 3: CONTENT OF THE NURSING MODEL

- How are human beings defined and described?
- How is environment defined and described?
- How is health defined? How are wellness and illness differentiated?
- How is nursing defined?
- What is the goal of nursing?
- How is nursing practice described?
- What statements are made about the relations among the four metaparadigm concepts?

QUESTIONS FOR EVALUATION

STEP 1: EXPLICATION OF ORIGINS

- Are the philosophical claims on which the nursing model is based explicit?
- Are the scholars who influenced the model author's thinking acknowledged and are bibliographic citations given?

(continued)

► ‹‹ **TABLE 3–1**
A FRAMEWORK FOR ANALYSIS AND EVALUATION OF NURSING MODELS *(continued)*

STEP 2: COMPREHENSIVENESS OF CONTENT

- Does the nursing model provide adequate descriptions of all four concepts of nursing's metaparadigm?
- Do the relational propositions of the nursing model completely link the four metaparadigm concepts?
- Is the researcher given sufficient direction about what questions to ask and what methodology to use?
- Does the educator have sufficient guidelines to construct a curriculum?
- Does the administrator have sufficient guidelines to organize and deliver nursing services?
- Is the practitioner given sufficient direction to be able to make pertinent observations, decide that an actual or potential need for nursing exists, and prescribe and execute a course of action that achieves the goal specified in a variety of practice situations?

STEP 3: LOGICAL CONGRUENCE

- Does the model reflect more than one world view?
- Does the model reflect characteristics of more than one category of nursing knowledge?
- Do the components of the model reflect logical translation or reformulation of diverse perspectives?

STEP 4: GENERATION OF THEORY

- What theories have been generated from the nursing model?

STEP 5: CREDIBILITY OF THE NURSING MODEL: SOCIAL
UTILITY, SOCIAL CONGRUENCE, SOCIAL SIGNIFICANCE

- Are education and special skill training required before applying the nursing model in nursing practice?
- Is it feasible to implement practice protocols derived from the nursing model and related theories?
- To what extent is the nursing model actually used to guide nursing research, education, administration, and practice?
- Does the nursing model lead to nursing activities that meet the expectations of the public and health professionals of various cultures and in diverse geographic regions?
- Does application of the nursing model, when linked with relevant theories and appropriate empirical indicators, make important and positive differences in the health conditions of the public?

STEP 6: CONTRIBUTIONS TO THE DISCIPLINE OF NURSING

- What is the overall contribution of the nursing model to the discipline of nursing?

 REFERENCES

Aggleton, P., & Chalmers, H. (1985). Critical examination. Nursing Times, 81(14), 38–39.

Barnum, B.J.S. (1998). Nursing theory: Analysis, application, evaluation (5th ed.). Philadelphia: Lippincott.

Christensen, P.J., & Kenney, J.W. (Eds.). (1995). Nursing process: Application of conceptual models (4th ed.). St. Louis: Mosby.

Cormack, D.F., & Reynolds, W. (1992). Criteria for evaluating the clinical and practical utility of models used by nurses. Journal of Advanced Nursing, 17, 1472–1478.

Duffey, M., & Muhlenkamp, A.F. (1974). A framework for theory analysis. Nursing Outlook, 22, 570–574.

Fawcett, J. (1980). A framework for analysis and evaluation of conceptual models of nursing. Nurse Educator, 5(6), 10–14.

Fawcett, J. (2003a). Conceptual models of nursing: International in scope and substance? The case of the Roy adaptation model. Nursing Science Quarterly, 16, 315–318.

Fawcett, J. (2003b). Theory and practice: A conversation with Marilyn E. Parker. Nursing Science Quarterly, 16, 131–136.

Fitzpatrick, J.J., & Whall, A.L. (1996). Conceptual models of nursing: Analysis and application (3rd ed.). Norwalk, CT: Appleton & Lange.

George, J.B. (Ed.). (2002). Nursing theories: The base for professional nursing practice (5th ed.). Upper Saddle River, NJ: Prentice Hall.

Grinnell, F. (1992). Theories without thought? Nursing Times, 88(22), 57.

Johnson, D.E. (1974). Development of theory: A requisite for nursing as a primary health profession. Nursing Research, 23, 372–377.

Johnson, D.E. (1987). Guest editorial: Evaluating conceptual models for use in critical care nursing practice. Dimensions of Critical Care Nursing, 6, 195–197.

Jones, S. (1989). Is unity possible? Nursing Standard, 3(1), 22–23.

Levine, M.E. (1988). Antecedents from adjunctive disciplines: Creation of nursing theory. Nursing Science Quarterly, 1, 16–21.

Levine, M.E. (1994). Some further thoughts on the ethics of nursing rhetoric. In J.F. Kikuchi & H. Simmons (Eds.), Developing a philosophy of nursing (pp. 104–109). Thousand Oaks, CA: Sage.

Levine, M.E. (1995). The rhetoric of nursing theory. Image: Journal of Nursing Scholarship, 27, 11–14.

Magee, M. (1994). Eclecticism in nursing philosophy: Problem or solution? In J.F. Kikuchi & H. Simmons (Eds.), Developing a philosophy of nursing (pp. 61–66). Thousand Oaks, CA: Sage.

Marriner-Tomey, A., & Alligood, M.R. (2002). Nursing theorists and their work (5th ed.). St. Louis: Mosby.

McLane, A. (1983). Book review of Fawcett, J. Analysis and evaluation of conceptual models of nursing. The Leading Edge (Newsletter of Delta Gamma Chapter of Sigma Theta Tau), 3(2), 15–16.

Meleis, A.I. (1997). Theoretical nursing: Development and progress (3rd ed.). Philadelphia: Lippincott.

Parse, R.R. (2002). Words, words, words: Meanings, meanings, meanings! Nursing Science Quarterly, 15, 183.

Reese, H.W., & Overton, W.F. (1970). Models of development and theories of development. In L.R. Goulet & P.B. Baltes (Eds.), Life span development psychology: Research and theory (pp. 116–145). New York: Academic Press.

See, E.M. (1986). Book review of George, J. (Ed.). Nursing theories: The base for nursing practice (2nd ed.). Research in Nursing and Health, 9, 355–356.

Silva, M.C., & Sorrell, J.M. (1992). Testing of nursing theory: Critique and philosophical expansion. Advances in Nursing Science, 14(4), 12–23.

Walker, L.O., & Nicholson, R. (1980). Criteria for evaluating nursing process models. Nurse Educator, 5(5), 8–9.

Whall, A.L. (1980). Congruence between existing theories of family functioning and nursing theories. Advances in Nursing Science, 3(1), 59–67.

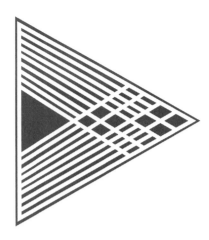

Chapter **4**

Johnson's Behavioral System Model

Dorothy Johnson presented the rudimentary ideas for the Behavioral System Model in her 1959 journal article, "A Philosophy of Nursing," and in her 1961 journal article, "The Significance of Nursing Care." However, Johnson did not present her entire conceptual model in the literature until she prepared a chapter for the second edition of Riehl and Roy's (1980) book, *Conceptual Models for Nursing Practice*. Before the publication of that book chapter, the only public records of the model were a widely cited paper that Johnson presented at Vanderbilt University in 1968 and an audiotape of her 1978a presentation at the Second Annual Nurse Educator Conference. Versions of the model had, however, been available to interested nurses since Grubbs published her interpretation of the Behavioral System Model in 1974 and Auger published her interpretation in 1976.

Johnson did not present any major revisions in her conceptual model after the 1980 book chapter, although she continued to discuss and provide more detail about various aspects of the model, especially the practice methodology, in her 1990a book chapter, "The Behavioral System Model for Nursing," and presented a very informative discussion of the origins of the model in her 1992 book chapter, "The Origins of the Behavioral System Model." Dorothy Johnson died on February 4, 1999.

Overview

Johnson's work focuses on human beings as behavioral systems, which are made up of all the patterned, repetitive, and purposeful ways of behavior that characterize life. Her work clearly fits the definition of conceptual model used in this book, and she has always classified it as such. The concepts of Johnson's Behavioral System Model and their dimensions are listed here, along with the goal of nursing and the components of her practice methodology. The concepts, their dimensions, and the methodology components are defined and described, and the goal of nursing is discussed in detail, later in this chapter.

Key Terms

HUMAN BEINGS
BEHAVIORAL SYSTEM
    Attachment or Affiliative Subsystem
    Dependency Subsystem
    Ingestive Subsystem
    Eliminative Subsystem
    Sexual Subsystem
    Aggressive Subsystem
    Achievement Subsystem
STRUCTURAL COMPONENTS
    Drive or Goal
    Set

Choice
  Action or Behavior
FUNCTIONAL REQUIREMENTS
  Protection
  Nurturance
  Stimulation
ENVIRONMENT
SYSTEM ENVIRONMENT
  Internal Environment
  External Environment
HEALTH
BEHAVIORAL SYSTEM BALANCE AND STABILITY
BEHAVIORAL SYSTEM IMBALANCE AND
  INSTABILITY
NURSING
EXTERNAL REGULATORY FORCE
  Impose External Regulatory or Control
    Mechanisms
  Change Structural Components
  Fulfill Functional Requirements

GOAL OF NURSING
  To Restore, Maintain, or Attain Behavioral
    System Balance and Dynamic Stability
    at the Highest Possible Level for the
    Individual
PRACTICE METHODOLOGY: THE NURSING
  DIAGNOSTIC AND TREATMENT PROCESS
    Determination of the Existence of a Problem
    Diagnostic Classification of Problems
      Internal Subsystem Problems
      Intersystem Problems
    Management of Nursing Problems
      Impose External Regulatory or Control
        Mechanisms
      Repair Damaged Structural Components
      Fulfill Functional Requirements
    Evaluation of Behavioral System Balance
      and Stability

ANALYSIS OF JOHNSON'S BEHAVIORAL SYSTEM MODEL

This section presents an analysis of Johnson's Behavioral System Model. The analysis relies heavily on Johnson's 1980 and 1990a publications, "The Behavioral System Model for Nursing," and also draws from her 1992 publication, "The Origins of the Behavioral System Model."

ORIGINS OF THE NURSING MODEL

Historical Evolution and Motivation

Johnson (1990a) noted that the Behavioral System Model "has been in the process of development for nearly the entire course of my professional life" (p. 23). The unique focus and content of the model evolved over a period of 20 years, beginning in the early 1940s when Johnson began to teach nursing. As she developed baccalaureate nursing courses, Johnson was motivated to ask several questions:

• What content is properly included in a course in nursing because it constitutes nursing knowledge?
• Knowledge for what purpose, to what end?
• What is the explicit, ideal goal of nursing? (Johnson, 1990a, p. 23)

In answering those questions, the task as Johnson saw it was to clarify nursing's social mission from the perspective of a theoretically sound view of human beings served by nursing and to identify the nature of the body of knowl-

edge needed to attain the goal of nursing. Johnson (1990a) stated that she approached that task historically, empirically, and analytically. The historical approach led her to accept from Nightingale nursing's traditional concern with human beings who are ill, rather than with diseases per se, as well as "a focus on the basic human needs of the person and a concern for the relationship between the person and the environment" (Johnson, 1992, p. 24). The empirical approach led to a review of studies of nursing tasks. Johnson noted that this approach, which defines nursing as what nurses do, was not fruitful. However, it kept the focus on human beings who are ill or who might be prevented from becoming ill. Finally, the analytical approach led Johnson to consider what reason suggests. This turned out to be the most useful approach.

"The work began," as Johnson (1992) noted, "with the effort to develop course content in the basic curriculum by focusing on common human needs, moving on to 'care and comfort' as organizing principles, and then to stress and tension reduction as the major principles" (p. 24). Through reasoning, Johnson (1980) finally came to conceive of nursing's specific contribution to patient welfare as "the fostering of efficient and effective behavioral functioning in the patient to prevent illness and during and following illness" (p. 207). That perspective led Johnson (1990a) to accept "a theoretical view of the client, the person, as a behavioral system in much the same way that physicians have accepted a theoretical view of the person as a biological system" (p. 24).

Elaborating, Johnson (1992) explained that the Behavioral System orientation leads nursing to fulfill its social mission through the special responsibility of promoting "the most effective and efficient behavioral system possible, as well as to prevent specific problems from occurring in the system. Meeting this responsibility would also contribute to healthier biologic and social systems" (pp. 26–27).

Philosophical Claims

Johnson presented the philosophical claims undergirding the Behavioral System Model in the form of beliefs, assumptions, premises, and a value system. Examination of those statements yielded fundamental values about behavior, beliefs about the nature and operation of the Behavioral System, and beliefs about nursing that are listed here.

Fundamental Values about Behavior

- There is a wide range of behavior which is tolerated in this society or any other, and only the middle section of the continuum can be said to represent the cultural norms (Johnson, 1968, p. 4).
- So long as behavior does not threaten the survival of society, either directly through the death or lack of productivity of individuals or indirectly through the creation of massive disorder or deviance from established social values, it appears to be acceptable (Johnson, 1968, p. 4).
- The outer limits of acceptable, and therefore tolerated, behavior are thus set for the professions by society, but in fact, the limits of acceptable behavior set by the health professions, including nursing, probably tend to be narrower in some areas and in some respects than those set by the larger society (Johnson, 1968, p. 4).
- Since the professions have an obligation which goes beyond accepting the current state of affairs to shaping the reality of the future, an additional facet of this problem of values is that of determining what is desirable, rather than simply acceptable, behavior. At least two closely related facts must be remembered in this connection. In the first place, forced change in behavior in one area of life may and often does require other behavioral modifications. The consequences may be unforeseen, unintended, and undesirable. Second, the current status of knowledge about man and his universe does not allow us to predict, with reasonable certainty, a configuration of behavioral responses which measured against some established standards could be said to be of a "better" or "higher" level in an absolute way (Johnson, 1968, p. 4).
- The final judgment of the desired level of functioning is the right of the individual, given that that level is within survival limits and that the individual has been provided with adequate understanding of the potential for and the means to obtain a more optimal level of behavioral functioning than is evident at the present time (Johnson, 1978a).

Beliefs about the Nature and Operation of the Behavioral System

- A system is a whole which functions as a whole (Johnson, 1980, p. 208).
- Parts or elements of a system are organized, interactive, interdependent, and integrated (Johnson, 1980, p. 208).
- The system tends to achieve a balance among various forces acting within and upon it (Johnson, 1980, p. 208).
- Man strives continually to maintain behavioral system balance and [a] steady state by more or less automatic adjustments and adaptations to the natural forces impinging upon him (Johnson, 1980, p. 208).
- Behavioral System balance represents adjustments and adaptations that are successful to some degree and in some way, even though observed behavior may not match cultural or biologic norms for acceptable or healthy behavior (Johnson, 1980, p. 208).
- Man actively seeks new experiences that may disturb balance, at least temporarily, and that may require small or large behavioral system modification to reestablish balance (Johnson, 1980, p. 208).
- Observed regularities and constancies in human behavior that result from behavioral system balance and stability are functionally significant for the individual and for social life (Johnson, 1980, p. 208).
- Living systems can and do operate at varying levels of efficiency and effectiveness; but in order for a system to operate at all, it must maintain a certain level of balance and stability internally and in its environmental interactions (Johnson, 1978a; 1990a, p. 25).
- Behavioral systems have sufficient flexibility to take account of the usual fluctuations in the impinging forces and enough stress tolerance for adjustment to many common, but extreme, fluctuations (Johnson, 1980, p. 209).
- When behavioral regularities are disturbed, integrity of the person is threatened and functions served by such order are less than adequately fulfilled (Johnson, 1978a).
- If extraordinarily strong impinging forces, or a lowered resistance to or capacity to adjust to more moderate forces disturb behavioral system balance, the integrity of the person is threatened (Johnson, 1968, p. 4).
- During their lives, most individuals probably experience a psychologic or social crisis or physical illness grave enough to disturb system balance and require external assistance (Johnson, 1980, p. 209).

- Insofar as behavioral system balance requires a minimum (for the moment at least and in reference to a particular individual) expenditure of energy, a larger supply of energy is available in the service of biologic processes and recovery (Johnson, 1968, p. 4).
- The attempt by man to preserve or re-establish behavioral system balance in the face of continuing excessive forces making for imbalance requires an extraordinary expenditure of energy (Johnson, 1968, p. 4).

Beliefs about Nursing

- My own educational experience had led me to believe that nursing was a profession, or at least an emerging one, and that as a profession nursing makes a unique and significant contribution to patients—a contribution that differs from but is complementary to those made by medicine and other health professions (Johnson, 1992, p. 24).
- Nursing is, or could be, the force that supplies assistance both when disturbances in system balance occur and at other times to prevent such disturbances (Johnson, 1980, p. 209).
- Nursing must not … purposefully support, certainly over a prolonged period or in the absence of other counteractive measures, behavioral responses which are so deviant that they are intolerant to society or constitute a threat to the survival of the individual, either socially or biologically, and thus ultimately are a threat to society (Johnson, 1968, pp. 4–5).
- While nursing has an obligation to [help the person] seek the highest possible level of behavioral functioning, and to contribute, through research, to the specification of what that level might be, we cannot afford to go very far beyond what is known. Quite specifically … nursing [cannot] presume to transform the values, beliefs, and norms of the individuals we serve to those in accordance with the culture of middle-class, urban, American society which we generally represent. We cannot, and must not, substitute our judgments at any given point in time for those of the individual or of the larger society (Johnson, 1968, p. 5).

Strategies for Knowledge Development

Johnson's conception of human beings as behavioral systems reflects a synthesis of knowledge from the literature of many disciplines, as well as from nursing's past. Her description of the development of the Behavioral System Model suggests that she used both inductive and deductive reasoning. She explained, "Over a period of some twenty years and in the light of my clinical experiences, thinking,

reading, and conversations with colleagues, I evolved the notion that one potentially useful way of viewing man is as a behavioral system" (Johnson, 1978b, pp. 7–8).

Influences from Other Scholars

Johnson acknowledged the influences of many scholars, starting with Florence Nightingale, on the development of the Behavioral System Model. She explained that she received a facsimile edition of Nightingale's (1859/1946) *Notes on Nursing* in 1946. The book "came just at the right time to have a profound influence on the course of my professional experience" (Johnson, 1992, p. 23). Johnson went on to explain that Nightingale's work "provided direction to my thinking" (p. 24). Two points in particular influenced the beginning of the development of the Behavioral System Model: "A focus on the basic human needs of the person and a concern for the relationship between the person and the environment" (p. 24).

Johnson (1988) commented that her teacher and subsequent colleague, Lulu Wolfe Hassenplug, convinced her that nursing is a profession. Moreover, she acknowledged the contributions made by her colleagues at the University of California, Los Angeles, to the continuing development of the Behavioral System Model.

The influence of nursing, behavioral, and biological scientists, as well as animal and human ethologists, on the development of the Behavioral System Model is evident in Johnson's many citations of interdisciplinary literature that focuses on the observable features and actions that make up social behavior and on behavior that has major adaptive significance. The acceptance of the idea of human beings as behavioral systems is, according to Johnson (1980), "made possible by the relatively recent development and rapid expansion of … an interdisciplinary literature … focused on the behavior of the individual as a whole—on what he does, why, and on the consequences of that behavior—not on why or how he has changed over time in an intraorganismic sense" (p. 207). Scholars whose writings influenced the identification and content of seven behavioral subsystems include Ainsworth (1964, 1972); Atkinson and Feather (1966); Crandal (1963); Feshbach (1970); Gewirtz (1972); Heathers (1955); Kagan (1964); Lorenz (1966); Mead (1953); Resnik (1972); Robson (1967); Rosenthal (1967); Sears, Maccoby, and Levin (1954); and Walike, Jordan, and Stellar (1969).

Johnson (1980, 1990a, 1992) also acknowledged the influence of general system theory, as set forth by Buckley (1968), Chin (1961), and Rapoport (1968), on her thinking. She explained that "although general system theory was in its infancy, it did seem valid enough to support the notion of humans as behavioral systems, developing and changing, reacting and adapting to their respective environments, including other behavioral systems in that environment" (1992, p. 25).

World View

The Behavioral System Model reflects the *reciprocal interaction* world view. The features of that world view that are evident in the Behavioral System Model are:

- The Behavioral System Model reflects a holistic view of human beings, with emphasis on the behavioral system as a whole.
- The behavioral system is active, not reactive (Johnson, personal communication cited in Brown et al., 1998).
- Human beings are regarded as active organisms who seek new experiences.
- Each subsystem strives to achieve a particular goal, and each human being makes certain behavioral choices.
- Individuals are active beings who adjust environments to ensure better functioning for themselves.
- Human beings determine and limit the interactions between themselves and the environment, and establish their relationship to the objects, events, and situations in the environment (Johnson, 1990a).
- Persistence is reflected in Johnson's emphasis on behavioral system balance and stability. "Interestingly, one of the first of the current nursing theorists, Dorothy Johnson, tried to head the profession in the direction of persistence. She takes equilibrium as a starting point in her original conception. The goal of nursing care, in her model, emphasizes balance, order, stability, and maintenance of the integrity of the patient" (Hall, 1981, p. 5).
- Change is postulated to occur only when necessary for survival. Behavior changes when it no longer is "functionally efficient and effective ... in managing the individual's relationship to the environment ... or when some more optimal level of functioning is perceived as desirable by the individual" (Johnson, 1990a, p. 25).

The focus on the behavioral system as a whole and emphasis on behavior, per se, indicate a holistic view of human beings. Subsystems are explicitly identified as parts of the whole behavioral system, rather than as discrete entities. Consistent with the reciprocal interaction world view, the Behavioral System Model incorporates elements of both persistence and change. As Johnson (1980) noted, the behavioral system "both requires and results in some degree of regularity and constancy in behavior. ... Behavioral system balance reflects adjustments and adaptations that are successful in some way and to some degree" (p. 208).

UNIQUE FOCUS OF THE NURSING MODEL

The unique focus of the Behavioral System Model is human beings as behavioral systems (Johnson, 1968, 1978a, 1980, 1990a). More specifically, the focus of the Behavioral System Model "is on social behavior—the observable features and actions of the person that take into account the actual or implied presence of other social beings. In particular, the focus is on those forms of behavior that have been shown to have major adaptive significance" (Johnson, 1990a, p. 25).

Particular attention is given to actual or potential structural or functional problems in the behavioral system as a whole and in the various subsystems and to behavioral functioning that is at a less than desired or optimal level (Johnson, 1980, 1990a). Two types of behavioral system disorders are particularly relevant—"those that are related tangentially or peripherally to disorder in the biological system; that is, they are precipitated simply by the fact of illness or the situational context of treatment, and those that are an integral part of a biological system disorder in that they are either directly associated with or a direct consequence of a particular kind of biological system disorder or its treatment" (Johnson, 1968, pp. 6–7).

Johnson (1990a) maintained, "The acceptance of the behavioral system as the client is the primary component of this nursing model" (p. 24). She claimed, "The conception of man as a behavioral system, or the idea that man's specific response patterns form an organized and integrated whole is original with me, so far as I know" (Johnson, 1980, p. 208). She further noted that the literature indicates that others support her idea. Indeed, Ackoff used the term Behavioral System in 1960.

Category of Knowledge

The Behavioral System Model is classified as a systems model by Barnum (1998), Marriner-Tomey (1989), and Riehl and Roy (1980). Meleis (1997) regards the Behavioral System Model as a prominent example of the outcome category of models and also classified the model as client focused. Although Barnum (1998) classified the Behavioral System Model as a systems model, she also placed it within the intervention category of her classification scheme. The appropriateness of the systems category classification is evident in the comparison of the Behavioral System Model content with the characteristics of the systems category of knowledge, as can be seen here.

- System: Human beings are behavioral systems.
- Integration of Parts: The parts are the subsystems, which are "linked and open, as is true in all systems, and a dis-

turbance in one subsystem is likely to have an effect on others" (Johnson, 1980, p. 210).

- Environment: Internal and external environments are mentioned but particular parameters are not identified (Johnson, 1980, 1990a).
- Boundary: Not addressed explicitly, although boundary permeability is alluded to: "There appears to be built into the system sufficient flexibility to take account of the usual fluctuations in the impinging forces and enough stress tolerance for the system to adjust to many common, but extreme fluctuations" (Johnson, 1980, p. 209).
- Tension, Stress, Strain, and Conflict: The "natural" forces impinging upon the behavioral system are regarded as the source of tension or stress, and lead to "more or less automatic adjustments and adaptations" required for continuing behavioral system balance and stability (Johnson, 1980, p. 208).
- Steady State: Steady state is associated with behavioral system balance (Johnson, 1980). Although the concept of behavioral system balance and stability implies that the system is at a fixed point or achieves equilibrium when stable, Johnson apparently regards stability as a dynamic equilibrium. That aspect of the conceptual model requires clarification.
- Feedback: According to Johnson (1978a), it is necessary to understand input, output, feedback, and regulatory control mechanisms to analyze behavioral system functioning. However, the nature of those system operations was not described.

CONTENT OF THE NURSING MODEL

Concepts

The metaparadigm concepts of human beings, environment, health, and nursing are reflected in the concepts of the Behavioral System Model. Each conceptual model concept is classified here according to its metaparadigm forerunner.

The metaparadigm concept of human beings is represented by the Behavioral System Model concepts of BEHAVIORAL SYSTEM, STRUCTURAL COMPONENTS, and FUNCTIONAL REQUIREMENTS. Each of those concepts is multidimensional. The concept of Behavioral System has seven dimensions, which are viewed as subsystems—Attachment or Affiliative Subsystem, Dependency Subsystem, Ingestive Subsystem, Eliminative Subsystem, Sexual Subsystem, Aggressive Subsystem, and Achievement Subsystem. The concept of Structural Components has four dimensions—Drive or Goal, Set, Choice, and Action or Behavior. The concept of Functional Requirements has three dimensions—Protection, Nurturance, and Stimulation.

The metaparadigm concept of environment is represented by the Behavioral System Model concept of SYSTEM ENVIRONMENT, which has two dimensions—Internal Environment and External Environment. The metaparadigm concept of health is represented by the Behavioral System Model concepts of BEHAVIORAL SYSTEM BALANCE AND STABILITY and BEHAVIORAL SYSTEM IMBALANCE AND INSTABILITY, both of which are unidimensional.

The metaparadigm concept of nursing is represented in the Behavioral System Model by the concept of EXTERNAL REGULATORY FORCE. That concept has three dimensions—Impose External Regulatory or Control Mechanisms, Change Structural Components, and Fulfill Functional Requirements.

Nonrelational Propositions

The definitions of the concepts of the Behavioral System Model are listed here. Those constitutive definitions are the nonrelational propositions of this nursing model.

BEHAVIORAL SYSTEM

- The whole individual is a behavioral system (Johnson, 1980, 1990a).
- The behavioral system is composed of "all patterned, repetitive, and purposeful ways of behaving that characterize each man's life" (Johnson, 1980, p. 209).

The concept of Behavioral System encompasses seven dimensions, which are viewed as subsystems (Johnson, 1980, 1990a)—the Attachment or Affiliative Subsystem, the Dependency Subsystem, the Ingestive Subsystem, the Eliminative Subsystem, the Sexual Subsystem, the Aggressive Subsystem, and the Achievement Subsystem. Each of the seven subsystems has a distinctive and specialized task or function needed to maintain the integrity of the whole behavioral system and manage its relationship to the environment (Johnson, 1980, 1990a). Each function evolves "to carry out its own specialized tasks for the system as a whole. ... [The] responses are differentiated, developed, and modified through maturation, experience, and learning. They are determined and are continuously governed by a multitude of physical, biological, psychological, and social factors operating in a complex and interlocking fashion" (p. 26). The functions of the seven subsystems are given here.

- Attachment or Affiliative Subsystem: Functions are attainment of the security needed for survival as well as social inclusion, intimacy, and the formation and maintenance of social bonds (Johnson, 1980, 1990a). This subsystem is "one of the first response systems to emerge developmentally . . .[and as] probably the most critical subsystem for it forms the basis for all social organization" (Johnson, 1990a, p. 27).

- **Dependency Subsystem:** Functions are succoring behavior that calls for a response of nurturance as well as approval, attention, or recognition, and physical assistance (Johnson, 1980, 1990a). Dependency subsystem behavior, according to Johnson (1990a), "in the socially optimum case evolves [developmentally] from almost total dependence on others to a greater degree of dependence on self, with a certain amount of interdependence essential to the survival of social groups" (p. 28).

- **Ingestive Subsystem:** Function is appetite satisfaction, with regard to when, how, what, how much, and under what conditions the individual eats, which is governed by social and psychological considerations as well as biological requirements for food and fluids (Johnson, 1980, 1990a). The ingestive subsystem extends beyond the biological function of ingestion of substances. "Ingestive behavior," in Johnson's (1990a) view, "serve[s] the broad function of appetitive satisfaction in its own right, [which] may be and all too often is at odds with biological requirements for [f]oods and fluids" (p. 28).

- **Eliminative Subsystem:** Function is elimination, with regard to when, how, and under what conditions the individual eliminates wastes (Johnson, 1980, 1990a). The eliminative subsystem, however, extends beyond the biological function of elimination of waste products. Although the function of the eliminative subsystem, Johnson (1990a) admitted, "is more difficult to differentiate from that of the biological system" (p. 28) than is the ingestive subsystem, "clearly all humans ... must learn expected modes of behavior in the excretion of wastes, and these behaviors often take precedence over or strongly influence otherwise purely biological acts" (p. 28).

- **Sexual Subsystem:** Functions are procreation and gratification, with regard to behaviors dependent on the individual's biological sex and gender role identity, including but not limited to courting and mating (Johnson, 1980, 1990a). The sexual subsystem, which as Johnson (1990a) pointed out, "has strong biological underpinnings ... probably originates with the development of a gender role identity and covers the broad range of those behaviors dependent upon that identity" (p. 28).

- **Aggressive Subsystem:** Function is protection and preservation of self and society (Johnson, 1980, 1990a). Johnson's (1990a) view of the aggressive subsystem "follows the thinking of animal behaviorists [and is in sharp contrast to] that of the behavioral reinforcement school, which maintains that aggressive behavior is not only learned, but has as its primary intent the injury of others" (p. 29).

- **Achievement Subsystem:** Function is mastery or control of some aspect of self or environment, with regard to intellectual, physical, creative, mechanical, social, and caretaking (of children, spouse, home) skills, and as measured against some standard of excellence (Johnson, 1980, 1990a). This subsystem, according to Johnson (1990a), probably develops through "exploratory behavior and attempts to manipulate the environment" (p. 29).

Johnson (1980) explained that the seven subsystems "are linked and open, ... and a disturbance in one subsystem is likely to have an effect on others" (p. 210). She further explained, "Although each subsystem has a specialized task or function, the system as a whole depends on an integrated performance" (p. 210).

Johnson (1980, 1990a) maintained that the subsystems are found cross-culturally and across a broad range of the phylogenetic scale, suggesting that they are genetically programmed. She also noted the significance of social and cultural factors involved in the development of the subsystems. The seven subsystems are not, however, to be regarded as a complete set, because "the ultimate group of response systems to be identified in the behavioral system will undoubtedly change as research reveals new systems or indicates changes in the structure, functions, or behavior pattern groupings in the original set" (Johnson, 1980, p. 212).

STRUCTURAL COMPONENTS

- Refers to the structural elements of the subsystems (Johnson, 1980).

The concept of **Structural Components** encompasses four dimensions (Johnson, 1980, 1990a)—Drive or Goal, Set, Choice, and Action or Behavior.

- **Drive or Goal:** Refers to motivation for behavior (Johnson, 1980, 1990a). The drive is "that which is a stimulant to action [whereas] the goal is that which is sought"(Johnson, 1990a, p. 27). Drive or goal is "perhaps the most significant structural component" (Johnson, 1990a, p. 27). The drive or goal of each subsystem is, in general, the same for all people, "but there are variations among individuals in the specific objects or events that are drive-fulfilling, in the value placed on goal attainment, and in drive strength" (Johnson, 1980, p. 210). This structural component cannot be observed directly but is inferred from the individual's action or behavior.

- **Set:** Refers to the individual's predisposition to act in certain ways, rather than in other ways, to fulfill the function of each subsystem (Johnson, 1990a). With regard to set, Johnson (1980) explained that "through maturation, experience, and learning, the individual comes to develop and use preferred ways of behaving under particular circumstances and with selected individuals" (p. 211). This structural component cannot be observed directly but is inferred from the individual's action or behavior.

- **Choice:** Refers to the individual's total behavioral repertoire for fulfilling subsystem functions and achieving particular goals (Johnson, 1980). The behavioral repertoire encompasses the scope of action alternatives from which individuals can choose (Johnson, 1980). With regard to choice, Johnson (1980) pointed out that people rarely use all of the alternatives in their behavioral repertoire, but rather choose certain preferred behaviors. However, the other behaviors are available if the preferred ones do not work in a certain situation. She also noted that people continuously acquire new choices and modify old ones, and that the most adaptable individuals are those with the largest repertoire of choices. This structural component cannot be observed directly but is inferred from the individual's action or behavior.

- **Action or Behavior:** Refers to the actual organized and patterned behavior in a situation (Johnson, 1980). Action or behavior is "A set of behavioral responses, responsive tendencies, or actions systems ... [that] are developed and modified over time through maturation, experience, and learning. They are determined developmentally and are continuously governed by a multitude of physical, biologic, psychologic, and social factors operating in a complex and interlocking fashion. These responses are reasonably stable, though modifiable, and regularly recurrent, and their action pattern is observable" (Johnson, 1980, p. 209). Behavior or action is instigated, inhibited, shaped, continued, or terminated by the complex biological, psychological, sociological, and physical factors that constitute the other structural components (Johnson, 1980). This is the only structural component that can be observed. Johnson (1990a) explained, "Only the actual behavior can be directly observed, but inferences can be made as to the [nature] of the components of the subsystems by studying the form the behavior takes (its organization and patterning), the significant ambient variables, and the consequences achieved by the behavior" (p. 27).

FUNCTIONAL REQUIREMENTS

- Refers to the requirements "that must be met through the individual's own efforts, or through outside assistance" so that the behavioral subsystems can fulfill their functions (Johnson, 1980, p. 212).

The concept of **Functional Requirements** encompasses three dimensions (Johnson, 1980, 1990a)—Protection, Nurturance, and Stimulation.

- **Protection:** Protection is needed from noxious influences with which the system cannot cope (Johnson, 1980).
- **Nurturance:** Nurturance is acquired through the input of appropriate supplies from the environment (Johnson, 1980).
- **Stimulation:** Stimulation is needed to enhance growth and prevent stagnation (Johnson, 1980).

The ability of the seven subsystems to fulfill their functions depends on those three functional requirements. If human beings are unable to provide adequate protection, nurturance, and stimulation to fulfill their subsystem functions, those requirements must be supplied by other human beings or institutions (Johnson, 1980).

SYSTEM ENVIRONMENT

- The environment is of the behavioral system.

Johnson (1980) did not provide an explicit definition for the concept of **System Environment**. She did, however, refer to the internal environment and the external environment of the system, as well as to "the interaction between the person and his environment" (p. 209). It can, therefore, be inferred that the concept of **System Environment** encompasses two dimensions—Internal Environment and External Environment (Johnson, 1980).

- **Internal Environment:** Not explicitly defined but it can be inferred that the components include, although they may not be limited to, "the composition, quantity, temperature, and distribution of body fluids" (Johnson, 1961, p. 64).
- **External Environment:** Not explicitly defined but it can be inferred that the components are objects, events, situations, and forces that impinge on the person and to which the person adjusts and adapts (Johnson, 1980).

BEHAVIORAL SYSTEM BALANCE AND STABILITY

- Demonstrated by observed behavior that is purposeful, orderly, and predictable (Johnson, 1978a).
  - Purposeful behavior is goal directed; that is, actions reveal a plan and cease at an identifiable point (Johnson, 1978a).
  - Orderly behavior is methodical and systematic, as opposed to diffuse and erratic; and encompasses actions that build sequentially toward a goal and form a recognizable pattern (Johnson, 1978a).
  - Predictable behavior is that which is repetitive under particular circumstances (Johnson, 1978a).

- Purposeful, orderly, and predictable behavior is maintained when it is efficient and effective in managing the individual's relationship to the environment. Individuals are said to achieve efficient and effective behavioral functioning when their behavior is commensurate with social demands, when they are able to modify their behavior in ways that support biological imperatives, when they are able to benefit to the fullest extent during illness from the physician's knowledge and skill, and when their behavior does not reveal unnecessary trauma as a consequence of illness (Johnson, 1978a, 1980).

BEHAVIORAL SYSTEM IMBALANCE AND INSTABILITY

- Not explicitly defined but can be inferred from the following statement to be a malfunction of the behavioral system: "The subsystems and the system as a whole tend to be self-maintaining and self-perpetuating so long as conditions in the internal and external environment of the system remain orderly and predictable, the conditions and resources necessary to their functional requirements are met, and the interrelationships among the subsystems are harmonious. If those conditions are not met, malfunction becomes apparent in behavior that is in part disorganized, erratic, and dysfunctional. Illness or other sudden internal or external environmental change is most frequently responsible for such malfunctions" (Johnson, 1980, p. 212).
- Occurs when efficiency and effectiveness of behavior are no longer evident or when a more optimal level of functioning is perceived as desirable (Johnson, 1978a, 1990a).

Johnson (1978b) commented that health, in its most global sense, is a concern of the members of all health professions, political scientists, agronomists, and others. Her particular focus, however, and one that she considered appropriate for nursing, is the health of the **Behavioral System**. This focus is reflected in Johnson's (1968) statement that "one or more of [the behavioral system] subsystems is likely to be involved in any episode of illness, whether in an antecedent or a consequence way, or simply in association, directly or indirectly, with the disorder or its treatment" (p. 3). In various presentations and publications, Johnson has mentioned behavioral system balance and stability, efficient and effective behavioral functioning, and behavioral system imbalance and instability.

Johnson (1980) also referred to physical and social health, but she did not explicitly define wellness. Moreover, she did not define illness, although she mentioned psychological and social crisis, physical illness, and the person who is ill. It may be inferred that wellness is **Behavioral System Balance and Stability** in the form of purposeful, orderly, and predictable behavior that supports efficient and effective behavioral functioning, and conversely, that illness is **Behavioral System Imbalance and Instability**. These inferences suggest that Johnson views health as a di-

chotomy rather than a continuum. Caution must be observed, however, when assessing the adequacy of those inferences. Indeed, Johnson (1990b) commented that health is neither a continuum nor a dichotomy, but she did not explain the meaning of her comment or identify her view of health.

EXTERNAL REGULATORY FORCE

- "Nursing acts to preserve the organization and integration of the patient's behavior at the highest possible level under those conditions in which behavior constitutes a threat to physical or social health, or in which illness is found" (Johnson, 1990a, p. 29).

The concept of **External Regulatory Force** encompasses three dimensions (Johnson, 1980, 1990a)—Impose External Regulatory or Control Mechanisms, Change Structural Components, and Fulfill Functional Requirements.

- **Impose External Regulatory or Control Mechanisms:** Nursing actions that are directed toward inhibition, stimulation, or reinforcement of certain behaviors (Johnson, 1990a).
- **Change Structural Components:** Nursing actions that involve "changes in the drive (goal), the set, the choices, and the behavior itself and [that require] such things as attitudinal changes, redirection of goals, and sometimes reduction in drive strength" (Johnson, 1990a, p. 31).
- **Fulfill Functional Requirements:** Nursing actions that "provide the [essential] conditions and resources [such as] information giving, role modeling, attention to the food being offered or the way in which it is being served, and seeing that infants or young children have access to their parents or elderly people to their pets" (Johnson, 1990a, p. 31).

"The need for nursing," according to Johnson (1990a), "arises when there are disturbances in the structure or function of the system as a whole or in one or more subsystems, or when behavioral functioning is at a less than desired level for the individual" (p. 29). Johnson (1992) also indicated that there is a need for nursing when prevention is the goal. In particular, she stated that nursing should concentrate on "developing preventive nursing to fulfill its social obligations" (p. 26). She went on to explain that "clarifying nursing's social mission through an explicit goal in client care and using a specific body of knowledge relevant to that goal therefore enables the discipline to work toward completing its special tasks in prevention, thus contributing to a high level of wellness in society" (p. 27).

Johnson (1980, 1990a) clearly distinguished nursing from medicine by stating that nursing views the client as a behavioral system and medicine views the client as a biological system. She views nursing as "a service that is complementary to that of medicine and other health professions, but which makes its own distinctive contribution to the health and well-being of people" (Johnson, 1980, p. 207).

The **GOAL OF NURSING** is "to restore, maintain, or attain behavioral system balance and dynamic stability at the highest possible level for the individual" (Johnson, 1980, p. 214; 1990a, p. 29). That goal may be expanded to include helping the person to achieve a more optimal level of balance and stability when that is possible and desired (Johnson, 1978a).

Johnson (1990a) referred to the nursing process as the **NURSING DIAGNOSTIC AND TREATMENT PROCESS.** That process, which is the **PRACTICE METHODOLOGY** for the Behavioral System Model, is outlined in Table 4–1.

▶ **TABLE 4–1**
JOHNSON'S PRACTICE METHODOLOGY: THE NURSING DIAGNOSTIC AND TREATMENT PROCESS

DETERMINATION OF THE EXISTENCE OF A PROBLEM

The nurse obtains data about the nature of behavioral system functioning in terms of the efficiency and effectiveness with which the client's goals are obtained, with special attention directed toward the amount of energy required to achieve desired goals, the compatibility of the client's behavior with survival imperatives and its congruence with the social situation, and the client's degree of satisfaction with the behavior.

The nurse obtains data to determine the degree to which the behavior is purposeful, orderly, and predictable.

The nurse interviews the client and family to determine the condition of the subsystem structural components and uses the obtained data to:

- Make inferences about drive strength, direction, and value.
- Make inferences about the solidity and specificity of the set.
- Make inferences about the range of behavior patterns available to the client.
- Make inferences about the usual behavior in a given situation.

The nurse assesses and compares the client's behavior with the following indices for behavioral system balance and stability:

- The behavior is succeeding to achieve the consequences sought.
- Effective motor, expressive, or social skills are evident.
- The behavior is purposeful—actions are goal directed, reveal a plan and cease at an identifiable point, and are economical in sequence.
- The behavior is orderly—actions are methodical and systematic, build sequentially toward a goal, and form a recognizable pattern.
- The behavior is predictable—actions are repetitive under particular circumstances.
- The amount of energy expended to achieve desired goals is acceptable.
- The behavior reflects appropriate choices—actions are compatible with survival imperatives and are congruent with the social situation.
- The client is sufficiently satisfied with the behavior.

The nurse makes inferences about the organization, interaction, and integration of the subsystems.

DIAGNOSTIC CLASSIFICATION OF PROBLEMS

Internal Subsystem Problems are present when:

- Functional requirements are not met.
- Inconsistency or disharmony among the structural components of subsystems is evident.
- The behavior is inappropriate in the ambient culture.

Intersystem Problems are present when:

- The entire behavioral system is dominated by one or two subsystems.
- A conflict exists between two or more subsystems.

MANAGEMENT OF NURSING PROBLEMS

The general goals of action are to:

- Restore, maintain, or attain the client's behavioral system balance and stability.
- Help the client achieve an optimum level of balance and functioning when that is possible and desired.

(continued)

The nurse determines what nursing is to accomplish on behalf of the behavioral system by determining who makes the judgment regarding the acceptable level of behavioral system balance and stability.

The nurse identifies the value system of the nursing profession.

The nurse identifies his or her own explicit value system.

The nurse negotiates with the client to select a type of treatment.

The nurse temporarily Imposes External Regulatory or Control Mechanisms by:

- Setting limits for behavior by either permissive or inhibitory means.
- Inhibiting ineffective behavioral responses.
- Assisting the client to acquire new responses.
- Reinforcing appropriate behaviors.

The nurse Repairs Damaged Structural Components in the desirable direction by:

- Reducing drive strength by changing attitudes.
- Redirecting goal by changing attitudes.
- Altering set by instruction or counseling.
- Adding choices by teaching new skills.

The nurse Fulfills Functional Requirements of the subsystems by:

- Protecting the client from overwhelming noxious influences.
- Supplying adequate nurturance through an appropriate input of essential supplies.
- Providing stimulation to enhance growth and to inhibit stagnation.

The nurse negotiates the treatment modality with the client by:

- Establishing a contract with the client.
- Helping the client to understand the meaning of the nursing diagnosis and the proposed treatment.

If the diagnosis or proposed treatment is rejected, the nurse continues to negotiate with the client until agreement is reached.

EVALUATION OF BEHAVIORAL SYSTEM BALANCE AND STABILITY

The nurse compares the client's behavior after treatment to indices of behavioral system balance and stability.

Constructed from Johnson, 1968, 1978a, 1980, 1990a.

Relational Propositions

The relational propositions of the Behavioral System Model are listed below. Relational propositions A and B link the metaparadigm concepts human beings and environment. The metaparadigm concepts human beings, environment, and health are linked in relational proposition C. The links among the metaparadigm concepts human beings, health, and nursing are specified in relational propositions D and E.

A. All the patterned, repetitive, and purposeful ways of behaving that characterize each man's life are considered to comprise his behavioral system. These ways of behaving form an organized and integrated functional unit that determines and limits the interaction between the person and his environment and establishes the relationship of the person to the objects, events, and situations in his environment (Johnson, 1980, p. 209).

B. The behavioral system has many tasks or missions to perform in maintaining its own integrity and in managing the system's relationship to its environment (Johnson, 1980, p. 209).

C. The subsystems and the system as a whole tend to be self maintaining and self perpetuating so long as conditions in the internal and external environment of the system remain orderly and predictable, the conditions and resources necessary to their functional requirements are met, and the interrelationships among the subsystems are harmonious. If these conditions are not met, malfunction becomes apparent in behavior that is in part disorganized, erratic, and dysfunctional. Illness or other sudden internal or external environmental change is most frequently responsible for such malfunctions (Johnson, 1980, p. 212).

D. Most individuals probably experience at one or more times during their lives a psychologic crisis or a physical illness grave enough to disturb the system balance and to require external assistance. Nursing is (or could be) the force that supplies assistance both at the time of occurrence and at other times to prevent such occurrences (Johnson, 1980, p. 209).

E. Nursing is thus seen as an external regulatory force which acts to preserve the organization and integration of the client's behavior at an optimal level under those conditions in which the behavior constitutes a threat to physical or social health, or in which illness is found (Johnson 1980, p. 214).

 ## EVALUATION OF JOHNSON'S BEHAVIORAL SYSTEM MODEL

This section presents an evaluation of the Behavioral System Model. The evaluation is based on the results of the analysis of the model, as well as on publications and presentations by others who have used or commented on Johnson's work.

EXPLICATION OF ORIGINS

Johnson explicated the origins of the Behavioral System Model clearly and concisely. She chronicled the development of the model over time and indicated what motivated her to formulate a conceptual model of nursing. Furthermore, she stated her philosophical claims explicitly in the form of beliefs about nursing, beliefs about the nature and operation of the behavioral system, and a comprehensive value system regarding what should be considered acceptable behavior.

Johnson stated that the use of the Behavioral System Model is based on the values of the nursing profession as well as those of the individual nurse. She valued a focus on each human being's behavior and viewed that behavior as a manifestation of the momentary condition of the whole behavioral system and the subsystems. Johnson also valued nursing intervention before, during, and following illness. Moreover, she valued the client's contributions to his or her care, as indicated by her recommendation that a contract for nursing intervention be negotiated between the nurse and the client.

Johnson explicitly acknowledged other scholars and cit-ed the knowledge she drew on from nursing and adjunctive disciplines. She was especially informative with regard to the influence of Nightingale's work and general system theory on the development of the Behavioral System Model.

COMPREHENSIVENESS OF CONTENT

The Behavioral System Model is sufficiently comprehensive with regard to depth of content, although clarity could

be enhanced in some instances. Johnson addressed all four concepts of nursing's metaparadigm—human beings, environment, health, and nursing. The human being is clearly defined and described as a **Behavioral System.** Johnson referred to human beings as patients in her early publications, but as clients in her later work. The reason for the change in terminology is not known. Although Johnson mentioned environment repeatedly in her publications, she never defined the term explicitly. Furthermore, she did not clearly specify the parameters of the relevant environment beyond references to the **Internal Environment** and the **External Environment.** Randell's (1991) work expanded the concept of environment through the specification of internal and external environmental regulators. "Regulators," Randell (1991) explained, "represent specific units of the environment that simultaneously influence and are influenced by behavior" (p. 157). The Internal Environment is composed of the biophysical regulator, the psychological regulator, and the developmental regulator. The External Environment is composed of the sociocultural, the family, and the physical environmental regulators.

Johnson also did not define health explicitly. As a consequence, inferences must be made about what she meant by wellness and illness, as well as how one is distinguished from the other. In particular, the relation of health to **Behavioral System Balance and Stability** versus **Behavioral System Imbalance and Instability** must be articulated. Furthermore, although **Behavioral System Balance and Stability** is clearly and comprehensively described, the description of **Behavioral System Imbalance And Instability** is not explicit. It must be inferred that this is the converse of **Behavioral System Balance and Stability.**

Other aspects of Johnson's discussion of health also require clarification. Although the model clearly focuses on behavior, Johnson uses the terms psychological and social crises and physical illness. The meaning of those terms in relation to the various subsystems of the **Behavioral System** is not clear. One interpretation of Johnson's statements about illness is that the condition is separate from **Behavioral System** functioning. Thus, it is not clear if illness (physical, psychological, or social) is an external condition that affects behavior in certain subsystems, or if illness is manifested when those subsystems are not functioning efficiently and effectively. Similarly, the meaning of the terms physical and social health and their relation to the condition of the **Behavioral System** require specification.

It must be pointed out, however, that Johnson (1978b) regarded health as "an extremely elusive state" (p. 6). It is not surprising, then, that her conceptual model does not include an explicit definition of health and that there is some lack of clarity about aspects of that concept.

Johnson adequately defined and described nursing, the

Goal of Nursing, and the **Practice Methodology.** She emphasized the need to base judgments about **Behavioral System** functioning on theoretical and empirical knowledge of systems, as well as on the scientific knowledge dealing with each subsystem (Johnson, 1980). Johnson did not present the **Practice Methodology** of the Behavioral System Model as a particularly dynamic activity, although some dynamism is evident in the negotiation of proposed treatment between nurse and client. Johnson's explication of her value system, her statement that the use of the model should be based on the values of the nursing profession as well as those of the individual nurse, and the inclusion of negotiation of treatment between client and nurse all attest to her concern for ethical standards for nursing practice.

The relational propositions of the Behavioral System Model link human beings and the environment; human beings, the environment, and health; and human beings, health, and nursing. No one statement links all four metaparadigm concepts, and there is no direct link between environment and nursing. That linkage was implied, however, when Johnson (1980) stated that nursing is "an external regulatory force … that operates through the imposition of external regulatory or control mechanisms" (p. 214). It may be inferred that nursing is part of the **External Environment.**

Some limitations of the Behavioral System Model, especially those related to the lack of comprehensive descriptions of some metaparadigm concepts, have been overcome by others who have extended the model. Auger (1976) provided an interpretation of the model that focused on the human being as a personality system (Johnson, personal communication, October 17, 1977), thus extending the model further into the psychological realm. Grubbs (1974, 1980) presented an interpretation of the model that expanded each of the metaparadigm concepts. Randell (1991) expanded the description of the environment. In addition, Holaday (2002) outlined a practice methodology for the Behavioral System Model that includes a detailed list of the elements of the model within the categories of behavioral assessment, environmental assessment, diagnostic analysis, planning and intervention, and evaluation, along with questions nurses should consider as they think critically about and apply the practice methodology.

The Behavioral System Model also is sufficiently comprehensive in breadth of content. Johnson has specified a broad goal for nursing that focuses attention on correction of existing behavioral system problems, as well as the prevention of problems. Sensitive to a criticism that the Behavioral System Model does not permit preventive nursing actions, Johnson (1990a) stated emphatically, "That is not true" (p. 31). Elaborating, she stated: "The fact is, however, that like medicine where problems in the biological system cannot be prevented until the nature of the problem is fully explained, preventive nursing is not possible until problems in the behavioral system are explicated. To the extent that any problem that might arise can be anticipated, and appropriate methodologies are available, preventive action is in order" (p. 31).

Moreover, Johnson (1990a) maintained that then-current knowledge supported her claim that the seven subsystems encompass all relevant behavior, despite others' attempts to add an eighth subsystem dealing with restorative behavior (e.g., Grubbs, 1974) and to interpret the functions of some of the subsystems in other ways (e.g., Auger, 1976). She stated that her discussion of the seven subsystems and their functions "is my original conception and the one to which I still subscribe. This point needs to be emphasized since major changes to the model have been made over the years by those using it, and these changes have appeared in the literature. The changes are such that they alter the fundamental nature of the behavioral system as originally proposed, and I do not agree with them" (Johnson, 1990a, p. 27).

The comprehensiveness of the breadth of the Behavioral System Model is further supported by the direction it provides for research, education, administration, and practice. Although guidelines for each area are not explicit in Johnson's writings, many can be extracted from Johnson's publications about the focus and content of the model. The developing guidelines for research, nursing education, administration of nursing services, and nursing practice are listed in the following paragraphs.

Nursing Research Guidelines

The guidelines for nursing research based on the Behavioral System Model, which were constructed from Johnson (1968, p. 6; 1980, 1990a, 1996), are:

- Purpose of the research
  - One focus of Behavioral System Model-based research is on problems in the structure or function of the behavioral system and its subsystems. The task is to identify, describe, and explain these problems.
  - The second focus of research is the prevention and treatment of problems in the structure or function of the behavioral system and its subsystems. The task is to develop the scientific bases for intervention, as well as specific methodologies for intervention.

- Phenomena of interest
  - The phenomena of interest are the behavioral system as a whole, as well as the structural components and the functional requirements of the behavioral subsystems.

- Problems to be studied
  - The precise problems to be studied are those that represent actual or potential imbalances and instability in the behavioral system and subsystems.

- Study participants
  - Study participants may be individuals of all ages in various settings.

- Research methods
  - Data may be collected via interview; observation, including participant observation, filming, and photographing; and projective techniques.
  - Data may be collected using research instruments and practice tools derived from the Behavioral System Model (see Table 4–2 on page 77).
  - Other guidelines for research methods, including designs and procedures, remain to be developed.

- Data analysis
  - Definitive guidelines for data analysis techniques remain to be developed.

- Contributions
  - Behavioral System Model-based research findings enhance understanding of factors that affect human behavioral system functioning.

Nursing Education Guidelines

The guidelines for nursing education based on the Behavioral System Model, which were constructed from Johnson (1980, p. 214; 1989, p. 4; 1990a), are:

- Focus of the curriculum
  - The focus of a Behavioral System Model-based nursing education program is the behavioral system and its subsystems.

- Nature and sequence of content
  - A thorough grounding in the underlying natural and social sciences is the first level of instruction.
  - Nursing's basic science—the study of the individual as a behavioral system, as well as the study of the pathophysiology of the biological system, of medicine's clinical science, and of the health system as a whole—is the second level of instruction.
  - Nursing's clinical science—the study of behavioral system problems in individuals, including relevant diagnostic and treatment rationales and methodologies—is the third level of instruction.

- Settings for nursing education
  - Basic education for professional nursing practice should be at the postbaccalaureate level: "The entry level for the practice of professional nursing [should]

be through graduate education. Even now the 4 or 5 years of college required is not a great enough time span to permit the acquisition of the knowledge and skill needed or the maturity and wisdom required for professional practice" (Johnson, 1989, p. 4).
  - Basic education for technical nursing practice should be at the associate degree level. Associate degree programs should be redesigned and "deprofessionalized" so that the focus of the curriculum is appropriately on "the knowledge and skill needed to follow prescriptions for nursing and medical care and document outcomes and to allow perceptive and intelligent observation" (Johnson, 1989, p. 4).

- Characteristics of students
  - Students interested in professional practice have to meet graduate school requirements.
  - Students interested in technical practice have to meet associate degree program requirements.

- Teaching-learning strategies
  - Definitive guidelines regarding teaching-learning strategies remain to be developed.

Administration of Nursing Services Guidelines

Guidelines for the administration of nursing services based on the Behavioral System Model, which were constructed from Johnson (1980; 1989, p. 3; 1990a), are:

- Focus of nursing in the health-care institution
  - The focus of nursing in health-care institutions is the individual behavioral system.

- Purpose of nursing services
  - The purpose of the administration of nursing services is to facilitate the delivery of nursing that will promote behavioral system balance and stability.

- Characteristics of nursing personnel
  - Nursing personnel include both professional nurses and technical nurses.
    - Professional nurses have caseloads of clients on both an inpatient and an outpatient basis. "Whether salaried or in solo or group practice, [professional nurses are] independent practitioners, licensed to practice nursing and solely responsible for professional decisions and actions" (Johnson, 1989, p. 3).
    - Technical nurses are "employed by hospitals or other institutions or by professionals including nurses, in private practice" (Johnson, 1989, p. 3).

- Settings for nursing services
  - Nursing services are located in medical centers, community hospitals, outpatient clinics, home health-care agencies, and group and individual nursing practices.

- Management strategies and administrative policies
  - Definitive guidelines for management strategies and formulation of administrative policies remain to be developed.

Nursing Practice Guidelines

Guidelines for nursing practice based on the Behavioral System Model, which were constructed from Johnson (1980, 1990a), are:

- Purpose of nursing practice
  - The purpose of nursing practice is to facilitate restoration, maintenance, or attainment of behavioral system balance and stability.

- Practice problems of interest
  - Practice problems of particular interest include all conditions in which behavior is a threat to health or in which illness is found.

- Settings for nursing practice
  - Nursing practice occurs in diverse settings, ranging from people's homes to practitioners' private offices to ambulatory clinics to the critical care units of tertiary medical centers.

- Characteristics of legitimate participants in nursing practice
  - Legitimate participants in nursing practice are those individuals who are experiencing actual or potential threats to behavioral system balance and stability.

- Nursing process
  - The nursing process for the Behavioral System Model is Johnson's **Nursing Diagnostic and Treatment Process.** The components of the process are as follows: Determination of the Existence of a Problem, Diagnostic Classification of Problems, Management of Nursing Problems, Evaluation of Behavioral System Balance and Stability (see Table 4–1).

- Contributions of nursing practice to participants' well-being
  - Behavioral System Model-based nursing practice contributes to the well-being of individuals by promoting behavioral system balance and stability.

LOGICAL CONGRUENCE

The Behavioral System Model is logically congruent. The content of the model clearly flows from Johnson's philosophical claims, and it reflects the reciprocal interaction world view. Although elements of the reaction world view are suggested by her references to forces that operate on the behavioral system and the characterization of nursing as an external regulatory force, Johnson (1980) reconciled the two world views in a satisfactory manner. She explained, "Man strives continually to maintain a behavioral system balance and steady states by more or less automatic adjustments and adaptations to the 'natural' forces impinging upon him. At the same time, … man also actively seeks new experiences that may disturb his balance" (p. 208). Furthermore, although nursing is defined as an external regulatory force, negotiation between the nurse and the client is an essential feature of Johnson's **Nursing Diagnostic and Treatment Process** (see Table 4–1).

The Behavioral System Model clearly reflects a systems approach. Although Johnson discussed some subsystem behavior in a developmental context, the systems approach is the dominant and overriding perspective.

GENERATION OF THEORY

Alligood (1997, 2002) identified three theories that she claimed have been derived from the Behavioral System Model. The **Theory of the Person as a Behavioral System**, Alligood (2002) explained, "is an implied grand theory … that has not been formalized" (p. 47). Commenting on the lack of formalization of a theory of the behavioral system as a whole, Johnson (1990a) stated:

> An empirical literature supporting the conception of a behavioral system composed of all of the person's patterned and purposeful behavior is largely to be developed. There has been considerable research and theoretical attention, however, directed toward specific response systems within what I consider to be the total complex of the whole behavioral system. This is not unlike the case of knowledge about the biological system where knowledge of parts, the subsystems, preceded knowledge of the whole. Fortunately, we can tentatively rely on a developing body of knowledge about systems in general and the laws that govern the operation of all systems until further knowledge of the behavioral system as a whole is developed (p. 25).

Alligood (1997, 2002) credited Grubbs (1974) with the development of the middle-range **Theory of a Restorative Subsystem**. The goals of the restorative subsystem, according to Grubbs (1974), are "to relieve fatigue and/or achieve a state of equilibrium by reestablishing or replenishing the energy distribution among the other subsystems; to redistribute energy" (p. 171). Whether Grubbs' work represents a middle-range theory or an extension of the Behavioral System Model is debatable. Johnson (1990a), however, never accepted the addition of the restorative subsystem to her original set of seven subsystems.

Alligood (1997, 2002) labeled Holaday, Turner-Henson, and Swan's (1996) explanatory theory of chronically ill children's achievement behavior as the **Theory of Sustenal Imperatives.** Holaday and colleagues indicated that they derived that middle-range theory directly from the Behavioral System Model. The theory asserts that:

> Children not receiving adequate amounts of protection, nurturance, and stimulation from [functional requirements] can be classified as being at risk for an imbalanced behavioral system or a deficiency in desirable life experiences. The more risk factors in a child's life and the longer the periods of time during which those factors are present, the more likely the child will experience a behavioral system imbalance (Holaday et al., 1996, p. 41).

The theory was tested empirically in a cross-sectional survey designed to examine factors related to chronically ill children's use of time outside of school. The sample included 365 children with chronic illnesses and a parent or caretaker of each child. Data were collected via interviews using a 59-item open-ended and multiple-choice child questionnaire, an 83-item open-ended and multiple-choice parent/caretaker questionnaire, and a medical background questionnaire. Demographic data for the children and the parents/caretakers also were collected. The child questionnaire items focused on the children's physical and nonphysical activities when alone and with friends. The parent/caretaker questionnaire items focused on socialization priorities, childbearing practices, and questions about the neighborhood and available services.

Holaday (personal communication, August 26, 1987) indicated that the long-range goal of the theory development work is to identify "the important [functional requirements] for each subsystem and how they influence choice and action." She went on to say that she and her colleagues "will attempt to see if there is a hierarchy of [functional requirements] for each subsystem."

Riegel (1989) derived an explanatory theory of the relation of social support, self-esteem, anxiety, depression, and perceptions of functional capacity to adjustment to coronary heart disease directly from the dependency subsystem, functional requirements, and structural components elements of the Behavioral System Model. She used several empirical indicators, including the UCLA Social Support Inventory, the Self-Perception Inventory, the Profile of Mood States, the General Health Perceptions Inventory, and the Interpersonal Dependency Inventory to test the theory in a sample of clients 1 and 4 months after myocardial infarction (Riegel, 1990).

Coward and Wilkie (2000) used the aggressive subsystem to guide their theory-generating study of behaviors reported by men and women with cancer and bone metastasis. Analysis of data collected via semi-structured interviews revealed a rudimentary theory of the meanings associated with self-report and self-management decision making about metastatic cancer bone pain. They concluded, "Consistent with the JBSM [Johnson Behavioral System Model], pain was perceived as protecting both men and women with bone metastasis by providing them with incentive to seek cancer treatment and preventing them from 'doing too much' and thus causing further harm to themselves" (Coward & Wilkie, 2000, p. 106).

In addition, the formation of conceptual-theoretical-empirical systems of nursing knowledge is evident in many of the applications of the Behavioral System Model listed in the Research and Practice sections of the chapter references and chapter bibliography (see CD-ROM for the chapter bibliography). In several instances, selected concepts of the model were linked with theories and empirical indicators borrowed from other disciplines. One example comes from Wilkie and colleagues' (1988) work. They linked the aggressive subsystem with the gate control theory of pain in their study of the relation of cancer pain control behaviors and pain intensity. The empirical indicators for that study were a Demographic Pain Data Form, which was adapted from existing pain assessment questionnaires, a Behavioral Observation-Validation Form, and a visual analog scale.

Another example comes from Lachicotte and Alexander's (1990) research. They linked the Behavioral System Model with the Nadler-Tushman Congruence Model to guide their study of the relationship between nurse administrators' attitudes toward nurse impairment and their method of dealing with the impairment. The empirical indicators were the Attitudes toward Nurse Impairment Inventory and the Methods for Dealing with Nurse Impairment Questionnaire.

CREDIBILITY OF THE NURSING MODEL

Social Utility

Johnson (1980) claimed that the Behavioral System Model "has already proved its utility in providing clear direction for practice, education, and research" (p. 215). Publications by proponents of the Behavioral System Model indicate that it also has provided useful guidelines for administration.

Johnson's Behavioral System Model is especially attractive to those nurses who are familiar with general system theory and the attendant vocabulary. Although Rawls (1980) regarded the complex and unique terminology used to explain the model as a disadvantage, this limitation is readily overcome by studying the model's vocabulary. Indeed, Johnson (1988) maintained that an understanding of the vocabulary of any science or framework is a prerequisite to description of relevant phenomena. In addition, study is required to fully understand the unique focus and content of the Behavioral System Model. Johnson (1980) explained:

> Adoption of this model for practice carries with it direct responsibilities in education [see Nursing Education Guidelines on page 73]. The user will need a thorough grounding in the underlying natural and social sciences. Emphasis should be placed in particular on the genetic, neurologic, and endocrine bases of behavior; psychologic and social mechanisms for the regulation and control of behavior; social learning theories; and motivational structures and processes. (p. 214)

Furthermore, Johnson (1990a) pointed out that the effective use of the Behavioral System Model in practice requires "intensive study of the rich literature available on the seven response [sub]systems" (p. 32). She went on to explain,

> The nurse must know, for example, how these [sub]systems develop over time, the many factors that influence that development, the cultural variations in the basic response [sub]systems to be expected, and much more. The nurse must also acquire an understanding of how living systems operate. Only with such knowledge and understanding is it possible for the practitioner to be aware of the kinds of data needed about the individual. Only with such knowledge can the practitioner analyze [those] data and intervene effectively (p. 32).

Johnson (1980) also stated that the user of the model must study the behavioral system as a whole and as a composite of subsystems, as well as pathophysiology, medicine's and nursing's clinical sciences, and the health-care system (see Nursing Education Guidelines on page 73). In addition, the potential user of the Behavioral System Model must understand Johnson's value system and accept as appropriate a wide range of behavior. In addition, the user of the model must be willing and have the interpersonal skills to negotiate nursing treatment options with the client (see Table 4–1).

The implementation of Behavioral System Model-based nursing practice is feasible. Herbert (1989) commented, "Considerable changes in education and resources would be necessary to allow general implementation" (p. 34). She did not, however, identify the specific changes that would be required. Dee (1990) maintained, "The challenge to nurse executives is to create environments that promote optimal professional practice so that the quality of client care can be sustained and further enhanced" (p. 41). Her description of the implementation of Behavioral System Model-based nursing practice at the University of California-Los Angeles (UCLA) Neuropsychiatric Institute and Hospital indicated that administrators at that institution committed the time and human and material re-

sources required to revise existing nursing assessment forms; develop teaching materials; conduct ongoing in-service education programs to orient staff to the model and provide a forum for ongoing dialogue on the refinement of the model; conduct orientation classes for new employees and supervise those employees in the application of the model; develop strategies to overcome resistance to change; develop a patient classification instrument that includes parameters to determine staffing needs; and develop standardized nursing care plans, model-based nursing diagnoses, and criteria to evaluate client outcomes.

Nursing Research. The utility of the Behavioral System Model for nursing research is documented by several studies that have been guided by the model. Instrument development research based on the Behavioral System Model is listed in Table 4–2. Published reports of descriptive and correlational studies that have been derived from the Behavioral System Model are listed in Table 4–3. Citations to published abstracts of doctoral dissertations and a master's thesis are listed in the Doctoral Dissertations and Master's Thesis sections of the chapter bibliography on the CD-ROM. Holaday (personal communication, August 26, 1987) reported that other master's theses based on the Behavioral System Model were conducted by Broering (1985), Dawson (1984), Kizpolski (1985), Miller (1987), Moran (1986), and Wilkie (1985).

Although much of the Behavioral System Model-based research is limited to a single study on a single topic, programmatic research has been conducted by Derdiarian; Holaday, and colleagues; and nurses at the UCLA Neuropsychiatric Institute and Hospital, including Poster, Dee, Randell, and their colleagues (see Tables 4–2 and 4–3). Derdiarian's collective research findings provide empirical support for Johnson's (1980) contention that the behavioral subsystems are "linked and open, ... and a disturbance in one subsystem is likely to have an effect on others" (p. 210). Commenting on Holaday's program of research, Johnson (1996) stated, "Through Holaday's long series of studies of achievement behavior in chronically ill children, she has [begun to build] a body of knowledge in this area. Her work, and that of her colleagues, exemplifies quite well the value of cumulative research in the development of a sound substantive base in a practice field" (p. 34). The program of research at the UCLA Neuropsychiatric Institute and Hospital has yielded empirical evidence of the effectiveness of Behavioral System Model-based nursing interventions on promotion of behavioral system balance and stability.

Nursing Education. The utility of the Behavioral System Model for nursing education is documented by its use as a guide for curriculum construction in nursing education

Instrument and Citation*	Description
RESEARCH INSTRUMENTS	
Derdiarian Behavioral System Model Instrument Self-Report Form (DBSM) (Derdiarian, 1983, 1984, 1988, 1990; Derdiarian & Forsythe, 1983)	Measures cancer patients' self-reported behavioral changes in all behavioral subsystems.
Derdiarian Behavioral System Model Observational Form (DBSM-O) (Derdiarian, 1990)	Recording form for nurses' observations of cancer patients' behavioral changes in all behavioral subsystems.
Johnson Model First-Level Family Assessment Tool (JFFA-J) (Lovejoy, 1982, 1983)	Measures the needs of members of families with a chronically ill child.
Sexual Behaviors Questionnaire (Wilmoth 1993; Wilmoth & Townsend, 1995)	Measures female sexual behaviors, including communication, appearance, desire, arousal, activity level, techniques, orgasm, and satisfaction.
Wilmoth Sexual Behaviors Questionnaire— Female (Wilmoth & Tingle, 2001)	Measures women's self-reported current sexual behaviors.
PRACTICE TOOLS	
Patient Classification Instrument (PCI) (Auger & Dee, 1983; Dee & Auger, 1983; Dee, 1986)	Provides a classification system for psychiatric patients based on behaviors in each behavioral subsystem and identifies appropriate nursing interventions for each classification level.
Behavioral System Assessment (Dee et al., 1998)	An extension of the PCI that includes an overall behavioral category rating of the patient's severity of illness based on the degree of effectiveness or ineffectiveness of each behavioral subsystem and the degree of overall system balance or imbalance, as well as a rating of the impact of biophysical, psychological, developmental, familial, sociocultural, and physical environmental regulators on the behavioral system and each subsystem.
Patient Indicators of Nursing Care Instrument (Majesky et al., 1978)	Measures the quality of nursing care in terms of the prevention of nursing care complications.
Quality Assurance Audit Tool (Bruce et al., 1980)	Measures outcome criteria for fluid and electrolyte balance in patients with end-stage renal disease.
Predicted Patient Outcome Instrument (Poster et al., 1997)	Tool to record medical record data on patient demographics, patient behavior acuity ratings, predicted outcomes, short- and long-term goals, and nursing interventions.
The Johnson Model and the Nursing Process (Holaday, 2002)	Tool to guide the Behavioral System Model Practice Methodology, with questions to guide the nurse's thinking about each element of the methodology.

*See Research Instruments and Practice Tools section of the chapter references for complete citations.

Research Topic	Study Participants	Citation*
DESCRIPTIVE STUDIES		
Dependency behaviors	Children who made numerous visits to an elementary school nurse	Stamler & Palmer, 1971
Differences in perceived body image and spatial awareness	Visually handicapped and normally sighted preschool children	Small, 1980
Differences in needs of visitors of patients in cancer research units	Visitors who did and did not maintain vigils at the patient's bedside	Lovejoy, 1985
Acquired immunodeficiency syndrome (AIDS) beliefs, behaviors, and informational needs	Clients with AIDS or AIDS-related complex	Lovejoy & Moran, 1988
Quality of nursing care	Nursing care plans for cancer patients	Derdiarian, 1991
Meaning of pain in the context of pain self-report and self-management decision making	Men and women with cancer and bone metastasis	Coward & Wilkie, 2000
Satisfaction with Behavioral System Model-based nursing care	Cancer patients Registered nurses	Derdiarian, 1990a
Perceived changes in the direction, quality, and relative importance of subsystem behaviors	Clients with AIDS	Derdiarian & Schobel, 1990
Differences in achievement behavior	Chronically ill and well children	Holaday, 1974
Mothers' responses to the crying behaviors of their chronically ill infants	Pairs of mothers and chronically ill infants	Holaday, 1982, 1987
Use of out-of-school time	Chronically ill children	Bossert et al., 1990 Holaday & Turner-Henson, 1987 Holaday et al., 1996
Frequency of use of Behavioral System Model-based diagnostic labels	Retrospective review of charts of hospitalized geriatric psychiatric patients	Lewis & Randell, 1991
Comparison of frequency of use of NANDA-based and Behavioral System Model-based diagnostic labels	Retrospective review of charts of hospitalized adult and geriatric psychiatric patients	Randell, 1991
Behavioral changes during hospitalization	Hospitalized adolescent psychiatric patients	Poster & Beliz, 1988, 1992
Nursing care needs, level of functioning, and length of hospital stay	Retrospective review of charts of inpatients under managed behavioral health care contracts	Dee et al., 1998
CORRELATIONAL STUDIES		
Relation of selected physiological disequilibria to behavioral disequilibria and relation of particular nursing diagnoses to effective nursing interventions	Clients with posttransfusion hepatitis	Damus, 1974
Relation of nurse administrators' attitudes toward nurse impairment and their method of dealing with nurses who were impaired by alcoholism or other drug dependency	Nurse administrators	Lachicotte & Alexander, 1990

* See the Research section of the chapter references for complete citations.

Relation between pain control behaviors and pain intensity	Adult patients with solid tumor malignancies	Wilkie et al., 1988
Relation of social support, self-esteem, anxiety, depression, and perceptions of functional capacity on adjustment to myocardial infarction	Clients who had a myocardial infarction	Riegel, 1990
Relation between the aggressive subsystem and the other subsystems of the Behavioral System Model	Cancer patients	Derdiarian, 1990b
Relation of degree of illness, infant's sex, and ordinal position on maternal response to infants' crying	Mothers of chronically ill children Mothers of well children	Holaday, 1981
Factors related to client outcomes	Retrospective review of charts of hospitalized child, adolescent, adult, and geriatric psychiatric patients	Poster et al., 1997

programs. Hadley (1970) described the use of the model at the University of Colorado in Denver. Harris (1986) explained how a modified version of the Behavioral System Model guided curriculum design at the University of California in Los Angeles. Fleming (1990) described its use by the Department of Nursing at California State University in Bakersfield. Carino (personal communication, January 24, 1990) explained how the model was operationalized in the curriculum at the University of Hawaii in Honolulu in the 1960s. The utility of the Behavioral System Model for nursing education also is documented by Derdiarian (1981), who discussed the application of the model to cancer nursing education. No literature was located that described the use of the Behavioral System Model to guide development of Johnson's proposal for postbaccalaureate programs to prepare professional nurses or associate degree programs to prepare technical nurses (see Nursing Education Guidelines on p. 73).

Nursing Administration. The utility of the Behavioral System Model for nursing administration is documented by its use as a guide for the nursing administrative structures of health-care institutions. Hackley (1987) reported the work she did to redesign nursing care processes within the context of the Behavioral System Model for the psychiatric unit at the United States Naval Hospital in Philadelphia, Pennsylvania. She noted that the model guided the practice of all health-care team members, from orderlies to nurses to the staff psychiatrist.

Dee (1990) presented a detailed description of the use of the model at the UCLA Neuropsychiatric Institute and Hospital in Los Angeles, California. She explained that the Behavioral System Model is implemented in the child and adult psychiatric inpatient services with clients ranging from 2 to over 90 years of age. Practice settings include a child and adolescent psychiatric unit, a child and adolescent developmental disabilities unit, general adult psychiatric units, and a geropsychiatry unit. The Patient Classification Instrument and the Predicted Patient Outcome Instrument (see Table 4–2) are used at the UCLA Neuropsychiatric Institute and Hospital, as is a Behavioral System Model-based nursing diagnostic system (Lewis & Randell, 1991). Dee (1990) explained that use of the Behavioral System Model at the UCLA Neuropsychiatric Institute and Hospital:

(1) provides a comprehensive and systematic method of assessing patient behaviors, (2) facilitates the identification of specific areas of patient strengths and weaknesses in ways that are observable and measurable, (3) enhances consistency and continuity of care, (4) promotes the organization of diverse data into meaningful segments, (5) prioritizes the provision of care on the basis of an understanding of subsystem interactions, (6) promotes a common language and unity in the practice environment, (7) facilitates a sense of professional identity, and (8) enhances the equitable allocation of resources according to variable patient care needs rather than allocation of resources merely by census. (pp. 38, 41)

Glennin (1980) developed Behavioral System Model-based standards of nursing practice for hospitalized clients receiving acute care from professional registered nurses. Emphasis was placed on psychosocial, rather than physiologic, management. Glennin classified the standards according to the generic nursing process areas of data gathering, assessment, diagnosis, prescription, implementation, and evaluation. In each area, specific standards were formulated for relevant concepts and propositions of the model.

Rogers (1973) proposed that the behavioral subsystems represent areas for clinical specialization in nursing. One could, for example, be a clinical specialist in the aggressive subsystem or the attachment subsystem. There is no evidence to indicate that her innovative proposal has ever been implemented.

In contrast, nurse administrators at the UCLA Neuropsychiatric Institute and Hospital developed and implemented the Behavioral System Model-based role of the "attending nurse" (Dee & Poster, 1995; Moreau, Poster, & Niemela, 1993; Niemela, Poster, & Moreau, 1992). The major focus of the new role is clinical case management. Role responsibilities include direct patient care; delegation and monitoring of selected aspects of nursing care; provision of leadership, consultation, and guidance to nursing staff; and collaboration with multidisciplinary team members. Moreau and colleagues (1993) reported that the new nursing role was well received by the nurses and members of the multidisciplinary team. Moreover, attending nurses reported an increase in job satisfaction and retention and a decrease in role conflict. Neimela and colleagues (1992) reported that the attending nurse role increased general satisfaction and role clarity and decreased role tension for the nurses, and increased their communication with patients' family members.

Additional empirical evidence supporting the utility of the Behavioral System Model for nursing administration is provided by the findings of Derdiarian's (1991) study of the effects of using two Derdiarian Behavioral System Model assessment instruments on the quality of nursing care. She found that when compared with routine nursing assessment, the use of the model-based instruments resulted in a statistically significant increase in the completeness of objective and subjective data gathered; the quality of the nursing diagnosis; the compatibility and specificity of nursing interventions with the nursing diagnoses; and the appropriateness and recording of follow-ups, evaluation of outcomes, and discharge plans.

Several of the practice tools derived from the Johnson Behavioral System Model are particularly useful to nurse administrators. Those tools are identified and described in Table 4–2.

Nursing Practice. Evidence supporting the utility of the Behavioral System Model in various practice settings is accumulating. The published reports listed in Table 4–4 indicate that the Behavioral System Model can be used in many different practice situations with clients of all ages. In particular, review of the publications cited in Table 4–4, as well as those listed in the Commentary: Practice section of the chapter bibliography on the CD-ROM, indicate that the Behavioral System Model has been used to guide the nursing of children and adults with such conditions as am-

putation, neurological problems, cardiac problems, cerebrovascular accident, renal problems, problems requiring surgery, cancer, and emotional problems. In addition, nursing practice has been directed toward caregivers of individuals with brain injuries and Alzheimer's disease. Moreover, the Behavioral System Model has been used to guide nursing practice for individuals who reside in the community and those who are hospitalized. Several of the research instruments, as well as the practice tools, listed in Table 4–2 are helpful guides for assessment of individuals and members of families and facilitate documentation of nursing practice.

Lobo (2002) maintained that although the use of the Behavioral System Model "can be generalized across the lifespan and across cultures, ... [its] focus ... may make it difficult for nurses working with physically impaired individuals to use the model" (p. 166). Lobo did not, however, give an explanation for why use of the model would be difficult when working with physically impaired individuals.

The Behavioral System Model emphasizes and focuses explicitly on the individual behavioral system. Lobo (2002) commented that families "can be considered only as the environment in which the individual presents behaviors and not as the focus of care" (p. 166). Johnson (1978a) suggested the use of Chin's (1961) intersystem model for nurses who are interested in the care of families and other groups. This approach permits consideration of each individual behavioral system and the interaction of those systems.

Social Congruence

The Behavioral System Model remains generally congruent with contemporary social expectations regarding nursing practice. Commenting on that criterion, Johnson (1980) stated, "Insofar as it has been tried in practice, the resulting nursing decisions and actions have generally been judged acceptable and satisfactory by clients, families, nursing staff, and physicians" (p. 215). Later, Johnson (1990a) noted that the Behavioral System Model "is commensurate with what nurses and the public perceive as nursing's function" (p. 31). Dee (1990) added, "The Johnson Model has provided nurses with a framework not only to describe phenomena, but also to explain, predict, and control clinical phenomena for the purpose of achieving desired patient outcomes. Levels of nursing care provided for the patient are, therefore, purposeful and nursing practice is more meaningful for the practitioner" (p. 41). Furthermore, Grubbs (1980) maintained that the role of the nurse, as described in this model, "is congruent

Practice Situation	Population	Citation*
Assessment of health status and development of nursing interventions	A 6-year-old child scheduled for surgery, a 12-year-old child with meningomyelocele and multiple urinary tract problems, and a 15-year-old retarded child with a discrepancy of the eliminative subsystem	Holaday, 1974
Promotion of the development of hope	The mother of a dying brain-injured 22-year-old man	Skolny & Riehl, 1974
Development of a nursing care plan	An adult amputee with a problem in body image	Rawls, 1980
	A 75-year-old woman with flaccid hemiplegia caused by a cerebrovascular accident	Herbert, 1989
Family-centered nursing care	Clients with ventricular tachycardia	McCauley et al., 1984
Pain management	Cancer patients	Wilkie, 1990
Development of a support group	Caregivers of patients with Alzheimer's disease	Fruehwirth, 1989
Assessment of quality of life	Clients with end-stage renal disease	Ma & Gaudet, 1997
Assessment of fear of crime and development of client-focused and community/ neighborhood-focused nursing interventions	Older adults residing in the community	Benson, 1997
Application of the Behavioral System Model	A 12-year-old boy with myelomeningocele and neurogenic bladder	Holaday, 1997, 2002
	A pregnant woman	Urh, 1998
	A 29-year-old woman with cervical cancer	Holaday, 1997, 2002
	A 58-year-old Navajo Indian with metastatic mandibular cancer	Derdiarian, 1993
	A 16-year-old male adolescent who had attempted suicide	Fawcett, 1997
	A 25-year-old woman who had attempted suicide	Poster, 1991
Application of Auger's interpretation of the Behavioral System Model	Long-term hemodialysis patients	Broncatello, 1980

*See the Practice section of the chapter references for complete citations.

with society's expectations of nursing and that nursing's contribution to health care is a socially valued service" (p. 218).

Empirical evidence supporting the claims made by Johnson, Dee, and Grubbs comes from Derdiarian (1990), who reported a statistically significant increase in both cancer patients' and nurses' satisfaction with the nursing process, including the comprehensiveness of assessment, the appropriateness and priority rank of diagnoses, the interventions, and the effectiveness of outcomes, when nursing assessments were structured according to the Behavioral System Model compared with routine assessment.

Johnson (1968) deliberately attempted to structure nursing practice so that it would be congruent with societal expectations. She maintained, "The value of the model does not lie so much in the fact that it leads to very different forms of action—if it did depart markedly from currently accepted practice, it would perhaps be open to greater question than it otherwise might be" (p. 6).

In contrast with her 1968 comment, 10 years later Johnson (1978a) indicated that in some situations, the nurse, the client, or both may accept a wider range of behavior than prescribed by cultural norms. In such cases, society would have to be helped to accept variances from the average. Additionally, society may have to be helped to accept the role of nursing in assisting people to maintain efficient and effective behavioral functioning when the threat of illness exists. This is because, although there is increased worldwide attention on primary health care with its emphasis on promotion of wellness and prevention of illness, some people still do not expect nursing care before the onset of illness.

Social Significance

Johnson (1980) claimed that the Behavioral System Model leads to nursing actions that are socially significant, stating that "resulting [nursing] actions have been thought to make a significant difference in the lives of the persons involved" (p. 215). Grubbs (1980) agreed with Johnson, noting that the model "provides the framework for categorizing all aspects of the nursing process so that the science of nursing, the personal satisfaction of the nurse, and ultimately the welfare of the patient will improve" (p. 249). Neither Johnson nor Grubbs, however, supported her claim with empirical evidence.

Rawls (1980) provided anecdotal evidence from practice of the social significance of the Behavioral System Model. She stated:

> Use of the Model allowed me to systematically assess the patient and facilitated identification of specific factors which influenced the effectiveness of nursing care. The assessment data allowed identification of interventions which had the desired effect and resulted in effective care for the patient. (p. 16)

Ma and Gaudet (1997) added anecdotal evidence from practice when they stated:

> The benefits of using [the Behavioral System Model] are highlighted in its effectiveness and user friendliness. The model provides nurses with a systematic framework for assessing clients from a behavioural perspective. … Using [the model] complements the application of the medical model and enables the nurse to conduct a more comprehensive assessment of the whole person. (p. 16)

Poster and Beliz (1988, 1992) provided empirical evidence from research of the social significance of the Behavioral System Model. Using the Patient Classification Instrument (see Table 4–2), they found that 90 percent of the 38 adolescent psychiatric inpatients studied had an adaptive change in at least one behavioral subsystem after one week of Behavioral System Model-based nursing care. Furthermore, on average, the patients demonstrated significant improvement in all behavioral subsystems during the discharge phase of hospitalization.

Dee, van Servellen, and Brecht (1998) added empirical research evidence of the social significance of the Behavioral System Model with their findings of improvement in all behavioral subsystems for inpatients under managed behavioral health-care contracts. More specifically, the study results revealed statistically significant differences in the dependency, affiliative, aggressive, and achievement subsystems from admission to discharge.

 ## CONTRIBUTIONS TO THE DISCIPLINE OF NURSING

Johnson certainly may be considered a pioneer in the development of distinctive nursing knowledge, despite the fact that she did not publish her model until 1980. The Behavioral System Model makes a substantial contribution to nursing knowledge by focusing attention on the individual's behavior, rather than on his or her health state or disease condition. Johnson used that distinction to clarify the different foci of nursing and medicine, a clarification that is especially important for continued development of nursing as a distinct discipline. However, she recognized the boundary overlaps that are inevitable in all disciplines. Elaborating, Johnson (1968) pointed out that "this model attempts to specify [the goal of nursing] in keeping with our historical concerns, and to reclarify nursing's mission and area of responsibility. In doing so, no denial of nursing's old relationship with medicine is intended. Nursing has, and undoubtedly always will play an important role in assisting medicine to fulfill its mission. We do this directly by taking on activities delegated by medicine, but also, and perhaps more importantly, we may contribute to the achievement of medicine's goals by fulfilling our own mission" (p. 9).

Johnson (1968) identified the advantages she saw in the Behavioral System Model. The list adequately summarizes the many contributions her conceptual model makes to the discipline of nursing:

1. The assumptions and values of the model are made explicit. This allows their examination and offers the possibility that those assumptions which have not been adequately verified can be logically and perhaps empirically tested.
2. The model offers a reasonably precise and limited ideal goal for nursing by stating the end product desired. Specification of this ideal state or condition is the first step in its operational definition in the concrete case. It thus offers promise for the establishment of standards against which to measure the effectiveness and significance of nursing actions.
3. The model directs our attention to those aspects of the patient, in all his complex reality, with which nursing is concerned, and provides a systematic way to approach the identification of nursing problems.
4. It provides us with clues as to the source of difficulty (i.e., either functional or structural stress).
5. It offers a focus for intervention and suggests the major modes of intervention which will be required.

6. It opens the door to focused research programs in nursing and the possibility that the findings of individual investigators will become cumulative and of theoretical as well as of practical significance. (pp. 7–8)

Commenting on the contributions of the Behavioral System Model in a later paper, Johnson (1992) added:

> Admittedly even now knowledge about the behavioral patterns in the response or action systems is greater than knowledge of the underlying structures, and knowledge about the parts or subsystems is greater than knowledge of the system as a whole. Nonetheless, the body of knowledge about the behavioral system and its subsystems is sufficiently substantial to allow pertinent observations and useful interpretations in practice. It also points to many possibilities for intervention as well as avenues for research. In this way a body of knowledge about disorders in the behavioral system and their prevention and treatment will be developed and expanded over time and will be known as nursing science. (p. 26)

In conclusion, the Behavioral System Model has been enthusiastically adopted by many nurses interested in a systematic approach to nursing. It has documented utility in nursing research, administration, and practice, and it provides direction for curriculum development. The credibility of the Behavioral System Model is beginning to be established by means of studies directly derived from several of its concepts and linked with relevant theories and appropriate empirical indicators. That empirical work must be expanded, and more systematic evaluations of the use of the model in various practice situations and educational settings are needed.

REFERENCES

Ackoff, R.L. (1960). Systems, organizations, and interdisciplinary research. General Systems, 5, 1–8.

Ainsworth, M. (1964). Patterns of attachment behavior shown by the infant in interaction with mother. Merrill-Palmer Quarterly, 10(1), 51–58.

Ainsworth, M. (1972). Attachment and dependency: A comparison. In J. Gewirtz (Ed.), Attachment and dependency (pp. 97–137). Englewood Cliffs, NJ: Prentice-Hall.

Alligood, M.R. (1997). Models and theories: Critical thinking structures. In M.R. Alligood & A. Marriner Tomey (Eds.), Nursing theory: Utilization and application (pp. 31–45). St. Louis: Mosby.

Alligood, M.R. (2002). Philosophies, models, and theories: Critical thinking structures. In M.R. Alligood & A. Marriner Tomey (Eds.), Nursing theory: Utilization and application (2nd ed., pp. 41–61). St. Louis: Mosby.

Atkinson, J.W., & Feather, N.T. (1966). A theory of achievement maturation. New York: Wiley.

Auger, J.R. (1976). Behavioral systems and nursing. Englewood Cliffs, NJ: Prentice-Hall.

Barnum, B.J.S (1998). Nursing theory: Analysis, application, evaluation (5th ed.). Philadelphia: Lippincott.

Broering, J. (1985). Adolescent juvenile status offenders' perceptions of stressful life events and self-perception of health status. Unpublished master's thesis, University of California, San Francisco.

Brown, V.M., Conner, S.S., Harbour, L.S., Magers, J.A., & Watt, J.K. (1998). Dorothy E. Johnson: Behavioral system model. In A. Marriner-Tomey & M.R. Alligood (Eds.), Nursing theorists and their work (4th ed., pp. 227–242). St. Louis: Mosby.

Buckley, W. (Ed.). (1968). Modern systems research for the behavioral scientist. Chicago: Aldine.

Chin, R. (1961). The utility of system models and developmental models for practitioners. In W.G. Bennis, K.D. Beene, & R. Chin (Eds.), The planning of change (pp. 201–214). New York: Holt, Rinehart & Winston.

Coward, D.D., & Wilkie, D.J. (2000). Metastatic bone pain: Meanings associated with self-report and self-management decision making. Cancer Nursing, 23, 101–108.

Crandal, V. (1963). Achievement. In H.W. Stevenson (Ed.), Child psychology (pp. 416–459). Chicago: University of Chicago Press.

Dawson, D.L. (1984). Parenting behaviors of mothers with hospitalized children under two years of age. Unpublished master's thesis, University of California, San Francisco.

Dee, V. (1990). Implementation of the Johnson model: One hospital's experience In M.E. Parker (Ed.), Nursing theories in practice (pp. 33–44). New York: National League for Nursing.

Dee, V., & Poster, E.C. (1995). Applying Kanter's theory of innovative change: The transition from a primary to attending model of nursing care delivery. Journal of the American Psychiatric Nurses Association, 1, 112–119.

Dee, V., van Servellen, G., & Brecht, M. (1998). Managed behavioral health care patients and their nursing care problems, level of functioning, and impairment on discharge. Journal of the American Psychiatric Nurses Association, 4, 57–66.

Derdiarian, A.K. (1981). Nursing conceptual frameworks: Implications for education, practice, and research. In D.L. Vredevoe, A.K. Derdiarian, L.P. Sarna, M. Eriel, & J.C. Shipacoff (Eds.), Concepts of oncology nursing (pp. 369–385). Englewood Cliffs, NJ: Prentice-Hall.

Derdiarian, A.K. (1990). Effects of using systematic assessment instruments on patient and nurse satisfaction with nursing care. Oncology Nursing Forum, 17, 95–101.

Derdiarian, A.K. (1991). Effects of using a nursing model-based assessment instrument on quality of nursing care. Nursing Administration Quarterly, 15(3), 1–16.

Feshbach, S. (1970). Aggression. In P. Mussen (Ed.), Carmichael's manual of child psychology (Vol. 2, 3rd ed., pp. 159–259). New York: Wiley.

Fleming, B.H. (1990). Use of the Johnson model in nursing education (Abstract). In Proceedings of the National Nursing Theory Conference (pp. 109–111). Los Angeles: UCLA Neuropsychiatric Institute and Hospital Nursing Department.

Gewirtz, J. (Ed.). (1972). Attachment and dependency. Englewood Cliffs, NJ: Prentice-Hall.

Glennin, C.G. (1980). Formulation of standards for nursing practice using a nursing model. In J.P. Riehl & C. Roy (Eds.), Conceptual models for nursing practice (2nd ed., pp. 290–301). New York: Appleton-Century-Crofts.

Grubbs, J. (1974). An interpretation of the Johnson Behavioral System Model. In J.P. Riehl & C. Roy (Eds.), Conceptual models for nursing practice (pp. 160–197). New York: Appleton-Century-Crofts.

Grubbs, J. (1980). An interpretation of the Johnson Behavioral System Model. In J.P. Riehl & C. Roy (Eds.), Conceptual models for nursing practice (2nd ed., pp. 217–254). New York: Appleton-Century-Crofts.

Hackley, S. (1987, February). Application of Johnson's behavioral system model. Paper presented at the University of Pennsylvania School of Nursing, Philadelphia.

Hadley, B.J. (1970, March). The utility of theoretical frameworks for curriculum development in nursing: The happening at Colorado. Paper presented at the Western Interstate Council of Higher Education in Nursing General Session, Honolulu, Hawaii.

Hall, B.A. (1981). The change paradigm in nursing: Growth versus persistence. Advances in Nursing Science, 3(4), 1–6.

Harris, R.B. (1986). Introduction of a conceptual nursing model into a fundamental baccalaureate course. Journal of Nursing Education, 25, 66–69.

Heathers, G. (1955). Acquiring dependence and independence: A theoretical orientation. Journal of Genetic Psychology, 87, 277–291.

Herbert, J. (1989). A model for Anna. Nursing, 3(42), 30–34.

Holaday, B. (2002). Johnson's behavioral system model in nursing practice. In M.R. Alligood & A. Marriner-Tomey (Eds.), Nursing theory: Utilization and application (2nd ed., pp. 149–171). St. Louis: Mosby.

Holaday, B., Turner-Henson, A., & Swan, J. (1996). The Johnson behavioral system model: Explaining activities of chronically ill children. In P. Hinton Walker & B. Neuman (Eds.), Blueprint for use of nursing models (pp. 33–63). New York: NLN Press.

Johnson, D.E. (1959). A philosophy of nursing. Nursing Outlook, 7, 198–200.

Johnson, D.E. (1961). The significance of nursing care. American Journal of Nursing, 61(11), 63–66.

Johnson, D.E. (1968, April). One conceptual model of nursing. Paper presented at Vanderbilt University, Nashville, TN.

Johnson, D.E. (1978a, December). Behavioral system model for nursing. Paper presented at the Second Annual Nurse Educator Conference, New York [Audiotape].

Johnson, D.E. (1978b). State of the art of theory development in nursing. In Theory development: What, why, how? (pp. 1–10). New York: National League for Nursing.

Johnson, D.E. (1980). The behavioral system model for nursing. In J.P. Riehl & C. Roy (Eds.), Conceptual models for nursing practice (2nd ed., pp. 207–216). New York: Appleton-Century-Crofts.

Johnson, D.E. (1988). The nurse theorists: Portraits of excellence—Dorothy Johnson. Athens, OH: Fuld Institute for Technology in Nursing Education [Videotape].

Johnson, D.E. (1989). Some thoughts on nursing [Editorial]. Clinical Nurse Specialist, 3, 1–4.

Johnson, D.E. (1990a). The behavioral system model for nursing. In M.E. Parker (Ed.), Nursing theories in practice (pp. 23–32). New York: National League for Nursing.

Johnson, D.E. (1990b, September). Response to V. Dee & B.P. Randell, The Johnson behavioral systems model: Conceptual issues and dilemmas. Paper presented at the National Nursing Theory Conference, UCLA Neuropsychiatric Institute and Hospital Nursing Department, Los Angeles, CA.

Johnson, D.E. (1992). The origins of the behavioral system model. In F.N. Nightingale, Notes on nursing: What it is, and what it is not (Commemorative ed., pp. 23–27). Philadelphia: Lippincott.

Johnson, D.E. (1996). Introduction to "The Johnson behavioral system model: Explaining activities of chronically ill children." In P. Hinton Walker & B. Neuman (Eds.), Blueprint for use of nursing models (pp. 33–34). New York: NLN Press.

Kagan, J. (1964). Acquisition and significance of sex typing and sex role identity. In M. Hoffman & L. Hoffman (Eds.), Review of child development research (Vol. 1, pp. 137–167). New York: Russell Sage Foundation.

Kizpolski, P.A. (1985). Family adaptation during the midstage of cancer. Unpublished master's thesis, University of California, San Francisco.

Lachicotte, J.L., & Alexander, J.W. (1990). Management attitudes and nurse impairment. Nursing Management, 21; 102–104, 106, 108, 110.

Lewis, C., & Randell, B.P. (1991). Alteration in self-care: An instance of ineffective coping in the geriatric patient. In R.M. Carroll-Johnson (Ed.), Classification of nursing diagnoses: Proceedings of the ninth conference: North American Nursing Diagnosis Association (pp. 264–265). Philadelphia: Lippincott.

Lobo, M.L. (2002). Behavioral system model: Dorothy E. Johnson. In J. B. George (Ed.), Nursing theories: The base for professional nursing practice (5th ed., pp. 155–169). Upper Saddle River, NJ: Prentice Hall.

Lorenz, K. (1966). On aggression. New York: Harcourt.

Ma, T., & Gaudet, D. (1997). Assessing the quality of life of our end-stage renal disease client population. Journal of the Canadian Association of Nephrology Nurses and Technicians, 7(2), 13–16.

Marriner-Tomey, A. (1989). Nursing theorists and their work (2nd ed). St. Louis: Mosby.

Mead, M. (1953). Cultural patterns and technical change. World Federation for Mental Health: UNESCO.

Meleis, A.I. (1997). Theoretical nursing. Development and progress (3rd ed.). Philadelphia: Lippincott.

Miller, M. (1987). Uncertainty, coping, social support and family functioning in parents of children with myelomeningocele. Unpublished master's thesis. University of California, San Francisco.

Moran, T.A. (1986). The effect of an AIDS diagnosis on the sexual practices of homosexual men. Unpublished master's thesis, University of California, San Francisco.

Moreau, D., Poster, E.C., & Niemela, K. (1993). Implementing and evaluating an attending nurse model. Nursing Management, 24(6); 56–58, 60, 64.

Niemela, K., Poster, E.C., & Moreau, D. (1992). The attending nurse: A new role for the advanced clinician—Adolescent inpatient unit. Journal of Child and Adolescent Psychiatric and Mental Health Nursing, 5(3), 5–12.

Nightingale, F.N. (1946). Notes on nursing: What it is, and what it is not (Facsimile ed.). Philadelphia: Lippincott. [Originally published in 1859.]

Poster, E.C., & Beliz, L. (1988). Behavioral category ratings of adolescents in an inpatient psychiatric unit. International Journal of Adolescence and Youth, 1, 293–303.

Poster, E.C., & Beliz, L. (1992). The use of the Johnson behavioral system model to measure changes during adolescent hospitalization. International Journal of Adolescence and Youth, 4, 73–84.

Randell, B.P. (1991). NANDA versus the Johnson behavioral systems model: Is there a diagnostic difference? In R.M. Carroll-Johnson (Ed.), Classification of nursing diagnoses: Proceedings of the ninth conference: North American Nursing Diagnosis Association (pp. 154–160). Philadelphia: Lippincott.

Rapoport, A. (1968). Foreword. In W. Buckley (Ed.), Modern systems research for the behavioral scientist (pp. xiii–xxii). Chicago: Aldine.

Rawls, A.C. (1980). Evaluation of the Johnson Behavioral Model in clinical practice. Image: Journal of Nursing Scholarship, 12, 13–16.

Resnik, H.L.P. (1972). Sexual behaviors. Boston: Little, Brown.

Riegel, B. (1989). Social support and psychological adjustment to chronic coronary heart disease: Operationalization of Johnson's behavioral system model. Advances in Nursing Science, 11(2), 74–84.

Riegel, B. (1990). Social support and cardiac invalidism following acute myocardial infarction: A test of Johnson's behavioral system model. In Proceedings of the National Nursing Theory Conference (pp. 12–14). Los Angeles: UCLA Neuropsychiatric Institute and Hospital Nursing Department.

Riehl, J.P., & Roy, C. (Eds.). (1980). Conceptual models for nursing practice (2nd ed.). New York: Appleton-Century-Crofts.

Robson, K.K. (1967). Patterns and determinants of maternal attachment. Journal of Pediatrics, 77, 976–985.

Rogers, C.G. (1973). Conceptual models as guides to clinical nursing specialization. Journal of Nursing Education, 12(4), 2–6.

Rosenthal, M. (1967). The generalization of dependency from mother to a stranger. Journal of Child Psychology and Psychiatry, 8, 177–183.

Sears, R., Maccoby, E., & Levin, H. (1954). Patterns of child rearing. White Plains, NY: Row, Peterson.

Walike, B., Jordan, H.A., & Stellar, E. (1969). Studies of eating behavior. Nursing Research, 18, 108–113.

Wilkie, D. (1985). Pain intensity and observed behaviors of adult cancer patients experiencing pain. Unpublished master's thesis, University of California, San Francisco.

Wilkie, D., Lovejoy, N., Dodd, M., & Tesler, M. (1988). Cancer pain control behaviors: Description and correlation with pain intensity. Oncology Nursing Forum, 15, 723–731.

RESEARCH

Bossert, E., Holaday, B., Harkins, A., & Turner-Henson, A. (1990). Strategies of normalization used by parents of chronically ill school age children, Journal of Child and Adolescent Psychiatric and Mental Health Nursing, 3, 57–61.

Coward, D.D., & Wilkie, D.J. (2000). Metastatic bone pain: Meanings associated with self-report and self-management decision making. Cancer Nursing, 23, 101–108.

Damus, K. (1974). An application of the Johnson behavioral system model for nursing practice. In J.P. Riehl & C. Roy, Conceptual models for nursing practice (pp. 218–233). New York: Appleton-Century-Crofts. [Reprinted in J.P. Riehl & C. Roy (Eds.). (1980). Conceptual models for nursing practice (2nd ed., pp. 274–289). New York: Appleton-Century-Crofts.]

Dee, V., van Servellen, G., & Brecht, M. (1998). Managed behavioral health care patients and their nursing care problems, level of functioning, and impairment on discharge. Journal of the American Psychiatric Nurses Association, 4, 57–66.

Derdiarian, A.K. (1990a). Effects of using systematic assessment instruments on patient and nurse satisfaction with nursing care. Oncology Nursing Forum, 17, 95–101.

Derdiarian, A.K. (1990b). The relationships among the subsystems of Johnson's behavioral system model. Image: Journal of Nursing Scholarship, 22, 219–225.

Derdiarian, A.K. (1991). Effects of using a nursing model-based assessment instrument on quality of nursing care. Nursing Administration Quarterly, 15(3), 1–16.

Derdiarian, A.K., & Schobel, D. (1990). Comprehensive assessment of AIDS patients using the behavioural systems model for nursing practice instrument. Journal of Advanced Nursing, 15, 436–446.

Holaday, B. (1974). Achievement behavior in chronically ill children. Nursing Research, 23, 25–30.

Holaday, B. (1981). Maternal response to their chronically ill infants' attachment behavior of crying. Nursing Research, 30, 343–348.

Holaday, B. (1982). Maternal conceptual set development: Identifying patterns of maternal response to chronically ill infant crying. Maternal-Child Nursing Journal, 11, 47–69.

Holaday, B. (1987). Patterns of interaction between mothers and their chronically ill infants. Maternal-Child Nursing Journal, 16, 29–45.

Holaday, B., & Turner-Henson, A. (1987). Chronically ill school-age children's use of time. Pediatric Nursing, 13, 410–414.

Holaday, B., Turner-Henson, A., & Swan, J. (1996). The Johnson behavioral system model: Explaining activities of chronically ill children. In P. Hinton Walker & B. Neuman (Eds.), Blueprint for use of nursing models (pp. 33–63). New York: NLN Press.

Lachicotte, J.L., & Alexander, J.W. (1990). Management attitudes and nurse impairment. Nursing Management, 21; 102–104, 106, 108, 110.

Lewis, C., & Randell, B.P. (1991). Alteration in self-care: An instance of ineffective coping in the geriatric patient. In R.M. Carroll-Johnson (Ed.), Classification of nursing diagnoses: Proceedings of the ninth conference: North American Nursing Diagnosis Association (pp. 264–265). Philadelphia: Lippincott.

Lovejoy, N. (1985). Needs of vigil and nonvigil visitors in cancer research units. In Fourth Cancer Nursing Research Conference Proceedings (pp. 142–164). Honolulu: American Cancer Society.

Lovejoy, N.C., & Moran, T. A. (1988). Selected AIDS beliefs, behaviors and informational needs of homosexual/bisexual men with AIDS or ARC. International Journal of Nursing Studies, 25, 207–216.

Poster, E.C., & Beliz, L. (1988). Behavioural category ratings of adolescents on an inpatient psychiatric unit. International Journal of Adolescence and Youth, 1, 293–303.

Poster, E.C., & Beliz, L. (1992). The use of the Johnson behavioral system model to measure changes during adolescent hospitalization. International Journal of Adolescence and Youth, 4, 73–84.

Poster, E.C., Dee, V., & Randell, B.P. (1997). The Johnson behavioral system model as a framework for patient outcome evaluation. Journal of the American Psychiatric Nurses Association, 3, 73–80.

Randell, B.P. (1991). NANDA versus the Johnson behavioral systems model: Is there a diagnostic difference? In R.M. Carroll-Johnson (Ed.), Classification of nursing diagnoses: Proceedings of the ninth conference: North American Nursing Diagnosis Association (pp. 154–160). Philadelphia: Lippincott.

Riegel, B. (1990). Social support and cardiac invalidism following acute myocardial infarction: A test of Johnson's behavioral system model [Abstract]. In Proceedings of the National Nursing Theory Conference (pp. 12–14). Los Angeles: UCLA Neuropsychiatric Institute and Hospital Nursing Department.

Small, B. (1980). Nursing visually impaired children with Johnson's model as a conceptual framework. In J.P. Riehl & C. Roy (Eds.), Conceptual models for nursing practice (2nd ed., pp. 264–273). New York: Appleton-Century-Crofts.

Stamler, C., & Palmer, J.O. (1971). Dependency and repetitive visits to the nurse's office in elementary school children. Nursing Research, 20, 254–255.

Wilkie, D., Lovejoy, N., Dodd, M., & Tesler, M. (1988). Cancer pain control behaviors: Description and correlation with pain intensity. Oncology Nursing Forum, 15, 723–731.

RESEARCH INSTRUMENTS AND PRACTICE TOOLS

Auger, J.A., & Dee, V. (1983). A patient classification system based on the behavioral system model of Nursing: Part 1. Journal of Nursing Administration, 13(4), 38–43.

Bruce, G.L., Hinds, P., Hudak, J., Mucha, A., Taylor, M.C., & Thompson, C.R. (1980). Implementation of ANA's quality assurance program for clients with end-stage renal disease. Advances in Nursing Science, 2(2), 79–95.

Dee, V. (1986). Validation of a patient classification instrument for psychiatric patients based on the Johnson model for nursing. Dissertation Abstracts International, 47, 4822B.

Dee V., & Auger, J.A. (1983). A patient classification system based on the behavioral system model of nursing: Part 2. Journal of Nursing Administration, 13(5), 18–23.

Dee, V., van Servellen, G., & Brecht, M. (1998). Managed behavioral health care patients and their nursing care problems, level of functioning, and impairment on discharge. Journal of the American Psychiatric Nurses Association, 4, 57–66.

Derdiarian, A.K. (1983). An instrument for theory and research using the behavioral systems model for nursing: The cancer patient (Part I). Nursing Research, 32, 196–201.

Derdiarian, A.K. (1984). An investigation of the variables and boundaries of cancer nursing: A pioneering approach using Johnson's behavioral systems model for nursing. In Proceedings of the 3rd International Conference on Cancer Nursing (pp. 96–102). Melbourne, Australia: The Cancer Institute/Peter MacCallum Hospital and the Royal Melbourne Hospital.

Derdiarian, A.K. (1988). Sensitivity of the Derdiarian behavioral system model instrument to age, site, and stage of cancer: A preliminary validation study. Scholarly Inquiry for Nursing Practice, 2, 103–121. Holaday, B. (1989). Response to "Sensitivity of the Derdiarian behavioral system model instrument to age, site, and stage of cancer: A preliminary validation study." Scholarly Inquiry for Nursing Practice, 2, 123–125.

Derdiarian, A.K. (1990). Effects of using systematic assessment instruments on patient and nurse satisfaction with nursing care. Oncology Nursing Forum, 17, 95–101.

Derdiarian, A.K., & Forsythe, A.B. (1983). An instrument for theory and research using the behavioral systems model for nursing: The cancer patient (Part II). Nursing Research, 32, 260–266.

Holaday, B. (2002). Johnson's behavioral system model in nursing practice. In M.R. Alligood & A. Marriner-Tomey (Eds.), Nursing theory: Utilization and application (2nd ed., pp. 149–171). St. Louis: Mosby.

Lovejoy, N.C. (1982). An empirical verification of the Johnson behavioral system model for nursing. Dissertation Abstracts International, 42, 2781B.

Lovejoy, N. (1983). The leukemic child's perception of family behaviors. Oncology Nursing Forum, 10(4), 20–25.

Majesky, S.J., Brester, M.H., & Nishio, K.T. (1978). Development of a research tool: Patient indicators of nursing care. Nursing Research, 27, 365–371.

Poster, E.C., Dee, V., & Randell, B.P. (1997). The Johnson behavioral system model as a framework for patient outcome evaluation. Journal of the American Psychiatric Nurses Association, 3, 73–80.

Wilmoth, M.C. (1993). Development and testing of the Sexual Behaviors Questionnaire. Dissertation Abstracts International, 54, 6137B–6138B.

Wilmoth, M.C., & Tingle, L.R. (2001). Development and psychometric testing of the Wilmoth Sexual Behaviors Questionnaire—Female. Canadian Journal of Nursing Research, 32, 135–151.

Wilmoth, M.C., & Townsend, J. (1995). A comparison of the effects of lumpectomy versus mastectomy on sexual behaviors. Cancer Practice, 3, 279–285.

PRACTICE

Benson, S. (1997). The older adult and fear of crime. Journal of Gerontological Nursing, 23(10), 24–31.

Broncatello, K.F. (1980). Auger in action: Application of the model. Advances in Nursing Science, 2(2), 13–24.

Derdiarian, A.K. (1993). Application of the Johnson behavioral system model in nursing practice. In M.E. Parker (Ed.), Patterns of nursing theories in practice (pp. 285–298). New York: National League for Nursing.

Fawcett, J. (1997). Conceptual models as guides for psychiatric nursing practice. In A.W. Burgess (Ed.), Psychiatric nursing: Promoting mental health (pp. 627–642). Stamford, CT: Appleton & Lange.

Fruehwirth, S.E.S. (1989). An application of Johnson's behavioral model: A case study. Journal of Community Health Nursing, 6(2), 61–71.

Herbert, J. (1989). A model for Anna. Nursing, 3(42), 30–34.

Holaday, B.J. (1974). Implementing the Johnson model for nursing practice. In J.P. Riehl & C. Roy (Eds.), Conceptual models for nursing practice (pp. 197–206). New York: Appleton-Century-Crofts. [Reprinted in J.P. Riehl & C. Roy (Eds.). (1980). Conceptual models for nursing practice (2nd ed., pp. 255–263). New York: Appleton-Century-Crofts.]

Holaday, B. (1997). Johnson's behavioral system model in nursing practice. In M.R. Alligood & A. Marriner-Tomey (Eds.), Nursing theory: Utilization and application (pp. 49–70). St. Louis: Mosby.

Holaday, B. (2002). Johnson's behavioral system model in nursing practice. In M.R. Alligood & A. Marriner Tomey (Eds.), Nursing theory: Utilization and application (2nd ed., pp. 149–171). St. Louis: Mosby.

Ma, T., & Gaudet, D. (1997). Assessing the quality of life of our end-stage renal disease client population. Journal of the Canadian Association of Nephrology Nurses and Technicians, 7(2), 13–16.

McCauley, K., Choromanski, J.D., Wallinger, C., & Liu, K. (1984). Current management of ventricular tachycardia: Symposium from the Hospital of the University of Pennsylvania. Learning to live with controlled ventricular tachycardia: Utilizing the Johnson model. Heart and Lung, 13, 633–638.

Poster, E.C. (1991). Quality assurance and treatment outcome: A psychiatric nursing perspective. In S.M. Mairin, J.T. Gossett, & M.C. Grob (Eds.), Psychiatric treatment: Advances in outcome research (pp. 279–292). Washington, DC: American Psychiatric Press.

Rawls, A.C. (1980). Evaluation of the Johnson Behavioral Model in clinical practice. Image: Journal of Nursing Scholarship, 12, 13–16.

Skolny, M.A., & Riehl, J.P. (1974). Solving patient and family problems by using a theoretical framework. In J.P. Riehl & C. Roy (Eds.), Conceptual models for nursing practice (pp. 206–218). New York: Appleton-Century-Crofts.

Urh, I. (1998). Dorothy Johnson's theory and nursing care of a pregnant woman. Obzornik Zkravstvene Nege, 32(5/6), 199–203. [Slovenian; English abstract.]

Wilkie, D. (1990). Cancer pain management: State-of-the-art care. Nursing Clinics of North America, 25, 331–343.

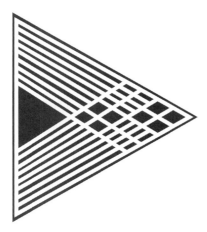

Chapter **5**

King's Conceptual System

Imogene M. King presented the foundation for her Conceptual System in her 1964 publication, "Nursing Theory—Problems and Prospect." She then identified several concepts of the Conceptual System in her 1968 article, "A Conceptual Frame of Reference for Nursing." The entire Conceptual System was presented in her 1971 book, *Toward a Theory for Nursing.* King went on to describe refinements in the Conceptual System in her 1978 speech at the Second Annual Nurse Educator Conference. She presented further refinements in the Conceptual System and introduced the Theory of Goal Attainment in her 1981 book, *A Theory for Nursing: Systems, Concepts, Process.* Subsequently, King published overviews of the Conceptual System and theory, with some refinements, in a book (King, 1986a), book chapters (King, 1986b, 1987b, 1989a, 1990b, 1995a, 1995b), and a journal article (King, 1992a). In 1987, King (personal communication, July 18, 1987) stated that her Conceptual System "will not change but will continue to generate theories." Later, King (2001) commented that "there has been no change in the conceptual system or theory except to add the concept of coping in the personal system" (p. 281). (In an earlier paper, King (1987a) had placed coping in the interpersonal system.) King (2001a) went on to note, "The word 'spiritual' was added to my assumptions about human beings. This was in my original manuscript in 1971 but was accidentally omitted in the publication" (p. 281).

Theories derived from the Conceptual System continue to be generated, and two other changes in the Conceptual System, not mentioned by King, are evident. Those changes are the addition of learning as a dimension of the concept of personal system and the addition of control as a dimension of the concept of social system (King, 1986a).

Overview

King's work focuses on the continuing ability of individuals to meet their basic needs so that they may function in their socially defined roles, as well as on individuals' interactions within three open, dynamic, interacting systems. King has always been very clear about the separation of her work into a conceptual framework or Conceptual System and a theory, which fit the definition of a conceptual model and a middle-range theory, respectively, used in this book. In accordance with King's (1999) preference, the term Conceptual System, rather than conceptual model or conceptual framework, will be used throughout this chapter.

King did not provide an explicit title for her Conceptual System until the late 1980s. In earlier editions of this book, the Conceptual System was referred to as the Open Systems Model (Fawcett, 1984) and the Interacting Systems Framework (Fawcett, 1989). King (1989a, 1992b) eventually titled her work the General

Systems Framework and then began to refer to the Conceptual System as King's Conceptual System (King, 1997a, 1997c). The title General Systems Framework was used in the previous edition of this book (Fawcett, 2000). Here, the title King's Conceptual System is used.

The concepts of King's Conceptual System and her Theory of Goal Attainment and their dimensions and subdimensions are listed here, along with the goals of nursing and the components of King's practice methodology. The concepts, their dimensions and subdimensions, and the methodology components are defined and described, and the goal of nursing is discussed in detail later in this chapter.

Key Terms

HUMAN BEINGS
PERSONAL SYSTEM
   Perception
   Self
   Growth and Development
   Body Image
   Time
   Personal Space
   Learning
INTERPERSONAL SYSTEM
   Interaction
   Communication
     Verbal Communication
     Nonverbal Communication
   Transaction
   Role
   Stress
   Coping

SOCIAL SYSTEM
   Organization
   Authority
   Power
   Status
   Decision Making
   Control
ENVIRONMENT
INTERNAL ENVIRONMENT
EXTERNAL ENVIRONMENT
HEALTH
HEALTH
ILLNESS
NURSING
ACTION, REACTION, AND INTERACTION PROCESS
GOAL OF NURSING
   Help Individuals, Families, Groups, and Communities Attain, Maintain, and Restore Health, So That They Can Function in Their Respective Roles, and to Help Individuals Die with Dignity
PRACTICE METHODOLOGY: THE INTERACTION-TRANSACTION PROCESS
   Perception
   Judgment
   Action
   Reaction
   Disturbance
   Mutual Goal Setting
   Exploration of Means to Achieve Goals
   Agreement on Means to Achieve Goals
   Transaction
   Attainment of Goals
THEORY OF GOAL ATTAINMENT

ANALYSIS OF KING'S CONCEPTUAL SYSTEM

This section presents an analysis of King's Conceptual System and her Theory of Goal Attainment. The analysis relies heavily on King's (1981) book, *A Theory for Nursing: Systems, Concepts, Process*; her book chapter (1990b), "King's Conceptual Framework and Theory of Goal Attainment;" and her journal article (1992a), "King's Theory of Goal Attainment;" and draws from other recent publications (King, 1995a, 1995b, 1997c).

ORIGINS OF THE NURSING MODEL

Historical Evolution and Motivation

King began to develop her Conceptual System at a time when nursing was striving for status as a science and hence as a legitimate profession. She, along with other writers of the 1960s (e.g., Moore, 1968, 1969), maintained that the delineation of a theoretical body of knowledge was necessary for the advancement of nursing. King (1964) voiced her concern that an existing "antitheoretical bias" in nursing had resulted in "nursing theory … based on practical techniques—the 'how' rather than the 'why'" (p. 395). She therefore deliberately set out to develop a conceptual frame of reference for nursing as a precursor to a theory that would explicate the "why" of nursing actions.

King (1988) stated that the specific motivation to develop her Conceptual System was the need to select essential content for a new master's degree program in nursing. She went on to explain:

In 1963 as I worked with a faculty committee to develop a new master of science in nursing program, I was challenged by a question from a philosophy professor who was familiar with my undergraduate philosophy courses. He asked: "Imogene, have you or any nurses defined the 'nursing act'?" I perceived this to be a philosophical type question and my response was

"Not that I know of, but first one needs to define a 'human act' because nurses and the clients they serve are first and foremost human beings." He chuckled and said that I had a good beginning and to continue to think about it (King, 1997c, p. 15).

King (1971) explained that the particular concepts of her Conceptual System were formulated in response to several questions emanating from her "personal concern about the changes influencing nursing, a conscious awareness of the knowledge explosion, and a hunch that some of the essential components of nursing have persisted" (p. 19). The questions were:

1. What are some of the social and educational changes in the United States that have influenced changes in nursing?
2. What basic elements are continuous throughout these changes in nursing?
3. What is the scope of the practice of nursing, and in what kind of settings do nurses perform their functions?
4. Are the current goals of nursing similar to those of the past half-century?
5. What are the dimensions of practice that have given the field of nursing a unifying focus over time?

King (1971) then noted, "These questions established a framework for thinking about nursing today, for reading about nursing in society, [and] for discussing ideas with nurses and other individuals" (p. 19). Later, King (1995a) explained, "In my initial thoughts about theory and nursing, I identified three major problems: (a) the lack of a professional language, (b) an antitheoretical bias, and (c) that the domain of nursing had not yet been identified" (p. 17).

King (1997c) continued by explaining the process she used to develop her Conceptual System. She stated:

> Initial thoughts were that the nursing act represents actions (not interventions) and a series of these actions represent nursing as a process. This led me to ask a few more questions, such as, where do nurses perform these acts and engage in this process? My next step was to conduct a comprehensive review of nursing literature (1923–1963). My review revealed that multiple concepts were being discussed as essential knowledge used by nurses. … From this analysis multiple concepts were listed from which I selected those that represented broad conceptualizations of knowledge. This resulted in formulating my initial conceptual framework which was published in Nursing Research (King, 1968). [Then, I audited] three formal classes in systems research. Learning the language of systems helped me design my conceptual framework represented by three dynamic interacting systems. (p. 15)

Reading and course work led King (1971) to the literature of systems analysis and general system theory, and hence to another set of questions:

1. What kind of decisions are nurses required to make in the course of their roles and responsibilities?
2. What kind of information is essential for them to make decisions?
3. What are the alternatives in nursing situations?
4. What alternative courses of action do nurses have in making critical decisions about another individual's care, recovery, and health?
5. What skills do nurses now perform and what knowledge is essential for nurses to make decisions about alternatives? (pp. 19–20)

In another recounting of the development of her Conceptual System, King (1990b) explained, "After studying the research on General System Theory, I was able to synthesize my analysis of the nursing literature and my knowledge from other disciplines into a conceptual framework" (p. 74). Later, she elaborated: "General system theory, which guides the study of organized complexity as whole systems … guided me to focus on knowledge as an information processing, goal seeking, and decision making system" (King, 1997b, pp. 19–20).

King (1985a) later commented that her perspective of nursing evolved in response to the two other questions:

1. What is the essence of nursing?
2. What is the human act?

Still later, King (1992a) stated that additional questions served as a guide for review and analysis of the nursing literature. The questions were: "(a) Who are nurses and how are they educated? (b) How and where is nursing practiced? (c) Who needs nursing in society? (d) What is the overall goal of nursing? (e) What is the nursing act? (f) What is the nursing process?" (p. 19).

Elaborating on the origin of her Conceptual System, King (1971) explained, "Concepts that consistently appeared in nursing literature, in research findings, in speeches by nurses, and were observable in the world of nursing practice were identified and synthesized into a conceptual framework" (pp. 20–21). That synthesis resulted in selection of four universal ideas—social systems, health, perception, and interpersonal relations. King (1971) maintained that those ideas formed a Conceptual System that "suggests that the essential characteristics of nursing are those properties that have persisted in spite of environmental changes" (p. ix). The four universal ideas then were used as a general frame of reference for identification of the other concepts of the Conceptual System.

Furthermore, King (1992a) stated that the literature review revealed three major ideas about nursing. "One idea was that nursing is complex because of the human variables found in nursing situations. … A second idea … was that nurses play different roles in health care organizations of varying sizes and organizational structure. Nurses are expected to perform many functions in these organizations. A third idea was that changes in society, changes in the role of women, and advancement in knowledge from research and technology have influenced changes in nursing" (pp. 19–20).

Philosophical Claims

King presented the philosophical claims undergirding her Conceptual System and the Theory of Goal Attainment in the form of a philosophical orientation to science and a philosophical orientation to nursing. King (1989a, 1990b, 1997b, 2001) has revealed that her philosophical orientation to science is general system theory. She explained,

> My philosophical position is rooted in General System Theory, which guides the study of organized complexity as whole systems. This philosophy gave me the impetus to focus on knowledge development as an information-processing, goal-seeking, and decision-making system. General System Theory provides a holistic approach to study nursing phenomena as an open system and frees one's thinking from the parts versus whole dilemma (King, 2001a, p. 277).

King (1990b) requested that her work be read "from the perspective of General System Theory and a science of wholeness, which is my philosophical position" (p. 74). Furthermore, King (1990b) maintained that her philosophical orientation to science is congruent with her philosophical orientation to nursing. All of King's philosophical claims, which are expressed as assumptions about open systems, human beings, and nurse-client interactions; beliefs about nursing; and propositions about nursing, are presented here.

Assumptions about Open Systems

- Open systems exhibit an exchange of energy and information and are goal directed (King, 1997a, p. 180; 1997b, p. 20).
- Open systems exhibit equifinality in that different means may be used to attain similar goals (King, 1997b, p. 20).
- A system is composed of at least five elements: goals, structure, functions, resources, and decision making (King, 1997a, p. 180).
- Resources flow into the system as inputs, activities indicate the use of resources, and outputs are generated (King, 1997b, p. 20).
- When inputs are converted to outputs, transformation takes place (King, 1997b, p. 20).
- Open systems are essential in studying the wholeness of nursing (King, 1997a, p. 181).
- The goal of the system is health (King, 1997a, p. 181).

Assumptions about Human Beings

- Characteristics that are common to human beings are that they are unique, holistic individuals of intrinsic worth who are capable of rational thinking and decision making in most situations (King, 1995b, p. 26).
- Individuals are sentient and social, as observed by their interactions with persons and objects in the environment (King, 1995b, p. 26).
- Individuals] are perceived as reacting beings who are controlling, purposeful, action-oriented, and time-oriented in their behavior (King, 1995b, p. 26).
- Individuals are social, spiritual, sentient, and rational human beings who act in situations by perceiving, controlling, and exhibiting purposeful action-oriented behavior over time (King, 1997b, p. 21).
- Individuals have the capacity to think, to know, to make choices, and to select alternative courses of actions (King, 1995b, pp. 26–27).
- Human beings have an intellect and by nature, they desire to know (King, 1997b, p. 21).
- Individuals differ in their needs, wants, and goals (King, 1995b, p. 27).
- Values form the basis of each person's goals (King, 1995b, p. 27).
- Because each person is unique, the nature of values emanates from the nature of human beings (King, 1995b, p. 27).
- [Values] are demonstrated in the standards of human conduct and have been handed down from one generation to another (King, 1995b, p. 27).
- Values are linked to cultures and, therefore, vary from person to person, family to family, and society to society (King, 1995b, p. 27).
- Human beings are open systems who think, who set goals, and who select means to achieve them (King, 1997b, p. 20).
- Human beings … are open systems in transaction with the environment (King, 1995b, p. 26).
- Individuals exhibit a sense of wonder about their world and ask questions, seek answers, identify problems, and seek resolution (King, 1997b, pp. 20–21).
- Individuals process selective inputs from the environment through the senses (King, 1981).
- Individuals are in continuous transaction with their internal and external environments (King, 1997b, p. 21).
- Transaction connotes that there is no separateness between human beings and environment (King, 1995b, p. 26).
- Individuals organize and relate information from the external environment with the internal environment (King, 1997b, p. 20).
- Human beings have the ability through their language

and other symbols to record their history and preserve their culture (King, 1995b, p. 27).

- Individuals generally wish to preserve life, avoid pain, procreate, gratify desires, and insure their security. In addition, individuals want to perform functions associated with activities of daily living (King, 1990a, p. 127).
- People and money are the key resources in achieving goals (King, 1997a, p. 181).

Beliefs about Nursing

- The focus of nursing is the human being and human acts (King, 1985a).
- The focus of nursing is human beings interacting with their environment leading to a state of health for individuals, which is an ability to function in social roles (King, 1981, p. 143).
- Nursing is perceived by me to be a complex, organized whole system transacting with a variety of whole systems (King, 1997b, p. 21).
- Nursing is a goal-seeking system (King, 1997b, p. 21).
- Nurses, in the performance of their roles and responsibilities, assist individuals and groups in society to attain, maintain, and restore health (King, 1971, p. 22).
- In the process of functioning in social institutions, nurses assist individuals to meet their basic needs at some point in time in the life cycle when they cannot do this for themselves (King, 1971, p. 22).
- An understanding of basic human needs in the physical, social, emotional, and intellectual realm of the life process from conception to old age, within the context of social systems of the culture in which nurses live and work, is essential and basic content for learning the practice of nursing (King, 1971, p. 22).

Propositions about Nursing

- The nursing process is conducted within a social system, the dimensions [of which] include: (a) the nursing process, (b) the individuals involved in the nursing process, (c) the individuals involved in the environment within which the nursing process is activated, (d) the social organization within which the process takes place, [and] (e) the community within which the social organization functions (King, 1964, p. 401).
- The nursing process will differ, dependent upon the individual nurse and each recipient of nursing service (King, 1964, p. 401).
- The nursing process will differ relative to all individuals in the environment (King, 1964, p. 401).
- The nursing process will differ relative to the social organization in which the nursing process takes place (King, 1964, p. 401).

- The relationships among the dimensions have an effect upon the nursing process (King, 1964, p. 401).
- Nursing includes specific components: (a) nursing judgment, (b) nurse action, (c) communication, (d) evaluation, (e) coordination (King, 1964, p. 402).
- The nursing judgment will vary relative to each nursing action (King, 1964, p. 402).
- The effectiveness of nursing action will vary with the extent to which it is communicated to those responsible for its implementation (King, 1964, p. 402).
- Nursing action is more effectively assured if the goals are communicated and standards of nursing performance have been established (King, 1964, p. 402).
- Nursing action is based on facts, which may change; thus, nursing judgments and action are evaluated and revised as the situation changes (King, 1964, p. 402).
- Nursing action is one component of health care; thus health care is affected by the coordination of nursing with health services (King, 1964, p. 402).

Assumptions about Nurse-Client Interactions

- Perceptions of nurse and of client influence the interaction process (King, 1981, p. 143).
- Goals, needs, and values of nurse and client influence the interaction process (King, 1981, p. 143).
- Individuals and families have a right to knowledge about their health (King, 1992a, p. 21).
- [Individuals and families] have a right to participate in decisions that influence their life, their health, and community services (King, 1992a, p. 21).
- Health professionals have a responsibility to share information that helps individuals make informed decisions about their health (King, 1992a, p. 21).
- [Individuals and families] have a right to accept or to reject health care (King, 1992a, p. 21).
- Goals of health professionals and goals of recipients of health care may be incongruent (King, 1981, p. 144).
- Health professionals have a responsibility to gather relevant information about the perceptions of the client so that their goals and the goals of the client are congruent (King, 1992a, p. 21).
- The assumption that individuals (nurse and client) are capable of interacting to set mutual goals and agree on means to achieve the goals has been extended to include mutual goal setting with family members in relation to clients and families (King, 1986b, p. 200).

Strategies for Knowledge Development

King used both inductive and deductive thought processes to formulate her Conceptual System and Theory of Goal

Attainment. Explaining her approach, King (1975) commented:

> My personal approach to synthesizing knowledge for nursing was to use data and information available from research in nursing and related fields and from my 25 years in active practice, teaching, and research. ... A search of the literature in nursing and other behavioral science fields, discussion with colleagues, attendance at numerous conferences, inductive and deductive reasoning, and some critical thinking about the information gathered, led me to formulate my own framework. (pp. 36–37)

Elaborating on the process she used to review the literature, King (1992a) stated, "The process used ... to identify relevant concepts began with a review of the literature. ... From the literature review, a list of words [was] recorded using content analysis. A reconceptualization of this list provided the comprehensive concepts for the King conceptual system. ... Subsequent to the review of literature and discussions with colleagues and with nurses giving direct care, and with critical thinking about the information gathered, [I] was led to formulate the conceptual system" (pp. 19–20).

Influences from Other Scholars

King (1971, 1975, 1981, 1989a, 1992a) has repeatedly mentioned the influence of the literature of nursing and adjunctive disciplines on the development of her Conceptual System and Theory of Goal Attainment. She explained:

> I know of no other discipline that deals with knowledge that is so vitally essential in the empirical world of application to practice as the knowledge we expect nurses to have for decision making for immediate action in many situations. If one analyzes the knowledge required for nurses to function in the complex world of practice, that knowledge is composed of concepts in every discipline in higher education. This is what motivated me to identify those concepts in other disciplines that give nurses specific knowledge that is applied in real world situations. (King, 1989a, p. 150)

Furthermore, although King (1981) cited the influence of general system theory on the formulation of her Conceptual System in the past, she has underscored that influence in more recent publications (King, 1989a, 1990b, 1997b, 2001).

Among the numerous authors from many disciplines whose works King cited are Benne and Bennis (1959), Boulding (1956), Bross (1953), Bruner and Krech (1968), Cherry (1966), DiVincenti (1977), Erikson (1950), Etzioni (1975), Fisher and Cleveland (1968), Fraser (1972), Freud (1966), Gesell (1952), Gibson (1966), Griffiths (1959), Haas (1964), Hall (1959), Hall and Fagen (1956), Havighurst (1953), Ittleson and Cantril (1954), Janis (1958), Jersild (1952), Katz and Kahn (1966), Klein (1970), Linton (1963), Lyman and Scott (1967), Monat and Lazarus (1977), Orme (1969), Parsons (1951), Piaget (1969), Ruesch and Kees (1972), Schilder (1951), Selye (1956), Shontz (1969), H.A. Simon (1957), Y.R. Simon (1962), Sommer (1969), von Bertalanffy (1956, 1968), Wapner and Werner (1965), Watzlawick, Beavin, and Jackson (1967), and Zald (1970). Moreover, King (1992a) revealed that the term transaction "came from a study of Dewey's theory of knowledge (Dewey & Bentley, 1949)" (p. 21).

King (1971, 1981) also acknowledged the influence of students, academic colleagues, nurse researchers, and practicing nurses on her thinking. During an interview conducted in the late 1980s, King (1988) highlighted the contributions to her thinking made by Kaufmann (1958), Orlando (1961), and Peplau (1952). King (1988) explained that Kaufmann's (1958) doctoral dissertation led her to explore the concepts of perception, time, and stress. She also noted that the research conducted at Yale University School of Nursing to test Orlando's (1961) theory of the deliberative nursing process influenced her thinking. King and Peplau (as cited in Takahashi, 1992) pointed out the connections between their works with regard to patient outcomes. Peplau commented, "When [King] talks about setting goals and I talk about beneficial outcomes for the patient in relation to the nurse's interventions in presenting phenomena, I think you have a very close connection" (p. 86). King responded by saying, "And I have to tell you all publicly that Dr. Peplau's [1952] work influenced my work" (p. 86).

Furthermore, King (1988) noted that a review of her 1971 book by Rosemary Ellis (1971) encouraged her to continue her work by deriving a theory from her Conceptual System. The result was the Theory of Goal Attainment.

Moreover, King (2001a) acknowledged the influence of the Howland Systems Model (Howland, 1976) and the Howland and McDowell conceptual framework (Howland & McDowell, 1964) on the development of her diagram of the interactions among the personal, interpersonal, and social systems concepts of her conceptual system. That diagram is displayed in Figure 5–1.

World View

King's Conceptual System reflects a *reciprocal interaction* world view. Particularly compelling is King's (1990b) philosophical allegiance to "a science of wholeness" (p. 74). Moreover, the focus of the Conceptual System on the personal, interpersonal, and social systems as wholes

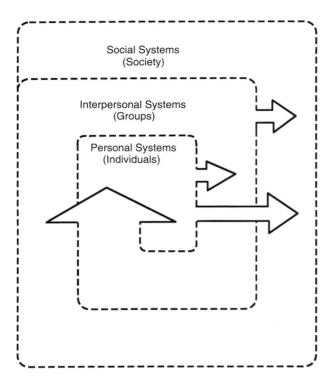

FIG. 5–1. A conceptual framework for nursing: dynamic interacting systems. (From King, I.M. (1981). A theory for nursing: Systems, concepts, process. New York: Wiley. [Reissued 1990. Albany, NY: Delmar, p. 11.] Reprinted with permission from Imogene M. King.)

indicates a holistic perspective. In keeping with the reciprocal interaction world view, King's Conceptual System emphasizes change. The features of the reciprocal interaction world view that are evident in King's Conceptual System are:

- The three interacting systems of King's Conceptual System—the personal system, the interpersonal system, and the social system—function as wholes (King, 1971, 1981, 1995a).
- [The focus is on] holism—that is, the total human being's interactions with another total human being in a specific situation (King, 1989a, p. 155).
- Human beings are active participants in interaction with one another (King, 1971, 1981, 1995a).
- Change is a central feature of King's Conceptual System. King's (1981) statement that health is a dynamic life experience implies continuous adjustment to environmental stressors. King's (1981) comment that normal changes in growth and development take place continu-

ously indicates that King views change as continuous, natural, and desirable.

UNIQUE FOCUS OF THE NURSING MODEL

The unique focus of King's Conceptual System is human beings (King, 1981). In particular, the Conceptual System focuses on human behavior, social interaction, and social movements (King, 1976). More specifically, the unique focus of King's Conceptual System is "human beings interacting with their environment" (King, 1989a, p. 150), or "individuals whose interactions in groups within social systems influence behavior within the systems" (King, 1989a, p. 152). Particular attention is given to the continuing ability of individuals to meet their basic needs so that they may function in their socially defined roles (King, 1971, 1981). Factors that contribute to problems in the individual's ability to function in social roles may be inferred to be stressors in the internal and external environment. Health is defined as "dynamic life experiences" of a human being, which implies continuous adjustment to stressors in the internal and external environment through optimum use of one's resources to achieve maximum potential for daily living (King, 1981, p. 5).

Category of Knowledge

Meleis (1997) classified King's Conceptual System as interaction focused, and Marriner-Tomey (1989) placed the Conceptual System in her interpersonal relationships category. Barnum (1998) did not place King's Conceptual System in any of the categories of her classification scheme. In an earlier edition of her book, she commented that King's work cannot be "categorized according to the classification of intervention, conservation, substitution, sustenance, and enhancement [because it] seems to desire interaction for its own sake rather than for the sake of a determined change (intervention), for conservation, for substitution, for sustenance, or for enhancement" (Stevens, 1984, p. 259).

King has maintained for many years that her Conceptual System is a derivative of systems thinking. She explained, "When I was studying systems research in the late 1960s, this movement in general [system] theory provided information for me to think about the complexities and variability in the field of nursing" (King, 1989a, p. 150). King (personal communication, May 12, 1980) also acknowledged the contributions of social psychology to her thinking, although she stated that she "never followed the symbolic interactionist school." Close examination of the content of the Conceptual System, however, revealed that characteristics of both the systems category and the interaction category of knowledge are evident, as can be seen here.

Systems Category of Knowledge

- System: "A system is defined as a set of elements connected by communication links that exhibits goal-directed behavior" (King, 1997a, p. 180). King's Conceptual System encompasses the personal, interpersonal, and social systems (King, 1971, 1981, 1995a).
- Integration of the Parts: The personal, interpersonal, and social systems are open, dynamic, and interacting (King, 1971, 1981, 1995a). The concepts associated with each system in no way represent parts or subsystems. Rather, they may be construed as global characteristics of the system.
- Environment: Environment is viewed as internal and external. The personal, interpersonal, and social systems interact with the environment and exchange matter, energy, and information (King, 1981). The interaction between open systems and the environment is dynamic: The nursing process is defined as a dynamic, ongoing interpersonal process in which the nurse and the patient are viewed as a system with each affecting the behavior of the other and both being affected by factors within the situation (Daubenmire & King, 1973, p. 513).
- Boundary: "Open systems, such as man interacting with the environment, exhibit permeable boundaries permitting an exchange of matter, energy, and information" (King, 1981, p. 69). "The structure of the theory [of goal attainment] indicates some semipermeable boundaries of two or more individuals interacting in a health-care system for a purpose that leads to goal attainment" (King, 1989a, p. 155). The "artificial boundaries of nursing [are] individuals and groups interacting with the environment" (King, 1981, p. 1).
- Tension, Stress, Strain, Conflict: "When transactions are made, tension or stress is reduced in a situation" (King, 1981, p. 82).
- Steady State: Steady state is not explicitly addressed. King's (1981) statement that the dynamic life experience of health involves continuous adjustment to environmental stressors suggests that King would accept the idea of a steady state, rather than a fixed point equilibrium.
- Feedback: Feedback is such that "perception of the nurse leads to judgments and to action by the nurse. Simultaneously, the perception of the patient leads to judgments and then to actions by the patient. This is a continuous dynamic process rather than separate incidents in which the action of one person influences the perceptions of the other and vice versa" (King, 1971, p. 92).

Interaction Category of Knowledge

- Social Acts and Relationship: The social act of human interaction occurs in the relationship between nurse and patient.
- Perception: Perception is a dimension of the personal system, and is a central aspect of the process of human interaction.
- Communication: Communication is a dimension of the interpersonal system and is used to establish and maintain relationships between human beings, and nurses and patients communicate to establish mutual goals and decide on the means to achieve these goals (King, 1981).
- Role: Role is a dimension of the interpersonal system and is addressed in the definition of health as "an ability to function in social roles" (King, 1981, p. 143).
- Self-Concept: Self-concept is addressed through the concept of self, which is a dimension of the personal system. King's definition of self as "a composite of thoughts and feelings which constitute a person's awareness of his individual existence, his conception of who and what he is" (Jersild, 1952, as cited in King, 1981, p. 9) coincides with Heiss' (1981) definition of self-concept as "the individual's thoughts and feelings about himself" (p. 83), which Heiss (1981) explicitly identified as a part of symbolic interactionism.

CONTENT OF THE NURSING MODEL

Concepts

The metaparadigm concepts of human beings, environment, health, and nursing are reflected in the concepts of King's Conceptual System. Each conceptual model concept is classified here according to its metaparadigm forerunner.

The metaparadigm concept of human beings is represented by King's Conceptual System concepts of **PERSONAL SYSTEM, INTERPERSONAL SYSTEM**, and **SOCIAL SYSTEM**. Each of those concepts is multidimensional. The concept of **Personal System** has seven dimensions—**Perception, Self, Growth and Development, Body Image, Time, Personal Space**, and **Learning**.

The concept of **Interpersonal System** has six dimensions—**Interaction, Communication, Transaction, Role, Stress**, and **Coping**. The dimension of **Communication** has two subdimensions—*Verbal Communication* and *Nonverbal Communication*. The concept of **Social System** has six dimensions—**Organization, Authority, Power, Status, Decision Making**, and **Control**.

King (1989a) explained that the placement of the dimensions within the concepts of **Personal System, Interpersonal System**, and **Social System** required arbitrary decisions because the three systems are "so interrelated in the interactions of human beings with their environment" (p. 151). King (1995a) went on to explain that the "dimensions … represent knowledge essential for understanding the interactions between the three systems" (p. 18). Indeed, although the dimensions of "all three systems [are] interrelated when one observe[s] any concrete nursing situation, the purpose for placing these [dimensions] in [a particular] system was to facilitate learning about self as an individual and about interactions with other individuals" (King, 1992a, p. 20). Knowledge of perception, for example, "is essential for nurses to understand self and to understand other individuals… Knowledge of interaction is essential for nurses to understand a fundamental process for gathering information about human beings… [And] knowledge of organization is essential for nurses to understand the variety of social systems within which individuals grow and develop" (King, 1989a, pp. 152–153).

The metaparadigm concept of environment is represented by King's Conceptual System concepts of **INTERNAL ENVIRONMENT** and **EXTERNAL ENVIRONMENT**. Both concepts are unidimensional. The metaparadigm concept of health is represented by King's Conceptual System concepts of **HEALTH** and **ILLNESS**, both of which are unidimensional. The metaparadigm concept of nursing is represented by King's Conceptual System concept of **ACTION, REACTION, AND INTERACTION PROCESS**, which also is unidimensional.

Nonrelational Propositions

The definitions of the concepts of King's Conceptual System and their dimensions and subdimensions are listed here. Those constitutive definitions are the nonrelational propositions of this nursing model.

PERSONAL SYSTEM

- Personal systems … are individuals (King, 1986a, p. 80).
- [The personal system is] a unified, complex whole self who perceives, thinks, desires, imagines, decides, identifies goals, and selects means to achieve them (King, 1981, p. 27).
- Personal systems encompass both healthy and ill individuals (King, 1992b).

The concept of **Personal System** encompasses seven dimensions—Perception, Self, Growth and Development, Body Image, Time, Personal Space, and Learning (King, 1995a).

- **Perception:** [Perception is] a process of organizing, interpreting, and transforming information from sense data and memory. It is a process of human transactions with the environment. It gives meaning to one's experience, represents one's image of reality, and influences one's behavior (King, 1981, p. 24). Perception is defined as each person's representation of reality. It is an awareness of persons, objects, and events (King, 1981, p. 146). Perception involves the following elements: (1) import of energy from the environment organized by information, (2) transformation of energy, (3) processing of information, (4) storing of information, [and] (5) export of information in overt behaviors (King, 1981, p. 146). Perception varies from one individual to another because each human being has different backgrounds of knowledge, skills, abilities, needs, values, and goals (King, 1989a, p. 152).

- **Self:** The self is a composite of thoughts and feelings which constitute a person's awareness of his individual existence, his conception of who and what he is. A person's self is the sum total of all he can call his. The self includes, among other things, a system of ideas, attitudes, values, and commitments. The self is a person's total subjective environment. It is a distinct center of experience and significance. The self constitutes a person's inner world as distinguished from the outer world consisting of all other people and things. The self is the individual as known to the individual. It is that to which we refer when we say "I" (Jersild, 1952, as cited in King, 1981, pp. 9–10). Self [is defined as] a personal system synonymous with the terms I, me, and person. Self is a unified, complex whole person who perceives, thinks, desires, imagines, decides, identifies goals and selects means to achieve them (King, 1986b, p. 201).

- **Growth and Development:** Growth and development include cellular, molecular, and behavioral changes in human beings (King, 1981, p. 30). Growth and development are defined as continuous changes in individuals at the cellular, molecular, and behavioral levels of activities (King, 1986b, p. 201). Growth and development are a function of genetic endowment, meaningful and satisfying experiences, and an environment conducive to helping individuals move toward maturity (King, 1981, p. 31).

- **Body Image:** [Body image is] a person's perceptions of his own body, others' reactions to his appearance, and is a result of others' reactions to self (King, 1981, p. 33).

- **Time:** [Time is] the duration between the occurrence of one event and the occurrence of another event (King, 1981, p. 44). Time is a sequence of events moving onward to the future; a continuous flow of events in successive order that implies change; a past and a future (King, 1986b, p. 201). [Time gives] order to events and [is used] to determine duration based on perceptions of each person's experiences (King, 1981, p. 45).

- **Personal Space:** [Personal space refers to the space that] exists to the extent that it is perceived by each person

(King, 1981, p. 36). [Space is defined as] existing in all directions and is the same everywhere … [and] as the physical area called territory and by the behavior of individuals occupying space (King, 1981, pp. 37–38). Space is that element that exists in all directions and is the same everywhere… [It is] a physical area called territory, and is defined by the behavior of individuals occupying space such as gestures, postures, and visible boundaries erected to mark off personal space (King, 1986b, p. 201). Spatial arrangements communicate role, position, and interactions with others. Marking off an area [of the invisible boundaries of personal space] for self gives individuals a sense of security and identity (King, 1981, p. 37). Space orients a person to his or her environment (King, 1981, p. 37). Space is unique to an individual and [is] influenced by needs, past experiences, and culture (King, 1981, p. 37).

- **Learning:** Learning is a process of sensory perception, conceptualization, and critical thinking involving multiple experiences in which changes in concepts, skills, symbols, habits, and values can be evaluated in observable behaviors and inferred from behavioral manifestations (King, 1986a, p. 24). Learning is self-activity; no one can learn from another individual (Gulitz & King, 1988, p. 129). Learning is dynamic, goal oriented, and self regulating in that reinforcement and feedback influence inputs and outputs (Gulitz & King, 1988, p. 129).

King (1981) summarized the connections among the dimensions of the concept of **Personal System**, with the exception of learning, in this statement:

> An individual's perceptions of self, of body image, of time and space influence the way he or she responds to persons, objects, and events in his or her life. As individuals grow and develop through the life span, experiences with changes in structure and function of their bodies over time influence their perceptions of self. (p. 19)

INTERPERSONAL SYSTEM

- [The interpersonal system is composed of] two, three, or more individuals interacting in a given situation (King, 1976, p. 54).
- Interpersonal systems … are dyads, triads, [and] small and large groups (King, 1986a, p. 80).

In regard to the **Interpersonal System,** King (1990a) explained that "individuals increase consciousness and are open to interpersonal perceptions in the communications and interactions with persons and things in the environment. Individuals have the potential to make transactions that include goal setting, and choosing means to attain goals to maintain their health and function in roles" (p. 127).

The concept of **Interpersonal System** encompasses six dimensions—Interaction, Communication, Transaction, Role, Stress, and Coping (King, 1986a, 1987a). The dimension of Communication encompasses two subdimensions—Verbal Communication and Nonverbal Communication (King, 1995a).

- **Interaction:** Interaction is a process of perception and communication between person and person and person and environment, represented by verbal and nonverbal behaviors that are goal directed (King, 1981, p. 145). [Interactions are defined as] the acts of two or more persons in mutual presence (King, 1981, p. 85). Interactions can reveal how one person thinks and feels about another person, how each perceives the other and what the other does to him, what his expectations are of the other, and how each reacts to the actions of the other (King, 1981, p. 85). The process of interaction between two or more individuals represents a sequence of verbal and nonverbal behaviors that are goal directed (King, 1981, p. 60). The process of interaction consists of each person's simultaneous perceptions and judgments about the other in the interaction, the taking of some mental actions based on the judgments, and reacting to the other's perceptions. Interaction follows those mental processes, and this is followed in turn by transaction (King, 1971, 1981). In the interactive process, two individuals mutually identify goals and the means to achieve them. When they agree to the means to implement the goals, they move toward transactions. Transactions are defined as goal attainment (King, 1981, p. 61).

- **Communication:** [Communication is] the vehicle by which human relations are developed and maintained (King, 1981, p. 79). Communication is a process whereby information is given from one person to another either directly in face-to-face meetings or indirectly through telephone, television, or the written word (King, 1986b, p. 201). All behavior is communication (King, 1981, p. 80). All human activities that link person to person and person to environment are forms of communication (King, 1981, p. 79).

The dimension Communication encompasses two subdimensions—*Verbal Communication* and *Nonverbal Communication* (King, 1981).

- *Verbal Communication*: Verbal communication, which is both intrapersonal and interpersonal in nature, encompasses verbal signs and symbols, including spoken and written words, used by individuals to express their goals and values (King, 1981).
- *Nonverbal Communication*: Nonverbal communication, which is both intrapersonal and interpersonal in nature, encompasses nonverbal signs and symbols,

including gestures and touch, used by individuals to express their goals and values (King, 1981). Nonverbal communication is use of space and defense of space (King, 1981, p. 38).

- **Transaction**: [Transaction is defined as] a process of interaction in which human beings communicate with environment to achieve goals that are valued. Transactions are goal directed human behaviors (King, 1981, p. 82). Transaction is defined as observable behavior of human beings interacting with their environment that leads to goal attainment (King, 1986b, p. 201). Transactions are viewed as a flow of information from the environment through coding, transformation, and processing of sensory, linguistic, and neurophysiologic elements resulting in decision making that leads to human actions (King, 1997b, p. 20).
- **Role**: Role is a set of behaviors expected when occupying a position in a social system (King, 1981, p. 93). Role is a set of behaviors expected of persons occupying a position in a social system; rules that define rights and obligations in a position; [and] a relationship with one or more individuals interacting in specific situations for a purpose (King, 1986b, p. 201). Role is a relationship with one or more individuals interacting in specific situations for a purpose (King, 1981, p. 93). [Roles involve] rules or procedures [that] define [the] rights and obligations [of] a position in an organization (King, 1981, p. 93).
- **Stress**: Stress is a dynamic state whereby a human being interacts with the environment to maintain balance for growth, development, and performance, which involves an exchange of energy and information between the person and the environment for regulation and control of stressors (King, 1981, p. 98). Stress is viewed as negative and positive as well as constructive and destructive (King, 1981). Stress is reduced when transactions are made (King, 1981).
- **Coping**: An essential area of knowledge related to the interpersonal system (King, 1987a). [Coping refers to] coping with stress (King, 1992a, p. 21).

SOCIAL SYSTEM

- [A social system is] an organized boundary system of social roles, behaviors, and practices developed to maintain values and the mechanisms to regulate the practices and rules (King, 1981, p. 115).
- Social systems … are the groups that form to achieve specific purposes within society, such as the family, the school, the hospital, industry, [social organizations,] and the church (King, 1986a, p. 80, 1989a).
- Social systems describe units of analysis in a society in

which individuals form groups to carry on activities of daily living to maintain life and health and, hopefully, happiness (King, 1976, p. 54).

King (1992b) commented that the inclusion of the **Social System** in her Conceptual System "reminds us that a variety of [such] systems provide[s] the background for each person's growth, and development, etc., and health professionals assess situations on that basis" (p. 604).

The concept of **Social System** encompasses six dimensions—Organization, Authority, Power, Status, Decision Making, and Control (King, 1986a).

- **Organization**: An organization is composed of human beings with prescribed roles and positions who use resources to accomplish personal and organizational goals (King, 1981, p. 119).
- **Authority**: Authority is a transactional process characterized by active, reciprocal relations in which members' values, background, and perception play a role in defining, validating, and accepting the authority of individuals within an organization. One person influences another, and he recognizes, accepts, and complies with the authority of that person (King, 1981, p. 124).
- **Power**: The process whereby one or more persons influence other persons in a situation. Power defines a situation in a way that people will accept what is being done while they may not agree with it (King, 1981, p. 127).
- **Status**: The position of an individual in a group or a group in relation to other groups in an organization (King, 1981, p. 129). Status is ascribed or achieved (King, 1981).
- **Decision Making**: Decision making in organizations is a dynamic and systematic process by which goal-directed choice of perceived alternatives is made and acted on by individuals or groups to answer a question and attain a goal (King, 1981, p. 132).
- **Control**: A dimension of the concept of **Social System** (King, 1986a).

The linkages among the **Personal System, Interpersonal System**, and **Social System** are explicated in King's (1989a) statement that the focus of her Conceptual System is "on individuals whose interactions in groups within social systems influence behavior within the systems" (p. 152). The linkages are illustrated in Figure 5–1. The figure clearly depicts the three "open systems in a dynamic interacting framework" (King, 1981, p. 10).

INTERNAL ENVIRONMENT

- Not explicitly defined, but it can be inferred that the internal environment is a source of stressors and energy (King, 1981).

EXTERNAL ENVIRONMENT

- Not explicitly defined, but it can be inferred that the external environment is a source of stressors and continuous changes (King, 1981).

King (1981, 1995a) has used the terms environment, social environment, health-care environment, internal environment, and external environment. With regard to the **Internal Environment** and the **External Environment**, King (1981) maintained that "the internal environment of human beings transforms energy to enable them to adjust to continuous external environmental changes" (p. 5). Moreover, King (1990a) noted that "environment is a function of balance between internal and external interactions" (p. 127). In particular, "the performance of activities of daily living … depends on one's external and internal environments working in some type of harmony and balance" (p. 125). She went on to say "the social milieu is an environmental factor that influences health" (p. 125). She also has noted that the **Personal System, Interpersonal System,** and **Social System** "are elements in the total environment" (King, 1992a, p. 20). Furthermore, King (1995a) stated that her Conceptual System "describes environments within which human beings grow, develop, and perform daily activities" (p. 18).

HEALTH

- [Health is] dynamic life experiences of a human being, which implies continuous adjustment to stressors in the internal and external environment through optimum use of one's resources to achieve maximum potential for daily living (King, 1981, p. 5).
- A state of health is an ability to function in social roles (King, 1986b, p. 200).
- Health is functional ability (King, 1985b).
- [Health is] a function of persons interacting with the environment, symbolized by the equation, $H = f(P \leftrightarrow E)$ (King, 1990a, p. 127).
- [Health is] a dynamic state of an individual in which change is a constant and an ongoing process (King, 1989a, p. 152).
- [Health can be related to] individuals and their health, to groups and their health, and to society and health (King, 1989a, p. 155).
- Health encompasses eight characteristics—genetic, subjective, relative, dynamic, environmental, functional, cultural, and perceptual (King, 1990a, p. 127).

ILLNESS

- [Illness is] a deviation from normal, that is, an imbalance in a person's biologic structure or in his psychological make-up, or a conflict in a person's social relationships (King, 1981, p. 5).
- Illness or disability is a disturbance in the dynamic state of the individual (King 1989a).
- Disease is one kind of illness (King, 1981).

King did not use the term wellness, and although she did mention illness, she "rejects a linear continuum of wellness-illness" (King, 1989a, p. 152). Elaborating on that point, King (1990a) explained that her concept of health "has been published since 1971. At that time [I] mentioned a continuum, and the definition indicated it was a dynamic process. [I have] deleted the word continuum from [my] concept as it represents a linear concept" (p. 127). It seems that King also would regard a dichotomy of health and illness as a linear concept that is inconsistent with the general system orientation of her Conceptual System.

ACTION, REACTION, AND INTERACTION PROCESS

- [Nursing is] a process of action, reaction, and interaction whereby nurse and client share information about their perceptions in the nursing situation. Through purposeful communication, they identify special goals, problems, or concerns. They explore means to achieve a goal and agree to [the] means to [achieve] the goal. When clients participate in goal setting with professionals, they interact with nurses to move toward goal attainment in most situations (King, 1981, p. 2).

King (1976) views nursing as a helping profession that "provides a service to meet a social need" (p. 52). This service extends to the care of individuals and groups who are ill and hospitalized, those who have chronic diseases and require rehabilitation, and those who require guidance for the maintenance of health. The domain of nursing, then, "includes promotion of health, maintenance and restoration of health, care of the sick and injured, and care of the dying" (King, 1981, p. 4).

According to King (1976), nurses are important figures in health-care delivery. She viewed nurses as "partners with physicians, social workers, and allied health professionals in promoting health, in preventing disease, and in managing patient care. They cooperate with physicians, families, and others to coordinate plans of health care" (p. 52).

The person seeks help from the nurse when he or she cannot perform usual daily activities (Daubenmire & King, 1973). Accordingly, the **GOAL OF NURSING** "is to help individuals maintain their health so they can function in their roles" (King, 1981, pp. 3–4). A related goal of nursing "is to help individuals and groups attain, maintain, and restore health" (King, 1981, p. 13; 1995a, p. 20). Another closely related goal is to help "individuals, families, groups, and communities maintain health" (King, 1997b, p. 21). King went on to say that if health is not possible, "nurses help individuals die with dignity" (King, 1981, p. 13). The various statements about the **Goal of Nursing** can be integrated into this statement:

> The goal of nursing is to help individuals, families, groups, and communities attain, maintain, and restore health, so that they can function in their respective roles, and to help individuals die with dignity.

King referred to the nursing process as an **INTERACTION-TRANSACTION PROCESS**. In particular, she labeled the nursing process an "interaction-transaction process model" (King, 1989a, p. 153), a "transaction model" (King, 1989a, p. 157), and a "transaction process" (King, 1997a, p. 181). This model, which is the **PRACTICE METHODOLOGY** for King's Conceptual System, is elaborated through the **Theory of Goal Attainment.** King (1992b) explained that the theory "has identified an interaction process that leads to transactions and then to goal attainment (p. 604). The components of the **Interaction-Transaction Process** (King, 1981, 1990b, 1992a, 1997a) are identified and described in Table 5–1 and depicted in Figure 5–2.

The **Interaction-Transaction Process** is "a dynamic, on-

▶ TABLE 5–1
KING'S PRACTICE METHODOLOGY: THE INTERACTION-TRANSACTION PROCESS

PERCEPTION

One aspect of the assessment phase of the interaction-transaction process.

The nurse and the client meet in some nursing situation and perceive each other.

Accuracy of perception will depend upon verifying [the nurse's] inferences with the client (King, 1981, p. 146).

The nurse can use the Goal-Oriented Nursing Record (GONR) to record perceptions (see Table 5–2 on p. 110).

JUDGMENT

Another aspect of the assessment phase of the interaction-transaction process.

The nurse and the client make mental judgments about the other.

The nurse can use the GONR to record judgments.

ACTION

Another aspect of the assessment phase of the interaction-transaction process.

Action is a sequence of behaviors of interacting persons, which includes (1) recognition of presenting conditions; (2) operatives or activities related to the condition or situation; and (3) motivation to exert some control over the events to achieve goals (King, 1971, pp. 90–91).

The nurse and the client take some mental action.

The nurse can use the GONR to record mental actions.

REACTION

Another aspect of the assessment phase of the interaction-transaction process.

The nurse and the client mentally react to each one's perceptions of the other.

The nurse can use the GONR to record mental reactions.

DISTURBANCE

The diagnosis phase of the interaction-transaction process.

The nurse and the client communicate and interact, and the nurse identifies the client's concerns, problems, and disturbances in health.

The nurse conducts a nursing history to determine the client's activities of daily living, using the Criterion-Referenced Measure of Goal Attainment Tool (CRMGAT) (see Table 5–2 on p. 110); roles; environmental stressors; perceptions; and values, learning needs, and goals. The nurse records the data from the nursing history on the GONR.

The nurse records the medical history and physical examination data, results of laboratory tests and radiographic examination, and information gathered from other health professionals and the client's family members on the GONR.

The nurse records diagnoses on the GONR.

MUTUAL GOAL SETTING

One aspect of the planning phase of the interaction-transaction process.

The nurse and the client interact purposefully to set mutually agreed on goals.

The nurse interacts with family members if the client cannot verbally participate in goal setting.

Mutual goal setting is based on the nurse's assessment of the client's concerns, problems, and disturbances in health; the nurse's and client's perceptions of the interference; and the nurse's sharing of information with the client and his/her family to help the client attain the goals identified.

Mutual goal setting includes consideration of the ethical aspects of the situation, including:

- Helping the client and family to sort out the values inherent in the situation and encouraging them to think through their own value system and the consequences of action they decide to take in the situation
- Helping the client and family to make decisions that take their value system into consideration by providing information that contributes to their decision, by emphasizing their reality as they have expressed it, and by not making decisions for them
- Becoming skillful in identifying options in every nursing situation and exploring those options with the client and family
- Identifying those elements in the situation that can be changed and controlled and those that cannot, and concentrating energy and efforts on control and change
- Being especially sensitive to the ethical issues that may arise when considering the right to life, the right to die, and the right to information required for informed choice

The nurse records the goals on the GONR.

EXPLORATION OF MEANS TO ACHIEVE GOALS

Another aspect of the planning phase of the interaction-transaction process.

The nurse and the client interact purposefully to explore the means to achieve the mutually set goals.

AGREEMENT ON MEANS TO ACHIEVE GOALS

Another aspect of the planning phase of the interaction-transaction process.

The nurse and the client interact purposefully to agree on the means to achieve the mutually set goals.

The nurse records the nursing orders with regard to the means to achieve goals on the GONR.

TRANSACTION

The implementation phase of the interaction-transaction process.

[Transaction refers to] the valuational components of the interaction (King, 1990a, p. 128).

The nurse and the client carry out the measures agreed upon to achieve the mutually set goals.

The nurse can use the GONR flow sheet and progress notes to record the implementation of measures used to achieve goals.

ATTAINMENT OF GOALS

The evaluation phase of the interaction-transaction process.

The nurse and the client identify the outcome of the interaction-transaction process. The outcome is expressed in terms of the client's state of health, or ability to function in social roles.

The nurse and the client make a decision with regard to whether the goal was attained and, if necessary, determine why the goal was not attained.

The nurse can use the CRMGAT to record the outcome and the GONR to record the discharge summary.

Constructed from King, 1981, pp. 59–63, 144–149, 164–176; 1985b; 1986b, p. 200; 1989b; 1992a, p. 22; 1995b; 1997a, p. 182; 1999, pp. 295–296.

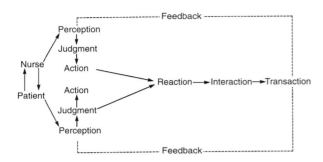

FIG. 5–2. King's model of the nursing process. (From King, I.M. (1981). A theory for nursing: Systems, concepts, process. New York: Wiley. [Reissued 1990. Albany, NY: Delmar, p. 145.] Reprinted with permission from Imogene M. King.)

going interpersonal process in which the nurse and the patient are viewed as a system with each affecting the behavior of the other and both being affected by factors within the situation" (Daubenmire & King, 1973, p. 513). The two arrows connecting the nurse and the patient seen in Figure 5–2 signify a dynamic, interactive process, rather than a linear process. King (1971) explained, "Perception of the nurse leads to judgments and to action by the nurse. Simultaneously, the perception of the patient lead to judgments and then to action by the patient. This is a continuous dynamic process rather than separate incidents in which the action of one person influences the perception of the other and vice versa" (p. 92)

King (2001a) referred to the generic nursing process of assessment, diagnosis, planning, intervention, and evaluation as "a method" (p. 280). She explained that the **Interaction-Transaction Process** "provides the theoretical knowledge base to implement [that] method" (p. 280).

In likening the **Interaction-Transaction Process** to all human processes, King (1976) pointed out that "the nursing act [is] as all other human acts, that is, a sequence of behaviors of interacting persons that occur in the following three phases: recognition of presenting conditions, operations or activities related to the conditions or situations, and motivation to exert some control over the events to achieve goals" (p. 54).

King (1981) initially noted that the perceptions, judgments, actions, and reactions of the individuals engaged in the **Interaction-Transaction Process** cannot be directly observed, but must be inferred from the directly observable interaction. Elaborating, she stated, "First, the informational component of interactions can be observed as communication. Second, the valuational component of interactions can be observed as transaction because one

obviously values a goal, identifies means to achieve it, and takes action to attain it" (p. 62). In later publications, however, King noted that inferences must be made about each person's perceptions and mental judgments, whereas all of the other behaviors encompassed by the **Interaction-Transaction Process** are directly observable in concrete situations in nursing practice" (King, 1992a, p. 22; 1996, p. 62).

Relational Propositions

The relational propositions of King's Conceptual System are listed here. Relational proposition A links the metaparadigm concepts human beings and environment. The metaparadigm concepts human beings, environment, and nursing are linked in relational proposition B. Relational proposition C links the metaparadigm concepts human beings, health, and nursing. All four metaparadigm concepts are linked in relational proposition D.

A. In open systems, such as human beings interacting with their environments, there is continuous and dynamic communication occurring (King, 1981, p. 66).
B. The artificial boundaries of nursing are individuals and groups interacting with the environment. Nurses function in their roles in a variety of health-care environments (King, 1981, p. 1).
C. As professionals, nurses deal with the behavior of individuals and groups in potentially stressful situations relative to health and illness and help people meet needs that are basic in performing activities of daily living (King 1976, p. 51).
D. The focus of nursing is human beings interacting with their environment leading to a state of health for individuals, which is an ability to function in social roles (King, 1981, p. 143).

 ### EVALUATION OF KING'S CONCEPTUAL SYSTEM

This section presents an evaluation of King's Conceptual System. The evaluation is based on the results of the analysis of the Conceptual System, as well as on publications and presentations by King and others who have used or commented on King's work.

EXPLICATION OF ORIGINS

King articulated the origins of her Conceptual System and the Theory of Goal Attainment clearly and concisely. She outlined the development of the Conceptual System and theory over time and indicated her motivation for the work. Furthermore, she explicated the philosophical claims undergirding the Conceptual System and theory in the form of assumptions about open systems, human beings, and nurse-client interactions; beliefs about nursing; and propositions about nursing.

The philosophical claims indicate that King values the client's participation in nursing. They also indicate that King values the client's right to accept or reject the services offered by nurses and other health-care professionals.

King's presentation of the **Interaction-Transaction Process** (see Table 5–1) indicates that she values equally the nurse's and the client's perceptions of any given situation. In addition, King (1999) has introduced the need for consideration of ethical issues, including understanding of the client's and family's value system, in the mutual goal-setting component of the **Interaction-Transaction Process.** Furthermore, a central feature of the **Interaction-Transaction Process** is the participation of both nurse and client in goal setting and determining the means to achieve the goals.

King explicitly acknowledged the influence of other scholars on her thinking and provided extensive bibliographic citations of relevant works. In addition, she underscored the influence of general system theory on the development of her Conceptual System and theory.

COMPREHENSIVENESS OF CONTENT

King's Conceptual System is sufficiently comprehensive regarding depth of content, although some inconsistencies are evident and some points require clarification. King provided a comprehensive discussion of the metaparadigm concept of person. Indeed, her descriptions of the dimensions of the concepts of **Personal System, Interpersonal System**, and **Social System** provide more specification of individuals, groups, and society than usually is found in a conceptual model.

An inconsistency evident in King's discussion of human beings is the designation of the human being as a client in most of her writings and the designation of the human being as a patient in others. Moreover, in some instances, she refers to the human being as a client and as a patient in the same paper (e.g., King, 1990b, 1999). In addition, definitions of the Coping dimension of the concept of **Interpersonal System** and the Control dimension of the concept of **Social System** are needed to enhance the clarity of King's Conceptual System.

In contrast to the comprehensive consideration of human beings, King's discussion of the concepts of **Internal Environment** and **External Environment** is vague. She did not define either concept, nor did she identify any

parameters. Although King (personal communication to R. Martone, July 25, 1989) claimed that her concept of **Social System** "explains environments and internal [environment] is explained in [the] communication concept," further explication of the concepts of **Internal Environment** and **External Environment** would provide clarification.

Health was clearly defined in King's Conceptual System. King revealed that she rejected the idea of health as a continuum of wellness to illness because that is a linear notion. Using the same reasoning, it may be inferred that she also rejects the idea of health as a dichotomy of wellness and illness. That inference, however, requires explicit commentary by King. King defined **Illness** and related that concept to the concept of **Health** by indicating that disturbances in the dynamic state that is health are regarded as illness or disability.

King defined and described nursing in a comprehensive manner and clearly identified the **Goal of Nursing.** Moreover, over the years, King has reinforced the one-to-one correspondence between her Theory of Goal Attainment and the **Interaction-Transaction Process.**

Furthermore, King defined and described the components of the **Interaction-Transaction Process** and has related those components to the steps of the generic nursing process (Yura & Walsh, 1983). There is, however, an inconsistency in her publications with regard to whether **Action** and **Reaction** are observable components of the process (King, 1981, 1992a, 1996). In addition, it is unclear whether the **Interaction-Transaction Process** can be used not only with individuals but also with groups and social organizations, and if so, how that might be accomplished. King (1983a, 1983b, 1983c) extended the nursing process to families, although explicit use of the **Interaction-Transaction Process** was not evident in the examples given. Indeed, King's extension of the nursing process to families contradicts her emphasis on the individual, as is evident in the following statement: "Although the primary point of interest in the [Theory of Goal Attainment] relates to interpersonal systems of an individual in the role of caregiver and an individual in the role of recipient of care, the goals to be attained relate to the individual receiving care" (King, 1989a, p. 155).

King deliberately related the concepts making up her Conceptual System to theoretical and empirical literature about human behavior. That is especially obvious in the strong scientific knowledge base used to describe each dimension of the concepts of **Personal System, Interpersonal System**, and **Social System.** Moreover, King underscored the need for an extensive base of knowledge on which to base judgments regarding nursing diagnoses and goals. She emphatically stated, "Judgments made by nurses will be influenced by their knowledge of the physical, psychological, and social components of man, by their system of values, and by their selected perceptions in the nursing situation" (King, 1971, p. 92). In particular, interaction is based on the perceptions, judgments, mental actions, and mental re-actions of the nurse and the client engaged in a nursing situation. Furthermore, the database requires collection of considerable information about the person for the identification of nursing diagnoses and goals.

King (1971) conceptualized human interaction as a dynamic process. She explained, "Perception of the nurse leads to judgments and to action by the nurse. Simultaneously, the perception of the patient leads to judgments and then to action by the patient. This is a continuous dynamic process rather than separate incidents in which the action of one person influences the perceptions of the other and vice versa" (p. 92).

Furthermore, the Goal-Oriented Nursing Record (GONR) suggests a dynamic nursing process inasmuch as that documentation tool fosters continual monitoring of changes in the status of nursing diagnoses and recording of the client's current health status, as well as frequent revisions in the nursing diagnoses and goal list on the basis of outcomes of nursing care (see Table 5–2, p. 110).

King's concern for ethical standards of nursing practice is evident in her insistence on consideration of the client's perception of a situation and explication of the client's and family's value system. Her concern for ethical standards also is evident in her insistence that the client or a designee participate in goal setting and identification of the means to attain the goals.

The relational propositions of King's Conceptual System link the metaparadigm concepts. Statements were located that link human beings and environment; human beings, the environment, and nursing; human beings, health, and nursing; and human beings, the environment, health, and nursing.

King's Conceptual System is sufficiently comprehensive in breadth of content. King has specified a relatively broad goal for nursing that focuses on the health of individuals, groups, and society. She has claimed that her concept of **Health** "includes health promotion, health maintenance, and regaining health when there is some interference along the life cycle—for example, an illness" (King, 1995b, p. 25). In addition, King (1981) maintained that "nurses play strategic roles in the process of human growth and development and in helping individuals cope with disturbances in their health. They have an essential role in community planning for the delivery of health services to the public. As professionals, nurses deal with behavior of individuals and groups in potentially stressful situations pertaining to health, illness, and crises [including death], and help people cope with changes in daily activities" (p. 13).

King's Conceptual System provides direction for nursing research, education, administration, and practice. Many guidelines can be extracted from King's publications about the Conceptual System. The guidelines for research, nursing education, administration of nursing services, and nursing practice are listed below.

Nursing Research Guidelines

The guidelines for nursing research based on King's Conceptual System, which were constructed from Byers (1985), Fawcett (2001, p. 314), and King (1968, 1971, 1981, 1989a), are:

- Purpose of the research
  - The ultimate purpose of King's Conceptual System-based research is to determine the effects of mutual goal setting and implementation of the nursing interventions related to goal attainment.

- Phenomena of interest
  - The phenomena of interest are transactions and health.
  - [Transaction is] a critical dependent variable in nurse-client interactions that lead to goal attainment (King, 1986b, p. 202).
  - Health—the ability to function in social roles—is an outcome variable (King, 1986b, p. 200).
  - Other phenomena are the set of variables that are predictors of nurse behaviors, including the nurse's education and experience, which can be used to predict effectiveness of nursing care.
  - Still other phenomena are the set of variables that influence the whole complex of behaviors entering the nursing process, such as patient perceptions and expectations, as well as the structure of the health-care organization.
  - Additional phenomena are the set of variables that focus on situational behaviors related to nurse-patient interaction, including communication and interpersonal relationships.
  - Other phenomena are the set of variables that encompass criteria of effectiveness of nursing care, such as the client's performance of activities of daily living and knowledge about health maintenance.

- Problems to be studied
  - The precise problems to be studied are actual or potential disturbances in the client's ability to function in social roles.

- Study participants
  - Study participants include individuals; dyads, triads, and other groups; and families, social organizations, and health-care systems.

- Research methods
  - Research designs may be qualitative or quantitative. The method used must relate to the problem to be studied.
  - The objective of qualitative, descriptive studies would be to gather information that is not already available. The qualitative methodology selected must adhere to the problem to be studied and the basic philosophic claims undergirding the Conceptual System and Theory of Goal Attainment.
  - Quantitative experimental studies measuring goal attainment can view goal attainment as a dichotomy—the goal is attained or not attained; can use the Criterion-Referenced Measure of Goal Attainment Tool, which yields ordinal scores; or can adapt the technique of goal attainment scaling developed in psychology.
  - Data may be collected using instruments derived from King's Conceptual System (see Table 5–2 on page 110).
  - Data may be gathered in health-care systems within society, the home of the individual, a school, an industry or a business, or another social setting.

- Data analysis
  - Definitive guidelines for data analysis remain to be developed.

- Contributions
  - King's Conceptual System-based research findings enhance understanding of factors that affect health as the ability to function in social roles.

Nursing Education Guidelines

The guidelines for nursing education based on King's Conceptual System, which were constructed from Daubenmire (1989, pp. 167–168), Fawcett (2001, pp. 313–314), and King (1986a, 1989a), are:

- Focus of the curriculum
  - The focus of a King's Conceptual System-based nursing education program is the dynamic interaction of the nurse-client dyad health.
  - The purposes of education are to facilitate the intellectual, emotional, and social growth of human beings; prepare individuals to be useful, productive, and relatively happy citizens; to prepare people to become professional practitioners and to assist them to acquire knowledge in the practice of nursing; and to provide a curriculum, a climate for lifelong learning, and resources whereby students acquire values, knowledge, and skills used in practicing theory-based nursing.
  - The ultimate goal of education is the pursuit and dissemination of truth.

- Education should demonstrate a balance between freedom and individual responsibility.
- Emphasis is placed on nursing student behavior, as well as client behavior.

- Nature and sequence of content
  - The content of a King's Conceptual System-based curriculum encompasses knowledge about and psychomotor skills related to the dimensions of the concepts of Personal System, Interpersonal System, and Social System.
  - Prerequisites to the nursing major encompass courses in the behavioral and biophysical sciences and the humanities. Courses in the behavioral sciences include sociology, psychology, anthropology, political science, and economics. Courses in the biophysical sciences include physics, biology, anatomy, physiology, biochemistry, microbiology, and immunology. Humanities courses include English, with an emphasis on communication; art and music appreciation; philosophy, including logic; and history.
  - The sequence of content emphasizes expansion of knowledge of individuals regarding each dimension of the personal, interpersonal, and social systems, and then knowledge about families and health-care systems.
  - The curriculum should include a sequence of related theory and practicum courses. The practicum courses that accompany the theory courses provide selected experiences for students to use the knowledge beginning with experiences with relatively healthy human beings, such as well-child clinics, children in the school system, and adults in industry and business. Then the knowledge can be used in experiences with individuals who have an interference in their ability to function in their usual roles and enter a health-care system for assistance.

- Settings for nursing education
  - Nursing education can occur in hospital-based diploma programs; in formal degree-granting programs in community colleges, senior colleges, or universities; and in continuing education programs.
  - Preparation for entry into professional nursing, however, should take place in universities in postbaccalaureate Doctor of Nursing (ND) programs.

- Characteristics of students
  - Students must meet the requirements for admission to a particular program.
  - Students must have the ability to acquire intellectual skills, interpersonal skills, and technical skills.
  - Students must be able to be active participants in their educational experiences and learn how to think, make

decisions, and act consistently and reasonably as members of a profession and a democratic society.

- Teaching-learning strategies
  - Teaching-learning strategies should be directed toward providing a climate conducive to individual growth and freedom to inquire into the nature of the environment.
  - Learning experiences should move the student from looking at the state of health to disturbances in the state of health, and back to health.
  - Specific strategies include lecture and discussion; group discussion; role playing; demonstrations of interviewing techniques, participant and nonparticipant observation techniques, and structured observations; and individual and group conferences between students and teachers.

Administration of Nursing Services Guidelines

Guidelines for the administration of nursing services based on King's Conceptual System, which were constructed from King (1986a, 1989b), are:

- Focus of nursing in the health-care institution
  - The distinct focus of King's Conceptual System-based nursing services in health-care organizations is the nurse and the client interacting for the purpose of mutual goal setting and goal attainment.

- Purpose of nursing services
  - The purpose of nursing services is to help clients attain their goals.

- Characteristics of nursing personnel
  - Nursing personnel include both technical and professional nurses, whose functions are clearly differentiated.
    - Technical nurses are prepared in associate degree programs and provide general nursing with supervision from professional nurses.
    - Professional nurses are prepared in postbaccalaureate Doctor of Nursing (ND) degree programs and are able to supervise and manage nursing practice, observe behaviors in the form of reactions and symptoms of disease and illness, record and report facts about clients and evaluate the total situation, implement nursing goals, direct nursing with individuals and groups, provide for essential health education to help them maintain their health, supervise nursing personnel, and implement physician's orders for treatments and medications based on nursing knowledge and understanding.

- Settings for nursing services
  - Nursing services are located in many different settings, including acute and chronic care facilities and ambulatory clinics.

- Management strategies and administrative policies
  - Nurse administrators restructure job descriptions to reflect differentiation in roles and functions of all nursing personnel and change the organizational chart to clearly show the lines of communication and responsibility for each level of nursing personnel.
  - Nursing personnel who are affected by any changes in the organizational structure are encouraged by nurse administrators to participate in decision making about the changes in the job descriptions and the organizational chart.
  - Nurse administrators recommend the use of the GONR to document nursing care and to measure the effectiveness of that care.

Nursing Practice Guidelines

Guidelines for nursing practice based on King's Conceptual System, which were constructed from Fawcett (2001, p. 314) and King (1981, p. 2; 1986b, 1989a), are:

- Purpose of nursing practice
  - The purpose of King's Conceptual System-based nursing practice is to perceive, think, relate, judge, and act vis-à-vis the behavior of individuals who come to a nursing situation.
  - More specifically, the purpose of nursing practice is to help individuals attain and maintain their health, and if there is some disturbance such as illness or disability, nurses' actions are goal directed to help individuals regain health or live with a chronic illness or a disability.

- Practice problems of interest
  - Practice problems encompass the client's activities of daily living related to the performance of social roles.

- Settings for nursing practice
  - A nursing situation is the immediate environment, the spatial and temporal reality, in which nurse and client establish a relationship to cope with health states and adjust to changes in activities of daily living if the situation demands adjustment.
  - Nursing practice can occur in acute and chronic care settings, as well as those appropriate to delivery of care for the maintenance of health.
  - Opportunities for health promotion exist wherever people are in their communities, regardless of their age and health state.

- Characteristics of legitimate participants in nursing practice
  - Legitimate participants in nursing are people who can actively participate in decisions that influence their care, as well as clients who have family members with whom nurses can make transactions until the clients can participate.

- Nursing process
  - The nursing process for King's Conceptual System is King's **Interaction-Transaction Process.** The components of that process are perception, judgment, action, reaction, disturbance, mutual goal setting, exploration of means to achieve goals, agreement on means to achieve goals, transaction, and attainment of goals (see Table 5–1).

- Contributions of nursing practice to participants' well-being
  - King's Conceptual System-based nursing practice contributes to the well-being of clients by enhancing their abilities to function in the activities of daily living associated with their social roles.

LOGICAL CONGRUENCE

King's Conceptual System is generally logically congruent. The content of the Conceptual System follows logically from King's philosophical claims. Despite the use of terms such as action and reaction, the Conceptual System does not reflect the reaction world view. King (1981) effectively translated those terms to conform to the reciprocal interaction world view by describing the process of interaction as a dynamic "sequence of verbal and nonverbal behaviors that are goal-directed" in which both individuals participate (p. 60). Perhaps it was the terms action and reaction that led Magan (1987) to regard the Conceptual System as mechanistic and consistent with the totality paradigm. But Parse's (1987) description of the totality paradigm suggests that it actually is a bridge between the mechanistic elements of the reaction world view and the organismic, holistic elements of the reciprocal interaction world view. Furthermore, although King cited Freud's and Selye's essentially reactive views of human beings, she provided definitions of growth and development and stress that depict human beings as active. Confusion about this element of logical congruence could be overcome if King replaced the references to Freud and Selye with those that reflect a transactional view.

King's Conceptual System reflects the characteristics of both the systems and interaction categories of nursing knowledge, but there is no evidence of logical incompatibility. The development of a Conceptual System combining all of those characteristics was accomplished by using an open-systems approach along with a perspective of active participation of individuals in human interactions. In effect, the characteristics of the interaction approach represent the dimensions of the concepts **Personal System, Interpersonal System,** and **Social System.**

GENERATION OF THEORY

Several explicit middle-range theories, including the **Theory of Goal Attainment,** have been directly derived from King's Conceptual System. Those middle-range theories are:

- Theory of Goal Attainment (King, 1981, 1995b, 1997a)
- Theory of Nursing Administration (King, 1989b)
- Theory of Departmental Power (Sieloff, 1995)
  - Retitled Theory of Group Power (Frey, Sieloff, & Norris, 2002)
- Theory of Families, Children, and Chronic Illness (Frey, 1989, 1995)
  - Also called the Theory of Social Support and Health (Alligood, 1997, 2001)
- Theory of Family Health (Wicks, 1995, 1997)
- Theory of Family Health (Doornbos, 1995, 2000)
- Theory of Intrapersonal Perceptual Awareness (Brooks & Thomas, 1997)
  - Also called the Theory of Perceptual Awareness (Alligood, 2001)
- Theory of Basic Empathy, Self-Awareness, and Learning Styles (May, 2000)
- Theory of Personal System Empathy (Alligood & May, 2000)
- Theory of Decision Making (Ehrenberger, 2000; Ehrenberger et al., 2002)
- Theory of Interaction Enhancement (Meighan, 2000)
- Theory of Asynchronous Development (Du Mont, 1998)
- Theory of Health and Social Support (Fries, 1998).

The **Theory of Goal Attainment** serves as the basis of King's **Interaction-Transaction Process** (see Table 5–1) (King, 1986b, pp. 203, 206; 1990b, pp. 81–82; 1997a, pp. 181, 184). The concepts of the theory are: Perception, Communication, Interaction, Transaction, Self, Role, Growth and Development, Stress/Stressors, Coping, Time, and Personal Space. The concept definitions are the same as the corresponding concepts of King's Conceptual System (see Analysis section of this chapter.). The relational propositions of the theory are:

- If perceptual accuracy is present in nurse-client interactions, transactions will occur.

- If nurse and client make transactions, goals will be attained.
- If goals are attained, effective nursing care will occur.
- If transactions are made in nurse-client interactions, growth and development will be enhanced for both.
- If nurses with special knowledge and skills communicate appropriate information to clients, mutual goal setting will occur.
- When mutual goals have been identified, means have been explored, and nurse and client agree on means to achieve goals, transactions will be made and goals achieved.
- If role expectations and role performance as perceived by nurse and client are congruent, transactions will occur.
- If role conflict is experienced by nurse, client, or both, stress in nurse-client interactions will occur.
- Accurate perception of time and space dimensions in nurse-client interactions leads to transactions.
- Knowledge of one's concept of self will help bring about a helping relationship with clients.
- King's Law of Nurse-Patient Interaction: Nurses and patients in mutual presence, interacting purposefully, make transactions in nursing situations based on each individual's perceptions, purposeful communication, and valued goals.

The hypotheses of the theory are:

- Functional abilities will be greater in patients who participate in mutual goal setting than in those who do not participate.
- Mutual goal setting will increase functional abilities in performance of activities of daily living.
- Goal attainment will be greater in patients who participate in mutual goal setting than in patients who do not participate.
- There is a positive relationship between functional abilities and goal attainment.
- Perceptual congruence in nurse-patient interactions increases mutual goal setting.
- Mutual goal setting will increase the morale of elderly patients.
- Mutual goal setting decreases stress in planning and implementing decisions about goals to be attained.
- Mutual goal setting increases transactions, which increases goal attainment, which leads to effective nursing care.
- Goal attainment in nursing situations leads to growth and development in nurse and client.
- Transactions increase nurses' and patients' self-awareness in goal attainment.
- Congruence in role expectations and role performance increases transactions in nurse-patient interactions.
- Accurate perceptions of time-space relations in nurse-

client interactions increase transactions and goal attainment.
- Goal attainment decreases stress and anxiety in nursing situations.
- Goal attainment increases patients' learning and coping abilities in nursing situations.

The amount of other middle-range theory development already accomplished is impressive. Noteworthy are scholars' efforts to derive theories that further specify the personal system, interpersonal system, or social system concepts of King's Conceptual System.

Fawcett and Whall (1995) pointed out that other works, which currently represent implicit middle-range theories, could easily be transformed into explicit theories by stating the concepts and propositions in a formal manner. Two examples they gave were the work on empathy by Alligood and colleagues (1995) and the work on intimate space, personal space, and social space by Rooke (1995a). In addition, Hobdell's (1995) report of her research included an explicit conceptual-theoretical-empirical structure that could serve as the basis for formal theory development.

Alligood and colleagues went on to formalize theories of empathy. Alligood and May (2000) developed the theory of personal system empathy, and May (2000) developed the theory of basic empathy, self-awareness, and learning styles. King (2001b) objected to Alligood and May's (2002) use of rational hermeneutic interpretation as the strategy for theory development, declaring, "They have taken my ideas out of context to fit their purpose and then attributed their ideas [about empathy] to me" (p. 81). Whelton (2001) also objected to the use of rational hermeneutic interpretation as the theory development strategy. She pointed out that because "empathy was within their tool of inquiry … they found empathy, but this is fallacious, circular reasoning. They began with what they wanted to find" (p. 82). Clearly, the value of rational hermeneutic interpretation as a strategy for development of theories of empathy within the context of King's Conceptual System requires much more dialogue.

CREDIBILITY OF THE NURSING MODEL

Social Utility

The social utility of King's Conceptual System and the Theory of Goal Attainment was highlighted by King's (1992a) statement that her Conceptual System and theory have been used "to generate hypotheses that have been tested, and some are being tested currently in research. … Moreover, [the Conceptual System and theory have] been used as a guide to help nurses organize the delivery of nursing services in hospitals and in the community. The concepts [and dimensions of the Conceptual System] have served as the knowledge base for using the nursing process of assessing, [diagnosing,] planning, implementing, and evaluating nursing care. The [conceptual system and theory have] helped teachers assist learners to organize a multitude of facts into meaningful wholes" (pp. 22–23). The social utility of King's Conceptual System and Theory of Goal Attainment are further documented by an entire book, which contains 21 chapters of extensions and tests of the Conceptual System and theory in nursing research, education, administration, and practice (Frey & Sieloff, 1995).

The knowledge required for application of King's Conceptual System and Theory of Goal Attainment comes from extensive study of the dimensions of the concepts of **Personal System, Interpersonal System**, and **Social System** through course work in nursing and adjunctive disciplines. King (1986a) identified several courses in the adjunctive disciplines as prerequisite to the nursing major (see Nursing Education Guidelines on pp. 105–106).

King (1986a) indicated that implementation of King's Conceptual System and Theory of Goal Attainment requires not only theoretical and empirical knowledge of the dimensions of the concepts **Personal System, Interpersonal System**, and **Social System**, but also the ability to use that knowledge with people of all ages, with a focus on their activities of daily living. In addition, use of the Conceptual System and theory requires the perceptual and psychomotor skills necessary to assess individuals' health states and the interpersonal and communication skills necessary to engage in mutual goal setting. Furthermore, the user of the Conceptual System and theory must learn to be sensitive to and accepting of the client's perception of what is happening. King (1992a) indicated that professional values also must be learned. Finally, King (1986a) identified four processes as essential nursing content that must be mastered in order to use the Conceptual System and theory—nursing process, teaching and learning processes, transaction process, and research process.

King (2001a) explained that the Conceptual System and theory are not applied directly. Rather, as she noted she has stated repetitively, "One cannot apply and abstraction, which is what conceptual frameworks, models, and theories represent. What one applies is the knowledge of the concepts of the structure and process proposed in the abstractions" (p. 281).

The many concepts that make up King's Conceptual System and Theory of Goal Attainment provide an extensive vocabulary. However, the concepts and their definitions were taken from well-known works. Thus, mastery of the vocabulary should not pose a major problem for potential users of the Conceptual System and theory.

Implementation of practice protocols derived from the knowledge of the content of King's Conceptual System and Theory of Goal Attainment certainly is feasible but, as with the implementation of any conceptual model or theory, requires considerable time and effort. Byrne-Coker and Schreiber (1990a, 1990b) identified several strategies that facilitate King's Conceptual System-based nursing practice in health-care organizations. One strategy is a 2-week orientation program that progresses from discussion of the **Personal System**, with emphasis on comparison of the new employee's values with those of the health-care organization, to the **Social System**, with emphasis on how the organization defines the role of the nurse, to the **Interpersonal System**, with emphasis on the nursing process. The orientation program concludes with a formal presentation of the Conceptual System. In addition, new nurses receive an exercise book "to help them practice applying the concepts in their clinical area" (Byrne-Coker & Schreiber, 1990b, p. 26).

Another strategy is 45-minute inservice education sessions offered on all shifts on all units to help continuing staff learn the content and processes of the Conceptual System and theory. Still another strategy is ongoing inservice education in the form of a "concept of the month." Byrne-Coker and Schreiber (1990a) explained that "each month, a concept [of the Conceptual System] was featured and information about the concept, taken from King's text, was posted. In addition, mini-discussions, 15 minutes each, highlighted the selected concept and encouraged nurses to begin thinking about it. Nurses thought about how the concept influenced their nursing care that particular month and were asked to write this on the perimeter of the poster" (p. 90).

Another strategy is to redesign existing nursing history and assessment forms, nursing diagnoses, patient teaching programs, and quality assurance programs so that they are consistent with King's Conceptual System. An additional strategy is to design computer software that is consistent with the Conceptual System and theory.

Finally, Byrne-Coker and Schreiber (1990a) drew attention to the need to use morale-boosting strategies during periods of waning enthusiasm for Conceptual System- and theory-based nursing. They cited the effectiveness of a visit to the health-care organization by King herself, as well as "Kingratulations" parties held at the completion of all the "concepts of the month."

Messmer (1992) described other strategies that make the implementation of King's Conceptual System and Theory of Goal Attainment feasible. She reported the effectiveness of case study presentations, a self-study module for staff nurses and newly employed nurses that carries 5 contact hours of continuing education credits, and "lunch and learn" inservice education sessions.

West (1991) described other strategies. She commented on the effectiveness of a video and "resources nurses" for each unit who helped their peer staff nurses to "internalize theory (as they understood it) and accept it as an every day part of nursing" (p. 29). In addition, a coordinator supervised the overall implementation process on all nursing units.

Clearly, the administrators of the health-care organization must be willing to underwrite the cost of such strategies, in terms of the required personnel time and materials. In addition, the nurses must be willing to expend the time and energy required to revise forms and implement changes.

Nursing Research. The utility of King's Conceptual System for nursing research is documented by the many studies that have been guided by this conceptual model of nursing. Instrument development research is listed in Table 5–2. Published reports of descriptive, correlational, and experimental studies are listed in Table 5–3. Published abstracts of doctoral dissertations and master's theses are listed in the Doctoral Dissertations and Master's Theses sections of the chapter bibliography on the CD-ROM.

(Text continues on page 114)

TABLE 5–2
RESEARCH INSTRUMENTS AND PRACTICE TOOLS DERIVED FROM KING'S CONCEPTUAL SYSTEM AND THEORY OF GOAL ATTAINMENT

Instrument and Citation[*]	Description
RESEARCH INSTRUMENTS	
Postpartum Satisfaction Inventory (PPSI) (Pfoutz, 1990)	Measures postpartum women's satisfaction with their maternity care
Killeen-King Patient Satisfaction with Nursing Care (KKPSNC) (Killeen, 1996)	Measures patient satisfaction with nursing care
Sieloff-King Assessment of Departmental Power (SKADP) (Sieloff, 1996); revised as the Sieloff-King Assessment of Group Power Within Organizations (Sieloff, personal communication, January 4, 1999)	Measures nursing's power within a hospital
PRACTICE TOOLS	
Criterion-Referenced Measure of Goal Attainment Tool (CRMGAT) (King, 1988; Young et al., 2001)	Used to assess, plan, and evaluate nursing in terms of the client's physical ability to perform activities of daily living (ADL), level of consciousness, hearing, vision, smell, taste, touch, speaking ability, listening ability, reading and writing abilities, nonverbal communication, and decision-making ability; response to the performance of ADL; and goals to be attained
Goal-Oriented Nursing Record (GONR) (King, 1981, 1984, 1989)	A documentation system used to record and evaluate the nurse's observations and actions and the client's responses to nursing. The GONR is composed of a database, nursing diagnoses, a goal list, nursing orders, flow sheets, progress notes, and a discharge summary
Assessment Format (Swindale, 1989)	Guides assessment of the minor surgery patient's anxieties, coping strategies, and nature of information needed
Nursing Process Tool (Norris & Frey, 2002)	Displays the relationship among the nursing process, critical thinking process, transaction process, and ethical decision-making process
Nursing Process Format for Families (Gonot, 1986)	Guides the use of a Theory of Goal Attainment-based nursing process for families
Family Needs Assessment Tool (Rawlins et al., 1990; Young et al., 2001)	Measures the special needs of the families of chronically ill children
Community Health Assessment (Hanchett, 1988)	Guides assessment of a community according to the dimensions of personal systems, interpersonal systems, and social systems

[*]See the Research Instruments and Practice Tools section of the chapter references for complete citations.

Research Topic	Study Participants	Citation[*]
DESCRIPTIVE STUDIES		
Process of scientific nursing knowledge development, epitomized through Imogene M. King's life and work	Imogene M. King King's family members, friends, and colleagues Correspondence Photographs Books and articles Videotape	Messmer, 1995
Power	Literature review	Hawks, 1991
Empathy	Literature review	Alligood et al., 1995
Theory of empathy derived from King's personal system	Hermeneutic interpretation of King's writings about the personal system concept in her Conceptual System	Alligood & May, 2000
Description of the image of nurses on Internet greeting cards	Greeting cards obtained from the Internet	Pierce et al., 2002
Perceptions of benefits of and barriers to use of oral contraceptives	Female adolescents	Hanna, 1994
Perceptions of the female domestic violence victim's experience in an emergency department	Women residing in a shelter for domestic violence victims	Mayer, 2000
Perceptions of living with chronic inflammatory bowel disease	Young adults	Daniel, 2002
Patients' satisfaction with their choice of walking or going by stretcher from a same-day surgery admitting area to the operating room	Adult surgical patients	Porteous & Tyndall, 1994
Types of space	Swedish nurses' written descriptions of critical situations related to the concept of space in a geriatric hospital	Rooke, 1995a
Nurses' interpretations of transaction, interaction, perception, and time	Swedish nurses' written descriptions of nursing situations	Rooke, 1995b
Nurses' self-esteem, gender identity, and personality characteristics	Members of the American Association of Critical Care Nurses	Levine et al., 1988
Nurses' perceptions of their competence and role expectations	Newly employed Norwegian nurses	Olsson & Forsdahl, 1996
Identification of the elements of transactions	Nurses Medical-surgical patients	King, 1981
Perceived needs of family members	Registered nurses working in neonatal or adult intensive care units Family members of patients in a neonatal or adult intensive care unit	Jacono et al., 1990
Description of interpersonal relationships with health professionals	Adults with hypertension who were not compliant with treatment	Moreira & Araújo, 2002
Identification of categories of nurse-patient interactions	Videotapes of nurses and surgical patients on high-dependency (intermediate or step-down) units	Rundell, 1991
Factors in nurse-patient interactions that interfere with transactions	Japanese nurses Orthopedic patients	Kusaka, 1991 Kameoka [nee Kusaka], 1995

[*]See the Research section of the chapter references for complete citations.

(continued)

Research Topic	Study Participants	Citation*
Perceptions of obesity	Medical and nursing students	Petrich, 2000
Perceptions of facial disfigurement	Staff nurses caring for male and female patients after surgery for head and neck cancer	Lockhart, 1999
Nurses' perceptions of the dimensions of nursing situations	Registered nurses	Houfek, 1992
Nurse-patient communication patterns	Videotapes of nurses' encounters with older patients residing in their own homes or in a home for older adults	Caris-Verhallen et al., 1998
Nurses' perceptions of their co-workers' responses to the nurses' attempts to quit smoking	Registered nurses	Kneeshaw, 1990
Categories of nurses' descriptions of problematic and meaningful nursing situations	Swedish nurses working on a geriatric ward	Rooke & Norberg, 1988
Differences in nurses' attitudes toward older persons	Registered nurses employed in visiting nurse associations, private home health agencies, nursing homes, and hospitals	Brower, 1981
Nursing diagnoses for mothers with a preterm infant in a neonatal intensive care unit	Staff nurses	Viera & Rossi, 2000
Classification of nursing diagnoses	Registered nurses	Byrne-Coker et al., 1990
Factors associated with clinical decision-making	Baccalaureate program senior nursing students	Brooks & Thomas, 1997
Attitudes and beliefs about organ donation and participation in an organ donation program	African-American individuals	Richard-Hughes, 1997
Clients' and family members' knowledge of common medical terms	Hospitalized surgical clients Family members	Spees, 1991
Parents' needs	Parents of critically ill hospitalized children	Scott, 1998
Use of coping strategies	Infertile women	Davis & Dearman, 1991

CORRELATIONAL STUDIES

Relation of adequacy of prenatal care to changes from pregnancy to postpartum depression, family functioning, social support, functional status, and life events	Low-income pregnant and postpartal women	Schiffman et al., 1995
Relations among menopausal stage, current life change, attitude toward women's roles, menopausal symptoms, use of hormone therapy, socioeconomic status, and perceived health status	Women 40 to 55 years of age	Sharts Engel, 1984, 1987; Sharts-Hopko, 1995
Relation of uncertainty, role, functioning, and social support to emotional health (hope and mood state) and relation of emotional health (hope and mood state) to treatment decision	Adult women with cancer eligible for a cancer clinical trial	Ehrenberger et al., 2002
Relation of social support and anomia to self-reported health	Older nursing home residents	Zurakowski, 2000
Relation between chronic sorrow and accuracy of parental perception of the child's cognitive development	Parents of children with a neural tube defect	Hobdell, 1995

Relation of exercise to severity of illness and current mood	Cardiac rehabilitation program clients	McGirr et al., 1990
Relations among general health behavior, illness management behavior, health status, and illness outcome	Children with diabetes or asthma	Frey, 1996
Relation of social support to child health and family health	Children with diabetes and their parents	Frey, 1989, 1993
	Children with diabetes or asthma and their parents	Frey, 1995
Relation of family health to time since diagnosis, perception of symptom severity, caregiver stress, and family stressors	Families with a member with chronic obstructive pulmonary disease	Wicks, 1995, 1997
Relation of family stressors, family coping, family perception of the ill member's level of health, and time since diagnosis to family health	Families with a young chronically mentally ill member	Doornbos, 1995
Relation of family stressors, family coping, family of the client's level of health, and time since diagnosis of mental illness to family health	Families of young adults with serious and persistent mental illness	Doornbos, 2000
Relation between nurses' perceptions of patients and patients' satisfaction with nursing	Registered nurses Patients with new ostomies	Jackson et al., 1993
Relation of client and nurse congruency of perception of the clients' illness situation and of nursing required to client satisfaction with nursing	Nurse-client pairs on medical and surgical units	Froman, 1995

EXPERIMENTAL STUDIES

Effect of attending behavior on mental status	Investigator Older people residing in a chronic care facility	Rosendahl & Ross, 1982
Effects of animal-assisted therapy on abstinence	Individuals recovering from chemical addictions	Campbell-Begg, 2000
Effect of a King's Conceptual System-based cancer awareness educational program on knowledge of and attitudes toward prostate and testicular cancer	White, Black, and Hispanic men 18 to 64 years of age	Martin, 1990
Effects of a Theory of Goal Attainment-based nursing intervention and a control intervention on pain sensation and distress, analgesic use, ambulation, complications, and satisfaction with nursing	Patients undergoing pyelolithotomy or nephrolithotomy	Hanucharurnkul & Vinya-nguag, 1991
Effect of a Theory of Goal Attainment-based nursing intervention and a control intervention on oral contraceptive adherence	Female adolescents	Hanna, 1993, 1995
Effect of a teaching program on medication-taking behavior	African-American patients 65 years of age or older receiving hemodialysis	Long et al., 1998
Effect of education about urinary incontinence on help-seeking behaviors	Community-dwelling older adults with urinary incontinence	Milne, 2000
Effects of individualized teaching on knowledge of physical changes, psychological problems, and home care of older adults	Family caregivers of older adults	Suresh, 2002
Effects of an experimental patient appointment guidebook and a control standard appointment reminder letter on patient participation in the health-care visit and perceptions of primary-care visit effectiveness	Veterans Health Administration patients	Wilkenson & Williams, 2002

(Text continued from page 110)

Much of King's Conceptual System-based research is limited to a single study on a single topic. Programs of research, however, are beginning to be developed. Especially noteworthy are the efforts of Brooks and Thomas, Doornbos, Frey, and Wicks to use research findings to revise and refine the theories they derived from King's Conceptual System (see Table 5–3).

Nursing Education. King (1989a) maintained that her Conceptual System and theory have been used "in curriculum development, for teaching in higher education, and with undergraduate and graduate students to plan, implement, and evaluate nursing care" (p. 155). The utility of King's Conceptual System and Theory of Goal Attainment for nursing education is documented. As shown below, published reports and a personal communication from King indicate that King's Conceptual System and Theory of Goal Attainment have been used as guides for curriculum construction in a few nursing education programs and a continuing nursing education program. The complete citations for the publications are given in the Education section of the chapter references.

- Ohio State University, Columbus, Ohio (Baccalaureate curriculum) (Daubenmire, 1989; Daubenmire & King, 1973)
- Loyola University of Chicago, Chicago, Illinois (Master's program) (King, personal communication, February 23, 1982)
- Olivet Nazarene College, Kankakee, Illinois (Asay & Ossler, 1984)
- Hospital-based school of nursing, Winnipeg, Manitoba, Canada (Fromen & Sanderson, 1985)
- Continuing nursing education (Brown & Lee, 1980)

In addition, Gulitz and King (1988) described a process of curriculum development using King's Conceptual System. King (1986a) also presented detailed descriptions of the nursing curriculum plans for a hypothetical associate degree program and a hypothetical baccalaureate program, including the philosophy of nursing education, curriculum Conceptual System, program objectives, prerequisite and concurrent courses in adjunctive disciplines, nursing courses, plan of study, and sample courses with course description, objectives, content, learning activities, teaching strategies, and strategies for formative and summative evaluation. She also outlined a curriculum to articulate associate degree and baccalaureate degree programs. In addition, King (1986a) shared her ideas, along with course titles and objectives, about undergraduate and graduate education in nursing for the future. Here she emphasized professional education and learning about nursing as an academic discipline.

Nursing Administration. The utility of King's Conceptual System and Theory of Goal Attainment for nursing administration is documented through their use as a guide for nursing administrative structures. King (1989a) noted that her Conceptual System and theory can be used "as a guide to help individuals organize the delivery of nursing services in health care systems" (p. 155). The practice tools that have been derived from King's Conceptual System and the Theory of Goal Attainment (see Table 5–2) are especially useful to the nurse administrator.

Elberson (1989) linked King's Conceptual System and Arndt and Huckabay's (1980) theory of nursing administration to create a conceptual-theoretical structure for nursing administration. Elberson explained that "For King, the unit of analysis is the individual. The focus is the individual nurse managing care for patients and small groups of clients. For Arndt and Huckabay, the unit of analysis is also the individual, but in this case the focus is the individual nurse administrator managing the care provided by individual nurses and groups of nurses. Both perspectives are models of health-care management" (p. 49).

Furthermore, Hampton (1994) described the use of the Theory of Goal Attainment in combination with CareMaps as a guide for nursing in managed care situations. In addition, Tritsch (1998) described the use of the Theory of Goal Attainment in combination with the Carondelet St. Mary's nursing case management model.

Published reports indicate that King's Conceptual System and Theory of Goal Attainment have been implemented in health-care organizations in the United States and Canada. Those health-care organizations are listed here. The complete citations for the publications are given in the Administration section of the chapter references.

- Tampa General Hospital, Tampa, Florida (LaFontaine, 1989; Messmer, 1992)
- A large teaching hospital in Florida (King, 1996)
- Mount Sinai Medical Center, Miami Beach, Florida (Jones et al., 1995)
- AID Atlanta, Inc. (An AIDS Service Organization), Atlanta, Georgia (Sowell & Lowenstein, 1994; Sowell & Meadows, 1994)
- A 52-bed rural hospital (Sowell & Fuszard, 1989)
- Centenary Hospital, Scarborough, Ontario, Canada (Byrne & Schreiber, 1989; Byrne-Coker & Schreiber, 1990a, 1990b; Byrne-Coker et al., 1990; Gill et al., 1995; Schreiber, 1991)
- Sunnybrook Health Science Centre, Toronto, Ontario, Canada (West, 1991)
- Hamilton Civic Hospitals, Hamilton, Ontario, Canada (Fawcett et al., 1995)

Nursing Practice. King (1992a) maintained that her Conceptual System and Theory of Goal Attainment provide a useful approach for nursing practice. She claimed that although any one Conceptual System theory "cannot cover every nursing situation [the nursing process of the Theory of Goal Attainment] can be used in most nursing situations" (p. 24). Indeed, King's Conceptual System and the Theory of Goal Attainment have documented utility in nursing practice with individuals of various ages and with many different conditions of health (Table 5–4).

TABLE 5–4
PUBLISHED REPORTS OF NURSING PRACTICE GUIDED BY KING'S CONCEPTUAL SYSTEM AND THEORY
OF GOAL ATTAINMENT

Practice Situation	Population	Citation[*]
Application of King's Conceptual System	A critically ill infant	Frey & Norris, 1997; Norris & Frey, 2002
	Couples who are infertile	Davis, 1987
	Women experiencing menopause	Heggie & Gangar, 1992
	A man receiving individual psychotherapy	DeHowitt, 1992
	A 29-year-old woman with cervical cancer	Frey & Norris, 1997; Norris & Frey, 2002
	A 41-year-old woman with breast cancer, toxic megacolon, and spinal osteomyelitis	Fawcett et al., 1995
	Alcohol-dependent women who were victims of sexual abuse	McKinney & Frank, 1998
	An older man with a leg ulcer	Lucas, 1998
	Patients scheduled for minor elective surgery	Swindale, 1989
	Patients with cardiac disease and their families	Sirles & Selleck, 1989
	A subcommunity of prostitutes working in a large community	Hanchett, 1988
	A community	Batra, 1996
Application of the Theory of Goal Attainment	Infants in a neonatal intensive care unit and their parents	Norris & Hoyer, 1993
	A 17-year-old high school student with an ankle injury admitted to an emergency department	Hughes, 1983
	A 25-year-old female victim of domestic violence admitted to an emergency department	Benedict & Frey, 1995
	A 17-year-old female accident victim with multiple fractures	Alligood, 1995
	Women participating in a self-esteem group	Laben et al., 1995
	A 30-year-old woman who had a cesarean birth	Smith, 1988
	A 40-year-old woman with chronic back pain	Alligood, 1995
	A man with AIDS-related lymphoma receiving outpatient chemotherapy	Porter, 1991
	A 43-year-old man who had coronary artery bypass surgery	King, 1986
	Individuals who have neurofibromatosis	Messner & Smith, 1986
	Adults with diabetes mellitus	Husband, 1988
	An older widower residing alone in an apartment complex	Kohler, 1988
	A 70-year-old hospitalized woman with diabetes mellitus	Jonas, 1987

[*]See the Practice section of the chapter references for complete citations.

(continued)

TABLE 5–4
PUBLISHED REPORTS OF NURSING PRACTICE GUIDED BY KING'S CONCEPTUAL SYSTEM AND THEORY OF GOAL ATTAINMENT *(continued)*

Practice Situation	Population	Citation
	Individuals who were scheduled to undergo gastroendoscopic examination	LaFontaine, 1989
	A psychotic man with HIV infection	Kemppainen, 1990
	Women receiving group psychotherapy	Calladine, 1996
	Juvenile sexual offenders receiving group psychotherapy	Laben et al., 1991
	Inmates at a state maximum security prison receiving group psychotherapy	Laben et al., 1991
	Parolees involved in a work-release program residing in a community halfway house and receiving group psychotherapy	Laben et al., 1991, 1995
	Filial caregivers of an older man with metastatic cancer and his wife	Temple & Fawdry, 1992
	A family with a member with diabetes mellitus and leukemia	King, 1983a
	A family with an older member	King, 1983b
	Workers subject to carpal tunnel syndrome and other repetitive stress injuries	Norgan et al., 1995
	A group of older clients residing in a nursing home	Woods, 1994
	A family composed of a mother, a stepfather, and a 17-year-old girl experiencing behavior problems	Gonot, 1986
Use of the Goal-Oriented Nursing Record	A comatose young girl	King, 1981
	A 60-year-old woman who had a cerebrovascular accident	
	Patients with end-stage renal disease	King, 1984
Intrusion of Personal Space	Clients with posttraumatic stress disorder	Brown & Yantis, 1996

George (2002) argued that a limitation of King's work "is the lack of development of application of the theory in proving nursing care to groups, families, or communities." She evidently ignored the family theory development work by Doornbos (1995, 2000) and Wicks (1995, 1997) and the growing literature documenting the use of King's Conceptual System and Theory of Goal Attainment with families and communities (see Table 5–4), as well as the practice tools for assessment of families and communities (see Table 5–2).

More specifically, review of the publications cited in Tables 5–2 and 5–4 and those listed in the Commentary: Practice section of the chapter bibliography on the CD-ROM reveals that King's Conceptual System and Theory of Goal Attainment are equally applicable to individuals, families, and communities. In particular, King's work has been used to guide nursing practice with children, adolescents, and adults with such conditions as ankle injury, infertility, cesarean birth, menopause, coronary artery bypass surgery, cerebrovascular accident, end-stage renal disease, neurofibromatosis, diabetes, and mental illness.

Furthermore, turning attention to groups other than families, Laben and her colleagues (1991) focused on group therapy for offenders in the criminal justice system. Moreover, King (1984) discussed the application of her work in community health nursing. And Hanchett (1988, 1990) provided informative discussions of the use of King's work when the client is the community.

Although a client's inability to communicate verbally may seem to limit the use of King's Conceptual System and Theory of Goal Attainment, King (1992a) explained that "when clients cannot communicate with a nurse, they can nonverbally send and receive messages. In some situations, nurses use their judgment and set goals for the patients and families when they are unable to do this for themselves. ... When working with patients who are comatose, nurses can verbally communicate and observe for nonverbal gestures such as muscle movement, the squeezing of the nurse's hand, or changes in facial expressions" (p. 24).

In a specific example, King (1986b) described the use of the Theory of Goal Attainment by a graduate student who was caring for a comatose patient. Because the patient could not communicate verbally, mutual goals were set with the patient's husband. The student, however, communicated verbally with the patient and observed and recorded her nonverbal responses. The student ascertained that goals set with the husband were attained after the patient regained consciousness and returned to her home.

Furthermore, practice tools have been developed to guide assessment of individuals, families, and communities, and to document nursing practice based on the Theory of Goal Attainment. Those tools are identified and described in Table 5–2.

In addition, King has pointed out that her Conceptual System and Theory of Goal Attainment can be used by family members and by teachers. She explained, "Families can be taught how to use the transaction process in their interactions, so that they are mutually setting goals with each other. A spouse can be taught to mutually set goals with his or her partner. A mother can be taught to mutually set goals with her children. Furthermore, the transaction process can be taught to teachers, who can mutually set goals with the students" (Fawcett, 2001, p. 314). Elaborating, King declared, "The key is that my work is based on general system theory; this means that the whole system of interest is identified. The concepts of my [Conceptual System] and theory can be used with any system because the knowledge of the concepts relate to human beings and environment" (Fawcett, 2001, p. 314).

Social Congruence

The social congruence of King's Conceptual System and the Theory of Goal Attainment is based, in part, on King's (1975) deliberate construction of the Conceptual System from "recurring ideas or ... concepts that were undergoing verification through systematic investigation" (p. 37) and systematic derivation of the theory from selected dimensions of the Conceptual System concepts. The resulting unique conceptual-theoretical system of nursing knowledge emphasizes nursing practice based on empirically ad-

equate scientific findings and enduring traditions deemed acceptable by society.

The **Interaction-Transaction Process**, with its emphasis on mutual goal setting, is particularly appealing to health-care consumers and nurses who believe that health care is a collaborative endeavor and to health-care consumers who wish to participate actively in their nursing care. Indeed, King (1992b) noted that the **Interaction-Transaction Process** "is based on knowledge of human interactions in which a critical human variable (coping) should be of concern in helping those we serve to build collaborative relationships and participate as informed decision makers in their own health care" (p. 604).

Bramlett, Gueldner, and Sowell (1990) pointed out that King's assumptions about human beings and her emphasis on mutual goal-setting support "a need to redefine the concept of advocacy to accommodate a more active and less dependent client role in decision making" (p. 160). They also pointed out that "King's focus on the information giving role of the nurse is consistent with the concept of consumer-centric advocacy" (p. 160). Health-care consumers and nurses who do not subscribe to such an approach to nursing practice would have to be persuaded to see its value. That is especially so when caring for clients with external locus of control. More specifically, King (1987a) noted that the use of the **Interaction-Transaction Process** may be limited to clients who have internal locus of control because it is difficult to set mutual goals with a client who has an external locus of control.

King's Conceptual System and Theory of Goal Attainment are appropriate for use with clients of various cultural backgrounds. Husting (1997) maintained that the Theory of Goal Attainment is congruent with international and multicultural nursing, and that use of the theory prevents cultural stereotypes. Frey and colleagues (1995) explicitly refuted charges by others (e.g., Meleis, 1985) that the Conceptual System and theory may not be appropriate for people of diverse cultures. They presented examples of the successful use of the Conceptual System and theory for many years in Japan and Sweden, as well as in the United States. Rooke (1995b) added that King's Conceptual System and Theory of Goal Attainment have been used successfully to guide nursing practice in Sweden. Furthermore, King's Conceptual System and Theory of Goal Attainment have been used by nurses in Thailand (King, as cited in Takahashi, 1992), and have been implemented successfully in health-care organization in Canada. Moreover, King's 1968 journal article and her 1971 and 1981 books were translated into Japanese (Frey et al., 1995), and her 1981 book was translated into Spanish (King, personal communication, May 7, 1992, as cited in Carter & Dufour, 1994).

In addition, Spratlen (1976) built on King's early work to develop "an approach to nursing education, research and practice which incorporates the cultural dimensions of attitudes and behavior in matters of health" (p. 23). Furthermore, Rooda (1992) described the conceptual model for multicultural nursing that she developed from the Theory of Goal Attainment. She noted that the model provides direction for nursing practice and research and prepares nurses to provide holistic nursing care in a global society.

King's Conceptual System and Theory of Goal Attainment are not, however, necessarily universally applicable. "Rather," as Frey and colleagues (1995) pointed out, "use and interpretation would vary based on cultural considerations of clients and nurses" (p. 128).

Jonas' (1987) experience using the Theory of Goal Attainment to guide nursing practice provides anecdotal evidence supporting social congruence. She reported that both she and the client were satisfied with the nursing provided.

West's (1991) experience with the implementation of King's Conceptual System and Theory of Goal Attainment provides empirical data regarding social congruence. She reported that a study of nurses' reactions to the implementation of King's Conceptual System and Theory of Goal Attainment-based practice at Sunnybrook Health Science Centre in Toronto revealed mixed results. Interviews with nursing unit directors and discussions with staff nurses indicated a clear dichotomy—approximately equal numbers of nurses were "adamantly for theory or vehemently against it. There seemed to be little ambivalence" (p. 30). Chart audits of the GONR using a quality assurance tool to ensure nonbiased, reliable, and valid assessments revealed "a wide range of comprehension and various levels of abilities to not only format a care plan reflecting the theory, but also to monitor the outcome of that theory and the patient's response to the plan" (p. 30). West (1991) concluded that greater attention must be paid to discussion of the value of conceptual model-based nursing practice before the selection and implementation of a particular model in a health-care organization.

Additional empirical evidence of social congruence comes from Messmer's (1995) report of an increase in female patients' satisfaction with nursing on a general surgical inpatient pilot unit that implemented King's Conceptual System-based practice, compared with the satisfaction of patients on two other units that were not yet using the Conceptual System.

Still other empirical evidence of social congruence comes from a study by Hanucharurnkul and Vinya-nguag (1991). They found that patients who received a nursing intervention based in part on the Theory of Goal Attainment reported greater satisfaction with nursing than those who did not receive the intervention.

Social Significance

King (1992b) claimed that the "use of my conceptual system and theory in nursing practice has shown cost containment, health care outcomes, and health team approach in using the same conceptual system" (p. 604). Later, King maintained that "Ninety-nine percent of the time, goals are achieved when [the **Interaction-Transaction Process**] is used. Achievement of goals represents an outcome, and outcomes demonstrate evidence-based nursing practice" (Fawcett, 2001, p. 314). She did not, however, provide any empirical or anecdotal evidence to support that claim.

Anecdotal evidence supporting the contention that use of King's Conceptual System and Theory of Goal Attainment leads to improvements in individuals' health status is beginning to accrue. In summarizing that evidence, Fawcett and Whall (1995) pointed to the comprehensiveness of assessments and the success of mutual goal setting in goal attainment reported by many nurses who have used the Conceptual System and theory in nursing practice (see Table 5–4).

Empirical evidence from research supporting the social significance of King's Conceptual System and Theory of Goal Attainment also is accruing. Fawcett and Whall (1995) noted the efficacy of interventions derived from the Conceptual System and theory that have been reported by investigators who have conducted studies guided by the Conceptual System and theory (see Table 5–3). Especially noteworthy is the evidence that supports the empirical adequacy of theories derived from King's Conceptual System. More specifically, although study findings have led to revision and refinement of some of the theories, the essential propositions of each theory have been supported. In addition, Wilkinson and Williams (2002) reported that, in a study guided by King's Conceptual System, patients regarded an experimental patient appointment guidebook positively, and more of those patients received influenza and pneumococcal vaccinations and gender-specific cancer screening than patients who received a standard appointment reminder letter before scheduled routine visits.

 ## CONTRIBUTIONS TO THE DISCIPLINE OF NURSING

King's Conceptual System and her Theory of Goal Attainment are substantial contributions to the discipline of nursing. The concepts and propositions of the Conceptual System, together with the content related to each dimension of the **Personal System, Interpersonal System, and Social System,** form the beginning of conceptual-theoretical systems of nursing knowledge needed for various nursing activities. Furthermore, the Theory of Goal

Attainment is a major contribution to the growing list of distinctive nursing theories. Noteworthy is the empirical testing of and initial support for the Theory of Goal Attainment. However, additional tests of the Theory of Goal Attainment are needed. Furthermore, the credibility of King's Conceptual System requires additional investigation by means of systematic tests of conceptual-theoretical-empirical structures derived from the Conceptual System, the Theory of Goal Attainment or other relevant theories, and appropriate empirical indicators.

The emphasis on client participation in King's Conceptual System and Theory of Goal Attainment, including mutual goal setting and exploration of means to achieve goals, should be attractive to the many nurses who are consumer advocates. The Conceptual System and theory also should be attractive to those clients who wish to actively participate in their health care.

King's Conceptual System, as King (1995a) pointed out, describes "a holistic view of the complexity in nursing, within various groups, [and] in different types of health care systems" (p. 21). More specifically, King's Conceptual System "provides a way of thinking about the 'real world' of nursing practice ... suggests one approach for selecting concepts from the literature that represent fundamental knowledge for the practice of professional nursing ... [and] shows a process for developing concepts that symbolize experiences within various environments in which nursing is practiced" (King, 1995a, p. 17).

Furthermore, the Theory of Goal Attainment and the **Interaction-Transaction Process** represent "a human process of interactions that lead to transactions and to goal attainment [which is] successful ... because it enables one to predict outcomes of sets of events in the concrete world of practice" (p. 62).

The scholarly work needed to continue to generate and evaluate empirical data about King's Conceptual System, the Theory of Goal Attainment, and other theories derived from the Conceptual System was advanced by several members of the King International Nursing Group (KING; King International Nursing Group, 2000) during its existence, as well as by other nurses who are interested in this perspective of nursing. The KING was founded in 1997 "to improve the quality of patient care, and to contribute to the science of nursing, through advancement of King's [Conceptual System] for Nursing ... [and] the Theory of Goal Attainment as well as other theoretical formulations derived from the [Conceptual System]" (Bylaws of the King International Nursing Group, April 17, 1998, p. 1). The KING published a newsletter, *King's Systems Update*, and sponsored annual educational conferences. At the request of Imogene King, the KING disbanded in 2002. The work to advance King's Conceptual System and Theory of Goal Attainment will, however, continue.

King's (1997c) vision for the future "is a dream that nurses will be at the center of health-care delivery systems in the next century. In addition, my conceptual system and theory of goal attainment will provide the structure for gathering information relative to access, quality, and cost for all human beings" (p. 16). Later, King (2001a) indicated that her vision for the future of nursing is that:

> ... nursing will provide access to health care of all citizens. The United States health-care system will be structured using my conceptual system. Entry into the system will be via nurses' assessment so individuals are directed to the right place in the system for nursing care, medical care, social services information, health teaching, or rehabilitation. My [Interaction-Transaction Process] will be used by every practicing nurse so that goals can be achieved to demonstrate quality care that is cost effective. My conceptual system, Theory of Goal Attainment and [Interaction-Transaction Process] will continue to serve a useful purpose in delivering professional nursing care (p. 284).

Given the widespread interest in King's work, her dream is likely to become a reality.

 ## REFERENCES

Alligood, M.R. (1997). Models and theories: Critical thinking structures. In M.R. Alligood & A. Marriner-Tomey (Eds.), Nursing theory: Utilization and application (pp. 31–45). St. Louis: Mosby.

Alligood, M.R. (2001). Philosophies, models, and theories: Critical thinking structures. In M.R. Alligood & A. Marriner-Tomey (Eds.), Nursing theory: Utilization and application (2nd ed., pp. 41–61). St. Louis: Mosby.

Alligood, M.R., Evans, G.W., & Wilt, D.L. (1995). King's interacting systems and empathy. In M.A. Frey & C.L. Sieloff (Eds.), Advancing King's systems framework and theory of nursing (pp. 66–78). Thousand Oaks, CA: Sage.

Alligood, M.R., & May, B.A. (2000). A nursing theory of personal system empathy: Interpreting a conceptualization of empathy in King's interacting systems. Nursing Science Quarterly, 113, 243–247.

Arndt, C., & Huckabay, L.M.D. (1980). Nursing administration: Theory for practice with a systems approach (2nd ed) St. Louis: Mosby.

Barnum, B.J.S. (1998). Nursing theory. Analysis, application, evaluation (5th ed.). Philadelphia: Lippincott.

Benne, R.D., & Bennis, W.G. (1959). The role of the professional nurse. American Journal of Nursing, 59, 380–383.

Boulding, K. (1956). General system theory—The skeleton of science. Yearbook of the Society for the Advancement of General System Theory, 1(1), 11–17.

Bramlett, M.H., Gueldner, S.H., & Sowell, R.L. (1990). Consumer-centric advocacy: Its connection to nursing frameworks. Nursing Science Quarterly, 3, 156–161.

Brooks, E.M., & Thomas, S. (1997). The perception and judgment of senior baccalaureate student nurses in clinical decision making. Advances in Nursing Science, 19(3), 50–69.

Bross, I. (1953). Design for decision. New York: Macmillan.

Bruner, I.S., & Krech, W. (Eds.). (1968). Perception and personality. New York: Greenwood Press.

Byers, P. (1985, August). Application of Imogene King's framework. Paper presented at conference on Nursing Theory in Action, Edmonton, Alberta, Canada. [Audiotape.]

Byrne-Coker, E., & Schreiber, R. (1990a). Implementing King's conceptual framework at the bedside. In M.E. Parker (Ed.), Nursing theories in practice (pp. 85–102). New York: National League for Nursing.

Byrne-Coker, E., & Schreiber, R. (1990b). King at the bedside. Canadian Nurse, 86(1), 24–26.

Carter, K.F., & Dufour, L.T. (1994). King's theory: A critique of the critiques. Nursing Science Quarterly, 7, 128–113.

Cherry, C. (1966). On human communication. Cambridge, MA: MIT Press.

Daubenmire, M.J. (1989). A baccalaureate nursing curriculum based on King's conceptual framework. In J.P. Riehl-Sisca (Ed.), Conceptual models for nursing practice (3rd ed., pp. 167–178). Norwalk, CT: Appleton & Lange.

Daubenmire, M.J., & King, I.M. (1973). Nursing process models: A systems approach. Nursing Outlook, 21, 512–517.

Dewey, J., & Bentley, A. (1949). Knowing and the known. Boston: Beacon Press.

DiVincenti, M. (1977). Administering nursing service (2nd ed.). Boston: Little, Brown.

Doornbos, M.M. (1995). Using King's systems framework to explore family health in the families of the young chronically mentally ill. In M.A. Frey & C.L. Sieloff (Eds.), Advancing King's systems framework and theory of nursing (pp. 192–205). Thousand Oaks, CA: Sage.

Doornbos, M.M. (2000). King's systems framework and family health: The derivation and testing of a theory. Journal of Theory Construction and Testing, 4, 20–26.

Du Mont, P.M. (1998). The effects of early menarche on health risk behaviors. Dissertation Abstracts International, 60, 3200B.

Ehrenberger, H.E. (2000). Testing a theory of decision making derived from King's systems framework in women eligible for a cancer clinical trail. Dissertation Abstracts International, 60, 3201B.

Ehrenberger, H.E., Alligood, M.R., Thomas, S.P., Wallace, D.C., & Licavoli, C.M. (2002). Testing a theory of decision-making derived from King's systems framework in women eligible for a cancer clinical trial. Nursing Science Quarterly, 15, 156–163.

Elberson, K. (1989). Applying King's model to nursing administration. In B. Henry, M. DiVincenti, C. Arndt, & A. Marriner (Eds.), Dimensions of nursing administration. Theory, research, education, and practice (pp. 47–53). Boston: Blackwell Scientific.

Ellis, R. (1971). Book review of King, I.M. (1971). Toward a theory for nursing: General concepts of human behavior. Nursing Research, 20, 462.

Erikson, E. (1950). Childhood and society. New York: Norton.

Etzioni, A.A. (1975). Comparative analysis of complex organizations (rev. ed.). New York: The Free Press.

Fawcett, J. (1984). Analysis and evaluation of conceptual models of nursing. Philadelphia: F.A. Davis.

Fawcett, J. (1989). Analysis and evaluation of conceptual models of nursing (2nd ed.). Philadelphia: F.A. Davis.

Fawcett, J. (2000). Analysis and evaluation of contemporary nursing knowledge: Nursing models and theories. Philadelphia: F.A. Davis.

Fawcett, J. (2001). The nurse theorists: 21st century updates—Imogene M. King. Nursing Science Quarterly, 14, 311–315.

Fawcett, J., & Whall, A.L. (1995). State of the science and future directions. In M.A. Frey & C.L. Sieloff (Eds.), Advancing King's systems framework and theory of nursing (pp. 327–334). Thousand Oaks, CA: Sage.

Fisher, S., & Cleveland, S. (1968). Body image and personality. New York: Dover.

Fraser, J.T. (Ed.). (1972). The voices of time. New York: George Braziller.

Freud, S. (1966). Introductory lectures on psychoanalysis (J. Strachey, Ed. and Trans.) New York: Norton.

Frey, M.A. (1989). Social support and health: A theoretical formulation derived from King's conceptual framework. Nursing Science Quarterly, 2, 138–148.

Frey, M.A. (1995). Toward a theory of families, children, and chronic illness. In M.A. Frey & C.L. Sieloff (Eds.), Advancing King's systems framework and theory of nursing (pp. 109–125). Thousand Oaks, CA: Sage.

Frey, M.A., Rooke, L., Sieloff, C., Messmer, P.R. & Kameoka, T. (1995). King's framework and theory in Japan, Sweden, and the United States. Image: Journal of Nursing Scholarship, 27, 127–130.

Frey, M.A., & Sieloff, C.L. (Eds.). (1995). Advancing King's systems framework and theory of nursing. Thousand Oaks, CA: Sage.

Frey, M.A., Sieloff, C.L., & Norris, D.M. (2002). King's conceptual system and theory of goal attainment: Past, present, and future. Nursing Science Quarterly, 15, 107–112.

Fries, J.E. (1998). Health and social support of older adults. Dissertation Abstracts International, 59, 6262B.

George, J.B. (2002). Systems framework and theory of goal attainment; Imogene M. King. In J. B. George (Ed.), Nursing theories: The base for professional nursing practice (5th ed.), pp. 241–267. Upper Saddle River, NJ: Prentice Hall.

Gesell, A. (1952). Infant development. New York: Harper.

Gibson, J. (1966). The senses considered as perceptual systems. Boston: Houghton Mifflin.

Griffiths, D. (1959). Administrative theory. Englewood Cliffs, NJ: Prentice-Hall.

Gulitz, E.A., & King, I.M. (1988). King's general systems model: Application to curriculum development. Nursing Science Quarterly, 1, 128–132.

Haas, J.E. (1964). Role conception and group consensus: A study of disharmony in hospital work groups. Columbus, OH: Ohio State University College of Commerce and Administration, Bureau of Business Research.

Hall, A.D., & Fagen, R.E. (1956). Definition of system. Yearbook of the Society for the Advancement of General System Theory, 1(1), 18–28.

Hall, E. (1959). The silent language. Greenwich, CT: Fawcett.

Hampton, D.C. (1994). King's theory of goal attainment as a framework for managed care implementation in a hospital setting. Nursing Science Quarterly, 7, 170–173.

Hanchett, E.S. (1988). Nursing frameworks and community as client: Bridging the gap. Norwalk, CT: Appleton & Lange.

Hanchett, E.S. (1990). Nursing models and community as client. Nursing Science Quarterly, 3, 67–72.

Hanucharurnku[l], S., & Vinya-nguag, P. (1991). Effects of promoting patients' participation in self-care on postoperative recovery and satisfaction with care. Nursing Science Quarterly, 4, 14–20.

Havighurst, R. (1953). Human development and education. New York: McKay.

Heiss, J. (1981). The social psychology of interaction. Englewood Cliffs, NJ: Prentice-Hall.

Hobdell, E.F. (1995). Using King's interacting systems framework for research on parents of children with neural tube defect. In M.A. Frey & C.L. Sieloff (Eds.), Advancing King's systems framework and theory of nursing (pp. 126–136). Thousand Oaks, CA: Sage.

Howland, D. (1976). An adaptive health system model. In H.H. Werley & J.C. Abbey (Eds.), Health research: The systems approach (p. 109). New York: Springer.

Howland, D., & McDowell, W. (1964). A measurement of patient care: A conceptual framework. Nursing Research, 13, 320–324.

Husting, P.M. (1997). A transcultural critique of Imogene King's theory of goal attainment. Journal of Multicultural Nursing and Health, 3(3), 15–20.

Ittleson, W., & Cantril, H. (1954). Perception: A transactional approach. Garden City, NY: Doubleday.

Janis, I. (1958). Psychological stress. New York: Wiley.

Jersild, A.T. (1952). In search of self. New York: Columbia University Teachers College Press.

Jonas, C.M. (1987). King's goal attainment theory: Use in gerontological nursing practice. Perspectives, 11(4), 9–12.

Katz, D., & Kahn, R.L. (1966). The social psychology of organizations. New York: Wiley.

Kaufmann, M.A. (1958). Identification of theoretical bases for nursing practice. Unpublished doctoral dissertation, University of California, Los Angeles.

King, I.M. (1964). Nursing theory—Problems and prospect. Nursing Science, 2, 394–403.

King, I.M. (1968). A conceptual frame of reference for nursing. Nursing Research, 17, 27–31.

King, I.M. (1971). Toward a theory for nursing: General concepts of human behavior. New York: Wiley.

King, I.M. (1975). A process for developing concepts for nursing through research. In P.J. Verhonick (Ed.), Nursing research I (pp. 25–43). Boston: Little, Brown.

King, I.M. (1976). The health care system: Nursing intervention subsystem. In H. Werley, A. Zuzich, M. Zajkowski, & A.D. Zagornik (Eds.), Health research: The systems approach (pp. 51–60). New York: Springer.

King, I.M. (1978, December). King's conceptual model of nursing. Paper presented at Second Annual Nurse Educator Conference, New York. [Audiotape.]

King, I.M. (1981). A theory for nursing: Systems, concepts, process. New York: Wiley. [Reissued 1990. Albany, NY: Delmar.]

King, I.M. (1983a). King's theory of nursing. In I.W. Clements & F.B. Roberts, Family health: A theoretical approach to nursing care (pp. 177–188). New York: Wiley.

King, I.M. (1983b). The family coping with a medical illness. Analysis and application of King's theory of goal attainment. In I.W. Clements & F.B. Roberts, Family health: A theoretical approach to nursing care (pp. 383–385). New York: Wiley.

King, I.M. (1983c). The family with an elderly member. Analysis and application of King's theory of goal attainment. In I.W. Clements & F.B. Roberts, Family health: A theoretical approach to nursing care (pp. 341–345). New York: Wiley.

King, I.M. (1984). A theory for nursing. King's conceptual model applied in community health nursing. In M.K. Asay & C.C. Ossler (Eds.), Conceptual models of nursing. Applications in community health nursing: Proceedings of the eighth annual community health nursing conference (pp. 13–34). Chapel Hill, NC: Department of Public Health Nursing, School of Public Health, University of North Carolina.

King, I.M. (1985a, May). Panel discussion with theorists. Nurse Theorist Conference, Pittsburgh, PA. [Audiotape.]

King, I.M. (1985b, August). Imogene King. Paper presented at conference on Nursing Theory in Action, Edmonton, Alberta, Canada. [Audiotape.]

King, I.M. (1986a). Curriculum and instruction in nursing. Norwalk, CT: Appleton-Century-Crofts.

King, I.M. (1986b). King's theory of goal attainment. In P. Winstead-Fry (Ed.), Case studies in nursing theory (pp. 197–213). New York: National League for Nursing.

King, I.M. (1987a, May). King's theory. Paper presented at Nurse Theorist Conference, Pittsburgh, PA. [Audiotape.]

King, I.M. (1987b). King's theory of goal attainment. In R.R. Parse, Nursing science. Major paradigms, theories, and critiques (pp. 107–113). Philadelphia: W.B. Saunders.

King, I.M. (1988). The nurse theorists: Portraits of excellence—Imogene King. Athens: OH: Fuld Institute for Technology in Nursing Education. [Videotape.]

King, I.M. (1989a). King's general systems framework and theory. In J.P. Riehl-Sisca (Ed.), Conceptual models for nursing practice (3rd ed., pp. 149–158). Norwalk, CT: Appleton & Lange.

King, I.M. (1989b). Theories and hypotheses for nursing administration. In B. Henry, M. DiVincenti, C. Arndt, & A. Marriner (Eds.), Dimensions of nursing administration. Theory, research, education, and practice (pp. 35–45). Boston: Blackwell Scientific.

King, I.M. (1990a). Health as the goal for nursing. Nursing Science Quarterly, 3, 123–128.

King, I.M. (1990b). King's conceptual framework and theory of goal attainment. In M.E. Parker (Ed.), Nursing theories in practice (pp. 73–84). New York: National League for Nursing.

King, I.M. (1992a). King's theory of goal attainment. Nursing Science Quarterly, 5, 19–26.

King, I.M. (1992b). Window on general systems framework and theory of goal attainment. In M. O'Toole (Ed.), Miller-Keane encyclopedia and dictionary of medicine, nursing, and allied health (p. 604). Philadelphia: W.B. Saunders.

King, I.M. (1995a). A systems framework for nursing. In M.A. Frey & C.L. Sieloff (Eds.), Advancing King's systems framework and theory of nursing (pp. 14–22). Thousand Oaks, CA: Sage.

King, I.M. (1995b). The theory of goal attainment. In M.A. Frey & C.L. Sieloff (Eds.), Advancing King's systems framework and theory of nursing (pp. 23–32). Thousand Oaks, CA: Sage.

King, I.M. (1996). The theory of goal attainment in research and practice. Nursing Science Quarterly, 9, 61–66.

King, I.M. (1997a). King's theory of goal attainment in practice. Nursing Science Quarterly, 10, 180–185.

King, I.M. (1997b). Knowledge development for nursing: A process. In I.M. King & J. Fawcett (Eds.), The language of nursing theory and metatheory (pp. 19–25). Indianapolis: Sigma Theta Tau International Center Nursing Press.

King, I.M. (1997c). Reflections on the past and a vision for the future. Nursing Science Quarterly, 10, 15–17.

King, I.M. (1999). A theory of goal attainment: Philosophical and ethical implications. Nursing Science Quarterly, 12, 292–296.

King, I.M. (2001a). Imogene M. King: Theory of goal attainment. In M.E. Parker (Ed.), Nursing theories and nursing practice (pp. 275–286). Philadelphia: F.A. Davis.

King, I.M. (2001b). Letter to the Editor. Nursing Science Quarterly, 14, 80–81.

King International Nursing Group. (2000). Theoria: Journal of Nursing Theory, 9(4), 11.

Klein, G. (1970). Perception, motivation and personality. New York: Alfred A. Knopf.

Laben, J.K., Dodd, D., & Sneed, L. (1991). King's theory of goal attainment applied in group therapy for inpatient juvenile sexual offenders, maximum security state offenders, and community parolees, using visual aids. Issues in Mental Health Nursing, 12(1), 51–64.

Linton, R. (1963). The study of man. New York: Appleton-Century-Crofts.

Lyman, S., & Scott, M. (1967). Territoriality: A neglected sociological dimension. Social Problems, 15, 236–249.

Magan, S.J. (1987). A critique of King's theory. In R.R. Parse (Ed.), Nursing science. Major paradigms, theories, and critiques (pp. 115–133). Philadelphia: Saunders.

Marriner-Tomey, A. (1989). Nursing theorists and their work (2nd ed). St. Louis: Mosby.

May, B.A. (2000). Relationships among basic empathy, self-awareness, and learning styles of baccalaureate pre-nursing students within King's person system. Dissertation Abstracts International, 61, 29991B.

Meighan, M.M. (2000). Testing a nursing intervention to enhance paternal-infant interaction and promote paternal role assumption. Dissertation Abstracts International, 60, 3204B.

Meleis, A.I. (1985). Theoretical nursing: Development and progress. Philadelphia: Lippincott.

Meleis, A.I. (1997). Theoretical nursing: Development and progress (3rd ed.). Philadelphia: Lippincott.

Messmer, P.R. (1992). Implementing theory based nursing practice. Florida Nurse, 40(3), 8.

Messmer, P.R. (1995). Implementation of theory-based nursing practice. In M.A. Frey & C.L. Sieloff (Eds.), Advancing King's systems framework and theory of nursing (pp. 294–304). Thousand Oaks, CA: Sage.

Monat, A., & Lazarus, R.S. (Eds.). (1977). Stress and coping. New York: Columbia University Press.

Moore, M.A. (1968). Nursing: A scientific discipline? Nursing Forum, 7, 340–348.

Moore, M.A. (1969). The professional practice of nursing: The knowledge and how it is used. Nursing Forum, 8, 361–373.

Orlando, I.J. (1961). The dynamic nurse-patient relationship. New York: G.P. Putnam's Sons.

Orme, J.E. (1969). Time, experience and behavior. New York: American Elsevier.

Parse, R.R. (Ed.). (1987). Nursing science. Major paradigms, theories, and critiques. Philadelphia: Saunders.

Parsons, T. (1951). The social system. Glencoe, IL: The Free Press.

Peplau, H.E. (1952). Interpersonal relations in nursing. New York: G.P. Putnam's Sons. [Reprinted 1991. New York: Springer.]

Piaget, J. (1969). The mechanisms of perception. New York: Basic Books.

Rooda, L.A. (1992). The development of a conceptual model for multicultural nursing. Journal of Holistic Nursing, 10, 337–347.

Rooke, L. (1995a). The concept of space in King's systems framework: Its implications for nursing. In M.A. Frey & C.L. Sieloff (Eds.), Advancing King's systems framework and theory of nursing (pp. 79–96). Thousand Oaks, CA: Sage.

Rooke, L. (1995b). Focusing on King's theory and systems framework in education by using an experiential learning model: A challenge to improve the quality of nursing care. In M.A. Frey & C.L. Sieloff (Eds.), Advancing King's systems framework and theory of nursing (pp. 278–293). Thousand Oaks, CA: Sage.

Ruesch, J., & Kees, W. (1972). Nonverbal communication. Los Angeles: University of California Press.

Schilder, P. (1951). The image and appearance of the human body. New York: International Universities Press.

Selye, H. (1956). The stress of life. New York: McGraw-Hill.

Shontz, F. (1969). Perceptual and cognitive aspects of body experience. New York: Academic Press.

Sieloff, C.L. (1995). Development of a theory of departmental power. In M.A. Frey & C.L. Sieloff (Eds.), Advancing King's systems framework and theory of nursing (pp. 46–65). Thousand Oaks, CA: Sage.

Simon, H.A. (1957). Administrative behavior (2nd ad.). New York: Macmillan.

Simon, Y.R. (1962). A general theory of authority. South Bend, IN: University of Notre Dame Press.

Sommer, R. (1969). Personal space. Englewood Cliffs, NJ: Prentice-Hall.

Spratlen, L.P. (1976). Introducing ethnic-cultural factors in models of nursing: Some mental health care applications. Journal of Nursing Education, 15(2), 23–29.

Stevens, B.J. (1984). Nursing theory. Analysis, application, evaluation (2nd ed.). Boston: Little, Brown.

Takahashi, T. (1992). Perspectives on nursing knowledge. Nursing Science Quarterly, 5, 86–91.

Tritsch, J.M. (1998). Application of King's theory of goal attainment and the Carondelet St. Mary's case management model. Nursing Science Quarterly, 11, 69–73.

von Bertalanffy, L. (1956). General system theory. Yearbook of the Society for the Advancement of General System Theory, 1(1), 1–10.

von Bertalanffy, L. (1968). General system theory. New York: George Braziller.

Wapner, S., & Werner, H. (Eds.). (1965). The body percept. New York: Random House.

Watzlawick, P. Beavin, J.H., & Jackson, D.D. (1967). Pragmatics of human communication. New York: Norton.

West, P. (1991). Theory implementation: A challenging journey. Canadian Journal of Nursing Administration, 4(1), 29–30.

Whelton, B.J.B. (2001). Letter to the Editor. Nursing Science Quarterly, 14, 81–82.

Wicks, M.N. (1995). Family health as derived from King's framework. In M.A. Frey & C.L. Sieloff (Eds.), Advancing King's systems framework and theory of nursing (pp. 97–108). Thousand Oaks, CA: Sage.

Wicks, M.N. (1997). A test of the Wicks family health model in families coping with chronic obstructive pulmonary disease. Journal of Family Nursing, 3, 189–212.

Wilkinson, C.R., & Williams, M. (2002). Strengthening patient-provider relationships. Lippincott's Case Management, 7, 86–102.

Yura, H., & Walsh, M. (1983). The nursing process. Norwalk: CT: Appleton-Century-Crofts.

Zald, M.N. (Ed.). (1970). Power in organization. Nashville, TN: Vanderbilt University Press.

RESEARCH

Alligood, M.R., Evans, G.W., & Wilt, D.L. (1995). King's interacting systems and empathy. In M.A. Frey & C.L. Sieloff (Eds.), Advancing King's systems framework and theory of nursing (pp. 66–78). Thousand Oaks, CA: Sage.

Alligood, M.R., & May, B.A. (2000). A nursing theory of personal system empathy: interpreting a conceptualization of empathy in King's interacting systems. Nursing Science Quarterly, 113, 243–247. King, I.M. (2001). Letter to the Editor. Nursing Science Quarterly, 14, 80–81. Whelton, B.J.B. (2001). Letter to the Editor. Nursing Science Quarterly, 14, 81–82.

Brooks, E.M., & Thomas, S. (1997). The perception and judgment of senior baccalaureate student nurses in clinical decision making. Advances in Nursing Science, 19(3), 50–69.

Brower, H.T. (1981). Social organization and nurses' attitudes toward older persons. Journal of Gerontological Nursing, 7, 293–298.

Byrne-Coker, E., Fradley, T., Harris, J., Tomarchio, D., Chan, V., & Caron, C. (1990). Implementing nursing diagnoses within the context of King's conceptual framework. Nursing Diagnosis, 1, 107–114. [Reprinted in Frey, M.A., & Sieloff, C.L. (Eds.). (1995). Advancing King's systems framework and theory of nursing (pp. 161–175). Thousand Oaks, CA: Sage.]

Campbell-Begg, T. (2000). A case study using animal-assisted therapy to promote abstinence in a group of individuals who are recovering from chemical addictions. Journal of Addictions Nursing, 12, 31–35.

Caris-Verhallen, W.M.C., Kerkstra, A., van der Heijden, P.G.M., & Bensing, J.M. (1998). Nurse-elderly patient communication in home care and institutional care: An exploratory study. International Journal of Nursing Studies, 35, 95–108.

Daniel, J.M. (2002). Young adults' perceptions of living with chronic inflammatory bowel disease. Gastroenterology Nursing, 25(3), 83–94.

Davis, D.C., & Dearman, C.N. (1991). Coping strategies of infertile women. Journal of Obstetric, Gynecologic, and Neonatal Nursing, 20, 221–228.

Doornbos, M.M. (1995). Using King's systems framework to explore family health in the families of the young chronically mentally ill. In M.A. Frey & C.L. Sieloff (Eds.), Advancing King's systems framework and theory of nursing (pp. 192–205). Thousand Oaks, CA: Sage.

Doornbos, M.M. (2000). King's systems framework and family health: The derivation and testing of a theory. Journal of Theory Construction and Testing, 4, 20–26.

Ehrenberger, H.E., Alligood, M.R., Thomas, S.P., Wallace, D.C., & Licavoli, C.M. (2002). Testing a theory of decision-making derived from King's systems framework in women eligible for a cancer clinical trial. Nursing Science Quarterly, 15, 156–163.

Frey, M.A. (1989). Social support and health: A theoretical formulation derived from King's conceptual framework. Nursing Science Quarterly, 2, 138–148.

Frey, M.A. (1993). A theoretical perspective of family and child health derived from King's conceptual framework of nursing: A deductive approach to theory building. In S.L. Feetham, S.B. Meister, J.M. Bell, & C.L. Gillis (Eds.), The nursing of families: Theory/research/ education/practice (pp. 30–37). Newbury Park, CA: Sage.

Frey, M.A. (1995). Toward a theory of families, children, and chronic illness. In M.A. Frey & C.L. Sieloff (Eds.), Advancing King's systems framework and theory of nursing (pp. 109–125). Thousand Oaks, CA: Sage.

Frey, M. (1996). Behavioral correlates of health and illness in youths with chronic illness. Applied Nursing Research, 9, 167–176.

Froman, D. (1995). Perceptual congruency between clients and nurses: Testing King's theory of goal attainment. In M.A. Frey & C.L. Sieloff (Eds.), Advancing King's systems framework and theory of nursing (pp. 223–238). Thousand Oaks, CA: Sage.

Hanna, K.M. (1993). Effect of nurse-client transaction on female adolescents' oral contraceptive adherence. Image: Journal of Nursing Scholarship, 25, 285–290. Beal, J.A. (1994). Critique of "Effect of nurse-client transaction on female adolescents' oral contraceptive use." Nursing Scan in Research, 7(2), 14.

Hanna, K.M. (1994). Female adolescents' perceptions of benefits of and barriers to using oral contraceptives. Issues in Comprehensive Pediatric Nursing, 17, 47–55.

Hanna, K.M. (1995). Use of King's theory of goal attainment to promote adolescents' health behavior. In M.A. Frey & C.L. Sieloff (Eds.), Advancing King's systems framework and theory of nursing (pp. 239–250). Thousand Oaks, CA: Sage.

Hanucharurnku[l], S., & Vinya-nguag, P. (1991). Effects of promoting patients' participation in self-care on postoperative recovery and satisfaction with care. Nursing Science Quarterly, 4, 14–20.

Hawks, J.H. (1991). Power: A concept analysis. Journal of Advanced Nursing, 16, 754–762.

Hobdell, E.F. (1995). Using King's interacting systems framework for research on parents of children with neural tube defect. In M.A. Frey & C.L. Sieloff (Eds.), Advancing King's systems framework and theory of nursing (pp. 126–136). Thousand Oaks, CA: Sage.

Houfek, J.F. (1992). Nurses' perceptions of the dimensions of nursing care episodes. Nursing Research, 41, 280–285.

Jackson, A.L., Pokorny, M.E., & Vincent, P. (1993). Relative satisfaction with nursing care of patients with ostomies. Journal of Enterostomal Therapy Nursing, 20, 233–238.

Jacono, J., Hicks, G., Antonioni, C., O'Brien, K., & Rasi, M. (1990). Comparison of perceived needs of family members between registered nurses and family members of critically ill patients in intensive care and neonatal intensive care units. Heart and Lung, 19, 72–78.

Kameoka [nee Kusaka], T. (1995). Analyzing nurse-patient interactions in Japan. In M.A. Frey & C.L. Sieloff (Eds.), Advancing King's systems framework and theory of nursing (pp. 251–260). Thousand Oaks, CA: Sage.

King, I.M. (1981). A theory for nursing: Systems, concepts, process (pp. 141–161). New York: Wiley. [Reissued 1990. Albany, NY: Delmar.]

Kneeshaw, M.F. (1990). Nurses' perceptions of co-worker responses to smoking cessation attempts. Journal of the New York State Nurses' Association, 21(9), 9–13.

Kusaka, T. (1991). Application of King's goal attainment theory in Japanese clinical settings. Journal of Japan Academy of Nursing Education, 1(1), 30–31.

Levine, C.D., Wilson, S.F., & Guido, G.W. (1988). Personality factors of critical care nurses. Heart and Lung, 17, 392–398.

Lockhart, J.S. (1999). Nurses' perceptions of head and neck oncology patients after surgery: Severity of facial disfigurement and patient gender. ORL-Head and Neck Nursing, 17(4), 12–25.

Long, J.M., Kee, C.C., Graham, M.V., Saethang, T.B., & Dames, F.D. (1998). Medication compliance and the older hemodialysis patient. American Nephrology Nurses Association Journal, 25, 43–49.

Martin, J.P. (1990). Male cancer awareness: Impact of an employee education program. Oncology Nursing Forum, 17, 59–64.

Mayer, B.W. (2000). Female domestic violence victims: Perspectives on emergency care. Nursing Science Quarterly, 13, 340–346.

McGirr, M., Rukholm, E., Salmoni, A., O'Sullivan, P., & Koren, I. (1990). Perceived mood and exercise behaviors of cardiac rehabilitation program referrals. Canadian Journal of Cardiovascular Nursing, 1(4), 14–19.

Messmer, P.R. (1995). Portrait in professionalism: Imogene M. King [Abstract]. In 1995 Scientific Sessions Abstracts. Indianapolis: Sigma Theta Tau International.

Milne, J. (2000). The impact of information on health behaviors of older adults with urinary incontinence. Clinical Nursing Research, 9, 161–176.

Moreira, T.M.M., & Araújo, T.L. (2002). Interpersonal system of Imogene King: The relationships among patient with no-compliance to the treatment of the hypertension and professionals of health. ACTA Paulista de Enfermagem, 15(3), 35–43. [Portuguese; English abstract.]

Olsson, H., & Forsdahl, T. (1996). Expectations and opportunities of newly employed nurses. Social Sciences in Health, 2, 14–22.

Petrich, B.E.A. (2000). Medical and nursing students' perceptions of obesity. Journal of Addictions Nursing, 12, 3–16.

Pierce, S., Grodal, K., Smith, L.S., Elia-Tyvoll, S., Miller, A., & Tallman, C. (2002). Image of the nurse on internet greeting cards. Journal for Undergraduate Nursing Scholarship, 4(1), 10 pages [Online journal].

Porteous, A., & Tyndall, J. (1994). Yes, I want to walk to the OR. Canadian Operating Room Nursing Journal, 12(2), 15–16, 18–19, 23.

Richard-Hughes, S. (1997). Attitudes and beliefs of Afro-Americans related to organ and tissue donation. International Journal of Trauma Nursing, 3, 119–123.

Rooke, L. (1995a). The concept of space in King's systems framework: Its implications for nursing. In M.A. Frey & C.L. Sieloff (Eds.), Advancing King's systems framework and theory of nursing (pp. 79–96). Thousand Oaks, CA: Sage.

Rooke, L. (1995b). Focusing on King's theory and systems framework in education by using an experiential learning model: A challenge to improve the quality of nursing care. In M.A. Frey & C.L. Sieloff (Eds.), Advancing King's systems framework and theory of nursing (pp. 278–293). Thousand Oaks, CA: Sage.

Rooke, L., & Norberg, A. (1988). Problematic and meaningful situations in nursing interpreted by concepts from King's nursing theory and four additional concepts. Scandinavian Journal of Caring Sciences, 2, 80–87.

Rosendahl, P.B., & Ross, V. (1982). Does your behavior affect your patient's response? Journal of Gerontological Nursing, 8, 572–575.

Rundell, S. (1991). A study of nurse-patient interaction in a high dependency unit. Intensive Care Nursing, 7, 171–178.

Schiffman, R.F., Omar, M.A., & Kaser, M. (1995). Changes in psychosocial characteristics of low income women from pregnancy to postpartum [Abstract]. In 1995 Scientific Sessions Abstracts. Indianapolis: Sigma Theta Tau International.

Scott, L.D. (1998). Perceived needs of parents of critically ill children. Journal of the Society of Pediatric Nurses, 3(1), 4–12.

Sharts Engel, N. (1984). On the vicissitudes of health appraisal. Advances in Nursing Science 7(1), 12–23.

Sharts Engel, N. (1987). Menopausal stage, current life change, attitude toward women's roles and perceived health status among 40- to 55-year-old women. Nursing Research, 36, 353–357.

Sharts-Hopko, N.C. (1995). Using health, personal, and interpersonal system concepts within King's systems framework to explore perceived health status during the menopause transition. In M.A. Frey & C.L. Sieloff (Eds.), Advancing King's systems framework and theory of nursing (pp. 147–160). Thousand Oaks, CA: Sage.

Sieloff, C.L. (1995). Development of a theory of departmental power. In M.A. Frey & C.L. Sieloff (Eds.), Advancing King's systems framework and theory of nursing (pp. 46–65). Thousand Oaks, CA: Sage.

Spees, C.M. (1991). Knowledge of medical terminology among clients and families. Image: Journal of Nursing Scholarship, 23, 225–229.

Suresh, K.N. (2002). The old age problems and care of senior citizens. Nursing Journal of India, 93, 225–226.

Viera, C.S., & Rossi, L. (2000). Nursing diagnoses from NANDA's taxonomy in women with a hospitalized preterm child and King's conceptual system. Revista Latino-Americana de Enfermagem, 8, 110–116. [Spanish; English abstract]

Wicks, M.N. (1995). Family health as derived from King's framework. In M.A. Frey & C.L. Sieloff (Eds.), Advancing King's systems framework and theory of nursing (pp. 97–108). Thousand Oaks, CA: Sage.

Wicks, M.N. (1997). A test of the Wicks family health model in families coping with chronic obstructive pulmonary disease. Journal of Family Nursing, 3, 189–212.

Wilkinson, C.R., & Williams, M. (2002). Strengthening patient-provider relationships. Lippincott's Case Management, 7, 86–102.

Zurakowski, T.L. (2000). The social environment of nursing homes and the health of older residents. Holistic Nursing Practice, 14(4), 12–23.

RESEARCH INSTRUMENTS AND PRACTICE TOOLS

Gonot, P.W. (1986). Family therapy as derived from King's conceptual model. In A.L. Whall, Family therapy theory for nursing. Four approaches (pp. 33–48). Norwalk, CT: Appleton-Century-Crofts.

Hanchett, E.S. (1988). Nursing frameworks and community as client: Bridging the gap. Norwalk, CT: Appleton & Lange.

Killeen, M.B. (1996). Patient-consumer perceptions and responses to professional nursing care: Instrument development. Dissertation Abstracts International, 57, 2479B.

King, I.M. (1981). A theory for nursing: Systems, concepts, process (pp. 164–176). New York: Wiley. [Reissued 1990. Albany, NY: Delmar.]

King, I.M. (1984). Effectiveness of nursing care: Use of a goal-oriented nursing record in end stage renal disease. American Association of Nephrology Nurses and Technicians Journal, 11(2); 11–17, 60.

King, I.M. (1988). Measuring health goal attainment in patients. In C.F. Waltz & O.L. Strickland (Eds.), Measurement of nursing outcomes. Vol. 1. Measuring client outcomes (pp. 108–127). New York: Springer.

King, I.M. (1989). Theories and hypotheses for nursing administration. In B. Henry, M. Di Vincenti, C. Arndt, & A. Marriner (Eds.), Dimensions of nursing administration. Theory, research, education, and practice (pp. 35–45). Boston: Blackwell Scientific.

Norris, D.M., & Frey, M.A. (2002). King's interacting systems framework and theory in nursing practice. In M.R. Alligood & A. Marriner-Tomey (Eds.), Nursing theory: Utilization and application (2nd ed., pp. 173–196). St. Louis: Mosby.

Pfoutz, S.K.K. (1990). Development of an instrument to measure satisfaction with patient care in the postpartum period. Dissertation Abstracts International, 52, 163B.

Rawlins, P.S., Rawlins, T.D., & Horner, M. (1990). Development of the family needs assessment tool. Western Journal of Nursing Research, 12, 201–214.

Sieloff, C.L. (1996). Development of an instrument to estimate the actualized power of a nursing department. Dissertations Abstracts International, 57, 2484B.

Swindale, J.E. (1989). The nurse's role in giving pre-operative information to reduce anxiety in patients admitted to hospital for elective minor surgery. Journal of Advanced Nursing, 14, 899–905.

Young, A., Taylor, S.G., & McLaughlin-Renpenning, K. (2001). Connections: Nursing research, theory, and practice. St. Louis: Mosby.

EDUCATION

Asay, M.K., & Ossler, C.C. (Eds.) (1984). Conceptual models of nursing: Applications in community health nursing: Proceedings of the eighth annual community health nursing conference. Chapel Hill, NC: Department of Public Health Nursing, School of Public Health, University of North Carolina.

Brown, S.T., & Lee, B.T. (1980). Imogene King's conceptual framework: A proposed model for continuing nursing education. Journal of Advanced Nursing, 5, 467–473.

Daubenmire, M.J. (1989). A baccalaureate nursing curriculum based on King's conceptual framework. In J.P. Riehl-Sisca (Ed.), Conceptual models for nursing practice (3rd ed., pp. 167–178). Norwalk, CT: Appleton & Lange.

Daubenmire, M.J., & King, I.M. (1973). Nursing process models: A systems approach. Nursing Outlook, 21, 512–517.

Fromen, D., & Sanderson, H. (1985, August). Application of Imogene King's framework. Paper presented at conference on Nursing Theory in Action, Edmonton, Alberta, Canada. [Cassette recording.]

ADMINISTRATION

Byrne, E., & Schreiber, R. (1989). Concept of the month: Implementing King's conceptual framework at the bedside. Journal of Nursing Administration, 19(2), 28–32.

Byrne-Coker, E., Fradley, T., Harris, J., Tomarchio, D., Chan, V., & Caron, C. (1990). Implementing nursing diagnoses within the context of King's conceptual framework. Nursing Diagnosis, 1, 107–114. [Reprinted in Frey, M.A., & Sieloff, C.L. (Eds.). (1995). Advancing King's systems framework and theory of nursing (pp. 161–175). Thousand Oaks, CA: Sage.]

Byrne-Coker, E., & Schreiber, R. (1990a). Implementing King's conceptual framework at the bedside. In M.E. Parker (Ed.), Nursing theories in practice (pp. 85–102). New York: National League for Nursing.

Byrne-Coker, E., & Schreiber, R. (1990b). King at the bedside. Canadian Nurse, 86(1), 24–26.

Fawcett, J.M., Vaillancourt, V.M., & Watson, C.A. (1995). Integration of King's framework into nursing practice. In M.A. Frey & C.L. Sieloff (Eds.), Advancing King's systems framework and theory of nursing (pp. 176–191). Thousand Oaks, CA: Sage.

Gill, J., Hopwood-Jones, L., Tyndall, J., Gregoroff, S., LeBlanc, P., Lovett, C., Rasco, L., & Ross, A. (1995). Incorporating nursing diagnosis and King's theory in the O.R. documentation. Canadian Operating Room Nursing Journal, 13(1), 10–14.

Jones, S., Clark, V.B., Merker, A., & Palau, D. (1995). Changing behaviors: Nurse educators and clinical nurse specialists design a discharge planning program. Journal of Nursing Staff Development, 11, 291–295.

King, I.M. (1996). The theory of goal attainment in research and practice. Nursing Science Quarterly, 9, 61–66.

LaFontaine, P. (1989). Alleviating patient's apprehensions and anxieties. Gastroenterology Nursing, 11, 256–257.

Messmer, P.R. (1992). Implementing theory based nursing practice. Florida Nurse, 40(3), 8.

Schreiber, R. (1991). Psychiatric assessment—a la King. Nursing Management, 22(5), 90–94.

Sowell, R.L., & Fuszard, B. (1989). Inpatient nursing case management as a strategy for rural hospitals: A case study. Journal of Rural Health, 5, 201–205.

Sowell, R.L., & Lowenstein, A. (1994). King's theory as a framework for quality: Linking theory to practice. Nursing Connections, 7(2), 19–31.

Sowell, R.L., & Meadows, T.M. (1994). An integrated case management model: Developing standards, evaluation, and outcome criteria. Nursing Administration Quarterly, 18(2), 53–64.

West, P. (1991). Theory implementation: A challenging journey. Canadian Journal of Nursing Administration, 4(1), 29–30.

PRACTICE

Alligood, M.R. (1995). Theory of goal attainment: Application to adult orthopedic nursing. In M.A. Frey & C.L. Sieloff (Eds.), Advancing King's systems framework and theory of nursing (pp. 209–222). Thousand Oaks, CA: Sage.

Batra, C. (1996). Nursing theory and nursing process in the community. In J.M. Cookfair (Ed.), Nursing care in the community (2nd ed., pp. 85–124). St. Louis: Mosby.

Benedict, M., & Frey, M.A. (1995). Theory-based practice in the emergency department. In M.A. Frey & C.L. Sieloff (Eds.), Advancing King's systems framework and theory of nursing (pp. 317–324). Thousand Oaks, CA: Sage.

Brown, P., & Yantis, J. (1996). Personal space intrusion and PTSD. Journal of Psychosocial Nursing and Mental Health Services, 34(7), 23–28.

Calladine, M.L. (1996). Nursing process for health promotion using King's theory. Journal of Community Health Nursing, 13, 51–57.

Davis, D.C. (1987). A conceptual framework for infertility. Journal of Obstetric, Gynecologic, and Neonatal Nursing, 16, 30–35.

DeHowitt, M.C. (1992). King's conceptual model and individual psychotherapy. Perspectives in Psychiatric Care, 28(4), 11–14.

Fawcett, J.M., Vaillancourt, V.M., & Watson, C.A. (1995). Integration of King's framework into nursing practice. In M.A. Frey & C.L. Sieloff (Eds.), Advancing King's systems framework and theory of nursing (pp. 176–191). Thousand Oaks, CA: Sage.

Frey, M.A., & Norris, D. (1997). King's systems framework and theory in nursing practice. In M.R. Alligood & A. Marriner-Tomey (Eds.), Nursing theory: Utilization and application (pp. 71–88). St. Louis: Mosby.

Gonot, P.W. (1986). Family therapy as derived from King's conceptual model. In A.L. Whall (Ed.), Family therapy theory for nursing. Four approaches (pp. 33–48). Norwalk, CT: Appleton-Century-Crofts.

Hanchett, E.S. (1988). Nursing frameworks and community as client: Bridging the gap. Norwalk, CT: Appleton & Lange.

Heggie, M., & Gangar, E. (1992). A nursing model for menopause clinics. Nursing Standard, 6(21), 32–34.

Hughes, M.M. (1983). Nursing theories and emergency nursing. Journal of Emergency Nursing, 9, 95–97.

Husband, A. (1988). Application of King's theory of nursing to the care of the adult with diabetes. Journal of Advanced Nursing, 13, 484–488.

Jonas, C.M. (1987). King's goal attainment theory: Use in gerontological nursing practice. Perspectives, 11(4), 9–12.

Kemppainen, J.K. (1990). Imogene King's theory: A nursing case study of a psychotic client with human immunodeficiency virus infection. Archives of Psychiatric Nursing, 4, 384–388.

King, I.M. (1981). A theory for nursing: Systems, concepts, process (pp. 169–176). New York: Wiley. [Reissued 1990. Albany, NY: Delmar.]

King, I.M. (1983a). The family coping with a medical illness. Analysis and application of King's theory of goal attainment. In I.W. Clements & F.B. Roberts (Eds.), Family health: A theoretical approach to nursing care (pp. 383–385). New York: Wiley.

King, I.M. (1983b). The family with an elderly member. Analysis and application of King's theory of goal attainment. In I.W. Clements & F.B. Roberts (Eds.), Family health: A theoretical approach to nursing care (pp. 341–345). New York: Wiley.

King, I.M. (1984). Effectiveness of nursing care: Use of a goal-oriented nursing record in end stage renal disease. American Association of Nephrology Nurses and Technicians Journal, 11(2); 11–17, 60.

King, I.M. (1986). King's theory of goal attainment. In P. Winstead-Fry (Ed.), Case studies in nursing theory (pp. 197–213). New York: National League for Nursing.

Kohler, P. (1988). Model of shared control. Journal of Gerontological Nursing, 14(7), 21–25.

Laben, J.K., Dodd, D., & Sneed, L. (1991). King's theory of goal attainment applied in group therapy for inpatient juvenile sexual offenders, maximum security state offenders, and community parolees, using visual aids. Issues in Mental Health Nursing, 12(1), 51–64.

Laben, J.K., Sneed, L.D., & Seidel, S.L. (1995). Goal attainment in short-term group psychotherapy settings: Clinical implications for practice. In M.A. Frey & C.L. Sieloff (Eds.), Advancing King's systems framework and theory of nursing (pp. 261–277). Thousand Oaks, CA: Sage.

LaFontaine, P. (1989). Alleviating patient's apprehensions and anxieties. Gastroenterology Nursing, 11, 256–257.

Lucas, J. (1998). Chronic venous leg ulcers: One client's experience. Whitireia Nursing Journal, 5, 16–24.

McKinney, N, & Frank, D.I. (1998). Nursing assessment of adult females who are alcohol dependent and victims of sexual abuse. Clinical Excellence for Nurse Practitioners, 2, 152–158.

Messner, R., & Smith, M.N. (1986). Neurofibromatosis: Relinquishing the masks; a quest for quality of life. Journal of Advanced Nursing, 11, 459–464.

Norgan, G.H., Ettipio, A.M., & Lasome, C.E.M. (1995). A program plan addressing carpal tunnel syndrome: The utility of King's goal attainment theory. American Association of Occupational Health Nurses Journal, 43, 407–411.

Norris, D.M., & Frey, M.A. (2002). King's interacting systems framework and theory in nursing practice. In M.R. Alligood & A. Marriner-Tomey (Eds.), Nursing theory: Utilization and application (2nd ed., pp. 173–196). St. Louis: Mosby.

Norris, D.M., & Hoyer, P.J. (1993). Dynamism in practice: Parenting within King's framework. Nursing Science Quarterly, 6, 79–85.

Porter, H.B. (1991). A theory of goal attainment (King 1981) and ambulatory care oncology nursing; An introduction. Canadian Oncology Nursing Journal, 1, 124–126.

Sirles, A.T., & Selleck, C.S. (1989). Cardiac disease and the family: Impact, assessment, and implications. Journal of Cardiovascular Nursing, 3(2), 23–32.

Smith, M.C. (1988). King's theory in practice. Nursing Science Quarterly, 1, 145–146.

Swindale, J.E. (1989). The nurse's role in giving pre-operative information to reduce anxiety in patients admitted to hospital for elective minor surgery. Journal of Advanced Nursing, 14, 899–905.

Temple, A., & Fawdry, K. (1992). King's theory of goal attainment. Resolving filial caregiver role strain. Journal of Gerontological Nursing, 18(3), 11–15.

Woods, E.C. (1994). King's theory in practice with elders. Nursing Science Quarterly, 7, 65–69.

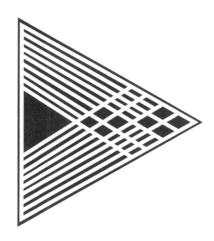

Chapter **6**

Levine's Conservation Model

Myra E. Levine presented the rudiments of the Conservation Model in her 1966a article, "Adaptation and Assessment: A Rationale for Nursing Intervention." Additional elements of the model were presented in two other articles, "The Four Conservation Principles of Nursing" (Levine, 1967), and "The Pursuit of Wholeness" (Levine, 1969b). A comprehensive discussion of the Conservation Model was presented in the first edition (1969a) and the second edition (1973) of Levine's book, *Introduction to Clinical Nursing*. Other features of the model were given in Levine's 1971 publication, "Holistic Nursing," and her presentations at conferences (Levine, 1978a, 1984a, 1986), as well as her responses to a videotaped interview (Levine, 1987). More recent explications of the Conservation Model are Levine's 1989b, 1990, and 1991 book chapters and her last publication, a 1996 journal article entitled "The Conservation Principles: A Retrospective." Levine (personal communication, July 15, 1987) regarded the 1989b chapter as "a significant restatement of the model ... a natural evolutionary statement of how the basic concepts are related to each other." Further refinements are evident in the 1990 and 1991 book chapters, and some clarification of the conservation principles is evident in the 1996 journal article. Myra Levine died on March 20, 1996.

Overview

Levine's work focuses on conservation of human beings' wholeness. Her work clearly fits the definition of a conceptual model of nursing used in this book. Moreover, Levine (1985, 1987) noted that her work is "a generalization" of nursing and agreed that it is indeed a conceptual model.

The concepts of Levine's Conservation Model and their dimensions are listed here, along with the goal of nursing and the components of her practice methodology. The concepts, their dimensions, and the methodology components are defined and described, and the goal of nursing is discussed in detail later in this chapter.

Key Terms

HUMAN BEINGS
HOLISTIC BEING
    System of Systems
    Wholeness
    Integrity
ENVIRONMENT
INTERNAL ENVIRONMENT
    Homeostasis
    Homeorrhesis
EXTERNAL ENVIRONMENT
    Perceptual Environment
    Operational Environment
    Conceptual Environment

HUMAN BEINGS AND ENVIRONMENT	NURSING
ADAPTATION	HUMAN INTERACTION
Historicity	GOAL OF NURSING
Specificity	Promotion of Wholeness for All People,
Redundancy	Well or Sick
ORGANISMIC RESPONSES	PRACTICE METHODOLOGY: NURSING PROCESS
Fight or Flight Response	AS CONSERVATION
Inflammatory-Immune Response	*Trophicognosis*
Stress Response	*Observation*
Perceptual Awareness	*Provocative Facts*
Basic Orienting System	*Testable Hypothesis*
Visual System	Intervention/Action
Auditory System	*Therapeutic Nursing Intervention*
Haptic System	*Supportive Nursing Intervention*
Taste-Smell System	*Principle of Conservation of Energy*
CONSERVATION	*Principle of Conservation of Structural*
Principle of Conservation of Energy	*Integrity*
Principle of Conservation of Structural	*Principle of Conservation of Personal*
Integrity	*Integrity*
Principle of Conservation of Personal Integrity	*Principle of Conservation of Social*
Principle of Conservation of Social Integrity	*Integrity*
HEALTH	Evaluation of Intervention/Action
CHANGE	THEORY OF THERAPEUTIC INTENTION
HEALTH	THEORY OF REDUNDANCY
DISEASE	THEORY OF CONSERVATION

 ## ANALYSIS OF LEVINE'S CONSERVATION MODEL

This section presents an analysis of Levine's Conservation Model. The analysis draws from several of Levine's publications, including three book chapters, "The Conservation Principles of Nursing: Twenty Years Later" (Levine, 1989b), "Conservation and Integrity" (Levine, 1990), and "The Conservation Principles: A Model for Health" (Levine, 1991), as well as her final publication, the 1996 journal article, "The Conservation Principles: A Retrospective."

ORIGINS OF THE NURSING MODEL

Historical Evolution and Motivation

Levine (1969a) commented that she was motivated to develop the Conservation Model as a starting point for the theory development needed to provide the "whys" of nursing activities. She stated, "The serious study of any discipline requires a theoretical baseline which gives it substance and meaning" (p. ix). Although Levine did not underestimate the importance of technical skills, she pointed out that "nursing … remain[s] characterized by a rigid dependence on procedures. The 'why' is not entirely neglected, but it is often applied after the fact, as if such jus-

tification invested the procedure with a special scientific holiness. Nurses cherish 'applied science principles' in an era when nursing is deeply involved in scientific research, but even the lessons learned from nurse researchers are too often ignored" (p. vii).

Levine's attention to the theoretical basis for nurses' actions came at a time when nursing was beginning to recognize the need for substantive knowledge (Newman, 1972). A major feature of her work is the explication of the scientific concepts underlying nursing processes. Indeed, Levine (1969a) deliberately set out to provide "an intellectual framework for analysis and understanding of the scientific nature of nursing activity" (p. viii).

Levine (1988b) maintained that the universal importance of conservation made it essential knowledge about human life that must be included in the nursing curriculum. She went on to explain:

> The development of the four conservation principles grew naturally out of my desire to organize nursing knowledge so that the student would have a strong organizing basis for interpreting all kinds of nursing situations. It was easy to work with, and in its simplicity it seemed to open many channels of thinking that had not been obvious before. … I adopted it as the basis for a textbook in beginning nursing, *Introduction to Clinical Nursing*. I never dreamed that others would see in it a new [conceptual model of] nursing. I was certain it would educate good nurses. That is all I ever wanted to do. (p. 227)

Philosophical Claims

Levine presented the philosophical claims undergirding the Conservation Model in the form of a value system, assumptions about human beings and nursing, and beliefs about nursing. Those philosophical claims are listed here. Review of Levine's assumptions about human beings indicates that she placed human beings within the context of their surroundings. Furthermore, Levine's values extend to her very deliberate choice of the term "patient" to describe the human being in need of nursing.

Levine's Value System

- The two moral imperatives of Western democratic societies are the sanctity of life and the prevention or alleviation of suffering (Levine, 1989a, 1989d).
- The fundamental belief of the sanctity of life provides the structure upon which all moral systems are based (Levine, 1989a, p. 125).
- All the efforts of the healing sciences are founded on the holiness and wholeness of the human being, and the special injunction this places on the caregiver to bring dignity and compassion to the tasks of caring for another person. … The sanctity of life … is the essence of the respectful relationship that one person must have for another. It is never more important than when a nurse-patient dyad is created whereby one individual enters dependency, willing or not, and places his trust in another person. … Every moment of a nurse-patient interaction requires recognition of the selfhood, the uniqueness of each individual: nurse and patient. … The nurse functions in the role of caregiver and assumes an additional moral burden to recognize, value, and defend the dependency of the patient (Levine, 1989a, p. 125).
- The fundamental moral responsibility of patient care is the limitation and relief of suffering (Levine, 1989c, pp. 4–5).
- The health care system is dedicated to the task of preventing or alleviating suffering. It is the individual who enters "patienthood" who is the sufferer. It is the moral duty of the nurse to confront the suffering individual and bring all the skills of hand, heart, and mind to alleviate it. It is equally binding that once the conditions of patienthood have been successfully overcome, the individual is free of his dependent role. He ceases to be a patient. His privacy is restored (Levine, 1989a, p. 126).
- The ultimate freedom of the individual is to make decisions. The patient's freedom must prohibit the imposition of the nurse's values into his decisions for his care (Levine, 1989a, p. 126).
- The word "patient" has been deliberately used whenever the care recipient [is] discussed [in my publications].

The widespread use of the substitute term "client" was just as deliberately excluded even though many nurses use it habitually. Its original purpose, to add some professional elegance to nursing practice, does not justify the moral failure it reflects. The word client comes from the Latin root that means "follower." That idea is a pure derivative of the paternalistic-parentalistic relationship and ought to be forbidden in nursing on moral grounds. The word "patient" comes from the Latin word for "suffering." Job, for example, is often credited with patience, not because he was willing to wait without complaint until his ordeal was over, but because he was suffering. He was not a quiescent sufferer; he argued, complained, lamented, and despised his undeserved misfortune (Levine, 1989a, p. 126).

- The labeling of persons as clients reinforces … dependency because a client is a follower. The provenance of the word patient is sufferer. It is the condition of suffering that makes it possible to set independence aside and accept the services of another person (Levine, 1990, p. 199).
- It is patients whose predicament of need sets the standards of ethical responsibility (Levine, 1989c, p. 5).
- It is the challenge of the nurse to provide the individual with appropriate care without losing sight of the individual's integrity, to honor the trust that the patient has placed in the nurse, and to encourage the participation of the individual in his or her own welfare. The patient comes in trust and dependence only for as long as the services of the nurse are needed. The nurse's goal is always to impart knowledge and strength so that the individual can resume a private life—no longer a patient, no longer dependent (Levine, 1990, p. 199).
- There are four guidelines for the personal responsibility that is the particular province of the caregivers, privileges of behavior that have been awarded by the community that licenses them to practice (Levine, 1989d, p. 88).
- Persons who require [care] enter with a contract of trust. They place their well being, and often their lives in the hands of caregivers. To respect that trust by the most vigorous effort is a moral responsibility (Levine, 1989d, pp. 88–89).
- It is not the task of the practitioner … to evaluate the social worth of the patient. Judgments as to the quality of life of individual patients are inappropriate and unsupportable and should never be used as a rationale for withholding or withdrawing essential care (Levine, 1989d, p. 89).
- The decisions for introducing treatments should be based (as they have been historically) on the physician's evaluation of the patient's condition and the consequent appropriate interventions. The interference of third party payers in which therapeutic decisions are dictated

by cost or any other extraneous factors is morally repugnant (Levine, 1989d, p. 89).

- Life or death decisions are not properly those of caregivers and never should be left to those whose mission is to protect life and relieve suffering. Decisions to use extraordinary means of sustaining life processes should be made in advance of the actual events by the informed wisdom of the physician whenever possible. The caregivers—physicians and nurses—should bring all their skills to bear to alleviate suffering, but that does not include hastening the death of another human being (Levine, 1989d, p. 89).
- The wholeness which is part of our awareness of ourselves is shared best with others when no act diminishes another person, and no moment of indifference leaves him with less of himself. Every moment of moral injustice extracts a price from both patient and nurse, just as every moment of moral responsibility gives each strength to grow in his wholeness (Levine, 1977, p. 849).
- True conservation demands that the nurse accept the patient the way he is (Levine, 1967, p. 55).
- Nursing intervention must deal with the rights and privileges of the individual in tangible ways. … The emphasis on patient teaching recognizes the individual's right to be assisted in understanding the implications of his disease, his treatment, and his care. He must also be assured that his medical and social problems will remain privileged and confidential (Levine, 1967, p. 54).

Assumptions about Human Beings

- Living things of every kind share the earth, and the multitude of environmental habitats exist in a vital, changing harmony. To understand the individual, the place and time of his or her living must also be understood (Levine, 1990, p. 196).
- The individual cannot be understood outside of the context of a place and time. The individual cannot be separated from the influence of everything that is happening around him or her, nor indeed, from all those events—remembered and forgotten—which have created the individual as he or she is at this precise moment. Nursing can succeed only when it recognizes that the person is not summarized by the immediate present, but is burdened by a lifetime of experience—recorded not only on the tissues of the body, but on the spirit and mind as well (Levine, 1990, p. 197).
- The human being responds to the forces in his environment in a singular yet integrated fashion (Levine, 1973, p. 6).
- Human beings are sentient, thinking, future-oriented and past-aware individuals (Levine, 1989b, p. 326).
- The human being is a sentient being, and the ability to

interact with the environment seems ineluctably tied to his sensory organs (Levine, 1973, p. 446).

Assumptions about Nursing

- A basic assumption of the Conservation Model is that nursing intervention is a conservation activity (Levine, 1973).
- The multidimensional unity of life must be conserved (Levine, 1973, p. 6).
- The holistic nature of the human response to the environment provides the rationale for substantive principles of nursing. A principle is a fundamental concept that forms the basis for a chain of reasoning. Formulated on a broad base, it establishes the relationships between apparently otherwise unrelated facts. Nursing principles are fundamental assumptions which provide a unifying structure for understanding a wide variety of nursing activities. Nursing principles are all "conservation" principles (Levine, 1973, p. 13).

Beliefs about Nursing

- Emphasizing the integrity of the patient brings integrity to the nursing profession and the individual nurse. Bringing together the best science and the most devoted humanism is the ultimate aim of nursing. In finding, valuing, and cherishing the integrity of the patient, the nurse's integrity is acknowledged and rewarded (Levine, 1990, p. 200).
- All nursing actions are moral statements. … Expectations [regarding care] must be realistic. Goals that are impossible are more than merely frustrating; they are also unethical. Nurses cannot promise good health and long life to everyone, and it is cruel to place the onus of failure on the individual. Nurses have long been expert at celebrating small victories with patients. It may be, finally, that such moments most truly reflect the moral burden of nursing practice. Moral judgments must be reserved and patients must be accepted as they are—for what they are—with dignity and honesty (Levine, 1989c, p. 6).

Strategies for Knowledge Development

Levine's use of knowledge from a variety of adjunctive disciplines indicates that she used a deductive approach to develop the Conservation Model. That approach is further illustrated in Levine's (1969a) comment that "the essential science concepts develop the rationale [for nursing actions], using ideas from all areas of knowledge that contribute to the development of the nursing process in the specific area of the model" (p. viii).

Influences from Other Scholars

Levine is known for her careful citations of the many scholars and scientists from nursing and adjunctive disciplines whose work influenced her thinking. Levine (personal communication, February 2, 1982) stated that she "did not invent the notion of Conservation—I simply live in a natural world where it is a characteristic of experience." Indeed, Levine (1988b, 1991, 1996) pointed out that conservation is a natural law of science and cited Feynman (1965), who described conservation "as one of the 'great general principles [which] all detailed laws ... seem to follow' [p. 59]" (Levine, 1991, p. 3). She went on to explain that "no sophisticated theorizing can displace the fundamental importance of natural law" (p. 3).

Levine (1990) commented that her use of concepts and theories from adjunctive disciplines "brings coherence to nursing problems, encouraging freedom of exploration in practice, research, and teaching without losing sight of the integrity of either the practitioner or the patient" (p. 196). She explicitly acknowledged the contributions to her thinking made by the work of Bates (1967), Beland (1971), Bernard (1865/1957), Cannon (1939), Cohen (1968), Dubos (1961, 1965), Erikson (1964, 1968), Gibson (1966), Goldstein (1963), Hall (1959, 1966), Hochachka and Somero (1984), Margulis (1971), Sacks (1985), Selye (1956), Sherrington (1906), Tillich (1961), Waddington (1968), and Wiener (1954). Moreover, Levine (1996) credited Gaylin for pointing out the distinction between the terms "patient" and "client" but, surprisingly, did not provide a citation for that work.

Levine (personal communication, February 2, 1982) disclaimed "even with some vigor," however, any dependence on Maslow and other more recent authors whose works focus on holism. Moreover, she decried Maslow's influence on nursing education (Levine, 1991).

Furthermore, Levine (1992) identified parallels between the Conservation Model and Nightingale's (1859) ideas about observation, environment, and nursing. She explained, "I quoted [Nightingale's] words on 'observation' in my text (Levine, 1973), and emphasized, as I believe she did, that observation was a guardian activity" (p. 41). Nightingale's emphasis on environment influenced Levine in that "the Conservation Model insists that the person can only be understood in the context of environment" (p. 41).

Levine (1992) went on to discuss the link between Nightingale and the Conservation Model concerning nursing:

> The nursing that Nightingale describes fits comfortably into the Conservation principles. She details the parameters of the conservation of energy. ... Although her physiology is very limited, Nightingale recognizes the importance of conservation of structural integrity. ... Those injunctions in *Notes on*

Nursing that describe the experience of the patient seem very personal, even though her own invalidism had hardly begun. She lists many of the behaviors basic to the personal integrity of the patient and the nurse. ... *Notes on Nursing* was directed at the social integrity, health, and well-being of the English people. (pp. 41–42)

World View

The Conservation Model clearly reflects the *reciprocal interaction* world view. Levine has always emphasized the wholeness of the human being, but she did not always embrace holism. Indeed, as she explained:

> When the first edition of *Introduction to Clinical Nursing* was published in 1969, I decided against using "holistic" in favor of "organismic," largely because the term "holistic" had been appropriated by pseudoscientists endowing it with the mythology of transcendentalism. I used holism in the second edition in 1973 because I realized it was too important to be abandoned to the mystics. (Levine, 1996, p. 39)

The features of the reciprocal interaction world view that are evident in Levine's Conservation Model are:

- The Conservation Model focuses on human beings as holistic beings who constantly strive to preserve wholeness and integrity (Levine, 1973, 1989a, 1990, 1991, 1996).
- Nursing intervention, traditionally directed by procedures or manifestations of disease symptoms, needs new directions if the holistic approach is to be utilized. The individual must be recognized in his wholeness, and the powerful influence of adaptation recognized as a dynamic and ever-present factor in evaluating his care. Instead of listing "needs" or "symptoms," it should be possible to identify for each individual the patterns of his adaptive response, and to tailor intervention to enhance their effectiveness (Levine, 1971, pp. 257–258).
- All nursing care is focused on man and the complexity of his relationships with his environment, both internal and external, and common experience emphasizes that every response to every environmental stimulus results from the integrated and unified nature of the human organism. In other words, every response is an organismic one—no other kind is possible—and every adaptive change is accomplished by the entire individual (Levine, 1967, p. 46).
- Human beings are regarded as active participants in interactions with the environment.
- The individual can ... never be passive. He is an active participant in his environment, not only altering it by his presence but also actively and constantly seeking information from it (Levine, 1969b, p. 96).
- The person is an active participant, exploring, seeking,

and testing understanding of the world he or she inhabits (Levine, 1992, p. 41).

- The perceptual systems provide information to the individual; usually this is knowledge sought by the individual (Levine, 1973, p. 450).
- Persistence is reflected in Levine's emphasis on homeostasis and conservation.
- Homeostasis is "a state of energy-sparing" (Levine, 1989b, p. 329); it even "might be called the state of conservation" (p. 329). The essence of conservation, in turn, is use of responses "that cost the least to the individual in expense of effort and demand on his or her well-being" (p. 329).
- Change also is evident in the content of the Conservation Model.
- Change is the essence of life, and it is unceasing as long as life goes on. ... here] Change is characteristic of life (Levine, 1973, p. 10).
- Change is characteristic of life, and adaptation is the method of change. The organism retains its integrity in both the internal and external environment through its adaptive capability. Adaptation is the process of change whereby the individual retains his integrity within the realities of his environments (Levine, 1973, pp. 10–11).

In keeping with the reciprocal interaction world view, the Conservation Model incorporates elements of both persistence and change. Despite the pervasiveness of change in a human being's life, however, conservation—and hence persistence—appear to be predominant. Apparently, Levine regarded the many changes that must occur as human beings face environmental challenges as necessary for survival. Conservation facilitates and maintains the patterns and routines of human behavior, and adaptive changes represent the invention of new routines to avoid extinction.

UNIQUE FOCUS OF THE NURSING MODEL

The unique focus of the Conservation Model is the conservation of the human being's wholeness (Levine, 1969b, 1973, 1989a, 1990, 1991). More specifically, the focus of the Conservation Model is on adaptation as the process by which human beings maintain their wholeness or integrity. Thus, the model emphasizes the effectiveness of human beings' adaptations (Levine, 1969b, 1973, 1989a, 1990, 1991, 1996).

Furthermore, the Conservation Model focuses the nurse's attention on human beings and the complexity of their relationships with the internal and external environments (Levine, 1969b, 1973, 1989a, 1990, 1991, 1996). The Conservation Model also emphasizes the nurse's responsibility for conservation of the patient's energy, as well as his

or her structural, personal, and social integrity (Levine, 1969b, 1973, 1989a, 1990, 1991, 1996).

Category of Knowledge

At one time, Levine (cited in Riehl-Sisca, 1989) apparently regarded the Conservation Model as an interaction model, and Riehl-Sisca (1989) classified it as such. The content of the model does not, however, address any of the characteristics of that category as described in Chapter 1 of this book. Certainly, the Conservation Model deals with the interaction between human beings and environment, but that is not the same as the symbolic interactionism emphasis of the interaction category of knowledge. When asked about the interaction classification, Levine (personal communication, August 13, 1987) agreed that her conceptual model does not reflect symbolic interactionism. She went on to say that hers is "an adaptation model."

Meleis (1997) regards the Conservation Model as a prominent example of the outcome category of models. She also placed the Conservation Model in her nursing therapeutics category, noting that Levine's work focuses on nursing activities and actions designed to care for people. Marriner-Tomey (1989) placed the Conservation Model within her energy fields category. Barnum (1998) classified the Conservation Model in the conservation category. Close examination of the content of the Conservation Model indicates that the systems category is the most appropriate classification. The appropriateness of the systems category classification is evident in the comparison of the Conservation Model content with the characteristics of the systems category of knowledge, as can be seen here:

- System: The human being, or organism, is a system.
- Integration of Parts: The parts are the organism's systems. The total life process of the entire organism is dependent upon the inter-relatedness of its component systems. In fact, the organism is a system of systems (Levine, 1973, pp. 8–9). Human life must be described in the language of "wholes" ... perceiving the "wholes" depends upon recognizing the organization and interdependence of observable phenomena (Levine, 1971, p. 255).
- Environment: The environment is viewed as both internal and external. However, "The person cannot be described apart from the specific environment in which he or she is found" (Levine, 1989b, p. 325).
- Open System: The idea of "wholeness" is associated with the idea of the open system (Levine, 1973). A whole is an open system (Levine, 1973). The unceasing interaction of the individual organism with its environments does represent an "open and fluid" system (Erikson, 1968, cited in Levine, 1973, p. 11).

- Boundary: The characteristic of boundary is explicitly addressed in the Conservation Model in the discussion of individual territoriality. "Every individual requires space, and both the establishment of his personal boundaries and their defense are essential components of his behavior" (Levine, 1973, p. 459). Boundary is related to the idea of territorial behavior, with its identification of the intimate, personal distance, social distance, and public distance zones maintained between people (Hall, 1966, cited in Levine, 1973).

- Tension, Stress, Strain, and Conflicts: The source of threats to human beings' wholeness or integrity is environmental challenge. Apparently, challenges may come from the internal or external environment. "The exquisite internal balance responds constantly to the external forces. ... There is an intimate relationship between the internal and the external environments, much of it vividly understood in recent years by research in physiological periodicity and the circadian cycles" (Levine, 1973, p. 8).

- Equilibrium and Steady State: Levine (1973) referred to a steady state when she discussed homeorrhesis, which denotes "a stabilized flow, rather than a static state" (p. 7). "The concept of stabilized flow more accurately reflects the reality of daily change as well as the alterations in physiological activity that characterize the processes of growth and development" (Levine, 1973, pp. 7–8). Levine (personal communication, August 13, 1987) indicated that homeostasis is the appropriate view of the internal environment because it captures the notion of the congruence of human beings with the environment. Homeostasis is a state that "provides the necessary baselines for a multitude of synchronized physiological and psychological factors" rather than a system of balance and quiescence (Levine, 1989b, p. 329).

- Feedback: Feedback is a method of controlling a system by reinserting into it the results of past performances (Wiener, 1954, as cited in Levine, 1996, p. 39). Positive feedback in the internal environment is manifested when pathological processes occur and can be responsible for pathology (Levine, 1973, 1989b). Negative feedback is associated with autoregulation of physiological systems (Levine, 1973, 1989b). "Negative feedbacks provide the mechanisms for successful adaptation. ... While there are hundreds of negative feedbacks in every living system—human and otherwise—they are not simple linear relationships, nor are they necessarily distinct and sequential. They are, instead, interactive. They have been compared to a cascade—the initial series of changes is still present when the final changes have begun" (Levine, 1996, p. 39). "Negative feedbacks provide the living system with the most economic, most energy-sparing systems. [They] are fundamental in assuring the viability of the individual." (Levine, 1996, p. 39)

Although Levine (1989b) discussed physiologic and behavioral responses, she regarded those responses as "one and the same—not merely parallel and not merely simultaneous—but essential portions of the same activity" (p. 330). Moreover, although she identified four principles of conservation, she views them as joined, not isolated or separate.

CONTENT OF THE NURSING MODEL

Concepts

The metaparadigm concepts of human beings, environment, health, and nursing are reflected in the concepts of the Conservation Model. Each conceptual model concept is classified here according to its metaparadigm forerunner.

The metaparadigm concept of human beings is represented by the Conservation Model concept of **HOLISTIC BEING**, which has three dimensions—**System of Systems, Wholeness**, and **Integrity**. The metaparadigm concept of environment is represented by the Conservation Model concepts of **INTERNAL ENVIRONMENT** and **EXTERNAL ENVIRONMENT**. The concept of **INTERNAL ENVIRONMENT** has two dimensions—**Homeostasis** and **Homeorrhesis**. The concept of **EXTERNAL ENVIRONMENT** has three dimensions—**Perceptual Environment, Operational Environment**, and **Conceptual Environment**.

The integral relationship between the metaparadigm concepts of human beings and environment is central to the Conservation Model. The Conservation Model concepts of **ADAPTATION, ORGANISMIC RESPONSES**, and **CONSERVATION** best represent that integral relation. The concept of **ADAPTATION** has three dimensions—**Historicity, Specificity**, and **Redundancy**. The concept of **ORGANISMIC RESPONSES** has four dimensions—**Fight or Flight Response, Inflammatory-Immune Response, Stress Response**, and **Perceptual Awareness**. The dimension of **Perceptual Awareness** itself has five subdimensions—*Basic Orienting System, Visual System, Auditory System, Haptic System*, and *Taste-Smell System*. The concept of **CONSERVATION** has four dimensions—**Conservation of Energy, Conservation of Structural Integrity, Conservation of Personal Integrity**, and **Conservation of Social Integrity**.

The metaparadigm concept of health is represented by the Conservation Model concepts of **CHANGE, HEALTH**, and **DISEASE**, each of which is unidimensional. The metaparadigm concept of nursing is represented by the Conservation Model concept of **HUMAN INTERACTION**, which also is unidimensional.

Nonrelational Propositions

The definitions of the concepts of the Conservation Model are given here. Those constitutive definitions are the non-relational propositions of this nursing model.

HOLISTIC BEING

• The individual is a holistic being (Levine, 1973, 1996).

The concept of **Holistic Being** encompasses three dimensions—System of Systems, Wholeness, and Integrity.

• **System of Systems:** The organism is a system of systems (Levine, 1973, pp. 8–9). The total life process of the entire organism is dependent upon the inter-relatedness of its component systems (Levine, 1973, p. 8).
• **Wholeness:** Wholeness emphasizes a sound, organic, progressive mutuality between diversified functions and parts within an entirety, the boundaries of which are fluid and open (Erikson, 1968, as cited in Levine, 1996, p. 39). Wholeness means that the boundaries between parts are open and fluid, such that the parts "have a yearning for each other" (Erikson, 1968, as cited in Levine, 1978a). Wholeness expresses the organization of all the contributing parts of the organism (Levine, 1973, p. 9). The experience of wholeness is the foundation of all human enterprise (Levine, 1991, p. 3). We know we are whole. Everything in our life experience reinforces our confidence in that certainty (Levine, 1996, p. 39).
Citing Erikson's (1964) definition of wholeness, Levine (1969b) stated, "From the moment of birth until the instant of death, every individual cherishes and defends his 'wholeness'" (p. 93). But wholeness, according to Levine (1989b), "can be used as a starting point of analysis only if it can be converted into manageable parts … but none of the isolated aspects of wholeness can have meaning outside of the context within which the individual experiences his or her life. … Only then are the 'open and fluid' boundaries established" (pp. 325–326).
• **Integrity:** Integrity is the equivalent of wholeness. Integrity is having the freedom to choose: to move without constraint, as slowly or as swiftly as desired, and to exercise decisions on all matters—trivial and otherwise—without apology, indebtedness, or guilt. Integrity is the experience of life, the sensations of the body and its limbs, the sensory recording of every place and time on the mind and in the spirit (Levine, 1990, p. 193).

INTERNAL ENVIRONMENT

• The "milieu interne"—the primordial seas, captured within the integument of the human body and providing the organism with a tightly regulated solution of sub-stances essential to its continuing well-being (Levine, 1973, p. 7).
• The integrated response of the individual aris[es] from the internal environment (Levine, 1973, p. 12).

Levine traced the development of the concept of **Internal Environment** from Claude Bernard's (1865/1957) mid-nineteenth century notion of milieu interne to Cannon's (1939) formulation of homeostasis and finally to Waddington's (1968) idea of homeorrhesis. More specifically, Levine (1973) explained:

> Man carried the essentials with him, safely packaged inside his skin. But it was apparent to Bernard, and to the army of investigators who followed him, that the internal environment [the milieu interne] was susceptible to constant change. In 1915, Walter Cannon … coined the word "homeostasis" (*homeo*, equal, and *stasis*, condition) to describe the remarkable equilibrium that was maintained in the internal environment in the face of constant change. … The concept of the "stable state," or homeostasis, has been extremely valuable in understanding the process of health and illness. But as so often happens, the enlargement of understanding that came from this concept suggests that even this important idea represents an oversimplification of reality. … Waddington has suggested that the process be called homeor[r]hesis (*homeo*, stable; *rhesis*, flow), a stabilized flow rather than a static state. (p. 7)

The concept of **Internal Environment** encompasses two dimensions—Homeostasis and Homeorrhesis (Levine, 1991).

• **Homeostasis:** A stable state (Levine, 1991, p. 5). A state of energy-sparing that also provides the necessary baselines for a multitude of synchronized physiological and psychological factors (Levine, 1989b, p. 329). Homeostasis reflects congruence of human beings with the environment (Levine, personal communication, August 13, 1987).
• **Homeorrhesis:** A stabilized flow (Levine, 1973, p. 7). Homeor[r]hesis emphasizes the fluidity of change within a space-time continuum and more nearly describes the remarkable patterns of adaptation which permit the individual's body to sustain its well-being within the vast changes which encroach upon it from the environment (Levine, 1973, p. 7).

The **Internal Environment** is subject to continuous change from the challenges of the **External Environment**, which always are a form of energy. The maintenance of the integration of bodily functions in the face of these changes depends on multiple negative feedback loops, which are control mechanisms that result in autoregulation of the **Internal Environment** (Levine, 1973). Collective synchronization of multiple negative feedback loops is accomplished through homeostasis and "creates the 'stable state' of the internal environment" (Levine, 1989b, p. 329).

EXTERNAL ENVIRONMENT

- [The external environment is not] a kind of stage setting against which the individual plays out his life (Levine, 1973, p. 12).
- [The external environment] is not a backdrop on a stage where life events are acted (Levine, 1990, p. 196).

The concept of **External Environment** encompasses three dimensions—Perceptual Environment, Operational Environment, and Conceptual Environment (Levine, 1973).

- **Perceptual Environment:** That portion of the environment to which the individual responds with his sense organs (Bates, 1967, as cited in Levine, 1973, p. 12). [The perceptual environment includes] those factors which can be recorded on the sensory system—the energies of light, sound, touch, temperature, and chemical change that is smelled or tasted, as well as position sense and balance (Levine, 1989b, p. 326).
  Acknowledgment of the Perceptual Environment dimension of the **External Environment** facilitates understanding that the human being "is not a passive recipient of sensory input. [Rather,] he seeks, selects, and tests information from the environment in the context of his definition of himself, and so constantly defends his safety, his identity, and in a larger sense, his purpose" (Levine, 1971, p. 262).
- **Operational Environment:** That [portion of the environment] which interacts with living tissues even though the individual does not possess sensory organs that can record the presence of these external factors (Bates, 1967, as cited in Levine, 1989b, p. 326). The operational environment is not directly perceived by the individual (Levine, 1973, 1989b). [The operational environment encompasses] every unseen and unheard aspect of the individual's life-space [including] all forms of radiation, microorganisms, [and] pollutants that are odorless and colorless (Levine, 1989b, p. 326).
  The Operational Environment dimension of the **External Environment** cannot be apprehended by the senses or anticipated symbolically, but it is of vital concern because of its potential danger to the well-being of the individual (Levine, 1971).
- **Conceptual Environment:** The environment of language, ideas, symbols, concepts, and invention (Bates, 1967, as cited in Levine, 1989b, p. 326). [The conceptual environment encompasses] the exchange of language, the ability to think and to experience emotion. … value systems, religious beliefs, ethnic and cultural traditions, and the individual psychological patterns that come from life experiences (Levine, 1973, p. 12).

The Conceptual Environment dimension takes into account Levine's assumption that "human beings are sentient, thinking, future-oriented and past-aware individuals" (Levine, 1989b, p. 326).

Levine (1973) mentioned the importance of both the **Internal Environment** and the **External Environment** and noted that the interface between the two is involved in **Adaptation.** She explained that:

> … separate consideration of either the internal or external environments can provide only a partial view of the complex interaction that is taking place between them. It is, in fact, at the interface where the exchange between internal and external environments occurs that the determinants for nursing intervention are found. In this broader sense, all adaptations represent the accommodation that is possible between the internal and external environments. (p. 12)

ADAPTATION

- The life process is the process of adaptation (Levine, 1989b, p. 326).
- The purpose of life is to maintain life: adaptation is life (Cohen, 1968, p. 8, as cited in Levine, 1989b, p. 326).
- The process of adaptation is acknowledged as a process of change (Levine, 1989b, p. 326).
- Adaptation is the process of change whereby the individual retains his integrity within the realities of his environments. Adaptation is basic to survival, and it is an expression of the integration of the entire organism (Levine, 1973, pp. 10–11).
- The way in which human beings and the environment become congruent over time (Levine, 1989b).
- The fit of the person with his or her predicament of time and space (Levine, 1989b, p. 326).
- The process by which individuals "fit" the environments in which they live (Levine, 1996, p. 38).
- The most successful adaptations are those that best fit the organism in its environment. A "best fit" is accomplished with the least expenditure of effort, and with sufficient protective devices built in so that the goal is achieved in as economic and expeditious a manner as possible (Levine, 1989b, p. 330).
- Adaptation is not an all or none process; rather, it is a matter of degree—some adaptations are successful and some are not; some work and some do not. There are, however, no maladaptations. Thus, adaptation has no value attached to it; it just is (Levine, 1973; 1989b, 1991).
- The measure of effective adaptation is compatibility with life. A poor adaptation may threaten life itself, but at the same time the degree of adaptive potential available to the individual may be sufficient to maintain life at a different level of effectiveness. … All the processes of living are processes of adaptation. Survival itself depends upon

the quality of the adaptation possible for the individual (Levine, 1973, p. 11).

The concept of **Adaptation** encompasses three dimensions—Historicity, Specificity, and Redundancy (Levine, 1989b, 1996).

- **Historicity:** [The fundamental nature of adaptation is] a consequence of a historical progression: the evolution of the species through time, reflecting the sequence of change in the genetic patterns that have recorded the change in the historical environments (Levine, 1989b, p. 327). [Refers to the information] conveyed by generations of genes that every living creature has inherited—but for each individual in a unique pattern—no two alike. Life experience creates further patterns for each person throughout the life span (Levine, 1996, p. 38).
- **Specificity:** Specificity is exemplified by the synchronized tasks of body systems—each body system has specific tasks involving biochemical changes in response to environmental challenges. Although the tasks are specific, they are synchronized with each other and serve the individual as a whole (Levine, 1989b). Specificity in biochemistry is dependent upon sequential change that occurs in cascades (Levine, 1989b). [The cascade] is characterized by the intermingling of the steps with each other—the precursor is not entirely exhausted when the intermediate forms develop and the final stage is congruent with the steps that precede it (Levine, 1989b, p. 328).
- **Redundancy:** [Refers to shared functions that] not only provide a "menu" of related activities but also spreads the energy cost (Levine, 1996, p. 39). Refers to the series of wave-like adaptive responses that are available to the individual when environmental challenges arise (Levine, 1989b). [Examples of redundancy in adaptation include the] ubiquitous … "fail-safe" options in the anatomy, physiology, and psychology of individuals (Levine, 1991, p. 6). Some redundant systems respond instantly to threatened shifts in physiological parameters. Others are corrective and utilize the time interval provided by the instantaneous response to correct imbalances. Still other redundant systems function by reestablishing a previously failed response (Levine, 1989b, 1991).

ORGANISMIC RESPONSES

- [Physiological and behavioral responses to environmental challenges that] are coexistent in a single individual, and in fact, often influence each other. They represent, however, an assembly of parts which have indeed entered into fruitful association and organization. Together they permit the person to protect and maintain his integrity as an individual (Levine, 1969b, p. 98, 1989b).

Organismic Responses are redundant. Levine (1989b) pointed out that because the responses are redundant, "they do not follow one another in a prescribed sequence, but are integrated in individuals by their cognitive abilities, the wealth of their previous experience, their ability to define their relationships to the events and the strengths of their adaptive capabilities" (p. 330). She further noted that although some responses can be considered physiological and some behavioral, "the integration of living processes argues that they are one and the same—not merely parallel and not merely simultaneous—but essential portions of the same activity" (p. 330).

The concept of **Organismic Responses** encompasses four dimensions—Fight or Flight Response, Inflammatory-Immune Response, Stress Response, and Perceptual Awareness.

- **Fight or Flight Response:** The most primitive level of organismic response (Levine, 1973, 1989b). An adrenocortical-sympathetic reaction that is an instantaneous response to a real or imagined threat (Levine, 1973, 1989b). Swiftly provides a condition of physiological and behavioral readiness for sudden and unexplained environmental challenges (Levine, 1973, 1989b).
- **Inflammatory-Immune Response:** The second level of organismic response (Levine, 1973, 1989b). A response to injury that is important for maintenance of structural continuity and promotion of healing (Levine, 1973, 1989b). Assures restoration of physical wholeness and the expectation of complete healing (Levine, 1989b, p. 330).
- **Stress Response:** The third level of organismic response (Levine, 1973, 1989b). [A response that is] recorded over time and is influenced by the accumulated experience of the individual (Selye, 1956, as cited in Levine, 1989b, p. 330).
- **Perceptual Awareness:** The fourth level of organismic response (Levine, 1973, 1989b). The response, which is mediated through the sense organs, is concerned with gathering information from the environment and converting it to meaningful experience (Levine, 1969b, 1989b). Individual identity arises out of information received through [five] intact and functional perceptual systems (Gibson, 1966, as cited in Levine, 1969b, p. 97).

The dimension of Perceptual Awareness encompasses five subdimensions—Basic Orienting System, Visual System, Auditory System, Haptic System, and Taste-Smell System (Levine, 1973, 1989b).

- *Basic Orienting System:* Provides a general orientation to the environment and is essential to the function of the other perceptual systems (Gibson, 1966, as cited in Levine, 1969b, 1973). The anatomical organ is the balancing portion of the inner ear, which responds to changes in gravity, acceleration, and movement (Gibson, 1966, as cited in Levine, 1969b, 1973).

- *Visual System*: Permits the human being to look (Gibson, 1966, as cited in Levine, 1969b, 1973).
- *Auditory System*: Permits listening to sounds as well as identifying the direction from which they are coming (Gibson, 1966, as cited in Levine, 1969b, 1973).
- *Haptic System*: Permits responses to touch through reception of sensations by the skin, joints, and muscles (Gibson, 1966, as cited in Levine, 1969b, 1973).
- *Taste-Smell System*: Provides information about chemical stimuli and facilitates safe nourishment (Gibson, 1966, as cited in Levine, 1969b, 1973).

Levine (1969b, 1973, 1989b) drew from Gibson (1966) to explain the subdimensions of the dimension of Perceptual Awareness. In particular, Levine (1989b) pointed out that for Gibson (1966), "individuals do not merely 'see'—they *look*; they do not merely 'hear'—they *listen*. Thus equipped with the ability to select information from the environment, the individual is an active, seeking participant in it— not merely reacting but influencing, changing, and creating the parameters of his or her life" (p. 330).

CONSERVATION

- Conservation is keeping together (Levine, 1989b, p. 331).
- Conservation is a universal concept (Levine, 1990, p. 192).
- Conservation is the guardian activity that defends and protects [wholeness, which is] the universal target of selfhood (Levine, 1991, p. 4).
- Conservation describes the way complex systems are able to continue to function even when severely challenged. They sustain themselves, not only in the face of immediate disruptive threats, but in such a way as to assure the vitality of future responses. This work is accomplished in the most economic way possible (Levine, 1990, p. 192).
- The … process of conservation is characteristic of the way that physiological functions are regulated in the body. Negative feedback is activated when something needs to be adjusted, but is quiescent otherwise (Levine, 1990, p. 192).
- Conservation defends the wholeness of living systems by ensuring their ability to confront change appropriately and retain their unique identity (Levine, 1990, p. 192).
- Every self-sustaining system monitors its own behavior by conserving the use of resources required to define its unique identity (Levine, 1991, p. 4).
- [The ultimate purpose of conservation is] to defend, sustain, maintain, and define the integrity of the system for which it functions (Levine, 1991, p. 3).

Conservation is the product of **Adaptation**. Levine (1989b) explained, "Survival depends on the adaptive ability to use responses that *cost the least* to the individual in expense of effort and demand on his or her well-being. That is, of course, the essence of *conservation*" (p. 329).

Levine (1989b, 1991) linked **Conservation** to both of the **Internal Environment** concept dimensions of Homeostasis and Homeorrhesis. With regard to Homeostasis, Levine (1989b) maintained, "Conservation is clearly the consequence of the multiple, interacting, and synchronized negative feedback systems that provide for the stability of the living organism. … [Indeed,] homeostasis might be called the state of conservation" (p. 329). Speaking of the link between Homeorrhesis and **Conservation**, Levine (1991) claimed, "Homeor[r]hesis … [is] a consequence of conservation: the frugal, economic, contained, and controlled use of environmental resources by the individual organism in his or her best interest. This is the achievement of adaptation" (p. 5).

The concept of **Conservation** encompasses four dimensions—the Principle of Conservation of Energy, the Principle of Conservation of Structural Integrity, the Principle of Conservation of Personal Integrity, and the Principle of Conservation of Social Integrity (Levine, 1967, 1973, 1989b, 1990, 1991, 1996).

- **Principle of Conservation of Energy**: Refers to balancing energy output and energy input to avoid excessive fatigue, that is, adequate rest, nutrition, and exercise (Levine, 1988b, p. 227). A natural law found to hold everywhere in the universe for all animate and inanimate entities (Levine, 1989b, p. 331). There are finite sources of energy available to human beings. Conservation of energy assures that "energy is spent carefully with essential priorities served first" (Levine, 1991, p. 7). Although individuals conserve their energy, the energy from life-sustaining activities, such as biochemical changes, is expended even at perfect rest (Levine, 1989b). Energy is not directly observable, although "the consequences of its exchange are predictable, manageable, and quantifiable. Instruments can monitor, measure, produce or capture energy" (Levine, 1991, p. 7). The conservation of energy is clearly evident in the very sick, whose lethargy, withdrawal, and self-concern are manifested while, in its wisdom, the body is spending its energy resource on the processes of healing (Levine, 1989b, p. 332).
- **Principle of Conservation of Structural Integrity**: Refers to maintaining or restoring the structure of the body, that is, preventing physical breakdown and promoting healing (Levine, 1988b, p. 227). Focuses on human beings' ability to move and choose activities freely (Levine, 1988b). Human beings expect and have confidence in the ability of their bodies to heal. Healing is the defense of

wholeness ... [and] a consequence of an effective immune system (Levine, 1989b, p. 333). Emphasizes that the individual's defense[s] against the hazards of the environment are achieved with the most economical expense of effort (Levine, 1991, p. 8). Results in repair and healing to sustain the wholeness of structure and function (Levine, 1991, p. 7).

- **Principle of Conservation of Personal Integrity**: [Refers to] the maintenance or restoration of the patient's sense of identity, self-worth, and acknowledgment of uniqueness (Levine, 1988b, p. 227). Emphasizes individuals' perseverance in retaining their identities. Everyone seeks to defend his or her identity as a self, in both that hidden, intensely private person that dwells within and in the public faces assumed as individuals move through their relationships with others (Levine, 1989b, p. 334). Every individual defends his unique personhood, the individual within known as the "self." Wholeness is summarized in that knowledge [of self] (Levine, 1991, p. 8). [The self is] much more than a physical experience of the whole body, although it is unquestionably a part of that awareness (Levine, 1989b, p. 334).

- **Principle of Conservation of Social Integrity**: Refers to the acknowledgment of the patient as a social being (Levine, 1988b, p. 227). Involves the recognition and presentation of human interaction, particularly with the patient's significant others (Levine, 1988b, p. 227). [States that each individual's identity places him or her] in a family, a community, a cultural heritage, a religious belief, a socioeconomic slot, an educational background, a vocational choice (Levine, 1989b, p. 335). [Emphasizes that] selfhood needs definition beyond the individual ... [and that] the individual is created by the environment and in turn creates within it (Levine, 1989b, p. 335). It is impossible to acknowledge the wholeness of the individual without placing him into his social context (Levine, 1991, p. 9).

Levine (1989b) pointed out that the **Principle of Conservation of Energy**, the **Principle of Conservation of Structural Integrity**, the **Principle of Conservation of Personal Integrity**, and the **Principle of Conservation of Structural Integrity** do not operate singly but rather are "joined within the individual as a cascade of life events, churning and changing as the environmental challenge is confronted and resolved in each individual's unique way" (p. 336). Elaborating on the integration of the four conservation principles, Levine (1991) stated:

> The conservation principles address the integrity of the individual ... from birth to death. Every activity requires an energy supply because nothing works without it. Every activity must respect the structural wholeness of the individual because well-being depends upon it. Every activity is chosen out of the abilities, life experience and desires of the "self" who makes the choices. Every activity is a product of the dynamic social systems to which the individual belongs. (p. 10)

CHANGE

- Change is the essence of life (Levine, 1973, p. 10).
- The life process is characterized as unceasing change (Levine, 1973).
- Change is directed, purposeful, and meaningful (Levine, 1973, p. 10).
- The organism represents a pattern of orderly, sequential change. Because it is both ordered and sequential, the pattern is a message. So long as the pattern is consistent, it is also understandable. ... The change which supports the well-being of the organism can be predicted, measured, and observed, and therefore is a cogent message (Levine, 1973, pp. 9–10).

HEALTH

- A pattern of adaptive change (Levine 1973, 1984a).
- A state of being described as "health" ... is inherent in the life experience (Levine, 1991, p. 4).
- Every individual defines health for himself or herself (Levine, 1991, p. 4).
- [Health] is not an entity, but rather a definition imparted by the ethos and beliefs of groups to which the individual belongs (Levine, personal communication to K.M. Schaefer, February 21, 1995, as cited in Schaefer, 1996, p. 187).
- Health is socially defined in the sense of "Do I continue to function in a reasonably normal fashion?" (Levine, 1984b).

Levine (1991) pointed out that **Health**, whole, and healing all share the same root. She explained:

> Healing is the avenue of return to the daily activities compromised by ill health. It is not only the insult or injury that is repaired—but the person himself or herself as whole and healing. Indeed, the expectation that healing will restore the conditions that existed before the intrusion persists even in situations where the therapeutic outcome leaves a loss of function or effectiveness. It is not merely the healing of an afflicted part. It is, rather, a return to selfhood, where the encroachment of the disability can be set aside entirely, and the individual is free to pursue once more his or her own interests without constraint. (p. 4)

Levine (1984b) indicated that she did not like the term wellness and preferred the word healthy. It may be inferred from her description of health as "wholeness" (Levine, 1973, p. 11) and as "successful adaptation" (Levine, 1966a, p. 2452) that she used the term **Health** to mean wellness.

It also may be inferred that wellness means social

well-being. This inference is supported by Levine's (1966a) statement that "one criterion of successful adaptation is the attainment of social well-being, but there is tremendous variation in the degree to which this is achieved" (p. 2452).

Levine's description of **Health** indicates that she conceptualized that concept as a continuum. This interpretation is supported by the following comment:

> Adaptation ... is susceptible to an infinite range within the limits of life compatibility. Within that range, there are numerous possible degrees of adaptation. Thus, the dynamic processes establishing balance along the continuum are adaptations (Levine, 1973, p. 11).

DISEASE

- A pattern of adaptive change (Levine, 1973, 1984a).
- Disease is undisciplined and unregulated change, a disruption in the orderly sequential pattern of change that is characteristic of life. This anarchy of pattern may not be successful in supporting life (Levine, 1973).
- Such anarchy, in fact, occurs in disease processes, and unless the pattern can be restored, the organism will die (Levine, 1973, p. 9).
- [The anarchy of disease processes is a positive feedback mechanism, which] results in an increasing rate of function without the regulatory control that restores balance. Thus, a "vicious cycle" is instituted which produces more and more disruption of function (Levine, 1973, p. 10).
- Disease represents efforts of the individual to protect his integrity (Levine, 1971, p. 257).

Levine (1971) used Wolf's (1961) conception of **Disease** as adaptation to noxious environmental forces for her description of illness. In a later publication, Levine (1991) noted that inasmuch as "illness challenges the integrity of the person, defending his health—his unique wholeness—is a continuing endeavor" (p. 4).

Levine (1973) pointed out that individuals acknowledge illness through their perceptual systems. She explained, "Physical well-being is dependent upon an experienced body which is communicating the "right" signals. The constancy of awareness of the internal feeling of the body is the baseline against which well-being is measured. ... Individuals can acknowledge "illness" only in recognizing an alteration in their perception of internal feelings" (p. 456).

HUMAN INTERACTION

- Nursing is a human interaction. It is a discipline rooted in the organic dependency of the individual human being on his relationships with other human beings (Levine, 1973, p. 1).

Levine (1973) emphasized the importance of scientific concepts and knowledge as the basis for nursing. She noted, "Nursing knowledge, thoroughly grounded in modern scientific concepts, allows for a sensitive and productive relationship between the nurse and the individual entrusted to her care. ... Nursing practice has always mirrored the prevailing theories of health and disease that pervade every culture" (p. 1).

Nursing is also based on the unique beliefs of nurses. Indeed, "nursing itself is a subculture, possessing ideas and values which are unique to nurses, even though they mirror the social template which created them" (Levine, 1973, p. 3).

The **GOAL OF NURSING**, according to Levine (1984a), is the promotion of wholeness for all people, well or sick. She maintained: "The goal of all nursing care should be to promote wholeness, realizing that for every individual that requires a unique and separate cluster of activities. The individual's integrity—his one-ness, his identity as an individual, his wholeness—is his abiding concern, and it is the nurse's responsibility to assist him to defend and to seek its realization" (Levine, 1971, p. 258).

For Levine, the nursing process of the Conservation Model is **Conservation**. Levine (1989b) stated that conservation—the "keeping together" function—should be the major guideline for all nursing intervention (p. 331). "Every nursing act," Levine (1991) maintained, "is dedicated to the conservation or the 'keeping together' of the wholeness of the individual" (p. 3). Although Levine did not identify an explicit nursing process, it was possible to extract a **PRACTICE METHODOLOGY** from several of her publications. The **NURSING PROCESS AS CONSERVATION**, which Levine (1966b) regards as a "scientific approach in the determination of nursing care" (p. 57), is outlined in Table 6–1.

In keeping with her view of nursing as a **Human Interaction**, Levine (1973) emphasized the roles of both nurse and patient in the **Nursing Process as Conservation**. She explained:

> "To keep together" means to maintain a proper balance between active nursing intervention coupled with patient participation on the one hand and the safe limits of the patient's ability to participate on the other. (p. 13)

Levine (1984b) stated that she regarded patients as partners or participants in nursing care. Levine viewed the human being who is a patient as being temporarily dependent on the nurse. The nurse's goal is to end the dependence, that is, the status of patient, as quickly as possible. More specifically:

> An individual who enters into the dependency of health care is a patient. The nurse provides whatever service is needed—even if it is only health counseling—but only for as long as the nurse's professional services are required. Then the depend-

TROPHICOGNOSIS

Observation

The nurse observes and collects data that will influence nursing practice rather than medical practice.

The nurse uses appropriate assessment tools derived from the Conservation Model.

The nurse uses data to establish an objective and scientific rationale for nursing practice.

The nurse fully understands his or her role in medical and paramedical prescriptions.

The nurse understands the basis for the prescribed medical regimen, including the medical diagnosis, the medical history, and the laboratory and x-ray reports—with specific reference to areas influencing the nursing care plan.

The nurse consults with the physician to share information and clarify nursing decisions.

The nurse understands the basis for the prescribed paramedical regimen, including paramedical diagnoses and prescriptions for care.

The nurse determines the nursing processes required by medical and paramedical treatment by observing the effects of the medical regimen on the patient's progress.

The nurse gathers additional data by consulting with family members or other individuals concerned with the patient, including the religious counselor.

The nurse conducts a nursing history with specific reference to aspects that will influence the nursing care plan.

The nurse assesses the patient's *Conservation of Energy* by determining his or her ability to perform necessary activities without producing excessive fatigue.
> Relevant observations include vital signs, the patient's general condition, the patient's behavior, and the patient's tolerance of nursing activities required by his or her condition, and allowable activity for the patient based on his or her energy resources.

The nurse assesses the patient's *Conservation of Structural Integrity* by determining his or her physical functioning.
> Relevant observations include status of any pathophysiological processes, status of healing processes, and effects of surgical procedures.

The nurse assesses the patient's *Conservation of Personal Integrity* by determining his or her moral and ethical values and life experiences.
> Relevant observations include the patient's life story, determining the patient's interest in participating in decision making, and identifying the patient's sense of self.

The nurse assesses the patient's *Conservation of Social Integrity* by taking the patient's family members, friends, and conceptual environment into account.
> Relevant observations include identification of the patient's significant others, participation in workplace or school activities, religion, and cultural and ethnic history.

The nurse understands the basis for implementation of the nursing care plan, including principles of nursing science, and how to adapt nursing techniques to the unique cluster of needs demonstrated in the individual patient.

Awareness of Provocative Facts

The nurse identifies the provocative facts within the data collected, that is, the data that provoke attention on the basis of knowledge of the situation.

Construction of a Testable Hypothesis

The provocative facts provide the basis for a hypothesis, or trophicognosis.

The nurse accurately records and transmits observations and the trophicognosis.

INTERVENTION/ACTION

A Test of the Hypothesis

The nurse implements the nursing care plan within the structure of administrative policy, availability of equipment, and established standards of nursing.

The nurse accurately records and transmits evaluation of the patient's response to implementation of the nursing care plan.

The nurse identifies the general type of nursing intervention required.

(continued)

TABLE 6–1
LEVINE'S PRACTICE METHODOLOGY: NURSING PROCESS AS CONSERVATION *(continued)*

Therapeutic Nursing Intervention
Nursing intervention that influences adaptation favorably, or toward renewed social well-being.

Supportive Nursing Intervention
Nursing intervention that cannot alter the course of the adaptation and that can only maintain the status quo or that fails to halt a downward course.

The nurse structures nursing intervention according to the four conservation principles.

Principle of Conservation of Energy
Nursing intervention is based on the conservation of the individual patient's energy through an adequate deposit of energy resource and regulation of the expenditure of energy.

The nurse helps the patient to balance energy output and energy input by preventing excessive fatigue and promoting adequate rest, nutrition, and exercise.

The nurse takes relevant scientific considerations into account:
   The ability of the human body to perform work is dependent upon its energy balance—the supply of energy-producing nutrients measured against the rate of energy-using activities.
   The energy required by alterations in physiological function during illness represents an additional demand made on the energy production systems.
   Fatigue, often experienced with illness, is an empiric measure of the additional energy demand.

Principle of Conservation of Structural Integrity
Nursing intervention is based on the conservation of the individual patient's structural integrity through maintenance or restoration of the structure of the body.

The nurse acts to prevent physical breakdown, promote healing, limit the amount of tissue involvement in infection and disease, and prevent trophicogenic (nurse-induced) disease by correct anatomical and physiologic positioning, maintenance of the patient's personal hygiene, and assisting the patient with range-of-motion exercises and passive exercises.

The nurse takes relevant scientific considerations into account:
   Structural change results in a change of function.
   Pathophysiological processes present a threat to structural integrity.
   Healing processes restore structural integrity.
   Surgical procedures are designed to restore structural integrity.
   Structural integrity is restored when the scar is organized and integrated into the continuity of the part affected.

Principle of Conservation of Personal Integrity
Nursing intervention is based on the conservation of the patient's personal integrity through maintenance or restoration of the patient's sense of identity, self-worth, and acknowledgment of uniqueness.

The nurse understands that respect from the nurse is essential to the patient's self-respect and accepts the patient the way he or she is.

The nurse recognizes and protects the patient's space needs, assures privacy during performance of body functions and therapeutic procedures, respects the importance the patient places on personal possessions, uses the appropriate mode of address when dealing with the patient, and supports the patient's defense mechanisms as appropriate.

The nurse takes relevant scientific considerations into account:
   There always is a privacy to individual life.
   Assumption of responsibility for one's own decisions develops with maturation.
   Self-identify and self-respect are the foundations of a sense of personal integrity.

Illness threatens self-identity and self-respect.
Hospitalization may compound and exaggerate the threat to personal integrity.
Individuals possess a lifetime commitment to the value systems and social patterns of their subcultural affiliations.

Principle of Conservation of Social Integrity
Nursing intervention is based on the conservation of the individual patient's social integrity through acknowledging the patient as a social being.

The nurse understands that a failure to consider the patient's family and friends is a failure to provide excellent nursing; the social system of the hospital is artificial; a concern for holistic well-being of individuals demands attention to community attitudes, resources, and provision of health care in the community; and the nurse-patient interaction is a social relationship that is disciplined and controlled by the professional role of the nurse.

The nurse considers patients' social needs when placing them in the nursing unit; positions each patient in bed to foster social interaction with other patients; avoids sensory deprivation for the patient; promotes the patient's use of newspapers, magazines, radio, and television as appropriate; provides family members with knowledgeable support and assistance; and teaches family members to perform functions for the patient as necessary.

The nurse takes relevant scientific considerations into account:
The social integrity of individuals is tied to the viability of the entire social system.
Individual life has meaning only in the context of social life.
The way in which individuals relate to various social groups influences their behavior.
Individual recognition of wholeness is measured against relationships with others.
Interactions with others become more important in times of stress.
The patient's family may be deeply affected by the changes resulting from illness.
Hospitalization is characterized by isolation from family and friends.

Evaluation of Intervention/Action
The nurse evaluates the effects of intervention and revises the trophicognosis as necessary.

An indicator of the success of nursing interventions is the patient's organismic response.

Source: Constructed from Levine, 1966b, pp. 57–60; 1967, 1973, pp. 13–18, 28; 1988b, p. 227; Schaefer, 1991a, p. 222.

ency must be ended. I want the patient to walk away from me. As participants in their care, individuals need to retain whatever portion of their independence they can, and they should not be defined as [clients, that is, as] followers. (Levine, 1996, p. 40)

Levine (1989b) noted that, as part of the patient's environment, the nurse brings to nursing care situations his or her "own cascading repertoire of skill, knowledge, and compassion. It is a shared enterprise and each participant is rewarded" (p. 336).

Within her **Nursing Process as Conservation**, Levine (1966b) presented **Trophicognosis** as an alternative to nursing diagnosis. Tracing the development of nursing diagnosis and its legal interpretation, Levine (1966b) pointed out that the term always referred to "diagnosis of disease made by a nurse" (p. 55). Then, citing the dictionary definition of diagnosis as "knowledge of disease," she maintained that it is "incorrect to use the term diagnosis as a synonym for observations, judgments, problems, needs or assessments" (pp. 56–57). In concluding her argument, Levine stated:

Because the term, nursing diagnosis, is now susceptible of legal interpretation, and other usages of the term are semantically incorrect, it is proposed that a new nursing term be used to describe the scientific approach in the determination of nursing care. Such a method of ascribing nursing care needs may be called trophicognosis (p. 57).

Levine (1966b) drew from Feiblemann's (1959) description of the scientific method to construct the steps involved in formulation of a **Trophicognosis**. Those steps are *Observation, Awareness of Provocative Facts,* and *Construction of a Testable Hypothesis* (see Table 6–1).

Observation, for Levine (1966b), focuses on the collection of data that is especially relevant to nursing. She explained:

The development of a trophicognosis requires a reorientation in the selection of data because the information required to project nursing care needs differs somewhat from the kind of information required to direct medical therapy. Although nurses are exhorted to observe from the first day of clinical practice, the focus of attention is almost invariably on collecting data for the physician's use. Too infrequently does the nurse observe with the primary purpose of illuminating her own role in the care of the patient. And yet the nurse does have responsibilities to the patient which she does *not* share with the physician. Thus her observations may be primarily useful to the physician, primarily useful to the nurse, or useful in some degree to both. In selecting observations to be used to construct the trophicognosis, emphasis should be placed on those which influence nursing care. (p. 58)

Levine (1966b) went on to say that "by its very nature, nursing responsibility involves gathering data which includes all the information available from every source involved in the care of the patient, including medical and paramedical information as well as [those] data which [are] specifically and uniquely the province of the nurse herself" (p. 58). Data that are particularly relevant to nursing are those observations about the status of the patient with regard to the conservation principles (see Table 6–1).

The hypothesis represents the **Trophicognosis**. As Levine (1966b) stated, "In developing the trophicognosis, the observations and assembled data provide the 'provocative facts.' The testable hypothesis formulated on the basis of the strength of this information is the trophicognosis" (pp. 57–58).

Levine (personal communication, August 13, 1987) stated that she and her colleagues were developing a taxonomy of trophicognoses. To date, no presentations or publications have given any details of the taxonomy, although Schaefer (1991a), citing a personal communication (September 21, 1989), reported that Levine "supports the development of [trophicognoses] from the clustering of provocative facts that recur in practice and become the focus of nursing intervention" (p. 221).

Intervention/Action, according to Levine (1973), "must be designed so that it fosters successful adaptation whenever possible" (p. 13). Thus, nursing must view individuals so that the best fit available to each human being can be sustained (Levine, 1989b). Interestingly, however, adaptation is impossible to measure or quantify. Levine (1991) explained that although "certain, generalized adaptations can be described—the required oxygen tension, [the] temperature tolerance of living cells, the effect of atmospheric pressure on physiological function, as examples—precise identification of the adaptive condition is not [yet] possible" (pp. 6–7). Inasmuch as adaptation cannot be directly observed, the goal of nursing intervention, Levine (1991) maintained, "must be on the consequences of care rather than on algorithms designed to display the adaptive patterns. ... The research necessary to describe adaptation patterns and the therapeutic interventions that will support them has yet to be done" (p. 7).

Levine (1988b) noted that the four conservation principles "apply equally to living things, and the derivative

meaning of 'conservation' as a 'keeping together' function seemed entirely appropriate as the essential goal of nursing care" (p. 227). Indeed, "Conserving the integrity of the individual is the hallmark of nursing intervention" (Levine, 1996, p. 40).

Levine (1966b) fully supported the need for **Evaluation** of the results of the **Intervention/Action**. She stated:

Like any hypothesis, the trophicognosis is continually evaluated in the light of the results of the action, and revised and changed in response to new information signalling the necessity for change. In the very nature of the disease process, the daily flux of events causes a continuing pattern of change, and to adequately reflect the dynamics of the events the nurse is witnessing, the system used to design patient care must be equally susceptible to revision. (p. 58)

Relational Propositions

The relational propositions of the Conservation Model are listed here. The metaparadigm concepts of human beings and environment are linked in relational propositions A, B, C, D, E, F, and G. Relational propositions H, I, and J assert the linkages between the metaparadigm concepts of human beings, environment, and health. Relational proposition K asserts the linkage of the metaparadigm concepts of human beings, environment, and nursing. The linkages among all four metaparadigm concepts are evident in relational propositions L and M.

A. [The Conservation Model] emphasizes that the environment is not a passive stage setting, but rather that the person is an active participant, exploring, seeking, and testing understanding of the world he or she inhabits (Levine, 1992, p. 41).

B. The individual is always within an environmental milieu, and the consequences of his awareness of his environment persistently influence his behavior at any given moment (Levine, 1973, p. 444).

C. [The person's] presence in the environment also influences it and thereby the kind of information available from it (Levine, 1973, p. 446).

D. The individual protects and defends himself within his environment by gaining all the information he can about it (Levine, 1973, p. 451).

E. The interaction at the interface between individual and environment is an orderly, sometimes predictable, but always limited process. The consequence of the interaction is invariably the product of the characteristics of the living individual and the external factors. ... The process of the interaction is adaptation (Levine, 1989b, p. 326).

F. The ability of every individual not only to survive but to flourish is a consequence of the competence of the person's interactions with the environments in which he or she functions (Levine, 1991, pp. 4–5).

G. The person cannot be described apart from the specific environment in which he or she is found. The precise environment necessarily completes the wholeness of the individual (Levine, 1989b, p. 325).

H. The goal of conservation is health (Levine, 1990, p. 193).

I. Conservation of the integrity of the person is essential to assuring health, and providing the strength to confront disability. Indeed, the importance of conservation in the treatment of illness is precisely focused on the reclamation of wholeness, of health (Levine, 1991. p. 3).

J. The environment is not always "user-friendly." Successful engagement with the environment depends upon the individual's repertoire—that store of adaptations which is either built into the genes or achieved through life experience. While there are redundant or back-up systems that offer options when the initial response is insufficient, health and safety are products of a competent conservation (Levine, 1990, p. 193).

K. The nurse cannot enter another person's environment without becoming an essential factor in it (Levine, 1992, p. 41).

L. The nurse participates actively in every patient's environment, and much of what she does supports his adaptations as he struggles in the predicament of illness (Levine, 1973, p. 13).

M. But even in the presence of disease, the organism responds wholly to the environmental interaction in which it is involved, and a considerable element of nursing care is devoted to restoring the symmetry of response—symmetry that is essential to the well-being of the organism (Levine 1969b, p. 98).

 ## EVALUATION OF LEVINE'S CONSERVATION MODEL

This section presents an evaluation of the Conservation Model. The evaluation is based on the results of the analysis of the model, as well as on publications and presentations by Levine and by others who have used or commented on the Conservation Model.

EXPLICATION OF ORIGINS

Levine explicated the origins of the Conservation Model clearly and concisely, and she identified the motivation for development of the model. In addition, Levine articulated her philosophical claims in the form of a reasoned discussion of assumptions, beliefs, and values. Levine's presenta-

tion of the Conservation Model indicates that she values a holistic approach to nursing of all human beings, well or sick. She also values the unique individuality of each human being, as noted in comments such as those given here:

> Ultimately, decisions for nursing intervention must be based on the unique behavior of the individual patient. ... A theory of nursing must recognize the importance of unique detail of care for a single patient within an empiric framework which successfully describes the requirements of all patients. (Levine, 1973, p. 6)

> Patient centered nursing care means individualized nursing care. It is predicated on the reality of common experience: every man is a unique individual, and as such he requires a unique constellation of skills, techniques, and ideas designed specifically for him. (Levine, 1973, p. 23)

Furthermore, although Levine (1973) noted that human beings are dependent on their relationships with other human beings, she values the patient's participation in nursing care. That is attested to by the comment here:

> "To keep together" means to maintain a proper balance between active nursing intervention coupled with patient participation on the one hand and the safe limits of the patient's ability to participate on the other. (p. 13)

Levine carefully cited the many scholars and scientists from nursing and adjunctive disciplines whose work influenced her thinking. With the single exception of her reference to Gaylin (Levine, 1996), she heeded her own mandate to provide proper bibliographic references to influential works (Levine, 1988a).

COMPREHENSIVENESS OF CONTENT

The Conservation Model is sufficiently comprehensive with regard to depth of content. Levine's descriptions of human beings, environment, health, and nursing are comprehensive and essentially complete.

Clarity could, however, be enhanced with regard to the most appropriate description of the concept of **Internal Environment**. Despite Levine's (personal communication, August 13, 1987) comment that homeostasis best reflects congruence of human beings with the environment, she continued to imply that homeorrhesis is the more appropriate descriptor of the internal environment (Levine, 1989b, 1991). Levine (1996) provided some illumination on this matter when she stated: "But [neither] of these terms [homeostasis and homeorrhesis] suffice because the labels simply do not fit the complexity of events as we have come to know them. There must be a bridge that allows ready movement from one environmental reality to another. Adaptation is the bridge" (p. 38).

Clarity also could be enhanced with regard to Levine's discussion of health. Levine herself (personal communication to K.M. Schaefer, February 21, 1995, as cited in Schaefer, 1996, p. 187) admitted that she "felt a little empty on [my] discussion of health."

Moreover, clarity could be enhanced concerning the assessment component of the **Nursing Process as Conservation**. Levine never explicitly identified the parameters of nursing assessment, although her various discussions of the conservation principles suggest that they can be used in the assessment, that is, the Trophicognosis component, of the **Nursing Process as Conservation** and the Intervention/Action component. Many nurses who have used the Conservation Model to guide nursing practice used the conservation principles as the framework for nursing assessment; some included the elements of the perceptual, operational, and conceptual environments as well. The levels of organismic response, which Schaefer (1991a) used in the evaluation phase of the nursing process, also could be a part of the assessment phase.

Levine repeatedly emphasized the importance of deriving trophicognoses and interventions from scientific knowledge (see Table 6–1), as well as from the messages given by the patient, as is evident in these comments:

> The modern nurse has available rich knowledge of human anatomy, physiology, and adaptability. (Levine, 1966a, p. 2453)

> Ultimately, decisions for nursing intervention must be based on the unique behavior of the individual patient. It is the nurse's task to bring a body of scientific principles on which decisions depend into the precise situation which she shares with the patient. (Levine, 1966a, p. 2452)

> The integrated response of the individual to any stimulus results in a realignment of his very substance, and in a sense this creates a message which others may learn to understand. Each message, in turn, is the result of observation, selection of relevant data, and assessment of the priorities demanded by such knowledge. ... Understanding the message and responding to it accurately constitute the substance of nursing science. (Levine, 1967, pp. 46–47)

The dynamic nature of the nursing process is evident in Levine's (1973) statement that nursing care plans "must allow for progress and change and project into the future the patient's response to treatment" (p. 46), as well as in Levine's (1989b) description of nursing practice as use of a "cascading repertoire of skill, knowledge, and compassion" (p. 326). Given Levine's explanation of cascades as nonlinear interacting and evolving processes, the nursing process clearly is dynamic. Levine's explication of her own value system, with its emphasis on the patient's freedom to make decisions, attest to her exceptional concern for ethical standards for nursing practice.

The propositions of the Conservation Model link all four metaparadigm concepts. In addition, the integral nature of the four conservation principles is specified clearly.

The Conservation Model also is sufficiently comprehensive in breadth of content. Levine has repeatedly and emphatically explained that her conceptual model is equally applicable for the nursing care of sick and healthy individuals. She stated:

> I have described energy conservation and the wholeness embodied in the integrity of structure, person, and society in broad terms in order to emphasize that the Conservation Principles are not limited only to the care of the sick in the hospital. I have borne the burden of that naive and foolish criticism for several years—ever since two misinformed graduate students wrote a chapter in which they made clear they knew more about what was in my mind than I did (Esposito & Leonard, 1980). They chose my textbook of medical-surgical nursing, *Introduction to Clinical Nursing* (Levine, 1969[a], 1973) as the text from which to critique my work. That text ... was begun in 1963. I was not writing a nursing theory. I was teaching medical-surgical nursing to students whose practice was in a hospital. That is the way it was in the early 60s. (Levine, 1990, p. 195)

Indeed, the Conservation Model represents a broad organizing framework "within which nursing practice in every environment can be anticipated, predicted, and performed. In acute care institutions, nursing homes, clinics, and community health programs and in their management and administration—everywhere nursing is essential—the rules of conservation and integrity hold" (Levine, 1990, p. 195).

Furthermore, the Conservation Model permits a focus on prevention through the principle of social integrity (Levine, 1990). Schaefer (1991a) pointed out that the principle of social integrity "provides a basis for the nurse to consider environmental factors that affect the patient and may indeed be far removed from the immediate environment. It is within this framework that nurses could consider more of the social, cultural, environmental, and political factors that might affect the human condition and over which they could have some control" (p. 220). Such factors also could be considered within the context of the conceptual environment.

The comprehensiveness of the breadth of the Conservation Model is further supported by the direction it provides for nursing research, education, administration, and practice. Although all guidelines are not explicit in Levine's writings, many can be extracted from the focus and content of the model and from the publications of nurses who have used the model. The developing guidelines for research, nursing education, administration of nursing services, and nursing practice are listed below.

Nursing Research Guidelines

The guidelines for nursing research based on the Conservation Model, which were constructed from Levine (1978a, 1991) and Schaefer (1991a, 1991c, 2001), are:

- Purpose of the research
  - The purpose of Conservation Model-based nursing research is to identify nursing interventions derived from the conservation principles that will maintain wholeness and support adaptation, within the context of the unique predicament of the individual, the family, or both.

- Phenomena of interest
  - The phenomena of interest are the conservation principles. Studies may address just one conservation principle, but ultimately all four principles must be considered.
  - Research and scholarly study must focus on discrete issues. But the integrity of the whole person cannot be violated. However narrowed the study problem may be, the influence of all four conservation principles must be acknowledged, and the wholeness of the person sustained (Levine, 1991, p. 10).
  - Other relevant phenomena are the levels of organismic response and the elements of the perceptual, operational, and conceptual environments.

- Problems to be studied
  - The precise problems to be studied are those dealing with the maintenance of the individual's wholeness and the interface between the internal and external environments of the person.

- Study participants
  - Study participants may be healthy or sick individuals of all ages in virtually any setting.

- Research methods
  - Both qualitative and quantitative designs are appropriate.
    - Qualitative research designs should focus on discovering how patients experience challenges to their internal and external environments.
    - Quantitative designs should focus on testing relations between study concepts and testing the effects of interventions on conservation of energy, structural integrity, personal integrity, and social integrity.
  - Ideally, research designs should combine qualitative and quantitative methodologies.
  - Research designs should take into account the linkage of specific variables to each conservation principle that have been identified.
- Variables that can be linked with the Conservation of Energy are:
  - Anxiety
  - Oxygen saturation
  - Blood glucose
  - Pulse
  - Temperature
  - Respirations
  - Blood pressure
  - Hemoglobin and hematocrit
  - Skin turgor
  - Fluid and electrolytes
  - Heat
  - Energy exchange
  - Diarrhea
  - Blood loss
  - Body weight
  - Wound drainage
- Variables that can be linked with the Conservation of Structural Integrity are:
  - White blood cell count
  - Healing (granulation tissue)
  - Skin integrity
  - Sedimentation rate
  - Body density
  - Muscle strength
  - End-organ damage (renal function, liver function)
- Variables that can be linked with the Conservation of Personal Integrity are:
  - Loneliness
  - Boredom
  - Helplessness
  - Fear
  - Self-esteem
  - Privacy
  - Listening
  - Empathy
  - Control
  - Meaning
  - Teaching
  - Learning
  - Role
  - Self-concept
- Variables that can be linked with the Conservation of Social Integrity are:
  - Socialization
  - Moral development
  - Group process
  - Interaction
  - Social isolation

- Practice tools derived from the Conservation Model may be used to collect data for research purposes (see Table 6–3 on page 155).
- A question that can be used to identify aspects of nursing directed toward the whole person is:
  - How has this predicament (illness, lifestyle change, new baby, marriage, change in job) affected your normal life-style? (Schaefer, 1991c, p. 52).
- Definitive guidelines for research procedures beyond those typically used for qualitative and quantitative designs remain to be developed.

- Data analysis
  - Techniques for data analysis should be appropriate to the particular qualitative and quantitative methodologies used.

- Contributions
  - Conservation Model-based research findings enhance understanding of factors and nursing interventions that promote adaptation and the maintenance of wholeness.

Nursing Education Guidelines

The guidelines for nursing education based on the Conservation Model, which were constructed from Barnum (1998), Grindley and Paradowski (1991), Levine (1990), and Schaefer (1991b), are:

- Focus of the curriculum
  - The focus of a Conservation Model-based nursing education program is the conservation principles and the preparation of students for the practice of holistic nursing.

- Nature and sequence of content
  - The content of a Conservation Model-based curriculum encompasses nursing courses that focus on the conservation principles, as well as courses in philosophy, theology, the humanities, physiology, microbiology, biochemistry, psychology, sociology, education, history, anthropology, mathematics, English, and research.
  - One approach to the sequence of content is separate, sequential courses for each of the four conservation principles.
  - Another approach is to organize the curriculum along the health-illness continuum and include appropriate content from all four conservation principles in each course.

- Settings for nursing education
  - Nursing education can occur in a variety of settings; no one type of nursing education program has been identified as most appropriate.

- Characteristics of students
  - Students should be able to think intuitively, critically, and creatively.
  - Students should appreciate the need for lifelong learning.

- Teaching-learning strategies
  - Teaching-learning strategies foster intuitive thinking, critical thinking, and creativity in practice. Such strategies include free association, in-class summaries of reactions to class discussions and required readings, videotapes of oral presentations, descriptions of responses to abstract art, and validating hypotheses in practice.

Administration of Nursing Services Guidelines

Guidelines for the administration of nursing services based on the Conservation Model, which were constructed from Levine (1969b) and Schaefer (1991a), are:

- Focus of nursing in the health-care organization
  - The distinctive focus of Conservation Model-based nursing services is the conservation of the patient's wholeness.

- Purpose of nursing services
  - One purpose of nursing services is to maintain the integrity of the nursing department and the individuals who function within that department, including both staff and patients.
  - Another purpose of nursing services is to promote the adaptation of the nursing department for social good.

- Characteristics of nursing personnel
  - Nursing personnel are required to understand that patients are in a temporary state of dependence, and therefore they must be committed to fostering the patient's freedom and encouraging decision making.

- Settings for nursing services
  - Nursing services are located in many different settings, including medical centers, ambulatory clinics, community agencies, and nursing centers.
  - Hospital units should be organized on the basis of the patients' perceptual system, especially their abilities to receive and interpret information and their territorial needs.

- Management strategies and administrative policies
  - The four conservation principles serve as a basis for specific management strategies and administrative policies.

- The conservation of energy focuses the administrator on productivity issues, which have a direct effect on cost.
- The conservation of structural integrity focuses the administrator on the equipment (technology), supplies, and human resources needed for the nursing department to function in a cost-effective manner.
- The conservation of personal integrity focuses the administrator on the need to run a department that considers the individual needs of the each staff member, measures to ensure job satisfaction, and the need for a management style (decentralized versus centralized; shared governance) that supports the human element of the department.
- The conservation of social integrity focuses the administrator on how well the nursing department is meeting the needs of the community or the social system, while at the same time considering the effect of the community and the social system on the nursing department.

Nursing Practice Guidelines

Guidelines for nursing practice based on the Conservation Model, which were constructed from Levine (1989c, 1990, 1991), are:

- Purpose of nursing practice
  - The purpose of Conservation Model-based nursing practice is conservation of the patient's wholeness.
  - Every nursing act is dedicated to the conservation, or "keeping together," of the wholeness of the individual (Levine, 1991, p. 3).
  - The practice of conservation in nursing is dedicated to providing the best possible health status available to the individual (Levine, 1990, p. 198).

- Practice problems of interest
  - Practice problems encompass conditions of health and disability reflected in the four conservation principles.
  - Every patient displays some problems in each of the areas [that] the Conservation Principles describe. Concerns for energy conservation and structural, personal, and social integrity are always present—though one area may present a more demanding problem than another. These areas can be explored individually, but they cannot be separated from the person (Levine, 1990, p. 199).

- Settings for nursing practice
  - The conservation principles have implications for every nursing situation (Levine, 1990, p. 199). Consequently, nursing practice occurs in virtually any setting, ranging from patients' homes to shelters for the homeless to ambulatory clinics to emergency departments to critical care units.

- Characteristics of legitimate participants in nursing practice
  - [Legitimate participants of nursing are] individuals [who] enter into a state of patienthood when they require the expert services that physicians and nurses can provide. [Patients may be sick or healthy.] Once individuals are restored, the dependent but willing partnership is dissolved. Their privacy restored to them, individuals cease to be patients (Levine, 1989c, pp. 4–5).

- Nursing Process
  - The nursing process for the Conservation Model is **Nursing Process as Conservation**. The components of the process are Trophicognosis, Intervention/Action, and Evaluation of Intervention/Action (see Table 6–1).

- Contributions of nursing practice to participants' well-being
  - Conservation Model-based nursing practice contributes to the well-being of individuals by promoting wholeness.

LOGICAL CONGRUENCE

The Conservation Model is logically congruent. The content of the model flows directly from Levine's philosophical claims. The overriding world view is that of reciprocal interaction. There is no evidence of the reaction world view in the Conservation Model. Levine (1971) explicitly rejected mechanism: "The mechanistic view of the body and mind does little to restore to the individual the wholeness he recognizes in himself" (p. 254). Although Levine (1966a) stated that "the human being responds to the forces in his environment in a singular yet integrated fashion" (p. 2452), she successfully translated the mechanistic idea of reaction to the environment by bringing in the idea of a more holistic, integrated response. However, Levine did cite Selye's mechanistic approach to stress within her description of the levels of organismic response. That potential threat to the logical consistency of the Conservation Model could be eliminated by the selection of a formulation of the stress response that reflects the reciprocal interaction world view.

GENERATION OF THEORY

Levine (1978a) stated that she was trying to develop two theories, which she called Therapeutic Intention and Redundancy. Work on the **Theory of Therapeutic**

Intention began in the early 1970s. Levine (personal communication to L. Criddle, July 22, 1987) indicated that she "was seeking a way of organizing nursing intervention growing out of the reality of the biological realities which nurses had to confront."

Schaefer (2001) has identified what she called the "guiding assumptions" for the **Theory of Therapeutic Intention** (p. 117). Those assumptions are:

- Conservation is the outcome of adaptation.
- Change associated with therapeutic intervention results in adaptation.
- The proper application of conservation (conservation principles) results in the restoration of health.
- Activities directed toward the preservation of health include health promotion, surveillance, illness prevention, and follow-up activities. (p. 117)

Levine's thinking about therapeutic intention is summarized in the seven areas of therapeutic intention listed here. Levine (personal communication, August 13, 1987) regarded the seven areas of therapeutic intention as an "imperfect list that is not yet complete."

- Therapeutic [regimens] that support the integrated healing processes of the body and permit optimal restoration of structure and function through natural response to disease.
- Therapeutic [regimens] that substitute an external servomechanism for a failure of autoregulation of an essential integrating system.
- Therapeutic [regimens] that focus on specific causes, and by surgical restructuring or drug therapy, restore individual integrity and well-being.
- Therapeutic [regimens] that cannot alter or substitute for the pathology so that only supportive measures are possible to promote comfort and humane concern.
- Therapeutic [regimens] that balance a significant toxic risk against the threat of the disease process.
- Therapeutic [regimens] that simulate physiological processes and reinforce or antagonize usual responses in order to create a therapeutic change in function.
- Therapeutic [regimens] that provide manipulation of diet and activity to correct metabolic imbalances related to nutrition and/or exercise. (Levine, personal communication to L. Criddle, July 22, 1987)

Although the **Theory of Therapeutic Intention** seems to extend the Levine's **Practice Methodology**, that is, the **Nursing Process as Conservation**, Levine (personal communication to L. Criddle, July 22, 1987) stated that she never associated the idea of therapeutic intention with the conservation principles. She explained, "I suppose it would be a claim to some greater wisdom to suggest that every idea I ever had was in some way associated with the Conservation Principles—but that is simply not true. My thought habits are fairly consistent but I have devoted them to many areas which are not organically related."

Schaefer (1991a) regarded the **Theory of Therapeutic Intention** as "very exciting" (p. 223). She commented, "Not only will the nurse have a repertoire of tested interventions, given that a theory provides specific information about care delivery, but also the nurse should have information about the expected organismic responses. With this in mind the theory provides direction for quality-assurance activities and measures of cost effectiveness" (p. 223). "The expected outcome of therapeutic intention," Schaefer (2001) explained, "would be a therapeutic response measured by the organismic change (e.g., adaptation resulting in conservation)" (p. 117).

Levine (1978a) noted that she and a colleague had been working on the **Theory of Redundancy** for some time. This "completely untested, completely speculative" theory has "redefined aging and almost everything else that has to do with human life." She proposed that "aging is the diminished availability of redundant systems necessary for effective maintenance of physical and social well-being" (Levine, 1978b). Later, Levine (1991) noted that "the possibility exists that aging itself is a consequence of failed redundancy of physiological and psychological processes" (p. 6). More specifically, the **Theory of Redundancy** postulates "that loss of redundant systems accounts for the process of aging. A critical loss of redundancy is not compatible with health and is often life-threatening" (Levine, 1996, p. 39). The theory clearly extends the discussion of the Redundancy dimension of the concept of Adaptation. Indeed, Schaefer (2001) commented that the **Theory of Redundancy** "is grounded in the concept of adaptation. Change is the process of adaptation and conservation is the outcome of adaptation" (p. 117).

Schaeffer (1991a) pointed out that the theory "is less clear than therapeutic intention because the thinking has not been related successfully to nursing practice. Continued work is needed before it can be considered for use" (p. 223). Citing a personal communication (September 21, 1989), Schaefer (1991a) reported that Levine "would like to continue to work on the development of [the] Theories [of Therapeutic Intention and Redundancy] but is unsure of the direction she will take" (p. 223). Unfortunately, Levine did not have the opportunity to continue her theoretical work before her death in 1996.

Schaefer, however, has continued the development of the theory by identifying statements that can be separated into an assumption undergirding the theory and three propositions about redundancy. The assumption is:

- The Theory of Redundancy assumes that there are fail-safe options available in the physiologic, anatomical, and psychological responses of individuals that are employed in the development of patient care (Schaefer, 2001, p. 117)

The propositions are:

- The body has more than one way for its function to be accomplished. It involves a series of adaptive responses (cascade of integrated responses—simultaneous, not separate) available when the stability of the organism is challenged.
- The selection of an option rests with the knowledge of the health-care provider in consultation with the patient.
- When redundant choices are lost, survival becomes difficult and ultimately fails for lack of fail-safe options—either those that the patient possess (e.g., two lungs) or those that can be employed on his or her behalf (e.g., medications or a pacemaker). (Schaefer, 2001, pp. 117-118)

Schaefer (1991a) commented that the **Theory of Redundancy** "may … explain the compensatory responses found in patients with congestive heart failure" (p. 223).

Alligood (1997, 2002) identified what she called the **Theory of Conservation**, which she regarded as a grand theory. Alligood indicated that the theory is implicit. Following Alligood's (1997) lead, Schaefer (2001) added that the theory "is based on the universal principle of conservation, which provides the foundation for the conservation principles in the model" (p. 117). She contributed statements about the theory that can be separated into assumptions and propositions. The assumptions are:

- All nursing actions are conservation.
- Conservation is natural law that is fundamental to many basic sciences.
- The purpose of conservation is to "keep together," … [which] means to maintain a proper balance between active nursing interventions coupled with patient participation on the one hand and the safe limits of the patients' abilities to participate on the other.
- Conservation assures wholeness, integrity, and unity. (Schaefer, 2001, p. 117)

Drawing from Levine's (1969b, 1973) work, Schaefer (2001) identified the major propositions of the **Theory of Conservation** as:

- Individual[s are] always within an environment milieu, and the consequences of [their] awareness of [their] environment persistently influence [their] behavior at any given moment.

- Individual[s protect] and defends [themselves] within [their] environment by gaining all the information [they] can about it.
- Nurse[s participate] actively in every patient's environment, and much of what [they do] supports his [or her] adaptations as he [or she] struggles in the predicament of illness.
- Even in the presence of disease, the organism responds wholly to the environment interaction in which it is involved, and considerable element of nursing care is devoted to restoring the symmetry of response—symmetry that is essential to the well-being of the organism (p. 117).

Levine (1991) denied that the so-called models included in her textbook *Introduction to Clinical Nursing* (vital signs; body movement and positioning; personal hygiene; pressure gradient systems—fluids; nutrition; pressure gradient systems—gases; heat and cold; medications; and asepsis) are a theory, as Pieper (1983) asserted. Rather, those so-called models "were intended to direct the nursing fundamentals essential to a beginning student of nursing. They were part of the textbook but were completely unrelated to the [Conservation Model], and only by stretching far beyond the text could they be construed as germane to the conservation principles" (Levine, 1991, p. 3).

The Conservation Model also has served as the basis for Schaefer's (1995, 1996) theory of struggling to maintain balance, which she generated from data about women's responses to fibromyalgia. In addition, the Conservation Model guided the development of Mock and colleagues' (1998, 2001) theory of the effects of walking exercise for women with breast cancer. A hallmark of Mock and colleagues' work is a diagram of the conceptual-theoretical-empirical structure for the study that was designed to test the theory.

CREDIBILITY OF THE NURSING MODEL

Social Utility

The utility of the Conservation Model for nursing research, education, administration, and practice is documented by the publication of the book *Levine's Conservation Model: A Framework for Nursing Practice* (Schaefer & Pond, 1991) and several journal articles and book chapters. The Conservation Model has a distinctive and extensive vocabulary that requires some study for mastery. Levine was, however, careful to provide adequate definitions of most terms so that there would be minimal confusion about the meaning of her ideas. As George (2002) pointed out, "Levine's careful use of words is … a strength. Her careful selection of terminology provides clarity to the reader" (p. 237).

A thorough understanding of the extensive and rich base of knowledge on which the Conservation Model is grounded requires considerable study in nursing and diverse adjunctive disciplines. Specific courses are identified in the Nursing Education Guidelines section on page 148.

Conservation Model-based nursing practice is feasible for many different patient populations in many different settings. George (2002) stated, "A major strength of Levine's work is its universality. Her concepts apply to all human beings wherever they may be. ... [T]he use of this work is not limited to any given setting but may be used wherever there is a nurse and a patient" (p. 237).

Cox's (1991) description of the use of the Conservation Model at the Alverno Health Care Facility (Clinton, Iowa) provides glimpses of the human and material resources needed to implement the model at the health-care organization level. The Alverno is a 136-bed intermediate care facility that provides long-term care to a patient population with an average age of 85 years. Staff members are taught to structure all nursing according to the conservation principles, and nursing goals have been established for each conservation principle. Parameters have been identified to determine the need to terminate activities because of excessive energy expenditure (conservation of energy) and to assess functional capability (structural integrity). Staff members learn to show respect for the residents by asking them how they wish to be addressed, and time is taken to learn the residents' former routines and to incorporate as much of that routine as possible into the plan of care (personal integrity). Residents and staff negotiate their roles and goals, and efforts are made to help the residents maintain ties with the local community (social integrity). Moreover, Cox (1991) commented that the conservation principles "allow each level of practitioner (nurse's aide, LPN, RN) to provide care based upon the knowledge appropriate for the level of practice" (p. 196).

Nursing Research. The utility of the Conservation Model for nursing research is documented by several studies. Published reports of descriptive, correlational, and experimental studies are listed in Table 6–2. Citations for those studies, as well as published abstracts of doctoral dissertations are listed in the Doctoral Dissertations section of the chapter bibliography on the CD-ROM. In addition, Levine (1989b) pointed out that Wong's (1968) master's thesis was derived from the Conservation Model.

Although much of the Conservation Model-based research is limited to a single study on a single topic, some programmatic research is evident. Burd and colleagues conducted a major program of pressure ulcer research derived from the principle of the conservation of structural integrity (see Table 6–2). In addition, Winslow and associates conducted a series of studies derived from the principle of the conservation of energy (see Table 6–2). Moreover, Foreman's research on confusion in older persons represents the beginning of a program of research, as do Schaefer's studies (see Table 6–2).

Noteworthy is Mock and colleagues' use of Levine's Conservation Model to guide a multisite study of the effects of an exercise intervention on fatigue among patients with cancer (see Table 6–2). The study was conducted as a central component of the Fatigue Initiative Through Research and Education (FIRE) project, which was a joint effort of the Oncology Nursing Foundation and the Oncology Nursing Society and funded by Ortho Biotech Incorporated (Haberman, 1998).

Nursing Education. The utility of the Conservation Model for nursing education is documented. Findings from surveys of baccalaureate nursing programs conducted by Hall (1979) and Riehl (1980) revealed that the Conservation Model was used as a guideline for curriculum development. In particular, Riehl found that Levine's model was "popular with faculty, especially in the Chicago area" (p. 396). The names of the schools of nursing using the Conservation Model were not given in the survey reports. However, Cox (1991) noted that the Conservation Model was used as a basis for course work in the master's degree medical-surgical nursing program at Loyola University of Chicago in the late 1960s.

Grindley and Paradowski (1991) presented a detailed description of the use of the Conservation Model as the curriculum guide for the baccalaureate nursing program at Allentown College of St. Francis de Sales in Center Valley, Pennsylvania. Schaefer (1991b) described the Conservation Model-based curriculum for the master's program in nursing at the same college.

In addition, Zwanger (personal communication, June 4, 1982) reported that Levine's Conservation Model was used in nursing education programs sponsored by Kapat-Holim, the Health Insurance Institution of the General Federation of Labour in Israel, based in Tel Aviv. Moreover, Stafford (personal communication, June 2, 1982) stated that she used the model "in teaching formal and informal classes such as the Critical Care Nursing course, Pacemaker Therapy, and The Nurse's Role in Electrocardiography" at the Hines Veterans Administration Medical Center in Hines, Illinois.

Nursing Administration. Levine's Conservation Model has documented utility for nursing service administration. Taylor developed a tool that can be used to evaluate the quality of nursing practice (Table 6–3). Stafford (personal communication, June 2, 1982) commented that she used Levine's Conservation Model to identify process and outcome criteria in the nursing care of patients with cardiovascular problems.

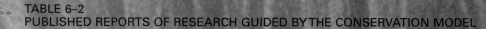
Research Topic	Study Participants	Citation*
Conservation of Energy: Energy utilization during toileting and bathing	Healthy adults Cardiac patients	Winslow et al., 1984, 1985 Personal communication to M.E. Levine from Winslow, October 6, 1982
Conservation of Energy: Energy expenditure during rest, occupied bedmaking, and unoccupied bedmaking	Healthy adults	Lane & Winslow, 1987
Conservation of Energy: Effects of boomerang and straight pillows on respiratory capacity	Healthy adult women	Roberts et al., 1994
Conservation of Energy: Sleep disturbances 1 week, 1 month, 3 months, and 6 months after surgery	Patients who had coronary artery bypass surgery	Schaefer et al., 1996
Conservation of Energy: Use of music therapy and other independent therapeutic nursing intervention in acute care	Hospitalized patients	Gagner-Tjellesen et al., 2001
Conservation of Energy: Effects of waterbeds on heart rate	Medically stable preterm infants	Deiriggi & Miles, 1995
Conservation of Structural Integrity: Prevalence and incidence of pressure ulcers	Hospice patients Patients in a nonacute rehabilitation center Patients in a skilled care nursing home Patients in an acute care hospital, a skilled care nursing home, a rehabilitation hospital, a home care agency, and a hospice	Hanson et al., 1991 Hunter et al., 1992 Burd et al., 1992 Langemo et al., 1993
Conservation of Structural Integrity: Incidence and prediction of pressure ulcers	Patients in an acute-care hospital, a skilled-care nursing home, a rehabilitation hospital, a home-care agency, and a hospice	Langemo et al., 1991
Conservation of Structural Integrity: Effect of pressure ulcer prevention and treatment protocols on prevalence of pressure ulcers	Hospice patients Patients in a nonacute rehabilitation hospital Patients in a skilled nursing home Patients in a skilled nursing home and a rehabilitation hospital	Hanson et al., 1994 Hunter et al., 1995 Burd et al., 1994 Langemo et al., 1993
Conservation of Structural Integrity: Incidence of and factors associated with intravenous site symptoms	Patients from two community hospitals, a large teaching hospital, and a government hospital	Dibble et al., 1991
Conservation of Energy and Structural Integrity: Identification of cues used by nurses for diagnosing activity intolerance related to an imbalance between oxygen supply and demand	Registered nurses	MacLean, 1987, 1988
Conservation of Energy and Structural Integrity: Effect of different body positions on transcutaneous oxygen tension	Infants 2 weeks to 2 years of age in a pediatric intensive care unit	Hader & Sorensen, 1988
Conservation of Energy and Social Integrity: Comparison of body temperature of infants placed on their mothers' chests immediately after birth and infants placed in a warmer	Newborn infants	Newport, 1984

*See the Research section of the chapter references for complete citations.

(continued)

Research Topic	Study Participants	Citation
Conservation of Energy and Structural Integrity: Effects of a boomerang pillow on respiratory capacity	Frail older women residing in nursing homes	Roberts et al., 1995
Conservation of Energy, Structural Integrity, Personal Integrity, and Social Integrity: Comparison of the effects of two bearing-down techniques during the second stage of labor on labor progress	Women in labor	Yeates & Roberts, 1984
Conservation of Energy, Structural Integrity, Personal Integrity, and Social Integrity: Integration of authors' previous research on perineal integrity	Women in labor	Roberts et al., 1991
Conservation of Energy, Structural Integrity, Personal Integrity, and Social Integrity: Description and causes of fatigue associated with congestive heart failure	Patients with congestive heart failure	Schaefer, 1990, 1991 Schaefer & Potylycki, 1993
Conservation of Energy, Structural Integrity, Personal Integrity, and Social Integrity: Relation of nutritional status, depression, and sleep-rest to fatigue	Chronically ill patients receiving long-term mechanical ventilation	Higgins, 1998
Conservation of Energy, Structural Integrity, Personal Integrity, and Social Integrity: Effects of a walking exercise intervention and a usual care control intervention on fatigue, physical functioning, emotional distress, social functioning, and quality of life	Women with breast cancer receiving chemotherapy or radiation therapy	Mock et al., 1998, 2001
Conservation of Energy, Structural Integrity, Personal Integrity, and Social Integrity: Incidence and onset of, andpsychophysiological variables associated with, the onset of acute confusional states (delirium)	Hospitalized older patients	Foreman, 1987, 1989, 1991
Conservation of Energy, Structural Integrity, Personal Integrity, and Social Integrity: Effects of Conservation Model-based nursing actions and control nursing actions on prevention of confusion	Hospitalized older patients	Nagley, 1986
Conservation of Energy, Structural Integrity, Personal Integrity, and Social Integrity: Effects of a Conservation Model-based dayroom program on complications from hospitalization and family satisfaction	Hospitalized confused geriatric patients	Clark et al., 1995
Maintaining wholeness: Living with fibromyalgia	Women with fibromyalgia	Schaefer, 1995, 1996
Identification of the nursing diagnosis of infection risk	Male and female patients scheduled for surgery	Piccoli & Galvão, 2001
Description of health needs of students with chronic health problems that require nursing interventions in the school setting and nature and extent of nursing services provided in schools in the late 1990s	School Nurse Organization of Minnesota members	Lowe & Miller, 1998

TABLE 6–3
PRACTICE TOOLS DERIVED FROM THE CONSERVATION MODEL

Practice Tool and Citation*	Description
Wound Assessment Instrument (Cooper, 1991)	Permits assessment of the conservation of structural integrity by documenting the visual characteristics of open, soft-tissue wounds.
Family Assessment Tool (Lynn-McHale & Smith, 1991)	Permits assessment of family members of patients in critical care units in terms of the conservation of energy (perception of the event, coping mechanisms, transportation logistics), conservation of structural integrity (nature of patient's illness, family functioning, current and future health needs), conservation of personal integrity (past experiences with illness, life events, ethnic/religious factors, family needs for solitude, information, meetings with physician or nurse), and conservation of social integrity (family support systems, visitation, work patterns).
Assessment Tool (McCall, 1991)	Permits identification of the nursing care needs of patients with seizures in terms of the conservation of energy (description of seizures and other medical problems), conservation of structural integrity (safety measures during seizures), conservation of personal integrity (effects of seizures on patient's feelings and functioning) and conservation of social integrity (patient's interactions with significant others, visitors during hospitalization, and other patients).
Nursing Diagnosis Assessment Guide (Taylor, 1987, 1989)	Permits assessment of neurological patients in terms of conservation of energy (oxygen supply, nutrition, activity/rest/sleep, illness-related energy expenditures), conservation of structural integrity (integument, musculoskeletal system, sensation/ perception, cerebral perfusion pressure, elimination, fluids and electrolytes, treatment-related risks), conservation of personal integrity (mental status, communication, image of self, adaptation), and conservation of social integrity (family/significant others, social situation). Assessment data are used to develop a comprehensive nursing care plan that lists the nursing diagnoses, expected outcomes, and interventions for each conservation principle.
Levine's Nursing Process Tool (Schaefer, 2001, 2002)	Provides guidelines for each component of Levine's Practice Methodology.
Levine's Nursing Process in the Community Tool (Schaefer, 2001)	Provides guidelines for each component of Levine's Practice Methodology, within the context of the community.
Evaluation of Quality of Care Tool (Taylor, 1974)	Permits evaluation of the quality of nursing care of neurological patients; the conservation principles serve as the goals of nursing care and are used as the frame of reference for defining commonly recurring nursing problems on the neurological service.

*See the Practice Tools section of the chapter references for complete citations.

The utility of Levine's conceptual model as a guide for the administration of nursing services is further documented by its use at The Alverno Health Care Facility (Cox, 1991). Here, the conservation principles structure the format of the nursing care plan and provide guidelines for staff development. The nursing care plan contains an extensive summary of the patient's trophicognosis, and nursing practice is organized according to the four conservation principles. The Conservation Model also was used to guide delivery of nursing services at the Temple Health Connection Neighborhood Nursing Center in Philadelphia, Pennsylvania (Pond, personal communications, 1995–1998).

Nursing Practice. Evidence supporting the utility of the Conservation Model for nursing practice is accumulating. Cooper, Lynn-McHale and Smith, McCall, and Taylor all have developed tools for assessment of patients with particular health problems, and Schaefer has developed tools to guide the application of Levine's **Nursing Process as Conservation** methodology for individuals and communities (Table 6–3). George (2002) commented, "A limitation [of Levine's Conservation Model] could be considered the need for each nurse to create his or her own assessment tool to use Levine's conservation principles. This could also be viewed a providing flexibility and allowing each nurse to create a personal fit with the principles" (p. 238). The first sentence in George's comment is especially puzzling, given the existence of the practice tools listed in Table 6–3.

The utility of the Conservation Model in many different settings and for patients with many different conditions is evident. The available published reports are listed in Table 6–4.

Review of the publications cited in Table 6–4 and those listed in the Commentary: Practice section of the chapter bibliography on the CD-ROM reveals that the principles of conservation have been used to guide nursing practice in inpatient settings for children and adults with conditions such as pneumonia, developmental delay, burn injuries, cancer, cardiac disease, failure of nervous system integration, cognitive impairment, confusion, hormonal disturbances, and fluid and electrolyte imbalances. The principles of conservation also have been used to guide nursing practice in emergency departments, operating rooms, obstetrical units, medical and surgical units, ambulatory clinics, a home for older adults, homeless shelters, and city streets.

Schaefer (2001) extended the Conservation Model to the community. She explained, "Using Levine's Conservation Model, community was initially defined as 'a group of people living together within a larger society, sharing common characteristics, interests, and location'" (pp.

111–112). She also developed a practice tool for use of Levine's **Nursing Process as Conservation** for communities (see Table 6–3), and identified areas for community-based assessment within each conservation principle. The assessment areas for the Principle of Conservation of Energy include hours of employment, water supply, and community budget. The assessment areas for the Principle of Conservation of Structural Integrity include city planning, availability of resources, transportation, and public services. The assessment areas for the Principle of Conservation of Structural Integrity include community identity, governmental mission, and political environment. The assessment areas for the Principle of Conservation of Social Integrity include recreation and social services.

Social Congruence

Although the Conservation Model was initially formulated many years ago, it is congruent with the present-day emphasis on holistic approaches to health care and consideration of each human being as a unique individuals. Levine developed her conceptual model at a time when nursing activities in acute care settings were becoming more mechanical as a result of the rapid increase in medical technology. More than 30 years ago, Levine (1966a) spoke out against the growing functionalism of nursing and reoriented nurses to the patient as a whole being:

> Discovering ways to perceive and cherish the essential wholeness of man becomes imperative with the rapid growth of automation in modern disciplines which possess a technology. Nursing is one of them, and nurses will not escape the sweeping changes that automation promises. But nurses do know that the integrated human being is not merely "programmed" to respond to life in automatic ways. ... It is the task of nursing to recognize and value the wondrous variety of all mankind while offering ministrations that conserve the unique and special integrity of every man. (p. 2453)

Levine (1973) noted that "the whole man is the focus of nursing intervention—in health and sickness, in tragedy and joy, in hospitals and clinics and in the community" (p. vii). Although little discussion of the use of the Conservation Model in health promotion and illness prevention situations is available, its broad focus is congruent with society's increasing interest in promotion of health and prevention of illness. Indeed, "The four conservation principles can be used in all nursing contexts" (Schaefer, 2002, p. 219).

The Conservation Model is acceptable to all members of the health-care team. Pond and Taney (1991) reported that the use of the Conservation Model effectively highlighted the nursing components of collaborative nurse-

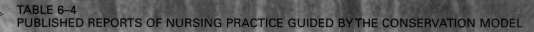

Practice Situation	Population	Citation*
Use of the haptic system as an information-gathering system	Older individuals with compromised perceptual systems	Gingrich, 1971
Development of trophicognoses	A 57-year-old man with end-stage heart disease	Fawcett et al., 1987
Development of nursing diagnoses based on the conservation principles	A 73-year-old woman who had a cerebrovascular accident	Taylor, 1987, 1989
Conservation of Energy	Patients who had a myocardial infarction and have a sleep disturbance	Littrell & Schumann, 1989
Conservation of Structural Integrity	Patients with soft-tissue wounds	Cooper, 1990 Neswick, 1997
Conservation of Personal Integrity and Social Integrity	Patients with chronic obstructive pulmonary disease	Dow & Mest, 1997
Conservation of Energy, Structural Integrity, Personal Integrity, and Social Integrity	An infant hospitalized with pneumonia	Dever, 1991
	A 16-month-old boy with multiple handicaps and severe developmental delay	Savage & Culbert, 1989
	A teenager with severe burn injuries	Bayley, 1991
	A 32-year-old woman with seizures of unknown etiology	McCall, 1991
	A 42-year-old man with epilepsy	McCall, 1991
	Patients with an ostomy	Neswick, 1997
	Patients with incontinence	Neswick, 1997
	Women with bladder dysfunction after radical hysterectomy for cervical cancer	O'Laughlin, 1986
	Patients with cardiac disease	Brunner, 1985
	Patients with congestive heart failure	Schaefer, 1991
	A woman undergoing reimplantation of digits of her hand	Crawford-Gamble, 1986
	A man who had undergone extensive bowel surgery resulting in a colostomy	Webb, 1993
	A 56-year-old woman with chronic pain from arthritis	Pasco & Halupa, 1991
	A 60-year-old man with chronic pain from metastatic prostate cancer	Pasco & Halupa, 1991
	Patients who are cognitively impaired as a result of illness	Hirschfeld, 1976
	Hospitalized confused older patients	Foreman, 1991
	Patients who had a cerebrovascular accident	Levine, 1973
	Patients with diabetes	Levine, 1973
	Patients with congestive circulatory failure	Levine, 1973
	Patients with a peptic ulcer	Levine, 1973
	Patients with emphysema	Levine, 1973
	Patients with anemia	Levine, 1973
	Patients with cancer	Herbst, 1981
Application of the Conservation Model	Patients with an acute infection	Levine, 1973
	Infants in an intensive care nursery	Levine, 1973
	A 29-year-old woman with cervical cancer	Langer, 1990
	A 44-year-old woman with fibromyalgia	Schaefer, 1997, 2002
	Women with fibromyalgia	Schaefer, 1997, 2002
	A 29-year-old white man with glomerulonephritis	Schaefer, 1996 Fawcett et al., 1992

*See the Practice section of the chapter references for complete citations.

(continued)

▶ ⋙ **TABLE 6–4**
PUBLISHED REPORTS OF NURSING PRACTICE GUIDED BY THE CONSERVATION MODEL *(continued)*

Practice Situation	Population	Citation
	A 20-year-old African-American woman with Guillain-Barré syndrome	Fawcett et al., 1992
	A 57-year-old African-American woman with diabetes, hypertension, lymphoma, and congestive heart failure	Schaefer & Pond, 1994
	Patients in the emergency department of the Hospital of the University of Pennsylvania in Philadelphia	Pond & Taney, 1991
	Homeless individuals at a clinic, shelters, day programs, feeding sites, and on the streets in Philadelphia, Pennsylvania	Pond, 1990, 1991
	Patients who have complications from a myocardial infarction	Molchany, 1992
	Older residents of The Alverno Health Care Facility in Clinton, Iowa	Cox, 1991

physician practice in an emergency department. Cox (1991) indicated that she had continued to use the conservation principles for more than 20 years in her work in the long-term care setting "because they are a natural fit for [that] setting" (p. 197). She also pointed out that the Conservation Model

> provides direction for nursing practice and staff development. The conservation principles provide an organizing framework, an easy-to-remember guide, for promoting wholeness within the limits imposed by the aging process and the consequences of chronic illness. … The model allows for the contributions made by all of the members of the interdisciplinary team. (p. 196)

Social Significance

The evidence supporting the social significance of the Conservation Model is both anecdotal, coming from reports of application of the model in nursing practice, and empirical, coming from reports of Conservation Model-based nursing research.

Anecdotal evidence from practice is evident in several published reports of the use of the Conservation Model in many settings. Hirschfeld (1976) noted that "Myra Levine's four principles of conservation are useful in deciding what will help the cognitively impaired aged person and determining what the priorities should be in his or her care" (p. 1981). She went on to describe application of the conservation principles to the care of several patients who had cognitive impairments. In concluding her article, Hirschfeld stated:

Surely, nursing care that incorporates Levine's four conservation principles can make a difference to the individual and family equilibrium that are disturbed by events as devastating as mental impairment. (p. 1984)

Lathrop (personal communication, May 5, 1982) used the Conservation Model to guide the nursing care of patients in the Intensive Treatment Unit for Mentally Ill Offenders at Saint Elizabeth's Hospital in Washington, D.C. She stated that nursing audits based on the American Nurses' Association Psychiatric/Mental Health Standards of Nursing Practice revealed that "treatment provided was more holistic in nature."

Cox (1991) reported that the four conservation principles provide a comprehensive focus for care and that "the identification of common recurring nursing problems and goals in long-term care gives direction and unity to nursing practice that fosters [high] quality care" (p. 196). Webb (1993) commented that the Conservation Model was useful in guiding postoperative nursing care "because of the emphasis it places on psychosocial nursing intervention, an area that is often neglected" (p. 128). Webb went on to say, "Nurses everywhere must redefine their attitude to psychological support and participate in truly holistic care that acknowledges all elements of the patient's environment" (p. 128).

Savage and Culbert (1989) pointed out that use of the conservation principles "allows the nurse to take a flexible, creative approach to caring for the family with a developmentally disabled child. Various approaches are incorporated into the nurse's role, moving the nurse from a peripheral position to a more central one on the early intervention multidisciplinary team. In turn, the nurse can contribute to the family's process of successful adaptation, which is the ultimate goal in the early intervention setting" (p. 345).

Pond and Taney (1991) maintained that the use of the Conservation Model

> ... strengthens communication among health care providers and improves the way nursing care is transmitted to and received by patients. In an atmosphere of collaboration each participant—health care provider and patient—is rewarded with respect and active contribution to the adaptation process. Both the internal and external environments of the patient are affected in such a way as to provide a move toward homeostasis. This is the goal called conservation or, from the medical model point of view, health maintenance. (p. 166)

Furthermore, Pond (1991) noted the difficulty of working with homeless patients but pointed to the success of Conservation Model-based nursing care. She commented, "As the conservation principles are used to assess each patient, a comprehensive picture develops. ... Many of our patients are easily managed and are integrated into the existing health care resources. Although it is never easy, many patients become independent in their health care and less dependent on our outreach services. We consider these many successes as reflective of the dedicated nursing interventions with these challenging situations" (p. 178).

In summarizing the empirical evidence, Schaefer (2001) pointed out that "studies support that energy can be conserved with nursing interventions and can be measured through the assessment of organismic responses" (p. 115). Empirical evidence from experimental studies of the effects of skin care strategies on pressure ulcer prevalence is especially compelling. Use of skin care prevention and intervention strategies, which were derived directly from the Principle of Conservation of Structural Integrity, resulted in a statistically significant and practically meaningful reduction in development of pressure ulcers in patients in a rehabilitation hospital and a skilled nursing home. More specifically, the prevalence of pressure ulcers declined 60 percent in the rehabilitation hospital (Hunter et al., 1995), and 54 percent in the nursing home (Burd et al., 1994).

Also compelling is the evidence from Mock and colleagues' (2001) multisite study of the effects of an exercise intervention on variables representing the four conservation principles in a sample of women receiving adjuvant treatment for breast cancer. They reported that women who exercised at least 90 minutes each week (the high-walk group) experienced less fatigue and emotional distress and higher functional ability and quality of life than women who exercised less (the low-walk group). Mock and colleagues (2001) explained:

The study results provide support for ... the Levine conservation model, with regard to each of its four conservation principles. High-walk subjects conserved energy as reflected in lower fatigue levels compared with low-walk subjects. The conservation of structural integrity for high-walk subjects was demonstrated by increased functional capacity. ... The conservation of personal integrity was reflected in lower mood distress scores ... and higher [quality of life] scores ... for high-walk subjects, while scores for low-walk subjects decreased over the course of their breast cancer treatment. (p. 126)

 ## CONTRIBUTIONS TO THE DISCIPLINE OF NURSING

The Conservation Model makes a substantial contribution to the discipline of nursing by focusing attention on the wholeness of each human being. Levine moved beyond the idea of the total person to the concept of the human being as a holistic being. Pointing to the limitations of the so-called total person approach, Levine (1969b) commented:

> Nurses have long known that patients are complete persons, not groups of parts. It is out of this realization that the attempts toward "comprehensive care" and "total care" have come, and it is because we have been frustrated by failing to achieve the ideal of completion that the search for a more definitive approach to bedside care has continued. (p. 94)

The Conservation Model is consistent in its approach to human beings as holistic beings. Wholeness is the central feature of the model. Indeed, Levine (1995a) stated, "I introduced the concept [wholeness] with the Conservation Principles in 1964, and it has remained a hallmark of my work ever since" (p. 262). Wholeness is evident in all aspects of the Conservation Model—physiological and behavioral responses are regarded as the same, and the conservation principles are joined. Moreover, the conservation principles provide a comprehensive framework for holistic nursing care and focus attention on the patient as an unique individual.

Grindley and Paradowski (1991) maintained that "the adaptability of the model is one of its greatest strengths. The conservation principles have easily stood the test of time and the impact of technology" (p. 207). They went on to say:

> Individuals continue to be unique; they cope with ever-increasing assaults on their energies. The constant barrage on their integrities by the world around them reinforces the fact that the nurse must be ever alert to the potential and actual impact of these assaults. Holistic care touches the individual, the family, and the community. Levine's principles are applicable not only to individuals but also to a larger group, the others who are significant to them. (pp. 207–208)

Noteworthy is the accurate use of knowledge from what Levine (1988a) called adjunctive disciplines. She credited the scholars of other disciplines from whose works she drew for the development of her conceptual model, and she heeded her own requirement to use that knowledge appropriately (Levine, 1995b).

Although documentation of the utility of the Conservation Model for nursing activities is increasing, additional empirical evidence of its credibility is warranted. Systematic evaluations of the use of the model in various nursing situations are needed, as are more studies that test conceptual-theoretical-empirical structures derived directly from the conservation principles. An excellent example of a Conservation Model-based conceptual-theoretical-empirical structure was provided by Mock and colleagues (1998, 2001). Perhaps the most important need is for more valid and reliable empirical indicators to measure the phenomena encompassed by the Conservation Model. The practice tools that already have been developed require systematic testing to determine intrarater and interrater reliability. Schaefer (1991a) pointed out, "An assessment tool is perhaps the most important measure of wholeness. Using the elements of trophicognosis, practitioners and researchers are encouraged to develop assessment measures based on Levine's Conservation Model and to test for a reliable and valid data base common to all patients presenting with a need for nursing care" (p. 221).

Myra Levine's death was not the end of the Conservation Model. Rather, the literature indicates that many nurses remain interested in using the Conservation Model as a guide for their nursing activities. Their collective works augur well for the continued development of this conceptual model of nursing. As Schaefer (2002) put it, the Conservation Model "has continued to have utility for nursing practice and research and is receiving increased recognition in this twenty-first century" (p. 219).

In conclusion, Levine's Conservation Model provides nursing with a logically congruent, holistic view of human beings. Theories related to the model have been formulated, but they require further development and empirical testing. The lack of major limitations suggests that the Conservation Model may be an effective and comprehensive guide for nursing actions in diverse settings.

 REFERENCES

Alligood, M.R. (1997). Models and theories: Critical thinking structures. In M.R. Alligood & A. Marriner-Tomey (Eds.), Nursing theory: Utilization and application (pp. 31–45). St. Louis: Mosby.

Alligood, M.R. (2002). Philosophies, models, and theories: Critical thinking structures. In M.R. Alligood & A. Marriner-

Tomey (Eds.), Nursing theory: Utilization and application (2nd ed., pp. 41–61). St. Louis: Mosby.

Barnum, B.J.S. (1998). Nursing theory: Analysis, application, evaluation (5th ed.). Philadelphia: Lippincott.

Bates, M. (1967). A naturalist at large. Natural History, 76(6), 8–16.

Beland, I. (1971). Clinical nursing: Pathophysiological and psychosocial implications (2nd ed.). New York: Macmillan.

Bernard, C. (1957). An introduction to the study of experimental medicine. New York: Dover. [Unabridged and unaltered reprint of the first English translation, published 1927. Originally published in French in 1865.]

Burd, C., Olson, B., Langemo, D., Hunter, S., Hanson, D., Osowski, K.F., & Sauvage, T. (1994). Skin care strategies in a skilled nursing home. Journal of Gerontological Nursing, 20(11), 28–34.

Cannon, W.B. (1939). The wisdom of the body. New York: Norton.

Cohen, Y. (1968). Man in adaptation: The biosocial background. Chicago: Aldine.

Cox, R.A., Sr. (1991). A tradition of caring: Use of Levine's model in long-term care. In K.M. Schaefer & J.B. Pond (Eds.), Levine's conservation model: A framework for nursing practice (pp. 179–197). Philadelphia: F.A. Davis.

Dubos, R. (1961). Mirage of health. New York: Doubleday.

Dubos, R. (1965). Man adapting. New Haven: Yale University Press.

Erikson, E.H. (1964). Insight and responsibility. New York: Norton.

Erikson, E.H. (1968). Identity: Youth and crisis. New York: Norton.

Esposito, C.H., & Leonard, M.K. (1980). Myra Estrin Levine. In Nursing Theories Conference Group, Nursing theories. The base for professional nursing practice (pp. 150–163). Englewood Cliffs, NJ: Prentice-Hall.

Feiblemann, J.K. (1959). The logical structure of the scientific method. Dialectica, 13, 209.

Feynman, R. (1965). The character of physical law. Cambridge, MA: M.I.T. Press.

George, J.B. (2002). The conservation principles, A model for health: Myra E. Levine. In J. B. George (Ed.), Nursing theories: The base for professional nursing practice (5th ed., pp. 2225–2240). Upper Saddle River, NJ: Prentice Hall.

Gibson, J.E. (1966). The senses considered as perceptual systems. Boston: Houghton-Mifflin.

Goldstein, K. (1963). The organism. Boston: Beacon Press.

Grindley, J., & Paradowski, M. (1991). Developing an undergraduate program using Levine's model. In K.M. Schaefer & J.B. Pond (Eds.), Levine's conservation model: A framework for nursing practice (pp. 199–208). Philadelphia: F.A. Davis.

Haberman, M. R. (1998). Implementing the FIRE® planning grant: Introduction. Oncology Nursing Forum, 25, 1389–1390.

Hall, E. (1959). Silent language. Greenwich, CT: Fawcett.

Hall, E. (1966). The hidden dimension. Garden City, NY: Doubleday.

Hall, K.V. (1979). Current trends in the use of conceptual frameworks in nursing education. Journal of Nursing Education, 18(4), 26–29.

Hirschfeld, M.J. (1976). The cognitively impaired older adult. American Journal of Nursing, 76, 1981–1984.

Hochachka, P.W., & Somero, G.H. (1984). Biochemical adaptation. Princeton, NJ: Princeton University Press.

Hunter, S.M., Langemo, D.K., Olson, B., Hanson, D., Cathcart-Silberberg, T., Burd, C., & Sauvage, T.R. (1995). The effectiveness of skin care protocols for pressure ulcers. Rehabilitation Nursing, 20, 250–255.

Levine, M.E. (1966a). Adaptation and assessment: A rationale for nursing intervention. American Journal of Nursing, 66, 2450–2453.

Levine, M.E. (1966b). Trophicognosis: An alternative to nursing diagnosis. In American Nurses' Association Regional Clinical Conference (Vol. 2, pp. 55–70). New York: American Nurses' Association.

Levine, M.E. (1967). The four conservation principles of nursing. Nursing Forum, 6, 45–59.

Levine, M.E. (1969a). Introduction to clinical nursing. Philadelphia: F.A. Davis.

Levine, M.E. (1969b). The pursuit of wholeness. American Journal of Nursing, 69, 93–98.

Levine, M.E. (1971). Holistic nursing. Nursing Clinics of North America, 6, 253–264.

Levine, M.E. (1973). Introduction to clinical nursing (2nd ed.). Philadelphia: F.A. Davis.

Levine, M.E. (1977). Nursing ethics and the ethical nurse. American Journal of Nursing, 77, 845–849.

Levine, M.E. (1978a, December). The four conservation principles of nursing. Paper presented at the Second Annual Nurse Educator Conference, New York. [Audiotape.]

Levine, M.E. (1978b, December). Application to education and practice. Paper presented at Second Annual Nurse Educator Conference, New York. [Audiotape.]

Levine, M.E. (1984a, August). Myra Levine. Paper presented at the Nurse Theorist Conference, Edmonton, Alberta, Canada. [Audiotape.]

Levine, M.E. (1984b, August). Concurrent sessions. M. Levine. Discussion at the Nurse Theorist Conference, Edmonton, Alberta, Canada. [Audiotape.]

Levine, M.E. (1985, August). Myra Levine. Paper presented at conference on Nursing Theory in Action, Edmonton, Alberta, Canada. [Audiotape.]

Levine, M.E. (1986, August). Myra Levine. Paper presented at Nursing Theory Congress: Theoretical Pluralism: Direction for a Practice Discipline, Toronto, Ontario, Canada. [Audiotape.]

Levine, M.E. (1987). The nurse theorists: Portraits of excellence—Myra Levine. Athens, OH: Fuld Institute for Technology in Nursing Education. [Videotape.]

Levine, M.E. (1988a). Antecedents from adjunctive disciplines: Creation of nursing theory. Nursing Science Quarterly, 1, 16–21.

Levine, M.E. (1988b). Myra Levine. In T.M. Schorr & A. Zimmerman, Making choices. Taking chances. Nurse leaders tell their stories (pp. 215–228). St. Louis: Mosby.

Levine, M.E. (1989a). Beyond dilemma. Seminars in Oncology Nursing, 5, 124–128.

Levine, M.E. (1989b). The conservation principles of nursing: Twenty years later. In J.P. Riehl (Ed.), Conceptual models for nursing practice (3rd ed., pp. 325–337). Norwalk, CT: Appleton & Lange.

Levine, M.E. (1989c). The ethics of nursing rhetoric. Image: Journal of Nursing Scholarship, 21, 4–6.

Levine, M.E. (1989d). Ration or rescue: The elderly patient in critical care. Critical Care Nursing Quarterly, 12(1), 82–89.

Levine. M.E. (1990). Conservation and integrity. In M.E. Parker (Ed.), Nursing theories in practice (pp. 189–201). New York: National League for Nursing.

Levine, M.E. (1991). The conservation principles: A model for health. In K.M. Schaefer and J.B. Pond (Eds.), Levine's conservation model: A framework for nursing practice (pp. 1–11). Philadelphia: F.A. Davis.

Levine, M.E. (1992). Nightingale redux. In F.N. Nightingale, Notes on nursing: What it is, and what it is not (Commemorative edition, pp. 39–43). Philadelphia: Lippincott.

Levine, M.E. (1995a). Myra Levine responds [Letter to the editor]. Image: Journal of Nursing Scholarship, 27, 262.

Levine, M.E. (1995b). The rhetoric of nursing theory. Image: Journal of Nursing Scholarship, 27, 11–14.

Levine, M.E. (1996). The conservation principles: A retrospective. Nursing Science Quarterly, 9, 38–41.

Margulis, L. (1971, August). Symbiosis and evolution, 225, 48–57.

Marriner-Tomey, A. (1989). Nursing theorists and their work (2nd ed.). St. Louis: Mosby.

Meleis, A.I. (1997). Theoretical nursing: Development and progress (3rd ed.). Philadelphia: Lippincott.

Mock, V., Pickett, M., Ropka, M.E., Lin, E.M., Stewart, K.J., Rhodes, V.A., McDaniel, R., Grimm, P.M., Krumm, S., & McCorkle, R. (2001). Fatigue and quality of life outcomes of exercise during cancer treatment. Cancer Practice, 9, 119–127.

Mock, V., Ropka, M.E., Rhodes, V.A., Pickett, M., Grimm, P.M., McDaniel, R., Lin, E.M., Allocca, P., Dienemann, J.A., Haisfield-Wolfe, M.E., Stewart, K.J., & McCorkle, R. (1998). Establishing mechanisms to conduct multi-institutional research—Fatigue in patients with cancer: An exercise intervention. Oncology Nursing Forum, 25, 1391–1397.

Newman, M.A. (1972). Nursing's theoretical evolution. Nursing Outlook, 20, 449–453.

Nightingale, F. (1859). Notes on nursing: What it is and what it is not. London: Harrison & Sons.

Pieper, B.A. (1983). Levine's nursing model. In J.J. Fitzpatrick & A.L. Whall (Eds.), Conceptual models of nursing: Analysis and application (pp. 101–115). Bowie, MD: Brady.

Pond, J.B. (1991). Ambulatory care of the homeless. In K.M. Schaefer & J.B. Pond (Eds.), Levine's conservation model: A framework for nursing practice (pp. 167–178). Philadelphia: F.A. Davis.

Pond, J.B., & Taney, S.G. (1991). Emergency care in a large university emergency department. In K.M. Schaefer & J.B. Pond (Eds.), Levine's conservation model: A framework for nursing practice (pp. 151–166). Philadelphia: F.A. Davis.

Riehl, J.P. (1980). Nursing models in current use. In J.P. Riehl & C. Roy (Eds.), Conceptual models for nursing practice (2nd ed., pp. 393–398). New York: Appleton-Century-Crofts.

Riehl-Sisca, J.P. (1989). Conceptual models for nursing practice (3rd ed.). Norwalk, CT: Appleton & Lange.

Sacks, O. (1985). The man who mistook his wife for a hat. Garden City, NY: Doubleday.

Savage, T.A., & Culbert, C. (1989). Early intervention: The unique role of nursing. Journal of Pediatric Nursing, 4, 339–345.

Schaefer, K.M. (1991a). Creating a legacy. In K.M. Schaefer & J.B. Pond (Eds.), Levine's conservation model: A framework for nursing practice (pp. 219–224). Philadelphia: F.A. Davis.

Schaefer, K.M. (1991b). Developing a graduate program in nursing: Integrating Levine's philosophy. In K.M. Schaefer & J.B. Pond (Eds.), Levine's conservation model: A framework for nursing practice (pp. 209–217). Philadelphia: F.A. Davis.

Schaefer, K.M. (1991c). Levine's conservation principles and research. In K.M. Schaefer & J.B. Pond (Eds.), Levine's conservation model: A framework for nursing practice (pp. 45–59). Philadelphia: F.A. Davis.

Schaefer, K.M. (1995). Struggling to maintain balance: A study of women living with fibromyalgia. Journal of Advanced Nursing, 21, 95–102.

Schaefer, K.M. (1996). Levine's conservation model: Caring for women with chronic illness. In P. Hinton Walker & B. Neuman (Eds.), Blueprint for use of nursing models: Education, research, practice, and administration (pp. 187–227). New York: NLN Press.

Schaefer, K.M. (2001). Myra Levine conservation model: A model for the future. In M.E. Parker (Ed.), Nursing theories and nursing practice (pp. 103–123). Philadelphia: F.A. Davis.

Schaefer, K.M. (2002). Myra Estrin Levine: The conservation model. In A. Marriner-Tomey & M.R. Alligood (Eds.), Nursing theorists and their work (5th ed., pp. 212–225). St. Louis: Mosby.

Schaefer, K.M., & Pond, J.B. (1991). Levine's conservation model: A framework for nursing practice. Philadelphia: F.A. Davis.

Selye, H. (1956). The stress of life. New York: McGraw—Hill.

Sherrington, A. (1906). Integrative function of the nervous system. New York: Scribner's.

Tillich, P. (1961). The meaning of health. Perspectives in Biology and Medicine, 5, 92–100.

Waddington, C.H. (Ed.). (1968). Towards a theoretical biology. I. Prolegomena. Chicago: Aldine.

Webb, H. (1993). Holistic care following a palliative Hartmann's procedure. British Journal of Nursing, 2, 128–132.

Weiner, N. (1954). The human use of human beings. New York: Avon Books.

Wolf, S. (1961). Disease as a way of life: Neural integration in systemic pathology. Perspectives in Biology and Medicine, 4, 288–305.

Wong, S. (1968). Rehabilitation of a patient following myocardial [infarction]. Unpublished master's thesis, Loyola University of Chicago School of Nursing.

RESEARCH

Burd, C., Langemo, D.K., Olson, B., Hanson, D., Hunter, S., & Sauvage, T. (1992). Skin problems: Epidemiology of pressure ulcers in a skilled care facility. Journal of Gerontological Nursing, 18(9), 29–39.

Burd, C., Olson, B., Langemo, D., Hunter, S., Hanson, D., Osowski, K.F., & Sauvage, T. (1994). Skin care strategies in a skilled nursing home. Journal of Gerontological Nursing, 20(11), 28–34.

Clark, L.R., Fraaza, V., Schroeder, S., & Maddens, M.E. (1995). Alternative nursing environments: Do they affect hospital outcomes? Journal of Gerontological Nursing, 21(11), 32–38.

Deiriggi, P.M., & Miles, K.E. (1995). The effects of waterbeds on heart rate in preterm infants. Scholarly Inquiry for Nursing Practice, 9, 245–262.

Dibble, S.L., Bostrom-Ezrati, J., & Bizzuto, C. (1991). Clinical predictors of intravenous site symptoms. Research in Nursing and Health, 14, 413–420.

Foreman, M. (1987). A causal model for making decisions about confusion in the hospitalized elderly. In K.J. Hannah, M. Reimer, W.C. Mills, & S. Letourneau (Eds.), Clinical judgment and decision making: The future with nursing diagnosis (pp. 427–429). New York: Wiley.

Foreman, M. (1989). Confusion in the hospitalized elderly: Incidence, onset, and associated factors. Research in Nursing and Health, 12, 21–29.

Foreman, M. (1991). Conserving cognitive integrity of the hospitalized elderly. In K.M. Schaefer & J.B. Pond (Eds.), Levine's conservation model: A framework for nursing practice (pp. 133–149). Philadelphia: F.A. Davis.

Gagner-Tjellesen, D., Yurkovich, E.E., & Gragert, M. (2001). Use of music therapy and other ITNIs in acute care. Journal of Psychosocial Nursing and Mental Health Services, 39(10), 26–37, 52–53.

Hader, C.F., & Sorensen, E.R. (1988). The effects of body position on transcutaneous oxygen tension. Pediatric Nursing, 14, 469–473.

Hanson, D.S., Langemo, D., Olson, B., Hunter, S., & Burd, C. (1994). Evaluation of pressure ulcer prevalence rates for hospice patients post-implementation of pressure ulcer protocols. American Journal of Hospice and Palliative Care, 11(6), 14–19.

Hanson, D.S., Langemo, D., Olson, B., Hunter, S., Sauvage, T.R., Burd, C., & Cathcart-Silberberg, T. (1991). The prevalence and incidence of pressure ulcers in the hospice setting: Analysis of two methodologies. American Journal of Hospice and Palliative Care, 8(5), 18–22.

Higgins, P.A. (1998). Patient perceptions of fatigue while undergoing long-term mechanical ventilation: Incidence and associated factors. Heart and Lung, 27, 177–183.

Hunter, S.M., Cathcart-Silberberg, T., Langemo, D.K., Olson, B., Hanson, D., Burd, C., & Sauvage, T.R. (1992). Pressure ulcer prevalence and incidence in a rehabilitation hospital. Rehabilitation Nursing, 17, 239–242.

Hunter, S.M., Langemo, D.K., Olson, B., Hanson, D., Cathcart-Silberberg, T., Burd, C., & Sauvage, T.R. (1995). The effectiveness of skin care protocols for pressure ulcers. Rehabilitation Nursing, 20, 250–255.

Lane, L.D., & Winslow, E.H. (1987). Oxygen consumption, cardiovascular response, and perceived exertion in healthy adults during rest, occupied bedmaking, and unoccupied bedmaking activity. Cardiovascular Nursing, 23(6), 31–36.

Langemo, D., Olson, B., Hanson, D., Hunter, S., Cathcart-Silberberg, T., & Sauvage, T. (1993). Pressure ulcer research: Incidence and evaluation of effectiveness of protocols. Prairie Rose, 62(2), 13–16.

Langemo, D.K., Olson, B., Hunter, S., Hanson, D., Burd, C., & Cathcart-Silberberg, T. (1991). Incidence and prediction of pressure ulcers in five patient care settings. Decubitus, 4(3), 25–26, 28, 30, 32, 36.

Lowe, J., & Miller, W. (1998). Health services provided by school nurses for students with chronic health problems. Journal of School Nursing, 14(5), 4–10, 12–16.

MacLean, S.L. (1987). Description of cues used by nurses when diagnosing activity intolerance. In K.J. Hannah, M. Reimer, W.C. Mills, & S. Letourneau (Eds.), Clinical judgment and decision making: The future with nursing diagnosis (pp. 161–163). New York: Wiley.

MacLean, S.L. (1988). Activity intolerance: Cues for diagnosis. In R.M. Carroll-Johnston (Ed.), Classification of nursing diagnoses: Proceedings of the eighth conference: North American Nursing Diagnosis Association (pp. 320–327). Philadelphia: Lippincott.

Mock, V., Pickett, M. Ropka, M.E., Lin, E.M., Stewart, K.J., Rhodes, V.A., McDaniel, R., Grimm, P.M., Krumm, S., & McCorkle, R. (2001). Fatigue and quality of life outcomes of exercise during cancer treatment. Cancer Practice, 9, 119–127.

Mock, V., Ropka, M.E., Rhodes, V.A., Pickett, M., Grimm, P.M., McDaniel, R., Lin, E.M., Allocca, P., Dienemann, J.A., Haisfield-Wolfe, M.E., Stewart, K.J., & McCorkle, R. (1998). Establishing mechanisms to conduct multi-institutional research—Fatigue in patients with cancer: An exercise intervention. Oncology Nursing Forum, 25, 1391–1397.

Nagley, S.J. (1986). Predicting and preventing confusion in your patients. Journal of Gerontological Nursing, 12(3), 27–31.

Newport, M.A. (1984). Conserving thermal energy and social integrity in the newborn. Western Journal of Nursing Research, 6, 176–197.

Piccoli, M. & Galvão, C.M. (2001). Perioperative nursing: Identification of the nursing diagnosis infection risk based on Levine's conceptual model. Revista Latino-Americana de Enfermagem, 9(4), 37–43. [Portuguese; English abstract]

Roberts, J.E., Fleming, N., & Yeates-Giese, D. (1991). Perineal integrity. In K.M. Schaefer & J.B. Pond (Eds.), Levine's conservation model: A framework for nursing practice (pp. 61–70). Philadelphia: F.A. Davis.

Roberts, K.L., Brittin, M., Cook, M., & deClifford, J. (1994). Boomerang pillows and respiratory capacity. Clinical Nursing Research, 3, 157–165.

Roberts, K.L., Brittin, M., & deClifford, J. (1995). Boomerang pillows and respiratory capacity in frail elderly women. Clinical Nursing Research, 4, 465–471.

Schaefer, K.M. (1990). A description of fatigue associated with congestive heart failure: Use of Levine's conservation model. In M.E. Parker (Ed.), Nursing theories in practice (pp. 217–237). New York: National League for Nursing.

Schaefer, K.M. (1991). Levine's conservation principles and research. In K.M. Schaefer & J.B. Pond (Eds.), Levine's conservation model: A framework for nursing practice (pp. 45–59). Philadelphia: F.A. Davis.

Schaefer, K.M. (1995). Struggling to maintain balance: A study of women living with fibromyalgia. Journal of Advanced Nursing, 21, 95–102.

Schaefer, K.M. (1996). Levine's conservation model: Caring for women with chronic illness. In P. Hinton Walker & B. Neuman (Eds.), Blueprint for use of nursing models (pp. 187–227). New York: NLN Press.

Schaefer, K.M., & Potylycki, M.J.S (1993). Fatigue associated with congestive health failure: Use of Levine's conservation model. Journal of Advanced Nursing, 18, 260–268.

Schaefer, K.M., Swavely, D., Rothenberger, C., Hess, S., & Williston, D. (1996). Sleep disturbances post coronary artery bypass surgery. Progress in Cardiovascular Nursing, 11, 5–14.

Winslow, E.H., Lane, L.D., & Gaffney, F.A. (1984). Oxygen consumption and cardiovascular response in patients and normal adults during in-bed and out-of-bed toileting. Journal of Cardiac Rehabilitation, 4, 348–354.

Winslow, E.H., Lane, L.D., & Gaffney, F.A. (1985). Oxygen consumption and cardiovascular response in control adults and acute myocardial infarction patients during bathing. Nursing Research, 34, 164–169.

Yeates, D.A., & Roberts, J.E. (1984). A comparison of two bearing-down techniques during the second stage of labor. Journal of Nurse-Midwifery, 29, 3–11.

PRACTICE TOOLS

Cooper, D.M. (1991). Development and testing of an instrument to assess the visual characteristics of open, soft tissue wounds. Dissertation Abstracts International, 51, 3320B.

Lynn-McHale, D.J., & Smith, A. (1991). Comprehensive assessment of families of the critically ill. AACN Clinical Issues in Critical Care Nursing, 2, 195–209.

McCall, B.H. (1991). Neurological intensive monitoring system: Unit assessment tool. In K.M. Schaefer & J.B. Pond (Eds.), Levine's conservation model: A framework for nursing practice (pp. 83–90). Philadelphia: F.A. Davis.

Schaefer, K.M. (2001). Myra Levine conservation model: A model for the future. In M.E. Parker (Ed.), Nursing theories and nursing practice (pp. 103–123). Philadelphia: F.A. Davis.

Schaefer, K.M. (2002). Levine's conservation model in nursing practice. In M.R. Alligood & A. Marriner-Tomey (Eds.), Nursing theory: Utilization and application (2nd ed., pp. 197–217). St. Louis: Mosby.

Taylor, J.W. (1974). Measuring the outcomes of nursing care. Nursing Clinics of North America, 9, 337–340.

Taylor, J.W. (1987). Organizing data for nursing diagnoses using conservation principles. In A.M. McLane (Ed.), Classification of nursing diagnoses: Proceedings of the seventh conference: North American Nursing Diagnosis Association (pp. 103–111). St. Louis: Mosby.

Taylor, J.W. (1989). Levine's conservation principles. Using the model for nursing diagnosis in a neurological setting. In J.P. Riehl-Sisca (Ed.), Conceptual models for nursing practice (3rd ed., pp. 349–358). Norwalk, CT: Appleton & Lange.

PRACTICE

Bayley, E.W. (1991). Care of the burn patient. In K.M. Schaefer & J.B. Pond (Eds.), Levine's conservation model: A framework for nursing practice (pp. 91–99). Philadelphia: F.A. Davis.

Brunner, M. (1985). A conceptual approach to critical care nursing using Levine's model. Focus on Critical Care, 12(2), 39–44.

Cooper, D.M. (1990). Optimizing wound healing. A practice within nursing's domain. Nursing Clinics of North America, 25, 165–180.

Cox, R.A., Sr. (1991). A tradition of caring: Use of Levine's model in long-term care. In K.M. Schaefer & J.B. Pond (Eds.), Levine's conservation model: A framework for nursing practice (pp. 179–197). Philadelphia: F.A. Davis.

Crawford-Gamble, P.E. (1986). An application of Levine's conceptual model. Perioperative Nursing Quarterly, 2(1), 64–70.

Dever, M. (1991). Care of children. In K.M. Schaefer & J.B. Pond (Eds.), Levine's conservation model: A framework for nursing practice (pp. 71–82). Philadelphia: F.A. Davis.

Dow, J.S., & Mest, C.G. (1997). Psychosocial interventions for patients with chronic obstructive pulmonary disease. Home Healthcare Nurse, 15, 414–420.

Fawcett, J., Archer, C.L., Becker, D., Brown, K.K., Gann, S., Wong, M.J., & Wurster, A.B. (1992). Guidelines for selecting a conceptual model of nursing: Focus on the individual patient. Dimensions of Critical Care Nursing, 11, 268–277.

Fawcett, J., Cariello, F.P., Davis, D.A., Farley, J., Zimmaro, D.M., & Watts, R.J. (1987). Conceptual models of nursing: Application to critical care nursing practice. Dimensions of Critical Care Nursing, 6, 202–213.

Foreman, M. (1991). Conserving cognitive integrity of the hospitalized elderly. In K.M. Schaefer & J.B. Pond (Eds.), Levine's conservation model: A framework for nursing practice (pp. 133–149). Philadelphia: F.A. Davis.

Gingrich, B. (1971). The use of the haptic system as an information-gathering system. In M. Duffey, E.H. Anderson, B.S. Bergersen, M. Lohr, & M.H. Rose (Eds.), Current concepts in clinical nursing (Vol. 3, pp. 235–246). St. Louis: Mosby.

Herbst, S. (1981). Impairments as a result of cancer. In N. Martin, N. Holt, & D. Hicks (Eds.), Comprehensive rehabilitation nursing (pp. 553–578). New York: McGraw-Hill.

Hirschfeld, M.J. (1976). The cognitively impaired older adult. American Journal of Nursing, 76, 1981–1984.

Langer, V.S. (1990). Minimal handling protocol for the intensive care nursery. Neonatal Network: Journal of Neonatal Nursing, 9(3), 23–27.

Levine, M.E. (1973). Introduction to clinical nursing (2nd ed.). Philadelphia: F.A. Davis.

Littrell, K., & Schumann, L.L. (1989). Promoting sleep for the patient with a myocardial infarction. Critical Care Nurse, 9(3), 44–49.

McCall, B.H. (1991). Neurological intensive monitoring system: Unit assessment tool. In K.M. Schaefer & J.B. Pond (Eds.), Levine's conservation model: A framework for nursing practice (pp. 83–90). Philadelphia: F.A. Davis.

Molchany, C.A. (1992). Ventricular septal and free wall rupture complicating acute MI. Journal of Cardiovascular Nursing, 6(4), 38–45.

Neswick, R.S. (1997). Myra E. Levine: A theoretic basis for ET nursing. Journal of Wound, Ostomy, and Continence Nursing, 24, 6–9.

O'Laughlin, K.M. (1986). Changes in bladder function in women undergoing radical hysterectomy for cervical cancer. Journal of Obstetric, Gynecologic, and Neonatal Nursing, 15, 380–385.

Pasco, A., & Halupa, D. (1991). Chronic pain management. In K.M. Schaefer & J.B. Pond (Eds.), Levine's conservation model: A framework for nursing practice (pp. 101–117). Philadelphia: F.A. Davis.

Pond, J.B. (1990). Application of Levine's conservation model to nursing the homeless community. In M.E. Parker (Ed.), Nursing theories in practice (pp. 203–215). New York: National League for Nursing.

Pond, J.B. (1991). Ambulatory care of the homeless. In K.M. Schaefer & J.B. Pond (Eds.), Levine's conservation model: A framework for nursing practice (pp. 167–178). Philadelphia: F.A. Davis.

Pond, J.B., & Taney, S.G. (1991). Emergency care in a large university emergency department. In K.M. Schaefer & J.B. Pond (Eds.), Levine's conservation model: A framework for nursing practice (pp. 151–166). Philadelphia: F.A. Davis.

Savage, T.A., & Culbert, C. (1989). Early intervention: The unique role of nursing. Journal of Pediatric Nursing, 4, 339–345.

Schaefer, K.M. (1991). Care of the patient with congestive heart failure. In K.M. Schaefer & J.B. Pond (Eds.), Levine's conservation model: A framework for nursing practice (pp. 119–131). Philadelphia: F.A. Davis.

Schaefer, K.M. (1996). Levine's conservation model: Caring for women with chronic illness. In P. Hinton Walker & B. Neuman (Eds.), Blueprint for use of nursing models (pp. 187–227). New York: NLN Press.

Schaefer, K.M. (1997). Levine's conservation model in nursing practice. In M.R. Alligood & A. Marriner-Tomey (Eds.), Nursing theory: Utilization and application (pp. 89–107). St. Louis: Mosby.

Schaefer, K.M. (2002). Levine's conservation model in nursing practice. In M.R. Alligood & A. Marriner-Tomey (Eds.), Nursing theory: Utilization and application (2nd ed., pp. 197–217). St. Louis: Mosby.

Schaefer, K.M., & Pond, J.B. (1994). Levine's conservation model as a guide to nursing practice. Nursing Science Quarterly, 7, 53–54.

Taylor, J.W. (1987). Organizing data for nursing diagnoses using conservation principles. In A.M. McLane (Ed.), Classification of nursing diagnoses: Proceedings of the seventh conference: North American Nursing Diagnosis Association (pp. 103–111). St. Louis: Mosby.

Taylor, J.W. (1989). Levine's conservation principles. Using the model for nursing diagnosis in a neurological setting. In J.P. Riehl-Sisca (Ed.), Conceptual models for nursing practice (3rd ed., pp. 349–358). Norwalk, CT: Appleton & Lange.

Webb, H. (1993). Holistic care following a palliative Hartmann's procedure. British Journal of Nursing, 2, 128–132.

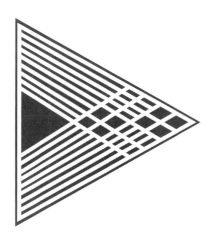

Chapter **7**

Neuman's Systems Model

Betty Neuman (2002b) traced the evolution of the Neuman Systems Model from its inception in 1970 to its current form. The Neuman Systems Model was first published in 1972, in an article entitled "A Model for Teaching Total Person Approach to Patient Problems" (Neuman & Young, 1972). A refinement of the model was published in the 1974 edition of Riehl and Roy's book *Conceptual Models for Nursing Practice* and reprinted in their 1980 edition (Neuman, 1974, 1980). Further refinements were presented in a chapter (Neuman, 1982a) of the first edition of Neuman's (1982b) book *The Neuman Systems Model: Application to Nursing Education and Practice*. Other refinements were included in the second edition of Neuman's (1989c) book *The Neuman Systems Model*. Still other refinements in the Neuman Systems Model were presented in a journal article (Neuman, 1990a) that was based on Neuman's presentation at the 1989 Nurse Theorist Conference and a book chapter (Neuman, 1990b) that was based on Neuman's presentation at a spring 1990 conference sponsored by Cedars Medical Center in Miami, Florida. Further refinements were presented in the third edition of Neuman's (1995b) book *The Neuman Systems Model*. The most recent refinements in the model were presented in the fourth edition of *The Neuman Systems Model* (Neuman & Fawcett, 2002).

Neuman's conceptual model has undergone changes in its title since its inception. The model originally was published under the title "A Model for Teaching Total Person Approach to Nursing Care" (Neuman & Young, 1972). The title was changed to "The Betty Neuman Health-Care Systems Model: A Total Person Approach to Patient Problems" in Neuman's 1974 and 1980 publications. Neuman's 1982a chapter carried the title "The Neuman Health-Care Systems Model: A Total Approach to Client Care," although her book (1982b) title was *The Neuman Systems Model*. In her 1985b journal article, Neuman referred to the model as "The Neuman Systems Model," and that title has been retained in subsequent publications.

Overview

Neuman's work focuses on the wellness of the client system in relation to environmental stressors and reactions to stressors. Neuman's work clearly fits the definition of a conceptual model of nursing. Indeed, Neuman (2002d) explicitly referred to her work as a conceptual model and a conceptual framework. The concepts of the Neuman Systems Model and their dimensions are listed here, along with the goal of nursing and the components of Neuman's practice methodology. The concepts, their dimensions, and the methodology components are defined and described, and the goal of nursing is discussed in detail later in this chapter.

ANALYSIS OF NEUMAN'S SYSTEMS MODEL

This section presents an analysis of the Neuman Systems Model. The analysis draws primarily from the fourth edition of *The Neuman Systems Model* (Neuman & Fawcett, 2002).

ORIGINS OF THE NURSING MODEL

Historical Evolution and Motivation

The development of the Neuman Systems Model was motivated by Neuman's desire to respond to the expressed needs of graduate students at the School of Nursing, University of California, Los Angeles (UCLA), for course content that would present the breadth of nursing problems before content emphasizing specific nursing problem areas (Neuman & Young, 1972). Neuman (2002b) claimed that she had no intention of creating a specific conceptual model for the nursing community when she developed the model. She commented, "It is important to state that neither was I knowledgeable about nursing models nor had a clear trend yet begun in nursing for developing models. The Neuman Systems Model was developed strictly as a teaching aid" (p. 327). The Neuman Systems Model was formulated at approximately the same time as other conceptual models of nursing (e.g., King, 1971; Orem, 1971; Rogers, 1970) and at the time when the criteria for National League for Nursing accreditation first stipulated that nursing education programs should be based on conceptual models (Peterson, 1977).

Neuman referred to human beings as patients and as clients in her 1974, 1980, and 1982a publications. Since 1989, she has used only the term client. She explained, "The initial term patient was changed ... to client to fulfill the need for a qualifying term that would indicate respect and imply a collaborative lateral relationship between caregivers and the clients they serve" (Neuman, 2002b, p. 330). She also commented that she uses the terms client or client system "out of respect for newer client-caregiver collaborative relationships, as well as wellness perspectives of the model" (Neuman, 2002d, p. 15).

Philosophical Claims

Neuman (2002d) declared,

> The philosophic base of the Neuman Systems Model encompasses wholism, a wellness orientation, client perception and motivation, and a dynamic systems perspective of energy and variable interaction with the environment to mitigate possible harm from internal and external stressors, while caregivers

167

and clients form a partnership relationship to negotiate desired outcome goals for optimal health retention, restoration, and maintenance. This philosophic base pervades all aspects of the model (p. 12).

Neuman has presented the philosophical claims undergirding the Neuman Systems Model in the form of a basic philosophy; beliefs about holism, reality, and wellness; and assumptions about human beings, spirituality, the environment, human beings and the environment, health, and nursing. All of Neuman's philosophical claims are presented here.

Neuman's Basic Philosophy

- Helping each other live (Neuman 2002b, p. 328).

Belief about Wholism

- Wholism is both a philosophical and a biological concept, implying relationships and processes arising from wholeness, dynamic freedom, and creativity in adjusting to stressors in the internal and external environments (Neuman, 2002d, p. 10).

Belief about Reality

- For a workable health creating philosophy based on systemic and holistic client perspectives, wellness can be defined in terms of the interrelationship of (a) system available energy, (b) influence of the client created environment, and (c) caregiver clarification of client health perception. These factors all coalesce into the *true reality* of the client's health experience and define the nature and quality of his or her life in the process, as related to socially and culturally accepted standards. Health, then, is more than the reality of client perceived experience, inasmuch as subjectivity usually distorts true reality (Neuman, 1990a, p. 130).

Beliefs about Wellness

- [Wellness is an] experienced energy based reality [that is] [e]lusive (Neuman, 1990a, p. 130).
- [The perception of wellness] is best defined and negotiated holistically between the client and the caregiver (Neuman, 1990a, pp. 130–131).
- Nurses as healers (wholistic themselves) have as a goal conservation of client energy in keeping the system harmonious, while facilitating change toward optimal wellness. Based on this assumption, causal factors must be discovered and carefully negotiated with clients for accountable health management (Neuman, 1990a, p. 131).

Assumptions about Human Beings

- Provided support factors are in place, the client, as a system, constantly monitors self by making adjustments as needed to retain, attain, and maintain stability for an optimal health state (Neuman, 1990a, p. 129).
- The client is an open system that interacts with the environment in order to promote harmony and balance between the internal and external environment. The client is a composite of physiologic, psychologic, sociocultural, developmental, and spiritual variables that are viewed as parts of the whole. Ideally the client as a system adjusts successfully to internal and external environmental stressors retaining the normal wellness level or system stability (Neuman, 1990b, p. 259).
- Each individual client or group as a client system is unique; each system is a composite of common known factors or innate characteristics within a normal, given range of response, contained within a basic structure (Neuman, 2002d, p. 14).

Assumptions about Spirituality

- It is assumed that each person is born with a spiritual energy force, or "seed," within the spiritual variable, as identified in the basic structure of the client system (Neuman, 2002d, p. 16).
- It is assumed that spiritual development in varying degrees empowers the client system toward well being by positively directing spiritual energy for use first by the mind and then by the body (Neuman, 2002d, p. 16).

Assumption about the Environment

- Environment contains both internal and external stressors and resistance factors. … Stressors are considered neutral; client encounter determines either a beneficial or noxious outcome (Neuman, 1990b, p. 259).

Assumption about Human Beings and Environment

- The client is in dynamic constant energy exchange with the environment (Neuman, 2002d, p. 14).

Assumption about Health

- Health represents a usual dynamic stability state of the normal line of defense. A reaction to stressors is caused as the normal line of defense is penetrated, causing illness symptoms. The client's position on his or her own wellness-illness continuum is related to the amount of available energy stored and/or used by the system in retaining, attaining, and maintaining system stability (Neuman, 1990b, p. 259).

Assumption about Nursing

- Nursing is concerned with reduction of potential or actual stressor reaction through use of primary, secondary, or tertiary prevention as intervention to retain, attain, and maintain an optimal wellness level. The goal of nursing is optimal client system stability or wellness. Perceptual distortions between client and nurse, as well as goal plans, are mutually negotiated and resolved (Neuman, 1990b, p. 259).

Strategies for Knowledge Development

The Neuman Systems Model arose from Neuman's observations, her practice and teaching experiences in mental health nursing, and her synthesis of knowledge from several adjunctive disciplines. As is evident in Neuman's (2002b) description of the development of the model, both inductive and deductive strategies were used:

> The development of the wholistic systemic perspective of the Neuman Systems Model was facilitated by my own basic philosophy of *helping each other live*, many diverse observations and clinical experiences in teaching and encouraging positive aspects of human variables in a wide variety of community settings, and theoretical perspectives of stress related to the interactive, interrelated, interdependent, and wholistic nature of systems theory. The significance of perception and behavioral consequences cannot be overestimated (p. 328).

Influences from Other Scholars

Neuman (2002b) acknowledged the support of colleagues and the influence of other scholars on the development of the Neuman Systems Model. She noted that the UCLA School of Nursing Curriculum Committee members selected her to develop and coordinate the course for which the model was initially formulated in 1970. She acknowledged the assistance of Rae Jean Young with the evaluation of the effectiveness of the model as a teaching tool, and noted that their collaboration led to the first publication about the model (Neuman & Young, 1972). Neuman (2002b) also paid tribute to UCLA School of Nursing Dean Lulu Wolfe Hassenplug and Nurse Continuing Education Director Marjorie Squaires "for providing many opportunities combined with a lack of constraints related to my functioning" (p. 328). Neuman (1989a) also expressed her "most sincere appreciation for all the fine people who in various ways have facilitated the mature status of the Neuman Systems Model" (p. 466).

In addition, Neuman (2002d) cited the influence of Putt's (1972) interpretation of system theory and Oakes' (1978) linkage of general system theory and the quality of client care. She also cited Beckstrand's (1980) proposal to advance nursing knowledge "by rigorous application of the methods of science, ethics, and philosophy to problems encountered in the professional experience of nurses" (p. 6).

Furthermore, Neuman (1974, 2002d) identified the knowledge from adjunctive disciplines that contributed to the content of the Neuman Systems Model. Scholars and works that were particularly influential include de Chardin's (1955) philosophical beliefs about the wholeness of life; Marxist philosophical views of the oneness of man and nature (Cornu, 1957); Gestalt and field theories of the interaction between human beings and environment (Edelson, 1970); a general system theory of the nature of living open systems (von Bertalanffy, 1968); Emery's (1969) and Lazarus's (1981, 1999) views of systems, stress, and perception of stressors; Caplan's (1964) articulation of levels of prevention; and Heslin's (1986) ideas about revitalization of living open systems.

World View

The Neuman Systems Model primarily reflects the *reciprocal interaction* world view. That world view is represented by Neuman's use of Gestalt and field theories, as well as philosophies that emphasize the unity of human beings. The features of the reciprocal interaction world view that are evident in Neuman's Systems Model are:

- The Neuman Systems Model reflects a holistic, multidimensional approach to the client as a system (Neuman, 1990b).
- All five variable areas constituting the client system (physiological, psychological, sociocultural, developmental, and spiritual) are considered together at any given time (Neuman, 2002d).
- The wholeness concept … is based upon the appropriate interrelationship of variables (Neuman, 1974, p. 103).
- The client system is regarded as active (Neuman, 2002d).
- Since [client system-]environment exchanges are reciprocal, both client and environment may be positively or negatively affected by each other (Neuman, 2002d, p. 12).
- Persistence is reflected in Neuman's emphasis on client system stability and her focus on protection of the client system basic structure by the lines of defense and resistance (Neuman, 2002d).
- Change is reflected in the contention that "the client is in constant change" (Neuman, 2002d, p. 12).

In keeping with the reciprocal interaction world view, the Neuman Systems Model incorporates elements of both persistence and change. Persistence and change are linked in Neuman's (2002d) statement that "a system implies dynamic energy exchange [with the environment], moving either toward or away from stability" (p. 10). Persistence and change, then, appear to be on a dual continuum of more or less persistence and more or less change at any time in the life of the client system. That interpretation of Neuman's work requires validation.

Although the primary world view of the Neuman Systems Model is reciprocal interaction, the *reaction world view* is introduced in Neuman's description of the created environment as an unconscious structure, which implies a psychoanalytic orientation. The psychoanalytic orientation associated with the reaction world view also is evident in Neuman's description of the spiritual variable as consciously developed. In the most recent version of her conceptual model, Neuman (2002d) has deleted earlier references to the closed system view of illness as entropy and Selye's (1950) mechanistic conceptualization of stress.

UNIQUE FOCUS OF THE NURSING MODEL

The unique focus of the Neuman Systems Model is the wellness of the client/client system in relation to environmental stress and reactions to stress (Neuman, 1974, 2002d). Neuman (2002d) pointed out that "The intent of the Neuman Systems Model is to set forth a structure that depicts the parts and subparts and their interrelationship for the whole of the client as a complete system. The same fundamental idea … would apply equally well to [the individual,] a small group or community, a larger aggregate, or even the universe" (p. 11).

The Neuman Systems Model pays particular attention to wellness retention and optimal client/client system wellness attainment and maintenance in the face of problems that originate in client system reactions to the intrapersonal, interpersonal, and extrapersonal stressors arising in the internal and external environments (Neuman, 2002d).

The Neuman Systems Model also focuses attention on variances from wellness and on nursing interventions directed toward retention, attainment, and maintenance of client system stability (Neuman, 2002d).

Category of Knowledge

Meleis (1997) regards the Neuman Systems Model as client focused. Barnum (1998) did not place the Neuman Systems Model within her classification scheme of intervention, conservation, substitution, sustenance/support, and enhancement categories. Otherwise, the Neuman

Systems Model always has been classified as a systems model (Barnum, 1998; Marriner-Tomey, 1989; Riehl & Roy, 1974, 1980; Riehl-Sisca, 1989). Neuman (personal communications, November 6 and 13, 1980) commented that she did not consider classification when formulating her model, but agrees that systems is the appropriate category. She stated, "The Neuman Systems Model is an open systems model that views nursing as being primarily concerned with defining appropriate action in stress-related situations or in possible reactions of the client/client system" (Neuman, 1995a, p. 11). The appropriateness of the systems category classification is evident in the comparison of the concepts and propositions of the Neuman Systems Model with the characteristics of the systems category of knowledge, as can be seen here.

- System: Individuals, families, communities, and social issues are considered client systems (Neuman, 2002d).
- Integration of Parts: The interacting open client system is a dynamic composite of the interrelationship of physiological, psychological, sociocultural, developmental, and spiritual variables (Neuman, 2002d).
- Environment: All factors affecting and affected by the system (Neuman, 2002d, p. 12). All internal and external factors or influences surrounding the identified client or client system (Neuman, 2002d, p. 18). The environment encompasses the internal, external, and created environments. The internal and external environments are regarded as the sources of stressors that influence the client system (Neuman, 2002d).
- Boundary: [Client system boundaries are] dynamic and constantly changing, presenting different appearances according to time, place, and the significance of events (Neuman, 2002d, p. 9). The flexible and normal lines of defense and the lines of resistance form boundaries between the central core of the client system and the environment; the outer boundary for the client as a system is the flexible line of defense (Neuman, 2002d). Boundary permeability is accounted for in the factors that influence stressor invasion and reactions to stressors (Neuman, 2002d).
- Tension, Stress, Strain, and Conflict: Stressors are defined as tension-producing stimuli with the potential for causing system instability (Neuman, 2002d, p. 21).
- Steady State: At the simplest level, a steady state, governed by a dynamic interaction of parts and subparts, is one of stability over time. At more complex levels, a steady state preserves the character of the system through growth and expansion (Neuman, 2002d, p. 11). A dynamic stability can exist within the system…. Stability implies a state of balance or harmony requiring energy exchange between the system and environment to cope adequately with imposing stressors (Neuman,

2002d, pp. 24–25). Stability preserves the character of the system. An adjustment in one direction is countered by a movement in the opposite direction, both movements being approximately rather than precisely compensatory. With opposing forces in effect, the process of stability is an example of the regulatory capacity of a system (Neuman, 2002d, p. 25).

• Feedback: Feedback of output into input makes the system self-regulatory in relation to either maintenance of a desired health state or goal outcome (Neuman, 2002d, p. 25).

CONTENT OF THE NURSING MODEL

Concepts

The metaparadigm concepts of human beings, environment, health, and nursing are evident in the concepts of the Neuman System Model. Each conceptual model concept is classified here according to its metaparadigm forerunner.

The metaparadigm concept of human beings is represented by the Neuman Systems Model concepts of CLIENT/CLIENT SYSTEM, INTERACTING VARIABLES, BASIC STRUCTURE, FLEXIBLE LINE OF DEFENSE, NORMAL LINE OF DEFENSE, and LINES OF RESISTANCE. The concept of CLIENT/CLIENT SYSTEM has four dimensions—Individual, Family, Community, and Social Issue. The concept of INTERACTING VARIABLES has five dimensions—Physiologic Variable, Psychological Variable, Sociocultural Variable, Developmental Variable, and Spiritual Variable. The concepts of BASIC STRUCTURE, FLEXIBLE LINE OF DEFENSE, NORMAL LINE OF DEFENSE, and LINES OF RESISTANCE are unidimensional.

The metaparadigm concept of environment is represented by the Neuman Systems Model concepts of INTERNAL ENVIRONMENT, EXTERNAL ENVIRONMENT, CREATED ENVIRONMENT, and STRESSORS. The concepts of INTERNAL ENVIRONMENT, EXTERNAL ENVIRONMENT, and CREATED ENVIRONMENT are unidimensional. The concept of STRESSORS has three dimensions—Intrapersonal Stressors, Interpersonal Stressors, and Extrapersonal Stressors.

The metaparadigm concept of health is represented by the Neuman Systems Model concepts of HEALTH/WELLNESS/OPTIMAL CLIENT SYSTEM STABILITY, VARIANCES FROM WELLNESS, ILLNESS, and RECONSTITUTION. Each concept is unidimensional.

The metaparadigm concept of nursing is represented in the Neuman Systems Model by the concept of PREVENTION AS INTERVENTION. That concept has three

dimensions—Primary Prevention as Intervention, Secondary Prevention as Intervention, and Tertiary Prevention as Intervention.

Nonrelational Propositions

The definitions of the concepts of the Neuman Systems Model are given here. Those constitutive definitions are the nonrelational propositions of this nursing model.

CLIENT/CLIENT SYSTEM

• The client is an interacting open system in interaction and total interface with both internal and external environmental forces or stressors (Neuman, 2002d, p. 12).

The concept of **Client/Client System** encompasses four dimensions—Individual, Family, Community, and Social Issue.

• **Individual:** The client as a system represents an "individual," a "person," or "man" (Neuman, 2002d, p. 15).
• **Family:** A type of group (Neuman, 2002d).
• **Community:** A type of group (Neuman, 2002d).
• **Social Issue:** A type of group (Neuman, 2002d).

INTERACTING VARIABLES

• The client system is a composite of five interacting variable areas (Neuman, 2002d, p. 16).
• Ideally, the five variables function harmoniously or are stable in relation to internal and external environmental stressor influences (Neuman, 2002d, p. 17).
• The client, whether in a state of wellness or illness, is a dynamic composite of the interrelationships of variables—physiologic, psychological, sociocultural, developmental, and spiritual (Neuman, 2002d, p. 14).

The concept of **Interacting Variables** encompasses five dimensions—Physiological Variable, Psychological Variable, Sociocultural Variable, Developmental Variable, and Spiritual Variable.

• **Physiological Variable:** Refers to bodily structure and internal function (Neuman, 2002d, p. 16).
• **Psychological Variable:** Refers to mental processes and interactive environmental effects, both internally and externally (Neuman, 2002d, p. 16).
• **Sociocultural Variable:** Refers to combined effects of social cultural conditions and influences (Neuman, 2002d, p. 16).
• **Developmental Variable:** Refers to age-related development[al] processes and activities (Neuman, 2002d, p. 17).

- **Spiritual Variable**: Refers to spiritual beliefs and influences (Neuman, 2002d, p. 17). [Spirituality] lies on a continuum of dormant, unacceptable, or undeveloped to recognition, development, and positive system influence (Neuman, 2002d, p. 16).

The five dimensions of the concept of **Interacting Variables** are interrelated in each **Client/Client System**. The interrelationships "determine the amount of resistance [a client system] has to any environmental stressors" (Neuman, 2002d, p. 22). Moreover, although all five dimensions of the concept of **Interacting Variables** are contained within each client system, each exhibits "varying degrees of development and a wide range of interactive styles and potential" (Neuman, 2002d, p. 16). Variability in development of the dimension Spiritual Variable is especially noted.

BASIC STRUCTURE

- The basic structure or central core consists of basic survival factors common to the species (Neuman, 2002d, p. 17).
- When the client is an individual, the basic survival factors are exemplified by maintenance of normal temperature range, genetic response patterns, and strength or weakness of body organs. Certain unique features or baseline characteristics, such as cognitive ability, also are contained within the central core (Neuman, 2002d).

Neuman (2002d) depicts **Client/Client System** as a **Basic Structure** surrounded by concentric rings called the **Flexible Line of Defense**, the **Normal Line of Defense**, and the **Lines of Resistance** (Fig. 7–1). The concentric rings are regarded as mechanisms that protect the **Basic Structure** from **Stressor** invasion. The outermost ring is the **Flexible Line of Defense**. The **Normal Line of Defense** lies between the **Flexible Line of Defense** and the **Lines of Resistance**. The innermost concentric rings are the **Lines of Resistance**.

FLEXIBLE LINE OF DEFENSE

- Forms the outer boundary of the defined client system (Neuman, 2002d, p. 17).
- [A mechanism that serves as] a protective buffer system for the client's normal or stable state (Neuman, 2002d, p. 17).
- Ideally, [the flexible line of defense] prevents stressor invasions of the client system, keeping the system free from stressor reactions or symptomatology (Neuman, 2002d, p. 17).
- The flexible line of defense protects the normal line of defense or usual wellness condition (Neuman, 2002d, p. 17).

- [The flexible line of defense] is accordionlike in function. As it expands away from the normal defense line, greater protection is provided; as it draws closer, less protection is available (Neuman, 2002d, p. 17).
- [The flexible line of defense] is dynamic rather than stable and can be rapidly altered over a relatively short time period or in a situation like a state of emergency or a condition like undernutrition, sleep loss, or dehydration (Neuman, 2002d, p. 17).

NORMAL LINE OF DEFENSE

- The client/client system's normal or usual wellness level (Neuman, 2002d).
- Each individual client/client system, over time, has evolved a normal range of response to the environment that is referred to as a normal line of defense, or usual wellness/stability state. It represents change over time through coping with diverse stress encounters (Neuman, 2002d, p. 14).
- [The normal line of defense] represents what the client has become, the state to which the client has evolved over time, or the usual wellness level (Neuman, 2002d, p. 17).
- The normal line of defense is the result of adjustment of the client system to environmental stressors, and of previous behavior of the client/client system (Neuman, 2002d).
- The normal line of defense defines the stability and integrity of the client/client system and its ability to maintain stability and integrity (Neuman, 2002d).
- The normal line of defense can be used as a standard from which to measure health deviation (Neuman, 2002d, p. 14).
- The normal line of defense is considered dynamic in that it can expand or contract over time. For example, the usual wellness level or system stability may remain the same, become reduced, or expand following treatment of a stressor reaction. [The normal line of defense] is also dynamic in terms of its ability to become and remain stabilized to deal with life stresses over time, thus protecting the basic structure and system integrity (Neuman, 2002d, p. 18).
- Expansion of the normal line of defense reflects an enhanced wellness state; contraction, a diminished state of wellness (Neuman, 1989d).

LINES OF RESISTANCE

- A protective mechanism that attempts to stabilize the client system and foster a return to the usual wellness level (Neuman, 2002d).
- [The lines of resistance] contain certain known and unknown internal and external resource factors that support the client's basic structure and normal defense line

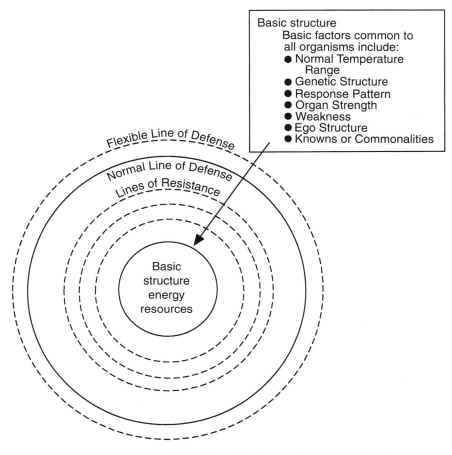

Basic structure
    Basic factors common to
    all organisms include:
    ● Normal Temperature
       Range
    ● Genetic Structure
    ● Response Pattern
    ● Organ Strength
    ● Weakness
    ● Ego Structure
    ● Knowns or Commonalities

Flexible Line of Defense

Normal Line of Defense

Lines of Resistance

Basic
structure
energy
resources

NOTE: Physiologic, psychologic, sociocultural,
developmental, and spiritual variables occur
and are considered simultaneously in each
client concentric circle.

FIG. 7–1. Diagram of the client system. (From Neuman, B. (2002). The Neuman systems model. In B. Neuman & J. Fawcett (Eds.), The Neuman Systems Model (4th ed., p. 15). Upper Saddle River, NJ: Prentice-Hall, with permission.)

[such as] mobilization of white blood cells or activation of immune system mechanisms,... thus protecting system integrity (Neuman, 2002d, p. 18).

- Implicit within each client system are internal resistance factors known as lines of resistance, which function to stabilize and return the client to the usual wellness state (normal line of defense) or possibly to a higher level of stability following an environmental stressor reaction (Neuman, 2002d, p. 14).
- The lines of resistance protect the basic structure and support return to wellness (Neuman, 1990b, p. 259).

The five **Interacting Variables** are considered to be inherent within the **Flexible Line of Defense**, the **Normal Line of Defense**, and the **Lines of Resistance**. Neuman (2002d) explained that the five **Interacting Variables** contained within the **Flexible Line of Defense** "ideally would protect the client system from possible instability caused by stressors. Determining factors would include the client's physiologic condition, sociocultural influences, developmental state, cognitive skills, and spiritual considerations" (p. 22). Similarly, the five **Interacting Variables** contained within the **Normal Line of Defense** can protect the **Client/Client System**. Here, influencing factors include "coping patterns, lifestyle factors, developmental and spiritual influences, and cultural considerations" (Neuman, 2002d, p. 18). Neuman did not identify any particular determining or influencing factors within the **Lines of Resistance**.

INTERNAL ENVIRONMENT

- Consists of all forces or interactive influences internal to or contained solely within the boundaries of the defined client/client system (Neuman, 2002d, p. 18).
- [The internal environment] correlates with Neuman Systems Model intrapersonal factors or stressors (Neuman, 2002d, p. 18).

EXTERNAL ENVIRONMENT

- Consists of all forces or interaction influences external to or existing outside the defined client/client system (Neuman, 2002d, p. 18).
- [The external environment] correlates with both the inter- and extrapersonal factors or stressors (Neuman, 2002d, p. 18).

CREATED ENVIRONMENT

- Represents an open system exchanging energy with both the internal and external environment (Neuman, 2002d, p. 19).
- The created environment is dynamic and represents the client's unconscious mobilization of all system variables (particularly the psycho-sociocultural), including the basic structure energy factors, toward system integration, stability and integrity. It is inherently purposeful. Though unconsciously developed, its function is to offer a protective coping shield (Lazarus, 1981) or safe arena for system function as the client is usually cognitively unaware of the host of existing psychosocial and physiological influences. It pervades all systems, large and small, at least to some degree; it is spontaneously created, increased, or decreased, as warranted by a special condition of need (Neuman, 2002d, pp. 19–20).
- [The created] environment [is] developed unconsciously by the client [as] a symbolic expression of system wholeness (Neuman, 2002d, p. 19).
- The created environment is based on unseen, unconscious knowledge, as well as self-esteem, beliefs, energy exchanges, system variables, and predisposition; it is a process-based concept of perpetual adjustment within which a client may either increase or decrease available energy affecting the wellness state (Neuman, 2002d, p. 21).

- [The created environment] acts as an immediate or long-range safe reservoir for existence or the maintenance of system integrity expressed consciously, unconsciously, or both simultaneously (Neuman, 2002d, p. 19).
- The created environment . . is intrapersonal, interpersonal, and extrapersonal in nature (Neuman, 2002d, p. 18).

The **Created Environment** plays an important role in determining the response to a **Stressor**. Neuman (1990a) explained that the created environment "is a self-help phenomenon that can reflect a temporary health state as a response to situational stressors on the client's flexible [and normal] line[s] of defense [and lines of resistance]" (p. 130). Although the client may be conscious of "the environmental reality that inexorably shapes the health condition" (p. 130), the created environment functions as a subjective safety mechanism that "may block conscious awareness of the true reality of the environment and the health experience [by structuring] a semblance or illusion of harmony in wellness" (p. 130) for the client system. More specifically, "the insulating effect of the created environment changes the response or possible response of the client to environmental stressors, for example, the use of denial or envy (psychological), physical rigidity or muscular constraint (physiological), life-cycle continuation of survival patterns (developmental), required social space range (sociocultural), and sustaining hope (spiritual)" (Neuman, 2002d, p. 20).

STRESSORS

- Tension producing stimuli or forces occurring within the internal and external environmental boundaries of the client/client system (Neuman, 2002d, p. 21).

The concept **Stressors** encompasses three dimensions—Intrapersonal Stressors, Interpersonal Stressors, and Extrapersonal Stressors.

- **Intrapersonal Stressors**: Internal environmental forces that occur within the boundary of the client/client system (e.g., conditioned response or autoimmune response) (Neuman, 2002d, p. 22).
- **Interpersonal Stressors**: External environmental forces that occur outside the boundaries of the client/client system at proximal range (e.g., between one or more role expectations or communication patterns) (Neuman, 2002d, p. 22).
- **Extrapersonal Stressors**: External environmental interaction forces that occur outside the boundaries of the client/client system at distal range (e.g., between one or more social policies or financial concerns) (Neuman, 2002d, p. 22).

The outcome of the **Client/Client System's** encounter with a **Stressor** is determined in part by natural and learned resistance, which is manifested by the strength of the **Flexible Line of Defense**, the **Normal Line of Defense**, and the **Lines of Resistance**. The amount of resistance, in turn, is determined by the interrelation of the five **Interacting Variables** of the **Client/Client System**.

The **Flexible Line of Defense** is immediately called into action when the **Client/Client System** encounters a **Stressor** and attempts to maintain stability. **Stressors** are inert or neutral, but the outcome of a reaction to a stressor may be beneficial or noxious, positive or negative (Neuman, 1985a, 2002d). If the **Flexible Line of Defense** cannot withstand the impact of one or more **Stressors**, the **Normal Line of Defense** is penetrated. A reaction, in the form of **Client/Client System Instability** or illness, occurs when the **Normal Line of Defense** is rendered ineffective in relation to the impact of the **Stressor(s)**. The **Lines of Resistance** are involuntarily activated when an environmental **Stressor** invades the **Normal Line of Defense**. "Effectiveness of the lines of resistance in reversing the reaction to stressors," Neuman (2002d) explained, "allows the system to reconstitute; ineffectiveness leads to energy depletion and death" (p. 18).

The nature and extent of the reaction to a **Stressor** also are influenced by such factors as "the time of stressor occurrence, past and present condition of the client, nature and intensity of the stressor, and the amount of energy required by the client to adjust … [as well as] past coping behavior or patterns in a similar situation" (Neuman, 2002d, p. 22). Other factors influencing reaction to a **Stressor** include idiosyncrasies in the **Basic Structure**, past and present conditions of the **Client/Client System**, available energy resources, and cognitive appraisal of the stressor (Neuman, 1974, 1985a, 2002d).

HEALTH/WELLNESS/OPTIMAL CLIENT SYSTEM STABILITY

- Health for the client is equated with optimal system stability, that is, the best possible wellness state at any given time (Neuman, 2002d, p. 23).
- Health is a manifestation of living energy available to preserve and enhance system integrity (Neuman, 2002d, p. 23).
- Health as energy is a result of system balance. Energy is regarded as the pervasive forces within the client that empower and regulate all systemic functions from cellular to motor. Energy, which acts as a primary and basic power resource for the client as a system, is innately or genetically acquired, generated and stored, used or spent, available or bound. The health condition reflects the amount of energy remaining following efforts made by the system to achieve balance during periods of instability (Neuman, 1990a).
- Health is reflected in the level of wellness: when system needs are met, a state of optimal wellness exists. Conversely, unmet needs reduce the client wellness condition (Neuman, 2002d, p. 12).
- Health and wellness [is] defined as the condition or the degree of system stability, that is, the condition in which all parts and subparts (variables) are in balance or harmony with the whole of the client/client system (Neuman, 2002d, p. 12).
- Wellness is a state of saturation or inertness, one free of disrupting needs (Neuman, 2002d, p. 25).
- Wellness is a stable condition in which system subparts are in harmony with the whole system (Neuman, 2002e, p. 324)
- Wellness is a matter of degree, a point on a continuum running from the greatest degree of wellness to severe illness or death (Neuman, 2002d, p. 3)
- Wellness is on a continuum of available energy to support the system in an optimal state of system stability (Neuman, 2002d, p. 14).
- [Wellness as energy] is a manifestation of the highest possible level of system stability, implying that energy is sufficient for necessary system function from the cellular level to gross motor participation in the life processes of adjustment and change (Neuman, 1990a, p. 129).
- Optimal wellness represents the greatest possible degree of system stability at a given point in time (Neuman, 2002d, p. 3).
- The degree of wellness is determined by the amount of energy required to return to and maintain system stability. When more energy is available than is being used, the system is stable (Neuman, 2002d, pp. 24–25).
- Optimal [client system stability] means the highest possible health condition achievable at a given point in time (Neuman, 2002d, p. 25).

For Neuman (2002d), **Health** "is envisioned as being at various, changing levels within a normal range, rising or falling throughout the life span because of basic structure factors and the satisfactory or unsatisfactory adjustment to environmental stressors" (p. 23). In keeping with the open systems perspective of the Neuman Systems Model, Neuman (2002d) conceptualized health as a continuum from wellness to illness or death.

Within the context of health as energy, Neuman views health as a continuum. She stated, "Health on a continuum is the degree of client wellness that exists at any point in time, ranging from an optimal wellness condition, with available energy at its maximum, to death, which represents total energy depletion" (Neuman, 1990a, p. 129).

VARIANCES FROM WELLNESS

• Varying degrees of system instability (Neuman, 2002d, p. 24).
• The difference from the normal or usual wellness condition (Neuman, 1995a, p. 39).
• A variance from wellness is determined by comparing the normal health state with that which is taking place at a given time (Neuman, 1985a).

ILLNESS

• Illness is a state of insufficiency with disrupting needs unsatisfied (Neuman, 2002d, p. 15).
• [Illness is an excessive expenditure of energy. In particular,] a violent energy flow occurs when a system is disrupted from its normal or stable state; that is, it expends energy to cope with disorganization. When more energy is used by the system in its state of disorganization than is built and stored, the outcome may be death (Neuman, 2002d, p. 24).
• Illness is on the opposite [end of the] continuum from wellness and represents instability and energy depletion among the system parts or subparts affecting the whole (Neuman, 2002e, p. 324).

RECONSTITUTION

• Reconstitution is the determined energy increase related to the degree of reaction [to a stressor] (Neuman, 2002d, p. 28).
• Reconstitution is identified as beginning at any point following treatment [for a stressor reaction] (Neuman, 2002d, p. 28).
• [Reconstitution depends on] the successful mobilization of client resources to prevent further stressor reaction or regression; it represents a dynamic state of adjustment to stressors and integration of all necessary factors towards optimal use of existing resources for client system stability or wellness maintenance (Neuman, 2002d, p. 28).
• Reconstitution may be viewed as feedback from the input and output of secondary intervention (Neuman, 2002d, p. 28).
• Complete reconstitution may progress well beyond the previously determined normal line of defense or usual wellness state, it may stabilize the system at a lower level, or it may return to the level prior to illness (Neuman, 2002d, p. 28).
• [If reconstitution does not occur,] death occurs as a result of failure of the basic structure (Neuman, 2002, p. 28).

PREVENTION AS INTERVENTION

• Nursing is prevention as intervention (Neuman, 2002d).

The concept **Prevention as Intervention** encompasses three dimensions—Primary Prevention as Intervention, Secondary Prevention as Intervention, and Tertiary Prevention as Intervention.

• **Primary Prevention as Intervention:** Primary prevention relates to general knowledge that is applied in client assessment and intervention in identification and reduction or mitigation of possible or actual risk factors associated with environmental stressors to prevent possible reaction. The goal of health promotion is included in primary prevention (Neuman, 2002d, p. 14). [The primary prevention as intervention] modality is used for primary prevention as wellness retention, that is, to protect the client system normal line of defense or usual wellness state by strengthening the flexible line of defense. The goal is to promote client wellness by stress prevention and reduction of risk factors ... [and to] reduce the possibility of stressor encounter or in some manner attempt to strengthen the client's flexible line of defense to decrease the possibility of a reaction (Neuman, 2002d, pp. 25–26). [Primary prevention as] intervention can begin at any point at which a stressor is either suspected or identified (Neuman, 2002d, p. 25). Primary prevention as intervention is provided when the degree of risk or hazard is known but a reaction has not yet occurred (Neuman, 2002d, p. 25).
• **Secondary Prevention as Intervention:** Secondary prevention relates to symptomatology following a reaction to stressors, appropriate ranking of intervention priorities, and treatment to reduce their noxious effects (Neuman, 2002d, p. 14). The secondary prevention as intervention modality is used for secondary prevention as wellness attainment, that is, to protect the basic structure by strengthening the internal lines of resistance. The goal is to provide appropriate treatment of symptoms to attain optimal client system stability or wellness and energy conservation (Neuman, 2002d, p. 26). Secondary prevention as intervention is provided when primary prevention as intervention was not provided or failed and a stressor reaction occurred (Neuman, 2002d). Treatment [using secondary prevention as intervention] could begin at any point following the occurrence of symptoms (Neuman, 2002d, p. 26).
• **Tertiary Prevention as Intervention:** Tertiary prevention relates to the adjustive processes taking place as reconstitution begins and maintenance factors move the client back in a circular manner toward primary prevention (Neuman, 2002d, p. 14). The tertiary prevention as inter-

vention modality is used for tertiary prevention as wellness maintenance, that is, to protect client system reconstitution or return to wellness following treatment [i.e., following secondary prevention as intervention]. ... The goal is to maintain an optimal wellness level by supporting existing strengths and conserving client system energy (Neuman, 2002d, p. 28). Tertiary prevention as intervention can begin at any point in client reconstitution following treatment, that is, when some degree of system stability has occurred (Neuman, 2002d, p. 28).

Neuman (1974) views nursing as a "unique profession [that] is concerned with all the variables affecting an individual's response to stressors" (p. 102). The three dimensions of the concept Prevention as Intervention actually are nursing intervention modalities that represent a typology of nursing actions. The typology identifies the client's entry point into the health-care system and the type of intervention needed. Neuman (2002d) pointed out that more than one prevention modality may be used simultaneously if the client's condition warrants such multilevel intervention. She stated, "Ideally, primary prevention is also considered concomitant with secondary and tertiary preventions as interventions" (p. 26). Moreover, "tertiary prevention tends to lead back, in circular fashion, toward primary prevention" (p. 29). Specific nursing functions or actions taken as part of Primary Prevention as Intervention, Secondary Prevention as Intervention, and Tertiary Prevention as Intervention include but are not limited to initiating, planning, organizing, monitoring, coordinating, implementing, integrating, advocating, supporting, and evaluating (Neuman, 2002d).

In keeping with the concept of **Prevention as Intervention** and its three dimensions, the **GOAL OF NURSING** is "to facilitate optimal wellness for the client through retention, attainment, or maintenance of client system stability" (Neuman, 1995a, p. 25). In particular, "nursing goals should enable the client in creating and shaping reality in a desired direction, related to retention, attainment, or maintenance of optimal system wellness, or a combination of these, through purposeful interventions [that] should mitigate or reduce stress factors and adverse conditions which affect or could affect optimal client functioning, at any given point in time" (Neuman, 1995a, p. 16). "The major goal for nursing," Neuman (1995a) declared, "is to reduce stressor impact, whether actual or potential, and to increase client resistance" (p. 36).

Neuman (2002d) presented the **NEUMAN SYSTEMS MODEL NURSING PROCESS FORMAT**, which is the **PRACTICE METHODOLOGY** for the Neuman Systems Model. The format is outlined in Table 7–1.

The **Neuman Systems Model Nursing Process Format**

takes into account the perceptions of both the client and the caregiver. Underscoring that point, Neuman (2002d) maintained that proper assessment requires consideration of both the client's and the caregiver's perceptions of the basic structure; the lines of resistance and defense; and the internal, external, and created environments. Neuman (1990a) pointed out that although identification of the relevant factors in the client's internal and external environments is relatively easy, determination of the created environment can be challenging:

> The familiar conscious level of internal (intrapersonal) and external (interpersonal and extrapersonal) environment factors of the model can be easily determined, whereas those of the unconsciously derived created environment are more [e]lusive and fragile, requiring discovery of causal as well as defining factors. These created environment factors can best be identified and defined as client patterned responses through caregiver use of intuition, empathy, inference, and clustering of response patterns to form mini-hypotheses for careful informal testing in client-nurse interaction (p. 130).

Relational Propositions

The relational propositions of the Neuman Systems Model are listed here. The relationship between the metaparadigm concepts human being and environment is mentioned repeatedly in the Neuman Systems Model. The reciprocal nature of that relationship is articulated in relational propositions A, B, C, D, and E. The linkage of the metaparadigm concepts human beings, environment, and health is asserted in relational propositions F and G. The integral relationship of the metaparadigm concepts human beings, environment, health, and nursing is evident in relational propositions H and I.

A. The client is a system capable of both input and output related to intrapersonal, interpersonal, and extrapersonal environmental influences, interacting with the environment by adjusting to it or, as a system, adjusting the environment to itself (Neuman, 2002d, pp. 23–24).

B. Input, output, and feedback between the client and the environment is of a circular nature; client and environment have a reciprocal relationship, the outcome of which is corrective or regulative for the system (Neuman, 2002d, p. 23).

C. Many known, unknown, and universal environmental stressors exist. Each differs in its potential for disturbing a client's usual stability level, or normal line of defense. The particular interrelationships of client variables—physiological, psychological, sociocultural, developmental, and spiritual—at any point in time can affect the degree to which a client is protected by the flexible line of defense against possible reaction to a single stressor or a combination of stressors (Neuman, 2002d, p. 14).

The nurse uses the Neuman Systems Model Assessment and Intervention Tool, the Neuman Systems Model Nursing Diagnosis Taxonomy, and any other relevant practice tools to guide collection of data and facilitate documentation of nursing diagnoses, nursing goals, and nursing outcomes (see Table 7–2).

NURSING DIAGNOSIS

The nurse establishes a database that includes the simultaneous consideration of the dynamic interactions of physiologic, psychological, sociocultural, developmental, and spiritual variables.

The nurse identifies the client/client system's perceptions and his or her own perceptions by:
Assessing the condition and strength of client/client system's basic structure factors and energy resources.
Assessing the characteristics of the client/client system's flexible and normal lines of defense, lines of resistance, degree of potential or actual reaction, and potential for reconstitution following a reaction.

Assessing the internal and external environmental stressors that threaten the stability of the client/client system by:
Identifying and evaluating potential or actual intrapersonal, interpersonal, and extrapersonal stressors that threaten the stability of the client/client system.
Classifying stressors that threaten the stability of the client/client system through deprivation, excess, change, or intolerance.
Identifying, classifying, and evaluating potential and actual intrapersonal, interpersonal, and extrapersonal interactions between the client/ client system and the environment, considering all five interacting variables.

Assessing the client/client system's created environment by discovering the nature of the client/client system's created environment. This is accomplished by:
Assessing the client/client system's perception of stressors.
Identifying the client/client system's major problem, stress areas, or areas of concern.
Identifying the client/client system's perceptions of how present circumstances differ from the usual pattern of living.
Identifying ways in which the client/ client system handled similar problems in the past.
Identifying what the client/client system anticipates for self in the future as a consequence of the present situation.
Determining what the client/client system is doing and what he or she can do to help himself or herself.
Determining what the client/client system expects caregivers, family, friends, or others to do for him or her.
Determining the degree of protection provided by the client/client system's created environment.
Uncovering the cause of the client/client system's created environment.
Evaluating the influence of past, present, and possible future life processes and coping patterns on client/client system stability.
Identifying and evaluating actual and potential internal and external resources for an optimal state of client/client system wellness.

The nurse compares the client/client system's and the nurse's perceptions by identifying similarities and differences in perceptions.

The nurse facilitates client awareness of major perceptual distortions.

The nurse and client/client system work to resolve differences in perceptions.

The nurse identifies variances from wellness by synthesizing the client database with relevant theories from nursing and adjunctive disciplines.

The nurse states a comprehensive nursing diagnosis that encompasses the client/client system's general condition or circumstances, including identification of actual or potential variances from wellness and available resources.

NURSING GOALS

The nurse proposes outcome goals and interventions that will facilitate the highest possible level of client/ client system stability or wellness, i.e., maintain the normal line of defense and retain the flexible line of defense.

The nurse negotiates the desired prescriptive change or outcome goals to correct variances from wellness

with the client/client system, taking client/client system needs and resources into account.

The nurse prioritizes goals by considering the client/client system wellness level, the meaning of the experience to the client/client system, system stability needs, and total available resources.

The nurse negotiates specific prevention as intervention modalities with the client/client system.

NURSING OUTCOMES

The nurse implements nursing interventions through the use of one or more of the three prevention as intervention modalities.

Primary Prevention as Intervention nursing actions to retain system stability are implemented by:
   Preventing stressor invasion.
   Providing resources to retain or strengthen existing client/client system strengths.
   Supporting positive coping and functioning.
   Desensitizing existing or possible noxious stressors.
   Motivating the client/client system toward wellness.
   Coordinating and integrating interdisciplinary theories and epidemiological input.
   Educating or reeducating the client/client system.
   Using stress as a positive intervention strategy.

Secondary Prevention as Intervention nursing actions to attain system stability are implemented by:
   Protecting the client/client system's basic structure.
   Mobilizing and optimizing the client/client system's internal and external resources to attain stability and energy conservation.
   Facilitating purposeful manipulation of stressors and reactions to stressors.
   Motivating, educating, and involving the client/client system in mutual establishment of health-care goals.
   Facilitating appropriate treatment and intervention measures.
   Supporting positive factors toward wellness.
   Promoting advocacy by coordination and integration.
   Providing primary preventive intervention as required.

Tertiary Prevention as Intervention nursing actions to maintain system stability are implemented by:
   Attaining and maintaining the highest possible level of client/client system wellness and stability during reconstitution.
   Educating, reeducating, and reorienting the client/client system as needed.
   Supporting the client/client system toward appropriate goals.
   Coordinating and integrating health services resources.
   Providing primary and secondary preventive intervention as required.

The nurse evaluates the outcome goals by:
   Confirming attainment of outcome goals with the client/client system.
   Reformulating goals as necessary with the client/client system.

The nurse and client/client system set intermediate and long-range goals for subsequent nursing action that are structured in relation to short-term goal outcomes.

Source: Adapted from Neuman, B. (1990). Health as a continuum based on the Neuman systems model. Nursing Science Quarterly, 3, 129–135; Neuman, B. (2002). The Neuman systems model. In B. Neuman & J. Fawcett, The Neuman systems model (4th ed., 29–30). Upper Saddle River, NJ: Prentice Hall; and Neuman, B. (2002). Assessment and intervention based on the Neuman systems model. In B. Neuman & J. Fawcett (Eds.), The Neuman systems model (4th ed., pp. 347–359). Upper Saddle River, NJ: Prentice Hall, with permission.

D. When the cushioning, accordion-like effect of the flexible line of defense is no longer capable of protecting the client/client system against an environmental stressor, the stressor breaks through the normal line of defense. The interrelationships of variables—physiological, psychological, sociocultural, developmental, and spiritual—determine the nature and degree of the system reaction or possible reaction to the stressor (Neuman, 2002d, p. 14).

E. Lines of resistance in the client (internal and external resources) are activated to combat potential or actual stressor reactions (Neuman, 1990b, p. 259).

F. The client is an interacting open system in total interface with both internal and external environmental forces or stressors. Furthermore, the client is in constant change, with reciprocal environmental interaction, at all times moving either toward a dynamic state of stability or wellness or toward one of illness in varying degrees (Neuman, 2002d, p. 12).

G. The process of interaction and adjustment results in varying degrees of harmony, stability, or balance between the client and the environment. Ideally, there is optimal client system stability (Neuman, 2002, p. 23).

H. The major concern for nursing is in keeping the client system stable through accuracy both in assessing the effects and possible effects of environmental stressors and in assisting client adjustments required for an optimal wellness level (Neuman, 2002d, p. 25).

I. In keeping the system stable, the nurse creates a linkage among the client, environment, health and nursing (Neuman, 2002d, p. 25).

 ## EVALUATION OF NEUMAN'S SYSTEMS MODEL

This section presents an evaluation of the Neuman Systems Model. The evaluation is based on the results of the analysis, as well as on publications and presentations by Neuman and by others who have used or commented on the model.

EXPLICATION OF ORIGINS

Neuman explicated the origins of the Neuman Systems Model clearly and concisely. She traced her own background and the evolution of the model from a teaching aid to a fully developed conceptual model of nursing in a concise, yet richly detailed manner (Neuman, 2002b), and she made clear the forces and circumstances that motivated her work. Furthermore, Neuman explicitly identified her basic philosophy, and she identified the philosophical claims undergirding the model. The philosophical statements, in the form of a basic philosophy, beliefs, and assumptions, indicate that Neuman values a holistic (which she spells as "wholistic"), systems-based approach to the care of clients. Neuman's choice of a systems approach to health care reflects her assumption that systems thinking is a comprehensive way of viewing clients and their environments. Neuman also values intervention before manifestations of variances from wellness or stressor reactions, as well as after they occur. She emphasized the need to consider both the client's and the caregiver's perceptions of stressors and resources. Furthermore, she assumes that nursing goals are established effectively when negotiated with the client. Those aspects of the Neuman Systems Model underscore Neuman's respect for the perceptions and rights of each client. Indeed, she stated that she deliberately labeled human beings as clients to denote her respect for those who participate in nursing and her concern for collaborative goal setting. Furthermore, Neuman values wellness; indeed, she always has regarded her work as a wellness model. Neuman assumes that the environment is the source of stressors but regards stressors as neutral. The outcome of encounters with stressors is what has a negative or positive valence. In addition, Neuman (2002d) assumes that every human being has at the very least an innate "seed" of spirituality (p. 16).

Neuman explicitly acknowledged nursing colleagues who supported her work, and she provided bibliographic citations for knowledge from adjunctive disciplines that she drew on for development of the Neuman Systems Model. Neuman has always cited the influence of systems thinking and has become increasingly clear about how she has integrated ideas from general system theory into the model (Neuman, 2002d).

COMPREHENSIVENESS OF CONTENT

The Neuman Systems Model is sufficiently comprehensive with regard to depth of content. The revisions and refinements evident in Neuman's (2002d) current version of the model have clarified several areas of confusion found in earlier versions and have improved the adequacy of concept definitions and descriptions (Neuman 2002d, 2002e). One remaining area of confusion, however, is the Family, Community, and Social Issue dimensions of the **Client/Client System.** These dimensions require definitions or descriptions that go beyond being described as kinds of groups. George (2002) added that "interpersonal and extrapersonal stressors need to be more clearly differentiated … [and] reaction needs to be defined" (p. 368). She also pointed out that identification of variances from wellness and levels of wellness requires greater specification. However, given the abstract and general nature of conceptual models, Neuman's descriptions of concepts representing the metaparadigm concepts human beings, environment, health, and nursing are generally adequate.

The revisions and refinements to date certainly suggest that Neuman has been responsive to critiques of her work, such as the chapter on analysis and evaluation of the model by Fawcett and associates (1982) published in the first edition of *The Neuman Systems Model* (Neuman, 1982b), and a similar chapter by Fawcett (1989) in the second edition of *The Neuman Systems Model* (Neuman, 1989c). Indeed, Stevens (1982) commended Neuman for the scholarly attitude and scientific detachment demonstrated by inclusion of the Fawcett et al. (1987) critique in the book. With regard to refinements, Neuman (personal communication, October 6, 1993) commented that "the model was originally set forth as a comprehensive guide for nursing practice, open to creative interpretation and implementation. However, the author of the model does not sanction structural changes which alter its basic intent, meaning, and purpose." A review of all versions of the Neuman Systems Model (Neuman, 1974, 1980, 1982a, 1989d, 1995a, 2002d; Neuman & Young, 1972) indicates that the basic intent, meaning, and purpose of the model have been retained.

Neuman's (2002a, 2002d) approach to the nursing process reflects systems thinking (see Table 7–1). She stated, "Using a wholistic systems approach to protect and promote client welfare, nursing action must be skillfully related to the meaningful and dynamic organization of … the whole" (Neuman, 1995a, pp. 10–11). She went on to say, "Both system processes and nursing actions are purposeful and goal directed. That is, nursing vigorously attempts to control variables affecting client care" (Neuman, 2002d, pp. 8).

The Neuman Systems Model is based on reputable scientific findings from several disciplines. Neuman has continuously emphasized the importance of basing nursing diagnoses on knowledge derived from a synthesis of theory with the database of client factors (see Table 7–1). The **Neuman Systems Model Nursing Process Format** is dynamic in that there is ongoing establishment of nursing goals, negotiation between nurse and client with regard to the goals and intervention strategies, and feedback from client outcomes to confirm goals or serve as a basis for reformulation of new goals (see Table 7–1). Dynamism also is evident in the circularity of the Prevention as Intervention modalities. As Neuman (2002d) noted, "Ideally, primary prevention is also considered concomitant with secondary and tertiary preventions as interventions [and] tertiary prevention tends to lead back, in circular fashion, toward primary prevention" (pp. 26, 29).

Neuman's (2002a) emphasis on the client's perception of the situation and the negotiation needed for identification of appropriate goals and interventions reflects a concern for ethical standards.

Some Neuman Systems Model relational propositions link the metaparadigm concepts human beings and environment and human beings, environment, and health. Two other relational propositions provide clear linkages between human beings, environment, health, and nursing.

The Neuman Systems Model is comprehensive in breadth of content. "The major goal for nursing," Neuman (2002d) asserted, "is to reduce stressor impact, whether actual or potential, and to increase client resistance" (p. 29). She went on to point out that the Neuman Systems Model encompasses both health promotion and illness care:

> Ideally, health promotion goals should work in concert with both secondary and tertiary preventions as interventions to prevent recidivism and to promote optimal wellness, since the Neuman Systems Model is wellness oriented. Health promotion, in general, and within the primary prevention concept, relates to activities that optimize the client wellness potential or condition (p. 29).

The comprehensiveness of the breadth of the Neuman Systems Model is further supported by the direction it provides for nursing research, education, administration, and practice. Guidelines have been explicated for each area. Although the guidelines presented here are targeted to nursing, Neuman's (2002d) interest in the interdisciplinary and multidisciplinary use of the Neuman Systems Model calls for the extrapolation of the guidelines to other disciplines concerned with the health of individuals, families, and communities. That work has begun. In their introduction to the guidelines for Neuman Systems Model-based nursing research, Louis, Neuman, and Fawcett (2002) declared, "These guidelines are applicable to Neuman Systems Model-based nursing research conducted by one or more members of any health care discipline" (p. 113). Newman, Neuman, and Fawcett (2002) presented "guidelines for Neuman Systems Model-based education for the health professions" (p. 193). Shambaugh, Neuman, and Fawcett (2002) explained, "As a systems approach, the Neuman Systems Model is easily adapted by nurse administrators for the management of nursing services. The Neuman Systems Model also can be used by the administrators of the fully array of other health care services … These guidelines are applicable to the administration of services in any health care discipline" (pp. 265–266). And Freese, Neuman, and Fawcett (2002) deliberately worded the Neuman Systems Model guidelines for practice in such a way that they "are applicable to clinical practice in any health care discipline" (p. 37).

The guidelines for research and those for practice stipulate a reciprocal relationship between research and practice, such that research and practice are linked to "through the use of research findings to direct practice. In turn, problems encountered in ... practice give rise to new research questions" (Freese, Neuman, & Fawcett, 2002, p. 38; Louis, Newman, & Fawcett, 2002, p. 114).

Research Guidelines

The guidelines for research based on Neuman's Systems Model, which were given by Louis, Newman, and Fawcett (2002, p. 114), based on previous work by Gigliotti (1997) and Grant, Kinney, and Davis (1993), are:

- Purpose of the research
  - One purpose of Neuman Systems Model-based research is to predict the effects of primary, secondary, and tertiary prevention interventions on retention, attainment, and maintenance of client system stability.
  - Another purpose of Neuman Systems Model-based research is to determine the cost, benefit, and utility of prevention interventions.

- Phenomena of interest
  - The phenomena of interest encompass the physiological, psychological, sociocultural, developmental, and spiritual variables; the properties of the central core of the client/client system; the properties of the flexible and normal lines of defense and the lines of resistance; the characteristics of the internal, external, and created environments; the characteristics of intrapersonal, interpersonal, and extrapersonal stressors; and the elements of primary, secondary, and tertiary prevention interventions.

- Problems to be studied
  - The precise problems to be studied are those dealing with the impact of stressors on client system stability with regard to physiological, psychological, sociocultural, developmental, and spiritual variables, as well as the lines of defense and resistance.

- Research methods
  - Research designs encompass both inductive and deductive research using qualitative and quantitative approaches and associated instrumentation.
  - Data encompass both the client system's and the investigator's perceptions, and may be collected in inpatient, ambulatory, home, and community settings.

- Study participants
  - Study participants can be the client systems of individuals, families, groups, communities, organizations, or

collaborative relationships between two or more individuals. The investigator also is a study participant.

- Data analysis
  - Data analysis techniques associated with both qualitative and quantitative methods are appropriate.
  - Quantitative methods of data analysis should consider the flexible line of defense as a moderator variable and the lines of resistance as a mediator variable.

- Contributions to knowledge development
  - Neuman Systems Model-based research findings advance understanding of the influence of prevention interventions on the relation between stressors and client system stability.

Education Guidelines

The guidelines for education based on Neuman's Systems Model, which were given by Newman et al. (2002, p. 194), are:

- Focus of the curriculum
  - The focus of a Neuman Systems Model-based educational program is on the client system's reaction to environmental stressors. The purpose of education for the health professions is to facilitate the design and use of primary, secondary, and tertiary prevention-as-intervention modalities by learners and teachers to assist client systems to retain, attain, and maintain optimal wellness.

- Nature and sequence of content
  - The content of a Neuman Systems Model-based curriculum encompasses all of the concepts of the model. The sequence of content may be guided by the complexity of interactions among the concepts or by the prevention-as-intervention modalities.

- Settings for education
  - Education can occur in vocational and technical programs, hospital-based nursing diploma programs, associate degree programs, baccalaureate programs, and graduate programs.

- Characteristics of learners
  - Learners who meet the requirements for any type of nursing education program must have the ability to engage in high-level critical thinking. Learners also must be willing to engage in both cooperative and independent learning.

- Teaching-learning strategies
  - Teaching-learning strategies include a variety of

modalities that foster critical thinking, as well as cooperative and independent learning.

Administration of Health-Care Services Guidelines

Guidelines for the administration of health-care services based on Neuman's Systems Model, which were given by Shambaugh, Newman, & Fawcett (2002, p. 267), are:

- Focus of health-care services
  - The focus of Neuman Systems Model-based health-care services is the client system, which can be individuals, families, groups, and communities. The administrator regards the collective staff as a client system that is a composite of physiological, psychological, sociocultural, developmental, and spiritual variables. The administrator also may regard each department of a health-care organization or the larger health-care organization as the client system.

- Purpose of administration of health-care services
  - The purpose of the administration of health-care services is to facilitate the delivery of the primary, secondary, and tertiary prevention interventions that will best help client systems to retain, attain, and maintain optimal stability.

- Characteristics of health-care personnel
  - Health-care personnel, including administrators and practitioners, must have knowledge of the content of the Neuman Systems Model, as well as the willingness to implement this conceptual model as a guide for administration and practice. Personnel also must appreciate systems thinking.

- Settings for health-care services
  - Health-care services are located in settings in which primary, secondary, and tertiary prevention is appropriate, including but not limited to ambulatory clinics, acute-care medical centers, community hospitals, rehabilitation units, elementary and secondary schools, colleges and universities, prisons, retirement communities, life-care communities, assisted-living facilities, nursing homes, hospices, clients' homes, community centers, and the streets and sidewalks of the community.

- Management strategies and administrative policies
  - Management strategies and administrative policies focus on the staff, the departments, or the total institution as the client system of the administrator, who uses management practices that promote optimal client system stability.

Practice Guidelines

Guidelines for practice based on Neuman's Systems Model, which were given by Freese, Newman, & Fawcett (2002, p. 38), are:

- Purpose of practice
  - The purpose of practice is to assist clients to retain, attain, or maintain optimal system stability.

- Practice problems of interest
  - Practice problems encompass actual or potential reactions to intrapersonal, interpersonal, and extrapersonal stressors.

- Settings for practice
  - Practice occurs in virtually any health-care or community-based setting, such as clinics, hospitals, hospices, homes, and the streets and sidewalks of the community.

- Characteristics of legitimate participants in practice
  - Legitimate participants in practice are those individuals, families, groups, and communities who are faced with actual or potential intrapersonal, interpersonal, and extrapersonal stressors.

- The practice process
  - The practice process is the **Neuman Systems Model Process Format,** which encompasses three components—Diagnosis, Goals, and Outcomes (see Table 7–1).
    - The Neuman Systems Model Process Format engages the client system and the caregiver in a mutual partnership to determine diagnosis, goals, and outcomes.
    - Diagnoses may be classified into a Neuman Systems Model diagnostic taxonomy that is organized according to client system (individual, family, group, community), level of response (primary, secondary, tertiary), client subsystem responding to the stressor (physiological, psychological, sociocultural, developmental, spiritual), source of the stressor (intrasystem, intersystem, extrasystem), and type of stressor (physiological, psychological, sociocultural, developmental, spiritual).
    - Interventions occur as primary, secondary, and tertiary prevention interventions, in accord with the degree to which stressors have penetrated the client system's lines of defense and resistance.
    - General outcomes are derived from the content of the Neuman Systems Model. Client system-specific outcomes involve application of the general outcomes to particular practice situations.

• Contributions of practice to participants' well-being
  • Neuman Systems Model-based practice contributes to client system well being by facilitating the highest possible level of stability achievable at a given point in time.

LOGICAL CONGRUENCE

The content of the Neuman Systems Model is not completely logically congruent. The model was developed primarily within the tradition of the reciprocal interaction world view. Despite refinements in content, elements of the reaction world view remain in Neuman's conceptualization of the **Created Environment**. To her credit, Neuman has attempted to translate the **Created Environment** in such a way that it reflects the reciprocal interaction world view. She explained that although the **Created Environment** is functionally at the unconscious level, "it exchanges energy with and encompasses the internal and external environments, making it congruent with the open system concept … of the Neuman System Model" (Neuman, 1990a, pp. 129–130). Still, however, the emphasis on the unconscious reflects a mechanistic, psychoanalytic orientation to the concept.

The logical problem found in Neuman's view of **Stressors** in previous versions of her conceptual model was resolved by incorporating Lazarus' (1981, 1999) view of stressors, which is more dynamic than Selye's (1950) view (Neuman, 2002d). Moreover, in the most recent version of her model, Neuman (2002d) eliminated any mention of wellness as negentropy and illness as entropy. That change in Neuman's conceptualization of health was needed because general system theory, on which Neuman based a substantial portion of her model, views the living open system as negentropic. Entropy, according to von Bertalanffy (1968), is a characteristic only of closed systems. Neuman now focuses on the flow of energy between the client and the environment and the amount of energy that is available to the client system at any time rather than referring to entropic or negentropic conditions.

In addition, in the most recent version of her model, Neuman (2002d) eliminated any mention of homeostasis, which was not logically compatible with her view of the client system as a living open system. Instead, she focuses on stability of the client system in a dynamic manner. Neuman (personal communication, October 6, 1993) explained, "The dynamic equilibrium or state of system stability equates with the degree of system wellness. The dynamism is inherent in the interactions [between client system and environment] and results in a particular degree of system stability or wellness."

The Neuman Systems Model clearly represents the systems category of knowledge. Although the model includes a developmental variable, development is viewed as change in the client system over time. Thus there is no evidence of logical incompatibility with regard to different categories of knowledge.

GENERATION OF THEORY

Neuman (2002d) explained that she and her colleague, Audrey Koertvelyessy, "jointly identified the major theory for the [Neuman Systems Model] as being the **Theory of Optimal Client System Stability**" (p. 30). The only proposition of that theory articulated to date is, "Stability represents health for the system" (Neuman, 2002d, p. 30).

In addition, a rudimentary **Theory of Prevention as Intervention** has begun to be generated from the Neuman Systems Model. Citing a personal communication in the fall of 1987 with Koertvelyessy, Neuman (2002d) explained:

> [Koertvelyessy] views the concept of prevention—whether primary, secondary, or tertiary—as prevalent and significant in the Neuman Systems Model, linked to each of the broad concepts of the model, that is, client, environment, health, and nursing. Inasmuch as the prevention strategies are the modes instituted to retain, attain, or maintain stability of the client's health status, she considers the development of a theory statement linking these concepts as a necessary next step (p. 31).

Alligood (2002) commented, "Both theories are useful in practice because nursing action is linked to a nursing outcome for the client. These broad theories have numerous applications when age, health status, and nature of stressors are specified" (p. 49).

Neuman (2002d) noted that "several other theories inherent within the model could be identified and clarified with the goal of optimizing health for the client" (p. 30). To date, three other explicit middle-range theories have been derived from the Neuman Systems Model. Lamb (1999) derived the Theory of Optimal Student System Stability, which addresses baccalaureate nursing students' perceptions of empathy and stress experienced in student-instructor interactions. Her study findings supported the hypothesis that the higher the levels of empathy baccalaureate nursing students perceive when interacting with clinical instructors, the less stressful students perceive the interaction to be.

Casalenuovo (2002) derived the Theory of Well-Being from the Neuman Systems Model. The theory addresses the relations among stress, well being, and fatigue. Her study findings supported the hypothesis that disruption in well being in adults living with the stress of diabetes mellitus leads to greater fatigue.

Stepans and Knight (2002) derived the Theory of Infant

Exposure to Environmental Tobacco Smoke from selected concepts of the Neuman Systems Model. They constructed an explicit conceptual-theoretical-empirical structure that linked extrapersonal stressors with environmental tobacco smoke, as measured by personal air monitoring, cigarette butt collection, and a Smoking Habits Questionnaire and the physiological variable in the flexible line of defense with the epithelium. They linked the physiological variable in the normal line of defense with the respiratory system, the circulatory system, the sympathoadrenal system, the hepatic system, and the renal system, as measured by urinary levels of nicotine and cotinine; and the physiological variable in the lines of resistance with increased carbon monoxide affinity for heme, increased carboxyhemoglobin, decreased oxygen availability, increased respiratory rate, decreased phagocytic functioning, decreased ciliary functioning, and increased biogenic amine release, as measured by carboxyhemoglobin, blood pressure, and the incidence of bronchitis, otitis media, and pneumonia. Finally, they linked the physiologic variable in the basic structure with sudden infant death syndrome (SIDS), lung function and impairment, asthma, and carcinogenesis, as measured by a pulmonary function test and the incidence of cancer, SIDS, and asthma.

Gigliotti's (2001) analysis of relational propositions found in Neuman Systems Model-based research reports is a major contribution to middle-range theory development. The next step in that work is to formalize the relational propositions and the concepts contained within those propositions as explicit middle-range theories.

Hoffman's (1982) translation of the abstract concepts of the Neuman Systems Model into more concrete middle-theory concepts is another major contribution to middle-range theory development. For example, she proposed that the internal environment could be represented by strength or weakness of various body parts or organs. Hoffman's attempt is a noteworthy first step, but it stops short of identifying the methods needed to empirically measure the concepts. Measurement of strength or weakness of body parts, for example, must be described in observable terms if the Neuman Systems Model concept of internal environment is to be empirically tested.

Breckenridge (1997, 2002) has contributed to theory generation within the context of the Neuman Systems Model by presenting an explicit conceptual-theoretical-structure for her qualitative studies of dialysis modality and prostate cancer treatment decision making. She linked the Neuman Systems Model emphasis on client perceptions with open-ended interview schedules, and then linked the themes identified in the responses of clients receiving hemodialysis or continuous ambulatory peritoneal dialysis and those receiving different forms of treatment for prostate cancer with the physiological, psychological, sociocultural, developmental and spiritual variables.

Lowry and Anderson (1993) also presented an explicit conceptual-theoretical-structure, in this case for their descriptive pilot study of reactions to mechanical ventilation. They linked selected concepts of the Neuman Systems Model (extrapersonal stressor; physiological, developmental, psychological, and spiritual variables; interpersonal factors) to the study variables (mechanical ventilation, disease state or injury, age, anxiety, control, level of hope, and social support), and then linked the study variables to appropriate empirical indicators (hospital chart documentation of multiple failed weaning attempts, medical diagnosis, chronological age, Anderson-Lowry Ventilation Scale, Multidimensional Health Locus of Control Scales, Hope Scale, and Norbeck Social Support Questionnaire).

Villarruel and colleagues (2001) added to the discussion of nursing middle-range theory development within the context of the Neuman Systems Model by describing a strategy for linking borrowed theories with the Neuman Systems Model. They claimed that linking a theory from another discipline with a nursing conceptual model and testing that middle-range theory within the context of the nursing conceptual model could, if the theory were found to be empirically adequate, yield a shared theory. They illustrated their strategy by linking the Neuman Systems Model with the theory of planned behavior, a middle-range theory developed within the discipline of social psychology (Ajzen, 1985, 1991; Doll & Ajzen, 1992). Simpson (2000) tested the linkage of the Neuman Systems Model and the theory of planned behavior in her study of condom use among Black women. She concluded that the theory was empirically adequate and may be considered a shared theory.

Latham (2002) rejected the strategy of linking theories borrowed from other disciplines with nursing conceptual models. She declared:

> Grafting a particular borrowed theory onto a nursing conceptual model may be a questionable exercise. ... Rather the emphasis could be placed on creating distinctive cognitive approaches with the parameters of nursing. ... investigating borrowed theories in the hope of sharing them may not be the most appropriate way forward. Nursing research will not advance knowledge if it continues to hang on the coattails of other disciplines (p. 264).

CREDIBILITY OF THE NURSING MODEL

Social Utility

The social utility of the Neuman Systems Model is thoroughly documented. Four editions of *The Neuman Systems Model* (Neuman, 1982b, 1989c, 1995b; Neuman & Fawcett, 2002), which contain numerous examples of the use of the model in nursing education, practice, administration, and research, have been published. Furthermore, a monograph addressing the use of the Neuman Systems Model in nursing education has been published (Lowry, 1998). Moreover, the number of book chapters and journal articles dealing with applications of the model continues to grow. The model is being used by nurses in many different educational and practice settings throughout the United States, and in Puerto Rico, Costa Rica, Brazil, Canada, Iceland, England, Wales, Holland, Denmark, Finland, Norway, Sweden, Portugal, Australia, New Zealand, Thailand, Japan, Taiwan, and South Korea, among other countries. Furthermore, International Neuman Systems Model Symposia have been held every 2 or 3 years since 1986.

The Neuman Systems Model has gained such wide acceptance due, at least in part, to "its flexibility for use with individuals, families, groups, and communities, and its emphasis on prevention as intervention. Furthermore, the sociocultural variable highlights the unique culture, values and beliefs, life patterns, infrastructure, economy, education, and health-care delivery system of each country and region of the world. [The model also] provides an ideal framework for international initiatives related to the World Health Organization goal of 'health for all by the year [2010]'" (Neuman et al., 1997, p. 20).

The content of the Neuman Systems Model comprises many terms, but most are familiar words; therefore, use of the model does not require mastery of an extensive new vocabulary. Craig and Beynon (1996) commented that they decided not to alter the language of the model during its implementation in a public health nursing agency, and found that "as staff began to think-through the model, its terminology, regarded initially as a limitation, became more meaningful" (p. 255).

Extensive study of the concepts of the Neuman Systems Model and relevant theories from nursing and adjunctive disciplines is, however, required before knowledgeable application in nursing research, education, administration, and practice. Indeed, as Neuman (1989b) pointed out:

> It is assumed that the professional nurse operates from a theoretical perspective as client data are gathered. It is most often in the interpretation of client data that theory is either not explicitly used or improperly related to client data, resulting in confusing and often faulty diagnoses. It is more common for theory to be related to interventions than to diagnoses. Professional nurses should (to be considered truly professional) be able to justify their diagnostic statement based upon specific theoretical relationships with available client data. [In addition,] when client data are specifically related to [nursing and] social sciences theories in developing the nursing diagnosis, nurses can present themselves as professional in a knowledgeable manner. It is a responsibility to one's self, profession, clients, colleagues, and other health disciplines to be able to present a logical and rational justification for such de-

cision making. Unless nurses can clearly articulate to others, particularly to the client, the why and how for arriving at a particular nursing diagnosis, they cannot claim the validity of their position; nor can they be certain of appropriate subsequent interventions (pp. 57–58).

Neuman Systems Model-based nursing practice is feasible for the health promotion and illness care of individuals, families, and communities experiencing many different health conditions. Caramanica and Thibodeau (1987) identified some of the human and material resources needed to implement the model at the health-care organization level. They cited the need for a formal action plan, a task force made up of nurses from all levels, and a consultant. Moreover, they maintained that the use of a conceptual model of nursing is especially important when resources are limited, commenting that in times of rapid change, a theory-based model which reflects staff's beliefs gives purpose, direction, and organization to a department of nursing. It profiles desired nursing practice and facilitates unified, goal-directed nursing care behaviors so vital in times of reduced resources and increased acuity (p. 71).

Capers and colleagues (1985) underscored the importance of thorough planning for the implementation of the Neuman Systems Model at the health-care organization level. Their strategies include the appointment of a planning committee to oversee the entire implementation project, with philosophy, nursing process, and implementation subcommittees; and the establishment of a timetable for implementation and evaluation, with target dates for a pilot implementation project, subsequent adoption of the model by several units, and evaluation of the project. Other strategies are a formal staff education program with collegiate courses, continuing education, and independent study options along with use of nurse preceptors, planning unit conferences, patient-centered unit conferences, and nursing grand rounds. Capers and colleagues (1985) cited the importance of including representatives from head nurse, coordinator, and staff nurse levels on the subcommittees and ascertaining that nurses from all three shifts are included in all aspects of the project. They also recommended hiring a project facilitator to coordinate the planning, implementation, and evaluation phases of the project and, whenever possible, seeking consultation from the faculty of a nearby college that uses the Neuman Systems Model. In addition, Capers and colleagues (1985) emphasized the importance of developing a comprehensive documentation package that is congruent with the Neuman Systems Model, including a nursing assessment form, a nursing care plan format, a nursing flow sheet, nursing progress notes, and a nursing discharge summary. Moreover, they noted the importance of adequate funding for the project and encouraged solicitation of funds from foundations or other extramural sources.

Moynihan (1990) emphasized the utility of a forced-choice Neuman Systems Model-based assessment tool for decreasing the missing data that frequently occur when an open-ended format is used and noted the effectiveness of self-directed learning using an educational booklet. Moreover, she highlighted the need for a surveillance or oversight committee to track progress toward full implementation of the model at the health-care organization level.

Craig and Beynon (1996) used many of the strategies mentioned previously and emphasized the importance of a strategic plan. They identified the keys to successful implementation of the Neuman Systems Model in a health-care organization given here:

- Plan the pace of the implementation project to reflect the workplace culture and revise the pace on the basis of regular feedback from participants.
- Maintain the momentum and sense of inquiry by routinely integrating opportunities to sustain ongoing commitment to the model and to theory-based practice.
- Use both structured and unstructured activities to encourage staff to use the model and critically analyze their practice.
- Rotate or share responsibility for scanning the literature for new resources and examples of how the Neuman Systems Model is being used in practice, education, administration, and research.
- Allocate staff development funds for purchase of resources and attendance at conferences.
- Use resources that encourage self-reliance and collegial peer networks.
- Establish a supportive and consultative network of model users within and outside the agency.
- Expand use of the model and develop expertise in areas such as program development and planning, administrative practice, and organizational development.

Nursing Research. Neuman Systems Model-based research continues to increase. Research instruments derived from the Neuman Systems Model are listed in Table 7–2. Gigliotti and Fawcett's (2002) review of research reports published in journals and book chapters yielded 121 different research instruments that have been used to measure middle-range theory concepts representing Neuman's Systems Model concepts. The 24 of those 121 instruments that were directly derived from the Neuman Systems Model are listed in Table 7–2. Gigliotti and Fawcett (2002) recommended that the review of research be extended to doctoral dissertations and master's theses, so that the instruments used in those studies can be identified. They also recommended that the utility of research instruments for practice be examined, as well as the utility of practice tools and educational tools (see Table 7–2) for research purposes. The Spiritual Care Scale was initially proposed as a practice tool (Carrigg & Weber, 1997); subsequently, Young and colleagues (2001) and Gigliotti and Fawcett (2002) identified its potential for use as a research instrument (see Table 7–2).

Published reports of Neuman Systems Model-based studies are listed in Table 7–3. Published abstracts of doctoral dissertations and master's theses are listed in the Doctoral Dissertations and Master's Theses sections of the chapter bibliography on the CD-ROM. Another master's thesis, which is not available in Master's Abstracts International, was completed by Collins (2000). Citations and abstracts for several unpublished studies conducted by graduate students and faculty, obtained from a survey of schools of nursing in the United States, Canada, and Europe, are given in Louis and Koertvelyessy (1989); Louis provided an updated list of largely unpublished studies in her 1995 book chapter.

A review of the research listed in Table 7–3, as well as the results of an integrative review of the Neuman Systems Model-based research published through 1997 (Fawcett & Giangrande, 2001, 2002) revealed that the Neuman Systems Model has guided a range of study designs, from descriptions of diverse Neuman Systems Model phenomena to experiments that tested effects of prevention interventions on a variety of client system outcomes. Most of the Neuman Systems Model-based research is limited to a single study on a single topic, although some programs of research are beginning to emerge. For example, Breckenridge (2002) described her research program, which focuses on decision making regarding treatment options. In addition, several studies have focused on the Neuman Systems Model phenomenon of client/client system perceptions of stressors, and several other studies have focused on prevention interventions (see Table 7–3).

Fawcett and Giangrande (2002) urged researchers to "explicate the linkages between the Neuman Systems Model concepts and propositions and their study variables in a clear and concise manner" (p. 135). They went on to say:

> It is not sufficient only to mention that the Neuman Systems Model guided the study. Rather, the Neuman Systems Model concepts and propositions selected to guide the study must be identified and explicitly linked to the study variables and hypotheses. Faculty supervising doctoral dissertations and master's theses, journal and book editors, and peer reviewers all are strongly encouraged to require an explicit statement of such linkages as a condition of acceptance of the manuscript. Furthermore, educators are strongly encouraged to include strategies for explicating the linkages in all nursing research courses (p. 135).

(Text continues on page 198)

Instrument or Tool and Citation*	Description
RESEARCH INSTRUMENTS	

Measurement of Stressors

Smoking Questionnaire (Cantin & Mitchell, 1989; Gigliotti & Fawcett, 2002)	Measures stressors in the form of nurses' age, gender, education, work area, and setting.
Smoking Habits Questionnaire (Stepans & Fuller, 1999; Stepans & Knight, 2002)	Measures the smoking habits of mothers as an indicator of their infants' exposure to environmental tobacco smoke.
Needs Assessment Interview Schedule (Decker & Young, 1991; Gigliotti & Fawcett, 2002)	Measures caregivers' (of home hospice patients) life situation.
Neuman Stressors Inductive Interviews (Blank, Clark, Longman, & Atwood, 1989; Gigliotti & Fawcett, 2002)	Measures home care needs and stressors of cancer patients and their caregivers.
Telephone Interview Schedule and Health Interview Schedule (Bowdler & Barrell, 1987; Gigliotti & Fawcett, 2002)	Measures physical, mental, social, economic, and general health of homeless persons and care providers.
Self-Identified Needs Questionnaire (Grant & Bean, 1992; Gigliotti & Fawcett, 2002)	Measures self-identified needs of caregivers of head-injured adults.
Hospital and Home Visits (Johnson, 1983; Gigliotti & Fawcett, 2002)	Measures stressors and coping patterns.
Semi-Structured Interview Guide (Maligalig, 1994; Gigliotti & Fawcett, 2002)	Measures parents' (of children who had day surgery) perceptions of stressors.
Logs of Problems, Solutions, Actions (Skipwith, 1994; Gigliotti & Fawcett, 2002)	Measures physical and psychological problems of caregivers of elders.
Cancer Survivors Questionnaire (Loescher et al., 1990; Gigliotti & Fawcett, 2002)	Measures physiologic, psychological, and sociocultural changes and problems/concerns of long-term cancer survivors.
Interview Schedule (Gries & Fernsler, 1988; Gigliotti & Fawcett, 2002)	Measures perception of the intubation experience of mechanically ventilated patients.
Neuman Model Nursing Assessment Guide (Hoch, 1987; Gigliotti & Fawcett, 2002)	Measures the impact of aging and retirement.
The Perceived Stress Level Tool (Open-Ended Stressor Rank) (Montgomery & Craig, 1990; Gigliotti & Fawcett, 2002)	Measures stressors of wives of alcoholics.
Patient Stressor Scale (Wilson, 1987; Gigliotti & Fawcett, 2002)	Measures patients' perceptions of surgical intensive care unit stressors.

Measurement of Lines of Defense and Resistance and Client System Response

Semi-Structured Interview Schedule (Semple, 1995; Gigliotti & Fawcett, 2002)	Measures stressors and experiences of family members of persons with Huntington's disease.
Cancer Survivors Questionnaire (Loescher et al., 1990; Gigliotti & Fawcett, 2002)	Measures needs of long-term cancer survivors.

Measurement of Prevention Interventions

Telephone Counseling Intervention (Skipwith, 1994; Gigliotti & Fawcett, 2002)	Protocol for telephone counseling primary, secondary, and tertiary prevention interventions for caregivers of elders.

*See the Research Instruments, Practice Tools, and Educational Tools section of the chapter references for complete citations.

Needs Assessment
Semi-Structured Interview Guide (Bass, 1991; Gigliotti & Fawcett, 2002) — Measures needs of parents of infants in a neonatal intensive care unit.

Measurement of Metaparadigm Concepts
The Safety Assessment Tool (Gellner et al., 1994; Gigliotti & Fawcett, 2002) — Records demographic data and risk factors, safety issues, and incident prevention/ intervention for community health nurses.

Measurement of Client System Perceptions
Semi-Structured Interview Guide (Cava, 1992; Gigliotti & Fawcett, 2002) — Measures long-term cancer survivors' major stress area, coping strategies, changes in lifestyle, views of the future, and expectations of support from others.

Patient Perception Interview Guide (Breckenridge, 1997b; Gigliotti & Fawcett, 2002) — Measures end-stage renal disease patients' perceptions of why, how, and by whom dialysis treatment modality was chosen

Measurement of the Spiritual Variable
Structured Interview Guide (Clark et al., 1991; Gigliotti & Fawcett, 2002) — Measures trust, support, respect

Measurement of the Five Client System Variables
Client Perception Interview Guide (Breckenridge, 1997a; Gigliotti & Fawcett, 2002) — Measures factors influencing dialysis treatment modality decision

Demographic Profile (Montgomery & Craig, 1990; Gigliotti & Fawcett, 2002) — Records demographic information

Documentation of Nursing Care
Spiritual Care Scale (Carrigg & Weber, 1997; Gigliotti & Fawcett, 2002) — Measures spiritual care and psychosocial care given by nurses

<h2 style="text-align:center">PRACTICE TOOLS</h2>

Individual as Client System

Neuman Systems Model Assessment and Intervention Tool (Mirenda, 1986; Neuman, 1989, 1995b, 2002a; Russell, 2002)	Guides client assessment and permits documentation of goals, intervention plan, and outcomes from the perspective of both clients and caregivers.
Nursing Assessment Guide (Beckman et al., 1998; Russell, 2002)	A modification of the Neuman Systems Model Assessment and Intervention Tool.
Nursing Assessment Form (Burke et al., 1989; Russell, 2002)	Guides identification of client's and nurse's perceptions of stressors and coping mechanisms, using open-ended questions.
Assessment Tool (Fulbrook, 1991; Russell, 2002)	Guides assessment and documentation of client's (or advocate's) and nurse's perceptions and provides a framework for nursing diagnoses; fosters assessment of client and family.
Assessment and Analysis Guideline Tool (McHolm & Geib, 1998; Russell, 2002)	Guides health assessment and formulation of nursing diagnoses.
Guide for Assessment of Structural Components of a System (Johnson et al., 1982; Russell, 2002)	Permits documentation of the status of the basic structure, and the lines of defense and resistance across variable areas for individuals, groups, families, or communities.
Maternal/Fetal Assessment Tool (Dunn & Trepanier, 1989; Trepanier et al., 1995; Russell, 2002)	Guides assessment of the pregnant woman and her fetus.
Perinatal Risk-Grading Tool (Trepanier et al., 1995; Russell, 2002)	Permits categorization of perinatal risks.
Early Weaning Risk Screening Tool (Murphy, 1990; Russell, 2002)	Permits identification of pregnant women at risk for early weaning from breast-feeding.

(continued)

Instrument or Tool and Citation	Description
Depression Symptom Assessment Checklist (Clark, 1982; Russell, 2002)	Guides assessment and documentation of depression.
Nursing Assessment of the Elderly Form (Gunter, 1982; Russell, 2002)	A modification of the Neuman Systems Model Assessment and Intervention Tool for use with elderly clients.
Systematic Nursing Assessment Tool for the CAPD Client (Breckenridge et al., 1982; Russell, 2002)	Guides assessment of continuous ambulatory peritoneal dialysis (CAPD) clients.
Grid for Stressor Identification (Johnson et al., 1982; Russell, 2002)	Guides assessment of types and sources of stressors.
Client Perception of Transfer as a Stressor Tool (Dunbar, 1982; Russell, 2002)	Measures the client's perception of readiness for transfer from a surgical intensive care unit.
Interdisciplinary High Risk Assessment Tool of Rehabilitation Inpatient Falls (Cotten, 1993; Russell, 2002)	Permits prediction of adult rehabilitation inpatients at risk for falling.
Occupational Health Nursing Risk Profile (McGee, 1995; Russell, 2002)	Guides assessment of environmental stressors and stressor impact on workers' lines of defense and resistance, along with calculation of relative risk and attributable risk.
Assessment/Intervention Tool (Beitler et al., 1980; Russell, 2002)	Guides assessment, using an interview format, and documents associated interventions.
Assessment/Intervention Tool for Postrenal Transplant Clients (Breckenridge, 1982; Russell, 2002)	Guides assessment of stressors and lists appropriate interventions for clients who have had a renal transplant.
Modified Assessment/Intervention Tool for Critical Care (Dunbar, 1982; Russell, 2002)	A modification of the Neuman Systems Model Assessment and Intervention Tool for use in the critical care setting.
Nursing Health Assessment Tool and Nursing Care Plan (Felix et al., 1995; Russell, 2002)	A modification of the Neuman Systems Model Assessment and Intervention Tool for use with elderly residents of chronic care facilities.
Guide for Data Synthesis to Derive Nursing Diagnosis (Johnson et al., 1982; Russell, 2002)	Permits documentation of client system responses to stressors and etiology of each stressor.
Neuman Systems Model Nursing Diagnosis Taxonomy (Ziegler, 1982; Russell, 2002)	Provides a taxonomy of nursing diagnoses directly derived from the Neuman Systems Model; permits documentation of nursing diagnoses based on the Neuman Systems Model.
Decision Matrix for Nursing Intervention (McGee, 1995; Russell, 2002)	Facilitates planning of nursing interventions.
Guide for Planning Theoretically Derived Nursing Practice (Johnson et al., 1982; Russell, 2002)	Permits documentation of nursing diagnoses; theoretically derived plan, goals, and intervention; and expected outcomes and evaluation.
Care Plan (Fulbrook, 1991; Russell, 2002)	Permits documentation of problems, goals, interventions, and evaluation of interventions.
Nursing Process Tool (Stepans & Knight, 2002)	Provides a structure for organizing and analyzing client assessment data in terms of client boundaries, a physiological variable within the boundaries, environmental stressors affecting the boundaries, the client's responses and reactions to the stressors affecting the boundaries, and the client's responses and reactions to the stressors in terms of variance from wellness, as well as a structure to record a nursing diagnosis, nursing goals and outcome criteria, nursing interventions, and evaluation of outcomes.

Summary of Practitioner-Client Goals and Rationale in Treating Depressed Clients (Clark, 1982; Russell, 2002	Presents a list of goals and associated prevention interventions goals for the depressed client.
Intervention Plan to Support Goals (Clark, 1982; Russell, 2002)	Presents a list of prevention interventions for the depressed client.
Minimum Data Set Format (Schlentz, 1993; Russell, 2002)	Presents a minimum data set for prevention interventions in long-term care facilities.
Patient Classification Worksheet (Hinton-Walker & Raborn, 1989; Russell, 2002)	Permits classification of patients in terms of personnel required for treatments within the context of physiological, psychological, sociocultural, and developmental variables.
Spiritual Care Scale (Carrigg & Weber, 1997; Russell, 2002; Young, et al., 2001)	Measures spiritual care for clients and distinguishes spiritual care from psychosocial care.
Format of Care Planning for the Acute Cardiac Surgical Client Using the Neuman Systems Model (McInerney, 1982; Russell, 2002)	Presents a comprehensive nursing care plan for clients who have had cardiac surgery.
Protocol of Potential Interventions for the Psychological Needs of the Patient with COPD (Baker, 1982; Russell, 2002)	Presents a list of psychological needs and associated nursing interventions for the client with chronic obstructive pulmonary disease.
Nursing Protocol for Management of Immobilization (Cardona, 1982; Russell, 2002)	Presents a list of goals and associated interventions, rationales, and outcomes for clients at risk for complications from immobilization due to skeletal traction for treatment of a hip fracture.
Nursing Protocol for Management of Mental Confusion (Cardona, 1982; Russell, 2002)	Presents a list of goals and associated interventions, rationales, and outcomes for clients who are mentally confused.
Protocol for Pain (Cunningham, 1982; Russell, 2002)	Presents a list of interventions, rationales, and outcomes for reduction of pain experienced by clients who do not request pain relief due to attitudes toward pain relief measures and cultural group affiliation.
Clinical Evaluation of the Nursing Care Plan Tool (Dunbar, 1982; Russell, 2002)	Measures the nurse's perception of a nursing care plan.
Theoretical Evaluation of the Nursing Care Plan (Dunbar, 1982; Russell, 2002)	Measures the nurse's perception of a nursing care plan in terms of the concepts of the Neuman Systems Model.
Format for Evaluation (McGee, 1995; Russell, 2002)	Permits documentation of evaluation of outcomes of nursing interventions.
Format for Evaluation of Theoretically Derived Nursing Practice (Johnson et al., 1982; Russell, 2002)	Permits documentation of evaluation of expected and actual outcomes in terms of each nursing diagnosis, goal, and intervention.
Guide to Critical Thinking with the Neuman Nursing Process (Sohier, 2002)	Provides specific nurse and client guidelines for assessment.

Family As Client System

Guide for Family Assessment (Reed, 1982; Russell, 2002)	A modification of Neuman Systems Model Assessment and Intervention Tool for use with families.
Neonatal/Family Assessment Tool (Dunn & Trepanier, 1989; Trepanier et al., 1995; Russell, 2002)	Guides assessment of the neonate and family.
FAMLI-RESCUE (Flannery, 1991; Russell, 2002)	Guides collection and evaluation of data on family functioning and resources for use by neuroscience nurses working in acute care settings.
Family Health Assessment/Intervention Tool (Mischke-Berkey et al., 1989; Russell, 2002)	Guides assessment and documentation of family and caregiver perceptions of family health.

(continued)

> ► ⚙ **TABLE 7–2**
> **RESEARCH INSTRUMENTS, PRACTICE TOOLS, AND EDUCATIONAL TOOLS DERIVED**
> **FROM THE NEUMAN SYSTEMS MODEL** *(continued)*

Instrument or Tool and Citation	Description
Family Systems Stressor-Strength Inventory: Family Form (Mischke-Berkey & Hanson, 1991; Russell, 2002)	Guides assessment of the family's perceptions of general and specific family system stressors and family system strengths.
Family Systems Stressor-Strength Inventory: Clinician Form (Mischke-Berkey & Hanson, 1991; Russell, 2002)	Guides assessment of the clinician's perceptions of general and specific family system stressors and family system strengths.
Community As Client System	
Community Assessment Guide (Benedict & Sproles, 1982; Russell, 2002)	Guides assessment of communities, including intracommunity, intercommunity, and extracommunity factors, and community's and health planner's perceptions of stressors.
Community-As-Client Assessment Guide (Beddome, 1989, 1995; Russell, 2002)	Guides collection of data about geopolitical and aggregate needs, community resources, and resource utilization patterns from the perspective of clients and caregivers.
Organization As Client System	
Neuman Systems-Management Tool for Nursing and Organizational Systems (Kelley & Sanders, 1995; Kelley et al., 1989; Neuman, 1995a; Russell, 2002)	Permits the nurse administrator to assess, resolve, prevent, and evaluate stressors in any type of administrative setting; measures the total system response to an environmental stressor.
A Systems-Based Assessment Tool for Child Day-Care Centers (Bowman, 1982; Russell, 2002)	Guides assessment of stressors in child day-care centers.
EDUCATIONAL TOOLS	
Format for Organization of Class Content (Tollett, 1982; Reed, 2002)	Facilitates organization of course content by variable areas and prevention interventions.
Nursing Assessment Guide (Beckman et al., 1998; Reed, 2002)	A modification of the Neuman Systems Model Assessment and Intervention Tool; helps students to collect and organize client system data.
Assessment and Analysis Guideline Tool (McHolm & Geib, 1998; Reed, 2002)	Guides health assessment and formulation of nursing diagnoses; may be used to teach students how to do a Neuman Systems Model-based assessment and analysis.
Clinical Evaluation Form Summary of Clinical Evaluation Form Profile of Clinical Evaluations Form (Strickland-Seng, 1995, 1998; Reed, 2002)	Three forms used to measure and document faculty and student perceptions of the student's progress toward achieving the expected level of performance in 25 behaviors exhibited in sophomore, junior, and senior year nursing courses.
Student Clinical Evaluation Tool (Beckman et al., 1998; Reed, 2002)	Permits assessment of cognitive, psychomotor, and affective student outcomes.
Lowry-Jopp Neuman Model Evaluation Instrument (LJNMEI) (Lowry, 1998; Lowry & Jopp, 1989; Lowry & Newsome, 1995; Reed, 2002)	Measures students' and new graduates' internalization of Neuman Systems Model concepts and application of the model to practice.

Research Focus and Topic	Study Participants	Citation*
	DESCRIPTIVE STUDIES	
Psychometric evaluation of the Levels of Cognitive Functioning Assessment Scale	Baccalaureate program senior nursing students Registered nurses Neuropsychologists Videotapes of clients with traumatic brain injury	Flannery, 1995
Comparison of smoking rates	Canadian registered nurses, registered psychiatric nurses, licensed practical nurses, and the Canadian population as a whole	Cantin & Mitchell, 1989
Use of alcohol, marijuana, over-the-counter drugs, and prescription drugs	Men and a women with traumatic spinal cord injuries and chronic pain	Radwanski, 1992
Real and perceived safety risks	Community health nurses	Gellner et al., 1994
Health needs	The homeless population of Richmond, Virginia	Bowdler & Barrell, 1987
Changes, problems, concerns, and needs related to long-term and late effects of cancer and cancer therapy	Adult cancer survivors	Loescher et al., 1990
Home care needs	Clients with metastatic cancer and their significant other caregivers	Blank et al., 1989
Perceptions of the mechanical ventilation experience	Men and women hospitalized in a critical care unit	Gries & Fernsler, 1988
Caregivers' needs	Informal caregivers of head-injured adults in the home setting	Grant & Bean, 1992
Caregivers' needs	Primary caregivers of terminally ill home-hospice clients	Decker & Young, 1991
Parents' perceptions of stressors	Parents of children undergoing day surgery	Maligalig, 1994
Parents' needs	Parents of infants in a neonatal intensive care unit	Bass, 1991
Description of online functional communication	Nursing students who were conducting a family nursing action research project	Molinari, 2001
Dialysis modality decision making	Clients with end-stage renal disease receiving hemodialysis or continuous ambulatory peritoneal dialysis	Breckenridge, 1997a, 1997b
Program of research about how, why, and by whom treatment modalities are chosen	Renal patients and prostate cancer patients	Breckenridge, 2002
Use of coping strategies	Adult cancer survivors	Cava, 1992
Comparison of use of, satisfaction with, and need for cancer education and support services	Younger (40–64 years of age) and older (≥65 years of age) cancer survivors	Narsavage & Romeo, 2003
Labeling and management of problematical behavior	Lay Black adults Black and White registered nurses	Capers, 1991
Feelings about mechanical ventilation, locus of control, and perceptions of hope and social support	Ventilator-dependent adults hospitalized in intensive care units	Lowry & Anderson, 1993
Family needs	Families with a critically ill member who had and those who did not have a "Do Not Resuscitate" order	Kahn, 1992

*See the Research section of the chapter references for complete citations.

(continued)

Research Focus and Topic	Study Participants	Citation
Spiritual needs	Adults who had surgery due to cancer or cardiac disease	Clark et al., 1991
Cultural stressors	A 36-year-old southern Black woman who experienced a hypertensive crisis	Johnson, 1983
Healing practices for common childhood illnesses	Hmong parents residing in California	Nuttall & Flores, 1997
Caregivers' needs	Family members and caregivers of individuals with Huntington's disease	Semple, 1995
Evaluation of health education programs	Elderly adults residing in a government-assisted apartment complex in Ohio	Imamura, 2002
Description of meaning of health and identification of stressors and stressor reactions	Thai elderly clients	Pothiban, 2002
Difference in ability to formulate nursing diagnoses with and without the use of the Neuman Systems Model	Baccalaureate program senior nursing students	Purushotham & Walker, 1994
Factors constraining or facilitating physical assessment	Registered nurse case managers, nurse administrators, and staff development coordinators working in continuing care facilities in Canada	Skillen et al., 2001
Comparison of maternal role development	Pregnant women who underwent or declined to undergo maternal serum screening	Denson & Komnenich, 2002
Description of problems identified and interventions utilized during postpartum home visits	Secondary analysis of Omaha assessment databases completed by student nurses for families with a mother no more than 6 months postpartum	Burns-Vandenberg & Jones, 1999
Assessment of patient flow and use of human resources	Observations in public health clinics	Lowry et al., 2001
Description of opinions about holistic care	Male patients in a detoxification unit	Norrish & Josste, 2001
CORRELATIONAL STUDIES		
Identification of beliefs that differentiate smokers and nonsmokers	African-American, Puerto Rican, and non-Hispanic White teenage females	Hanson, 1999
Relation of demographic characteristics to safety restraint use and alcohol use	Motor vehicle crash victims	Bueno et al., 1992
Relation between inclusion of perioperative nursing theory and clinical experience in a baccalaureate nursing program and selection of the perioperative setting for clinical practice following program completion	Registered nurses holding a baccalaureate degree	Roggensack, 1994
Relation between job stress and burnout, as mediated by spiritual well-being and hardiness	Registered nurses	Marsh et al., 1999
Relation between month of hospital admission and diagnosis of cerebrovascular accident	Charts of individuals who had experienced a cerebrovascular accident	Gifford, 1996
Relation between psychological responses to the surgical intensive care unit and identification of stressors	Clients in a surgical intensive care unit	Wilson, 1987

Relation of psychological maternal and student role involvement and perceived social support to perception of multiple role stress	Mothers attending college	Gigliotti, 1999
Relations among perception of infant health, preparation for caregiving, confidence in caregiving, and caregiver burden	Mothers of low and normal birthweight infants	May & Hu, 2000
Relation between perceived stress and health practices	Wives of alcoholics	Montgomery & Craig, 1990
Relation between stressors and changes in level of stress	Male and female caregivers of a traumatic head-injured family member	Jones, 1996
Relations between stress, coping, and health status	Family caregivers of individuals with hepatoma	Lin et al., 1996
Relation between mood symptoms and daytime ambulatory blood pressure	Black female caregivers and noncaregivers	Picot et al., 1999
Relation of prognosis, surgery, current radiation therapy, performance status, self-control skills, preference for information, and age to quality of life	Men and women with lung cancer	Hinds, 1990
Relation of health, function, family status, psychological status, spiritual status, socioeconomic status, age, gender, income, marital status, work status, occupation, monthly treatment costs, and type of insurance to quality of life	Adults with chronic pain	Gerstle & Wallace, 2001
Relation of social, emotional, and physical impact of arthritis, learned resourcefulness, and spirituality to general health perception	Older adults with arthritis	Potter & Zauszniewski, 2000
Relation of cognitive style to the first semester final grade	Diploma nursing program first-semester students	Nortridge et al., 1992
Relation of demographic variables, organizational characteristics, and role orientation to job satisfaction	Nurse faculty in institutions offering a doctoral degree in nursing	Moody, 1996
Relation between demographic variables and perceived autonomy	Registered nurses working in a clinical agency with shared governance	George, 1997
Relation of personality hardiness to job stress and burnout	Hospital staff nurses	Collins, 1996

EXPERIMENTAL STUDIES

Effects of type of audiometry on identification of hearing loss and middle ear disease	Elementary school children	Mannina, 1997
Effects of four combinations of antiseptics and dressings on skin bacterial growth	Hospitalized children with cancer who had a central venous line	Freiberger et al., 1992
Effects of public health clinic prenatal care and tertiary multidisciplinary clinic prenatal care on client satisfaction and pregnancy outcomes	Low socioeconomic status pregnant women	Lowry et al., 1997
Effect of an experimental structured demonstration about breast-feeding techniques and a control intervention on breast-feeding knowledge and skill and nipple pain and trauma	Postpartum women	Vijaylakshmi, & Raman, 2002
Effects of maternal smoking on infant urinary nicotine and cotinine levels, temperature, pulse, respiratory rate, blood pressure, and oxygen saturation	Infants of mothers do did and did not smoke	Stepans & Fuller, 1999

(continued)

Research Focus and Topic	Study Participants	Citation
Effects of a cardiovascular health fair	Participants in church-based health fairs	Wilson, 2000
Effects of radiant heat alone or in combination with pharmacological intervention on postanesthesia shivering	Adults who had surgery	Heffline, 1991
Effect of structured preoperative instruction on preoperative and postoperative anxiety	Patients scheduled for cataract surgery	Morrell, 2001
Effects of preparation for bronchial fibroscopy on anxiety	Patients scheduled to undergo bronchial fibroscopy	Leophonte et al., 2000
Effects of preoperative information versus a control intervention on postoperative complications	Adult men and women who had abdominal surgery	Ziemer, 1983
Effect of a preoperative psychoeducational intervention on postoperative state anxiety	Egyptian men and women with bladder cancer	Ali & Khalil, 1989
Effects of changes in body position every 2 hours versus maintenance of the supine position for the first 24 hours on atelectasis, other postoperative complications, and length of stay in the surgical critical care unit and in the hospital	Clients who had coronary artery bypass graft surgery	Gavigan et al., 1990
Effect of an ocean sounds (white noise) intervention versus usual environment sounds on night sleep pattern following transfer from an intensive care unit	Clients who had coronary artery bypass graft surgery	Williamson, 1992
Effects of planned surgery for hip replacement versus emergency surgery for hip fracture on incidence of delirium, sleep satisfaction, pain perceptions, and psychological concerns	Elderly persons who had undergone orthopedic hip surgery	Bowman, 1997
Effect of guided-imagery discharge teaching versus a control intervention on depression scores 1 week after hospital discharge	Adults ≥ 65 years of age hospitalized for surgery	Leja, 1989
Effect of an educational program about alternatives to physical restraints on use of physical restraints	Acute care patients with documented restraint use	Smith et al., 2003
Effects of a partial psychiatric hospitalization program on fear of fear, severity of psychological impairment, and general emotional distress	Participants in a 5-week partial psychiatric hospitalization program	Waddell & Demi, 1993
Effect of psychiatric nurse home visits versus standard care on readmission rates	Patients with depression, discharged from a mental health unit	Barker et al., 1999
Effect of transitional case management services versus traditional care on depression, cognitive status, patient and caregiver satisfaction (case management services only), and costs related to utilization of services	Discharged psychiatric patients	Chiverton et al., 1999
Effects of a fiber and fluid nursing intervention on maintenance of bowel movements and elimination aid withdrawal	Residents of a long-term health-care facility	Rodrigues-Fisher et al., 1993

Effects of comfort touch on self-esteem, well-being and social processes, health status, life satisfaction and self-actualization, faith or belief, and self-responsibility	Elderly female residents of a nursing home	Butts, 2001
Effects of a Neuman Systems Model-based treatment protocol, a Roy Adaptation Model-based treatment protocol, and a treatment protocol not based on an explicit conceptual model on depression and life satisfaction	Retired persons attending a senior citizens center	Hoch, 1987
Effect of a telephone counseling intervention on caregiver burden	Female caregivers of elderly family members	Skipwith, 1994
Effects of a worksite wellness/health promotion program on health awareness and health behaviors	Black American employees of a minority-owned industry	Fowler & Risner, 1994
Effect of progressive muscle relaxation versus control intervention on the stress response	Insurance company clerical workers	Vaughn et al., 1989
Effects of an experimental back school exercise regimen on back strength, back flexibility, psychological well-being, and anxiety	Municipal workers who had experienced back injuries	Sirles et al., 1991
Effects of an experimental back school rehabilitation program on lost work time, lost time cost, medical cost, and number of injuries	Municipal workers who had experienced back injuries and who participated in or did not participate in the back school program	Brown et al., 1992
Effects of counseling on severity of back pain	Municipal workers who experienced low back pain, attended a back school, and who received or did not receive the counseling intervention	Koku, 1992
Effect of a Neuman Systems Model-based curriculum and a medical model-based curriculum on role deprivation	Senior generic baccalaureate nursing students	Carroll, 1989
Effect of administering or not administering cyclosporin A on symptoms	Registered nurses	Courchene et al., 1991
Effects of guided imagery versus a control intervention on anxiety, stress, performance time, and performance score	Baccalaureate nursing students performing their first injection	Speck, 1990
Effects of 8- and 12-hour shifts on critical thinking and fatigue	Critical care nurses	Fields & Loveridge, 1988
Effect of a short-term (four 1-hour meetings) low-intensity nurse-led mutual help group and a control no group meetings on anxiety	Nurses working with long-term care clients in public health and rehabilitation settings	Louis, 1989
Effects of a death education program versus no education on attitudes and behavioral intentions toward dying patients and their families	Nurses who care for hospitalized terminally ill adults and their families	Hainsworth, 1996
Effects of a medical or nursing database on number and quality of diagnostic statements	Master's degree nursing program students	Andersen & Briggs, 1988
Effects of a medical or nursing database on number and quality of diagnostic statements	Public health nurses	Mackenzie & Laschinger, 1995
Effect of an inservice educational program on attitudes toward theory-based nursing	Nurse managers working in a public health department in Canada	Beynon & Laschinger, 1993

(Text continued from page 187)

Nursing Education. The utility of the Neuman Systems Model for nursing education is well documented in the literature. Practice tools and educational tools (see Table 7–2) have been developed for use by students to guide their activities related to all components of the **Neuman Systems Model Nursing Process Format** (see Table 7–1). Other educational tools have been developed for use by faculty to structure evaluation of students' practice performance and evaluation of the curriculum (see Table 7–2).

Reed's (2002) review of Neuman Systems Model-based educational tools (see Table 7–2) led her to conclude that:

> None of the descriptions of the educational tools discussed in this chapter included any information about validity and reliability testing. The development and testing of valid and reliable educational tools certainly requires considerable time. Given the many demands on faculty, tool development and psychometric testing rarely is a priority, unless linked to a research project. Yet educational tools are a valuable technique to help students to learn and faculty to evaluate the students' learning and the curriculum. Furthermore, lack of adequate psychometric properties severely limits any conclusions that may be drawn from administration of the tool. Educators are, therefore, encouraged to make the time for development and psychometric testing of educational tools that will provide meaningful information for evaluation of the students and the curriculum.
>
> Furthermore, if nursing educators are willing to expend the time and effort to develop a curriculum that is based on a conceptual model of nursing, and if they expect students to use that model to guide practice, then evaluation of the students' knowledge and clinical skills should be based on the same conceptual model. More specifically, time and effort need to be devoted to development and psychometric testing of educational tools that are based on the same conceptual model as the curriculum. Attention to the details of educational tool development and testing certainly will increase the continuity and quality of the educational process, which is the ultimate goal of evaluation (p. 242).

Lowry (2002) pointed out that her integrated review of the Neuman Systems Model-based educational literature "provides evidence that the Neuman Systems Model has been and continues to be a very useful guide for education" (p. 231). On the basis of her literature review, Lowry (2002) concluded:

> Although the trend is toward eclecticism in nursing education today, the Neuman Systems Model has served many programs well throughout the years. The faculty of those programs that have moved away from exclusive use of the model claim that they retained some of the broad concepts of the model. The faculty of the programs that have continued to use the model claim that they "think Neuman" and their graduates find the Neuman Systems Model useful as an organizing tool. The teaching strategies used to facilitate student learning are a tribute to faculty creativity. As nursing education in other countries moves from an apprentice style process to theory-based curricula, the Neuman Systems Model frequently is selected to

guide curriculum development. The Neuman Systems Model-based programs that have been described in the literature serve as prototypes for programs throughout the world (p. 231).

Published reports indicate that the Neuman Systems Model has been used successfully as a basis for curriculum construction and revision in practical nursing, associate degree, baccalaureate, and master's programs, as well as a guide for continuing education and in-service education programs. The names of the schools in which those programs are located are listed here. The complete citations for the publications are given in the Education section of the chapter references. The Neuman Systems Model also has been used to guide the development of a curriculum in physical therapy (Lowry, 2002; Toot & Schmoll, 1995).

- Practical Nursing Programs
  - Santa Fe Community College, Gainesville, Florida (Neuman, 1995)
  - Texas Woman's University, Houston (Gerontic Nursing) (Gunter, 1982; Lowry, 2002)
- Associate Degree Nursing Programs
  - Athens Area Technical Institute, Athens, Georgia (Lowry, 2002; Lowry & Newsome, 1995)
  - Cecil Community College, North East, Maryland (Johnson, 1989; Lowry, 1986, 1988, 1998, 2002; Lowry & Green, 1989; Lowry & Jopp, 1989; Lowry & Newsome, 1995; Strickland-Seng et al., 1996)
  - Central Florida Community College, Ocala, Florida (Lowry, 2002)
  - Contra Costa College, San Pablo, California (personal communication, Rita Ruderman, April 20, 2001)
  - Indiana University-Purdue University at Fort Wayne (Beckman et al., 1998a, 1998b; Freiburger, 1998; Lowry, 2002; Lowry & Green, 1989; Lowry & Newsome, 1995)
  - Los Angeles County Medical Center School of Nursing, Los Angles, California (Bloch & Bloch, 1995; Hilton & Grafton, 1995; Lowry, 2002)
  - Santa Fe Community College, Gainesville, Florida (Lowry, 2002; Lowry & Green, 1989; Lowry & Newsome, 1995; Neuman, 1995; Sutherland & Forrest, 1998)
  - Southern Adventist University, Collegedale, Tennessee (Lowry, 2002)
  - University of Nevada, Las Vegas (Louis et al., 1989; Lowry, 2002; Lowry & Green, 1989)
  - Yakima Valley Community College, Yakima, Washington (Evans, 1998; Lowry, 2002; Lowry & Newsome, 1995)
- Baccalaureate Nursing Programs
  - Aarhus University, Aarhus, Denmark (Johansen, 1989; Lowry, 2002)
  - Avon and Gloucestershire College of Health, School of Nursing, Avon, England (Child care curriculum) (Vaughan & Gough, 1995)

- Brandon University, Brandon, Manitoba, Canada (Practicum courses) (Craig, 1995; Lowry, 2002)
- California State University in Fresno (Lowry, 2002; Stittich et al., 1989, 1995)
- Dutch Reformed University Department of Nursing, Zwolle, Holland (de Kupier, 2002)
- Escola Superior De Enfermagem De Maria Fernanda Resende, Lisbon, Portugal (Neuman, 1995)
- Fitchburg State College, Fitchburg, Massachusetts (Nursing Process with Families/Groups in Communities course) (Cammuso & Wallen, 2002)
- Lander University, Greenwood, South Carolina (Hassell, 1998; Lowry, 2002; Reed-Sorrow et al., 1989; Sipple & Freese, 1989)
- Minnesota Intercollegiate Nursing Consortium: College of St. Catherine, St. Paul; Gustavus Adolphus College, St. Peter; St. Olaf College, Northfield (Glazebrook, 1995; Mrkonich, Hessian et al., 1989; Lowry, 2002; Mrkonich, Miller et al., 1989; Reed-Sorrow et al., 1989)
- Neumann College, Aston, Pennsylvania (Lowry, 2002; Mirenda, 1986; Strickland-Seng et al., 1996)
- North Dakota-Minnesota Nursing Education Consortium (Tri-College University): Moorhead State University, Moorhead, Minnesota; Concordia College, Moorhead, Minnesota; North Dakota State University, Fargo (Lowry, 2002; Nelson et al., 1989)
- Okanagan University, British Columbia, Canada (Beddome, 1995; Lowry, 2002)
- Queens University, Kingston, Ontario, Canada (Laschinger et al., 1989; Lowry, 2002)
- Ryerson Polytechnical Institute, Toronto, Ontario, Canada (Community Health Nursing course) (Craig, 1995)
- Saint Anselm College, Manchester, New Hampshire (Beyea & Matzo, 1989; Bruton & Matzo, 1989; Busch & Lynch, 1998; Lowry, 2002)
- Saint Xavier College, Chicago, Illinois (Lebold & Davis, 1980, 1982; Lowry, 2002)
- Simmons College, Boston, Massachusetts (Edwards & Kittler, 1991)
- State University of New York at Brockport (Weitzel & Wood, 1998)
- Texas Women's University, Houston, Texas (Gerontic Nursing)(Gunter, 1982; Lowry, 2002)
- Union College, Lincoln, Nebraska (Beitler et al., 1980)
- University College of Caring Sciences, Eskilstuna, Sweden (Primary Health in Nursing courses) (Engberg, 1995; Lowry, 2002)
- University College of Health Sciences, Jönköping, Sweden (Primary Health in Nursing courses) (Engberg, 1995; Lowry, 2002)

- University of Calgary, Calgary, Alberta, Canada (Craig, 1995; Lowry, 2002)
- University of Missouri-Kansas City (Conners, 1982, 1989; Lowry, 2002)
- University of Moncton, Moncton, New Brunswick, Canada (Craig, 1995; Lowry, 2002)
- University of Nevada, Las Vegas (Louis et al., 1989; Lowry, 2002)
- University of Ottawa, Ottawa, Ontario, Canada (Community Health Nursing, Occupational Health Nursing, Nursing Management of the At Risk Gravida During Antepartum and Intrapartum, Nursing Management of the Neonate at Risk courses) (Bourbonnais & Ross, 1985; Craig, 1995; Lowry, 2002; Ross et al., 1987; Story & Ross, 1986)
- University of Pittsburgh, Pittsburgh, Pennsylvania (Knox et al., 1982; Kilchenstein & Yakulis, 1984; Lowry, 2002)
- University of Prince Edward Island, Charlottetown, Prince Edward Island, Canada (Craig, 1995; Lowry, 2002)
- University of Saskatchewan, Saskatoon, Saskatchewan, Canada (Psychiatric Nursing course) (Craig, 1995; Dyck et al., 1989; Lowry, 2002; Peternelj-Taylor & Johnson, 1996)
- University of South Australia, Adelaide, Australia (Lowry, 2002; McCulloch, 1995)
- University of Tennessee at Martin (Strickland-Seng, 1995, 1998; Lowry, 2002)
- University of Texas at Tyler (Klotz, 1995; Lowry, 2002)
- University of Toronto, Toronto, Ontario, Canada (Craig, 1995; Lowry, 2002)
- University of Western Ontario, London, Ontario, Canada (Community Health Nursing course) (Craig, 1995)
- University of Windsor, Windsor, Ontario, Canada (Family and Community Health Nursing courses) (Craig, 1995; Lowry, 2002)
- University of Wyoming, Laramie (Dale & Savala, 1990; Nichols et al., 1989)

- Master's Degree Nursing Programs
  - California State University, Fresno (Lowry, 2002; Nuttall et al., 1998; Stittich et al., 1989)
  - Fitchburg State College, Fitchburg, Massachusetts (Master's program in forensic nursing) (Cammuso & Wallen, 2002)
  - Ohio University, Athens, Ohio (Nursing Service Administration Program) (Lowry, 2002; Neuman & Wyatt, 1980)
  - Northwestern State University, Shreveport, Louisiana (Lowry, 2002; Moxley & Allen, 1982)

- Texas Woman's University, Dallas and Houston, Texas (Conners et al., 1982; Johnson et al., 1982; Lowry, 2002; Neuman, 1995; Tollett, 1982)
- University of Missouri-Kansas City (Conners, 1982, 1989; Lowry, 2002)
- University of Nevada, Las Vegas (Louis et al., 1989; Lowry, 2002)
- University of Texas at Tyler (Klotz, 1995; Lowry, 2002)

- Continuing Nursing Education/Inservice Nursing Education (Baker, 1982a, 1982b; Capers, 1986; Engberg et al., 1995; Harty, 1982; Roberts, 1994; Story & DuGas, 1988)

Nursing Administration. The utility of the Neuman Systems Model in nursing service administration is well documented. Sanders and Kelley's (2002) review of the literature revealed that "The clarity, simplicity, and generalizability of the Neuman Systems Model is demonstrated by the frequency with which it has been implemented in clinical agencies as a framework for both administrative and clinical practice. ... The use of the Neuman Systems Model in clinical practice agencies has been as pervasive in other countries as in the United States. Second only to the United States, Canada has adopted the Neuman Systems Model as the nursing model of choice for guiding nursing practice in a variety of health care agencies" (pp. 280, 283).

Mann and colleagues (1993) explained how the Neuman Systems Model guided the development and implementation of the orthopedic case manager role within a large county health system. They noted that the new role was designed to improve the coordination and delivery of care for orthopedic trauma clients.

Published reports indicate that the model has been implemented successfully at the unit or organization level in the United States, Canada, Iceland, England, Wales, Holland, Slovenia, and Sweden. The health-care organizations in which Neuman Systems Model-based nursing practice has been implemented, as described in the available literature, are listed here. The complete citations for the publications are given in the Administration section of the chapter references.

- Mount Sinai Hospital, Hartford, Connecticut (Caramanica & Thibodeau, 1987, 1989; Craig & Beynon, 1996; Moynihan, 1990)
- Senior Health Service Community Nursing Center, University of Rochester, Rochester, New York (Dwyer et al., 1995)
- Francis Ashbury Manor United Methodist Homes, Ocean Grove, New Jersey (Schlentz, 1993)
- Friends Hospital, Philadelphia, Pennsylvania (Scicchitani et al., 1995)

- Chester Community Nursing Center, Chester, Pennsylvania (Reitano, 1997)
- Collington Episcopal Life Care Community, Mitchellville, Maryland (Rodriguez, 1995)
- Children's Hospital of Michigan, Detroit, MI (Torakis, 2002; Torakis & Smigielski, 2000)
- Jefferson Davis Memorial Hospital, Natchez, Mississippi (Craig & Beynon, 1996; Hinton Walker & Raborn, 1989)
- Allied Home Health Association, San Diego, California (Pinkerton, 1974)
- Kuakini Health Care System, Honolulu, Hawaii (Craig & Beynon, 1996)
- Hospice of Windsor, Windsor, Ontario, Canada (Echlin, 1982)
- Whitby Psychiatric Hospital, Whitby, Ontario, Canada (Craig & Beynon, 1996; Craig & Morris-Coulter, 1995)
- Geriatric Day Hospital, Parkwood Hospital, London, Ontario, Canada (Neuman, 1995)
- Middlesex-London Health Unit, Public Health Nursing Division, Ontario, Canada (Beynon, 1995; Craig, 1995; Craig & Beynon, 1996; Drew et al., 1989; Mytka & Beynon, 1994)
- Elgin-St. Thomas Health Unit, Public Health Nursing Division, St. Thomas, Ontario, Canada (Craig, 1995)
- Regional Neonatal Education Program of Eastern Ontario, Ottawa, Ontario, Canada (Dunn & Trepanier, 1989)
- Elizabeth Bruyere Health Centre, Ottawa, Ontario, Canada (Craig & Beynon, 1996; Felix et al., 1995; Neuman, 1995)
- Manitoba Department of Health, Manitoba, Canada (Drew et al., 1989)
- St. Joseph Hospital, Reykjavik, Iceland (Craig & Beynon, 1996)
- Burford Community Hospital, Oxfordshire, England (Johns, 1991)
- Queen Alexandra Hospital, Intensive Therapy Unit, Portsmouth, England (Fulbrook, 1991)
- Paediatric Unit, Royal Infirmary, Blackburn, Lancashire, England (Kenyon & Barnett, 2001)
- Community Psychiatric Nursing Practice: Breconshire, Powys, Wales; Ystradgynlais, Powys, Wales (Davies, 1989; Davies & Proctor, 1995)
- Emergis, The Institute for Mental Health Care, Zeeland, Holland (de Munck & Merks, 2002)
- Riagg Zuid Hollandse Eilanden (An agency for ambulatory mental health patients), Holland (Verbeck, 1995)
- World Health Organization Collaborative Center for Primary Health Care Nursing, Maribor, Slovenia (Neuman, 1995)

- Rykov Hospital, Jönköping, Sweden (Craig & Beynon, 1996)
- Primary Health Care Center, Savsjo, Sweden (Engberg, 1995)

Nursing Practice. The utility of Neuman's conceptual model for nursing practice is exceedingly well documented. Many practice tools (see Table 7–2) have been developed, collectively encompassing all components of the **Neuman Systems Model Nursing Process Format** (see Table 7–1). Moreover, Quayhagen and Roth (1989) identified existing psychometrically sound research instruments for use as assessment tools for the physiological, psychological, sociocultural, developmental, and spiritual variables and the external environment. Russell's (2002) review of the practice tools led her to conclude that:

> The Neuman Systems Model [practice] tools are practical and effectively guide wholistic assessment and prevention interventions for individual, family, community, and organization client systems. Collectively, the tools guide … practice with a wide array of client systems in diverse health-care settings.

> The review of the [practice] tools … provides direction for future work. First, the validity and reliability of the existing [practice] tools need to be determined, so that users can determine when and under what conditions each tool is most effectively used. Next, many tools have been developed for use with individuals, but many more are needed for use with families, communities, and organizations. Finally, [practice] tools that focus on portions of the content of the Neuman Systems Model are needed. For example, a tool is needed for assessment of individuals' internal, external, and created environments. Given the broad scope of the Neuman Systems Model, the creation of new [practice] tools is limitless. Commitment to the task is all that is required (p. 70).

The Neuman Systems Model has been used to guide nursing practice in so many different settings with diverse populations that "it would be difficult to identify a setting where this model could not be applied" (George, 2002, p. 359) (Table 7–4). In concluding her integrative review of the Neuman Systems Model-based literature about practice, Amaya (2002) pointed out that "The Neuman Systems Model is widely perceived to encompass a philosophy and values compatible with acknowledged roles and functions of nursing. Various authors described how the Neuman Systems Model provides a distinctive frame of reference to address particular health conditions within the context of clinical specialties and/or distinct settings. The publications specified client, environment, nursing, and health according to Neuman Systems Model concepts. Many centered on how the model guided wholistic approaches to patient care. Clearly, the Neuman Systems Model is capable of addressing actual and potential client needs within a broad spectrum of … situations. International use of the Neuman Systems Model provides additional evidence of its broad applicability" (p. 54) Amaya (2002) went on to declare "The systems approach holds the promise envisioned by Neuman (1982) for increasing self-determination, creativity, and adaptive ability of the profession by providing a tangible structure within which change can take place" (p. 55).

Review of the publications cited in Table 7–4 and those listed in the Commentary: Practice section of the chapter bibliography on the CD-ROM reveals that the Neuman Systems Model has been used for nursing practice targeted to the individual, the family, or the community as the client system. More specifically, nursing practice has taken place in both inpatient and outpatient settings. Client systems include children with acute conditions requiring hospitalization and children with chronic conditions such as cancer, mental and physical impairments, psychiatric disorders, and hyperkinesis. Other client systems encompass well adults and adults at risk for injury or illness who are in need of primary prevention interventions; adults with such acute conditions as cancer, multisystem failure, trauma, spinal cord injuries, cardiac disease, cerebrovascular accidents, and orthopedic problems; and adults, including the elderly, with chronic conditions such as substance abuse, cognitive impairment, diabetes, HIV disease, cancer, kidney disease, chronic obstructive pulmonary disease, multiple sclerosis, hypertension, and psychiatric illnesses.

Following from Neuman's (1983) explanation of how the Neuman Systems Model is used when the family is the client/client system, reports of nursing practice with the family as the client system have focused on childbearing families and families with an acutely ill or chronically ill member. Nursing practice with communities as the client system also has been reported, as has nursing practice with the nurse as the client system. To date, however, no reports of the use of the Neuman Systems Model to guide nursing practice with a social issue as the client system have been located.

Social Congruence

Although Neuman (1974, 2002d) has asserted for many years that nursing is a unique profession, she also always has considered her model to be appropriate for use by members of all health-care disciplines. Indeed, the multidimensional nature of the Neuman Systems Model is attractive to the many health-care professionals who recognize the complex nature of humans and their interactions with the environment. In particular, Toot and Schmoll (1995) described the application of the Neuman Systems Model to

(Text continues on page 204)

Practice Situation	Population	Citation*

APPLICATION OF THE NEUMAN SYSTEMS MODEL

Individual as the Client System

Well Children

	Adolescent school children	Cook, 1999
	Children at risk	
	Infants exposed to environmental tobacco smoke	Stepans & Knight, 2002

Children with Acute Conditions

	Hospitalized preschool-age children	Orr, 1993
	A young boy with tonsillitis	Wormald, 1995

Children with Chronic Conditions

	A mentally and physically impaired infant	Galloway, 1993
	An 8-year-old child with leukemia	Piazza et al., 1992; Wright et al., 1994
	A young boy with linear scleroderma	Fuller & Hartley, 2000
	Children who require psychiatric services	Herrick et al., 1991
	Children with hyperkinesis	Herrick et al., 1992

Well Adults

	Women seeking information about oral contraceptives	Lindell & Olsson, 1991
	A 29-year-old primipara making a decision regarding method of infant feeding	Gigliotti, 1998
	A man with learning disabilities	Spencer, 2002
	Older women residing in a home for the aged	Gibson, 1996

Adults at Risk for Illness/Injury

	Postpartal women at risk for domestic violence	Bullock, 1993
	Homeless women residing in an urban shelter	Sohier, 1997, 2002
	Women at risk for coronary heart disease	Lile, 1990

Adults with Acute Conditions

	Adults hospitalized for medical or surgical treatment	Robichaud-Ekstand & Delisle, 1989
	A 29-year-old woman who had undergone surgery for cervical cancer	Sohier, 1997, 2002
	A 40-year-old man having surgery for bladder cancer	Cheung, 1997
	A 41-year-old man with complications from radiation therapy for pancreatic cancer	Beitler et al., 1980
	Critically ill trauma clients	Bueno & Sengin, 1995
	A 19-year-old male with unrelieved pain due to chest trauma	Cunningham, 1982
	Adults with hypermetabolism in multisystem organ failure	Bergstrom, 1992
	A 42-year-old man admitted to the emergency department with symptoms of myocardial infarction	Redheffer, 1985

*See the Practice section of the chapter references for complete citations.

Adults with myocardial infarction and other cardiac disease	Fawcett et al., 1987, 1992
	McInerney, 1982
	Ross & Bourbonnais, 1985
	Smith, 1989
A 19-year-old malr with a cerebral aneurysm	Fawcett et al., 1987
A 40-year-old man experiencing sleep deprivation following coronary artery bypass graft surgery	Kido, 1991
A 78-year-old man hospitalized for a cerebrovascular accident	Rice, 1982
A 77-year-old Cree Indian with gangrene	Baerg, 1991
Adults with acute and chronic phase spinal cord injuries	Foote et al., 1990
	Hoeman & Winters, 1990
	Sullivan, 1986
Adults with orthopedic problems	Shaw, 1991
A 75-year-old woman recovering from surgery for a hip fracture	Neal, 1982
An 85-year-old man hospitalized due to a hip fracture and transurethral prostatectomy	Cardona, 1982

Adults with Chronic Conditions

Clients seeking treatment for substance abuse	Waters, 1993
A 22-year-old pregnant woman with a history of substance abuse	Poole & Flowers, 1995
Adults with a chemical dependency	Mynatt & O'Brien, 1993
A 19-year-old male with cognitive impairment due to a head injury	Chiverton & Flannery, 1995
A 31-year-old pregnant woman with diabetes	Mirenda, 1986
Women with postpartum mood disorders	Fashinpaur, 2002
Clients with HIV disease	Mill, 1997; Miner, 1995
	Pierce & Hutton, 1992
Adults with colon cancer	Weinberger, 1991
Adults with chronic obstructive pulmonary disease	Baker, 1982; Hiltz, 1990
	Narsavage, 1997
Adults with kidney disease	Breckenridge, 1982, 1989
Adult females with irritable bowel syndrome	Gigliotti, 2002
A 22-year-old woman with multiple sclerosis	Knight, 1990
Adults with hypertension	Mayers & Watson, 1982;
	Utz, 1980
Adults with depression	Hassell, 1996
A 34-year-old woman with manic-depressive disorder	F. Clark, 1982
A woman with Down syndrome	Owens, 1995
A 47-year-old woman residing in a rehabilitation center following a cerebrovascular accident	Cunningham, 1983
Elderly clients residing in their own homes and requiring mental health nursing	Fawcett, 1997
	Moore & Munro, 1990
Hospice clients	Echlin, 1982
The 63-year-old wife of a man who had a cerebrovascular accident	Ross & Helmer, 1988
Primary caregivers of homebound clients	Russell et al., 1995

(continued)

▶ ⋘ **TABLE 7–4**
PUBLISHED REPORTS OF NURSING PRACTICE GUIDED BY THE NEUMAN SYSTEMS MODEL *(continued)*

Practice Situation	Population	Citation
	Assessment of Nutritional Status	
Family as the Client System	A 3-month-old infant	Torkington, 1988
	Individuals across the life span	Gavan et al., 1988
	Pregnant women and their fetuses	Trepanier et al., 1995
	Parents of infants in a neonatal intensive care unit	Ware & Shannahan, 1995
	A family with a 2-month-old infant	J. Clark, 1982
	A family requiring child and adolescent psychiatric nursing services	Herrick & Goodykoontz, 1989
	A middle-class suburban family requiring family therapy	Goldblum-Graff & Graff, 1982
	A Spanish-American family with a mentally ill member	Neuman, 1983
	Family of a neurologically impaired and dying child	Wallingford, 1989
	A family with a critically ill member admitted to an emergency department	Picton, 1995
	Families of critically ill clients	Bueno & Sengin, 1995
	A family with a member who had a cerebrovascular accident	Ross & Helmer, 1988
	An elderly couple residing in their own home; husband has Parkinson's disease	Millard, 1992
	Elderly families experiencing crisis	Beckingham & Baumann, 1990
	A family at risk for elder abuse	Delunas, 1990
Community as the Client System	A community	Anderson et al., 1986 Cookfair, 1996
	A city	Benedict & Sproles, 1982
	An aggregate of postnatal parents residing in a suburban community	Beddome, 1989
Nurse as the Client System	Nurses working in high-dependence (intensive-care) units	Biley, 1989
	nurses at risk for latex allergy	Cowperthwaite et al., 1997
APPLICATION OF THE NEUMAN SYSTEMS MODEL WITH AN INTERDISCIPLINARY TEAM		
	Older adults recovering from hip fracture	Kain, 2000

(Text continued from page 201)

physical therapy education in the context of accreditation evaluative criteria and tracking of instructional units in an existing curriculum. They indicated their intent to extend their efforts to curriculum development based on the model and commented, "Students, faculty, and practitioners will benefit in the utilization of [a] ... systems model not only to master content unique to physical therapy but also to understand the Gestalt of the provision of health care. Such knowledge is crucial as we come upon the crossroads of health care reform" (p. 245).

Moreover, Neuman and colleagues (1997) reported that the Neuman Systems Model has been "combined with a health policy analysis model to create a framework for health policy research for community-based health care" (p. 20). They went on to comment that that framework is being used to guide a survey of the similarities and differences among nursing, medicine, psychology, social work, dentistry, podiatry, optometry, osteopathy, and veterinary medicine. To date, no published reports of the results of the survey have been located.

The adoption of the Neuman Systems Model by other health-care disciplines is, however, a two-edged sword.

More specifically, the applicability of the model to all health-care disciplines can foster a common perspective, but in doing so, it may fail to point out the distinct contribution of nursing to health care.

The Neuman Systems Model is generally congruent with current societal expectations of nursing practice. The increased emphasis on primary prevention and health promotion seen in the news media and in numerous self-help books and articles is increasing consumers' awareness of the contributions of all health-care workers, including nurses, to the promotion of wellness and prevention of illness. As more nurses move into ambulatory care settings, their roles in primary prevention are becoming a typical expectation of consumers. Neuman (2002d) maintained that "Primary prevention as intervention with inherent health promotion is an expanding futuristic, proactive concept with which the nursing field must become increasingly concerned. It has unlimited potential for major role development that could shape the future image of nursing as world health care reform continues to evolve into the twenty-first century" (p. 29).

The Neuman Systems Model's emphasis on consideration of both the client's and the nurse's perception of stressors and resources and negotiation of nursing goals and prevention interventions between client and caregiver enhances its congruence with those members of society who desire input into nursing. Neuman and colleagues (1997) pointed out that the Neuman Systems Model's "emphasis on both the client's and the nurse's perceptions of stressors and negotiated outcome goals are consonant with current and projected health mandates" (p. 20). Later, Neuman (2002d) commented, "These characteristics follow current mandates within the health care system for client rights in health care issues" (p. 30). Paradoxically, however, the emphasis on client participation may limit the congruence of Neuman Systems Model-based practice with the expectations for nursing held by individuals whose personal or culturally derived beliefs lead to the lack of desire to play an active part in nursing.

Social Significance

Neuman and colleagues (1997) noted that "The future of the Neuman Systems Model looks bright. The holistic, comprehensive, and flexible nature of the [model] can readily accommodate such future changes in healthcare delivery as increased interdisciplinary collaboration and home care" (p. 20). Moreover, Neuman (2002b, 2002c) has maintained that use of the model may resolve cross-cultural differences and improve health care in the many countries where it has been successfully applied.

Considerable anecdotal evidence supporting the social significance of the Neuman Systems Model in nursing education, nursing administration, and nursing practice exists. The success of the Neuman Systems Model as a guide for nursing curricula is documented in several reports. For example, Mirenda (1986) commented, "The nursing faculty at Neumann College have reported their satisfaction with this systems approach to the curriculum and to client care, and nursing students have demonstrated both professional growth and personal maturity" (p. 148). Furthermore, Dale and Savala (1990), who described a collaborative demonstration project between the University of Wyoming and the Veterans Administration Medical Center in Cheyenne for a baccalaureate nursing program senior practicum, reported that the staff, who acted as preceptors, became more aware of documentation, holistic nursing care, and the rationale for nursing practice, and students gained confidence, became responsible and self-motivated, and became more proficient with time management and decision making. Cammuso and Wallen (2002) added that the Neuman Systems Model-based baccalaureate and master's degree education at Fitchburg State University "offers direction for truly collaborative practice that can create a better world for clients and health professionals alike" (p. 251). And, in her report of the implementation of a Neuman Systems Model-based at the Dutch Reformed University in Holland, de Kuiper (2002) concluded, "Success is evident at the present time—the students are happy, and the affiliated institutes are satisfied with the students' level of competence" (pp. 261–262). She also noted that since the implementation of the Neuman Systems Model-based curriculum, the Dutch Reformed University has been "on the top of the list [of the 19 nursing schools evaluated by a national Visitation Committee] for three consecutive years" (p. 262).

The success of the Neuman Systems Model as a guide for delivery of nursing services also is documented in several reports. For example, Beynon (1995) commented that the flexibility of the model readily accommodated the shifting emphasis in public health nursing in Canada from an individual-based to a population-based approach, with greater focus on "groups and aggregates and an acknowledged need for different strategies and modes of intervention … [including] community development, social marketing, and healthy public policy" (p. 543). Beynon (1995) went on to report that the Neuman Systems Model Assessment and Intervention Tool "is used effectively as a community development tool with focus groups to assist communities in identifying areas of concern and determining possible solutions" (p. 543). de Munck and Merks (2002) added that at Emergis Institute for Mental Health Care in Holland, the Neuman Systems Model "has served not only as a model for practice but also guided the design of the implementation and research projects" (p. 314).

And, Torakis (2002) explained that although the process of implementing the Neuman Systems Model at the Children's Hospital in Detroit, Michigan, "has been lengthy and often tiresome … the positive outcome is proof of a newly created healthy and stable professional environment" (p. 298). She went on to explain:

> The use of the Neuman Systems Model in a pediatric hospital setting has many benefits. The Neuman Systems Model systems perspective provides an ideal framework for working closely with families. Therefore, the unique needs of children and their families together can be assessed by nurses; the illness episode as well as the hospitalization may only partially represent the stressors experienced by the child and family. Through the use of the Neuman Systems Model, nursing staff have greatly improved their ability to recognize and wholistically assess and care for the entire client system while greatly increasing their professionalism (p. 298).

Nurses who have described the use of the Neuman Systems Model in practice generally have indicated their own satisfaction with the resultant nursing practice in terms of comprehensiveness. Millard (1992), for example, indicated that use of the model facilitated achievement of the primary health-care team's short- and medium-term objectives for an elderly couple. Knight's (1990) comment that the outcomes of a client- and nurse-negotiated plan of care were "found to be largely congruent with the expected outcomes" (p. 455) suggests that satisfaction with Neuman Systems Model-based nursing practice extends to the client.

Galloway (1993) offered an informative Neuman Systems Model-based self-analysis of her practice with a mentally and physically impaired infant. She stated:

> Through analyzing my role as a student nurse in a difficult clinical situation, I learned that I not only adapted well but also experienced personal growth. I did not avoid the reality of my situation; rather, I worked within the difficulties it presented. Understanding the importance of identifying and expressing emotions, I did not deny my positive and negative feelings. By using effective coping mechanisms and introducing alternative methods as necessary to deal with stressors, I achieved a positive result. Although my flexible line of defense contracted slightly due to the influence of specific negative variables, it buffered effectively so that my underlying normal line of defense was not penetrated (p. 36).

Crawford and Tarko (2002) collected and analyzed narratives from 20 Canadian psychiatric nurses, who explained how their practice changed as a result of using the Neuman Systems Model. They commented, "The Neuman Systems Model and its utility with client populations enables psychiatric nurses to provide comprehensive, wholistic psychiatric nursing care, working as an integral part of the interdisciplinary health-care team. The notion of advanced psychiatric nursing practice is realized when psychiatric nurses base their practice on a conceptual model of nursing" (p. 107). They reported that although the nurses' narratives indicated their understanding of most components of the Neuman Systems Model, they "struggle with such components as the created environment and the process of reconstitution" (p. 107). Nevertheless, Crawford and Tarko (2002) concluded that "Documentation from the literature and the nurses' narratives further supports the utility of the Neuman Systems Model for theory-based psychiatric nursing practice in Canada, to enhance and strengthen the mental health system and services to client systems" (p. 107).

Speaking of the success of the Neuman Systems Model as a guide to nursing practice in a changing health-care environment, Bueno and Sengin (1995) pointed out:

> The dramatically increased use of inpatient technology, compressed length of stay, and increasing demand for family-centered services will influence the delivery of nursing care. To facilitate this evolutionary health care system, a paradigm shift will be necessary to provide a comprehensive structure that guides and directs critical care nursing practice. The Neuman Systems Model provides a framework that will work extremely well (p. 290).

The empirical evidence related to the social significance of the Neuman Systems Model is mixed. In the realm of nursing education, Lowry and Newsome (1995) reported that a formal evaluation of the graduates of the associate degree program at Cecil Community College revealed that they "internalize the model concepts very well. Graduates use the model most of the time when fulfilling the roles of care provider and teacher" (p. 205). In the realm of nursing administration, Beynon (1995) reported that annual surveys of the staff of the Middlesex-London Health Unit Public Health Nursing Division, in Ontario, Canada, revealed increasing acceptance and use of the Neuman Systems Model "when assessing individuals, families, and groups; when formulating nursing diagnoses, expected outcomes, and nursing interventions; in recording; and in case consultations with supervisors" (p. 539).

In the realm of nursing research, the findings of some studies support the effectiveness of preventive interventions, but the results of other studies do not. Fawcett and Giangrade (2002) found that just 10 of 62 (16%) studies they included in their integrative review yielded statistically significant findings, whereas 7 (11%) of the studies yielded nonsignificant findings, and 19 (31%) yielded some statistically significant and some statistically nonsignificant findings. Statistical significance was not reported for 5 (8%) of the studies, and statistical significance was not relevant for 21 (34%) descriptive studies. In addition, more than one half ($n = 15$, 54%) of the 28 experimental studies they reviewed yielded some statistically significant and some statistically nonsignificant findings. Six (21%) of the 28 experimental studies yielded statistically significant findings, 4 (14%) yielded nonsignificant findings, and statistical significance was not reported for 3 (11%) of the experimental studies. Additional research clearly is warranted.

CONTRIBUTIONS TO THE DISCIPLINE OF NURSING

The Neuman Systems Model reflects nursing's interest in people as holistic systems, whether well or ill, and in environmental influences on health. The use of terms such as variances from wellness and primary prevention underscores the emphasis Neuman places on wellness. Furthermore, Neuman's clear emphasis on clients' perceptions of stressors and resources, and the central part that clients play in setting goals and identifying relevant prevention interventions, underscore the importance of the client system in the nursing situation.

The primary contribution of the Neuman Systems Model has been pragmatic, in that it is an exceptionally useful guide for nursing education and nursing practice in various settings in several countries. The model is readily translatable to other cultures and, therefore, has the potential to facilitate resolution of universal nursing concerns (Neuman, 2002c). Despite the large number of studies already conducted, programs of targeted Neuman Systems Model-based research are needed to determine the credibility of the model beyond pragmatic considerations.

Neuman's (2002d) words best summarize the overall contributions of the Neuman Systems Model. She stated:

> The Neuman Systems Model fits well with the wholistic concept of optimizing a dynamic yet stable interrelationship of spirit, mind, and body of the client in a constantly changing environment and society (Neuman & Young, 1972). The Neuman Systems Model has fulfilled the World Health organization mandate for the year 2000 and reaches far beyond, seeking unity in wellness states—wellness of spirit, mind, body, and environment. The Neuman Systems Model also is in accord with the views of the American Nursing Association, sharing its concern about potential stressors and its emphasis on primary prevention, as well as world health care reform concern for preventing illness (p. 32).

Neuman (2002f) explained that she ensured the continued evolution of her conceptual model through establishment of the Neuman Systems Model Trustees Group in 1988. Trustees and Group members from the United States and several other countries are committed to supporting and promoting the Neuman Systems Model through scholarly work and professional forums. Furthermore, the establishment of the Neuman Systems Model Archives at Neumann College in Aston, Pennsylvania, has facilitated access to important documents. And, the establishment of the Neuman Systems Model Institute (Gigliotti, 2003; Smith & Edgil, 1995) should enhance the continuation of Neuman Systems Model-based scholarly work for many years to come.

REFERENCES

Alligood, M.R. (2002). Philosophies, models, and theories: Critical thinking structures. In M.R. Alligood & A. Marriner-Tomey (Eds.), Nursing theory: Utilization and application (2nd ed., pp. 41–61). St. Louis: Mosby.

Ajzen, I. (1985). From intentions to actions: A theory of planned behavior. In J. Kuhland & J. Beckman (Eds.), Action-control: From cognitions to behavior (pp.11–39). Heidelberg, Germany: Springer.

Ajzen, I. (1991). The theory of planned behavior. Organizational Behavior and Human Decision Processes, 50, 179–211.

Amaya, M.A. (2002). The Neuman systems model and clinical practice: An integrative review, 1974–2000. In B. Neuman & J. Fawcett (Eds.), The Neuman systems model (4th ed., pp. 43–60). Upper Saddle River, NJ: Prentice Hall.

Barnum, B.J.S. (1998). Nursing theory: Analysis, application, evaluation (5th ed.). Philadelphia: Lippincott.

Beckstrand, J. (1980). A critique of several conceptions of practice theory in nursing. Research in Nursing and Health, 3, 69–79.

Beynon, C.E. (1995). Neuman-based experiences of the Middlesex-London health unit. In B. Neuman, The Neuman systems model (3rd ed., pp. 537–547). Norwalk, CT: Appleton & Lange.

Breckenridge, D.M. (1997). Decisions regarding dialysis treatment modality: A holistic perspective. Holistic Nursing Practice, 12(1), 54–61.

Breckenridge, D.M. (2002). Using the Neuman systems model to guide nursing research in the United States. In B. Neuman & J. Fawcett (Eds.), The Neuman systems model (4th ed., pp. 176–182). Upper Saddle River, NJ: Prentice Hall.

Bueno, M.M., & Sengin, K.K. (1995). The Neuman systems model for critical care nursing: A framework for practice. In B. Neuman, The Neuman systems model (3rd ed., pp. 275–291). Norwalk, CT: Appleton & Lange.

Cammuso, B.S., & Wallen, A.J. (2002). Using the Neuman systems model to guide nursing education in the United States. In B. Neuman & J. Fawcett (Eds.), The Neuman systems model (4th ed., pp. 244–253). Upper Saddle River, NJ: Prentice Hall.

Capers, C.F., O'Brien, C., Quinn, R., Kelly, R., & Fenerty, A. (1985). The Neuman systems model in practice. Planning phase. Journal of Nursing Administration, 15(5), 29–39.

Caplan, G. (1964). Principles of preventive psychiatry. New York: Basic Books.

Caramanica, L., & Thibodeau, J. (1987). Nursing philosophy and the selection of a model for practice. Nursing Management, 10(10), 71.

Carrigg, K.C., & Weber, R. (1997). Development of the spiritual care scale. Image: Journal of Nursing Scholarship, 29, 293.

Casalenuovo, G.A. (2002). Fatigue in diabetes mellitus: Testing a middle-range theory of well-being derived from the Neuman's theory of optimal client system stability and the Neuman systems model. Dissertation Abstracts International, 63, 2301B.

Collins, T.J. (2000). Adherence to hypertension management recommendations for patient follow-up care and lifestyle modifications made by military health care providers. Unpublished master's thesis, Uniformed Services University of the Health Sciences, Bethesda, Maryland.

Cornu, A. (1957). The origins of Marxian thought. Springfield, IL: Charles C Thomas.

Craig, D., & Beynon, C. (1996). Nursing administration and the Neuman systems model. In P. Hinton Walker & B. Neuman (Eds.), Blueprint for use of nursing models (pp. 251–274). New York: NLN Press.

Crawford, J.A., & Tarko, M.A. (2002). Using the Neuman systems model to guide nursing practice in Canada. In B. Neuman & J. Fawcett (Eds.), The Neuman systems model (4th ed., pp. 90–110). Upper Saddle River, NJ: Prentice Hall.

Dale, M.L., & Savala, S.M. (1990). A new approach to the senior practicum. Nursing Connections, 3(1), 45–51.

de Chardin, P.T. (1955). The phenomenon of man. London: Collins.

de Kuiper, M. (2002). Using the Neuman systems model to guide nursing education in Holland. In B. Neuman & J. Fawcett (Eds.), The Neuman systems model (4th ed., pp. 254–262). Upper Saddle River, NJ: Prentice Hall.

de Munck, R., & Merks, A. (2002). Using the Neuman systems model to guide administration of nursing services in Holland: The case of Emergis, Institute for Mental Health Care. In B. Neuman & J. Fawcett (Eds.), The Neuman systems model (4th ed., pp. 300–315). Upper Saddle River, NJ: Prentice Hall.

Doll, J. & Ajzen, I. (1992). Accessibility and stability of predictors in the theory of planned behavior. Journal of Personality and Social Psychology, 63, 754–765.

Edelson, M. (1970). Sociotherapy and psychotherapy. Chicago: University of Chicago Press.

Emery, F. (Ed.). (1969). Systems thinking. Baltimore: Penguin Books.

Fawcett, J. (1989). Analysis and evaluation of the Neuman systems model. In B. Neuman, The Neuman systems model (2nd ed., pp. 65–92). Norwalk, CT: Appleton & Lange.

Fawcett, J., Botter, M.L., Burritt, J., Crossley, J.D., & Fink, B.B. (1989) Conceptual models of nursing and organization theories. In B. Henry, M. DiVincenti, C. Arndt, & A. Marriner-Tomey (Eds.), Dimensions of nursing administration. Theory, research, education, and practice (pp. 143–154). Boston: Blackwell Scientific.

Fawcett, J., Carpenito, J.J., Efinger, J., Goldblum-Graff, D., Groesbeck, M.J.V., Lowry, L.W., McCreary, C.S., & Wolf, Z.R. (1982). A framework for analysis and evaluation of conceptual models of nursing with an analysis and evaluation of the Neuman systems model: In B. Neuman, The Neuman systems model: Application to nursing education and practice (pp. 30–43). Norwalk, CT: Appleton-Century-Crofts.

Fawcett, J., & Giangrande, S.K. (2001). Neuman systems-based research: An integrative review project. Nursing Science Quarterly, 14, 231–238.

Fawcett, J., & Giangrande, S.K. (2002). The Neuman systems model and research: An integrative review. In B. Neuman & J. Fawcett (Eds.), The Neuman systems model (4th ed., pp. 120–149). Upper Saddle River, NJ: Prentice Hall.

Freese, B.T., Neuman, B., & Fawcett, J. (2002). Guidelines for Neuman systems model-based clinical practice. In B. Neuman & J. Fawcett (Eds.), The Neuman systems model (4th ed., pp. 37–42). Upper Saddle River, NJ: Prentice Hall.

Galloway, D.A. (1993). Coping with a mentally and physically impaired infant: A self-analysis. Rehabilitation Nursing, 18, 34–36.

George, J.B. (2002). The Neuman systems model: Betty Neuman. In J.B. George (Ed.), Nursing theories: The base for professional nursing practice (5th ed., pp. 339–384). Upper Saddle River, NJ: Prentice Hall.

Gigliotti, E. (1997). Use of Neuman's lines of defense and resistance in nursing research: Conceptual and empirical considerations. Nursing Science Quarterly, 10, 136–143.

Gigliotti, E. (2001). Empirical tests of the Neuman systems model: Relational statement analysis. Nursing Science Quarterly, 14, 149–157.

Gigliotti, E. (2003). The Neuman Systems Model Institute: Testing middle-range theories. Nursing Science Quarterly, 16, 201–206.

Gigliotti, E., & Fawcett, J. (2002). The Neuman systems model and research instruments. In B. Neuman & J. Fawcett (Eds.), The Neuman systems model (4th ed., pp. 150–175). Upper Saddle River, NJ: Prentice Hall.

Grant, J.S., Kinney, M.R., & Davis, L.L. (1993). Using conceptual frameworks of models to guide nursing research. Journal of Neuroscience Nursing, 25, 52–56.

Heslin, K. (1986). A systems analysis of the Betty Neuman model. Unpublished student paper, University of Western Ontario, London, Ontario, Canada.

Hoffman, M.K. (1982). From model to theory construction: An analysis of the Neuman Health-Care systems model: In B. Neuman, The Neuman systems model: Application to nursing education and practice (pp. 44–54). Norwalk, CT: Appleton-Century-Crofts.

King, I.M. (1971). Toward a theory for nursing. New York: Wiley.

Knight, J.B. (1990). The Betty Neuman systems model applied to practice: A client with multiple sclerosis. Journal of Advanced Nursing, 15, 447–455.

Lamb, K.A. (1999). Baccalaureate nursing students' perception of empathy and stress in their interactions with clinical instructors: Testing a theory of optimal student system stability according to the Neuman systems model. Dissertation Abstracts International, 60, 1028B.

Latham, L. (2002). Letter to the Editor. Nursing Science Quarterly, 15, 264.

Lazarus, R. (1981). The stress and coping paradigm. In C. Eisdorfer, D. Cohen, A. Kleinman, & P. Maxim (Eds.), Models for clinical psychopathology (pp. 177–214). New York: SP Medical and Scientific Books.

Lazarus, R. (1999). Stress and emotion: A new synthesis. New York: Springer.

Louis, M. (1995). The Neuman model in nursing research: An update. In B. Neuman, The Neuman systems model (3rd ed., pp. 473–495). Norwalk, CT: Appleton & Lange.

Louis, M., & Koertvelyessy, A. (1989). The Neuman model in research. In B. Neuman, The Neuman systems model (2nd ed., pp. 93–114). Norwalk, CT: Appleton & Lange.

Louis, M., Neuman, B., & Fawcett, J. (2002). Guidelines for Neuman systems model-based nursing research. In B. Neuman & J. Fawcett (Eds.), The Neuman systems model (4th ed., pp. 113–119). Upper Saddle River, NJ: Prentice Hall.

Lowry, L. (Ed.). (1998). The Neuman systems model and nursing education: Teaching strategies and outcomes. Indianapolis: Sigma Theta Tau International Center Nursing Press.

Lowry, L.W. (2002). The Neuman systems model and education: An integrative review. In B. Neuman & J. Fawcett (Eds.), The Neuman systems model (4th ed., pp. 216–237). Upper Saddle River, NJ: Prentice Hall.

Lowry, L.W., & Anderson, B. (1993). Neuman's framework and ventilator dependency: A pilot study. Nursing Science Quarterly, 6, 195–200.

Lowry, L.W., & Newsome, G.G. (1995). Neuman-based associate degree programs: Past, present, and future. In B. Neuman, The Neuman systems model (3rd ed., pp. 197–214). Norwalk, CT: Appleton & Lange.

Mann, A.H., Hazel, C., Geer, C., Hurley, C.M., & Podrapovic, T. (1993). Development of an orthopaedic case manager role. Orthopaedic Nursing, 12(4), 23–27, 62.

Marriner-Tomey, A. (1989). Nursing theorists and their work (2nd ed.). St. Louis: Mosby.

Meleis, A.I. (1997). Theoretical nursing: Development and progress (3rd ed.). Philadelphia: Lippincott.

Millard, J. (1992). Health visiting an elderly couple. British Journal of Nursing, 1, 769–773.

Mirenda, R.M. (1986). The Neuman systems model: Description and application. In P. Winstead-Fry (Ed.), Case studies in nursing theory (pp. 127–166). New York: National League for Nursing.

Moynihan, M.M. (1990). Implementation of the Neuman systems model in an acute care nursing department. In M.E. Parker (Ed.), Nursing theories in practice (pp. 263–273). New York: National League for Nursing.

Neuman, B. (1974). The Betty Neuman health-care systems model: A total person approach to patient problems. In J.P. Riehl & C. Roy (Eds.), Conceptual models for nursing practice (pp. 99–114). New York: Appleton-Century-Crofts.

Neuman, B. (1980). The Betty Neuman Health-Care Systems Model: A total person approach to patient problems. In J.P. Riehl & C. Roy (Eds.), Conceptual models for nursing practice (2nd ed., pp. 119–134). New York: Appleton-Century-Crofts.

Neuman, B. (1982a). The Neuman health-care systems model: A total approach to client care. In B. Neuman, The Neuman systems model: Application to nursing education and practice (pp. 8–29). Norwalk, CT: Appleton-Century-Crofts.

Neuman, B. (1982b). The Neuman systems model. Application to nursing education and practice. Norwalk, CT: Appleton-Century-Crofts.

Neuman, B. (1983). Family intervention using the Betty Neuman health care systems model. In I.W. Clements & F.B. Roberts (Eds.), Family health: A theoretical approach to nursing care (pp. 239–254). New York: Wiley.

Neuman, B. (1985a, August). Betty Neuman. Paper presented at conference on Nursing Theory in Action, Edmonton, Alberta, Canada. [Audiotape.]

Neuman B. (1985b). The Neuman systems model. Senior Nurse, 5(3), 20–23.

Neuman, B. (1989a). In conclusion—In transition. In B. Neuman, The Neuman systems model (2nd ed., pp. 453–470). Norwalk, CT: Appleton & Lange.

Neuman, B. (1989b). The Neuman nursing process format: Family. In J.P. Riehl-Sisca (Ed.), Conceptual models for nursing practice (3rd ed., pp. 49–62). Norwalk, CT: Appleton & Lange.

Neuman, B. (1989c). The Neuman systems model (2nd ed.). Norwalk, CT: Appleton & Lange.

Neuman, B. (1989d). The Neuman systems model. In B. Neuman, The Neuman systems model (2nd ed., pp. 3–63). Norwalk, CT: Appleton & Lange.

Neuman, B. (1990a). Health as a continuum based on the Neuman systems model. Nursing Science Quarterly, 3, 129–135.

Neuman, B. (1990b). The Neuman systems model: A theory for practice. In M.E. Parker (Ed.), Nursing theories in practice (pp. 241–261). New York: National League for Nursing.

Neuman, B. (1995a). The Neuman systems model. In B. Neuman, The Neuman systems model (3rd ed., pp. 3–61). Norwalk, CT: Appleton & Lange.

Neuman, B. (1995b). The Neuman systems model (3rd ed.). Norwalk, CT: Appleton & Lange.

Neuman, B. (2002a). Assessment and intervention based on the Neuman systems model. In B. Neuman & J. Fawcett (Eds.), The Neuman systems model (4th ed., pp. 347–359). Upper Saddle River, NJ: Prentice Hall.

Neuman, B. (2002b). Betty Neuman's autobiography and chronology of the development and utilization of the Neuman systems model. In B. Neuman & J. Fawcett (Eds.), The Neuman systems model (4th ed., pp. 325–346). Upper Saddle River, NJ: Prentice Hall.

Neuman, B. (2002c). The future and the Neuman systems model. In B. Neuman & J. Fawcett (Eds.), The Neuman systems model (4th ed., pp. 319–321). Upper Saddle River, NJ: Prentice Hall.

Neuman, B. (2002d). The Neuman systems model. In B. Neuman & J. Fawcett (Eds.), The Neuman systems model (4th ed., pp. 3–33). Upper Saddle River, NJ: Prentice Hall.

Neuman, B. (2002e). The Neuman systems model: Definitions. In B. Neuman & J. Fawcett (Eds.), The Neuman systems model (4th ed., pp. 322–324). Upper Saddle River, NJ: Prentice Hall.

Neuman, B. (2002f). The Neuman Systems Model Trustees Group, Inc. In B. Neuman & J. Fawcett (Eds.), The Neuman Systems model (4th ed., pp. 360–363). Upper Saddle River, NJ: Prentice Hall.

Neuman, B. Chadwick, P.L., Beynon, C.E., Craig, D.M., Fawcett, J., Chang, N.J., Freese, B.T., & Hinton-Walker, P. (1997). The Neuman systems model: Reflections and projections. Nursing Science Quarterly, 10, 18–21.

Neuman, B., & Fawcett, J. (Eds.). (2002). The Neuman systems model (4th ed.). Upper Saddle River, NJ: Prentice-Hall.

Neuman, B., & Young, R.J. (1972). A model for teaching total person approach to patient problems. Nursing Research, 21, 264–269.

Newman, D.M.L., Neuman, B., & Fawcett, J. (2002). Guidelines for Neuman systems model-based education for the health professions. In B. Neuman & J. Fawcett (Eds.), The Neuman systems model (4th ed., pp. 193–215). Upper Saddle River, NJ: Prentice Hall.

Oakes, D.L. (1978). A critique of general systems theory. In A. Putt (Ed.), General systems theory applied to nursing. Boston: Little, Brown.

Orem, D. (1971). Nursing: Concepts of practice. New York: McGraw-Hill.

Peterson, C.J. (1977). Questions frequently asked about the development of a conceptual framework. Journal of Nursing Education, 16(4), 22–32.

Putt, A. (1972). Entropy, evolution and equifinality in nursing. In J. Smith (Ed.), Five years of cooperation to improve curricula in western schools of nursing. Boulder, CO: Western Interstate Commission for Higher Education.

Quayhagen, M.P., & Roth, P.A. (1989). From models to measures in assessment of mature families. Journal of Professional Nursing, 5, 144–151.

Reed, K.S. (2002). The Neuman systems model and educational tools. In B. Neuman & J. Fawcett (Eds.), The Neuman systems model (4th ed., pp. 238–243). Upper Saddle River, NJ: Prentice Hall.

Riehl, J.P., & Roy, C. (Eds.). (1974). Conceptual models for nursing practice. New York: Appleton-Century-Crofts.

Riehl, J.P., & Roy, C. (Eds.). (1980). Conceptual models for nursing practice (2nd ed.). New York: Appleton-Century-Crofts.

Riehl-Sisca, J.P. (Ed.). (1989). Conceptual models for nursing practice (3rd ed.). Norwalk, CT: Appleton & Lange.

Rogers, M.E. (1970). An introduction to the theoretical basis of nursing. Philadelphia: F.A. Davis.

Ross, M.M., Bourbonnais, F.F., & Carroll, G. (1987). Curricular design and the Betty Neuman systems model: A new approach to learning. International Nursing Review, 34, 75–79.

Russell, J. (2002). The Neuman systems model and clinical tools. In B. Neuman & J. Fawcett (Eds.), The Neuman systems model (4th ed., pp. 61–73). Upper Saddle River, NJ: Prentice Hall.

Sanders, N.F., & Kelley, J.A. (2002). The Neuman systems model and administration of nursing services: An integrative review. In B. Neuman & J. Fawcett (Eds.), The Neuman systems model (4th ed., pp. 271–287). Upper Saddle River, NJ: Prentice Hall.

Selye, H. (1950). The physiology and pathology of exposure to stress. Montreal: ACTA.

Shambaugh, B.F., Neuman, B., & Fawcett, J. (2002). Guidelines for Neuman systems model-based administration of health care services. In B. Neuman & J. Fawcett (Eds.), The Neuman systems model (4th ed., pp. 265–270). Upper Saddle River, NJ: Prentice Hall.

Simpson, E.M. (2000). Condom use among black women: A theoretical basis for HIV prevention guided by Neuman systems model and theory of planned behavior. Dissertation Abstracts International, 61, 5240B.

Smith, M.C., & Edgil, A.E. (1995). Future directions for research with the Neuman systems model. In B. Neuman, The Neuman systems model (3rd ed., pp. 509–517). Norwalk, CT: Appleton & Lange.

Stepans, M.B.F., & Knight, J.R. (2002). Application of Neuman's framework: Infant exposure to environmental tobacco smoke. Nursing Science Quarterly, 15, 327–334.

Stevens, B.J. (1982). Foreword. In B. Neuman, The Neuman systems model: Application to nursing education and practice (pp. xiii–xiv). Norwalk, CT: Appleton-Century-Crofts.

Toot, J.L., & Schmoll, B.J. (1995). The Neuman systems model and physical therapy educational curricula. In B. Neuman, The Neuman systems model (3rd ed., pp. 231–246). Norwalk, CT: Appleton & Lange.

Torakis, M.L. (2002). Using the Neuman systems model to guide administration of nursing services in the United States: Redirecting nursing practice in a freestanding pediatric hospital. In B. Neuman & J. Fawcett (Eds.), The Neuman systems model (4th ed., pp. 288–299). Upper Saddle River, NJ: Prentice Hall.

Villarruel, A.M., Bishop, T.L., Simpson, E.M., Jemmott, L.S., & Fawcett, J. (2001). Borrowed theories, shared theories, and the advancement of nursing knowledge. Nursing Science Quarterly, 14, 158–163.

von Bertalanffy, L. (1968). General system theory. New York: George Braziller.

Young, A., Taylor, S.G., & McLaughlin-Renpenning, K. (2001). Connections: Nursing research, theory, and practice. St. Louis: Mosby.

 RESEARCH

Ali, N.S., & Khalil, H.Z. (1989). Effect of psychoeducational intervention on anxiety among Egyptian bladder cancer patients. Cancer Nursing, 12, 236–242.

Andersen, J.E., & Briggs, L.L. (1988). Nursing diagnosis: A study of quality and supportive evidence. Image: Journal of Nursing Scholarship, 20, 141–144.

Barker, E., Robinson, D., & Brautigan, R. (1999). The effect of psychiatric home nurse follow-up on readmission rates of patients with depression. Journal of the American Psychiatric Nurses Association, 5, 111–116.

Bass, L.S. (1991). What do parents need when their infant is a patient in the NICU? Neonatal Network, 10(4), 25–33.

Beynon, C., & Laschinger, H.K. (1993). Theory-based practice: Attitudes of nursing managers before and after educational sessions. Public Health Nursing, 10, 183–188.

Blank, J.J., Clark, L., Longman, A.J., & Atwood, J.R. (1989). Perceived home care needs of cancer patients and their caregivers. Cancer Nursing, 12, 78–84.

Bowdler, J.E., & Barrell, L.M. (1987). Health needs of homeless persons. Public Health Nursing, 4, 135–140.

Bowman, A.M. (1997). Sleep satisfaction, perceived pain and acute confusion in elderly clients undergoing orthopaedic procedures. Journal of Advanced Nursing, 26, 550–564.

Breckenridge, D.M. (1997a). Decisions regarding dialysis treatment modality: A holistic perspective. Holistic Nursing Practice, 12(1), 54–61.

Breckenridge, D.M. (1997b). Patients' perception of why, how, and by whom dialysis treatment modality was chosen. Association of Nephrology Nurses Journal, 24, 313–321.

Breckenridge, D.M. (2002). Using the Neuman systems model to guide nursing research in the United States. In B. Neuman & J. Fawcett (Eds.), The Neuman systems model (4th ed., pp. 176–182). Upper Saddle River, NJ: Prentice Hall.

Brown, K.C., Sirles, A.T., Hilyer, J.C., & Thomas, M.J. (1992). Cost-effectiveness of a back school intervention for municipal employees. Spine, 17, 1224–1228.

Bueno, M.N., Redeker, N., & Norman, E.M. (1992). Analysis of motor vehicle crash data in an urban trauma center: Implications for nursing practice and research. Heart and Lung, 21, 558–567.

Burns-Vandenberg, J., & Jones, E. (1999). Evaluating postpartum home visits by student nurses. Journal for Undergraduate Nursing Scholarship, 1(1), 5 pp.

Butts, J.B. (2001). Outcomes of comfort touch in institutionalized elderly female residents. Geriatric Nursing, 22, 180–184.

Cantin, B., & Mitchell, M. (1989). Nurses' smoking behavior. The Canadian Nurse, 85(1), 20–21.

Capers, C.F. (1991). Nurses' and lay African Americans' views about behavior. Western Journal of Nursing Research, 13, 123–135.

Carroll, T.L. (1989). Role deprivation in baccalaureate nursing students pre and post curriculum revision. Journal of Nursing Education, 28, 134–139.

Cava, M.A. (1992). An examination of coping strategies used by long-term cancer survivors. Canadian Oncology Nursing Journal, 2, 99–102.

Chiverton, P., Tortoretti, D., LaForest, M., & Walker, P.H. (1999). Bridging the gap between psychiatric hospitalization and community care: Cost and quality outcomes. Journal of the American Psychiatric Association, 5, 46–53.

Clark, C.C., Cross, J.R., Deane, D.M., & Lowry, L.W. (1991). Spirituality: Integral to quality care. Holistic Nursing Practice, 5, 67–76.

Collins, M.A. (1996). The relation of work stress, hardiness, and burnout among full-time hospital staff nurses. Journal of Nursing Staff Development, 12, 81–85.

Courchene, V.S., Patalski, E., & Martin, J. (1991). A study of the health of pediatric nurses administering Cyclosporine A. Pediatric Nursing, 17, 497–500.

Decker, S.D., & Young, E. (1991). Self-perceived needs of primary caregivers of home-hospice clients. Journal of Community Health Nursing, 8, 147–154.

Denson, V.L., & Komnenich, P. (2002). Maternal serum screening: Women's experiences. Communicating Nursing Research, 35, 394.

Fields, W.L., & Loveridge, C. (1988). Critical thinking and fatigue: How do nurses on 8- and 12-hour shifts compare? Nursing Economics, 6, 189–191.

Flannery, J. (1995). Cognitive assessment in the acute care setting: Reliability and validity of the Levels of Cognitive Functioning Assessment Scale (LOCFAS). Journal of Nursing Measurement, 3, 43–58.

Fowler, B.A., & Risner, P.B. (1994). A health promotion program evaluation in a minority industry. Association of Black Nursing Faculty Journal, 5(3), 72–76.

Freiberger, D., Bryant, J., & Marino, B. (1992). The effects of different central venous line dressing changes on bacterial growth in a pediatric oncology population. Journal of Pediatric Oncology Nursing, 9, 3–7.

Gavigan, M., Kline-O'Sullivan, C., & Klumpp-Lybrand, B. (1990). The effect of regular turning on CABG patients. Critical Care Nursing Quarterly, 12(4), 69–76.

Gellner, P., Landers, S., O'Rourke, D., & Schlegel, M. (1994). Community health nursing in the 1990s: Risky business? Holistic Nursing Practice, 8(2), 15–21.

George, J. (1997). Nurses' perceived autonomy in a shared governance setting. Journal of Shared Governance, 3(2), 17–21.

Gerstle, D.S., & Wallace, D.C. (2001). Quality of life and chronic pain management. Pain Management Nursing, 2, 98–109.

Gifford, D.K. (1996). Monthly incidence of stroke in rural Kansas. Kansas Nurse, 71(5), 3–4.

Gigliotti, E. (1999). Women's multiple role stress: Testing Neuman's flexible line of defense. Nursing Science Quarterly, 12, 36–44.

Grant, J.S., & Bean, C.A. (1992). Self-identified needs of informal caregivers of head-injured adults. Family and Community Health, 15(2), 49–58.

Gries, M., & Fernsler, J. (1988). Patient perceptions of the mechanical ventilation experience. Focus on Critical Care, 15, 52–59.

Hainsworth, D.S. (1996). The effect of death education on attitudes of hospital nurses toward care of the dying. Oncology Nursing Forum, 23, 963–967.

Hanson, M.J.S. (1999). Cross-cultural study of beliefs about smoking among teenaged females. Western Journal of Nursing Research, 21, 635–651.

Heffline, M.S. (1991). A comparative study of pharmacological versus nursing interventions in the treatment of postanesthesia shivering. Journal of Post Anesthesia Nursing, 6, 311–320.

Hinds, C. (1990). Personal and contextual factors predicting patients' reported quality of life: Exploring congruency with Betty Neuman's assumptions. Journal of Advanced Nursing, 15, 456–462.

Hoch, C.C. (1987). Assessing delivery of nursing care. Journal of Gerontological Nursing, 13, 1–17.

Imamura, E. (2002). Amy's chat room: Health promotion programmes for community dwelling elderly adults. International Journal of Nursing Practice, 8, 61–64.

Johnson, P. (1983). Black hypertension: A transcultural case study using the Betty Neuman model of nursing care. Issues in Health Care of Women, 4, 191–210.

Jones, W.R. (1996). Stressors in the primary caregivers of traumatic head injured persons. AXON, 18, 9–11.

Kahn, E.C. (1992). A comparison of family needs based on the presence or absence of DNR orders. Dimensions of Critical Care Nursing, 11, 286–292. Schare, B.L. (1993). Commentary on "A comparison of family needs based on the presence or absence of DNR orders." Nursing Scan in Research, 6(2), 16.

Koku, R.V. (1992). Severity of low back pain: A comparison between participants who did and did not receive counseling. American Association of Occupational Health Nurses Journal, 40, 84–89.

Leja, A.M. (1989). Using guided imagery to combat postsurgical depression. Journal of Gerontological Nursing, 15(4), 6–11.

Leophonte, P., Delon, S., Dalbiès, S., Fontes-Carrère, M., Concalves de Carvalho, E., & Lepage, S. (2000). Effects of the preparation on axiety befoe bronchial fibrescopy. Recherche En Soins Infirmiers, March (60), 50–66. [English abstract]

Lin, M, Ku, N., Leu, J., Chen, J., & Lin, L. (1996). An exploration of the stress aspects, coping behaviors, health status and related aspects in family caregivers of hepatoma patients. Nursing Research (China), 4, 171–185. [Chinese, English abstract.]

Loescher, L.J., Clark, L., Atwood, J.R., Leigh, S., & Lamb, G. (1990). The impact of the cancer experience on long-term survivors. Oncology Nursing Forum, 17, 223–229.

Louis, M. (1989). An intervention to reduce anxiety levels for nursing working with long-term care clients using Neuman's model. In J.P. Riehl-Sisca (Ed.), Conceptual models for nursing practice (3rd ed., pp. 95–103). Norwalk, CT: Appleton & Lange.

Lowry, L.W., & Anderson, B. (1993). Neuman's framework and ventilator dependency: A pilot study. Nursing Science Quarterly, 6, 195–200.

Lowry, L.W., Callahan, A.L., & Phillippe, T. (2001). Using computer simulations and focus groups for planned change in prenatal clinics. Outcomes Management for Nursing Practice, 5, 134–139.

Lowry, L.W., Saeger, J., & Barnett, S. (1997). Client satisfaction with prenatal care and pregnancy outcomes. Outcomes Management for Nursing Practice, 1(1), 29–35.

Mackenzie, S.J., & Laschinger, H.K.S. (1995). Correlates of nursing diagnosis quality in public health nursing. Journal of Advanced Nursing, 21, 800–808.

Maligalig, R.M.L. (1994). Parents' perceptions of the stressors of pediatric ambulatory surgery. Journal of Post Anesthesia Nursing, 9, 278–282.

Mannina, J. (1997). Finding an effective hearing testing protocol to identify hearing loss and middle ear disease in school-aged children. Journal of School Nursing, 13(5), 23–28.

Marsh, V., Beard, M.T., & Adams, B.N. (1999). Job stress and burnout: The mediational effect of spiritual well-being and hardiness among nurses. Journal of Theory Construction and Testing, 3, 13–19.

May, K.M., & Hu, J. (2000). Caregiving and help seeking by mothers of low birthweight infants and mothers of normal birthweight infants. Public Health Nursing, 17, 273–279.

Molinari, D.L. (2001). Asynchronous online group decision making: A qualitative study. Communicating Nursing Research, 34(9), 318.

Montgomery, P., & Craig, D. (1990). Levels of stress and health practices of wives of alcoholics. Canadian Journal of Nursing Research, 22, 60–70.

Moody, N.B. (1996). Nurse faculty job satisfaction: A national survey, Journal of Professional Nursing, 12, 277–288.

Morrell, G. (2001). Effect of structured preoperative teaching on anxiety levels of patients scheduled for cataract surgery. Insight: The Journal of the American Society of Ophthalmic Registered Nurses, 26(1), 4–9.

Narsavage, G., & Romeo, E. (2003). Education and support needs of young and older cancer survivors. Applied Nursing Research, 16, 103–109.

Norrish, M.E., & Josste, K. (2001). Nursing care of the patient undergoing alcohol detoxification. Curationis: South African Journal of Nursing, 24(3), 36–48.

Nortridge, J.A., Mayeux, V., Anderson, S.J., & Bell, M.L. (1992). The use of cognitive style mapping as a predictor for academic success of first semester diploma nursing students. Journal of Nursing Education, 31, 352–356.

Nuttall, P., & Flores, F.C. (1997). Hmong healing practices used for common childhood illnesses. Pediatric Nursing, 23, 247–251.

Picot, S.J.F., Zauszniewski, J.A., Debanne, S.M., & Holston, E.C. (1999). Mood and blood pressure responses in Black female caregivers and noncaregivers. Nursing Research, 48, 150–161.

Pothiban, L. (2002). Using the Neuman systems model to guide nursing research in Thailand. In B. Neuman & J. Fawcett (Eds.), The Neuman systems model (4th ed., pp. 183–190). Upper Saddle River, NJ: Prentice Hall.

Potter, M.L., & Zauszniewski, J.A. (2000). Spirituality, resourcefulness, and arthritis impact on health perception of elders with rheumatoid arthritis. Journal of Holistic Nursing, 18, 311–336.

Purushotham, D., & Walker, G. (1994). The Neuman systems model: A conceptual framework for clinical teaching/learning process. In R.M. Carroll-Johnson & M. Paquette (Eds.),

Classification of nursing diagnoses: Proceedings of the Tenth Conference (pp. 271–273). Philadelphia: Lippincott.

Radwanski, M. (1992). Self-medicating practices for managing chronic pain after spinal cord injury. Rehabilitation Nursing, 17, 312–318.

Rodrigues-Fisher, L., Bourguignon, C., & Good, B.V. (1993). Dietary fiber nursing intervention: Prevention of constipation in older adults. Clinical Nursing Research, 2, 464–477.

Roggensack, J. (1994). The influence of perioperative theory and clinical in a baccalaureate nursing program on the decision to practice perioperative nursing. Prairie Rose, 63(2), 6–7.

Semple, O.D. (1995). The experiences of family members of persons with Huntington's Disease. Perspectives, 19(4), 4–10.

Sirles, A.T., Brown, K., & Hilyer, J.C. (1991). Effects of back school education and exercise in back injured municipal workers. American Association of Occupational Health Nursing Journal, 39, 7–12.

Skillen, D.L., Anderson, M.C., & Knight, C.L. (2001). The created environment for physical assessment by case managers. Western Journal of Nursing Research, 23, 72–89.

Skipwith, D.H. (1994). Telephone counseling interventions with caregivers of elders. Journal of Psychosocial Nursing and Mental Health Services, 32(3), 7–12, 34–35.

Smith, N.H., Timms, J., Parker, V.G., Reimels, E.M., & Hamlin, A. (2003). The impact of education on the use of physical restraints in the acute care setting. Journal of Continuing Education in Nursing, 34(1), 26–33, 46–47.

Speck, B.J. (1990). The effect of guided imagery upon first semester nursing students performing their first injections. Journal of Nursing Education, 29, 346–350.

Stepans, M.B.F., & Fuller, S.G. (1999). Physiological effects of infant exposure to environmental tobacco smoke: A passive observation study. Journal of Perinatal Nursing, 8, 10–21.

Vaughn, M., Cheatwood, S., Sirles, A.T., & Brown, K.C. (1989). The effect of progressive muscle relaxation on stress among clerical workers. American Association of Occupational Health Nurses Journal, 37, 302–306.

Vijaylakshmi, S., & Raman, A.V. (2002). Breastfeeding technique in prevention of nipple sore—A study. Nursing Journal of India, 93, 173–174.

Waddell, K.L., & Demi, A.S. (1993). Effectiveness of an intensive partial hospitalization program for treatment of anxiety disorders. Archives of Psychiatric Nursing, 7, 2–10.

Williamson, J.W. (1992). The effects of ocean sounds on sleep after coronary artery bypass graft surgery. American Journal of Critical Care, 1, 91–97.

Wilson, L.C. (2000). Implementation and evaluation of church-based health fairs. Journal of Community Health Nursing, 17, 39–48.

Wilson, V.S. (1987). Identification of stressors related to patients' psychological responses to the surgical intensive care unit. Heart and Lung, 16, 267–273.

Ziemer, M.M. (1983). Effects of information on postsurgical coping. Nursing Research, 32, 282–287.

RESEARCH INSTRUMENTS, PRACTICE TOOLS, AND EDUCATIONAL TOOLS

Baker, N.A. (1982). Use of the Neuman model in planning for the psychological needs of the respiratory disease patient. In B. Neuman, The Neuman systems model: Application to nursing education and practice (pp. 241–251). Norwalk, CT: Appleton-Century-Crofts.

Bass, L.S. (1991). What do parents need when their infant is a patient in the NICU? Neonatal Network, 10(4), 25–33.

Beckman, S.J., Boxley-Harges, S., Bruick-Sorge, C., & Eichenauer, J. (1998). Evaluation modalities for assessing student and program outcomes. In L. Lowry (Ed.), The Neuman systems model and nursing education: Teaching strategies and outcomes (pp. 149–160). Indianapolis: Sigma Theta Tau International Center Nursing Press.

Beddome, G. (1989). Application of the Neuman systems model to the assessment of community-as-client. In B. Neuman, The Neuman systems model (2nd ed., pp. 363–374). Norwalk, CT: Appleton & Lange.

Beddome, G. (1995). Community-as-client assessment: A Neuman-based guide for education and practice. In B. Neuman, The Neuman systems model (3rd ed., pp. 567–579). Norwalk, CT: Appleton & Lange.

Beitler, B., Tkachuck, B., & Aamodt, D. (1980). The Neuman model applied to mental health, community health, and medical-surgical nursing. In J.P. Riehl & C. Roy (Eds.), Conceptual models for nursing practice (2nd ed., pp. 170–178). New York: Appleton-Century-Crofts.

Benedict, M.B., & Sproles, J.B. (1982). Application of the Neuman model to public health nursing practice. In B. Neuman, The Neuman systems model: Application to nursing education and practice (pp. 223–240). Norwalk, CT: Appleton-Century-Crofts.

Blank, J.J., Clark, L., Longman, A.J., & Atwood, J.R. (1989). Perceived home care needs of cancer patients and their caregivers. Cancer Nursing, 12, 78–84.

Bowdler, J.E., & Barrell, L.M. (1987). Health needs of homeless persons. Public Health Nursing, 4, 135–140.

Bowman, G.E. (1982). The Neuman assessment tool adapted for child day-care centers. In B. Neuman, The Neuman systems model: Application to nursing education and practice (pp. 324–334). Norwalk, CT: Appleton-Century-Crofts.

Breckenridge, D.M. (1982). Adaptation of the Neuman systems model for the renal client. In B. Neuman, The Neuman systems model: Application to nursing education and practice (pp. 267–277). Norwalk, CT: Appleton-Century-Crofts.

Breckenridge, D.M. (1997a). Decisions regarding dialysis treatment modality: A holistic perspective. Holistic Nursing Practice, 12(1), 54–61.

Breckenridge, D.M. (1997b). Patients' perception of why, how, and by whom dialysis treatment modality was chosen. Association of Nephrology Nurses Journal, 24, 313–321.

Breckenridge, D.M., Cupit, M.C., & Raimondo, J.M. (1982,

January/February). Systematic nursing assessment tool for the CAPD client. Nephrology Nurse, 24, 26–27, 30–31.

Burke, M.E., Sr., Capers, C.F., O'Connell, R.K., Quinn, R.M., & Sinnott, M. (1989). Neuman-based nursing practice in a hospital setting. In B. Neuman, The Neuman systems model (2nd ed., pp. 423–444). Norwalk, CT: Appleton & Lange.

Cantin, B., & Mitchell, M. (1989). Nurses' smoking behavior. The Canadian Nurse, 85(1), 20–21.

Cardona, V.D. (1982). Client rehabilitation and the Neuman model. In B. Neuman, The Neuman systems model: Application to nursing education and practice (pp. 278–290). Norwalk, CT: Appleton-Century-Crofts.

Carrigg, K.C., & Weber, R. (1997). Development of the Spiritual Care Scale. Image: Journal of Nursing Scholarship, 29, 293.

Cava, M.A. (1992). An examination of coping strategies used by long-term cancer survivors. Canadian Oncology Nursing Journal, 2, 99–102.

Clark, C.C., Cross, J.R., Deane, D.M., & Lowry, L.W. (1991). Spirituality: Integral to quality care. Holistic Nursing Practice, 5, 67–76.

Clark, F. (1982). The Neuman systems model: A clinical application for psychiatric nurse practitioners. In B. Neuman, The Neuman systems model: Application to nursing education and practice (pp. 335–353). Norwalk, CT: Appleton-Century-Crofts.

Cotten, N.C. (1993). An interdisciplinary high risk assessment tool for rehabilitation inpatient falls. Master's Abstracts International, 31, 1732.

Cunningham, S.G. (1982). The Neuman model applied to an acute care setting: Pain. In B. Neuman, The Neuman systems model: Application to nursing education and practice (pp. 291–296). Norwalk, CT: Appleton-Century-Crofts.

Decker, S.D., & Young, E. (1991). Self-perceived needs of primary caregivers of home-hospice clients. Journal of Community Health Nursing, 8, 147–154.

Dunbar, S.B. (1982). Critical care and the Neuman model. In B. Neuman, The Neuman systems model: Application to nursing education and practice (pp. 297–307). Norwalk, CT: Appleton-Century-Crofts.

Dunn, S.I., & Trepanier, M.J. (1989). Application of the Neuman model to perinatal nursing. In B. Neuman, The Neuman systems model (2nd ed., pp. 407–422). Norwalk, CT: Appleton & Lange.

Felix, M., Hinds, C., Wolfe, S.C., & Martin, A. (1995). The Neuman systems model in a chronic care facility: A Canadian experience. In B. Neuman, The Neuman systems model (3rd ed., pp. 549–565). Norwalk, CT: Appleton & Lange.

Flannery, J. (1991). FAMLI-RESCUE: A family assessment tool for use by neuroscience nurses in the acute care setting. Journal of Neuroscience Nursing, 23, 111–115.

Fulbrook, P.R. (1991). The application of the Neuman systems model to intensive care. Intensive Care Nursing, 7, 28–39.

Gellner, P., Landers, S., O'Rourke, D., & Schlegel, M. (1994). Community health nursing in the 1990s: Risky business? Holistic Nursing Practice, 8(2), 15–21.

Gigliotti, E., & Fawcett, J. (2002). The Neuman systems model and

research instruments. In B. Neuman & J. Fawcett (Eds.), The Neuman systems model (4th ed., pp. 150–175). Upper Saddle River, NJ: Prentice Hall.

Grant, J.S., & Bean, C.A. (1992). Self-identified needs of informal caregivers of head-injured adults. Family and Community Health, 15(2), 49–58.

Gries, M., & Fernsler, J. (1988). Patient perceptions of the mechanical ventilation experience. Focus on Critical Care, 15, 52–59.

Gunter, L.M. (1982). Application of the Neuman systems model to gerontic nursing. In B. Neuman, The Neuman systems model: Application to nursing education and practice (pp. 196–210). Norwalk, CT: Appleton-Century-Crofts.

Hinton-Walker, P., & Raborn, M. (1989). Application of the Neuman model in nursing administration and practice. In B. Henry, C. Arndt, M. DiVincenti, & A. Marriner-Tomey (Eds.), Dimensions of nursing administration. Theory, research, education, and practice (pp. 711–723). Boston: Blackwell Scientific.

Hoch, C.C. (1987). Assessing delivery of nursing care. Journal of Gerontological Nursing, 13, 1–17.

Johnson, M.N., Vaughn-Wrobel, B., Ziegler, S., Hough, L., Bush, H.A., & Kurtz, P. (1982). Use of the Neuman Health-Care systems model in the master's curriculum: Texas Woman's University. In B. Neuman, The Neuman systems model: Application to nursing education and practice (pp. 130–152). Norwalk, CT: Appleton-Century-Crofts.

Johnson, P. (1983). Black hypertension: A transcultural case study using the Betty Neuman model of nursing care. Issues in Health Care of Women, 4, 191–210.

Kelley, J.A., & Sanders, N.F. (1995). A systems approach to the health of nursing and health care organizations. In B. Neuman, The Neuman systems model (3rd ed., pp. 347–364). Norwalk, CT: Appleton & Lange.

Kelley, J.A., Sanders, N.F., & Pierce, J.D. (1989). A systems approach to the role of the nurse administrator in education and practice. In B. Neuman, The Neuman systems model (2nd ed., pp. 115–138). Norwalk, CT: Appleton & Lange.

Loescher, L.J., Clark, L., Atwood, J.R., Leigh, S., & Lamb, G. (1990). The impact of the cancer experience on long-term survivors. Oncology Nursing Forum, 17, 223–229.

Lowry, L. (1998). Efficacy of the Neuman systems model as a curriculum framework: A longitudinal study. In L. Lowry (Ed.), The Neuman systems model and nursing education: Teaching strategies and outcomes (pp. 139–147). Indianapolis: Sigma Theta Tau International Center Nursing Press.

Lowry, L.W., & Jopp, M.C. (1989). An evaluation instrument for assessing an associate degree nursing curriculum based on the Neuman systems model. In J.P. Riehl-Sisca (Ed.), Conceptual models for nursing practice (3rd ed., pp. 73–85). Norwalk, CT: Appleton & Lange.

Lowry, L.W., & Newsome, G.G. (1995). Neuman-based associate degree programs: Past, present, and future. In B. Neuman, The Neuman systems model (3rd ed., pp. 197–214). Norwalk, CT: Appleton & Lange.

Maligalig, R.M.L. (1994). Parents' perceptions of the stressors of pediatric ambulatory surgery. Journal of Post Anesthesia Nursing, 9, 278–282.

McGee, M. (1995). Implications for use of the Neuman systems model in occupational health nursing. In B. Neuman, The Neuman systems model (3rd ed., pp. 657–667). Norwalk, CT: Appleton & Lange.

McHolm, F.A., & Geib, K.M. (1998). Application of the Neuman systems model to teaching health assessment and nursing process. Nursing Diagnosis: Journal of Nursing Language and Classification, 9, 23–33.

McInerney, K.A. (1982). The Neuman systems model applied to critical care nursing of cardiac surgery clients. In B. Neuman, The Neuman systems model: Application to nursing education and practice (pp. 308–315). Norwalk, CT: Appleton-Century-Crofts.

Mirenda, R.M. (1986). The Neuman model in practice. Senior Nurse, 5(3), 26–27.

Mischke-Berkey, K., & Hanson, S.M.H. (1991). Pocket guide to family assessment and intervention. St. Louis: Mosby.

Mischke-Berkey, K., Warner, P., & Hanson, S. (1989). Family health assessment and intervention. In P.J. Bomar (Ed.), Nurses and family health promotion: Concepts, assessment, and interventions (pp. 115–154). Baltimore: Williams & Wilkins.

Montgomery, P., & Craig, D. (1990). Levels of stress and health practices of wives of alcoholics. Canadian Journal of Nursing Research, 22, 60–70.

Murphy, N.G. (1990). Factors associated with breastfeeding success and failure: A systematic integrative review (Infant nutrition). Masters Abstracts International, 28, 275.

Neuman, B. (1989). The Neuman systems model. In B. Neuman, The Neuman systems model (2nd ed., pp. 3–63). Norwalk, CT: Appleton & Lange.

Neuman, B. (1995a). In conclusion—Toward new beginnings. In B. Neuman, The Neuman systems model (3rd ed., pp. 671–703). Norwalk, CT: Appleton & Lange.

Neuman, B. (1995b). The Neuman systems model. In B. Neuman, The Neuman systems model (3rd ed., pp. 3–61). Norwalk, CT: Appleton & Lange.

Neuman, B. (2002a). Assessment and intervention based on the Neuman systems model. In B. Neuman & J. Fawcett (Eds.), The Neuman systems model (4th ed., pp. 347–359). Upper Saddle River, NJ: Prentice Hall.

Reed, K. (1982). The Neuman systems model: A basis for family psychosocial assessment. In B. Neuman, The Neuman systems model: Application to nursing education and practice (pp. 188–195). Norwalk, CT: Appleton-Century-Crofts.

Reed, K.S. (2002). The Neuman systems model and educational tools. In B. Neuman & J. Fawcett (Eds.), The Neuman systems model (4th ed., pp. 238–243). Upper Saddle River, NJ: Prentice Hall.

Russell, J. (2002). The Neuman systems model and clinical tools. In B. Neuman & J. Fawcett (Eds.), The Neuman systems model (4th ed., pp. 61–73). Upper Saddle River, NJ: Prentice Hall.

Schlentz, M.D. (1993). The minimum data set and the levels of prevention in the long-term care facility. Geriatric Nursing, 14, 79–83.

Semple, O.D. (1995). The experiences of family members of persons with Huntington's Disease. Perspectives, 19(4), 4–10.

Skipwith, D.H. (1994). Telephone counseling interventions with caregivers of elders. Journal of Psychosocial Nursing and Mental Health Services, 32 (3), 7–12, 34–35.

Sohier, R. (2002). Neuman's systems model in nursing practice. In M.R. Alligood & A. Marriner-Tomey (Eds.), Nursing theory: Utilization and application (2nd ed., pp. 219–238). St. Louis: Mosby.

Stepans, M.B.F., & Fuller, S.G. (1999). Measuring infant exposure to environmental tobacco smoke. Clinical Nursing Research, 8, 198–221.

Stepans, M.B.F., & Knight, J.R. (2002). Application of Neuman's framework: Infant exposure to environmental tobacco smoke. Nursing Science Quarterly, 15, 327–334.

Strickland-Seng, V. (1995). The Neuman systems model in clinical evaluation of students. In B. Neuman, The Neuman systems model (3rd ed., pp. 215–225). Norwalk, CT: Appleton & Lange.

Strickland-Seng, V. (1998). Clinical evaluation: The heart of clinical performance. In L. Lowry (Ed.), The Neuman systems model and nursing education: Teaching strategies and outcomes (pp. 129–134). Indianapolis: Sigma Theta Tau International Center Nursing Press.

Tollett, S.M. (1982). Teaching geriatrics and gerontology: Use of the Neuman systems model. In B. Neuman, The Neuman systems model: Application to nursing education and practice (pp. 1159–1164). Norwalk, CT: Appleton-Century-Crofts.

Trepanier, M.J., Dunn, S.I., & Sprague, A.E. (1995). Application of the Neuman systems model to perinatal nursing. In B. Neuman, The Neuman systems model (3rd ed., pp. 309–320). Norwalk, CT: Appleton & Lange.

Wilson, V.S. (1987). Identification of stressors related to patients' psychological responses to the surgical intensive care unit. Heart and Lung, 16, 267–273.

Young, A., Taylor, S.G., & McLaughlin-Renpenning, K. (2001). Connections: Nursing research, theory, and practice. St. Louis: Mosby.

Ziegler, S.M. (1982). Taxonomy for nursing diagnosis derived from the Neuman systems model. In B. Neuman, The Neuman systems model: Application to nursing education and practice (pp. 55–68). Norwalk, CT: Appleton-Century-Crofts.

EDUCATION

Baker, N.A. (1982a). The Neuman systems model as a conceptual framework for continuing education in the work place. In B. Neuman, The Neuman systems model: Application to nursing education and practice (pp. 260–264). Norwalk, CT: Appleton-Century-Crofts.

Baker, N.A. (1982b). Use of the Neuman model in planning for the psychological needs of the respiratory disease patient. In B. Neuman, The Neuman systems model: Application to nursing education and practice (pp. 241–251). Norwalk, CT: Appleton-Century-Crofts.

Beckman, S.J., Boxley-Harges, S., Bruick-Sorge, C., & Eichenauer, J. (1998a). Critical thinking, the Neuman systems model, and associate degree education. In L. Lowry (Ed.), The Neuman systems model and nursing education: Teaching strategies and outcomes (pp. 53–58). Indianapolis: Sigma Theta Tau International Center Nursing Press.

Beckman, S.J., Boxley-Harges, S., Bruick-Sorge, C., & Eichenauer, J. (1998b). Evaluation modalities for assessing student and program outcomes. In L. Lowry (Ed.), The Neuman systems model and nursing education: Teaching strategies and outcomes (pp. 149–160). Indianapolis: Sigma Theta Tau International Center Nursing Press.

Beddome, G. (1995). Community-as-client assessment: A Neuman-based guide for education and practice. In B. Neuman, The Neuman systems model (3rd ed., pp. 567–579). Norwalk, CT: Appleton & Lange.

Beitler, B., Tkachuck, B., & Aamodt, D. (1980). The Neuman model applied to mental health, community health, and medical-surgical nursing. In J.P. Riehl & C. Roy (Eds.), Conceptual models for nursing practice (2nd ed., pp. 170–178). New York: Appleton-Century-Crofts.

Beyea, S., & Matzo, M. (1989). Assessing elders using the functional health pattern assessment model. Nurse Educator, 14(5), 32–37.

Bloch, C., & Bloch, C. (1995). Teaching content and process of the Neuman systems model. In B. Neuman, The Neuman systems model (3rd ed., pp. 175–182). Norwalk, CT: Appleton & Lange.

Bourbonnais, F.F., & Ross, M.M. (1985). The Neuman systems model in nursing education: Course development and implementation. Journal of Advanced Nursing, 10, 117–123.

Bruton, M.R., & Matzo, M. (1989). Curriculum revisions at Saint Anselm College: Focus on the older adult. In B. Neuman, The Neuman systems model (2nd ed., pp. 201–210). Norwalk, CT: Appleton & Lange.

Busch, P., & Lynch, M.H. (1998). Creative teaching strategies in a Neuman-based baccalaureate curriculum. In L. Lowry (Ed.), The Neuman systems model and nursing education: Teaching strategies and outcomes (pp. 59–69). Indianapolis: Sigma Theta Tau International Center Nursing Press.

Cammuso, B.S., & Wallen, A.J. (2002). Using the Neuman systems model to guide nursing education in the United States. In B. Neuman & J. Fawcett (Eds.), The Neuman systems model (4th ed., pp. 244–253). Upper Saddle River, NJ: Prentice Hall.

Capers, C.F. (1986). Some basic facts about models, nursing conceptualizations, and nursing theories. Journal of Continuing Education, 16, 149–154.

Conners, V., Harmon, V.M., & Langford, R.W. (1982). Course development and implementation using the Neuman systems model as a framework: Texas Woman's University (Houston Campus). In B. Neuman, The Neuman systems model: Application to nursing education and practice (pp. 153–158). Norwalk, CT: Appleton-Century-Crofts.

Conners, V.L. (1982). Teaching the Neuman systems model: An approach to student and faculty development. In B. Neuman, The Neuman systems model: Application to nursing education and practice (pp. 176–181). Norwalk, CT: Appleton-Century-Crofts.

Conners, V.L. (1989). An empirical evaluation of the Neuman systems model: The University of Missouri–Kansas City. In B. Neuman, The Neuman systems model (2nd ed., pp. 249–258). Norwalk, CT: Appleton & Lange.

Craig, D.M. (1995). The Neuman model: Examples of its use in Canadian educational programs. In B. Neuman, The Neuman systems model (3rd ed., pp. 521–527). Norwalk, CT: Appleton & Lange.

Dale, M.L., & Savala, S.M. (1990). A new approach to the senior practicum. NursingConnections, 3(1), 45–51.

de Kuiper, M. (2002). Using the Neuman systems model to guide nursing education in Holland. In B. Neuman & J. Fawcett (Eds.), The Neuman systems model (4th ed., pp. 254–262). Upper Saddle River, NJ: Prentice Hall.

Dyck, S.M., Innes, J.E., Rae, D.I., & Sawatzky, J.E. (1989). The Neuman systems model in curriculum revision: A baccalaureate program, University of Saskatchewan. In B. Neuman, The Neuman systems model (2nd ed., pp. 225–236). Norwalk, CT: Appleton & Lange.

Edwards, P.A., & Kittler, A.W. (1991). Integrating rehabilitation content in nursing curricula. Rehabilitation Nursing, 16, 70–73.

Engberg, I.B. (1995). Brief abstracts: Use of the Neuman systems model in Sweden. In B. Neuman, The Neuman systems model (3rd ed., pp. 653–656). Norwalk, CT: Appleton & Lange.

Engberg, I.B., Bjalming, E., & Bertilson, B. (1995). A structure for documenting primary health care in Sweden using the Neuman systems model. In B. Neuman, The Neuman systems model (3rd ed., pp. 637–651). Norwalk, CT: Appleton & Lange.

Evans, B. (1998). Fourth-generation evaluation and the Neuman systems model. In L. Lowry (Ed.), The Neuman systems model and nursing education: Teaching strategies and outcomes (pp. 117–127). Indianapolis: Sigma Theta Tau International Center Nursing Press.

Freiburger, O.A. (1998). The Neuman systems model, critical thinking, and cooperative learning in a nursing issues course. In L. Lowry (Ed.), The Neuman systems model and nursing education: Teaching strategies and outcomes (pp. 79–84). Indianapolis: Sigma Theta Tau International Center Nursing Press.

Glazebrook, R.S. (1995). The Neuman systems model in cooperative baccalaureate nursing education: The Minnesota Intercollegiate Nursing Consortium experience. In B. Neuman, The Neuman systems model (3rd ed., pp. 227–230). Norwalk, CT: Appleton & Lange.

Gunter, L.M. (1982). Application of the Neuman systems model to gerontic nursing. In B. Neuman, The Neuman systems model: Application to nursing education and practice (pp. 196–210). Norwalk, CT: Appleton-Century-Crofts.

Harty, M.B. (1982). Continuing education in nursing and the Neuman model. In B. Neuman. The Neuman systems model: Application to nursing education and practice (pp. 100–106). Norwalk, CT: Appleton-Century-Crofts.

Hassell, J.S. (1998). Critical thinking strategies for family and community client systems. In L. Lowry (Ed.), The Neuman systems model and nursing education: Teaching strategies and outcomes (pp. 71–77). Indianapolis: Sigma Theta Tau International Center Nursing Press.

Hilton, S.A., & Grafton, M.D. (1995). Curriculum transition based on the Neuman systems model: Los Angeles County Medical Center School of Nursing. In B. Neuman, The Neuman systems model (3rd ed., pp. 163–174). Norwalk, CT: Appleton & Lange.

Johansen, H. (1989). Neuman model concepts in joint use—Community health practice and student teaching—School of Advanced Nursing Education, Aarhus University, Aarhus, Denmark. In B. Neuman, The Neuman systems model (2nd ed., pp. 334–362). Norwalk, CT: Appleton & Lange.

Johnson, M.N., Vaughn-Wrobel, B., Ziegler, S., Hough, L., Bush, H.A., & Kurtz, P. (1982). Use of the Neuman Health-Care systems model in the master's curriculum: Texas Woman's University. In B. Neuman, The Neuman systems model: Application to nursing education and practice (pp. 130–152). Norwalk, CT: Appleton-Century-Crofts.

Johnson, S.E. (1989). A picture is worth a thousand words: Helping students visualize a conceptual model. Nurse Educator, 14(3), 21–24.

Kilchenstein, L., & Yakulis, I. (1984). The birth of a curriculum: Utilization of the Betty Neuman health care systems model in an integrated baccalaureate program. Journal of Nursing Education, 23, 126–127.

Klotz, L.C. (1995). Integration of the Neuman systems model into the BSN curriculum at the University of Texas at Tyler. In B. Neuman, The Neuman systems model (3rd ed., pp. 183–195). Norwalk, CT: Appleton & Lange.

Knox, J.E., Kilchenstein, L., & Yakulis, I.M. (1982). Utilization of the Neuman model in an integrated baccalaureate program: University of Pittsburgh. In B. Neuman, The Neuman systems model: Application to nursing education and practice (pp. 117–123). Norwalk, CT: Appleton-Century-Crofts.

Laschinger, S.J., Maloney, R., & Tranmer, J.E. (1989). An evaluation of student use of the Neuman systems model: Queen's University, Canada. In B. Neuman, The Neuman systems model (2nd ed., pp. 211–224). Norwalk, CT: Appleton & Lange.

Lebold, M., & Davis, L. (1980). A baccalaureate nursing curriculum based on the Neuman health systems model. In. J.P. Riehl & C. Roy (Eds.), Conceptual models for nursing practice (2nd ed., pp 151–158). New York: Appleton-Century-Crofts.

Lebold, M.M., & Davis, L.H. (1982). A baccalaureate nursing curriculum based on the Neuman systems model: Saint Xavier College. In B. Neuman, The Neuman systems model: Application to nursing education and practice (pp. 124–129). Norwalk, CT: Appleton-Century-Crofts.

Louis, M., Witt, R., & LaMancusa, M. (1989). The Neuman systems model in multilevel nurse education programs: University of Nevada, Las Vegas. In B. Neuman, The Neuman systems model (2nd ed., pp. 237–248). Norwalk, CT: Appleton & Lange.

Lowry, L. (1986). Adapted by degrees. Senior Nurse, 5(3), 25–26.

Lowry, L. (1988). Operationalizing the Neuman systems model: A course in concepts and process. Nurse Educator, 13(3), 19–22.

Lowry, L. (1998). Efficacy of the Neuman systems model as a curriculum framework: A longitudinal study. In L. Lowry (Ed.), The Neuman systems model and nursing education: Teaching strategies and outcomes (pp. 139–147). Indianapolis: Sigma Theta Tau International Center Nursing Press.

Lowry, L.W. (2002). The Neuman systems model and education: An integrative review. In B. Neuman & J. Fawcett (Eds.), The Neuman systems model (4th ed., pp. 216–237). Upper Saddle River, NJ: Prentice Hall.

Lowry, L., & Green, G.H. (1989). Four Neuman—ased associate degree programs: Brief description and evaluation. In B. Neuman, The Neuman systems model (2nd ed., pp. 283–312). Norwalk, CT: Appleton & Lange.

Lowry, L.W., & Jopp, M.C. (1989). An evaluation instrument for assessing an associate degree nursing curriculum based on the Neuman systems model. In J.P. Riehl-Sisca (Ed.), Conceptual models for nursing practice (3rd ed., pp. 73–85). Norwalk, CT: Appleton & Lange.

Lowry, L.W., & Newsome, G.G. (1995). Neuman-based associate degree programs: Past, present, and future. In B. Neuman, The Neuman systems model (3rd ed., pp. 197–214). Norwalk, CT: Appleton & Lange.

McCulloch, S.J. (1995). Utilization of the Neuman systems model: University of South Australia. In B. Neuman, The Neuman systems model (3rd ed., pp. 591–597). Norwalk, CT: Appleton & Lange.

Mirenda, R.M. (1986). The Neuman systems model: Description and application. In P. Winstead-Fry (Ed.), Case studies in nursing theory (pp. 127–166). New York: National League for Nursing.

Moxley, P.A., & Allen, L.M.H. (1982). The Neuman systems model approach in a master's degree program: Northwestern State University. In B. Neuman, The Neuman systems model: Application to nursing education and practice (pp. 168–175). Norwalk, CT: Appleton-Century-Crofts.

Mrkonich, D., Miller, M., & Hessian, M. (1989). Cooperative baccalaureate education: The Minnesota intercollegiate nursing consortium. In B. Neuman, The Neuman systems model (2nd ed., pp. 175–182). Norwalk, CT: Appleton & Lange.

Mrkonich, D.E., Hessian, M., & Miller, M.W. (1989). A cooperative process in curriculum development using the Neuman health-are systems model. In J.P. Riehl-Sisca (Ed.), Conceptual models for nursing practice (3rd ed., pp. 87–94). Norwalk, CT: Appleton & Lange.

Nelson, L.F., Hansen, M., & McCullagh, M. (1989). A new baccalaureate North Dakota-Minnesota nursing education consortium. In B. Neuman, The Neuman systems model (2nd ed., pp. 183–192). Norwalk, CT: Appleton & Lange.

Neuman, B. (1995). In conclusion—Toward new beginnings. In B. Neuman, The Neuman systems model (3rd ed., pp. 671–703). Norwalk, CT: Appleton & Lange.

Neuman, B., & Wyatt, M. (1980). The Neuman Stress/Adaptation systems approach to education for nurse administrators. In J.P. Riehl & C. Roy (Eds.), Conceptual models for nursing practice (2nd ed., pp. 142–150). New York: Appleton-Century-Crofts.

Nichols, E.G., Dale, M.L., & Turley, J. (1989). The University of Wyoming evaluation of a Neuman—ased curriculum. In B. Neuman, The Neuman systems model (2nd ed., pp. 259–282). Norwalk, CT: Appleton & Lange.

Nuttall, P., Stittich, E.M., & Flores, F.C. (1998). The Neuman systems model in advanced practice nursing. In L. Lowry (Ed.), The Neuman systems model and nursing education: Teaching strategies and outcomes (pp. 109–114). Indianapolis: Sigma Theta Tau International Center Nursing Press.

Peternelj-Taylor, C.A., & Johnson, R. (1996). Custody and caring: Clinical placement of student nurses in a forensic setting. Perspectives in Psychiatric Care, 32(4), 23–29.

Reed-Sorrow, K., Harmon, R.L., & Kitundu, M.E. (1989). Computer-assisted learning and the Neuman systems model. In B. Neuman, The Neuman systems model (2nd ed., pp. 155–160). Norwalk, CT: Appleton & Lange.

Roberts, A.G. (1994). Effective inservice education process. Oklahoma Nurse, 39(4), 11.

Ross, M.M., Bourbonnais, F.F., & Carroll, G. (1987). Curricular design and the Betty Neuman systems model: A new approach to learning. International Nursing Review, 34, 75–79.

Sipple, J.A., & Freese, B.T. (1989). Transition from technical to professional-level nursing education. In B. Neuman, The Neuman systems model (2nd ed., pp. 193–200). Norwalk, CT: Appleton & Lange.

Stittich, E.M., Avent, C.L., & Patterson, K. (1989). Neuman-based baccalaureate and graduate nursing programs, California State University, Fresno. In B. Neuman, The Neuman systems model (2nd ed., pp. 163–174). Norwalk, CT: Appleton & Lange.

Stittich, E.M., Flores, F.C., & Nuttall, P. (1995). Cultural considerations in a Neuman-based curriculum. In B. Neuman, The Neuman systems model (3rd ed., pp. 147–162). Norwalk, CT: Appleton & Lange.

Story, E.L., & DuGas, B.W. (1988). A teaching strategy to facilitate conceptual model implementation in practice. Journal of Continuing Education in Nursing, 19, 244–247.

Story, E.L., & Ross, M.M. (1986). Family centered community health nursing and the Betty Neuman systems model. Nursing Papers, 18(2), 77–88.

Strickland-Seng, V. (1995). The Neuman systems model in clinical evaluation of students. In B. Neuman, The Neuman systems model (3rd ed., pp. 215–225). Norwalk, CT: Appleton & Lange.

Strickland-Seng, V. (1998). Clinical evaluation: The heart of clinical performance. In L. Lowry (Ed.), The Neuman systems model and nursing education: Teaching strategies and outcomes (pp. 129–134). Indianapolis: Sigma Theta Tau International Center Nursing Press.

Strickland-Seng, V., Mirenda, R., & Lowry, L.W. (1996). The Neuman systems model in nursing education. In P. Hinton Walker & B. Neuman (Eds.), Blueprint for use of nursing models (pp. 91–140). New York: NLN Press.

Sutherland, R., & Forrest, D.L. (1998). Primary prevention in an associate of science curriculum. In L. Lowry (Ed.), The Neuman systems model and nursing education: Teaching strategies and outcomes (pp. 99–108). Indianapolis: Sigma Theta Tau International Center Nursing Press.

Tollett, S.M. (1982). Teaching geriatrics and gerontology: use of the Neuman systems model. In B. Neuman, The Neuman systems model: Application to nursing education and practice (pp. 1159–1164). Norwalk, CT: Appleton-Century-Crofts.

Vaughan, B., & Gough, P. (1995). Use of the Neuman systems model in England: Abstracts. In B. Neuman, The Neuman systems model (3rd ed., pp. 599–605). Norwalk, CT: Appleton & Lange.

Weitzel, A., & Wood, K. (1998). Community health nursing: Keystone of baccalaureate education. In L. Lowry (Ed.), The Neuman systems model and nursing education: Teaching strategies and outcomes (pp. 91–98). Indianapolis: Sigma Theta Tau International Center Nursing Press.

ADMINISTRATION

Beynon, C.E. (1995). Neuman-based experiences of the Middlesex-London health unit. In B. Neuman, The Neuman systems model (3rd ed., pp. 537–547). Norwalk, CT: Appleton & Lange.

Caramanica, L., & Thibodeau, J. (1987). Nursing philosophy and the selection of a model for practice. Nursing Management, 10(10), 71.

Caramanica, L., & Thibodeau, J. (1989). Developing a hospital nursing philosophy and selecting a model for practice. In B. Neuman, The Neuman systems model (2nd ed., pp. 441–443). Norwalk, CT: Appleton & Lange.

Craig, D., & Beynon, C. (1996). Nursing administration and the Neuman systems model. In P. Hinton Walker & B. Neuman (Eds.), Blueprint for use of nursing models (pp. 251–274). New York: NLN Press.

Craig, D.M. (1995). Community/public health nursing in Canada: Use of the Neuman systems model in a new paradigm. In

B. Neuman, The Neuman systems model (3rd ed., pp. 529–535). Norwalk, CT: Appleton & Lange.

Craig, D.M., & Morris-Coulter, C. (1995). Neuman implementation in a Canadian psychiatric facility. In B. Neuman, The Neuman systems model (3rd ed., pp. 397–406). Norwalk, CT: Appleton & Lange.

Davies, P. (1989). In Wales: Use of the Neuman systems model by community psychiatric nurses. In B. Neuman, The Neuman systems model (2nd ed., pp. 375–384). Norwalk, CT: Appleton & Lange.

Davies, P., & Proctor, H. (1995). In Wales: Using the model in community mental health nursing. In B. Neuman, The Neuman systems model (3rd ed., pp. 621–627). Norwalk, CT: Appleton & Lange.

de Munck, R., & Merks, A. (2002). Using the Neuman systems model to guide administration of nursing services in Holland: The case of Emergis, Institute for Mental Health Care. In B. Neuman & J. Fawcett (Eds.), The Neuman systems model (4th ed., pp. 300–315). Upper Saddle River, NJ: Prentice Hall.

Drew, L.L., Craig, D.M., & Beynon, C.E. (1989). The Neuman systems model for community health administration and practice: Provinces of Manitoba and Ontario, Canada. In B. Neuman, The Neuman systems model (2nd ed., pp. 315–342). Norwalk, CT: Appleton & Lange.

Dunn, S.I., & Trepanier, M.J. (1989). Application of the Neuman model to perinatal nursing. In B. Neuman, The Neuman systems model (2nd ed., pp. 407–422). Norwalk, CT: Appleton & Lange.

Dwyer, C.M., Walker, P.H., Suchman, A., & Coggiola, P. (1995). Opportunities and obstacles: Development of a true collaborative practice with physicians. In B. Murphy (Ed.), Nursing centers: The time is now (pp. 135–155). New York: National League for Nursing.

Echlin, D.J. (1982). Palliative care and the Neuman model. In B. Neuman, The Neuman systems model: Application to nursing education and practice (pp. 257–259). Norwalk, CT: Appleton-Century-Crofts.

Engberg, I.B. (1995). Brief abstracts: Use of the Neuman systems model in Sweden. In B. Neuman, The Neuman systems model (3rd ed., pp. 653–656). Norwalk, CT: Appleton & Lange.

Felix, M., Hinds, C., Wolfe, S.C., & Martin, A. (1995). The Neuman systems model in a chronic care facility: A Canadian experience. In B. Neuman, The Neuman systems model (3rd ed., pp. 549–565). Norwalk, CT: Appleton & Lange.

Hinton Walker, P., & Raborn, M. (1989). Application of the Neuman model in nursing administration and practice. In B. Henry, C. Arndt, M. DiVincenti, & A. Marriner-Tomey (Eds.), Dimensions of nursing administration. Theory, research, education, and practice (pp. 711–723). Boston: Blackwell Scientific.

Johns, C. (1991). The Burford Nursing Development Unit holistic model of nursing practice. Journal of Advanced Nursing, 16, 1090–1098.

Kenyon, E., & Barnett, N. (2001). Partnership in nursing care (PINC): The Blackburn model. Journal of Child Health Care, 5, 35–38.

Moynihan, M.M. (1990). Implementation of the Neuman systems model in an acute care nursing department. In M.E. Parker (Ed.), Nursing theories in practice (pp. 263–273). New York: National League for Nursing.

Mytka, S., & Beynon, C. (1994). A model for public health nursing in the Middlesex-London, Ontario, schools. Journal of School Health, 64, 85–88.

Neuman, B. (1995). In conclusion—Toward new beginnings. In B. Neuman, The Neuman systems model (3rd ed., pp. 671–703). Norwalk, CT: Appleton & Lange.

Pinkerton, A. (1974). Use of the Neuman model in a home health-care agency. In J.P. Riehl & C. Roy (Eds.), Conceptual models for nursing practice (pp. 122–129). New York: Appleton-Century-Crofts.

Reitano, J.K. (1997). Learning through experience—Chester Community Nursing Center: A Healthy Partnership. Accent Magazine [Neumann College], Fall, 11.

Roberts, A.G. (1994). Effective inservice education process. Oklahoma Nurse, 39(4), 11.

Rodriguez, M.L. (1995). The Neuman systems model adapted to a continuing care retirement community. In B. Neuman, The Neuman systems model (3rd ed., pp. 431–442). Norwalk, CT: Appleton & Lange.

Schlentz, M.D. (1993). The minimum data set and the levels of prevention in the long-term care facility. Geriatric Nursing, 14, 79–83.

Scicchitani, B., Cox, J.G., Heyduk, L.J., Maglicco, P.A., & Sargent, N.A. (1995). Implementing the Neuman model in a psychiatric hospital. In B. Neuman, The Neuman systems model (3rd ed., pp. 387–395). Norwalk, CT: Appleton & Lange.

Torakis, M.L. (2002). Using the Neuman systems model to guide administration of nursing services in the United States: Redirecting nursing practice in a freestanding pediatric hospital. In B. Neuman & J. Fawcett (Eds.), The Neuman systems model (4th ed., pp. 288–299). Upper Saddle River, NJ: Prentice Hall.

Torakis, M.L., & Smigielski, C.M. (2000). Documentation of model-based practice: One hospital's experience. Pediatric Nursing, 26, 394–399.

Verberk, F. (1995). In Holland: Application of the Neuman model in psychiatric nursing. In B. Neuman, The Neuman systems model (3rd ed., pp. 629–636). Norwalk, CT: Appleton & Lange.

PRACTICE

Anderson, E., McFarlane, J., & Helton, A. (1986). Community-as-Client: A model for practice. Nursing Outlook, 34, 220–224.

Baerg, K. L. (1991). Using Neuman's model to analyze a clinical situation. Rehabilitation Nursing, 16, 38–39.

Baker, N.A. (1982). Use of the Neuman model in planning for the psychological needs of the respiratory disease patient. In B. Neuman, The Neuman systems model: Application to nursing education and practice (pp. 241–251). Norwalk, CT: Appleton-Century-Crofts.

Beckingham, A.C., & Baumann, A. (1990). The ageing family in crisis: Assessment and decision-making models. Journal of Advanced Nursing, 15, 782–787.

Beddome, G. (1989). Application of the Neuman systems model to the assessment of community-as-client. In B. Neuman, The Neuman systems model (2nd ed., pp. 363–374). Norwalk, CT: Appleton & Lange.

Beitler, B., Tkachuck, B., & Aamodt, D. (1980). The Neuman model applied to mental health, community health, and medical-surgical nursing. In J.P. Riehl & C. Roy (Eds.), Conceptual models for nursing practice (2nd ed., pp. 170–178). New York: Appleton-Century-Crofts.

Benedict, M.B., & Sproles, J.B. (1982). Application of the Neuman model to public health nursing practice. In B. Neuman, The Neuman systems model: Application to nursing education and practice (pp. 223–240). Norwalk, CT: Appleton-Century-Crofts.

Bergstrom, D. (1992). Hypermetabolism in multisystem organ failure: A Neuman systems perspective. Critical Care Nursing Quarterly, 15(3), 63–70.

Biley, F.C. (1989). Stress in high dependency units. Intensive Care Nursing, 5, 134–141.

Breckenridge, D.M. (1982). Adaptation of the Neuman systems model for the renal client. In B. Neuman, The Neuman systems model: Application to nursing education and practice (pp. 267–277). Norwalk, CT: Appleton-Century-Crofts.

Breckenridge, D.M. (1989). Primary prevention as an intervention modality for the renal client. In B. Neuman, The Neuman systems model (2nd ed., pp. 397–406). Norwalk, CT: Appleton & Lange.

Bueno, M.M., & Sengin, K.K. (1995). The Neuman systems model for critical care nursing: A framework for practice. In B. Neuman, The Neuman systems model (3rd ed., pp. 275–291). Norwalk, CT: Appleton & Lange.

Bullock, L.F.C. (1993). Nursing interventions for abused women on obstetrical units. AWHONN's Clinical Issues in Perinatal and Women's Health Nursing, 4(3), 371–377.

Cardona, V.D. (1982). Client rehabilitation and the Neuman model. In B. Neuman, The Neuman systems model: Application to nursing education and practice (pp. 278–290). Norwalk, CT: Appleton-Century-Crofts.

Cheung, Y.L. (1997). The application of Neuman System Model to nursing in Hong Kong? Hong Kong Nursing Journal, 33(4), 17–21.

Chiverton, P., & Flannery, J.C. (1995). Cognitive impairment; use of the Neuman systems model. In B. Neuman, The Neuman systems model (3rd ed., pp. 249–261). Norwalk, CT: Appleton & Lange.

Clark, F. (1982). The Neuman systems model: A clinical application for psychiatric nurse practitioners. In B. Neuman, The Neuman systems model: Application to nursing education and practice (pp. 335–353). Norwalk, CT: Appleton-Century-Crofts.

Clark, J. (1982). Development of models and theories on the concept of nursing. Journal of Advanced Nursing, 7, 129–134.

Cook, K.R. (1999). Assessment of potential inhalant use by students. Journal of School Nursing, 15(5), 20–23.

Cookfair, J.M. (1996). Community as client. In J.M. Cookfair (Ed.), Nursing care in the community (2nd ed., pp. 19–37). St. Louis: Mosby.

Cowperthwaite, B., LaPlante, K., Mahon, B., & Markowski, T. (1997). Latex allergy in the nursing population. Canadian Operating Room Nursing Journal, 15(2), 23–24, 26–28, 30–32.

Cunningham, S.G. (1982). The Neuman model applied to an acute care setting: Pain. In B. Neuman, The Neuman systems model: Application to nursing education and practice (pp. 291–296). Norwalk, CT: Appleton-Century-Crofts.

Cunningham, S.G. (1983). The Neuman systems model applied to a rehabilitation setting. Rehabilitation Nursing, 8(4), 20–22.

Delunas, L.R. (1990). Prevention of elder abuse: Betty Neuman health care systems approach. Clinical Nurse Specialist, 4, 54–58.

Echlin, D.J. (1982). Palliative care and the Neuman model. In B. Neuman, The Neuman systems model: Application to nursing education and practice (pp. 257–259). Norwalk, CT: Appleton-Century-Crofts.

Fashinpaur, D. (2002). Using the Neuman systems model to guide nursing practice in the United States: Nursing prevention interventions for postpartum mood disorders. In B. Neuman & J. Fawcett (Eds.), The Neuman systems model (4th ed., pp. 74–89). Upper Saddle River, NJ: Prentice Hall.

Fawcett, J. (1997). Conceptual models as guides for psychiatric nursing practice. In A.W. Burgess (Ed.), Psychiatric nursing: Promoting mental health (pp. 627–642). Stamford, CT: Appleton & Lange.

Fawcett, J., Archer, C.L., Becker, D., Brown, K.K., Gann, S., Wong, M.J., & Wurster, A.B. (1992). Guidelines for selecting a conceptual model of nursing: Focus on the individual patient. Dimensions of Critical Care Nursing, 11, 268–277.

Fawcett, J., Cariello, F.P., Davis, D.A., Farley, J., Zimmaro, D.M., & Watts, R.J. (1987). Conceptual models of nursing: Application to critical care nursing practice. Dimensions of Critical Care Nursing, 6, 202–213.

Foote, A.W., Piazza, D., & Schultz, M. (1990). The Neuman systems model: Application to a patient with a cervical spinal cord injury. Journal of Neuroscience Nursing, 22, 302–306.

Fuller, C.C., & Hartley, B. (2000). Linear scleroderma: A Neuman nursing perspective. Journal of Pediatric Nursing, 15, 168–174.

Galloway, D.A. (1993). Coping with a mentally and physically impaired infant: A self-analysis. Rehabilitation Nursing, 18, 34–36.

Gavan, C.A.S., Hastings-Tolsma, M.T., & Troyan, P.J. (1988). Explication of Neuman's model: A holistic systems approach to nutrition for health promotion in the life process. Holistic Nursing Practice, 3(1), 26–38.

Gibson, M. (1996). Health promotion for a group of elderly clients. Perspectives, 20(3), 2–5.

Gigliottti, E. (1998). You make the diagnosis. Case study:

Integration of the Neuman systems model with the theory of nursing diagnosis in postpartum nursing. Nursing Diagnosis: Journal of Nursing Language and Classification, 9, 14, 34–38.

Gigliotti, E. (2002). A theory-based clinical nurse specialist practice exemplar using Neuman's systems model and nursing's taxonomies. Clinical Nurse Specialist, 16, 10–16.

Goldblum-Graff, D., & Graff, H. (1982). The Neuman model adapted to family therapy. In B. Neuman, The Neuman systems model: Application to nursing education and practice (pp. 217–222). Norwalk, CT: Appleton-Century-Crofts.

Hassell, J.S. (1996). Improved management of depression through nursing model application and critical thinking. Journal of the American Academy of Nurse Practitioners, 8, 161–166.

Herrick, C.A., & Goodykoontz, L. (1989). Neuman's systems model for nursing practice as a conceptual framework for a family assessment. Journal of Child and Adolescent Psychiatric and Mental Health Nursing, 2, 61–67.

Herrick, C.A., Goodykoontz, L., & Herrick, R.H. (1992). Selection of treatment modalities. In P. West & C.L. Evans (Eds.), Psychiatric and mental health nursing with children and adolescents (pp. 98–115). Gaithersburg, MD: Aspen.

Herrick, C.A., Goodykoontz, L., Herrick, R.H., & Hackett, B. (1991). Planning a continuum of care in child psychiatric nursing: A collaborative effort. Journal of Child and Adolescent Psychiatric and Mental Health Nursing, 4, 41–48.

Hiltz, D. (1990). The Neuman systems model: An analysis of a clinical situation. Rehabilitation Nursing, 15, 330–332.

Hoeman, S.P., & Winters, D.M. (1990). Theory-based case management: High cervical spinal cord injury. Home Healthcare Nurse, 8, 25–33.

Kain, H.B. (2000). Care of the older adult following hip fracture. Holistic Nursing Practice, 14(4), 24–39.

Kido, L.M. (1991). Sleep deprivation and intensive care unit psychosis. Emphasis: Nursing, 4(1), 23–33.

Knight, J.B. (1990). The Betty Neuman systems model applied to practice: A client with multiple sclerosis. Journal of Advanced Nursing, 15, 447–455.

Lile, J.L. (1990). A nursing challenge for the 90s: Reducing risk factors for coronary heart disease in women. Health Values: Achieving High-Level Wellness, 14(4), 17–21.

Lindell, M., & Olsson, H. (1991). Can combined oral contraceptives be made more effective by means of a nursing care model? Journal of Advanced Nursing, 16, 475–479.

Mayers, M.A., & Watson, A.B. (1982). Nursing care plans and the Neuman systems model: In B. Neuman, The Neuman systems model: Application to nursing education and practice (pp. 69–84). Norwalk, CT: Appleton-Century-Crofts.

McInerney, K.A. (1982). The Neuman systems model applied to critical care nursing of cardiac surgery clients. In B. Neuman, The Neuman systems model: Application to nursing education and practice (pp. 308–315). Norwalk, CT: Appleton-Century-Crofts.

Mill, J.E. (1997). The Neuman systems model: Application in a Canadian HIV setting. British Journal of Nursing, 6, 163–166.

Millard, J. (1992). Health visiting an elderly couple. British Journal of Nursing, 1, 769–773.

Miner, J. (1995). Incorporating the Betty Neuman systems model into HIV clinical practice. AIDS Patient Care, 9(1), 37–39.

Mirenda, R.M. (1986). The Neuman systems model: Description and application. In P. Winstead-Fry (Ed.), Case studies in nursing theory (pp. 127–166). New York: National League for Nursing.

Moore, S.L., & Munro, M.F. (1990). The Neuman systems model applied to mental health nursing of older adults. Journal of Advanced Nursing, 15, 293–299.

Mynatt, S.L., & O'Brien, J. (1993). A partnership to prevent chemical dependency in nursing using Neuman's systems model. Journal of Psychosocial Nursing and Mental Health Services, 31(4), 27–34.

Narsavage, G.L. (1997). Promoting function in clients with chronic lung disease by increasing their perception of control. Holistic Nursing Practice, 12(1), 17–26.

Neal, M.C. (1982). Nursing care plans and the Neuman systems model: II. In B. Neuman, The Neuman systems model: Application to nursing education and practice (pp. 85–93). Norwalk, CT: Appleton-Century-Crofts.

Neuman, B. (1983). The family experiencing emotional crisis. Analysis and application of Neuman's health care systems model. In I.W. Clements & F.B. Roberts, Family health: A theoretical approach to nursing care (pp. 353–367). New York: Wiley.

Orr, J.P. (1993). An adaptation of the Neuman systems model to the care of the hospitalized preschool child. Curationis, 16(3), 37–44.

Owens, M. (1995). Care of a woman with Down's syndrome using the Neuman systems model. British Journal of Nursing, 4, 752–758.

Piazza, D., Foote, A., Wright, P., & Holcombe, J. (1992). Neuman systems model used as a guide for the nursing care of an 8-year-old child with leukemia. Journal of Pediatric Oncology Nursing, 9(1), 17–24.

Picton, C.E. (1995). An exploration of family-centered care in Neuman's model with regard to the care of the critically ill adult in an accident and emergency setting. Accident and Emergency Nursing, 3(1), 33–37.

Pierce, J.D., & Hutton, E. (1992). Applying the new concepts of the Neuman systems model. Nursing Forum, 27, 15–18.

Poole, V.L., & Flowers, J.S. (1995). Care management of pregnant substance abusers using the Neuman systems model. In B. Neuman, The Neuman systems model (3rd ed., pp. 377–386). Norwalk, CT: Appleton & Lange.

Redheffer G. (1985). Application of Betty Neuman's Health Care Systems Model to emergency nursing practice: Case review. Point of View, 22(2), 4–6.

Rice, M.J. (1982). The Neuman systems model applied in a hospital medical unit. In B. Neuman, The Neuman systems model: Application to nursing education and practice (pp. 316–323). Norwalk, CT: Appleton-Century-Crofts.

Robichaud-Ekstrand, S., & Delisle, L. (1989). Neuman en medecine-chirurgie [The Neuman model in medical-surgical settings]. The Canadian Nurse, 85(6), 32–35.

Ross, M., & Bourbonnais, F. (1985). The Betty Neuman systems model in nursing practice: A case study approach. Journal of Advanced Nursing, 10, 199–207.

Ross, M.M., & Helmer, H. (1988). A comparative analysis of Neuman's model using the individual and family as the units of care. Public Health Nursing, 5, 30–36.

Russell, J., Hileman, J.W., & Grant, J.S. (1995). Assessing and meeting the needs of home caregivers using the Neuman systems model. In B. Neuman, The Neuman systems model (3rd ed., pp. 331–341). Norwalk, CT: Appleton & Lange.

Shaw, M.C. (1991). A theoretical base for orthopaedic nursing practice: The Neuman systems model. Canadian Orthopaedic Nurses Association Journal, 13(2), 19–21.

Smith, M.C. (1989). Neuman's model in practice. Nursing Science Quarterly, 2, 116–117.

Sohier, R. (1997). Neuman's systems model in nursing practice. In M.R. Alligood & A. Marriner-Tomey (Eds.), Nursing theory: Utilization and application (pp. 109–127). St. Louis: Mosby.

Sohier, R. (2002). Neuman's systems model in nursing practice. In M.R. Alligood & A. Marriner-Tomey (Eds.), Nursing theory: Utilization and application (2nd ed., pp. 219–238). St. Louis: Mosby.

Spencer, P. (2002). Support system. Learning Disability Practice, 5(7), 16–20.

Stepans, M.B.F., & Knight, J.R. (2002). Application of Neuman's framework: Infant exposure to environmental tobacco smoke. Nursing Science Quarterly, 15, 327–334.

Sullivan, J. (1986). Using Neuman's model in the acute phase of spinal cord injury. Focus on Critical Care, 13(5), 34–41.

Torkington, S. (1988). Nourishing the infant. Senior Nurse, 8(2), 24–25.

Trepanier, M.J., Dunn, S.I., & Sprague, A.E. (1995). Application of the Neuman systems model to perinatal nursing. In B. Neuman, The Neuman systems model (3rd ed., pp. 309–320). Norwalk, CT: Appleton & Lange.

Utz, S.W. (1980). Applying the Neuman model to nursing practice with hypertensive clients. Cardiovascular Nursing, 16, 29–34.

Wallingford, P. (1989). The neurologically impaired and dying child: Applying the Neuman systems model. Issues in Comprehensive Pediatric Nursing, 12, 139–157.

Ware, L.A., & Shannahan, M.K. (1995). Using Neuman for a stable parent support group in neonatal intensive care. In B. Neuman, The Neuman systems model (3rd ed., pp. 321–330). Norwalk, CT: Appleton & Lange.

Waters, T. (1993). Self-efficacy, change, and optimal client stability. Addictions Nursing Network, 5(2), 48–51.

Weinberger, S.L. (1991). Analysis of a clinical situation using the Neuman System Model. Rehabilitation Nursing, 16, 278, 280–281.

Wormald, L. (1995). Samuel—The boy with tonsillitis: A care study. Intensive and Critical Care Nursing, 11, 157–160.

Wright, P.S., Piazza, D., Holcombe, J., & Foote, A. (1994). A comparison of three theories of nursing used as a guide for the nursing care of an 8-year-old child with leukemia. Journal of Pediatric Oncology Nursing, 11, 14–19.

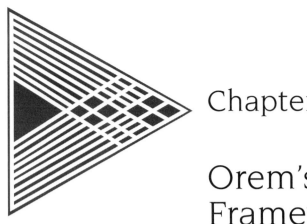

Chapter **8**

Orem's Self-Care Framework

Dorothea E. Orem formulated a definition of nursing in her 1956 report, *Hospital Nursing Service: An Analysis*. In 1959, she introduced the basic ideas undergirding her Self-Care Framework in the report, *Guides for Developing Curricula for the Education of Practical Nurses*. Orem continued her work with fellow members of the Nursing Model Committee of The Catholic University of America Nursing Faculty in the 1960s. The final report of that committee was submitted to the School of Nursing in May 1968. Orem then continued her work on the Self-Care Framework with a group of colleagues who formed the Nursing Development Conference Group in September 1968. In 1971, Orem published the first edition of her book *Nursing: Concepts of Practice*. The next publication dealing with the Self-Care Framework was written by the Nursing Development Conference Group and appeared in 1973 under the title *Concept Formalization in Nursing: Process and Product*. Revisions in the Self-Care Framework were presented by Orem in her 1978 speech at the Second Annual Nurse Educator Conference, as well as in the second editions of the books by the Nursing Development Conference Group (1979) and Orem (1980). Orem introduced three theories associated with the Self-Care Framework in her 1980 book. Refinements in the Self-Care Framework and the three theories were evident in the third edition of Orem's (1985) book and in Orem and Taylor's 1986 book chapter, "Orem's General Theory of Nursing." Further refinements are evident in the fourth, fifth, and sixth editions of Orem's (1991, 1995, 2001) book.

Overview

Orem's work focuses on patients' deliberate actions to meet their own and dependent others' therapeutic self-care demands and nurses' deliberate actions to implement nursing systems designed to assist individuals and multiperson units who have limitations in their abilities to provide continuing and therapeutic self-care or care of dependent others. Orem has referred to her work as the Self-Care Deficit Theory of Nursing, the Self-Care Nursing Theory, and a general theory of nursing. In various explications of the structure of her work, Orem (1990, 1995, 1997, 2001) has stated that the general theory of nursing is a conceptual framework or conceptual model or frame of reference that contains three parts—the Theory of Self-Care, the Theory of Self-Care Deficit, and the Theory of Nursing System. The concepts and propositions of the general theory of nursing are written at the level of abstraction and generality usually seen in a conceptual model. Because of that and to avoid confusion with grand and middle-range theories, the general theory of nursing, that is, the Self-Care Deficit Theory of Nursing or the Self-Care Deficit Nursing Theory, is referred to as the Self-Care Framework in this chapter.

The concepts of Orem's Self-Care Framework and their dimensions are listed here, along with the goal of nursing and the components of her practice methodology. The concepts, their dimensions, and the methodology components are defined and described, and the goal of nursing is discussed in detail, later in this chapter.

Key Terms

HUMAN BEINGS
PATIENT
    Individual
    Multiperson Unit
THERAPEUTIC SELF-CARE DEMAND
    Universal Self-Care Requisites
    Developmental Self-Care Requisites
    Health Deviation Self-Care Requisites
SELF-CARE
SELF-CARE AGENT
DEPENDENT- CARE
DEPENDENT-CARE AGENT
SELF-CARE AGENCY
    Development
    Operability
    Adequacy
DEPENDENT-CARE AGENCY
BASIC CONDITIONING FACTORS
POWER COMPONENTS
    Self-Care Agency Power Components
    Nursing Agency Power Components
SELF-CARE DEFICIT
DEPENDENT-CARE DEFICIT

ENVIRONMENT
ENVIRONMENTAL FEATURES
    Physical, Chemical, and Biologic Features
    Socioeconomic-Cultural Features
HEALTH
HEALTH STATE
WELL-BEING
NURSING
NURSING AGENCY
    Social System
    Interpersonal System
    Professional-Technological System
GOAL OF NURSING AGENCY
    To Compensate for or Overcome Known
        or Emerging Health-Derived or Health-
        Associated Limitations of Legitimate
        Patients for Self-Care or Dependent-Care
PRACTICE METHODOLOGY: PROFESSIONAL-
   TECHNOLOGIC OPERATIONS OF NURSING
   PRACTICE
    Case Management Operations
    Diagnostic Operations
    Prescriptive Operations
    Regulatory Operations: Design of Nursing
        Systems for Performance of Regulatory
        Operations
        Wholly Compensatory Nursing System
        Partly Compensatory Nursing System
        Supportive-Educative Nursing System
        Methods of Helping
    Regulatory Operations: Planning for
        Regulatory Operations
    Regulatory Operations: Production of
        Regulatory Care
    Control Operations
THEORY OF SELF-CARE
THEORY OF SELF-CARE DEFICIT
THEORY OF NURSING SYSTEM
GENERAL THEORY OF NURSING ADMINISTRATION

 ANALYSIS OF OREM'S SELF-CARE FRAMEWORK

This section presents an analysis of the Self-Care Framework. The analysis draws primarily from the sixth edition of Orem's (2001) book, *Nursing: Concepts of Practice*, a book chapter entitled "A Nursing Practice Theory in Three Parts, 1956–1989" (Orem, 1990), and the journal article "Views of Human Beings Specific to Nursing" (Orem, 1997).

ORIGINS OF THE NURSING MODEL

Historical Evolution and Motivation

Orem began to develop the Self-Care Framework in the 1950s, a time when most nursing education programs were based on conceptual models more representative of other

disciplines such as medicine, psychology, and sociology than of nursing (Phillips, 1977). Thus, Orem may be considered a pioneer in the development of distinctive nursing knowledge.

The development of the Self-Care Framework has been described in considerable detail (Nursing Development Conference Group, 1979; Orem, 2001; Orem & Taylor, 1986). The initial impetus for public articulation of the Self-Care Framework apparently was the need to develop a curriculum for a practical nursing program (Orem, 1959). Orem (1978) commented that that task required identification of the domain and boundaries of nursing as a science and an art. Continued work on the Self-Care Framework was motivated by "dissatisfaction and concern due to the absence of an organizing framework for nursing knowledge and … the belief that a concept of nursing would aid in formalizing such a framework"

(Nursing Development Conference Group, 1973, p. ix). In particular, the Self-Care Framework was formulated as a solution to the problem of "the lack of specification of, and agreement about, the general elements of nursing that give direction to (1) the isolation of problems that are specifically nursing problems and (2) the organization of knowledge accruing from research in problem areas" (Nursing Development Conference Group, 1973, p. 6).

Ideas that helped to shape the Self-Care Framework were formulated as Orem experienced a period of intensive exposure to nurses and their endeavors from 1949 to 1957, during her tenure as a nursing consultant in the Division of Hospital and Institutional Services of the Indiana State Board of Health. Her observations led to the idea that "nursing involved both a mode of thinking and a mode of communication" (Orem & Taylor, 1986, p. 41). Orem's "interest in and insights about the domain and boundaries of nursing" progressed from a global focus on "preventive health care" to a formal search "to know nursing in a way that would enlarge and deepen its meaning" and to identify "a proper nursing focus" (Orem, 1991, p. 60; Orem & Taylor, 1986, p. 39). Her search for the meaning of nursing was structured by six questions:

- What do nurses do and what should nurses do as practitioners of nursing? (Orem & Taylor, 1986, p. 39)
- Why do nurses do what they do? (Orem & Taylor, 1986, p. 39)
- What results from what nurses do as practitioners of nursing? (Orem & Taylor, 1986, p. 39)
- What human conditions and circumstances are associated with persons' requirements for the service of nursing? (Orem, 2001, p. 15)
- What brings the human conditions and circumstances associated with requirements for nursing outside the domain of personal and family responsibilities and into the domain of a publicly available service, nursing? (Orem, 2001, p. 15)
- What is the nature and structure of the service, the product that nurses make for persons who have requirements for nursing? (Orem, 2001, p. 15)

The answers to those questions began to emerge when Orem (1956, 1959) first articulated a definition of nursing, followed by rudimentary elements of the Self-Care Framework. Orem's 1956 report contained the following definition of nursing.

> Nursing is an art through which the nurse, the practitioner of nursing, gives specialized assistance to persons with disabilities of such a character that more than ordinary assistance is necessary to meet daily needs for self-care and to intelligently participate in the medical care they are receiving from the physician. The art of nursing is practiced by "doing for" the person with the disability, by "helping him to do for himself" and/or by "helping him to learn how to do for himself." Nursing is also practiced by helping a capable person from the patient's family or a friend of the patient to learn how "to do for" the patient. Nursing the patient is thus a practical and a didactic art (p. 85).

In her 1959 report, Orem stated that human limitations for self-care associated with health situations give rise to a requirement for nursing. Orem (2001) regards that statement as the articulation of the "proper object of nursing considered as a field of knowledge and a field of practice" (p. 489). She then identified areas of daily self-care, conditions that limit individuals' self-care capabilities, and methods of assisting those whose self-care abilities are limited. Orem (2001) pointed out that her 1959 report represents the formal beginning of her work of theorizing about nursing.

The questions were answered more fully as Orem first worked with the Catholic University of America Nursing Model Committee and then with the Nursing Development Conference Group. The theoretical concept of nursing system was expressed in 1970. Orem (2001) explained, "All of the conceptual elements [of the Self-Care Framework] were formalized and validated as static concepts by 1970. Since then, some refinement of expression and further development of substantive structure and continued validation have occurred, but no change of conceptual elements has been made" (p. 492).

Indeed, the structure and components of the Self-Care Framework have undergone various interpretations and refinements over time. In the first edition of her book *Nursing: Concepts of Practice*, Orem (1971) referred to dimensions of self-care and dimensions of nursing. By the second edition, she regarded her work as a "general comprehensive theory of nursing," which was made up of three "theoretical constructs" or theories—self-care deficit, self-care, and nursing system (Orem, 1980, p. 26). This structure was maintained in the third edition of Orem's (1985) book. A slight digression from the structure was noted in Orem and Taylor's 1986 book chapter, in which the theory of nursing system was referred to as "the general theory of nursing, because it explains the product made by nurses in nursing practice situations in relation to two conceptualized properties of individuals who need nursing, as these properties are expressed and related in the theory of self-care deficit" (p. 44).

Returning to the earlier structure in the fourth, fifth, and sixth editions of her book, Orem (1991, 1995, 2001) gave a title to the general theory of nursing and provided a hierarchical structure for the theories of self-care, self-care deficit, and nursing system. She explained, "The named theories in their articulations with one another express the whole that is self-care deficit nursing theory. The theory of nursing system subsumes the theory of self-care deficit and through it the theory of self-care. Self-care deficit theory [the general theory] subsumes the theory of self-care" (Orem, 2001, p. 141).

Further refinements in the structure of the Self-Care Framework are anticipated. Orem (2001) noted, "Each concept continues to undergo development through the identification and organization of secondary concepts that constitute its substantive structure" (p. 492).

Philosophical Claims

Orem has presented the philosophical claims undergirding the Self-Care Framework in the form of assumptions, premises, and presuppositions. Examination of those statements yielded assumptions about human beings, nursing-specific views of human beings, premises about human beings, presuppositions about self-care, assumptions about self-care requisites, assumptions about deliberate action, assumptions about human beings and deliberate action, assumptions about nursing, a philosophical claim about human beings and nursing, and an assumption about deliberate action and nursing. All of Orem's philosophical claims are listed here.

Assumptions About Human Beings

- Men, women, and children are unitary beings. They are embodied persons [who have] biological and psychobiological features (Orem, 1997, p. 29).
- [A] human being [is] a unity that can be viewed as functioning biologically, symbolically, and socially (Orem, 1991, p. 181).
- Each human being, like other living things, is a *substantial* or *real unity* whose parts are formed and attain perfection through the differentiation of the whole during processes of development (Orem, 2001, p. 187).

Nursing-Specific Views of Human Beings

- The view of [the human being] as person: Individual human beings are viewed as embodied persons with inherent rights that become sustained public rights who live in coexistence with other persons. A mature human being "is at once a self and a person with a distinctive I and me ... with private, publicly viable rights and able to process changes and pluralities without endangering his [or her] constancy or unity" (Weiss, 1980, p. 128, as cited in Orem, 1997, p. 28).
- The person view is central to and an integrating force for understanding the other ... views [of the human being]. All other views are subsumed by the person view (Orem, 1997, p. 29).
- The person view also is the view essential to understanding nursing as a triad of action systems. It is the view that nurses use (or should use) in all interpersonal contacts with individuals under nursing care and with their family and friends (Orem, 1997, p. 29).
- The view of [the human being as] agent: Individual human beings are viewed as persons who can bring about conditions that do not presently exist in humans or in their environmental situations by deliberately acting using valid means or technologies to bring about foreseen and desired results (Orem, 1997, p. 28).
- The person-as-agent view is the essential operational view in understanding nursing (Orem, 1997, p. 29).
- The view [of the human being as] user of symbols: Individual human beings are viewed as persons who use symbols to stand for things and attach meaning to them, to formulate and express ideas and to communicate ideas and information to others through language and other means of communication (Orem, 1997, p. 29).
- The view of person as user of symbols is essential in understanding the nature of interpersonal systems of interaction and communication between nurses and persons who seek and receive nursing (Orem, 1997, p. 29).
- The age and developmental state, culture and experiences of persons receiving nursing care affect their use of symbols and the meaning they attach to events internal and external to them (Orem, 1997, p. 29).
- The ability of nurses to be with and communicate effectively with persons receiving care and their families incorporates the use of meaningful language and other forms of communication, knowledge of appropriate social-cultural practices, and willingness to search out the meaning of what persons receiving care are endeavoring to communicate (Orem, 1997, p. 29).
- The user-of-symbol view is relevant to how persons who are nurses communicate with other nurses and other health care workers. Ideally persons who are nurses use the language of nursing and at the same time understand and can use the language of disciplines that articulate with nursing (Orem, 1997, p. 29).
- The view of [the human being as] organism: Individuals are viewed as unitary living beings who grow and develop, exhibiting biological characteristics of Homo sapiens during known stages of the human life cycle (Orem, 1997, p. 29).
- Viewing human beings as organisms brings into focus the internal structure, the constitution and nature of those human features that are the foci of the life sciences (Orem, 1997, p. 29).
- The view of [the human being as] object: Individual human beings are viewed as having the status of object subject to physical forces whenever they are able to act to protect themselves against such forces. Inability of individuals to surmount physical forces such as wind

or forces of gravity can arise from both the individual and prevailing environmental conditions (Orem, 1997, p. 29).

- The object view of individual human beings is a view taken by nurses whenever they provide nursing of infants, young children, or adults unable to control their positions and movement in space and contend with physical forces in their environment (Orem, 1997, p. 29).
- Taking the object view carries with it a requirement for protective care of persons subject to such forces (Orem, 1997, p. 29).

Premises About Human Beings

- Human beings require continuous deliberate inputs to themselves and their environments in order to remain alive and function in accord with natural human endowments (Orem, 2001, p. 140).
- Human agency, the power to act deliberately, is exercised in the form of care of self and others in identifying needs for and in making needed inputs (Orem, 2001, p. 140).
- Mature human beings experience privations in the form of limitations for action in care of self and others involving the making of life-sustaining and function-regulating inputs (Orem, 2001, p. 140).
- Human agency is exercised in discovering, developing, and transmitting to others ways and means to identify needs for and make inputs to self and others (Orem, 2001, p. 140).
- Groups of human beings with structured relationships cluster tasks and allocate responsibilities for providing care to group members who experience privations for making required deliberate input to self and others (Orem, 2001, p. 140).

Presuppositions About Self-Care

- Self-care is understood as conduct, as voluntary behavior guided by principles that give direction to action. In terms of ego psychology, it is ego-processed behavior (Orem, 2001, p. 45).
- Self-care as conduct reflects the essence of the concept [self-care]: self-care is behavior, it exists in reality situations (Orem, 1991, p. 119).
- Self-care is understood as learned activity, learned through interpersonal relations and communications (Orem, 2001, p. 45).
- Adult persons are viewed as having the right and responsibility to care for themselves to maintain their own rational life and health, and as having such responsibilities for persons socially dependent on them (Orem, 2001, p. 45).
- Giving, assisting with, or supervising the self-care of an-

other are components of infant and child care, care of the aged, and care of adolescents (Orem, 2001, p. 45).

- Adult persons require assistance from persons in social services or health care services whenever they are unable to obtain needed resources and maintain conditions necessary for the preservation of life and promotion of health for themselves or for their dependents; assistance may be needed for the accomplishment or the supervision of care of self or care of dependents (Orem, 2001, p. 45).

Assumptions About Self-Care Requisites

- Human beings, by nature, have common needs for the intake of materials (air, water, foods) and for bringing about and maintaining living conditions that support life processes, the formation and maintenance of structural integrity, and the maintenance and promotion of functional integrity (Orem, 2001, p. 48).
- Human development, from intrauterine life to adult maturation, requires the formation and maintenance of conditions that promote known developmental processes at each period of the life cycle (Orem, 2001, p. 48).
- Genetic and constitutional defects and deviations from normal structural and functional integrity and well-being bring about requirements for (1) their prevention and (2) regulatory action to control their extension and to control and mitigate their effects (Orem, 2001, p. 48).

Assumptions About Deliberate Action

- The *agent*, the person performing the actions, has incoming *sensory knowledge and awareness* of the reality of the situation of action. The agent *reflects* on the meaning of existent conditions and circumstances for the set or series of actions in process and for attainment of results toward purpose achievement. Reflection terminates in a particular productive situation with the agent's *decision* about the action that will be taken (Orem, 2001, p. 62).
- Accepting the [assumption] that deliberate action involves reflection as well as judgment and decision making requires the acceptance of human beings as having intrinsic activity rather than passivity or strict reactivity to stimuli (Orem, 2001, p. 65).
- Persons must have available the knowledge necessary to distinguish something as good or desirable from bad and undesirable and to reflect on its desirability or undesirability. The goal and ways to achieve it must be conceptualized or imagined (Orem, 2001, p. 65).
- Reasons for selecting certain actions to attain what has been appraised as good or desirable and afforded the tentative status of a goal should be known (Orem, 2001, p. 65).

- Time as well as knowledge is required for persons to form ideas about particular actions or to form images of how each action relates to the goal (Orem, 2001, p. 65).
- Reflection should be directed to these questions: Is this way of acting good or desirable? Is it more desirable or less desirable than other ways of acting to achieve the goal? (Orem, 2001, p. 65).
- Reflection about choosing a way of action could go on indefinitely; therefore, reflection should be brought to a close with a decision when the ways of action have been conceived as clear ideas or clear images are formed (Orem, 2001, p. 66).
- A person owns his or her appraisal of possible ways of action to attain a goal and his or her decision to act according to one or a combination of these ways, when this way of acting is formalized and incorporated into the person's self-image or self-concept (Orem, 2001, p. 66).

Assumptions About Human Beings and Deliberate Action

- Human beings know and appraise objects, conditions, and situations in terms of their effects on ends being sought (Orem, 2001, p. 65).
- Human beings know directly by sensing; but they also reflect, reason, and understand (Orem, 2001, p. 65).
- Human beings are capable of self-determined actions, even when they feel an emotional pull in the opposite direction (Orem, 2001, p. 65).
- Human beings can prolong reflection indefinitely in deliberations about what action to take by raising questions about and directing attention toward different aspects of a situation and different possibilities for action (Orem, 2001, p. 65).
- To act, human beings must concentrate on a suitable course of action and exclude other courses of action (Orem, 2001, p. 65).
- Purposive action requires not only that human beings be aware of objects, conditions, and situations but also that they have the ability to contend with them and treat them in some way (Orem, 2001, p. 65).
- Persons, as unitary beings, are the agents who act deliberately to attain ends or goals (Orem, 2001, p. 65).

Assumptions About Nursing

- Nursing is a form of help or assistance given by nurses to persons with a legitimate need for it (Orem, 1985, p. 31).
- Nurses are characterized by their knowledge of nursing and their capabilities to use their knowledge and specialized skills to produce nursing for others in a variety of types of situations (Orem, 1985, p. 31).

- Persons with a legitimate need for nursing are characterized (a) by a demand for discernible kinds and amounts of self-care or dependent-care and (b) by health-derived or health-related limitations for the continuing production of the amount and kind of care required. In dependent-care situations the limitations of dependent-care givers are associated with the health state and the care requirements of the dependent person (Orem, 1985, p. 31).
- Results of nursing are associated with the characterizing conditions of persons in need of nursing and include (a) the meeting of existent and emerging demands for self-care and dependent care and (b) the regulation of the exercise or development of capabilities for providing care (Orem, 1985, p. 31).
- Not all people under health care, for example, from physicians, are under nursing care nor does it follow that they should be (Orem, 2001, p. 489).
- [The answer to the question,] "What condition exists in a person when that person or a family member or the attending physician or a nurse makes the judgment that the person should be under nursing care?" (Orem, 1985, p. 19), [represents the assumption that identifies the proper object of nursing.] *Object* means that toward which or because of which action is taken. *Proper* means that which belongs to the field. Object is used in the philosophic or scientific sense as that which is studied or observed, that to which action is directed to obtain information about it or to bring about some new condition. Object is not used in the sense of something tangible. … The expressed proper object of the specialized health service nursing is identified as a *subclass* of the *class of persons who are unable to care for themselves* (Orem, 2001, pp. 20–21).
- [The proper object of nursing is expressed in the conditions of adults and children that validate a requirement for nursing.] [That] condition … in an adult *is the health associated absence of the ability to maintain continuously that amount and quality of self-care that is therapeutic in sustaining life and health, in recovering from disease or injury, or in coping with their effects*. With children, the condition is the *inability of the parent (or guardian) associated with the child's health state to maintain continuously for the child the amount and quality of care that is therapeutic* (Orem, 2001, p. 82).
- The word *therapeutic* is used to mean supportive of life processes, remedial or curative when related to malfunction due to disease processes, and contributing to personal development and maturing (Orem, 2001, p. 82).
- *Nursing is a direct human health service* (Orem, 2001, p. 15).

- Nursing as a human service has its foundations, on the one hand, in persons with needs for self-care of a positive, therapeutic quality and limitations for its management or maintenance and, on the other, in the specialized knowledge, skills, and attitudes of persons prepared as nurses (Orem, 2001, p. 83).
- [Nursing as a helping service is] a creative effort of one human being to help another human being (Orem, 1985, p. 132).
- [Nursing as a helping service] facilitates regulation of a patient's functioning through meeting the therapeutic self-care demand as well as movement by the patient under enabling conditions toward fulfillment of responsibilities for self-care (Orem, 2001, p. 190).
- Nursing relationships in society are based on a state of imbalance between the *abilities of nurses to prescribe, design, manage, and maintain systems* of therapeutic self-care for individuals and the *abilities of these individuals or their families to do so.* In other words, the nurses' abilities exceed those of other individuals. When the imbalance is in the opposite direction or when there is no imbalance, there is no valid basis for a nursing relationship (Orem, 2001, p. 95).
- Nursing practice has not only technologic aspects but also moral aspects because nursing decisions affect the lives, health, and welfare of human beings. Nurses must ask is it right for the patient as well as if it will work (Orem, 2001, p. 95).
- Solutions proposed to problems of the management and maintenance of therapeutic self-care for patients and families with limited ability to maintain their own care may give rise to other problems, solutions to which may be difficult if not impossible (Orem, 2001, p. 95).

Philosophical Claim About Human Beings and Nursing

- The [Self-Care Framework] assumes that nursing is a response of human groups to one recurring type of incapacity for action to which human beings are subject, namely, the incapacity to care for oneself or one's dependents when action is limited because of one's health state or the health care needs of the care recipient. From a nursing point of view, human beings are viewed as needing continuous self-maintenance and self-regulation through a type of action named *self-care* (Orem, 2001, p. 149).

Assumption About Deliberate Action and Nursing

- Nursing in every instance of its practice is action deliberately performed by some members of a social group to bring about events and results that benefit others in specified ways. Thinking about and conceptualizing

nursing as *deliberate action* is the most general approach that one can take to understand nursing (Orem, 1991, p. 79).

Additional philosophical claims undergird the Theory of Self-Care, the Theory of Self-Care Deficit, the Theory of Nursing System, and the General Theory of Nursing Administration. Those claims, which are stated in the form of presuppositions, are listed here.

Presuppositions for the Theory of Self-Care

- All things being equal, mature and maturing persons through learning develop and exercise intellectual and practical skills and manage themselves to sustain motivation essential for continuing daily care of themselves and their dependents with some degree of effectiveness (Orem, 2001, p. 143).
- Self-care and care of dependents require the availability, procurement, preparation, and use of resources for determining what care is needed and for its provision (Orem, 2001, p. 143).
- Available and known means and procedures of self-care and dependent-care are culture elements that vary within families, culture groups, and societies (Orem, 2001, p. 143).
- Individuals' action repertoires and their predilections for taking actions under certain conditions affect what persons do and do not do with respect to self-care or dependent-care within the context of stable or changing life situations (Orem, 2001, p. 143).
- Experiences of persons in the provision of self-care or dependent-care enable them to accumulate and structure bodies of experiential knowledge about kinds of care, when care is needed, and methods of providing care (Orem, 2001, p. 143).
- Scientific knowledge available and communicated to persons in communities is added to their experiential knowledge about self-care and dependent-care (Orem, 2001, p. 143).

Presuppositions for the Theory of Self-Care Deficit: Set One

- Engagement in self-care requires ability to manage self within a stable or changing environment (Orem, 2001, p. 146).
- Engagement in self-care or dependent-care is affected by persons' valuation of care measures with respect to life, development, health, and well-being (Orem, 2001, p. 146).
- The quality and completeness of self-care and dependent-care in families and communities rests on the

culture, including scientific attainments of groups and the educability of group members (Orem, 2001, p. 146).

- Engagement in self-care and dependent-care are affected, as is engagement in all forms of practical endeavor, by persons' limitations in knowing what to do under existent conditions and circumstances or how to do it (Orem, 2001, p. 146).

Presuppositions for the Theory of Self-Care Deficit: Set Two

- Societies provide for the human state of social dependency by instituting ways and means to aid persons according to the nature of and the reasons for their dependency (Orem, 2001, p. 146).
- When they are institutionalized, direct helping operations of members of social groups become the means for aiding persons in states of social dependency (Orem, 2001, p. 146).
- The direct helping operations of members of social groups may be classified into those associated with states of age-related dependency and those not so associated (Orem, 2001, p. 146).
- Direct helping services instituted in groups to provide assistance to persons irrespective of age include the health services (Orem, 2001, p. 146).
- Nursing is one of the health services of Western civilization (Orem, 2001, p. 146).

Presuppositions for the Theory of Nursing System

- Nursing is practical endeavor, a human health service (Orem, 2001, p. 147).
- Nursing can be understood as art, an intellectual quality of nurses designing and producing nursing for others (Orem, 2001, p. 147).
- Nursing has result-achieving operations that must be articulated with the interpersonal and societal features of nursing (Orem, 2001, p. 147).
- The results sought by nurses through nursing can be expressed as forms of care that ideally and ultimately result in movement to positive health or well-being (Orem, 2001, p. 148).

Presuppositions for the General Theory of Nursing Administration

- Health service institutions or health units of other types of institutions have purposes or missions that can be fulfilled at least in part through the provision of nursing to persons served by the institution (Orem, 1989, p. 58).
- Health service institutions or units serve persons who constitute describable changing populations (Orem, 1989, p. 59).

- Nursing administration is an organizational body, a component part of a health service institution or a unit of another type of institution (Orem, 1989, p. 59).
- Nursing administration in organized enterprises receives its managerial power from persons charged with institutional governance or with institutional administration (Orem, 1989, p. 59).
- Health-service institutions where nursing is provided as a continuously available service employ nursing practitioners or contract with them for their services, or grant them the privilege of practicing nursing within the institution (Orem, 1989, p. 59).

Strategies for Knowledge Development

Orem's description of the development of the Self-Care Framework indicates that she made extensive use of inductive reasoning. She explained that "The answer to the question [regarding conditions that exist in a person when a judgment is made of the need for nursing care] came spontaneously with images of situations in which such judgments were made and the idea that a nurse is 'another self' in a figurative sense, for the person under nursing care" (Orem, 2001, p. 489). Orem (1978) added that she looked to her personal and professional experiences for examples of judgments regarding the need for nursing care and the conditions of the persons when those judgments were made. The answer, she stated, finally came as a "flash of insight, an understanding that the reason why individuals could benefit from nursing was the existence of … self-care limitations." Inductive reasoning also is evident in the comment that the Self-Care Framework is "successful … because it is constituted from conceptualizations of the constant elements and relationships of nursing practice situations" (Orem & Taylor, 1986, p. 38).

Adding to her explanation of strategies used to develop the Self-Care Framework, Orem (1997) stated, "It is posited that the life experiences of nursing theorists, their observations and judgment about the world of nurses, can and do result in insights about nursing that can lead to descriptions and explanations of the human healthcare service, nursing. … What comes first, the view of humankind or the view of nursing in the cognitional processes of theorists, is a moot question. [My] position is that a theorist's life experiences in and accumulated knowledge of nursing practice situations support the recognition and naming of nursing-specific views of human beings" (p. 31).

Deductive reasoning is evident in Orem's (2001) discussion of her use of knowledge from adjunctive disciplines. For example, she noted that "Arnold's position about deliberate action and motivation led in 1987 to the expression of [several] conditions that may encourage action tendencies for self-care" (p. 65). (See Assumptions About Deliberate Action in the Philosophical Claims section of this chapter.)

Influences from Other Scholars

Orem has always cited the works of scholars in several adjunctive disciplines and has acknowledged the contributions to her thinking from her educational experiences. She commented that she read in a "wide range of fields, from organization and administration to social philosophy, including the philosophic notions of points of order in wholes composed of parts and different kinds of wholes; from hygiene and sanitation to cultural anthropology; from the philosophic notion of human acts to action theory as developed in sociology, psychology, and philosophy; and from action theory to a concept of systems and the constructs of cybernetics" (Orem & Taylor, 1986, p. 43).

Orem explicitly acknowledged the influences of Arnold (1960) and Kotarbinski (1965) on her ideas about deliberate human action and of Parsons (1937, 1951) on her ideas about the context of action. She also acknowledged Lonergan's (1958) influence on her thinking. She commented that her ability to express her ideas "required self-knowledge toward clarification of my own reality of knowing nursing in a dynamic way. B.J.F. Lonergan's (1958) work, *Insight*, was a helpful though difficult guide to self-knowledge" (Orem & Taylor, 1986, p. 43). She also has cited Black (1962), Harré (1970), Wallace (1983, 1996), and Weiss (1980), among other scholars.

In addition, Orem (1991, 1995, 2001) acknowledged the contributions of the members of the Nursing Development Conference Group to the development and refinement of much of the content of the Self-Care Framework. Over the years of its existence, the group included Sarah E. Allison, Joan E. Backscheider, Cora S. Balmat, Judy Crews, Mary B. Collins, M. Lucille Kinlein, Janina B. Lapniewski, Melba Anger Malatesta, Sheila M. McCarthy, Joan Nettleton, Louise Hartnett Rauckhorst, Helen A. St. Denis, and Dorothea Orem. The product of their combined effort to formalize a concept of nursing was the publication of two editions of the book, *Concept Formalization in Nursing: Process and Product* (Nursing Development Conference Group, 1973, 1979). Furthermore, Orem (1997) explicitly acknowledged the contributions of Hartnett-Rauckhorst's (1968) thesis work to the development of nursing-specific views of human beings. Moreover, Orem (1995, 2001) explicitly acknowledged her collaboration with Janet L. Fitzwater and Evelyn Vardiman in the conduct of a survey of nursing home residents about reasons for admission and

factors affecting the kind and amount of nursing required. Orem (1995, 2001) also acknowledged the contributions of Susan Taylor and graduate students at the University of Missouri, Columbia, School of Nursing, and of Evelyn Vardiman to the development and refinement of a nursing history form. And, Orem (1995, 2001) acknowledged the faculty of Incarnate Word College in San Antonio, Texas, who added the notions of dependent-care, dependent-care agency, and dependent-care agent to the developing Self-Care Framework in the 1970s.

Most recently, Orem (2001) has acknowledged the contributions of the members of Orem Study Group, including Gerd Bekel, Mary Denyes, George Evers, Elizabeth Geden, Marcella Hart, Donna Hartweg, Marjorie Isenberg, Bonnie Neuman, Kathie Renpenning, and Susan Taylor. Dorothea Orem herself also is a member of the Study Group. In addition, Orem (2001) acknowledged the contributions of Barbara E. Banfield, whose philosophic inquiry of Orem's framework "addresses the philosophic foundations for my work, expressed or implicit views of humankind, and the compatibility of [the Self-Care Framework] with various research paradigms" (p. 495).

There is no evidence to support contentions that the Self-Care Framework is based on earlier works by Frederick and Northam (1938) or Henderson (1955). Indeed, although the idea of patient as care agent was put forth by Frederick and Northam, the idea of self-care originated with and was formalized by Orem (Nursing Development Conference Group, 1979). Moreover, Orem explicitly denied that her Self-Care Framework was derived from Henderson's 1955 definition of nursing (Orem & Taylor, 1986), although she recognized the similarities between her 1959 idea of the proper object of nursing and Henderson's 1955 statement about nursing (Orem, 1995, 2001).

World View

Banfield (2001) reported that her philosophic inquiry revealed that Orem's Self-Care Framework "rests on a coherent philosophic system. Her views regarding the nature of reality, the nature of human beings, and nursing as a practice science all reflect the philosophic system of moderate realism" (p. xvi).

Within the context of the world views considered in this book, Orem's view of the relationship between the person and the environment clearly reflects the *reciprocal interaction* world view. In keeping with the reciprocal interaction world view, the Self-Care Framework reflects elements of both persistence and change. The features of the reciprocal interaction world view that are evident in Orem's Self-Care Framework are given here:

- The Self-Care Framework reflects a holistic view of the person, with emphasis on individuals as unitary beings (Orem, 1997, 2001).
- Human beings are never isolated from their environments. They exist in them (Orem, 2001, p. 79).
- Person and environment are identified as a unity characterized by human-environmental interchanges and by the impact of one on the other. Person-environment constitutes a functional type of unity with a concrete existence (Orem, 1991, p. 143).
- Although human beings have structural parts (e.g., arms, legs, stomach, lungs) and functional parts (e.g., urinary system, neuroendocrine system, neural circuits), the parts are viewed within the unity of human structure and functioning (Orem, 1995, 2001).
- If there is acceptance of the real unity of individual human beings, there should be no difficulty in recognizing structural and functional differentiations within the unity (Orem, 2001, p. 187).
- The person is viewed as an active agent who is capable of taking deliberate action to maintain self-care and to seek health care when faced with an imbalance between the current therapeutic demand for self-care or dependent-care and existing self-care agency or dependent-care agency (Orem, 2001).
- Persistence is reflected in the emphasis on maintenance of self-care agency. Stability of therapeutic self-care agency is the desired goal in the Self-Care Framework. Loss of self-care results from health-derived or health-related limitations and is not considered desirable (Orem, 2001).
- Change is evident in the developmental and health-related changes that occur in the demand for continuing therapeutic care and in self-care agency and dependent-care agency. Those changes are necessary for survival as the person matures (Orem, 2001).

UNIQUE FOCUS OF THE NURSING MODEL

The unique focus of the Self-Care Framework is the nurse's deliberate action related to the operations necessary to design, plan, implement, and evaluate systems of therapeutic self-care for individuals and multiperson units who have limitations in their abilities to provide continuing therapeutic self-care or care of dependent others. Limitations in abilities to provide complete and effective self-care or dependent-care stem from the individual's or the dependent other's health state or developmental stage or health care–related conditions (Orem, 1997, 2001).

Orem (1995) pointed out that "the reason why people need and can be helped through nursing defines the universe or domain of nursing as a socially institutionalized

human [health] service. The elements of nursing's domain are conceptualized and expressed as the [Self-Care Framework]" (p. v). The domain of nursing, for Orem, is individuals and multiperson units who have limitations in their abilities to provide continuing and therapeutic self-care or dependent-care.

Category of Knowledge

Meleis (1997) regarded the Self-Care Framework as an example of the needs category of models and also placed it in her nursing therapeutics category. Marriner-Tomey (1989) placed Orem's work in her humanistic category. Barnum (1998) regarded the Self-Care Framework as a good example of the substitution category of her classification scheme. The Self-Care Framework was classified as a systems model by Riehl and Roy (1980). Riehl-Sisca (1989) changed the classification to the interaction category. No rationale for its classification as either a systems or an interaction model was provided. Furthermore, close examination of the Self-Care Framework failed to reveal any evidence of a match between its content and the characteristics of systems or interaction models as those categories of knowledge are interpreted in this book. Instead, the Self-Care Framework is most appropriately placed in the developmental category of knowledge. The justification for that classification is evident in the comparison of the content of the Self-Care Framework with the characteristics of the developmental category of knowledge given here.

- Growth, Development, and Maturation: Those characteristics are addressed by the notion of developmental self-care requisites and by the consideration of the individual's self-care agency adjusted for age and developmental state (Orem, 2001).
- Change: Changes in self-care agency occur throughout life. Direction of change is viewed as toward higher levels of integration and assumption of self-care and dependent-care agency. "The point of view of human beings as persons is a moving rather than a static one. It is the view of personalization of the individual, that is, movement toward maturation and achievement of the individual's human potential. This process of coming to be a person involves individuals in communications with their worlds; in action; in the exercise of the human desire to know, to seek the truth; and in the giving of themselves in the doing of good for themselves and others. … Personalization proceeds as individuals live under conditions favorable or unfavorable to human developmental processes. … There is a striving by individuals to achieve the potential of their natural endowments for physical and rational functioning while living a life of faith with respect to things hoped for, and there is striving to per-

fect themselves as responsible human beings who raise questions, seek answers, reflect, and come to awareness of the relationship between what they know and what they do" (Orem, 2001, pp. 187–188).

- Identifiable State: Differences in self-care agency occur throughout life. The child is viewed as being in a stage of dependent-care, and the healthy adult is in a stage of total self-care and dependent-care agency. Socially dependent adults, including ill and disabled persons, are in a stage of dependent-care. "Infants and children require care from others because they are in the early stages of development physically, psychologically, and psychosocially. The aged person requires total care or assistance whenever declining physical and mental abilities limit the selection or performance of self-care actions. The ill or disabled person requires partial or total care from others (or assistance in the form of teaching or guidance) depending on his or her health state and immediate or future requirements for self-care. Self-care is an adult's continuous contribution to his or her own continued existence, health, and well-being. Care of others is an adult's contribution to the health and well-being of dependent members of the adult's social group" (Orem, 2001, pp. 43–44).

- Form of Progression of Development: Cycles of change occur in self-care agency; although the overall direction is toward increasing ability for self-care and dependent-care, loss of some agency does occur at various times throughout life, such as when illness or disability imposes limitations on self-care and dependent-care agency (Orem, 2001).

- Forces that Produce Growth and Development: Self-care and dependent-care agency naturally increase as the person matures, and people have an inherent, overt potential for development of self-care agency (Orem, 2001).

CONTENT OF THE NURSING MODEL

Concepts

The metaparadigm concepts of human beings, environment, health, and nursing are reflected in the concepts of the Self-Care Framework. Each conceptual model concept is classified here according to its metaparadigm forerunner.

The metaparadigm concept of human beings is represented by the Self-Care Framework concepts PATIENT, THERAPEUTIC SELF-CARE DEMAND, SELF-CARE, SELF-CARE AGENT, DEPENDENT-CARE, DEPENDENT-CARE AGENT, SELF-CARE AGENCY, DEPENDENT-CARE AGENCY, BASIC CONDITIONING FACTORS, POWER COMPONENTS, SELF-CARE DEFICIT, and DEPENDENT-CARE DEFICIT. The con-

cept of PATIENT has two dimensions—Individual and Multiperson Unit. The concept of THERAPEUTIC SELF-CARE DEMAND has three dimensions—Universal Self-Care Requisites, Developmental Self-Care Requisites, and Health Deviation Self-Care Requisites. The concept of SELF-CARE AGENCY has three dimensions—Development, Operability, and Adequacy. The concept of POWER COMPONENTS has two dimensions—Self-Care Agency Power Components and Nursing Agency Power Components. The remaining concepts are unidimensional.

The metaparadigm concept of environment is represented by the Self-Care Framework concept ENVIRONMENTAL FEATURES. That concept has two dimensions—Physical, Chemical, and Biologic Features; and Socioeconomic-Cultural Features.

The metaparadigm concept of health is represented by the Self-Care Framework concepts of HEALTH STATE and WELL-BEING. Each of these concepts is unidimensional.

The metaparadigm concept of nursing is represented in the Self-Care Framework by the concept of NURSING AGENCY. This concept has three dimensions—Social System, Interpersonal System, and Professional-Technologic System.

Nonrelational Propositions

The definitions of the concepts of the Self-Care Framework are given here. These constitutive definitions are the nonrelational propositions of this nursing model.

PATIENT

- A receiver of care, someone who is under the care of a health care professional at this time, in some place or places (Orem, 2001, p. 70).

The concept of Patient specifies who is the unit of service for nursing practice. The concept encompasses two dimensions—Individual and Multiperson Unit.

- Individual: Refers to the person as an individual or an individual member of a multiperson unit as the unit of service for nursing practice (Taylor & Renpenning, 2001).

- Multiperson Unit: Made up of more than a single person and [is] regarded as a whole—as "we" (Taylor & Renpenning, 2001, p. 397). [Refers to situations with more than one person as the unit of service for nursing practice where the] health and well-being of each person are subject to the effects of the interactions between and among the persons in the situation and the system of living within the unit (Taylor & Renpenning, 2001, p. 398). Taylor and Renpenning (2001) identified two types of multiperson units: (1) those in which the nursing system is designed for a number of persons who make up a collective or aggregate by virtue of something in common, such as a shared space, situation, or relationship, as well as a common concern that is within the domain of nursing, and (2) multiperson units, such as families and communities, where the unit itself is the object of nursing (p. 395).

Taylor and Renpenning (2001) explained that when the unit of service is the two or more persons who make up a Multiperson Unit, "each individual has his or her own set of operations and requisites ... the identification of these is important to understanding the functioning of the whole, the unit. Nevertheless, understanding the operations and requisites of each individual does not provide understanding of the functioning of the whole" (p. 397).

THERAPEUTIC SELF-CARE DEMAND

- The totality of required regulatory care measures (Orem, 2001, p. 23).
- A summation of measures of self-care required at moments in time and for some time duration by individuals in some location to meet self-care requisites particularized for individuals in relation to their conditions and circumstances (Orem, 2001, p. 491).
- The summation of care measures necessary at specific times or over a duration of time for meeting all of an individual's known self-care requisites, particularized for existent conditions and circumstances (Orem, 2001, p. 523).

The **Therapeutic Self-Care Demand** is an integral part of each individual's life because varied amounts and kinds of self-care requisites are present through the life cycle. Orem (2001) considers the human life cycle to encompass the intrauterine stages of life and the process of birth; the neonatal stage of life, including premature birth or term birth of normal or low birth weight; infancy; the developmental stages of childhood, including adolescence and entry into adulthood; the developmental stages of adulthood; and pregnancy in either childhood or adulthood.

The concept of **Therapeutic Self-Care Demand** has three dimensions—**Universal Self-Care Requisites, Developmental Self-Care Requisites,** and **Health-Deviation Self-Care Requisites.** Self-care requisites "have their origins in the anatomic and functional features of human beings" (Orem, 1991, p. 139). Denyes, Orem, and Bekel (2001) explained, "Self-care requisites are formalized expressions of kinds of action (named self-care) to achieve conditions that have some established or presumed effectiveness in individuals' regulation of their own functioning, development, and well-being on a day-to-day basis as

they live with other human beings in stable or changing environments" (p. 51). In particular, self-care requisites are "the reasons for doing actions that constitute self-care" (Orem, 1995, p. 108).

- **Universal Self-Care Requisites:** [Self-care requisites that] are common to all human beings during all stages of the life cycle, adjusted to age, developmental state, and environmental and other factors. They are associated with life processes, with the maintenance of the integrity of human structure and functioning, and with general well-being (Orem, 2001, p. 48). The eight universal self-care requisites are:
  1. The maintenance of a sufficient intake of air.
  2. The maintenance of a sufficient intake of water.
  3. The maintenance of a sufficient intake of food ... [in the form of nutrients, including] proteins and the amino acids of which they are composed [fats and fatty acids, carbohydrates, minerals, and vitamins].
  4. The provision of care associated with elimination processes and excrements.
  5. The maintenance of a balance between activity and rest.
  6. The maintenance of a balance between solitude and social interaction.
  7. The prevention of hazards to human life, human functioning, and human well-being.
  8. The promotion of human functioning and development within social groups in accord with human potential, known human limitations, and the human desire to be normal. Normalcy [refers to] that which is essentially human and that which is in accord with the genetic and constitutional characteristics and the talents of individuals. (Orem, 2001, p. 225)

- **Developmental Self-Care Requisites:** [Self-care requisites that] are associated with human developmental processes and with conditions and events occurring during various stages of the life cycle ... and events that can adversely affect development (Orem, 2001, p. 48). [Three sets of developmental self-care requisites have been identified. They encompass] provision of conditions that promote development, engagement in self-developments, and prevention of or overcoming effects of human conditions and life situations that can adversely affect human development (Orem, 2001, p. 231).

  [Developmental self-care requisites addressing conditions that promote development] are met by dependent care agents in the early stages of the human life cycle. When older children and adults are subjected to disasters, seriously ill, or in states of fear and anxiety, persons in helping roles ... may need to provide the ... conditions (Orem, 2001, p. 231). The conditions are:

1. Provide and maintain an adequacy of materials, such as water and food, and conditions essential for development of the human body at stages when foundations for bodily features are laid down and dynamic developments occur, and at later stages.
2. Provide and maintain physical, environmental, and social conditions that ensure feelings of comfort and safety, the sense of being close to another, and the sense of being cared for.
3. Provide and maintain conditions that prevent both sensory deprivation and sensory overload.
4. Provide and maintain conditions that promote and sustain affective and cognitional development.
5. Provide conditions and experiences to facilitate beginning and advances in skill development essential for life in society, including intellectual, perceptual, practical, interactional, and social skills.
6. Provide conditions and experiences to foster awareness that one possesses a self and of being a person within the world of the family and community.
7. Regulate the physical, biologic, and social environment to prevent development of states of fear, anger, or anxiety (Orem, 2001, p. 231).

[Developmental self-care requisites addressing engagement in self-development] demand the deliberate involvement of the self in processes of development (Orem, 2001, p. 231). Those self-care requisites are:

1. Seek to understand and form habits of introspection and reflection to develop insights about self, one's perception of others, relationships to others, and attitudes toward them.
2. Seek to accept feelings and emotions as leading, after reflection on them, to insights about self and about relationships to others, to objects, or to life situations.
3. Use talents and interests in preparing for and in maintaining and supporting engagement in productive work in society.
4. Engage in clarification of goals and values in situations that demand personal involvement.
5. Act with responsibility in life situations in accord with one's role or roles and with a developed or developing self-ideal.
6. Seek to understand the value of positive emotions in development of firm emotional dispositions that give rise to habits we call virtues. Positive emotions and action impulses include the desire to know; variations of human love, love of beauty, joy of making and doing, mirth and laughter, religious emotions, [and] happiness.
7. Seek to understand that negative emotions and action impulses are experienced when conduct is in discord with one's life goals and self-ideal. Negative emotions include guilt and guilt feelings, states of guilt, and unconscious conflict.
8. Promote positive mental health through deliberate efforts to (a) function within a veridical (reality) frame of reference, (b) function to bring about and maintain order in daily living, (c) function with integrity and self awareness, (d) function as a person in community, (e) function with increasing understanding of one's own humanity (Orem, 2001, pp. 231–232).

[Developmental self-care requisites addressing interferences with development are those] that adversely affect human development at the various stages of the life cycle. The two goals of those development self-care requisites are:

1. Provide conditions and promote behaviors that will prevent the occurrence of deleterious effects on development.
2. Provide conditions and experiences to mitigate or overcome existent deleterious effects on development. The conditions and problems referred to include (a) educational deprivation, (b) problems of social adaptation, (c) failures of healthy individuation, (d) loss of relatives, friends, associates, (e) loss of possessions, loss of occupational security, (f) abrupt change of residence to an unfamiliar environment, (g) status-associated problems, (h) poor health or disability, (i) oppressive living conditions, and (j) terminal illness and impending death (Orem, 2001, p. 232).

- **Health-Deviation Self-Care Requisites:** [Self-care requisites that] are associated with genetic and constitutional defects and human structural and functional deviations and with their effects and with medical diagnostic and treatment measures and their effects (Orem, 2001, p. 48). Self-care requisites [that] exist for persons who are ill or injured, have specific forms of pathology including defects and disabilities, and who are under medical diagnosis and treatment (Orem, 2001, p. 233). One category of health-deviation self-care requisites arises directly from disease, injury, disfigurement, and disability. Another category arises from the medical care measures that physicians perform or prescribe (Orem, 2001).

The six actions that need to be performed in relation to genetic and constitutional defects, human structural and functional deviations and their effects, and medical diagnostic and treatment measures prescribed or performed by physicians are:

1. Seeking and securing appropriate medical assistance when there is exposure to specific physical or biologic agents or environmental conditions associated with human pathologic events and states, or when there is

evidence of genetic, physiologic, or psychologic conditions known to produce or to be associated with human pathology.

2. Being aware of and attending to the effects and results of pathologic conditions and states, including effects on development.

3. Effectively carrying out medically prescribed diagnostic, therapeutic, and rehabilitative measures directed to preventing specific types of pathology, to the pathology itself, to the regulation of human integrated functioning, to the correction of deformities or abnormalities, or to compensation for disabilities.

4. Being aware of and attending to or regulating the discomforting or deleterious effects of medical care measures performed or prescribed by the physician, including effects on development.

5. Modifying the self-concept (and self-image) in accepting oneself as being in a particular state of health and in need of specific forms of health care.

6. Learning to live with the effects of pathologic conditions and states and the effects of medical diagnostic and treatment measures in a life-style that promotes continued personal development (Orem, 2001, p. 235).

The self-care requisites have been divided into those that are essential enduring elements and those that are situation-specific elements (Denyes et al., 2001). Universal self-care requisites and those developmental self-care requisites that are required by every human being are classified as essential enduring elements. Health-deviation self-care requisites and those developmental self-care requisites that are required in the event of development disorders and disabilities are classified as situation-specific elements.

The Universal Self-Care Requisites and the Developmental Self-Care Requisites, "particularized for the person by age, gender, developmental stage, pattern of living, and environmental conditions and circumstances," represent the baseline for the calculation of the **Therapeutic Self-Care Demand** (Orem, 2001, p. 247). Any Health-Deviation Self-Care Requisites are then added to the **Therapeutic Self-Care Demand.**

SELF-CARE

• Action of mature and maturing persons who have the powers and who have developed or developing capabilities to take use appropriate, reliable, and valid measures to regulate their own functioning and development in stable or changing environments. (Orem, 2001, p. 43).

• The practice of activities that individuals initiate and perform on their own behalf in maintaining life, health, and well-being (Orem, 2001, p. 43).

• Learned, goal-oriented activity of individuals (Orem, 2001, p. 490).

• Behavior that exists in concrete life situations directed by persons to self or to the environment to regulate factors that affect their own development and functioning in the interests of life, health, or well-being (Orem, 2001, p. 491).

Orem (1995) pointed out that **Self-Care** "carries the dual connotation of care 'for oneself' and 'given by oneself'" (p. 43).

SELF-CARE AGENT

• The provider of self-care (Orem, 2001, p. 43).

• [Mature or maturing persons who] have the capability to (1) determine the presence and characteristics of specific requirements for regulating their own functioning and development, including prevention and amelioration of disease processes and injuries (identification and particularization of self-care requisites); (2) make judgments and decisions about what to do; and (3) perform care measures to meet specific self-care requisites in time and over time (Orem & Taylor, 1986, p. 52).

In the concept of **Self-Care Agent**, "The term agent is used in the sense of *the person taking action*" (Orem, 2001, p. 43).

DEPENDENT CARE

• Activity [to regulate factors that affect development and functioning in the interests of life, health, or well-being] performed by responsible adults for socially dependent individuals (Orem, 2001, p. 491).

DEPENDENT-CARE AGENT

• The provider of infant care, child care, or dependent adult care (Orem, 1995, p. 104).

In the concept of **Dependent-Care Agent**, just as it is in the concept of **Self-Care Agent**, "The term agent is used in the sense of the *person taking action*" (Orem, 2001, p. 43).

SELF-CARE AGENCY

• The complex acquired capability to meet one's continuing requirements for *care of self* that regulates life processes, maintains or promotes integrity of human structure and functioning and human development, and promotes well-being (Orem, 2001, p. 254).

• The complex developed capability that enables adults and maturing adolescents to discern factors that must be controlled or managed in order to regulate their own functioning and development, to decide what can and should be done with respect to regulation, to lay out the components of their therapeutic self-care demands (self-care requisites, technologies, care measures), and finally to perform the care measures designed to meet their self-care requisites over time (Orem, 2001, p. 492).

Self-care agency, according to Orem (2001), "varies over a range with respect to its development from childhood through old age. It varies with health state, with factors that influence educability, and with life experiences as they are enabling for learning, for exposure to cultural influences, and for use of resources in daily living" (p. 254).

The concept of **Self-Care Agency** has three dimensions—**Development**, **Operability**, and **Adequacy**.

- **Development**: Identified in terms of the kinds of self-care operations individuals can consistently and effectively perform (Orem, 2001, p. 256).
- **Operability**: Identified in terms of the kinds of self-care operations individuals can consistently and effectively perform (Orem, 2001, p. 256).
- **Adequacy**: Measured in terms of the relationship of the number and kinds of operations that persons can engage in and the operations required to calculate and meet an existing or projected therapeutic self-care demand (Orem, 2001, p. 256).

DEPENDENT-CARE AGENCY

- The complex developed capability of responsible adults to [discern factors that must be controlled or managed in order to regulate functioning and development, to decide what can and should be done with respect to regulation, to lay out the components of therapeutic self-care demands (self-care requisites, technologies, care measures), and finally to perform the care measures designed to meet self-care requisites over time] for dependents (Orem, 2001, p. 492).
- The complex, acquired ability of mature or maturing persons to know and meet some or all of the self-care requisites of adolescent or adult persons who have health-derived or health-associated limitations of self-care agency, which places them in socially dependent relationships for care. With respect to infants and children, dependent-care agency is the complex acquired ability to incorporate knowing and meeting health-deviation self-care requisites of infants and children and needed adjustments in universal and developmental self-care requisites into ongoing systems of infant care, child care, and parenting activities (Orem, 2001, pp. 284–285).

BASIC CONDITIONING FACTORS

[The 10] factors internal or external to individuals that affect their abilities to engage in self-care or affect the kind and amount of self-care required (Orem, 2001, p. 245). The 10 basic conditioning factors, which "should be amended whenever a new factor is identified" (Orem, 2001, p. 245), are:

1. Age
2. Gender
3. Developmental state
4. Health state
5. Sociocultural orientation
6. Health-care system factors; for example, medical diagnostic and treatment modalities
7. Family system factors
8. Patterns of living including activities regularly engaged in
9. Environmental factors
10. Resource availability and adequacy (Orem, 2001, p. 245).

The concept of **Basic Conditioning Factors** is related to the concept of **Self-Care Agency**, such that the person's ability to perform self-care and the kind and amount of self-care that is required are influenced by certain internal and external factors that constitute the **Basic Conditioning Factors**.

POWER COMPONENTS

- Refers to the initiation of trains of events that enable the performance of required actions (Orem, 2001).

Orem (2001) explained that the terms power and capabilities are used interchangeably. Drawing from Harré (1970), Orem pointed out that power is not the same as activity, in the sense that power means the activity *can be* performed but does not mean that the activity *will be* performed.

The concept of **Power Components** has two dimensions—Self-Care Agency Power Components and Nursing Agency Power Components.

- **Self-Care Agency Power Components**: The 10 human powers that enable the performance of actions required for self-care (Orem, 2001). The 10 self-care agency power components are:
  1. Ability to maintain attention and exercise requisite vigilance with respect to self as self-care agent and internal and external conditions and factors significant for self-care.
  2. Controlled use of available physical energy that is sufficient for the initiation and continuation of self-care operations.
  3. Ability to control the position of the body and its parts in the execution of the movements required for the initiation and completion of self-care operations.
  4. Ability to reason within a self-care frame of reference.
  5. Motivation (i.e., goal orientations for self-care that are in accord with its characteristics and its meaning for life, health, and well-being).

6. Ability to make decisions about care of self and to operationalize these decisions.
7. Ability to acquire technical knowledge about self-care from authoritative sources, to retain it, and to operationalize it.
8. A repertoire of cognitive, perceptual, manipulative, communication, and interpersonal skills adapted to the performance of self-care operations.
9. Ability to order discrete self-care actions or action systems into relationships with prior and subsequent actions toward the final achievement of regulatory goals of self-care.
10. Ability to consistently perform self-care operations, integrating them with relevant aspects of personal, family, and community living (Orem, 2001, p. 265).

The Self-Care Agency Power Components dimension of the concept of **Power Components** is related to the concept of **Self-Care Agency**, such that the person's ability to perform self-care is influenced by the 10 power components. Orem (2001) explained, "Power components [enable] performance of self-care operations" (p. 257).

• **Nursing Agency Power Components**: The eight human powers that enable the performance of actions required for nursing (Orem, 2001). The eight nursing agency power components are:
   1. Valid and reliable knowledge of all three areas of nursing operation (social, interpersonal, professional-technologic).
   2. Intellectual and practical skills specific to the three areas [of nursing operation].
   3. Sustaining motives.
   4. Willingness to provide nursing.
   5. Ability to unify different action sequences toward result achievement.
   6. Consistency in performance of nursing operations.
   7. Making adjustments in [nursing operations] because of prevailing or emerging conditions.
   8. Ability to manage self as the essential professional operative element in nursing practice situations (Orem, 2001, p. 290).

SELF-CARE DEFICIT

• Refers to the relationship between self-care agency and therapeutic self-care demands of individuals in which capabilities for self-care, because of existent limitations, are not equal to meeting some or all of the components of their therapeutic self-care demands (Orem, 2001, p. 282).
• Self-care deficits are associated with the kinds of components that make up the therapeutic self-care demand and with the number and variety of self-care limitations (Orem, 2001, p. 282).

DEPENDENT-CARE DEFICIT

• Refers to the relationship between dependent-care agency and the therapeutic self-care demands of dependent others in which capabilities for dependent-care, because of existent limitations, are not equal to meeting some or all of the components of the therapeutic self-care demand (Orem, 2001).

A **Self-Care Deficit or a Dependent-Care Deficit** may be associated with functional and structural disorders, but neither is a disorder per se (Orem, 2001). Rather, a deficit signifies that the action demand for self-care or dependent-care is greater than the person's current capability for self-care or dependent-care (Orem, 2001). A **Self-Care Deficit or a Dependent-Care Deficit**, then, is a relational entity; each expresses a relation of inadequacy between **Self-Care Agency** or **Dependent-Care Agency**—the action capabilities—and the **Therapeutic Self-Care Demand**—the set of action requirements for engaging in **Self-Care** or **Dependent-Care** (Orem & Taylor, 1986). In other words, the **Therapeutic Self-Care Demand** exceeds the person's **Self-Care Agency** or **Dependent-Care Agency**. A deficit exists if the person does not yet have the ability to perform required self-care or dependent-care actions or if the person cannot or does not perform those actions due to health-related or situational circumstances.

A **Self-Care Deficit or a Dependent-Care Deficit** may be complete or partial. Orem (2001) explained that a complete deficit "means no capability to meet a therapeutic self-care demand" (p. 283). In contrast, partial deficits "may be extensive or may be limited to an incapacity for meeting one or several self-care requisites within a therapeutic self-care demand" (p. 282).

ENVIRONMENTAL FEATURES

• Features of the environment that are of interest are those that are "relevant to the values or presence of self-care requisites" (Orem, 2001, p. 80).

The concept of **Environmental Features** encompasses two dimensions—**Physical, Chemical, and Biologic Features** and **Socioeconomic-Cultural Features**.

• **Physical, Chemical, and Biologic Features**: Physio-chemical environmental features include the atmosphere of the earth, gaseous composition of air, solid and gaseous pollutants, smoke, weather conditions, and geologic stability of the earth's crust (Orem, 2001).

Biologic environmental features include pets, wild animals, and infectious organisms or agents along with their human and animal hosts (Orem, 2001).

- **Socioeconomic-Cultural Features:** Socioeconomic-cultural environmental features focus on the family and the community. Socioeconomic-cultural environmental family features include composition by roles and ages; cultural prescriptions of authority, responsibilities, and rights for the family unit; dominant family member and other members; positions of members within families and their culturally prescribed relationships; time-place localizations of family members; family dynamics; familial, contractual, and/or coercive nature of family relationships; the system of family living; resources of the individual members and of the family unit; cultural prescriptions for securing, managing, and using resources; and cultural elements specifying patterns of self-care and dependent-care and selection and use of care measures (Orem, 2001). Socioeconomic-cultural environmental community features include the population and its composition by family units, by other functional, collaborating social units, and by governmental organs; the availability of resources for community members' daily living and for special needs of the community as a whole; and the kind, localization, availability, openness to individuals and families, accessibility, cultural practices and prescriptions about use, cost, and methods of financing of health services (Orem, 2001).

Orem (2001) pointed out that **Environmental Features** "can be isolated, identified, and described, and [that] some environmental features are subject to regulation or control" (p. 79). She also noted that the two dimensions of the concept of **Environmental Features**—Physical, Chemical, and Biologic Features and Socioeconomic-Cultural Features—"may be interactive" (p. 79).

Orem (2001) underscored the potential contribution of **Environmental Features** to the person's development. She explained, "It is the total environment, not any single part of it, that makes it developmental" (p. 58).

HEALTH STATE

- A state of the person that is characterized by soundness or wholeness of developed human structures and of bodily and mental functioning (Orem, 2001, p. 186).
- A person's manifestation to self and others of features of his or her existence including the circumstances under which he or she exists (Orem & Vardiman, 1995, p. 165).
- Health state is made up of inseparable anatomic, physical, physiological, psychological, interpersonal, and social aspects (Orem, 2001).

Orem (2001) differentiated **Health State** from disease, which she defined as "an abnormal biologic process with characteristic symptoms" (p. 390). Orem (2001) also differentiated between illness, which she variously referred to as acute, chronic, and disabling, and **Health State**. In addition, Orem (2001) differentiated between **Health State** and sickness or poor health, as well as injury, disorder, or disability. The distinctions between **Health State** and disease, illness, injury, and disability are especially evident in Orem's (2001, p. 204) classification of nursing situations by health focus. The classification is given here.

Group 1: Life Cycle

- The health focus is oriented to events and circumstances in relation to the *life cycle* that give rise to anatomic, physiologic, or psychologic changes associated with periods of growth and development, maturity, parenthood, aging, and old age.
  - General health state is within the range of excellent to good.

Group 2: Recovery

- The health focus is oriented to the process of *recovery* from a specific disease … or injury … or to overcoming or compensating for the effects of the disease or injury.
  - Permanent *dysfunction, disfigurement,* or *disability* may or may not be present or expected.
  - General health state is within the range of excellent to good.

Group 3: Illness of Undetermined Origin

- The health focus is oriented to *illness or disorder of undetermined origin,* with concern for the degree of illness, specific effects of the disorder, and effects of specific diagnostic or therapeutic measures used.
  - General health state is within the range of good to fair.

Group 4: Genetic and Developmental Defects and Biologic Immaturity

- The health focus is oriented to *defects of a genetic or developmental nature,* or the *biological state of the premature infant,* or the *low-birth-weight infant.*
  - The state of general health may be affected by the direct or indirect effects of the defect or the biological state.

Group 5: Cure or Regulation

- The health focus is oriented to *regulation through active treatment of a disease or disorder or injury of determined origin,* with concern for the degree of illness; the specific

effects of the disease, disorder, or injury; and the specific effects of the therapeutic measures used. Temporary or permanent disfigurement or disability may or may not be present or expected.
  • The state of general health is or may be affected by direct or indirect effects of the disease, disorder, or injury.

Group 6: Stabilization of Integrated Functioning

• The health focus is oriented to the *restoration, stabilization, or regulation of integrated functioning.* A vital process may have stopped or be seriously disrupted, or in a newborn infant, breathing may not have started.
  • [General health state is directly affected by the lack of integrated functioning.]

Group 7: Quality of Life Irreversibly Affected or Terminal Illness

• The health care focus is oriented to the regulation of effects of processes that have disrupted human integrated functioning to the degree that quality of life is gravely affected or that life cannot long continue. Rational processes may be disturbed or relatively unaffected.
  • [General health state is directly affected by the disruption in integrated functioning.]

WELL-BEING

• Individuals' perceived condition of existence (Orem, 2001, p. 186).
• A state characterized by experiences of contentment, pleasure, and kinds of happiness; by spiritual experiences; by movement toward fulfillment of one's self-ideal; and by continuing personalization (Orem, 2001, p. 186).

Orem (2001) explained that **Health State** and **Well-Being** are associated. The experience of **Well-Being** may, however, occur for an individual under adverse conditions, including disorders in human structure and function.

Orem's discussion of the various health-related terms and her categories of health-related nursing situations suggest that she views health both as a continuum from excellent to poor and as a dichotomy of presence or absence. In addition, Orem apparently views disease, illness, sickness, injury, and disability as separate dichotomies of presence or absence. She commented, "[A]ny deviation from normal structure or functioning is properly referred to as an absence of health in the sense of wholeness or integrity" (Orem, 2001, p. 182).

NURSING AGENCY

• A power developed by maturing or mature persons through specialized education, training of self to master the cognitive and practical operations of nursing practice, clinical experiences in nursing practice situations under the guidance of advanced nursing practitioners, and clinical nursing experiences in providing nursing to persons representing some range of types of nursing cases (Orem, 2001, p. 289).
• A set of developed and developing capabilities that persons who are nurses exercise in the providing of nursing for individuals or groups (Orem, 2001, p. 289).
• A complex power of persons educated and trained as nurses that is enabling when exercised for knowing and helping others know their therapeutic self-care demands, for helping others meet or in meeting their therapeutic self-care demands, and in helping others regulate the exercise or development of their self-care agency or their dependent-care agency (Orem, 2001, pp. 491).

The concept of **Nursing Agency** is related to the Nursing Agency Power Components dimension of the concept of **Power Components**, such that the nurse's ability to perform nursing is influenced by the eight power components. Orem (2001) explained, "The operations of nursing practice to know and meet patients' therapeutic self-care demands and to protect and to regulate the exercise of development of patients' self-care agency requires enabling capabilities or power components" (p. 290).

The concept of **Nursing Agency** encompasses three interrelated action systems or dimensions—the **Social System**, the **Interpersonal System**, and the **Professional-Technological System**.

• **The Social System**: Establishes and legitimates the contractual relationship of nurses and persons who require nursing care (Orem, 1997, p. 28). An action system made up of one type of desirable nurse characteristics (Orem, 2001). Desirable nurse characteristics constituting the social system of nursing are:
1. Is well informed about and accepts the general social and legal dimensions of nursing situations; has specialized knowledge of the particular social and legal dimensions of types of nursing situations in his or her practice area.
2. Has knowledge of cultural differences among groups and among members of groups and understands the significance of persons' cultural orientations in their contacts and communications with others.
3. Has a repertoire of social skills, including communication skills, sufficient for effecting and maintaining contacts with individuals and multiperson units from a range of social classes and culture groups.

4. Accepts and respects himself or herself and others as developing persons, recognizing that each person has characteristic ways of conducting himself or herself in interpersonal situations.
5. Is courteous and considerate of others.
6. Is responsible in the provision of nursing to individuals or multiperson units within defined types of nursing situations.
7. Understands nursing with its domain and boundaries as one of the health services provided for by society.
8. Understands the nature of contractual and professional relationships and is able to perform the operations of nursing practice within limits set by these relationships (Orem, 2001, p. 291).

- **The Interpersonal System:** Constituted from series and sequences of interactions and communications among legitimate parties necessary for the design and production of nursing in time-place frames of reference (Orem, 1997, p. 28). An action system made up of one type of desirable nurse characteristics (Orem, 1995). Desirable nurse characteristics constituting the interpersonal system of nursing are:
1. Is well informed about the psychosocial dimensions of human functioning.
2. Has knowledge of factors that facilitate or impede interpersonal functioning.
3. Has knowledge of conditions necessary for the development of helping relationships.
4. Is interested in identifying and resolving human problems that interfere with satisfying relationships with others and produce emotional pain or suffering.
5. Has a repertoire of interpersonal skills that can be adjusted to infants, children, and adults, including those who are ill, disabled, or debilitated, and that enable the nurse to: (a) be an active participant in relationships with patients and their significant others, (b) be a participant observer in interpersonal relationships with patients and their significant others with the goal of identifying personality characteristics ... significant in the relationship, ... (c) reduce patients' emotional pain and physical discomfort and pain by effecting conditions that increase patients' comfort and satisfaction within the nurse-patient relationship, [and] (d) increase awareness of the interpersonal situation in terms of the desirable or undesirable factors that affect meeting patients' therapeutic self-care demands and regulating their self-care agency.
6. Is able to relate to patients and their significant others in a manner that conforms to the conventional form for human interactions.
7. Has a repertoire of communication skills (adjusted to the age and developmental state of individuals, their cultural practices, and communication problems resulting from genetic defects and pathological processes) sufficient for effecting and maintaining relationships essential in the production of wholly compensatory, partly compensatory, and supportive-educative nursing systems for patients.
8. Accepts persons who are under nursing care and works with them in accordance with their roles in self-care and dependent-care.
9. Identifies broader social and legal aspects of interpersonal situations ... and is able to represent these in a prudent way to patients or their significant others (Orem, 2001, pp. 291–292).

- **The Professional-Technological System:** The system of action productive of nursing (Orem, 1997, p. 28). An action system made up of one type of desirable nurse characteristics (Orem, 1995). Desirable nurse characteristics constituting the professional-technological system of nursing are:
1. Has mastery of valid and reliable techniques for nursing diagnosis and prescription; for meeting the therapeutic self-care demands of individuals with various mixes of universal, developmental, and health-deviation self-care requisites; and for regulating the exercise of self-care agency of individuals, its protection, and its development.
2. Is experienced or becoming experienced in using valid and reliable techniques in performing the technologic operations of nursing practice in defined types and subtypes of nursing situations and in producing nursing systems within these situations.
3. Is able to integrate the use of methods of helping with the technologic operations toward the production and management of effective nursing systems for individuals and multiperson units.
4. Is alert, at ease, and confident in nursing situations; is relaxed but able to mobilize for immediate and effective action to protect patients' well-being and to regulate the variables of nursing systems and the relationships among them.
5. Seeks nursing practice experience and supervision as well as specialized education and training to extend or deepen his or her area of nursing practice with respect to nursing populations.
6. Works toward the formulation and testing of methods and techniques for technologic operations of nursing practice within his or her nursing specialization.
7. Strives to increase ability to apprehend those factors in nursing situations that condition the values of the patient variables, self-care agency, and therapeutic self-care demand and thus set up requirements that nursing agency be of a particular value.

8. Identifies the results obtained in specific nursing situations from the use of specific methods in meeting patients' therapeutic self-care demands and in regulating their self-care agency, compiles results over time by types of nursing situations, isolates factors associated with types of results, and compares results in the different types of nursing situations (Orem, 2001, pp. 292–293).

Nursing, for Orem (1997), is "a triad of interrelated action systems" (p. 28). Those action systems constitute the three dimensions of the concept of Nursing Agency—the Social System, the Interpersonal System, and the Professional-Technological System. Orem (1997) explained that the existence of the Professional-Technological System is dependent on the existence of the Interpersonal System, which, in turn, is dependent on the existence of the Social System. More specifically, actions taken in the Social System lead to a contract between the nurse and the patient that "legitimates the interpersonal relationships of nurses and persons seeking nursing and their next of kin or their legitimate guardians" (p. 28). A contractual relationship is established between the nurse and the patient for the purpose of obtaining nursing care when an actual or potential self-care or dependent-care deficit is evident. The contract specifies that "the relation of the nurse to the patient is *complementary*. This means that nurses act to help patients act responsibly for their health-related self-care [or dependent-care] by making up for existent health-related deficiencies in the patients' capabilities for self-care [or dependent-care], and by maintaining or increasing capabilities for self-care [or dependent-care]" (Orem, 2001, p. 89).

Furthermore, the Professional-Technological System "is dependent upon the initial and continuing production of an effective interpersonal system" (Orem, 1997, p. 28). The Interpersonal System highlights the interpersonal relationship between the nurse and the patient. The essential elements of the interpersonal relationship are contact, association, and communication. Orem (1991) explained that "interpersonal contact and communication require effort and energy expenditure by both patient and nurse. ... Patients vary in their tolerance for contact and associations in accord with their temperament, their degree of illness, and their available energy" (p. 230). Orem (1991) went on to say, "Ideally, the interpersonal relationship between a nurse and a patient contributes to the alleviation of the patient's stress and that of the family, enabling the patient and the family to act responsibly in matters of health and health care. A relationship that permits a patient to develop and maintain confidence in the nurse and in himself or herself is the foundation for a deliberate process of nursing that contributes positively to the patient's achievement of present and future health goals" (p. 230).

Orem (2001) pointed out that the word nursing "is used as a noun, as an adjective, and as a verbal auxiliary derived from the verb to nurse" (p. 18). She went on to explain:

> Used as a noun and an adjective *nursing* signifies the kind of care or service that nurses provide. It is the work that persons who are nurses do. The word *nursing* as used in the statement *I am nursing* is a verbal auxiliary, a participle. *To nurse* literally means (1) to attend to and serve and (2) to provide close care of a person, an infant or a sick or disabled person, unable to care for self with the goal of helping the person become sound in health and "self-sufficient" (p. 18).

Orem (2001) distinguished nursing from medicine by noting that the physician focuses on the patient's life processes as they have been disrupted by injury or illness, and the nurse focuses on the patient's requirements for continuing therapeutic care. In particular, "Nurses view health states of persons they nurse as a basic conditioning factor influencing what persons need to do and what they can do with respect to self-care. [In contrast,] physicians view the health states of persons under their care as a central concern because the focus of medicine is the human potential of persons for health and their subjectivity to ill health, injury, and disability" (Orem, 2001, p. 81).

More specifically, nursing's special concern is "the individual's need for self-care action and the provision and management of it on a continuous basis in order to sustain life and health, recover from disease or injury, and cope with their effects" (Orem, 1985, p. 54). The nurse's focus, then, goes beyond the physician's focus or even the patient's immediate focus, to encompass (1) the patient's perspective of his or her own health situation; (2) the physician's perspective of the patient's health situation; (3) the patient's state of health; (4) the health results sought for the patient, which may be life, normal or near-normal functioning, or effective living despite disability; (5) the therapeutic self-care demand emanating from universal, developmental, and health-deviation self-care requisites; and (6) the patient's present abilities to engage in self-care and his or her health-related disabilities in giving self-care (Orem, 2001). Nursing is required, according to Orem (1997), "when individuals' developed and operational powers and capabilities to know and meet their own therapeutic self-care demands, in whole or part, in time-place frames of reference (that is, their self-care agency), are not adequate because of health state or health care-related conditions" (pp. 26–27).

The **GOAL OF NURSING AGENCY**, which Orem (2001) articulated as the "broad purpose of nursing," is "to compensate for or overcome known or emerging health-derived or health-associated limitations of legitimate patients … for self-care (or dependent-care)" (p. 289). The three components of this goal are:

1. Helping the patient accomplish therapeutic self-care
2. Helping the patient move toward responsible self-care, which may take the form of (a) steadily increasing independence in self-care actions, (b) adjustment to interruptions in self-care capabilities, or (c) steadily declining self-care capacities
3. Helping members of the patient's family or other persons who attend the patient become competent in providing and managing the patient's care using appropriate nursing supervision and consultation (Orem, 1985).

The **Goal of Nursing Agency** requires consideration of who are legitimate patients of nurses and, by extension, who are legitimate nurses. Legitimate patients of nurses "are persons whose self-care agency or dependent-care agency, because of their own or their dependents' health states or health care requirements, is not adequate or will become inadequate for knowing or meeting their own or their dependents' therapeutic self-care demands" (Orem, 2001, p. 490). Legitimate nurses "are persons who have the sets of qualities symbolized by the term *nursing agency* to the degree that they have the capability and the willingness to exercise it in knowing and meeting the existent and emerging nursing requirements of persons with health-associated, self-care or dependent-care deficits" (Orem, 2001, p. 491).

Orem lodged the nursing process within the Professional-Technological System dimension of the concept of **Nursing Agency**. Orem (2001) explained that she uses the term process "in the sense of a continuous and regular sequence of goal-achieving, deliberately performed actions of particular kinds carried out in a definite manner" (p. 309). Orem's version of the nursing process, which is the **PRACTICE METHODOLOGY** for the Self-Care Framework, is outlined in Table 8–1.

Orem (2001) noted that nursing practice may occur at three levels of prevention: primary, secondary, and tertiary. Universal self-care and developmental self-care, when therapeutic, constitute the primary level of prevention. Nursing care at this level includes assisting the patient to learn self-care practices that "promote and maintain health and development and [that] prevent specific disease" (p. 201). Health-deviation self-care, when therapeutic, constitutes the secondary or tertiary level of prevention. Nursing care at these levels focuses on helping the patient learn self-care practices that "regulate and prevent adverse effects of the disease, prevent complicating diseases, prevent prolonged disability, or adapt or adjust functioning to overcome or compensate for the adverse effects of permanent or prolonged disfigurement or dysfunction" (p. 202).

(Text continues on page 249)

TABLE 8–1
OREM'S PRACTICE METHODOLOGY: PROFESSIONAL-TECHNOLOGICAL OPERATIONS OF NURSING PRACTICE

CASE MANAGEMENT OPERATIONS

The nurse uses a case management approach to control, direct, and check each of the nursing diagnostic, prescriptive, regulatory, and control operations.

The nurse maintains an overview of the interrelationships between the social, interpersonal, and professional-technological systems of nursing.

The nurse uses the Nursing History and other appropriate practice tools for collection of information, documentation of information, and measurement of the quality of nursing (see Table 8–2).

The nurse records appropriate information in the patient's chart.

The nurse records progress notes as appropriate.

DIAGNOSTIC OPERATIONS

The nurse identifies the unit of service for nursing practice as an individual, an individual member of a multiperson unit, or a multiperson unit.

The nurse determines why the person needs nursing in collaboration with the patient or family and with continued review of decisions by the patient or family.

The nurse collects demographic data about the patient and information about the nature and boundaries of the patient's health-care situation and nursing's jurisdiction within those boundaries.

(continued)

> TABLE 8-1
> OREM'S PRACTICE METHODOLOGY: PROFESSIONAL-TECHNOLOGICAL OPERATIONS
> OF NURSING PRACTICE (continued)

DIAGNOSTIC OPERATIONS

The nurse calculates the person's present and future therapeutic self-care demand by:

- Identifying, formulating, and expressing each universal self-care requisite, developmental self-care requisite, and health-deviation self-care requisite in its relation to some aspect(s) of human functioning and development, including particularizing the values and frequency with which each requisite should be met.
- Identifying the presence of human and environmental conditions that are enabling for meeting each requisite, and those that are not enabling and constitute obstacles to or interference with meeting each requisite.
- Determining the methods or technologies that are known or hypothesized to have validity and reliability in meeting each requisite under prevailing human and environmental conditions and circumstances.
- Specifying the sets and sequences of actions to be performed when a particular method or technology or some combination is selected for use as the means through which each particularized requisite will be met under existent and emerging conditions and circumstances.

The nurse determines the person's self-care agency or dependent-care agency by:

- Identifying the person's self-care or dependent-care abilities by ascertaining the degree of development, the operability, and the adequacy of his or her ability to:
  - Attend to specific things and exclude other things.
  - Understand the characteristics and meaning of the characteristics of specific things.
  - Apprehend the need to change or regulate the things observed.
  - Acquire knowledge of appropriate courses of action for regulation.
  - Decide what to do.
  - Act to achieve change or regulation.

The nurse identifies the influence of power components on the exercise and operability of self-care or dependent-care agency by:

- Identifying the person's ability to maintain attention and exercise requisite vigilance with respect to self as self-care or dependent-care agent and internal and external conditions and factors significant for self-care or dependent-care.
- Identifying the person's use of available physical energy for the initiation and continuation of self-care or dependent-care operations.
- Identifying the person's ability to control body position and parts in the execution of the movements required for the initiation and completion of self-care or dependent-care operations.
- Identifying the person's ability to reason within a self-care or dependent-care frame of reference.
- Identifying the person's motivation for self-care or dependent-care.
- Identifying the person's ability to make decisions about self-care or dependent-care and to operationalize those decisions.
- Identifying the person's ability to acquire technical knowledge about self-care or dependent-care from authoritative sources, to retain it, and to operationalize it.
- Identifying the person's repertoire of cognitive, perceptual, manipulative, communication, and interpersonal skills for self-care or dependent-care operations.
- Identifying the person's ability to order discrete self-care or dependent-care actions systems into relationships with prior and subsequent actions toward the achievement of goals of self-care or dependent- care.
- Identifying the person's ability to consistently perform self-care or dependent-care operations, integrating them with relevant aspects of personal, family, and community living.

The nurse identifies the influence of basic conditioning factors on the exercise and operability of self-care or dependent-care agency by:

- Identifying the influence of the person's age, gender, developmental state, and health state.
- Identifying the influence of sociocultural orientation.
- Identifying the influence of health care system, family system, and environmental factors.
- Identifying the influence of the pattern of activities of daily living.
- Identifying the influence of resource availability and adequacy.

The nurse determines whether the person should be helped to refrain from self-care actions or dependent-care actions for therapeutic purposes.

The nurse determines whether the person should be helped to protect already developed self-care or dependent-care capabilities for therapeutic purposes.

The nurse determines the person's potential for self-care or dependent-care agency in the future by:

- Identifying the person's ability to increase or deepen self-care or dependent-care knowledge.
- Identifying the person's ability to learn techniques of care.
- Identifying the person's willingness to engage in self-care or dependent-care.
- Identifying the person's ability to effectively and consistently incorporate essential self-care or dependent-care measures into daily living.

The nurse calculates the self-care deficit or dependent-care deficit by:

- Determining the qualitative or quantitative inadequacy of self-care agency or dependent-care agency in relation to the calculated therapeutic self-care demand.
- Determining the nature of and reasons for the existence of the self-care deficit or dependent-care deficit.
- Specifying the extent of the self-care deficit or dependent-care deficit as complete or partial.

The nurse states the nursing diagnosis for the individual or a multiperson unit within the context of four levels:

- Level 1: Focuses on health and well-being, with emphasis on the relationship of self-care and self-care management to the overall life situation.
- Level 2: Deals with the relationship between the therapeutic self-care demand and self-care agency.
- Level 3: Expresses the relationship of the action demand by particular self-care requisites to particular self-care operations as influenced by the power components.
- Level 4: Expresses the influence of the basic conditioning factors on the therapeutic self-care demand and self-care agency.

PRESCRIPTIVE OPERATIONS

The nurse specifies the means to be used to meet the therapeutic self-care demand, in collaboration with the patient or family.

The nurse specifies all care measures needed to meet the entire therapeutic self-care demand, in collaboration with the patient or family.

The nurse specifies the roles to be played by the nurse(s), patient, and dependent-care agent(s) in meeting the therapeutic self-care demand, in collaboration with the patient or family.

The nurse specifies the roles to be played by the nurse(s), patient, and dependent-care agent(s) in regulating the patient's exercise or development of self-care agency or dependent-care agency, in collaboration with the patient or family.

(continued)

▶≪   **TABLE 8–1**
OREM'S PRACTICE METHODOLOGY: PROFESSIONAL-TECHNOLOGICAL OPERATIONS
OF NURSING PRACTICE *(continued)*

REGULATORY OPERATIONS: DESIGN OF NURSING SYSTEMS
FOR PERFORMANCE OF REGULATORY OPERATIONS

The nurse designs a nursing system, which is a series of coordinated, deliberate, practical actions performed by the nurse and the patient directed toward meeting the patient's therapeutic self-care demand and protecting and regulating the exercise or development of the patient's self-care agency or dependent-care agency, in collaboration with the patient or family.

The nursing system includes one or more methods of helping, which are sequential series of actions that will overcome or compensate for the health-associated limitations of patients to regulate their own or their dependents' functioning and development.

The selection of the appropriate nursing system is based on the answer to the question of who can or should perform self-care actions, and the determination of the patient's role (no role, some role) in the production and management of self-care.

- The wholly compensatory nursing system is selected when the patient cannot or should not perform any self-care actions, and thus the nurse must perform them.
- The partly compensatory nursing system is selected when the patient can perform some, but not all, self-care actions.
- The supportive-educative nursing system is selected when the patient can and should perform all self-care actions.

A single patient may require one or a sequential combination of the three types of nursing systems. All three nursing systems are most appropriately used with individuals.

Multiperson units usually require combinations of the partly compensatory and supportive-educative nursing systems, although it is possible that such multiperson units as families or residence groups would need wholly compensatory nursing systems under some circumstances.

- *Wholly compensatory nursing system:*
  The nurse accomplishes the patient's therapeutic self-care, compensates for the patient's inability to engage in self-care, and supports and protects the patient.
  The nurse selects wholly compensatory nursing system subtype 1 for persons unable to engage in any form of deliberate action, including:
  - Persons who are unable to control their position and movement in space.
  - Persons who are unresponsive to stimuli or responsive to internal and external stimuli only through hearing and feeling.
  - Persons who are unable to monitor the environment and convey information to others because of loss of motor ability.
  - The nurse selects this *method of helping:*
    - Acting for or doing for the patient.

The nurse selects wholly compensatory nursing system subtype 2 for persons who are aware and who may be able to make observations, judgments, and decisions about self-care and other matters but cannot or should not perform actions requiring ambulation and manipulative movements, including:
  - Persons who are aware of themselves and their immediate environment and able to communicate with others normally or in a restricted manner.
  - Persons who are unable to move about and perform manipulative movements because of pathologic processes or the effects or results of injury, immobilizing measures of medical treatment, or extreme weakness or debility.
  - Persons who are under medical orders to restrict movement.
  - The nurse selects one or more of these *methods of helping:*
    - Providing a developmental environment.
    - Acting for or doing for the patient.

- Supporting the patient psychologically.
- Guiding the patient.
- Teaching the patient.

The nurse selects wholly compensatory nursing system subtype 3 for persons who are unable to attend to themselves and make reasoned judgments and decisions about self-care and other matters but who can be ambulatory and may be able to perform some measures of self-care with continuous guidance and supervision, including:

- Persons who are conscious but unable to focus attention on themselves or others for purposes of self-care or care of others.
- Persons who do not make rational or reasonable judgments and decisions about their own care and daily living without guidance.
- Persons who can ambulate and perform some measures of self-care with continuous guidance and supervision.
- The nurse selects one or more of these *methods of helping:*
  - Providing a developmental environment.
  - Guiding the patient.
  - Providing support for the patient.
  - Acting for or doing for the patient.

- *Partly compensatory nursing system:*
  The nurse performs some self-care measures for the patient, compensates for self-care limitations of the patient, assists the patient as required, and regulates the patient's self-care agency; the patient performs some self-care measures, regulates self-care agency, and accepts care and assistance from the nurse.
  When the nurse selects partly compensatory nursing system subtype 1, the patient performs universal measures of self-care and the nurse performs medically prescribed measures and some universal self-care measures.
  - The nurse selects one or more of these *methods of helping:*
    - Acting for or doing for the patient.
    - Guiding the patient.
    - Supporting the patient.
    - Providing a developmental environment.
    - Teaching the patient.

When the nurse selects partly compensatory nursing system subtype 2, the patient learns to perform some new care measures.
  - The nurse selects one or more of these *methods of helping:*
    - Acting for or doing for the patient.
    - Guiding the patient.
    - Supporting the patient.
    - Providing a developmental environment.
    - Teaching the patient.

- *Supportive-educative nursing system:*
  The nurse regulates the exercise and development of the patient's self-care agency or dependent-care agency; the patient accomplishes self-care or dependent-care and regulates the exercise and development of self-care agency or dependent-care agency.
  The nurse selects supportive-educative nursing system subtype 1 if the patient can perform care measures and the appropriate *methods of helping* are guiding the patient and supporting the patient.
  The nurse selects supportive-educative nursing system subtype 2 if the patient can perform care measures and the appropriate *method of helping* is teaching the patient.
  The nurse selects supportive-educative nursing system subtype 3 if the patient can perform care measures and the appropriate *method of helping* is providing a developmental environment.
  The nurse selects supportive-educative nursing system subtype 4 if the patient is competent in self-care and the appropriate *method of helping* is guiding the patient periodically.

(continued)

TABLE 8–1
**OREM'S PRACTICE METHODOLOGY: PROFESSIONAL-TECHNOLOGICAL OPERATIONS
OF NURSING PRACTICE** *(continued)*

REGULATORY OPERATIONS: PLANNING FOR REGULATORY OPERATIONS

The nurse specifies what is needed to produce the nursing system(s) selected for the patient, including:

- The time during which the nursing system will be produced.
- The place where the nursing system will be produced.
- The environmental conditions necessary for the production of the nursing system.
- The equipment and supplies required.
- The number and the qualifications of nurses and other health care providers necessary to produce the nursing system and to evaluate its effects.
- The organization and timing of tasks to be performed.
- The designation of who (nurse or patient) is to perform the tasks.

REGULATORY OPERATIONS: PRODUCTION OF REGULATORY CARE

Nursing systems are produced by means of the actions of nurses and patients during nurse-patient encounters.

The nurse produces and manages the designated nursing system(s) and method(s) of helping for as long as the patient's self-care deficit or dependent-care deficit exists.

The nurse provides these direct nursing care operations:

- Performs and regulates the self-care or dependent-care tasks for patients or assists patients with their performance of self-care or dependent-care tasks.
- Coordinates self-care or dependent-care task performance so that a unified system of care is produced and coordinated with other components of health care.
- Helps patients, their families, and others bring about systems of daily living for patients that support the accomplishment of self-care or dependent-care and are, at the same time, satisfying in relation to patients' interests, talents, and goals.
- Guides, directs, and supports patients in their exercise of, or in the withholding of the exercise of, their self-care agency or dependent-care agency.
- Stimulates patients' interests in self-care or dependent-care by raising questions and promoting discussions of care problems and issues when conditions permit.
- Is available to patients at times when questions are likely to arise.
- Supports and guides patients in learning activities and provides cues for learning, as well as instructional sessions.
- Supports and guides patients as they experience illness or disability and the effects of medical care measures and as they experience the need to engage in new measures of self-care or change their ways of meeting ongoing self-care requisites.

The nurse carries out these decision-making operations regarding the continuation of or need for changes in direct nursing care:

- Monitors patients and assists patients to monitor themselves to determine if self-care or dependent-care measures were performed and to determine the effects of self-care or dependent-care, the results of efforts to regulate the exercise or development of self-care agency or dependent-care agency, and the sufficiency and efficiency of nursing action directed to these ends.
- Makes judgments about the sufficiency and efficiency of self-care or dependent-care, the regulation of the exercise or development of self-care agency or dependent-care, and nursing assistance.
- Makes judgments about the meaning of the results derived from nurses' performance when monitoring patients and judging outcomes of self-care or dependent -care for the well-being of patients.
- Makes or recommends adjustments in the nursing care system through changes in nurse and patient roles.

CONTROL OPERATIONS

The nurse performs control operations concurrently with or separate from the production of regulatory care.

The nurse makes observations and evaluates the nursing system to determine whether:

- The nursing system that was designed is actually produced.
- There is a fit between the current prescription for nursing and the nursing system that is being produced.
- Regulation of the patient's functioning is being achieved through performance of care measures to meet the patient's therapeutic self-care demand.
- Exercise of the patient's self-care agency or dependent-care agency is being properly regulated.
- Developmental change is in process and is adequate.
- The patient is adjusting to any declining powers to engage in self-care or dependent- care.

Constructed from Orem, 1985, 1991, 1995, 2001; Taylor, 1991.

(Text continued from page 243)

Relational Propositions

The relational propositions of the Self-Care Framework are given here. The link between the metaparadigm concepts of human beings and environment is specified in relational proposition A. The metaparadigm concepts of **Human Beings, Environment,** and **Health** are linked in relational proposition B. The linkage of the metaparadigm concepts of **Human Beings, Environment,** and **Nursing** is articulated in relational proposition C. The linkage of the metaparadigm concepts of **Human Beings, Health,** and **Nursing** is specified in relational propositions D and E. Relational proposition F links the metaparadigm concepts of **Human Beings, Environment, Health,** and **Nursing.**

A. Certain environmental features are continuously or periodically interactive with men, women, and children in their time-place localizations (Orem, 2001, p. 79).
B. Environmental conditions can positively or negatively affect the lives, health, and well-being of individuals, families, [and] communities; under conditions of war or natural disaster, whole societies are subject to disruption or destruction (Orem, 2001, p. 79).
C. Nurses in concrete nursing practice situations seek nursing-relevant information about both persons who seek or need nursing and their environmental situations (Orem, 2001, p. 79).
D. Nursing has as its special concern the individual's need for self-care action and the provision and management of it on a continuous basis in order to sustain life and health, recover from disease or injury, and cope with their effects (Orem, 1985, p. 54).
E. Nurses act deliberately to produce systems of nursing for persons who have health-related action deficits for knowing and continually meeting their own or their dependents' therapeutic self-care demands (Orem, 1995, p. 162).
F. Nursing is made or produced by nurses. It is a service, a mode of helping human beings. ... Nursing's form or structure is derived from actions deliberately selected and performed by nurses to help individuals or groups under their care to maintain or change conditions in themselves or their environments. This may be done by individuals or groups through their own actions under the guidance of a nurse or through the actions of nurses when persons have health-derived or health-related limitations that cannot be immediately overcome (Orem, 1980, p. 5).

 ## EVALUATION OF OREM'S SELF-CARE FRAMEWORK

This section presents an evaluation of the Self-Care Framework. The evaluation is based on the results of the analysis, as well as on publications and presentations by Orem and by others who have used or commented on her work.

EXPLICATION OF ORIGINS

Orem explicated the origins of the Self-Care Framework clearly. She traced the development and refinement of her work from the 1950s to the early 2000s in the sixth edition of her book (Orem, 2001). The fourth (1991), fifth (1995), and sixth (2001) editions of Orem's book are especially informative in that they include much of the content of the out-of-print text by the Nursing Development Conference Group (1979) along with the content of the Self-Care Framework and the Theory of Self-Care, the Theory of Self-Care Deficit, and the Theory of Nursing System.

Orem identified the philosophical claims undergirding her work in the form of assumptions and presuppositions. Taken together, Orem's philosophical claims indicate that she values individuals' abilities to care for themselves and dependent others, with intervention from health-care professionals only when actual or potential self-care deficits or dependent-care deficits arise. Furthermore, Orem expects people to be responsible for themselves and to seek help when they cannot maintain therapeutic self-care or dependent-care. Orem also values the person's perspective of his or her health status, as well as the physician's perspective of the person's health status. Consequently, she does not expect nursing to be based solely on the nurse's view of the patient's situation.

With regard to her philosophical claims, Orem pointed out that "many nurses are trying to get the answers in philosophy. But, although philosophy will help you to think about things, no philosophy will tell you your subject matter" (Fawcett, 2001, p. 36). The subject matter of nursing, from Orem's point of view, is encompassed by the concepts and propositions of the Self-Care Framework and the Theory of Self-Care, the Theory of Self-Care Deficit, and the Theory of Nursing System.

Orem acknowledged the contributions of her colleagues in the Nursing Development Conference Group to the evolution and refinement of her ideas about nursing. She also acknowledged and cited the work of scholars from adjunctive disciplines, emphasizing the importance of the work on deliberate human action to the development of the Self-Care Framework.

COMPREHENSIVENESS OF CONTENT

The Self-Care Framework is sufficiently comprehensive in depth of content. The person is fully defined and described as he or she relates to nursing. Orem (2001) was very clear about the correct label for the nursing participant. She rejected the term client for the human being, preferring instead the term **Patient**. She noted, "Some nurses use the term client in place of the term *patient*. This effort seems to be directed toward recognition of the contractual nature of the relationships of nurses to persons under their care and to avoid the philosophical use of the word *patient* to mean *that which is acted upon.* It is customary to use the term *client* in the practice of law, in business, and trade. ... *Client* also means a customer who *regularly* buys from another or receives services from another. ... Persons who are regular

seekers of the services of—that is, who are clients of—this or that nurse may not be under nursing care at particular times and, therefore, would not have patient status. ... The terms *patient* or *nurse's patient* will be used to refer to persons under the care of nurses" (p. 70).

Orem also is very clear about who are the legitimate recipients of nursing. She is not clear, however, about whether the **Self-Care Agency** concept dimensions of Development, Operability, and Adequacy also refer to the concept of **Dependent-Care Agency**.

Orem's description of environment is comprehensive, although environment, per se, is never explicitly defined. Instead, the concept of **Environmental Features** and a list of the components of the two dimensions of that concept were extracted from Orem's (2001) book.

The concepts of **Health State** and **Well-Being** are clearly defined, but illness is not. The person's **Health State** is regarded as a factor that may impose new or different demands for self-care on the person. In particular, illness, disability, and disease may impose **Therapeutic Self-Care Demands** that exceed the person's **Self-Care Agency** or **Dependent-Care Agency** and therefore create a **Self-Care Deficit** or a **Dependent-Care Deficit**.

Nursing is defined clearly and described in terms of scope and appropriate actions to be taken in relation to patients. Orem's description of the nursing process has, however, become more difficult to understand. In the first, second, and third editions of *Nursing: Concepts of Practice*, Orem (1971, 1980, 1985) presented a readily comprehensible three-step nursing process of diagnosis and prescription, designing and planning, and producing care to regulate therapeutic self-care demand and self-care agency. In the fourth edition, Orem (1991) mentioned three steps but gave an explicit number to only the third step, then called regulatory care or regulatory and treatment operations. In addition, confusion about the number of steps in the nursing process was introduced in the fourth edition with the inclusion of a section on control operations. Moreover, the language used to describe the process became obtuse in the fourth edition, with increased emphasis placed on discussion of technological operations and the dimensions of professional and case management operations. The revisions evident in the fifth (Orem, 1995) and sixth (2001) editions resulted in some clarification in the various components of the nursing process and elimination of any mention of steps of the nursing process, although the language remains obtuse. Furthermore, there is some inconsistency in the terms used for the various operations in the 1995 and 2001 editions. In particular, Orem (2001) variously identified the professional-technological operations of nursing practice as "nursing diagnosis, nursing prescription, nursing regulation or treatment, evaluation and control, and case management" (p. 289); "diagnostic operations" (p. 308), "prescriptive operations" (p. 308), "treatment or regulatory operations" (p. 308), and "case management operations" (p. 312); and "nursing diagnosis" (p. 312), "prescriptive operations" (p. 313), "regulation or treatment operations" (p. 318), "designs for performance of regulatory operations" (p. 321), "planning for regulatory operations" (p. 321), "production of regulatory care" (p. 322), and "control operations" (p. 324). The **Practice Methodology** (see Table 8–1) presented in this chapter finally resulted from a synthesis of Orem's discussions about the nursing process in the 1985, 1991, 1995, and 2001 editions of her book.

The Self-Care Framework is based on philosophical, theoretical, and scientific knowledge about human behavior, with emphasis placed on theories of deliberate action. Orem (2001) noted that nursing agency is based in large part on knowledge of nursing, sciences, arts, and humanities, and that the design of a nursing system is based on the nurse's factual knowledge about the patient, accumulated information about various therapeutic self-care demands and methods of helping, and knowledge about self-care as deliberate action.

The dynamic nature of the nursing process is evident in the following quotations from Orem's (2001) book:

> Case management is concerned with the integration of technologic operations to form a dynamic system of health service that is effective and judicious in the use of resources and that minimizes both psychological and physical stress for persons seeking and receiving the health service (p. 309).

> Development of designs for the production of regulatory nursing care [is done] with attention to continuing nursing diagnosis and prescription (p. 295).

> Nursing diagnosis precedes nursing prescription but the nursing diagnostic operation is not necessarily complete before prescriptions are made and regulatory care provided (p. 309).

> Nurses [should] avoid conceptualizing the provision of nursing as a linear process moving from a complete, definitive nursing diagnosis to nursing regulation and evaluation (p. 310).

> Control operations ... can be performed concurrently with regulatory or treatment operations of nursing practice (p. 325).

Orem's inclusion of the patient's perspective of health status, her emphasis on determining the extent of the patient's willingness to collaborate with nurses and participate in nursing, and her emphasis on obtaining sufficient information for an accurate diagnosis all reflect her concern with ethical standards. This concern is underscored by

Orem's (2001) characterization of nursing as having a moral component: "Nursing practice has not only technologic aspects but also moral aspects, because nursing decisions affect the lives, health, and welfare of human beings. Nurses must ask is it right for the patient as well as if it will work" (p. 95). She went on to say, "Closely allied to nurses' capabilities to produce nursing for others are the good habits (or virtues) of art and prudence. ... The proper interest of prudence is the morality, the goodness of individual human actions in concrete situations of daily living. Prudence is right reason about things to be done. ... Prudence is a virtue of the mind and of the character of individuals" (p. 293).

The criterion for the linkage of concepts requires that the propositions of the conceptual model link all four metaparadigm concepts. This criterion was met only by recourse to a quotation found in the second edition of Orem's (1980) book.

The Self-Care Framework is sufficiently comprehensive concerning breadth of content. The framework has been used in a wide variety of nursing situations and with individuals and multiperson units with many different states of health. For Orem (1991; Taylor & Renpenning, 1995, 2001), multiperson units include families, residence groups, work groups, self-help groups, prenatal or postnatal groups, weight control groups, and groups of patients in nursing clinics, as well as communities. Taylor and Renpenning's (1995, 2001) chapters in the fifth and sixth editions of Orem's book brought some clarification to the Individual and Multiperson Unit dimensions of the concept of **Patient**.

The comprehensiveness of the breadth of the Self-Care Framework is further supported by the direction it provides for nursing research, education, administration, and practice. Although guidelines for each area are not explicit in Orem's publications, many can be extracted from the content of the Self-Care Framework and various publications about its use. The developing guidelines for research, nursing education, administration of nursing services, and nursing practice are listed below.

Nursing Research Guidelines

The guidelines for nursing research based on the Self-Care Framework, which were constructed from Banfield (1998), Geden (1985, p. 265), Orem (2001), and Smith (1979), are:

- Purpose of the research
  - The purpose of Self-Care Framework-based nursing research is to develop knowledge for the practical

sciences of nursing, including *theoretically or speculatively practical sciences* and *practically practical science*. The knowledge gained from the *theoretically* or *speculatively practical sciences* brings unity and meaning to the universe of action of a practice field and to its elements. This kind of knowledge encompasses concepts and theories. The six speculatively or theoretically practical nursing sciences include *three nursing practice sciences* (wholly compensatory nursing science, partly compensatory nursing science, and supportive-developmental nursing science) and *three foundational nursing sciences* (the science of self-care, the science of the development and exercise of self-care agency in the absence or presence of limitations for deliberate action, and the science of human assistance for persons with health-associated self-care deficits). The knowledge gained from *practically practical science* deals with the details of cases, but always within the universal conceptualizations of the practice field, including its domain, elements, and types of results sought. This kind of knowledge encompasses the rules and standards of practice, the knowledge necessary for taking action.

- Phenomena of interest
  - Specific variables that make up nursing knowledge from the perspective of the Self-Care Framework are in the categories of basic conditioning factors, self-care practices, self-care requisites, health state, health results sought, the therapeutic self-care demand, self-care deficits, nursing requirements, health focus, nursing situations, nursing systems, nursing technologies, ways of assisting, and outcomes of nursing.

- Problems to be studied
  - The precise problems to be studied are those that reflect actual or predictable self-care or dependent-care deficits.

- Study participants
  - Study participants are the individuals and multiperson units who are considered legitimate patients of nurses, that is, people with deficit relationships between their current or projected capability for providing self-care or dependent- care and the qualitative and quantitative demand for care due to the health state or health-care needs of those requiring care.

- Research methods
  - Data may be collected from individuals and multiperson units in the person's home, in hospitals, clinics, and resident-care facilities, and in various other settings in which nursing occurs, using one or more Self-Care Framework-based research instruments (see Table 8–2).

- Descriptive, descriptive-correlational, case study, and quasi-experimental methods associated with the empiricist research paradigm are most consistent with Orem's Self-Care Framework. Furthermore, ethnographic, grounded theory, and phenomenological methods associated with the interpretive research paradigm may be consistent with Orem's theory. In contrast, methods associated with the critical theory research paradigm, "have limited [usefulness] for the development of the practical science of nursing" (Banfield, 1998, p. 178) related to the Self-Care Framework, due to the focus of that paradigm on emancipation of the study participants "from the ideologies that function to constrain or oppress them" (p. 152), as well as to the fact that Orem does not address such major issues in the critical theory paradigm as power, control, and domination. Other guidelines for research designs and procedures remain to be developed.

- Data analysis
  - Definitive guidelines for data analysis techniques remain to be developed.

- Contributions
  - Self-Care Framework-based research findings enhance understanding of patient and nurse variables that affect the exercise of continuing therapeutic self-care and dependent-care.

Nursing Education Guidelines

The guidelines for nursing education based on the Self-Care Framework, which were constructed from Orem (1991, 1995, 1997, 2001), Riehl-Sisca (1985a), and Taylor (1985a, 1985b), are:

- Focus of the curriculum
  - The distinctive focus of the curriculum is the Self-Care Framework and associated theories. Self-Care Framework-based curricula prepare *nursing practitioners* at the entry and advanced levels of professional nursing practice. A *nursing practitioner* is a person professionally educated and qualified to practice nursing and who is engaged in its provision. A *nursing practitioner* is *not* the same as a *nurse practitioner*, who is a nurse with a technical to technological level of preparation for performing selected tasks of managing certain subsystems of operations traditionally within the domain of medical practice.

- Nature and sequence of content
  - Nursing course content is based on the understanding of nursing as a practical science, with speculatively

or theoretically practical and practically practical components.

- Professional nursing component course content encompasses components of self-care, dependent-care, self-care agency, dependent-care agency, self-care deficits, dependent-care deficits; the social system, interpersonal system, and professional-technological system dimensions of nursing agency; and elements of the wholly compensatory, partly compensatory, and supportive-educative nursing systems, including methods of helping.

- Nursing practicum courses provide experiential knowledge of social and interpersonal situations; opportunities for development of the social and interpersonal skills needed to work with adults and children individually and in multiperson units; and opportunities for the development of personal knowledge arising from direct insights into self and others in personal relationships.

- Other nursing courses address nursing as a field of knowledge and practice, including nursing's domain and boundaries as defined by the proper object of nursing, nursing's social field, the profession and occupation of nursing, nursing jurisprudence, nursing ethics, and nursing economics.

- Nursing courses are not to be based on content primarily from the biologic, behavioral, and medical sciences.

- The curriculum also requires a preprofessional component, with courses addressing the arts and humanities, the history of health care and nursing in western and eastern civilizations, languages and cultural elements of specific cultural groups, foundational and basic sciences (such as human physiology, environmental physiology, and pathology), and applied medical and public health sciences.

- Programs of professional nursing education follow a sequence of a preprofessional component, a professional component, and a continuing education component.
  - Undergraduate nursing education focuses on the operations of information giving and acquiring, reflection on the information received, making some judgments, and problem solving.
  - At the master's level, emphasis is placed on acquiring specialized areas of information, increasing abilities to reflect and make judgments, and developing some facility with the operations of investigation and meaning.
  - At the doctoral level, emphasis is placed on the advanced understanding of the operations of investigation and meaning.
  - Continuing professional education focuses on content that will help nursing practitioners to maintain currency with scientific and technological developments, guidelines for nursing practice, changes in health service needs of populations, and relevant environmental and social conditions associated with needs for changes in nursing practice.

- Settings for nursing education
  - Professional nursing education occurs in senior colleges and universities.

- Characteristics of students
  - Students interested in professional nursing education have to meet requirements for admission to senior colleges or universities.
  - Nursing students must have the ability to achieve mastery "of a general comprehensive [conceptual model] of nursing [so that they will] become able to maintain awareness of the relationship between what they know and what they do as nursing practitioners" (Orem, 1991, p. 339). Nursing students also must have the ability to develop themselves as persons who can (1) establish contacts, negotiate agreements, and maintain contacts with persons who need nursing and those who seek it for them; (2) interact and communicate with persons under nursing and their significant others, with other nurses and caregivers under ranges of conditions and circumstances that facilitate or hinder interactions and communication; (3) direct interactions and communications toward the development of interpersonal and functional unities; (4) perform with increasing developing skills professional-technological operations of nursing, including observation, reasoning, judgment and decision making, and production of practical results in interpersonal and group situations; (5) seek nursing consultation as needed with respect to the professional-technological operations of nursing; and (6) maintain a dynamic sense of duty in all nursing practice situations.

- Teaching-learning strategies
  - Teaching-learning strategies are predicated on the assumption that the faculty understand the Self-Care Framework and have the required skills in its use.
  - Students are presented initially with an overview of the structure of the framework. Then, as students progress through the educational program, specific linkages can be made between the framework and new content. By the completion of the program, the student should have seen the overall structure of the Self-Care Framework, examined its elements in detail, related the elements back to the overall framework, and applied the framework in practice settings.

- Students' abilities to process information develop by starting with more concrete elements of the Self-Care Framework, such as self-care requisites and basic conditioning factors, and progressing to more abstract elements, such as the power components.
- Faculty should develop nursing systems for various situations that students can use as examples. Faculty should provide opportunities for students to test nursing systems and to reflect on their efficacy for particular patients.

Administration of Nursing Services Guidelines

Guidelines for the administration of nursing services based on the Self-Care Framework, which were constructed from Orem (1989, 1991, 1995, 2001), are:

- Focus of nursing in the health-care institution
  - The general focus of Self-Care Framework-based nursing administration is "the complement of persons for whom a health service agency has contracted to or in the process of contracting to provide nursing or agrees to admit on an ad hoc basis for purposes of receiving nursing (and other health services)" (Orem, 2001, p. 458).
  - The distinctive focus of Self-Care Framework-based nursing services is to provide regulatory nursing care to individuals with health-derived or health-associated self-care deficits.
- Purpose of nursing services
  - The purpose of nursing services is to help people to enhance their abilities to provide continuing, therapeutic self-care and dependent-care.
- Characteristics of nursing personnel
  - Nursing personnel include nurses, nursing practitioners, and nursing administrators.
  - Nurses are women and men prepared either through high-level technical education or professional level education. Nurses prepared through high-level technical education work with nursing practitioners or work under established nursing protocols.
  - Nursing practitioners are professionally educated nurses working at the entry or advanced level of nursing practice.
  - Nursing administrators are "persons who function in situational contexts to collectively manage courses of affairs enabling for the provision of nursing to the population currently served by an organized health service institution or agency and to populations to be served at future times" (Orem, 2001, p. 451).

- Settings for nursing services
  - Nursing services are located in many different settings. "Nurses may go to where patients are, in their homes, in hospitals, or other types of resident-care institutions. Or patients may come to clinics or other types of facilities where nurses are available to provide nursing" (Orem, 1989, p. 56).
- Management strategies and administrative policies
  - One managerial task is "the proper ordering of persons and material resources so that a functioning whole is continuously created as organizational members fulfill their positional role responsibilities" (Orem, 1989, p. 61). Managerial work operations associated with that task include (1) setting objectives in relation to the population to be served and to the health-care enterprise; (2) analyzing and organizing work to achieve objectives; (3) establishing standards for selection of nurses, assistants to nurses, and other support personnel; (4) motivating and communicating with nursing personnel; (5) producing designs for measuring performance of nursing care; and (6) measuring performance of nursing practice and using the results for the entire nursing department and its component parts.
  - Another managerial task is "to ensure that the current decisions and actions incorporate or are in harmony with future requirements of the enterprise" (Orem, 1989, p. 61). Managerial work operations associated with that task include (1) establishing and using standards and criteria for selection of individuals for operational and managerial positions; (2) identifying costs of continuing operations and sources of capital to finance them; (3) identifying new operational methods or extension of current methods; and (4) developing self and others within as managers.

Nursing Practice Guidelines

Guidelines for nursing practice based on the Self-Care Framework, which were constructed from Orem (1991, 1995, 2001), are:

- Purpose of nursing practice
  - The distinctive purpose of Self-Care Framework-based nursing practice is to help individuals and multiperson units who seek and can benefit from nursing because of the presence of existent or predicted health-derived or health-related self-care or dependent-care deficits.
  - The domain of nursing practice encompasses five areas of activity: (1) entering into and maintaining nurse-patient relationships with individuals, families, or groups until patients can legitimately be discharged

from nursing; (2) determining if and how patients can be helped through nursing; (3) responding to patients' requests, desires, and needs for nurse contacts and assistance; (4) prescribing, providing, and regulating direct help to patients (and their significant others) in the form of nursing; and (5) coordinating and integrating nursing with the patient's daily living, other health care needed or being received, and social and educational services needed or being received (Orem, 1991, p. 340).

- Practice problems of interest
  - Practice problems of interest are the individuals' self-care deficits and dependent-care deficits. Those problems occur when the health focus is people across the life cycle, people in recovery, people with illnesses of undetermined origin, people with genetic and developmental defects or biologic immaturity, people experiencing cure or regulation of disease, people experiencing stabilization of integrated functioning, people whose quality of life is irreversibly affected, and people who have a terminal illness.

- Settings for nursing practice
  - Nursing practice occurs in diverse settings, including people's homes, neighborhoods, group residential facilities, meeting places of various community-based groups, ambulatory clinics, rehabilitation and nursing home facilities, and tertiary medical centers.

- Characteristics of legitimate participants in nursing practice
  - An adult requires nursing when he or she does not have the ability to continuously maintain the amount and quality of self-care that is therapeutic in sustaining life and health, in recovering from disease or injury, or in coping with their effects. A child requires nursing when his or her parent or guardian cannot continuously maintain the amount and quality of care that is therapeutic.

- Nursing process
  - The nursing process for the Self-Care Framework is Orem's **Professional-Technological Operations of Nursing Practice.** The components of the process are case management operations, diagnostic operations, prescriptive operations, regulatory operations, and control operations (see Table 8–1).

- Contributions of nursing practice to participants' well-being
  - Self-Care Framework-based nursing practice contributes to the well-being of nursing participants by regulating self-care agency or dependent-care agency and meeting the therapeutic self-care demand.

LOGICAL CONGRUENCE

The Self-Care Framework is logically congruent. The content of the Self-Care Framework flows directly from Orem's philosophical claims. Just one world view—reciprocal interaction—is evident. Smith (1987) claimed that Orem's work "fits with the totality paradigm" (p. 97). To the extent that the totality paradigm reflects the reaction world view or even a bridge between the reaction and reciprocal interaction world views, there is no evidence of the reaction world view in the content of Orem's Self-Care Framework.

Furthermore, although the Self-Care Framework has been classified as a systems model (Riehl & Roy, 1980) and an interaction model (Riehl-Sisca, 1989), its classification as a developmental model, with no evidence of the characteristics of other categories of knowledge, is supported.

GENERATION OF THEORY

Orem views the **Theory of Self-Care,** the **Theory of Self-Care Deficit,** and the **Theory of Nursing System** as the constituent elements of the more general Self-Care Deficit Nursing Theory, that is, what is referred to in this chapter as the Self-Care Framework. Accordingly, an attempt was made to incorporate the three theories into the analysis of the framework. That attempt yielded a cumbersome and confusing structure. Consequently, the decision was made to treat the broad concepts of Patient, Therapeutic Self-Care Demand, Self-Care, Dependent-Care, Self-Care Agency, Self-Care Agent, Dependent-Care Agency, Dependent-Care Agent, Basic Conditioning Factors, Power Component, Self-Care Deficit, Dependent-Care Deficit, Environmental Features, Health State, Well-Being, and Nursing Agency as the concepts of the Self-Care Framework, and to discuss the central ideas and propositions of the three theories here. Continued refinement of Orem's work is required to clarify its structure with regard to the conceptual and theoretical elements.

An analysis of the **Theory of Self-Care,** the **Theory of Self-Care Deficit,** and the **Theory of Nursing System** revealed that each one may be regarded as a grand theory. The decision to classify the three theories as grand theories was based on Orem's (2001) comments that the propositions of each theory are not logically related but represent suggested guides for the formulation of hypotheses and the further development of that theory, as well as on an analysis of several studies that were guided by Orem's work. For example, Moore and her colleagues have conducted a series of studies that were guided explicitly by the Theory of Self-Care Deficit and yielded successive refinements of a middle-range theory of the relation between concepts representing the basic conditioning factors and concepts representing the self-care agency and dependent-care agency of school-age children and their mothers (Gaffney & Moore, 1996; Moore, 1993; Moore & Mosher, 1997; Mosher & Moore, 1998). In addition, McQuiston and Campbell (1997) presented an explicit conceptual-theoretical-empirical structure for a study that tested hypotheses derived from the Theory of Self-Care Deficit proposition asserting that the basic conditioning factors are associated with individuals' abilities to engage in self-care or dependent-care.

The central idea, concepts, and propositions of each theory are given here. The central idea of the **Theory of Self-Care** is that "Self-care is a human regulatory function that individuals must, with deliberation, perform for themselves or have performed for them (dependent-care) to supply and maintain a supply of materials and conditions to maintain life; to keep physical and psychic functioning and development within norms compatible with conditions essential for life; and for integrity of functioning and development" (Orem, 2001, p. 143). The concepts of the theory are: **Self-Care, Dependent-Care, Universal Self-Care Requisites,** and **Power Components**—Self-Care Agency Power Components dimension. The concept definitions are the same as the corresponding concepts of the Self-Care Framework. The propositions of the Theory of Self-Care are:

- Propositions: Set One
  - The materials continuously provided or sustained through self-care or dependent-care are materials essential for life, namely air, water, and food (Orem, 2001, p. 144).
  - Conditions that are provided or maintained through self-care or dependent-care are concerned with safe engagement in human excretory functions, sanitary disposal of human excrements, personal hygienic care, maintenance of normal body temperature, protection from environmental and self-imposed hazards, and what is needed for unhampered physical, cognitional, emotional, interpersonal, and social developments and functioning of individuals in their life situations (Orem, 2001, p. 144).
  - The quality and quantity of materials and the conditions provided or sustained through self-care or dependent-care must be within a range that is known to be compatible with what is biologically required for human life, for integrity of human development, and for integrity of human structure and function (Orem, 2001, p. 144).
  - Self-care or dependent-care performed by persons with the intention of doing good for self or others may fall short of the focal conditions and goals sought because of their lack of knowledge and skills or other action limitations (Orem, 2001, p. 144).

- Propositions: Set Two
  - Engagement in self-care or dependent-care involves performance of operations to estimate or establish what can and should be done, to decide what will be done and the operations to produce care (Orem, 2001, p. 144).
  - Self-care or dependent-care is work or labor that requires time, expenditure of energy, financial resources, and continued willingness of persons to engage in the operations of self-care or dependent-care (Orem, 2001, p. 144).
  - Self-care or dependent-care performed over time can be understood (intellectualized) as an action system (self-care system, dependent-care system) whenever there is valid and reliable information about care measures performed and the connecting links among them (Orem, 2001, p. 144).
  - Care measures selected and performed in self-care and dependent-care are specified by the technologies or methods selected for use to meet known or estimated requirements for regulation of functioning or development (self-care requisites). When this is understood and skills are developed, care measures become performance habits (Orem, 2001, p. 144).

The central idea of the **Theory of Self-Care Deficit** is that "Requirements of persons for nursing are associated with the subjectivity of mature and maturing persons to health-derived or health care–related action limitations associated with their own or their dependents' health states that render them completely or partially unable to know existent and emerging requisites for regulatory care for themselves or their dependents and to engage in the continuing performance of care measures to control or in some way manage factors that are regulatory of their own or their dependents' functioning and development" (Orem, 2001, p. 146). The concepts of the Theory of Self-Care Deficit are **Self-Care Agency, Power Components**—Self-Care Agency Power Components dimension, **Dependent-Care Agency, Basic Conditioning Factors, Therapeutic Self-Care De-mand, Self-Care Deficit, Dependent-Care Deficit, Nursing Agency,** and **Methods of Helping**. The concept definitions are the same as the corresponding concepts of the Self-Care Framework. The propositions of the theory are:

- Persons who take action to provide their own self-care or care for dependents have specialized capabilities for action (Orem, 2001, p. 147).
- Individuals' abilities to engage in self-care or dependent-care are conditioned by age, developmental state, life experience, sociocultural orientation, health, and available resources (Orem, 2001, p. 147).
- Relationship of individuals' abilities for self-care or

dependent-care to the qualitative and quantitative self-care or dependent-care demand can be determined when the value of each is known (Orem, 2001, p. 147).

- The relationship between care abilities and care demand can be defined in terms of *equal to, less than,* and *more than* (Orem, 2001, p. 147).
- Nursing is a legitimate service when (1) care abilities are less than those required for meeting a known self-care demand (a deficit relationship); and (2) self-care or dependent-care abilities exceed or are equal to those required for meeting the current self-care demand, but a future deficit relationship can be foreseen because of predictable decreases in care abilities, qualitative or quantitative increases in the care demand, or both (Orem, 2001, p. 147).
- Persons with existing or projected care deficits are in, or can expect to be in, states of social dependency that legitimate a nursing relationship (Orem, 2001, p. 147).
- A self-care deficit may be relatively permanent or it may be transitory (Orem, 2001, p. 147).
- A self-care or a dependent-care deficit may be wholly or partially eliminated or overcome when persons with deficits have the necessary human capabilities, dispositions, and willingness (Orem, 2001, p. 147).
- Self-care deficits, when expressed in terms of persons' limitations for engagement in the estimative (intentional) or production operations of self-care, provide guides for selection of methods of helping and understanding patient roles in self-care (Orem, 2001, p. 147).

The central idea of the **Theory of Nursing System** is that "All action systems that are nursing systems are formed (designed and produced) by nurses for legitimate recipients of nursing by exercising their powers of nursing agency. These systems compensate for or overcome existent or emerging health-derived or health-associated limitations of the recipients' powers of self-care agency or dependent-care agency in meeting their own or their dependents' known, existent, or projected therapeutic self-care demands in relatively stable or changing life situations. Nursing systems may be produced for individuals, for persons who constitute a dependent-care unit, for groups whose members have therapeutic self-care demands with similar components or who have similar limitations for engagement in self-care or dependent-care, or for families or for other multiperson units" (Orem, 2001, p. 148). The concepts of the Theory of Nursing System are **Patient, Therapeutic Self-Care Demand, Self-Care Agency, Dependent-Care Agency, Nursing Agency**—Professional-Technological System and Interpersonal System dimensions, and **Power Components**—Nursing Agency Power Components dimension. The concept definitions are the same as the corresponding concepts of the Self-Care Framework. The propositions of the theory are:

- Legitimate recipients of nursing are persons, as individuals or members of groups, with powers of self-care agency or dependent-care agency that are rendered totally or partially inadequate by their own or their dependents' states of health or by the nature of health care requirements (Orem, 2001, p. 148).
- In the design and production of the nursing system, nurses seek and confirm information needed to make judgments about the components (some or all) of therapeutic self-care demands and powers of self-care agency or dependent-care agency of persons under their care (Orem, 2001, p. 148).
- The compensatory nature of nursing systems for individuals in their time-place localizations is specified by the immediacy of their need to meet components of their therapeutic self-care demands and by their existent inabilities for taking the required kinds of action (Orem, 2001, p. 148).
- The action limitation overcoming nature of nursing systems is specified by persons' limitations of self-care agency that can be overcome by learning, by skill development and exercise, and by developing, enhancing, or adjusting skills in self-direction and self-management (Orem, 2001, p. 148).
- The structure of nursing systems vary with what legitimate recipients of nursing can and cannot do in knowing and meeting their own or their dependents' therapeutic self-care demands and in overcoming existent or projected action limitations (Orem, 2001, p. 148).
- The structure, content, and results of nursing systems in operation in concrete life situations vary with nurses' developed powers of nursing agency, with their willingness to exercise these powers, and with factors internal to nurses or with external circumstances and conditions that facilitate or impede nurses' exercise of their powers of nursing agency (Orem, 2001, p. 149).
- The linkages of nursing systems (as here described) to more encompassing interpersonal systems vary with the powers of legitimate recipients of nursing to interact and communicate with nurses and with nurses' powers of interaction and communication (Orem, 2001, p. 149).

Orem (1989) also developed a rudimentary **General Theory of Nursing Administration**. This theory also may be regarded as a grand theory. The propositions of the theory are:

- All actions that are proper to nursing administration are actions that are produced by persons with foreknowledge of: (1) nursing as a field of knowledge and practice, (2) the purpose or mission of the institution of which they are an organic part, (3) how nursing contributes to mission fulfillment, and (4) the domain and boundaries of their received powers to manage courses of affairs that ensure the continuing provision of nursing to populations served (Orem, 1989, p. 57).

- All actions that are proper to nursing administration regardless of situational location have a sequential order related to the purposes and the forms of the actions (Orem, 1989, pp. 57–58).
- Courses of action to provide continuous descriptions from a nursing perspective of populations to be provided with nursing are prior to courses of action to provide continuous calculation of what is required to provide nursing to the populations served at this time and at future times (Orem, 1989, p. 58).
- These two courses of action are prior to and provide the substructure or foundation for as well as the linkages with the continuous management of all courses of affairs that ensure the continuing availability and provision of nursing to present and future populations served by the institution (Orem, 1989, p. 58).

Dependent care is, of course, a concept of the Self-Care Framework. Until recently, however, little work had been done beyond defining the concept. Development of the Theory of Dependent-Care is a major contribution to understanding the concept (Taylor et al., 2001). The theory, which is regarded as parallel with Orem's Theory of Self-Care, proposes that:

- Responsible maturing and mature persons initiate and perform care activities, termed DC [dependent care], on behalf of socially dependent persons.
- This care is provided for some period of time on a continuing or intermittent basis.
- The purposes of DC are meeting the TSCD [therapeutic self-care demand] of the dependent, promoting development through the period of dependency, providing materials to sustain life, maintaining or developing positive relationships during the period of dependency, supporting the individual through period of dependency, and in some instances, facilitating peaceful death.
- [The purposes of DC are [accomplished] through the DC agent meeting the SC [self-care] requisites and/or regulating the exercise or development of SCA [self-care agency].
- DC is provided in response to a dependent care demand (DCD) through a system consisting of the actions of two or more persons, including the person in a state of social dependency unable to meet his or her own requirements for SC and one or more responsible persons or DC agents (Taylor et al., 2001, p. 41)

Another theory derived from the Self-Care Framework is the Middle-Range Theory of Testicular Self-Examination (Fessenden, 2003). That theory proposes that social support, age, health state, socioeconomic status, family influence on health behavior, and optimism are related to

self-care agency; that self-care agency is related to decisional balance and self-efficacy for testicular self-examination; and that decisional balance and self-efficacy for testicular self-examination are related to performance of testicular self-examination. A test of the theory with a sample of 167 men yielded evidence of its empirical adequacy.

CREDIBILITY OF THE NURSING MODEL

Social Utility

The social utility of the Self-Care Framework is extremely well documented. Orem (2001) noted that "nurses provide help or care in the form of nursing for persons of different ages, in different stages of development, in different health states, and in different time-place localizations" (p. 357). The framework and theories are being used by nurses to guide research and practice throughout the United States and in Mexico, Brazil, Canada, Belgium, The Netherlands, Germany, Switzerland, Norway, Finland, Denmark, Sweden, Australia, Thailand, and Japan. Books related to the Self-Care Framework of nursing have been published by Munley and Sayers (1984), Riehl-Sisca (1985c), and Dennis (1997).

In addition, the Self-Care Framework and the theories of Self-Care Deficit, Self-Care, and Nursing System have been the focus of many institutes and national and international nursing conferences. The annual Summer Self-Care Deficit Nursing Theory Institutes, sponsored by the School of Nursing at the University of Missouri-Columbia, were held from 1984 to 1992. The Fall Self-Care Deficit Nursing Theory Conferences, also sponsored by the School of Nursing at the University of Missouri-Columbia, were held from 1982 to 1988. The biennial International Self-Care Deficit Nursing Theory Conferences began in 1989. In recent years, the international conferences have been sponsored by the Sinclair School of Nursing at the University of Missouri-Columbia and the International Orem Society for Nursing Science and Scholarship. Those conferences, which have attracted large audiences of nurses from many countries, have been held in the United States, Belgium, Thailand, and Germany.

Before using the Self-Care Framework, considerable study is required to fully understand its unique focus and content. Nurses and nursing students have to learn the particular "style of thinking and communicating nursing" (Orem, 2001, p. 137) that is reflected in the Self-Care Framework. The framework has an extensive and relatively unique vocabulary that requires mastery for full understanding of its content. Foster and Bennett (2002) pointed out that the "magnitude of terms ... can be very confusing initially until the essence of each concept is understood" (p. 148). Orem and Taylor (1986) explained that "the terminology used to name the elements of the [framework] and the theories and their elements has its origin in the language traditionally used to describe and explain deliberate result-seeking action of human beings" (p. 49). Thus familiarity with the language of the theories of deliberate human action enhances understanding of Orem's work. In particular, "nurses must understand the actions that constitute self-care and dependent-care, as well as the capabilities that are enabling for performing these kinds of actions" (Orem, 1991, p. 145). Furthermore, the vocabulary of the Self-Care Framework reflects Orem's distinctive view of those features of Individuals and Multiperson Units that are specific to nursing. It is clear that even though Orem's terminology is at times obtuse, her work has overcome the handicap represented by "the lack of a nursing language … in nurses' communications about nursing to the public as well as to persons with whom they work in the health field" (Orem, 1997, p. 29). Confusion about the meaning and measurement of each concept of the Self-Care Framework, which has been noted in the past (Anna et al., 1978; Foster & Janssens, 1985), has decreased as appropriate research instruments and practice tools become available (see Table 8–2).

The use of the Self-Care Framework requires understanding of the preprofessional and professional components of nursing. Understanding the relations between the social, interpersonal, and professional-technological systems of nursing agency also is required. Furthermore, nurses must develop "the diagnostic skill to identify the self-care deficits of adult patients in meeting their current or projected therapeutic self-care demands. A related diagnostic skill [to be developed] is that of determining the infant or child care or dependent adult care competencies of responsible adults who seek nursing for socially dependent family members" (Orem, 2001, p. 251). Most of all, "nurses must be knowledgeable about and skilled in investigating and calculating individuals' therapeutic self-care demands, in determining the degrees of operability of self-care agency, and in estimating persons' potential for regulation of the exercise or development of their powers of self-care agency" (Orem, 1997, p. 27).

The implementation of Self-Care Framework-based nursing practice is feasible for patients of virtually all ages who are found in diverse practice situations ranging from health promotion practices to critical care units (Foster & Bennett, 2002; Young, Taylor, & Renpenning, 2001). Indeed, Foster and Bennett (2002) declared that the Self-Care Framework "applies to all of those who need nursing care" (p. 144). The framework may not, however, be appropriate for use in special hospitals for the criminally insane. Mason and Chandley (1990) pointed out that the framework "produces a fundamental conflict between the patient and society according to the clash of values embroiled with the special hospital setting" (p. 670).

Taylor (1990) noted that the implementation of Self-Care Framework-based nursing practice requires consideration of "the philosophy, goals, and objectives; the standards and quality assurance program; and the documentation, job description, and personnel evaluation systems" of the institution (p. 65). The array of human and material resources required for such an undertaking are evident in the comprehensive plans for the implementation of Self-Care Framework-based nursing practice described by Nunn and Marriner-Tomey (1989) and by Fernandez, Hebert, and Bliss-Holtz (1996). The strategies that can be used to implement the Self-Care Framework in nursing practice settings, which are taken from recommendations and suggestions given by Nunn and Marriner-Tomey (1989), Fernandez et al. (1996), Hooten (1992), and Paternostro (1992), are presented here.

- **Phase 1: Identification (2–8 months).** In this phase, various conceptual models of nursing are reviewed and the decision is made to select the Self-Care Framework. In addition, a nursing care delivery model that has built-in accountability is selected. Primary nursing or collaborative practice is regarded as appropriate for use with the Self-Care Framework. Team nursing also could be effective if a permanent team leader can assure continuity and accountability for care; however, neither team nursing with rotating team leaders nor functional nursing is effective.

- **Phase 2: Education (2–4 years).** All members of the nursing department are educated so that they have a clear understanding of the focus and content of the Self-Care Framework. Education is initially directed to the key people, including the nurse administrators, nurse educators, and quality assurance staff. At this point, a show of support by the nurse administrators can be demonstrated by hiring a consultant and sponsoring a retreat devoted to the framework. Next, education spreads to the staff nurses. Then the key people participate with the staff nurses in the development of plans for implementation and provide leadership in revisions of the nursing philosophy, objectives of nursing service, care plans, standards of care, and evaluation mechanisms. Development of new practice tools or any needed modifications in existing practice tools for use in the particular health-care institution is undertaken. As education of key people and staff nurses continues, the Self-Care Framework is introduced to the health-care workers who are responsible for services external to nursing, including but not limited to the hospital administrator, physicians, physical therapists, occupational therapists, and respiratory therapists. If the institution is affiliated with one or more schools of nursing, the faculty is informed that Self-Care Framework-based nursing practice is being implemented. In addition, the Self-Care Framework is introduced to patients and key community members. Throughout the education phase, articles about the framework could be published in the health-care institution's newsletter

- **Phase 3: Transition (4–6 years).** A pilot unit is selected to begin the implementation of the framework. Staff on the pilot unit are prepared for the transition to the Self-Care Framework by means of structured classes, reading assignments, and discussion groups. The Self-Care Framework then is implemented on other units. The transition phase could be launched with an "Orem Day" celebration, which could be in the form of a conference keynoted by a well-known nurse and a demonstration of a Self-Care Framework-based computer software package.
- **Phase 4: Implementation (6–8 years).** Practice tools are refined and the Self-Care Framework is fully operational throughout the nursing department and changes in nursing practice and patient outcomes are evident. Staff nurses practice nursing according to the Self-Care Framework, and true integration of the framework begins to occur. A Self-Care Framework-based computerized documentation system should be used to encourage and facilitate continued efforts after the Self-Care Framework is incorporated into daily nursing practice.
- **Phase 5: Evaluation.** Although evaluation is dynamic and ongoing, a formal, systematic evaluation of the implementation project is undertaken after completion of the implementation phase. At the patient level, evaluation includes patient and family teaching accomplished, patient and family understanding, goal attainment, progress or lack of progress toward patient goals, and discharge planning to support continuing care after discharge where necessary. Patient and family satisfaction are measured through the use of a questionnaire at the time of discharge. Patient outcomes are evaluated at the time of discharge and thereafter. At the unit level, nurse and physician satisfaction are measured. At the unit and nursing departmental levels, changes in nursing practice and movement toward full integration of the Self-Care Framework are evaluated. The ultimate product of evaluation is further refinement of the Self-Care Framework as a guide for nursing practice.

Wagnild, Rodriguez, and Pritchett's (1987) survey yielded factors that enhanced and inhibited the use of the Self-Care Framework by graduates of a baccalaureate program that was based on the framework. Use of the framework was enhanced in practice settings that encouraged self-care, prioritized early discharge planning, subscribed to a whole person concept of care, and placed a high expectation on patient teaching. Factors that inhibited use included time constraints, inability to adapt the framework to the prac-

tice setting, and difficulties in communicating with other staff nurses due to the terminology of the framework, along with patient preferences for dependence on the nurse and lack of interest in self-care.

Implementation of the Self-Care Framework, like any conceptual model of nursing, can occur at the level of the nursing unit or the entire health-care organization. Taylor (1990) noted that implementation of the Self-Care Framework at the unit rather than the organization level "works well when units are decentralized and relatively independent" (p. 65).

Nursing Research. Nursing research is the "careful, systematic study and investigation within a field of knowledge [i.e., nursing] of unanswered questions and hypothesized answers to them" (Orem, 2001, p. 521). Following the cautionary words of Orem and Taylor (1986), an attempt was made to locate published reports of nursing research that were based on Orem's approach to self-care rather than self-care in a general sense. The utility of the Self-Care Framework for nursing research is documented by a large number of studies that meet this criterion.

Published reports of the several research instruments that have been developed to measure concepts of the Self-Care Framework in diverse populations are listed in Table 8–2. Many of the research instruments now available measure patients' or nurses' perceptions of the patient's self-care agency or actual self-care or dependent-care activities performed by patients. Some of these instruments are appropriate for people of various ages with diverse health conditions; others are for particular populations or people of a particular age. In addition, some instruments are appropriate for populations in various countries.

Published reports of the plethora of Self-Care Framework-based descriptive, correlational, and experimental studies that have been conducted are listed in Table 8–3. And, as can be seen in the Doctoral Dissertations and Master's Theses sections of the chapter bibliography on the CD-ROM, numerous master's and doctoral students have used the Self-Care Framework to guide their research. Another master's thesis, not published in Master's Abstracts International, was conducted by Shanks (2001).

Descriptive studies guided by the Self-Care Framework have focused on the meaning of self-care, the level of patients' self-care agency, or the number and kind of self-care behaviors performed by diverse populations. Several of the correlational studies have examined variables associated with the exercise of self-care agency. Experimental studies have tested the effects of Self-Care Framework–based nursing interventions on various patient outcomes. Although much of the Self-Care Framework-based research is limited to a single study on a single topic (Taylor et al., 2000), an impressive amount of programmatic research has been

(Text continues on page 284)

Instrument and Citation*	Description
RESEARCH INSTRUMENTS	
Exercise of Self-Care Agency Scale (Kearey & Fleischer, 1979; McBride, 1987, 1991; Riesch & Hauck, 1988; Robichaud-Ekstrand & Loiselle, 1998; Whetstone, 1987; Whetstone & Hansson, 1989; Yamashita, 1998; Young et al., 2001)	Measures the patient's self-care agency in United States, French, Swedish, East German, and Japanese populations.
Perception of Self-Care Agency Questionnaire (Hanson, 1981; Bickel, 1982; Hanson & Bickel, 1985; Weaver, 1987; Bottorff, 1988; Cleveland, 1989; McBride, 1991; Young et al., 2001)	Measures adults' perception of their self-care agency; items reflect the 10 power components. May not be appropriate for use with older adults.
Children's Self-Care Performance Questionnaire (Mosher & Moore, 1998; Young et al., 2001)	Measures performance of self-care activities in the areas of universal, developmental, and health-deviation self-care requisites by children with cancer.
Child and Adolescent Self-Care Practice Questionnaire (Moore, 1995; Moore & Mosher, 1997; Young et al., 2001)	Measures children's and adolescents' performance of self-care activities in the areas of universal, developmental, and health-deviation self-care requisites.
Dependent Care Agency Questionnaire (Moore & Gaffney, 1989; Young et al., 2001)	Measures mothers' performance of their children's self-care activities.
Denyes Self-Care Agency Scale (DSCAI) (Denyes, 1980, 1982; Gaut & Kieckhefer, 1988; McBride, 1991; Young et al., 2001)	Measures adolescents' self-care agency.
Denyes Self-Care Practice Instrument (DSCPI) (Denyes 1980, 1988; Gast et al., 1989; Young et al., 2001)	Measures self-care actions taken by adolescents.
Self-As-Carer Inventory (SCI) (Geden & Taylor, 1991; Lukkarinen & Hentinen, 1994; Young et al., 1002)	Measures perceived capacity to care for self in diverse ethnic groups, including American Indians, Asian/Pacific Islanders, Hispanics, Black, and White populations residing in the United States, as well as Finnish patients scheduled for coronary artery bypass graft surgery.
Heart Failure Self-Care Behavior Scale (Artinian et al., 2002; Jaarsma et al., 2000)	Measures heart failure-related self-care activities.
Self-Care Agency Inventory (Lantz et al., 1995)	Measures enactment of self-care; scores identify those who and who will not enact self-care due to lack of knowledge or lack of motivation
Maieutic Dimensions of Self-Care Agency (O'Connor, 1995)	Measures selected capabilities and dispositions foundational to self-care agency.
Self-Care Limitations Tool (Beech et al., 1996)	Measures limitations in self-care.
Appraisal of Self-Care Agency Scale (ASA-A Form) (ASA-B Form) (van Achterberg et al., 1991; Evers, et al., 1993; Fok et al., 2002; Halfens et al., 1999; Lorensen et al., 1993; Söderhamn & Cliffordson, 2001; Söderhamn, Ek et al., 1996; Söderhamn, Evers et al., 1996; Söderhamn, Lindencrona et al., 1996; Sonninen, 1999; Young et al., 2001)	Measures self-reported (ASA-A Form) and nurse-reported (ASA-B Form) self-care agency of elderly populations in the United States, The Netherlands, Norway, Denmark, Finland, Sweden, and Hong Kong, China.

*See the Research Instruments and Practice Tools section in the chapter references for complete citations.

(continued)

Instrument and Citation	Description
RESEARCH INSTRUMENTS	
Lorensen's Self-Care Capability Scale (LSCS) (Lorensen, 1998)	Measures the degree of the elderly person's self-care capability to manage everyday life; items represent the universal, developmental, and health-deviation self-care requisites.
Mental Health Related Self-Care Agency Scale (West & Isenberg, 1997; Young et al., 2001)	Measures individuals' capabilities to perform mental health–related self-care.
Self-Care Ability Scale for the Elderly (Söderhamn, Ek, et al., 1996; Söderhamn, Lindencrona et al., 1996)	Measures perceived self-care ability of elderly individuals.
Biggs Elderly Self-Care Assessment Tool (BESCAT) (Biggs, 1990)	Measures family caregiver-rated self-care abilities of the elderly; items are based on the universal, developmental, and health-deviation self-care requisites.
Self-Care Needs Inventory (Page & Ricard, 1996)	Measures the self-care requisites of women being treated for depression.
Nursing Assessment of Readiness for Instruction of Breast Self-Examination Instrument (NARIB) (Eith, 1983)	Measures young women's readiness for breast self-examination instruction, in the areas of knowledge, perceived susceptibility, and perceived severity.
Danger Assessment Tool (Campbell, 1986)	Measures the extent to which battered women are in danger of homicide.
Functional Status Instrument (FSI) (Willard, 1990)	Measures the functional status of patients hospitalized for total hip or knee replacement.
CAPD Self-Efficacy Scale (Lin et al., 1998)	Measures the self-efficacy of individuals receiving continuous ambulatory peritoneal dialysis.
Stressors Questionnaire (Hayward et al., 1989)	Measures stressors experienced by new renal transplant patients; stress is viewed as a self-care deficit.
Self-Care Assessment Tool (SCAT) (McFarland et al., 1992)	Permits assessment of the cognitive and functional skills needed for self-care in persons with spinal cord injuries, including skills in bathing, grooming, nutritional management, taking medications, bowel management, and dressing.
Activities of Daily Living (ADL) Self-Care Scale (Gulick, 1987, 1988)	Measures activities of daily living of persons diagnosed with multiple sclerosis and other chronic neurological illnesses.
MS-Related Symptom Checklist (Gulick, 1989)	Rates symptoms related to multiple sclerosis; scale scores are used to determine potential self-care deficits for universal self-care requisites.
Risk Factor Self-Care Assessment Instrument (Carlisle et al., 1993)	Measures caregivers' knowledge of cardiovascular risk factors in children and self-care activities performed by caregivers to facilitate their children's cardiovascular health.
Oucher Scale—Hispanic and African-American Versions (Villarruel & Denyes, 1991)	Measures young children's perception of pain.
Children's Self-Care Behaviors Instrument (CSCB) (Rew, 1987)	Measures parents' rating of self-care behaviors performed by children with chronic illness, including general daily health behaviors and behaviors specific to long-term implications of coping with chronic illness
Self-Care Behavior Questionnaire (SCBQ) (Hanucharurnkul, 1989)	A self-report instrument that measures the self-care behaviors performed by patients receiving radiation therapy.

Self-Care Behavior Questionnaire (Dodd, 1982)	A self-report instrument that measures side effects of chemotherapy, severity of side effects, self-care behaviors used to manage the side effects, effectiveness of self-care behaviors, and source of information for each self-care behavior.
Self-Care Behaviors Log (Dodd, 1984)	A self-report instrument that measures side effects of radiation therapy, date of onset of side effects, severity of side effects, self-care behaviors used to manage the side effects and date used, effectiveness of self-care behaviors, and source of information for each self-care behavior.
Radiation Side Effects Profile (RSEP) (Hagopian, 1990)	Measures patients' self-report of the severity of side effects from radiation therapy and the helpfulness of self-care activities used to manage the side effects.

PRACTICE TOOLS

Patient Information Letter (Fernandez & Wheeler, 1990)	A letter given to hospitalized patients explaining basic care needs that are universal to all self-care agents.
Steps in Orem's Nursing Process (Dennis, 1997)	Provides a format for documentation of each component of the professional-technological operations of nursing practice.
Nursing History (Orem, 1995)	Guides the assessment of changes in a patient's therapeutic self-care demand and the patient's self-care agency, as well as the patient's conditions and pattern of living.
Development of Self-Care Agency Scale (Nursing Development Conference Group, 1979)	Guides assessment of degree of development of self-care agency in relation to a known therapeutic self-care demand.
Operability of Self-Care Agency Scale (Nursing Development Conference Group, 1979)	Guides assessment of degree of operability of self-care agency in relation to a known therapeutic self-care demand.
Adequacy of Self-Care Agency Scale (Nursing Development Conference Group, 1979)	Guides assessment of adequacy of self-care agency in relation to a known therapeutic self-care demand.
Guide for Nursing Assistance (GNA)—Step A (Herrington & Houston, 1984)	Guides collection of information regarding the patient's present health state and ability to perform self-care.
Guide for Nursing Assistance (GNA)—Step B (Herrington & Houston, 1984)	Permits documentation of the nursing system required, including significant data from the GNA—Step A, potential for self-care, nursing diagnosis, patient goals, nursing prescriptions, and evaluation of nursing.
Nursing Assessment Tool (Fernandez & Wheeler, 1990)	Guides the nursing history and assessment in the areas of the basic conditioning factors and universal self-care requisites.
Nursing Checklist (Guerrero Gamboa, 2000)	Used to evaluate neonatal units and families of newborn infants.
Nursing Data Base and Admission Assessment Form (Rossow-Sebring et al., 1992)	Guides assessment of universal self-care requisites for hospitalized patients.
Structured Data Collection Tool (Laschinger, 1990)	Guides assessment of patients in relation to the Self-Care Framework.
Assessment Format (Swindale, 1989)	Guides assessment of the minor surgery patient's anxieties, coping strategies, and nature of information needed.
Postoperative Self-Assessment Form (Graff et al., 1992)	A self-assessment form for use by patients recovering from surgery; the information obtained is used to determine the need for home care nursing.
Self-Care Assessment Instrument (Johannsen, 1992)	A self-assessment instrument for use by cardiac patients; the information obtained is used by the nurse to develop individualized teaching and discharge plans.

(continued)

Instrument and Citation	Description
Self-Care Assessment Tool for Hospitalized Patients with Chronic Obstructive Pulmonary Disease (Michaels, 1985, 1986)	Guides assessment of self-care for hospitalized patients with chronic obstructive pulmonary disease in the areas of respiratory status, level of function, complexity of the care plan, and familiarity with the care plan.
Chemotherapy Learning Needs Assessment Tool and Contract (Hiromoto & Dungan, 1991)	Guides assessment of learning needs of patients receiving chemotherapy, in the areas of universal, development, and health deviation self-care requisites. Provides a contract statement regarding use of self-care measures to be signed by both patient and nurse.
Massey Bedside Swallowing Screen (Massey & Jedlicka, 2002)	Assesses the swallowing function of patients who have had a stroke.
Self-Care Assessment Tool for the Psychiatric Patient (Davidhizar & Cosgray, 1990)	Permits assessment of psychiatric patients' self-care in the areas of air, food, and fluid; elimination; body temperature and personal hygiene; rest and activity; and solitude and social interaction, using a question and answer format.
Assessment Tool for Students with Disabilities (Hedahl, 1983)	Guides initial assessment of individual strengths, self-care deficits, and goals of adolescents with physical disabilities by college health nurses.
Nursing Evaluation of Neurological Function (Mitchell & Irvin, 1977)	Guides assessment of function in the areas of consciousness, mentation, motor function, and sensory function for patients with neurological and neurosurgical disorders.
Self-Care of Older Persons Evaluation (SCOPE) (Dellasega, 1995)	Provides a structured, brief format for assessment of the actual self-care abilities of institutionalized older adults.
Self-Management Inventory (Snyder et al., 1991)	Guides assessment of universal, developmental, and therapeutic demands of individuals hospitalized with complex health care problems; particularly useful for elderly individuals with chronic conditions.
Assessment-Classification Instrument (Leatt et al., 1981)	Guides assessment and classification of type of long-term care required by chronically ill patients.
Medication Knowledge Tool (Taira, 1991)	Guides assessment of chronically ill independent-living older persons' knowledge about their prescribed medications.
Medication Regimen Assessment (MacSweeney, 1992)	Permits documentation of self-administration of medications for patients with Parkinson's disease.
Facts on Osteoporosis Quiz (Ailinger et al., 1998, 2003)	Measures women's knowledge of osteoporosis. Revised version published in 2003.
Health Education Questionnaire (Baldwin & Davis, 1989)	Measures parents' perceptions of themselves as health educators for their school-age children.
The Self-Care Manual for Patients (Kyle & Pitzer, 1990)	A manual of information about self-care for hospitalized patients. The sections of the manual are entitled (1) Philosophy of self-care, (2) What does self-care mean? (3) What are patients' and nurses' roles? (4) How will the nursing staff assist you? and (5) How can you and your family help?

Teaching Tool for Renal Transplant Patients (Fridgen & Nelson, 1992)	Permits assessment of renal transplant patients' learning needs, based on Orem's power components, and development of individualized teaching plans.
Teaching Tool for Patients with Chronic Obstructive Pulmonary Disease (Brundage et al., 1993)	A teaching tool to prepare patients with chronic obstructive pulmonary disease for self-care at home.
Preoperative Education for Ambulatory Gynecological Surgery (Videotape) (Lisko, 1995)	A videotape of preoperative instruction for women scheduled for ambulatory gynecological surgery.
Documentation of Patient Education Tool (O'Connor, 1990)	Used to document patient education with regard to self-care deficits in knowledge and behaviors/skills.
Patient-Nurse Contract (Fernandez & Wheeler, 1990)	A formal contractual agreement between the patient and the nurse documenting level of participation in care and expected outcomes.
Standards of Care (Fernandez & Wheeler, 1990)	A document that identifies the standards of care applicable to self-care agents and dependent care agents in the area of universal self-care requisites.
Standards of Practice (Fernandez & Wheeler, 1990)	A document that identifies the standards for nursing practice in the area of universal self-care requisites; includes nurse agency responsibilities and scientific rationale.
Self-Care Nursing Plan (Eichelberger et al., 1980)	Permits documentation of universal, developmental, and health- deviation self-care demands, self-care agency, parent agency, nurse agency, and evaluation of agency for children.
Patient Care Flow Sheet (Fernandez & Wheeler, 1990)	Permits documentation of nursing actions in the area of universal self-care requisites.
Horn and Swain Measure of Quality of Nursing Care (Horn & Swain, 1976, 1977; Horn, 1978; Clinton et al., 1977)	Measures the quality of nursing practice in terms of the universal self-care requisites.
Quality of Medication Teaching Measure (Hageman & Ventura, 1981)	Measures the quality of nursing with regard to effects of medication teaching regimens; adapted from the medication-related items of the Horn and Swain measure.
Clinical Assessment Units of Care (UOCs) Package (Kaufman & Paulanka, 1994)	Permits documentation of nursing diagnosis, long-term goals, objectives/outcomes (short-term goals), nursing orders/ interventions, and specific instructions to encourage autonomy for nursing assistants.
Outcome Criteria Tools—Patient Self-Rating Sheet Outcome Achievement Rating Sheet for Use by Nurse Observers (Gallant & McLane, 1979)	A list of outcomes that are the result of nursing agency and achievable by patients.
Outcome Standards for Clients with Chronic Congestive Heart Failure (Fukuda, 1990)	A list of nursing outcome standards in the areas of universal, developmental, and health-deviation self-care requisites for clients with chronic congestive heart failure.
Classification of Patient Outcomes (Micek et al., 1996)	A patient outcome classification system based on Orem's Self-Care Framework and the Nursing Intervention Classification taxonomy.

(continued)

> ▶▷ TABLE 8–2
> RESEARCH INSTRUMENTS AND PRACTICE TOOLS DERIVED FROM THE SELF-CARE FRAMEWORK
> *(continued)*

Instrument and Citation	Description
Nursing System Design for New Spinal Cord Injury Patients (Allison & Renpenning, 1999a)	resents a detailed nursing system design for new spinal cord–injured patients.
Nursing Documentation Forms for Rehabilitation (Allison & Repenning, 1999b)	The forms used for documentation of Self-Care Framework-based nursing practice in a rehabilitation setting.
Nursing Documentation Form for Community Settings (Allison & Renpenning, 1999c)	The form used for documentation of Self-Care Framework-based nursing practice in a community health clinical agency.

Self-Care

Instrument and Citation	Description
Deficit Nursing Theory Outcome Categories (Allison & Renpenning, 1999d)	A list of outcomes for patients and nurses.
Self-Care Deficit Nursing Theory Outcome Categories in Rehabilitation (Allison & Renpenning, 1999e)	A list of outcomes for patients receiving rehabilitation nursing services.
Patient Self-Care Classification (Allison & Renpenning, 1999f)	A patient classification system in terms of patient capabilities, limitations, self-care deficits, conditioning factors, and nursing assistance needed.
Self-Care Deficit Nursing Theory Care Map (Allison & Renpenning, 1999g)	A care map for universal self-care requisites.
Nursing Systems International Computer Software (Bliss-Holtz, 1995; Bliss-Holtz & Riggs, 1996; Paternostro, 1992; Marvulli et al., 1992; Marvulli & Trofino, 1992; Mulvey et al., 1992; Brennan & Duffy, 1992)	A computer software package for documentation of Orem Self-Care Framework-based nursing practice.
NICU Skills Checklist (Angeles, 1991)	Used to evaluate the new neonatal intensive care nurse's skills in the use of Orem's Self-Care Framework.
Home Help Activities Registration Form (Arts et al., 1996)	Permits documentation of activities carried out by home health workers in The Netherlands.
Therapeutic Nursing Function (TNF) Indicator (Kitson, 1986)	Permits identification of nurses who provide more patient-centered or therapeutic nursing and those who provide routine-centered or nontherapeutic nursing.
Community Health Assessment (Hanchett, 1988)	Guides assessment of a community according to universal, developmental, and health-deviation self-care requisites for members of high-risk populations.

Research Topic	Study Participants	Citation*
	DESCRIPTIVE STUDIES	
Quality of life	Swedish patients who have a pacemaker	Malm et al., 1998
Meaning of health and quality of life	Liver transplant recipients 1 year after transplantation	Forsberg, 2002
Symptoms, side effects, and quality of life during and following treatment with radiation therapy	Women with breast cancer	Wengström et al., 2000
Description of the Pro-Self Program	Cancer patients undergoing chemotherapy or radiation therapy	Larson et al., 1998
Identification of health beliefs and values, perceptions of self-care abilities, and perceived barriers to health promotion	Male and female older adults	Whetstone & Reid, 1991
Desire for normalcy	Secondary analysis of data from studies of men and women with serious mental illness	Pickens, 1999
Meaning of health	Older women	Maddox, 1999
Meaning of self-care	American, East German, and Swedish people	Whetstone, 1987 Whetstone & Hansson, 1989
Self-care ability	Home-dwelling elderly individuals in Sweden	Söderhamn et al., 2000
Self-care ability and meaning of actualizing self-care ability into self-care activity	Home-dwelling elderly individuals in Sweden	Söderhamn, 1998
Meaning of rest	Adult men	Allison, 1971
Children's worries about their battered mothers	Children of battered women	Humphreys, 1991
Dependent-care activities to protect their children	Battered women	Humphreys, 1995
Comparison of perceived self-care agency	Pregnant low-socioeconomic adolescents who had and had not been abused or neglected	Warren, 1998
Responses to potential preterm labor symptoms hypothetically encountered at 24 weeks of gestation	Pregnant women at 20 to 32 weeks of gestation	Freston et al., 1997
Extent of concern for learning dependent-care of infants	Primiparous women	Bliss-Holtz, 1988
Interest in learning about labor and delivery	Primiparous women	Bliss-Holtz, 1991
Comparison of needs for information about self-care and infant care	Adolescent and young adult mothers	Degenhart-Leskosky, 1989
Level of self-care agency	Members of an Al-Anon group	Neil, 1984
Self-care behaviors	Individuals who participated in a smoking cessation program	Utz et al., 1994

*See the Research section of the chapter references for complete citations.

(continued)

Research Topic	Study Participants	Citation
Self-care behaviors used to stay well	Older adults, 57–83 years of age	Clark, 1998
Interpretation and use of health information in the practice of self-care related to weight management	White middle-class and working-class women	Allen, 1988
Health-seeking behaviors in relation to perimenstrual symptoms	Young adult Asian, Black, White, Native American, and Hispanic women	Woods et al., 1992
Self-care agency with regard to menarche	Black premenarcheal girls	Dashiff, 1992
Self-care practices related to menstruation	Adult women	Patterson & Hale, 1985
Use of information regarding hormone replacement therapy	Perimenopausal women	Rothert et al., 1990
Perceived demand for or change in universal and health-deviation self-care activity and the degree of difficulty ascribed to meeting that demand	Women with HIV disease	Anastasio et al., 1995
Universal and illness-related self-care activities used	Young adult married women	Woods, 1985
Self-care actions	Middle-aged women	Hartweg, 1993
The experience of urinary incontinence	Women 58 to 79 years of age	Dowd, 1991
Self-care practices	Noninstitutionalized women with urinary incontinence	Klemm & Creason, 1991
Self-care responses to respiratory illness	Vietnamese persons residing in Texas	Hautman, 1987
Adherence to appointment and medication taking for preventive therapy for latent tuberculosis infection	Latino immigrants	Ailinger & Dear, 1998
Knowledge, actions, and decisions required to manage medications	Older adults and their caregivers	Conn et al., 1995
Levels of self-care	Chinese children with nephrotic syndrome	Zhimin, 2003
Pain intensity and home pain management techniques	Children with sickle cell disease	Conner-Warren, 1996
Comparison of self-care agency	Healthy adolescents Adolescents with spina bifida	Monsen, 1992
Changes in self-care agency	Expectant parents attending childbirth education classes	Riesch, 1988
Description of use of the Young Parents Project	Adolescent mothers	Hudson et al., 1999
Side effects and self-care actions	Cancer patients receiving inpatient chemotherapy	Foltz et al., 1996
Self-care behaviors in response to fatigue	Cancer patients receiving chemotherapy	Richardson & Ream, 1997
Self-care behaviors	Cancer patients receiving chemotherapy or radiation therapy	Dodd, 1982, 1984b, 1988b

Therapeutic self-care demands	Cancer patients receiving radiation therapy	Kubricht, 1984
Self-care and dependent-care activities	Mexican-American individuals who experienced pain	Villarruel, 1995 Villarruel & Denyes, 1997
Conditions that make work or tasks difficult or easier	Adults with multiple sclerosis	Gulick et al., 1989
Categories of self-care needs	Adults with diabetes mellitus	Miller, 1982
Desires, concerns, and experiences regarding retention of self-management activities	Hospitalized adults with diabetes mellitus	Germain & Nemchik, 1988
Knowledge of diabetes mellitus, knowledge about diabetes mellitus management procedures and routines, performance of procedures	Ambulatory clinic patients with diabetes mellitus	Allison, 2003
Self-care home health education program	Adults with diabetes mellitus	Watson et al., 1996
Experiences of and attitudes toward subcutaneous infusions of gamma globulin	Adult women and men with primary antibody deficiencies	Gardulf et al., 1995
Self-care needs	Individuals diagnosed with mitral valve prolapse	Utz et al., 1993 Utz & Ramos, 1993
Perceived health state and body image	Individuals diagnosed with mitral valve prolapse	Utz et al., 1990
Self-care limitations	Individuals who had experienced a myocardial infarction	Beach et al., 1996
Problems and informational needs	Individuals who had experienced a myocardial infarction or coronary artery bypass graft surgery	Jaarsma et al., 1994
Differences in quality of life and life satisfaction among urinary management modality groups	Spinal cord–injured individuals	Brillhart, 2002
Perceptions of communication with health-care providers	Independent elderly women and men	Frank, 2003
Self-care factors that facilitate and inhibit adherence to cardiac therapy	Men with coronary artery disease	Baird & Pierce, 2001
Knowledge of congestive heart failure disease process and treatment	Individuals with congestive heart failure admitted to home health care after hospitalization	Hubbard, 2002
Changes in self-care agency, self-efficacy expectations, and performance of self-care/recovery behaviors	Individuals who had coronary artery bypass graft surgery	Carroll, 1995
Knowledge and beliefs about hypertension	Jamaican women	Grant & Hezekiah, 1996
Recognition of alcoholism	Military wives	McConnell, 2000
Universal self-care requisites	Homeless men	Harris & Williams, 1991
Relations between perception of power, self-care agency, self-care, basic conditioning factors, and health	Women living in urban squatter settlements in Karachi, Pakistan	Lee, 1999
Mental health status	Older adults	Reed, 1989
Management of self-care activities	Older adults at home following hospital discharge	Jopp et al., 1993

(continued)

Research Topic	Study Participants	Citation
Health habits, lifestyle practices, and perception of need for dependent-care agents	Older men and women	Schafer, 1989
Health status, satisfaction with lifestyle, and needs for nursing	Community-dwelling elderly Norwegian persons	Dahlen, 1997
Postprandial blood pressure changes	Healthy elderly persons	Lilley, 1997
Self-care activities related to health maintenance and symptom management	Young adult women	Lawrence & Schank, 1995
Self-care behaviors used to manage cold and influenza episodes	Adults 65 to 94 years of age	Conn, 1991
Self-care strategies to function in culturally prescribed roles during illness	Women with chronic pelvic pain	Zadinsky & Boyle, 1996
Medication-taking behaviors	White non-Hispanic and Hispanic frail elderly individuals	Lile & Hoffman, 1991
Perceptions of health, wellness, and self-care	Mexican-American women living in Texas	Mendias et al., 2001
Description of diet-related behaviors and beliefs	Elderly Hispanic women residing in New Mexico	Shuster et al., 2001
Frequency of and indications used for total feeding assistance and tube feeding	National representative sample of Belgian hospital patients included in the 1990 national minimum nursing data set	Evers et al., 2000
Changes in mental status and functional abilities	Elderly female nursing home residents	Hamilton & Creason, 1992
Obstacles to meeting universal self-care requisites	Nursing home residents	Orem, 1995
Capacity for self-care	Individuals with mental illness living in community residences	Getty et al., 1998
Capacity for dependent-care	Staff of community residences	
Self-care actions related to solitude and social interaction	Individuals with schizophrenia	Harris, 1990
Perception of indicators of mental illness	Individuals with schizophrenia	Hamera et al., 1992
Self-help strategies used for coping with auditory hallucinations	Individuals with schizophrenia	Frederick & Cotanch, 1995
Comparison of self-care practices used for coping	Adults with and without psychiatric illness	Crockett, 1982
Comparison of value ascribed to self-care requisites	Women with and without depression	Page & Ricard, 1995
Morning care behaviors	Patients with dementia and their nurses	Sandman et al., 1986
Caregivers' knowledge of and self-care activities related to cardiovascular risk factors	Caregivers and their 2- and 3-year-old children	Carlisle et al., 1993
Factors influencing opportunities for people with cancer to die at home	Primary caregivers of people with cancer who died at home	Grov, 1999

Family behavior patterns	Siblings of children with cystic fibrosis	Kruger et al., 1980
Comparison of knowledge, attitudes, confidence, and practice of breast self-examination	Hospital-employed female nurses and female non-nurses	Edgar et al., 1984
Problems and helpful interventions	Patients discharged from a rehabilitation unit who received follow-up telephone calls	Closson et al., 1994
Strategies used to establish preventive diabetic and hypertension programs in a Chinese community	Chinese men and women with diabetes mellitus and/or hypertension	Wang & Abbott, 1998
Comparison of women's self-diagnoses and advanced practice nurses' clinical diagnoses of vaginitis and cystitis	Women in the military and advanced practice nurses	Lowe & Ryan-Wenger, 2000
Pre-conception health teaching	Nurse practitioners	Barron et al., 1987
Description of words and approaches used when discussing young adults' contraceptive use	Nurse practitioners	Guthrie et al., 2001
Role intensity of rehabilitation nurses in home care	Members of the Association of Rehabilitation Nurses Home Health Special Interest Group	Brillhart et al., 2001
Characteristics of preoperative nursing assessments	Staff nurses	Takahashi & Bever, 1989
Nurses' perspectives of encouraging clients to care for themselves	Staff nurses	Singleton, 2000
Nursing actions used to prevent and alleviate pain in hospitalized children	Nurses with expertise in caring for children with pain Staff nurses	Denyes et al., 1991
Emotional reactions to self-destructive behavior	Nurses with experience and interest in self-mutilating patients	Brodtkorb, 2001
Nursing interventions used to prevent or relieve postoperative nausea and vomiting	Hospital records of patients who underwent cholecystectomy	Hinojosa, 1992
Moving and handling practices	Staff nurses working on medical units	Green, 1996
Nursing process and intervention related to discharge preparation	Case study of a family with a child requiring complex home care	Steele & Sterling, 1992
Nursing actions to prepare for hospital discharge	Case study of a 41-year-old woman with multiple sclerosis discharged to home on a mechanical ventilator	Storm & Baumgartner, 1987
Nursing protocol	Case study of two patients with acute lymphoblastic leukemia receiving outpatient consolidation chemotherapy	Palmer & Meyers, 1990
Preparation of stoma patients for self-management of the appliance	Staff nurses	Ewing, 1989
Experiences with individuals who have attempted suicide	Staff nurses working in emergency departments	Pallikkathayil & Morgan, 1988
Nursing interventions during home visits to the elderly	Community nurses and community nursing auxiliaries in The Netherlands	Kerkstra et al., 1991
Home care nurses' productivity	Registered nurses working in home health-care agencies	Spoelstra, 1996

(continued)

Research Topic	Study Participants	Citation
Description of the application of a self-care philosophy in practice	Staff nurses	Furlong, 1996
Facilitators and inhibitors to clinical application of the Self-Care Framework	Case study of a 73-year-old woman	Clark, 1986
Exploration of construct of thriving as an integration of nutritional, psychosocial, and lifestyle concerns of childbearing	Secondary analysis of data from women during the 12 months after childbirth	Walker & Grobe, 1999
Identification of Orem's self-care model-based nursing diagnoses	High-risk pregnant women	Farias & Nóbrega, 2000
Defining characteristics of the nursing diagnosis knowledge deficit in the third trimester of pregnancy	Staff nurses Third trimester pregnant women	Aukamp, 1989
Identification of nursing diagnoses	Case study of a pregnant adolescent	Torres et al., 1999
Defining characteristics of the nursing diagnosis self-care deficit, bathing/hygiene	Staff nurses	McKeighen et al., 1991
Integration of North American Nursing Diagnosis Association nursing diagnoses and Orem's Self-Care Framework	Registered nurse students in a baccalaureate nursing program	Jenny, 1991
Comparison of operable self-care agency	Patients in district nursing caseloads who did and did not self-neglect	Lauder, 1999b
Perceptions of self-neglect	Professionals, patients, and relatives	Lauder, 1999a
Comparison of judgments of self-neglect	Psychiatric nurses, general nurses, and student nurses	Lauder et al., 2001
Knowledge, attitudes, treatment practices, and health behaviors regarding blood cholesterol	Registered nurses	Ienatsch, 1999
How nurses describe patients' problems and possible effects of using different nursing models (Orem's Self-Care Framework and Roper's Activities of Daily Living Model) on the descriptions	Registered nurses	Griffiths, 1998
Perianesthesia nursing research from 1994 to 1999	Literature review	Fetzer & Hand, 2001
Criterion behaviors of positive mental health	Literature written by scholars in philosophy, psychology, clinical psychology, psychiatry, and human behavior	Orem & Vardiman, 1995
CORRELATIONAL STUDIES		
Relations between autonomy, locus of control, and self-care agency	Fifth-grade school children	Moore, 1987a
Relations between child's age, health state, self-care agency, performance of self-care activities, and mother's performance of dependent-care activities	Children and adolescents and their mothers	Moore, 1993

Relation of maternal age, child age, child gender, only child status, marital status, number of children, child status (adopted, biologic, stepchild), birth order, ethnic group, socioeconomic status, maternal employment status, and child health problems to mother's performance of dependent-care activities	Mothers of children ages 1 to 16 years	Gaffney & Moore, 1996
Relation of child's age, gender, health state (on or off therapy), socioeconomic status, and sociocultural orientation to child's state-trait anxiety, mother's state-trait anxiety, child's performance of self-care activities, and mother's performance of dependent-care activities	Children and adolescents with cancer and their mothers	Moore & Mosher, 1997
Relations among child's age, gender, sociocultural orientation, health state (on or off therapy; impairment from cancer and cancer treatment), self-concept, and performance of self-care activities, and mother's performance of dependent-care activities	Children and adolescents with cancer and their mothers	Mosher & Moore, 1998
Relation of social support to mothers' self-care and dependent care agency	Mothers of infants and children with developmental disabilities	Beauchesne, 1997
Relation of self-concept and sociocultural characteristics to self-care practices	Healthy adolescents	McCaleb & Edgil, 1994
General self-care practices	Middle adolescents	McCaleb & Cull, 2000
Relation of age, sex, child's health locus of control, and mother's and father's health locus of control to child's self-care behaviors	Children with asthma	Rew, 1987b
Relation between illness behaviors and health locus of control	Children with asthma	Rew, 1987a
Relation of age, outside activities, attendance at a summer camp for diabetics, sex, race, duration of diabetes mellitus, family history of diabetes mellitus, and self-concept to self-care diabetic management activities	School-age children with diabetes	Saucier, 1984
Relation of diabetes mellitus self-care to universal self-care, health status, and metabolic control	Children and adolescents with diabetes	Frey & Fox, 1990
Relations between basic conditioning factors, universal self-care, health-deviation self-care, health, and control of pathology	Adolescents with diabetes	Frey & Denyes, 1989
Relation between self-care agency and self-care practice	Adolescents	Slusher, 1999
Relation of physical abuse, social support, and self-care agency to infant birth weight and pregnancy complications	Pregnant adolescents 18–19 years of age	Renker, 1999
Relation of source of support to universal and health-deviation self-care	Adults with non–insulin-dependent diabetes mellitus	Wang & Fenske, 1996

(continued)

Research Topic	Study Participants	Citation
Relation of sociodemographic characteristics, educational level, and perception of health to universal and diabetes mellitus–related self-care activities	Chinese people with diabetes mellitus residing in Taiwan	Wang, 1997
Relations among age, marital status, social class, perceived health, self-care agency, health-promoting lifestyle, and well-being	Elderly Taiwanese women residing in a rural area	Wang, 2001
Relations among demographic variables, social class, perceived health, social support, self-care agency, health-promotion self-care behavior, and perceived well-being	Elderly Taiwanese women residing in a rural area	Wang & Laffrey, 2001
Relation of age, education, duration of illness, and arthritis severity to self-care agency	Adults with rheumatoid arthritis	Ailinger & Dear, 1993
Relation of age, gender, and health state to self-care needs	Adults with rheumatoid arthritis	Ailinger & Dear, 1997
Relation of self-care agency and social support from family and friends to contraceptive practices	Unmarried pregnant teenagers	Mapanga & Andrews, 1995
Relation of availability and adequacy of health-care resources, family system support, and self-care agency to initiation of prenatal care	Pregnant adolescents	Baker, 1996
Relation of gravidity, socioeconomic status, resource availability, family system, and age to self-care agency	Pregnant women attending childbirth education classes or a prenatal clinic	Hart & Foster, 1998
Relation of gravidity, weeks of gestation, prenatal risk designation, self-care agency, basic prenatal care actions, and foundations for dependent-care agency to maternal hemoglobin and infant birth weight	Pregnant women	Hart, 1995, 1996
Relation of age, race, socioeconomic status, health state, patterns of living, and influence of decision making to self-care agency related to sexually transmitted disease	Unmarried women at risk for sexually transmitted disease	McQuiston & Campbell, 1997
Relations among health-promoting self-care behaviors, self-care self-efficacy, and self-care agency	Healthy male and female adults	Callaghan, 2003
Relation of age, health, dyad gender, family behavior, and caregiver reciprocity to collaborative care system	Community living adult couples, at least one of whom had a self-labeled health problem	Geden & Taylor, 1999
Relation of symptoms, employment, and sex-role orientation to illness-related self-care practices	Young adult women	Maunz & Woods, 1988

Relations between locus of control, health values, health status, satisfaction with health, and exercise of self-care agency	Women faculty members at a midwestern university	Lakin, 1988
Relation of models of grief and learned helplessness to women's responses to battering	Women who had and had not been battered	Campbell, 1989
Relation of physical and nonphysical abuse and self-care agency to physical and emotional health	Well-educated, economically heterogeneous urban battered women	Campbell & Soeken, 1999
Relation of age, education, and culture to relational conflict, self-care agency, injury, physical symptoms, and depression	Women who had experienced battering in an intimate or marital relationship	Campbell & Weber, 2000
Relation between learned helplessness and self-care agency	Working women and men	McDermott, 1993
Relations among social support, self-esteem, and codependency	African-American women attending a women's support group	Cook & Barber, 1997
Relation of knowledge, beliefs, and health practices about breast cancer to breast self-examination	Women residing in Delhi, India	Malik, 1992
Relations among self-care, self-care agency, and well-being, controlling for basic conditioning factors	Homeless adults	Anderson, 2001
Relation of symptom recognition and management and self-care agency to symptom management	Individuals with mood disorders	Cutler, 2001
Relation of visual acuity, tactile sensitivity, and mobility of the upper extremities to proficiency in breast self-examination	Women 65 years of age and older	Baulch et al., 1992
Relation of demographic and health variables to participation in fecal occult blood screening	Elderly persons attending Council on Aging congregate meal sites in central South Carolina	Weinrich, 1990
Relation between self-concept and perception of self-care ability	Elderly persons residing in a hostel in Hong Kong	Ip et al., 1996
Relations among self-care agency, therapeutic self-care demand, and basic conditioning factors	Secondary analysis of data from individuals 65 years of age and older living in Sweden	Söderhamm & Cliffordson, 2001
Relations among years of schooling, word recognition, and reading comprehension of discharge instructions	Patients receiving discharge instructions from a gastroenterology department	Watkins, 1995
Relation between patient's exercise of self-care agency prior to hospitalization and satisfaction with nursing care during hospitalization	Adult medical-surgical patients	Lucas et al., 1988
Relation between medication regimen complexity and adherence to the medication regimen	Older adults recently discharged from hospital and older adults not recently hospitalized	Conn et al., 1991
Relation of knowledge of performance of self-care and actual performance of self-care	Individuals with heart failure	Artinian et al., 2002
Relation of appreciation of and motivation for self-care, age, sex, socioeconomic status, employment status, health behaviors, and health status to self-care agency	Finnish patients with coronary heart disease	Lukkarinen & Hentinen, 1997

(continued)

Research Topic	Study Participants	Citation
Relation of symptom distress and social support to self-care behaviors	Chinese patients who were recipients of a heart transplant	Wang et al., 1998
Relation of psychosocial characteristics, autonomy, attitudes about end-stage renal disease and dialysis, and self-care agency to occurrence of infectious complications	Patients receiving continuous ambulatory peritoneal dialysis	Pressley, 1995
Factors affecting self-care	Well adults and adults with end-stage renal disease	Horsburgh 1999
Relation between self-esteem and hope	Patients receiving a renal transplant	Frieson & Frieson, 1996
Relation of age, education, occupation, source of family livelihood, perception of health condition, social support, and motivation for self-care to self-care abilities	Taiwanese patients who had a colostomy	Kao & Ku, 1997
Relations among personality traits, health state, self-care abilities, and behaviors	Canadian adults awaiting renal transplant	Horsburgh et al., 2000
Gender differences in relations among health-related hardiness, patient attitude toward compliance, and self-care adherence to physical activity	Men and women with diabetes	Navuluri, 2000
Relations of income, education, current alcohol use, perceived support, barriers to medication taking, intention to adhere, and capacity for self-care to adherence to antituberculosis therapy	Individuals with TB and HIV disease	McDonnell et al., 2001
Relation of demographic variables to patient's choice of treatment	Review of hospital charts of women with stage I breast cancer	Graling & Grant, 1995
Relation of cancer patients' quality of life, symptoms, moods, and self-care self-efficacy to family caregivers' depression, role strain, and health outcomes	Female and male adults with cancer and their family caregivers	Lev & Owen, 2002
Relation of demographic variables, performance status, affective state, social support, ability to manage a situation, self-care ability, and prior health-promoting activities to self-care behavior	Adults with cancer who were to receive the first dose of chemotherapy	Dodd & Dibble, 1993
Relation of illness factors, age, gender, education, socioeconomic status, family hardiness, universal and health deviation self-care burden, and stress appraisal to mood	Patients receiving radiotherapy	Oberst et al., 1991
Relation of age, marital status, living arrangements, socioeconomic status stage and site of cancer, and social support to self-care behaviors	Thai adults receiving radiation therapy	Hanucharurnkul, 1989
Relation of symptoms, including tiredness and weakness to self-care activities	Adults receiving chemotherapy	Rhodes et al., 1988

Relation of patients', family members', and nurses' perception of the patient's fatigue to biological response modifier dosage and fatigue-related self-care activities	Patients receiving biological response modifier therapy, family members, and registered nurses	Robinson & Posner, 1992
Relation between self-care and ability to cope with cancer	Cancer patients	Gammon, 1991
Relations among age, gender, symptom severity, self-care and other's care, perception of the extent of problem solution, satisfaction with problem solution, and perception of control over health	Chronically ill women and men	Spitzer et al., 1996a, 1996b
Relation between self-care agency and quality of life	Individuals with inflammatory bowel disease	Smolen & Topp, 2001
Relation between patients' and partners' views of asthma self-management and family environment	Adults with asthma and their partners	Geden et al., 2002
Relation of demographic and disease-related variables to compliance with lithium therapy	Individuals with bipolar affective disorder and their relatives	Jose et al., 2003
Relation between self-concept and exercise of self-care agency	Independently living older adults	Smits & Kee, 1992
Relation of age, gender, educational level, health status, locus of control, support network, social participation, and economic status to institutionalization status	Community dwelling and institutionalized elderly persons	Brock & O'Sullivan, 1985
Relation of perception of choice and amount of choice preferred to self-care ability and functional ability	Nursing home residents	Jirovec & Maxwell, 1993
Relation of environmental constraints and personal characteristics to self-appraised self-care agency	Female and male nursing home residents 60 to 100 years of age	Jirovec & Kasno, 1990
Relation of age, sex, education, race, previous occupation, marital status, number of children, number of monthly visits, functional health, morale, perception of nursing home in terms of fostering dependence, and insurance type (Medicare vs. Medicaid) to self-appraised self-care agency	Female and male nursing home residents 60 to 100 years of age	Jirovec & Kasno, 1993
Relation of self-care agency, self-care actions, length of time in caregiver role, number of roles, and types of caregiving tasks to caregiver strain	Female family caregivers of elderly parents	Baker, 1997
Relation of health-related hardiness, caregiver burden, and dependent care to self-care agency	Spouses of radiation oncology patients and chemotherapy patients	Schott-Baer, 1993 Schott-Baer et al., 1995
Relation between clients' and nurses' perceptions of client self-care agency	Elderly clients and nurses in community health agencies	Ward-Griffin & Bramwell, 1990
Factors related to nurses' attitudes toward and knowledge of organ donation	Nurses working in critical care units	Bidigare & Oermann, 1991

(continued)

Research Topic	Study Participants	Citation
Relation between self-care agency and job satisfaction	Public health nurses	Behm & Frank, 1992
Relation between perceived and actual knowledge of diabetes mellitus	Registered nurses	Baxley et al., 1997
Relation of knowledge and attitudes about sex, empathy, and homophobia to attitudes about AIDS care	Registered nurses	Bennett et al., 1993
Relation of congruent societal and health care values, commonalities of patient needs, and primacy of caring through knowing the patient to individualized care	Registered nurses	Evans, 1996
Relation of family structure information on perception of a preschool-age child	Baccalaureate program nursing students	Siebert et al., 1986
Factors related to the use of the Self-Care Framework in nursing practice	Graduates of a liberal arts college baccalaureate nursing program based on the Self-Care Framework	Wagnild et al., 1987
EXPERIMENTAL STUDIES		
Effects of an educational program on knowledge of car safety and behaviors while riding in a car	Preschool-age children attending a day care center	Arneson & Triplett, 1990
Effect of an experimental self-care instruction program and a control health discussion on health locus of control	Fifth-grade school children	Blazek & McClellan, 1983
Effects of first-aid and assertion training on autonomy and self-care agency	Fifth-grade school children	Moore, 1987b
Effect of a planned teaching program on knowledge of menstrual hygiene	Pre-adolescent girls living in India	George, 2003
Effects of experimental and control nursing interventions on child's enuresis and self-esteem, and parents' behaviors toward the child	Turkish children with enuresis and their parents	Terakye & Bulduko-lu, 1997
Effects of an asthma education program on knowledge, behavior modification, and self-care management	Individuals with asthma and their family members	Alexander et al., 2000
Effects of clinical nurse specialist or hospital clinic pediatric resident care on outpatient department and emergency department visits, and allergy physician contacts	Low-income children with chronic asthma	Alexander et al., 1988
Effect of experimental computer-assisted instruction plus traditional instruction and control traditional instruction only on adherence to implementing house dust mite avoidance measures	Adults with atopic asthma	Huss et al., 1991
Effects of an educational program on premenstrual signs and physical, mental, emotional, and behavioral discomforts	Korean women with premenstrual syndrome	Min, 2002

Effects of an experimental parenting enhancement program and a control treatment on self-esteem, self-care agency, and perception of the infant	Egyptian mothers registered in a well-baby clinic	Porter et al., 1992
Effect of teaching scald burn prevention practices on burn-related home-safety practices	Parents of young children	Corrarino et al., 2001
Effects of a postpartum telephone call after discharge, a predischarge postpartum visit, and a control no intervention on appointment keeping at a family planning clinic	Non–high-risk obstetric patients	Buckley, 1990
Effect of experimental and control preoperative teaching methods on parents' postoperative knowledge and compliance levels	Parents of children experiencing tonsillectomy	McCord, 1990
Effects of an educational intervention and a control treatment on use of perimenstrual syndrome (PMS) self-care measures and PMS symptoms	Women who had one or more PMS symptoms	Kirkpatrick et al., 1990
Effects of experimental and control educational programs on number and severity of premenstrual symptoms and number of premenstrual days with symptoms	Employed women	Seideman, 1990
Effects of congruency of teaching strategy and learning style on accuracy and frequency of performance of breast self-examination	Women 20 to 40 years of age	Hartley, 1988
Effects of T'ai Chi on self-assessed health and self-reported benefits	Women aged 72 to 96 years	Taggert, 2001
Effects of location [non-dominant hand, dominant hand, dominant forearm; non-dominant forearm] of peripheral intravenous catheter on complications, pain, and self-care activities;	Hospitalized, non-critically ill adults	Marsigliese, 2001
Effects of an experimental nursing intervention targeting factors influencing delirium and a control nursing intervention on functional status	Elderly hospitalized patients	Wanich et al., 1992
Effect of experimental structured preoperative teaching and postoperative discharge preparation for mastectomy/hysterectomy and a control treatment on postoperative self-care behaviors	Women who had a mastectomy or hysterectomy	Williams et al., 1988
Effects of experimental procedure-specific instructions and control existing generic educational instructions on postoperative recovery and self-management of symptoms	Patients having day surgery	Young et al. 2000
Effects of experimental structured preoperative teaching and control usual and customary informal patient education on the incidence of postoperative atelectasis and patient satisfaction with education	Adults scheduled for first-time elective general surgery, urological surgery, or colon-rectal surgery	Meeker et al., 1992

(continued)

Research Topic	Study Participants	Citation
Effects of an experimental self-care plus usual care nursing intervention and a control usual care intervention on pain sensation and distress, analgesic use, ambulation, complications, and satisfaction with care	Thai adult patients undergoing pyelolithotomy or nephrolithotomy	Hanucharurnkul & Vinya-nguag, 1991
Effects of types of nurse-patient interaction on power, control, satisfaction, and agreement with prescribed treatment	Adults in a simulated clinical setting	Krouse & Roberts, 1989
Effects of an experimental programmed instruction booklet and a control treatment on knowledge, self-care, and postoperative recovery	Adults who had surgery for bronchogenic carcinoma	Goodwin, 1979
Effect of group education classes on self-care agency	Adults with chronic obstructive pulmonary disease	Stockdale-Woolley, 1984
Effect of structured and unstructured pretransfer information on posttransfer anxiety	Individuals who experienced a myocardial infarction and were being transferred from a coronary care unit	Toth, 1980
Effect of experimental and control nutrition programs on eating habits	Men and women who had experienced a myocardial infarction	Aish, 1996
Effects of an experimental Orem Self-Care Framework-based nursing intervention and a control intervention on self-care agency and self-efficacy for healthy eating	Individuals who had experienced a myocardial infarction	Aish & Isenberg, 1996
Effects of an experimental educational program about using a fluid volume management journal and weight change parameters on adherence to use of the journal, hospital readmission, and length of hospital stay	Adults with congestive heart failure who were clients of a hospital-based home health agency	Hubbard, 2001
Effect of a supportive-educative nursing system on promotion and maintenance of a prescribed medication regimen	Patients with congestive heart failure	Fujita & Dugan, 1994
Effect of an experimental medication discharge planning program and a control usual informal discharge planning program on hospital readmission	Patients with congestive heart failure	Schneider et al., 1993
Effects of an experimental supportive educational nursing intervention and control routine care on self-care abilities, self-care behavior, and quality of life	Patients with advanced heart failure	Jaarsma et al., 2000
Effects of a hemodialysis educational and support program (HESP) and a control treatment on self-care agency, functional status, compliance to the hemodialysis regimen, social functioning, and alienation	Adults receiving hemodialysis	Korniewicz & O'Brien, 1994

Effects of experimental and control nursing interventions on number of office visits, hospitalizations, use of medications, ADL functioning, symptom prevalence, and use of assistive devices	Individuals with multiple sclerosis	Gulick, 1991
Effects of relaxation training by audiotapes, live relaxation training by nurses, and no relaxation training on subjective pain and analgesic intake	Hospitalized oncology patients	Sloman et al., 1994
Effects of an experimental telephone call intervention and usual care and control usual care on anxiety, severity of side effects, helpfulness of self-care strategies used to manage side effects, and use of coping strategies	Patients receiving radiation therapy	Hagopian & Rubenstein, 1990
Effects of experimental structured nursing consultation and control health education or usual care on anxiety, side effects, and helpfulness of self-care strategies use to manage side effects	Patients receiving radiation therapy	Weintraub & Hagopian, 1990
Effects of an experimental weekly structured patient educational information newsletter on knowledge, severity of side effects, and helpfulness of self-care measures to manage side effects	Cancer patients receiving radiation therapy	Hagopian, 1991
Effects of experimental informational audiotapes and control standard care on number and severity of side effects, self-care measures used to manage side effects, and helpfulness of the self-care measures	Cancer patients receiving radiation therapy	Hagopian, 1996
Effects of experimental side effects management technique (SMET) information and a control treatment on self-care behaviors and severity and distress of experienced side effects, anxiety, and cancer health locus of control	Cancer patients receiving radiation therapy	Dodd, 1987
Effects of type of information (drug information [DI], self-effect management techniques [SMET], DI and SMET, and control conversation about disease-related topics) on self-care behavior	Cancer patients receiving chemotherapy	Dodd, 1983
Effect of type of information (DI, -SMET, DI and SMET, and control conversation about disease-related topics) on chemotherapy knowledge, self-care behavior, and affective state	Cancer patients receiving chemotherapy	Dodd, 1984a
Effects of experimental side effects management (SEM) information and control standard information on self-care behaviors, anxiety, and health locus of control	Cancer patients receiving chemotherapy	Dodd, 1988a
Effects of a nurse-initiated systematic oral hygiene teaching program (PRO-Self: Mouth Aware [PSMA]) and two types of mouth wash on prevention of chemotherapy-induced oral mucositis	Patients receiving mucositis-inducing chemotherapy	Dodd et al., 1996

(continued)

Research Topic	Study Participants	Citation
Effects of experimental progressive muscle relaxation and guided imagery on anxiety, depression, and quality of life	Individuals with advanced cancer	Sloman, 2002
Effects of an experimental efficacy-enhancing intervention and a control usual preparation treatment on quality of life, self-care self-efficacy, mood distress, and symptom distress	Cancer patients receiving chemotherapy	Lev, 1995
Effects of experimental guided imagery and standard antiemetic regimen and control standard antiemetic regimen only on chemotherapy-related nausea, vomiting, and retching	Patients receiving chemotherapy	Troesch et al., 1993
Effects of experimental aerobic interval training, placebo group interaction, and control normal activities on functional capacity	Women with stage II breast cancer receiving chemotherapy	MacVicar et al., 1989
Effects of telephone calls and oral and written self-care measures versus standard care on self-care for chemotherapy side effects	Women receiving chemotherapy for breast cancer	Craddock et al., 1999
Effects of an experimental social dramatics program and a control no social dramatics treatment on performance of social skills	Hospitalized patients with schizophrenia	Whetstone, 1986
Effects of an experimental family-patient teaching program and control no education on patients' functional level and readmission rate	Hospitalized patients with schizo-affective disorders	Youssef, 1987
Effects of a self-help group experience and no self-help group experience on feelings of hopelessness and helplessness	Hospitalized patients with reactive depression	Rothlis, 1984
Effect of an individually focused, guided decision-making intervention on perception of self-care ability	Individuals who were participating in a stroke rehabilitation program	Folden, 1993
Effects of an educational course on depression, hope, and ways of coping	Stroke survivors	Johnson & Pearson, 2000
Effects of use of Orem's Self-Care Framework-based nursing practice and no specific nursing framework–based nursing practice on nursing assessments and patient-care goals	Nursing records of residents of a Veterans Administration Nursing Home Care Unit and licensed nursing staff	Faucett et al., 1990
Effects of an experimental range-of-motion exercise program and a control no exercise treatment on independence in self-care activities	Elderly residents of an intermediate care facility	Karl, 1982
Effects of the Program of All-Inclusive Care for the Elderly (PACE) and nursing home care on frail elders' satisfaction and caregivers' burden and sources of stress	Frail elders residing in the community or a nursing home and their caregivers	Anderson & Campbell, 1993

Effects of animal-assisted therapy on well-being and blood pressure	Homebound elderly persons	Harris et al., 1993
Effect of high and low levels of components of care (technical quality, psychosocial care, and patient participation in planning care) on patient satisfaction with a hypothetical encounter with a health care provider	Elderly women attending senior citizen nutrition sites	Chang et al., 1984
Effect of high and low levels of components of care (technical quality, psychosocial care, and patient participation in planning care) on hypothetical intent to adhere to the health care plan	Elderly women attending senior citizen nutrition sites	Chang et al., 1985
Effect of an experimental educational program about the importance of mediation and consequences of not taking the prescribed dosage versus on compliance with the prescribed drug regimen	Individuals with hypertension	Saounatsou et al., 2001
Effects of an experimental medication self-care program and a control hypertension education program on knowledge of medications, self-care behaviors, medication errors, and systolic and diastolic blood pressure	Elderly African-American women with hypertension	Harper, 1984
Effects of mechanical lift, rocking axillary, self-lift, shoulder-assist, and straight-pull lifting techniques on oxygen consumption, heart rate, respiratory rate, and blood pressure	Female nursing students	Geden, 1982
Effect of information about a pediatric patient's diagnosis, family structure, and gender on students' stereotyping behaviors	Female students in a baccalaureate nursing program	Glanz et al., 1989
Effect of information about a client's marital status on students' stereotyping behaviors	Female students in a baccalaureate nursing program	Ganong & Coleman, 1992
Effect of curriculum on changes in self-care attitudes	Nursing students in an Orem Self-Care Framework-based baccalaureate program General university students	Hartweg & Metcalfe, 1986
Effect of an experimental career awareness program and a control no career awareness program on success rate	Practical nursing students	Belcher, 1992
Effect of a self-learning module on learning to care for hospitalized children with tracheostomies	Registered nurses	Kang, 2002
Effects of the implementation of Orem's Self-Care Framework on nurses' attitudes and charting behavior	Registered nurses working in an acute care hospital	Rossow-Sebring et al., 1992
Effects of implementation of an Orem's Self-Care Framework-based nursing protocol on client receptivity and self-care agency and implementation problems	Registered nurses Adult day care agency staff Aftercare clients attending an adult day care program	Loveland-Cherry et al., 1985

(continued)

▶ TABLE 8–3
PUBLISHED REPORTS OF RESEARCH GUIDED BY THE SELF-CARE FRAMEWORK *(continued)*

Research Topic	Study Participants	Citation
Effects of a gerontological nursing continuing education program on nurses' knowledge of and attitudes toward the elderly and patients' satisfaction with and perceptions of nursing	Registered nurses Hospitalized elderly patients	Harrison & Novak, 1988
Effects of a decision support system versus control procedures on elicitation of elderly patients' preferences for self-care capability, nurses' care priorities, and patient outcomes of preference achievement and patient satisfaction	Nurses and elderly patients	Ruland, 1999

(Text continued from page 260)

conducted by nurse researchers, especially by Campbell, Dodd, Hagopian, Jirovec, Moore, Söderhamm, and their respective colleagues (see Table 8–3). Dodd's work, which has been ongoing since 1978, is an outstanding example of Self-Care Framework-based programmatic research. She and her colleagues designed correlational studies, based on the findings of early descriptive studies, and experimental studies, based on descriptive and correlational study findings. Furthermore, Dodd returned to descriptive work when moving from a focus on cancer patients receiving chemotherapy to those receiving radiation therapy and when expanding from a focus on patients to patients and their family members. Dodd (1997) explained that the descriptive and correlational studies were important "because [they] documented the therapeutic self-care demand and served as a basis for subsequent work that looked at specific self-care behaviors and health-deviation self-care requisites. As a result of this work, [Self-Care Framework]-based interventions were developed to promote self-care" (p. 984). The experimental intervention studies now have progressed to the level of randomized controlled clinical trials, and outcomes include not only self-care activities but also chemotherapy-related morbidity.

Hanucharurnkul and colleagues (2003) reported the results of a meta-analysis of self-care research conducted in Thailand, including master's theses and doctoral dissertations, as well as research conducted by nursing program faculty members. Most studies were guided by Orem's Self-Care Framework. The investigators reported that the collective study findings support the relation between variables representing the basic conditioning factors and self-care agency or dependent-care agency, with effect sizes ranging from moderate to large. They also reported that interventions designed to promote self-care had positive, moderate to large effects on various patient-focused outcomes, such as patient satisfaction, pain, and fasting blood sugar, and small effects on organization-focused outcomes, such as length of hospital stay.

Nursing Education. The Self-Care Framework, according to Orem, "is useful in all levels of education" (Fawcett, 2001, p. 36). Nursing education encompasses preprofessional, professional, and continuing education components, as well as beginning, advanced, and scientific levels (Orem, 2001). "Professional nursing programs preparatory for entrance to practice and for movement toward the professional (scientific) form of practice have as their organizing center human beings and the range of types of conditions and problems of persons who can benefit from nursing" (Orem, 2001, p. 440).

The utility of the Self-Care Framework for nursing education is evident. Citing an unpublished survey by Karb and Von Cannon, Berbiglia (1991) noted that "of the four nursing [models] most frequently used by [National League for Nursing] accredited baccalaureate programs that adopted a single [model], the [Self-Care Framework] ranked second in use" (p. 1159). Berbiglia (1991) went on to explain that the Self-Care Framework has guided the curriculum "for more than a decade and has emphasized educator competency in the use of this [framework in] a parochial liberal arts college in the south-west United States," but she did not identify the school by name (p. 1160).

As can be seen below, published reports indicate that the Self-Care Framework has been used as a guide for curriculum construction in diploma, associate degree, and baccalaureate nursing programs, as well as in continuing education and inservice education programs. The complete citations for the publications are given in the Education section of the chapter references. The use of the Self-Care Framework in many other nursing education programs is documented in a list published by the International Orem Society for Nursing Science and Scholarship (1994).

- Diploma Nursing Program
  - Methodist Medical Center of Illinois, Peoria, Illinois (Woolley et al., 1990)

- Associate Degree Nursing Program
  - Thornton Community College, South Holland, Illinois (Fenner, 1979)

- Baccalaureate Degree Nursing Programs
  - Georgetown University, Washington, DC (Piemme & Trainor, 1977)
  - Illinois Wesleyan University, Bloomington, Illinois (Woolley et al., 1990)
  - University of Missouri–Columbia (Taylor, 1985)
  - University of Southern Mississippi, Hattiesburg, Mississippi (Herrington & Houston, 1984; Richeson & Huch, 1988)
  - Wichita State University, Wichita, Kansas (Kurger, 1988)
  - University of Quebec in Hull, Hull, Quebec, Canada (Family nursing theory and practice courses) (deMontigny et al., 1997)
  - University of Ottawa, Ottawa, Ontario, Canada (Junior year nursing course) (Story & Ross, 1986)
  - Robert Gordon University, Foresterhill Campus, Aberdeen, Scotland (Adult Branch Program of a Diploma in Higher Education Nursing Course) (Gordon & Grundy, 1997)

- Continuing Education and Inservice Education
  - Binghamton General Hospital, Binghamton, New York (Orientation Program for New Graduates) (Feldsine, 1982)
  - Riverview Medical Center, Red Bank, New Jersey (Management Education Program for Staff Nurses, Unit-based and Hospital-wide Educational Programs) (O'Brien et al., 1992; Hooten, 1992)
  - Veterans Administration Medical Center, Salem, Virginia (Surgical Unit Staff Education Program) (McCoy, 1989)
  - University of Missouri-Columbia (Continuing Education Course in Gerontological Nursing) (Langland & Farrah, 1990)
  - Bessemer Carraway Medical Center, Bessemer, Alabama (Staff Development Program) (Romine, 1986)
  - Toronto General Hospital, Toronto, Ontario, Canada (Staff Education Programs) (Harman et al., 1989; Reid et al., 1989)

In addition, Berbiglia and Saenz (2002) described an undergraduate elective course, Nursing Concepts: Self-Care, that is based on the content of the Self-Care Framework. They did not, however, identify the school at which the course was offered. In an unpublished paper, Mullin and Weed (1980) outlined the use of the Self-Care Framework as a guide for the baccalaureate nursing curriculum at George Mason University in Fairfax, Virginia.

Nursing Administration. Orem (2001) defined nursing administration as "the body of persons who function in situational contexts to collectively manage courses of affairs enabling for the provision of nursing to the population currently served by an organized health service institution or agency and to populations to be served at future times" (p. 451). The utility of the Self-Care Framework for administration of nursing services is evident.

Allison and Renpenning (1999) developed a model for nursing administration derived from the Self-Care Framework and Orem's General Theory of Nursing Administration. They reasoned that nurse administrators must know and think nursing to achieve nursing goals, and that the Self-Care Framework provides the requisite mental model. Their model elaborates on the governing functions, executive functions, and essential operations functions that Orem (1989, 1995) identified as components of nursing administration.

A particularly innovative application of the Self-Care Framework in nursing administration was the *Professional Care System*, a computer software package for nursing documentation (Bliss-Holtz et al., 1992). Software development was initiated by Patricia Sayers, the founder and president of Nursing Systems International Incorporated of Columbus, New Jersey. The software package "is an information system based in [the Self-Care Framework] that supports nursing practice and management of nursing services" (McLaughlin et al., 1990, p. 175). The input to the computer is clinical data from patients, structured within the context of the Self-Care Framework. "Output from the system includes production of individualized patient care plans, a chronological record of patient care, reports in narrative or chart form relating patient variables with nurse action and patient outcomes, quality assurance reports, and other periodic management reports" (Bliss-Holtz, McLaughlin, & Taylor, 1990, p. 175). The software also can generate personalized critical paths and care maps. Placement of computers or terminals at the patient's bedside facilitates comprehensive documentation (Paternostro, 1992). Furthermore, the software can be used on portable computers that permit nurses to follow patients from their homes through inpatient stays back to their homes.

In addition, various paper and pencil practice tools have been developed to document nursing practice, measure the quality of Self-Care Framework-based practice, and evaluate nurses themselves. Those tools are identified and described in Table 8–2.

The use of the Self-Care Framework to structure nursing practice at a pediatric rehabilitation facility, Children's Seashore House, when it was located in Atlantic City, New Jersey, is documented in a videotape produced by Hale and Rhodes (1985). Another videotape documents the use of Orem's Self-Care Framework at the Vancouver, British Columbia, Department of Health and the Veterans Administration Medical Center in Fresno, California (Orem, 1993).

Publications document the use of the Self-Care Framework as an administrative and management guide in several health-care organizations in the United States, Canada, England, and Australia. Those health-care organizations are listed here. The complete citations for the publications are given in the Administration section of the chapter references.

- Medical Center Hospital, Burlington, Vermont (Cooperative Care Unit) (Weis, 1988)
- Supervised Environmental Living Facility (SELF), Waterbury, Connecticut (Dibner & Murphy, 1991)
- Binghamton General Hospital, Binghamton, New York (Feldsine, 1982)
- St. Luke's/Roosevelt Hospital Center, New York, New York (Senior Citizens Nurse-Managed Stay Well Center) (Smith & Sorrell, 1989)
- Newark Beth Israel Hospital, Newark, New Jersey (Fernandez & Wheeler, 1990; Fernandez et al., 1990; Fernandez et al., 1996; Scherer, 1988)
- Saint Elizabeth's Hospital, Elizabeth, New Jersey (Fernandez & Wheeler, 1990)
- Betty Bachrach Rehabilitation Hospital, Pomona, New Jersey (Derstine, 1992)
- Overlook Hospital, Summit, New Jersey (Hospice Unit) (Murphy, 1981)
- Riverview Medical Center, Red Bank, New Jersey (Barth, 1992; Brady & Cadamuro, 1992; Brennan & Duffy, 1992; Duffy, 1992; Farwell & Gossett, 1992; Fernandez et al., 1990; Gossett & DeTata, 1992; Hamm-Vita, 1990; Kane & O'Brien, 1992; Lantz, 1992; Strickland et al., 1992; Trofino, 1992)
- Phoenixville Hospital, Phoenixville, Pennsylvania (Husted & Strzelecki, 1985)
- Delaware State Hospital, New Castle, Delaware (Kaufman & Paulanka, 1994)

- Johns Hopkins Hospital, Baltimore, Maryland (Diabetic Nurse Management Clinic) (Allison, 1973; Bachscheider, 1974)
- Johns Hopkins Hospital, Baltimore, Maryland (Cardiac Nurse-Managed Clinics) (Crews, 1972)
- Georgetown University Hospital, Washington, DC (Van Eron, 1985)
- Veterans Administration Medical Center, Salem, Virginia (McCoy, 1989)
- Dorn Veterans Hospital, Columbia, South Carolina (Oncology and Acute Care Units) (Roach & Woods, 1993)
- William F. Bowld Hospital, University of Tennessee, Memphis (Renal Transplant Unit) (Hathaway & Strong, 1988)
- Veterans Affairs Medical Center, Gainesville, Florida (Lott et al., 1992; MacLeod & Sella, 1992; Sella & MacLeod, 1991)
- Bessemer Carraway Medical Center, Bessemer, Alabama (Romine, 1986)
- Mississippi Methodist Hospital and Rehabilitation Center, Jackson, Mississippi (Allison, 1985)
- Veterans Administration Medical Center, Indianapolis, Indiana (Nunn & Marriner-Tomey, 1989)
- Neighborhood Family Service Center, Scottsbluff, Nebraska (McVay, 1985)
- Veterans Administration Medical Center, Minneapolis, Minnesota (Snyder et al., 1991)
- National Jewish Center for Immunology and Respiratory Medicine, Denver, Colorado (Barnes, 1991)
- Presbyterian Health Plan, New Mexico (Calhoun & Casey, 2002)
- Tucson Medical Center, Tucson, Arizona (Del Togno-Armanasco et al., 1989)
- Veterans Administration Medical Center, Roseburg, Oregon (O'Connor, 1990)
- Loma Linda University Medical Center, Loma Linda, California (Neonatal Intensive Care Unit) (Angeles, 1991)
- Veterans Administration Medical Center, Fresno, California (Rossow-Sebring et al., 1992)
- Sir Mortimer B. Davis–Jewish General Hospital, Montreal, Quebec, Canada (Nursing Clinic for Rheumatoid Arthritis) (Porter & Shamian, 1983)
- Scarborough General Hospital, Toronto, Ontario, Canada (Fitch et al., 1991)
- Mississauga Hospital, Toronto, Ontario, Canada (Fitch et al., 1991)
- Toronto General Hospital, Toronto, Ontario, Canada (Campbell, 1984; Harman et al., 1989; Laurie-Shaw & Ives, 1988a, 1988b; Reid et al., 1989)
- Vancouver Health Department, Vancouver, British Columbia, Canada (Duncan & Murphy, 1988; McWilliams et al., 1988; Walker, 1993)

- The Patient-Family Learning Centre, Queen Elizabeth II Health Sciences Centre, Halifax, Nova Scotia, Canada (Lanigan, 2000)
- St. Thomas' Hospital, St. John's Dermatology Centre Outpatient Department, London, England (Hunter, 1992)
- Manchester Royal Infirmary, Manchester, England (Renal Unit) (Turner, 1989)
- Worthing Hospital, Day Hospital, Worthing, England (Dyer, 1990)
- Birmingham Children's Hospital, Birmingham, England (Clark & Bishop, 1988)
- Prince Henry Hospital, Sydney, Australia (Avery, 1992)

The implementation of the Self-Care Framework in all of the agencies listed here certainly is noteworthy. Of special note to contemporary health-care delivery is Calhoun and Casey's (2002) innovative ambulatory case management model, which they based on Orem's Self-Care Framework and the Case Management Society of America's Standards of Practice. The model was implemented in the Presbyterian Health Plan in New Mexico. Calhoun and Casey (2002) reported cost savings, but concluded that the reduction in costs was due to a reduction in personnel rather than use of the model, per se.

Nursing Practice. A nursing practitioner is a person "professionally educated and qualified to practice nursing who [is] engaged in its regular provision ... working at the entry or advanced level of professional practice" (Orem, 2001, p. 69). Orem noted that nursing practitioners may use the Self-Care Framework in "any nursing situation, because [the framework] ... is an explanation of what is common to all nursing situations, not just an explanation of an individual situation" (Fawcett, 2001, p. 37). The utility of the Self-Care Framework for use by nursing practitioners is fully documented (Table 8–4).

Review of the publications cited in Table 8–4 and those listed in the Commentary: Practice section of the chapter bibliography on the CD-ROM reveals that the Self-Care Framework has been used to guide nursing practice for individuals across the life span and for families and communities in many different inpatient and outpatient settings. Publications present descriptions of the use of the framework in such inpatient settings as intensive care and critical care units, neonatal intensive care units, operating rooms, acute care units, medical-surgical units, obstetrical units, psychiatric units and institutions, rehabilitation units, pediatric residential treatment facilities, and nursing homes. Self-Care Framework-based nursing practice also occurs in such outpatient settings as persons' homes and the community, emergency departments, ambulatory clinics, pediatric interdisciplinary phenylketonuria clinics, college health programs, industry, and hospices.

In those and other settings, the Self-Care Framework has been used to guide the nursing care of well children and adults, childbearing women, and individuals with various acute and chronic health conditions such as substance abuse, asthma, upper respiratory infections, gastroenteritis, diabetes, cancer, cardiac and circulatory problems, cerebrovascular accidents, neurologic problems, multiple sclerosis, Parkinson's disease, Guillain-Barré syndrome, end-stage renal disease, emotional problems and mental illness, and terminal illness. In addition, Self-Care Framework–based nursing has been described for patients who have had elective minor surgery, cataract surgery, head and neck surgery, coronary artery bypass surgery, renal transplant, hip arthroplasty, and hysterectomy. Furthermore, the Self-Care Framework has been successfully adapted for use with people of diverse cultures, including Native Americans, African-Americans, Spanish-Americans, Puerto Ricans, and the Chinese.

The Self-Care Framework also has been extended for use with multiperson units, including the family and the community (see Table 8–4). Hanchett (1990) explained how the Self-Care Framework is used when the community is viewed as an aggregate of individuals. Taylor and McLaughlin (1991) explained that Orem's work is compatible with views of the community as an aggregate or collection, an entity having meaning and purpose beyond the individual, and as relationships among groups of people. Taylor and Renpenning (1995, 2001) extended the discussion of use of the Self-Care Framework to individuals versus multiperson units as the unit of service for nursing practice.

Social Congruence

The Self-Care Framework is generally congruent with contemporary expectations regarding nursing practice. Riehl-Sisca (1985b) noted that the self-care label associated with the Self-Care Framework is appealing to nurses and to potential and actual patients. She pointed out that Orem's approach to nursing "appeared on the scene when the general public was becoming more knowledgeable about medical treatment and disenchanted with physicians' care and motivation. ... In some cases, the patient seems to know as much about his or her condition as does the physician. This encourages the taking care of oneself" (p. 308).

The Self-Care Framework is congruent with society's expectations that individuals should have decision-making responsibility regarding their health care. Indeed, Bramlett, Gueldner, and Sowell (1990) noted that Orem's

(Text continues on page 291)

Practice Situation	Population	Citation*

APPLICATION OF THE SELF-CARE FRAMEWORK

INDIVIDUALS

Well Children
	Normal newborns	Dennis & Jesek-Hale, 2003
	An 8-year-old girl seen in a family practice clinic	Eichelberger et al., 1980
	10-year-old school children	Gantz, 1980
	Children and adolescents	Gast, 1992
	Children of mentally ill parents	Atkins, 1992

Children with Acute Health Conditions
	An infant in a neonatal intensive care unit	Tolentino, 1990
	A hospitalized infant, toddler, preschooler, and school-age child	Facteau, 1980
	Children experiencing pain and their parents	Knigge-Demal, 1998

Children with Chronic Health Conditions
	Children with asthma	Walsh, 1989
	Mentally and physically handicapped children	Hitejc, 2000
	Children with physical, emotional, cognitive, or behavioral problems due to abuse or neglect	Titus & Porter, 1989
	Children with autistic spectrum disorder	Oliver, 2003
	An 8-year-old child with leukemia	Foote et al., 1993; Wright et al., 1994
	Children with Down syndrome	Steele et al., 1989
	Adolescents who abuse alcohol	Kerr, 1985
		Michael & Sewall, 1980
	An adolescent who received a renal transplant	Norris, 1991
	An adolescent with a corneal dystrophy	Stevens, 1994
	Adolescents with cystic fibrosis	McCracken, 1985
	Adolescents with physical disabilities	Hedahl, 1983

Well Adults
	Employees in an industry	Ruddick-Bracken & Mackie, 1989
	Women seeking contraceptives at a family planning clinic	Oakley et al., 1989
	A 35-year-old married woman who sought counseling about sexuality	Cohen, 1985
	A health education group	Jewell & Sullivan, 1996
	Women experiencing labor and delivery	Fields, 1987
	Women attempting vaginal birth after a cesarean delivery	Catanese, 1987
	Postpartum women and their infants	Dunphy & Jackson, 1985
	Patients seeking facial rejuvenation	LeRoy, 1998
	85-year-old women living in their own homes	Finnegan, 1986; Langley, 1989
	Noninstitutionalized elderly persons	Eliopoulos, 1984; Garvan et al., 1980
	A healthy elderly man	García Velázquez, 2002

Adults at Risk for Illness/injury
	Indigent transient and migrant farmworkers	Stein, 1993
	Homeless persons	Park, 1989

Adults with Acute Health Conditions
	Pregnant women with gestational diabetes mellitus	Keohane & Lacey, 1991
	A pregnant woman with multiple obstetric problems	Woolery, 1983

*See the Practice section of the chapter references for complete citations.

A woman who underwent an emergency cesarean delivery	Harris, 1980
Women who underwent hysterectomy	Berbiglia, 1997; Thomas et al., 1992
	Weir, 1993
A 23-year-old woman who attempted suicide	Calley et al., 1980
A 38-year-old woman with multiple health problems who had been in a house fire	Fawcett et al., 1992
A 25-year-old woman with an acute asthmatic attack	Miller, 1989
A 64-year-old man with acute exacerbation of chronic obstructive pulmonary disease	Taylor, 1990
Adults scheduled for minor elective surgery	Swindale, 1989
A 32-year-old woman receiving chemotherapy for non-Hodgkin's lymphoma	Whenery-Tedder, 1991
Women with breast cancer	Marten, 1978; Meriney, 1990
A 64-year-old woman with metastatic cancer	Morse & Werner, 1988
Adults undergoing autologous bone marrow transplant for treatment of cancer	Mack, 1992
Adults undergoing head and neck surgery for treatment of cancer	Dropkin, 1981
Patient with hepatocellular carcinoma after extended right hepatectomy	Cheung, 2002
A 42-year-old man with shortness of breath seen in an outpatient clinic	Runtz & Urtel, 1983
Adults who had a myocardial infarction	Garrett, 1985; Gibson, 1980
Adults with severe cardiac illness	Dumas, 1992
	Jaarsma et al., 1998
Adults undergoing coronary artery bypass graft surgery	Campuzano, 1982; Fawcett et al., 1992
Adults with head injuries or cranial surgery	James, 1992
Adults with complex wounds and multiple health problems	Ogden, 1996
A 62-year-old man with multiple health problems and postoperative complications	Fawcett et al., 1987
A 68-year-old woman admitted to a hospital with multiple acute and chronic health problems	Hewes & Hannigan, 1985
Adults with acute pancreatitis	Noone, 1995
Adult women and men undergoing total hip arthroplasty	Boon & Graham, 1992; Craig, 1989
	Mehta, 1993
A 68-year-old man with multiple sclerosis admitted to a hospital due to urinary retention	Robichaud-Ekstrand, 1990
An elderly woman undergoing cataract surgery	Beed, 1991
Elderly surgical patients	Priddy, 1989
An elderly person with hypothermia	Smith, 1996
Hospitalized elderly patients with acute confusional syndrome	Cámara González et al., 2002
Adults with chronic health conditions	
Adults with developmental and learning disabilities	Boulter, 1995; Mann, 1994
	Raven, 1988–1989, 1989
	Rice, 1994
A 29-year-old woman with cervical cancer	Berbiglia, 2002
Adults who are alcohol dependent	Dunn, 1990
Adults who abuse drugs	Compton, 1989
Persons with HIV	Phillips & Morrow, 1998
Women with hypertension	Cade, 2001

(continued)

Practice Situation	Population	Citation
	Adults with Chronic Health Conditions	
	An adult with asthma	Monteiro et al., 2002
	Woman with diabetes mellitus	Payne, 1987
	Adults with diabetes mellitus	Clang, 1985
		Clark, 1985
		Fitzgerald, 1980
		Mulkeen, 1989
	Adults with diabetic ocular sequelae	Zach, 1982
	Adults with diabetic peripheral neuropathy	Petrlik, 1976
	Adults with urinary incontinence	Bernier, 2002
	Elderly individuals with urgency urinary incontinence	Barajas Román et al., 2002
	Adults with rheumatoid arthritis	Dear & Keen, 1982
		Smith, 1989
		Stewart & Basset, 1992
	A 64-year-old woman with rheumatoid arthritis receiving home health-care nursing services	Berbiglia, 2002
	Patients with chronic lower extremity edema	Shebel, 2002
	A patient with tetraplegia	Dornik, 2001
	Paraplegic patient at home	Fialho et al., 2002
	Adults undergoing rehabilitation for fractures	Strong et al., 1995
	Elderly persons requiring rehabilitation services	Bracher, 1989
	Adults with psychiatric illnesses	Underwood, 1980
	Adults with borderline personality disorder	Eagan, 1998
	A man with suspected Parkinson's disease	Kelly, 1995
	A 50-year-old woman with Huntington's disease	van der Weyden, 1994
	A 53-year-old man with amyotrophic lateral sclerosis	Taylor, 1988
	A person with Guillain-Barré syndrome	Anderson, 1992
	A 64-year-old woman with multiple sclerosis	MacLellan, 1989
	Adults with leg ulcers	Eagle, 1996; Flanagan, 1991
	Adults with an ostomy	Blaylock, 1991; Bromley, 1980
	Adults with end-stage renal failure	Harris, 1996
		Perras & Zappacosta, 1982
		Summerton, 1995; Zinn, 1986
	Adults recovering from a stroke	Redfern, 1990
	A 64-year-old woman with multiple health problems receiving home care	Berbiglia, 1997
	An elderly person	Best, 1998
	Elderly persons attending ambulatory nursing clinics	Alford, 1985
	Elderly persons requiring long-term care	Sullivan & Monroe, 1987; Walsh & Judd, 1989
	Elderly nursing home residents	Whelan, 1984; Anna et al., 1978
	Elderly persons with chronic mental illness	Sullivan & Munroe, 1986
		Duffey et al., 1993
		MacDonald, 1991; Moore, 1989
		O'Donovan, 1990a, 1990b, 1992; Wright, 1988

Elderly persons with depression	Whall, 1994
Elderly persons with dementia	Roper et al., 1991;
	Roy & Collin, 1994
	Sandman et al., 1986
Dying persons receiving hospice care	Leferriere, 1995;
	Walborn, 1980

FAMILIES

Siblings of a premature or ill infant	Doll-Speck et al., 1993
A family experiencing pertussis	Logue, 1997
An African-American family living in an urban low-income housing project	Chin, 1985
A Spanish-American family with a mentally ill member	Orem, 1983b
A family with a member with diabetes mellitus and leukemia	Orem, 1983a
A family with a member who is dying	Jones, 1996

COMMUNITIES

A community	Batra, 1996
A small urban community	Abraham & Fallon, 1997
An urban community	Nowakowski, 1980
An affluent residential community	Hanchett, 1988

assumptions about human beings and the overall focus of the Self-Care Framework lead to the consumer-centric form of nursing advocacy. They commented, "Although Orem's framework does not explicitly admonish paternalistically based advocacy, [it] specifies that advocacy activities should be limited to only those instances when an individual is incapable of complete self-care, and that such behaviors should be temporary, and patients should be provided with as much information regarding their health as possible" (p. 160).

Similarly, the Self-Care Framework is congruent with the primary health-care focus of the "Health for All by the Year 2010" initiative and other similar initiatives. Dier (1987) pointed to that congruence and proposed a collaborative project between Canada and Thailand that "combines the Canadian experience in using Orem's Self-Care Framework with the extensive Thai knowledge about nursing in primary health settings" (p. 326).

The emphasis on self-care agency during times of illness is, however, not completely congruent with some people's expectations of nursing practice. Moreover, attention must be given to expectations of people of different regional and cultural groups. For example, Anna and associates (1978) found that the nursing goal of self-care agency for the patient was not well accepted by either patients or staff of a nursing home. In that situation, a more dependent sick role view, with the nurse doing for and acting for the patient,

had been adopted by both patients and staff. Anna and colleagues (1978) also noted that a Mexican-American patient in the nursing home "did not see the relevance of performing self-care activities, and he functioned with the expectation that the staff would do everything for him" (p. 11). Similarly, Roach and Woods (1993) reported that although physicians and many patients had positive responses to an Orem Self-Care Framework-based cooperative care program that encourages patient self-care and family involvement in caregiving, the program "was not attractive to all patients" (p. 28). They attributed the lack of acceptance of cooperative care by patients at a veterans' hospital in South Carolina "in part to the fact that many of our patients were older men from traditional southern backgrounds who were cared for by spouses and female relatives" even when the men were functionally able to care for themselves (p. 29).

Orem (2001) noted that when the person is able but reluctant to engage in self-care, he or she must be helped to view himself or herself as a self-care agent. Elaborating, she stated, "Self-care is performed largely out of habit, but individuals who have not thought about their self-care role may need to be helped to look at themselves as self-care agents in order to understand the values to which their habits commit them and to appraise the adequacy of their self-care" (p. 256). Roach and Woods (1993) added that "in such instances, patients were encouraged to learn to care for themselves in case their spouse became unavailable or unable to do care giving" (p. 29).

Patients can be assisted to understand self-care and to become willing to participate actively in their care through the use of *The Self-Care Manual for Patients*, which was developed by Kyle and Pitzer (1990). They commented, "The key to the success of self-care is the transformation of individuals from passive, dependent patients to active partners" (p. 39).

In discussing the constraints on use of the Self-Care Framework of nursing in the United Kingdom, Behi (1986) stated, "Perhaps the most fundamental constraint in this country is society's attitude. Self-care as a concept, and more importantly, as a value, is stronger in American society where control of an individual's health is seen as that person's responsibility" (p. 35). Behi (1986) concluded, however, that the Self-Care Framework could be used in general wards of the National Health Service in the United Kingdom.

The primary prevention aspect of the Self-Care Framework is another area where attention to congruence with societal expectations must be given. Although consumers are becoming increasingly aware of the value of health promotion and the nurse's role in promoting wellness, they still may need to be helped to accept that nursing role and use nursing services in that area.

Anecdotal and empirical evidence supports the speculative claims that the Self-Care Framework is generally congruent with the expectations of patients and health-care team members for nursing care. Orem's (2001) list of nurses' reactions to use of the Self-Care Framework provides some anecdotal evidence of its social congruence. Particularly relevant points from the list are given here:

- Nurses develop their personal styles of practice within the domain and boundaries of nursing set by the [framework].
- Nurses (and physicians more slowly) recognize the need for nursing discharge of patients separate from medical discharge.
- Nurses recognize that they have a theoretical base that serves them in performing the professional function of design of systems of nursing care. The design function is retained by and specific to the professional person.
- Nurses through their design of systems of nursing bring into focus their own role responsibilities and role functions, as well as those of other nurses, their patients, and members of patients' families who are dependent-care agents. (Orem, 2001, p. 447)

An addition to the anecdotal evidence comes from Doherty (1992), who commented that the Self-Care Framework

made important contributions to her thinking about nursing care plans. Furthermore, Roach and Woods (1993) noted that "requests for [Orem Self-Care Framework-based] cooperative care were made by patients on repeat hospital admissions" (p. 29). Moreover, Scherer (1988) reported that use of the Self-Care Framework at the Beth Israel Medical Center in Newark, New Jersey, was associated with enhanced patient satisfaction with nursing care, less staff turnover, and reduced costs.

Empirical evidence was provided by Nunn and Marriner-Tomey (1989), who reported that in one survey at the Veterans Administration Medical Center in Indianapolis, Indiana, "30 out of 39 nurses perceived that [framework]-based practice would increase their job satisfaction, five said it wouldn't, and four were uncertain" (p. 67). In a survey of nursing attendants, 34 indicated that they believed patients would benefit from Self-Care Framework-based nursing practice, two did not believe patients would benefit, and three were uncertain (Nunn & Marriner-Tomey, 1989). Moreover, Rossow-Sebring, Carrieri, and Seward (1992) reported that the evaluation of the implementation of the Self-Care Framework at the Veterans Administration Medical Center in Fresno, California, revealed "increase[d] staff nurses' satisfaction with nursing and enhanced [nursing] perception of the value of patient teaching" (p. 212).

Social Significance

Orem (2001) claimed that Self-Care Framework-based nursing practice compensates for or overcomes "health-associated human limitations for engagement in self-care or dependent-care" (p. 81). By doing so, nurses contribute to "maintaining health, preventing disease and disability and restoring or maintaining life processes" (p. 81). The empirical evidence for that claim continues to accrue.

For example, Buckwalter and Kerfoot's (1982) work suggested that psychiatric patient discharge teaching that emphasizes self-care was effective in areas such as compliance with psychotropic medication regimens and appropriate use of community resources. The emphasis on self-care agency and recognition of the person's ability to care for self could lead to more efficient use of health-care services. Indeed, Gulick's (1991) study findings revealed that an intervention focusing on self-assessment and monitoring of functioning and symptom prevalence resulted in less frequent use of professional health services by the experimental group of multiple sclerosis patients than by the control group during a 27-month period.

Thus, if people are helped to recognize and improve their self-care abilities and to use health services only when they identify potential or actual self-care deficits, less inappropriate use of the services occurs. Furthermore, emphasis on self-care agency could reduce the length of time the person requires health-care services. This may be especially important in the continuing milieu of cost containment.

The empirical evidence related to the social significance of the Self-Care Framework is, however, equivocal. Some study results reveal beneficial effects of framework-based nursing interventions, but other results fail to support the hypothesized benefits. Dodd (1997), for example, reported that her experimental studies have not always yielded the expected beneficial effects on self-care. Consequently, additional research that builds on the knowledge gained from past research is warranted. As Dodd (1997) pointed out, "through testing of Orem's [Self-Care Framework], we have learned from the propositions that were supported and those that were not supported" (p. 987). Furthermore, sufficient research addressing particular topics now exists to support a meta-analysis that could determine the magnitude of effects and identify design and other study characteristics that may enhance understanding of the conflicting findings (Rosenthal, 1991).

CONTRIBUTIONS TO THE DISCIPLINE OF NURSING

The Self-Care Framework and the Theory of Self-Care, the Theory of Self-Care Deficit, and the Theory of Nursing System represent a substantial contribution to nursing knowledge by providing an explicit and specific focus for nursing actions that is different from that of other health-care professions. Orem has fulfilled her goal of identifying the domain and boundaries of nursing as a science and an art. The Self-Care Framework has, as Orem (2001) pointed out, been widely accepted "by nursing practitioners, by nursing curriculum designers, by teachers of nursing, by nursing researchers and scholars as a valid general comprehensive [nursing model]. It also [unfortunately] has been denigrated and rejected by some nurses since its inception" (p. 420). "Clearly," as Isenberg (2001) declared, the Self-Care Framework "is playing, and is expected to continue to play, a pivotal role in the advancement of nursing science and professional practice" (p. 187)

The emphasis on self-care agency in the Self-Care Framework and the consideration given to the patient's perspective of health status underscore the importance of the person in the nursing care situation. The wide acceptance of the Self-Care Framework suggests that these features are especially attractive to nurses who view the person as capable of deliberate and independent action. Moreover, the use of the framework in many different settings and with different age groups suggests that Orem's

view of the person who is the patient is an appropriate one for nursing.

Perhaps the most important contribution of the Self-Care Framework is its explicit focus on what matters to nurses and how that focus helps nurses to retain a nursing perspective in the multidisciplinary milieu of health care. Dodd (1997) explained that "Orem's [framework] provides a nursing-based focus and systematic guidelines for examining the balance between a person's needs, capabilities, and limitations in exercising self-care actions to enhance personal health. ... Although we have incorporated knowledge from other disciplines (e.g., physiology, pharmacology, dentistry), Orem's [framework] assisted us in maintaining a focus on issues salient to nursing practice" (p. 987).

Orem has continued to develop aspects of the Self-Care Framework and the Theory of Self-Care, the Theory of Self-Care Deficit, and the Theory of Nursing System. In 1987, Orem (personal communication, August 6, 1987) stated that her future work would focus specifically on "development of practice models, development of rules for practice when certain conditions prevail, continued study of 'foundational capabilities and dispositions' in their relationship to action, and development of ... models for each of the power components of self-care agency."

In the fifth edition of her book, published in 1995, Orem explained that advances in those areas had been made by "teachers of generic undergraduate nursing students, registered nurses and nursing assistants, nursing practitioners in specialty areas of nursing, nursing researchers, nursing scholars, and theorists. Some developments, [however,] are scattered, awaiting the efforts of scholars of [the Self-Care Framework] to organize specific developments and research findings within the structure provided by the [framework]" (p. 437).

In the sixth edition of her book, published in 2001, Orem explained that her work can be organized into six main themes. Those themes are:

- Why persons need and can be helped through nursing
- The tridimensional relationship between person who need nursing and persons who produce nursing, including a social relationship, an interpersonal relationship, and a technologic or clinical relationship
- The unitary nature of human beings who function as persons in their life situations
- Deliberate action, or actions that are deliberately selected and deliberately performed by persons to achieve a foreseen and desired result or condition that does not presently exist
- The methods that one person can use in the process of assisting or helping a person or persons do what should be done but which the person is unable to do because of

limited powers or capabilities for engaging in some or all of the process operations of deliberate action
- Nursing as practical science with [speculatively or] theoretically practical and practically practice content components (Orem, 2001, pp. vii–viii)

Orem "added an introductory chapter on human services [to the sixth edition of her book] to set forth what is common to all of the human health services. This is one of the things we forget; we sometimes think we are moving from outer space rather than from real life situations" (Fawcett, 2001, p. 35). In addition, Orem (2001) introduced a conceptualization of nursing science as six speculatively or theoretically practical nursing sciences, which "are based on the nature of the way or form in which nurses provide care to person who require nursing (nursing practice sciences) and the kinds of knowledge required by nurses to understand these forms of care (foundational nursing sciences)" (p. 493). (See the Nursing Research Guidelines section of this chapter.) Orem regards the nursing practice sciences as "in a sense … analogous to medicine's practice sciences, such as internal medicine, surgery, and so forth; they are the way you practice" (Fawcett, 2001, p. 35).

Despite the vast amount of Self-Care Framework-based research (Table 8–3), even more studies are needed, including systematic study of nursing practice outcomes (Taylor et al., 2000). Moreover, reliable and valid measures of the basic conditioning factors are needed (Moore & Pichler, 2000). The needed instrument development work and other research should be ensured by two organizations devoted to the study of self-care. The Self-Care Institute was established at George Mason University School of Nursing in Fairfax, Virginia, to promote self-care research and to develop, compile, and maintain a database consisting of individuals and organizations united across disciplines by a common interest in self-care. The interests of the Institute extend beyond Orem's approach to self-care to a consideration of self-care in a general manner. The International Orem Society for Nursing Science and Scholarship was founded in the late 1980s to "advance nursing science and scholarship through the use of Dorothea E. Orem's nursing conceptualizations in nursing education, practice, and research" (Bylaws of the International Orem Society for Nursing Science and Scholarship, April 1992, p. 1). The Society published a newsletter from 1989 to 2002 that extended the *Self-Care Deficit Nursing Theory Newsletter*, which had been published by the School of Nursing at the University of Missouri–Columbia between 1980 and 1989. In 2002, the Society newsletter was expanded to a peer-reviewed journal entitled *Self-Care, Dependent-Care, and Nursing*. Furthermore, the volume and quality of nursing research

dealing with self-care, including Orem's framework, was increased by the federally funded predoctoral and postdoctoral fellowship program that was established in 1992 at Wayne State University in Detroit, Michigan. In addition, the work of the members of the Orem Study Group should result in continued refinement of the Self-Care Framework and recommendations for targeted research projects.

The Self-Care Framework has been adopted enthusiastically by many nurses. It presents an optimistic view of patients' contributions to their health care that is in keeping with currently evolving social values. Despite the many advantages of the Self-Care Framework, potential users are encouraged to continue to evaluate the effectiveness of the Self-Care Framework in nursing situations through systematic research so that its cross-cultural credibility may be more fully determined.

 ### REFERENCES

Allison, S.E., & Renpenning, K. (1999). Nursing administration in the 21st century. Thousand Oaks, CA: Sage.

Anna, D.J., Christensen, D.G., Hohon, S.A., Ord, L., & Wells, S.R. (1978). Implementing Orem's conceptual framework. Journal of Nursing Administration, 8(11), 8–11.

Arnold, M.B. (1960). Deliberate action. In Emotion and Personality. Vol. 11, Neurological and Physiological Aspects (pp. 193–204). New York: Columbia University Press.

Banfield, B.E. (1998). A philosophical inquiry of Orem's self-care deficit nursing theory. Dissertation Abstracts International, 58, 5885B.

Banfield, B.E. (2001). Philosophic foundations of Orem's work. In D.E. Orem (Ed.), Nursing: Concepts of practice (6th ed., pp. xi–xvi). St. Louis: Mosby.

Barnum, B.J.S (1998). Nursing Theory: Analysis, Application, Evaluation (5th ed.). Philadelphia: Lippincott.

Behi, R. (1986). Look after yourself. Nursing Times, 82(37), 35–37.

Berbiglia, V.A. (1991). A case study: Perspectives on a self-care deficit nursing theory–based curriculum. Journal of Advanced Nursing, 16, 1158–1163.

Berbiglia, V., & Saenz, J. (2002). Teaching strategies for fostering concept attainment and student responsibility. Self-Care and Dependent-Care Nursing, 10(1), 3–7.

Black, M. (1962). Models and metaphors. Ithaca, NY: Cornell University Press.

Bliss-Holtz, J., McLaughlin, K., & Taylor, S.G. (1990). Validating nursing theory for use within a computerized nursing information system. Advances in Nursing Science, 13(2), 46–52.

Bliss-Holtz, J., Taylor, S.G., McLaughlin, K., Sayers, P., & Nickle, L. (1992). Development of a computerized information system based on self-care deficit nursing theory. In J.M. Arnold & G.A. Pearson, Computer applications in nursing education and practice (pp. 87–93). New York: National League for Nursing.

Bramlett, M.H., Gueldner, S.H., & Sowell, R.L. (1990). Consumer-centric advocacy: Its connection to nursing frameworks. Nursing Science Quarterly, 3, 156–161.

Buckwalter, K.C., & Kerfoot, K.M. (1982). Teaching patients self care: A critical aspect of psychiatric discharge planning. Journal of Psychiatric Nursing and Mental Health Services, 20(5), 15–20.

Calhoun, J., & Casey, P. (2002). Redesigning case management in managed care—An eclectic approach: From city to ranch. Lippincott's Case Management, 7, 180–191.

Dennis, C.M. (1997). Self-care deficit theory of nursing: Concepts and applications. St. Louis: Mosby.

Denyes, M.J., Orem, D.E., & Bekel, G. (2001). Self-care: A foundational science. Nursing Science Quarterly, 14, 48–54.

Dier, K.A. (1987). A model for collaboration in nursing practice: Thailand and Canada. In K.J. Hannah, M. Reimer, W.C. Mills, & S. Letourneau (Eds.), Clinical judgment and decision making: The future with nursing diagnosis (pp. 323–327). New York: Wiley.

Dodd, M.J. (1997). Self-care: Ready or not! Oncology Nursing Forum, 24, 981–990.

Doherty, S. (1992). Care plans—A personal view. British Journal of Theatre Nursing, 2(5), 4–5.

Fawcett, J. (2001). The nurse theorists: 21st century updates—Dorothea E. Orem. Nursing Science Quarterly, 14, 34–38.

Fernandez, R.D., Hebert, G.J., & Bliss-Holtz, J. (1996). Application of self-care deficit theory. In P. Hinton Walker & B. Neuman (Eds.), Blueprint for use of nursing models (pp. 228–235). New York: NLN Press.

Fessenden, C.C. (2003). Adoption of testicular self-examination. Dissertation Abstracts International, 63, 5157B.

Foster, P.C., & Bennett, A.M. (2002). Self-care deficit nursing theory: Dorothea E. Orem. In J. B. George (Ed.), Nursing theories: The base for professional nursing practice (5th ed., pp. 125–154). Upper Saddle River, NJ: Prentice Hall.

Foster, P.C., & Janssens, N.P. (1985). Dorothea E. Orem. In J.B. George (Ed.), Nursing theories: The base for professional nursing practice (2nd ed., pp. 124–139). Englewood Cliffs, NJ: Prentice-Hall.

Frederick, H.K., & Northam, E. (1938). A textbook of nursing practice (2nd ed.). New York: Macmillan.

Gaffney, K.F., & Moore, J.M. (1996). Testing Orem's theory of self-care deficit: Dependent care agent performance for children. Nursing Science Quarterly, 9, 160–164.

Geden, E.A. (1985). The relationship between self-care theory and empirical research. In J. Riehl-Sisca (Ed.), The science and art of self-care (pp. 265–270). Norwalk, CT: Appleton-Century-Crofts.

Gulick, E.E. (1991). Self-assessed health and use of health services. Western Journal of Nursing Research, 13, 195–219.

Hale, M., & Rhodes, G. (1985). Care with a concept. Chapel Hill, NC: Health Sciences Consortium. [Videotape.]

Hanchett, E.S. (1990). Nursing models and community as client. Nursing Science Quarterly, 3, 67–72.

Hanucharurnkul, S., Wittaya-sooporn, J., Luecha, Y., & Maneesriwongul, W. (2003). An integrative review and meta-analysis of self-care research in Thailand: 1988–1999. In K.M Renpenning & S.G. Taylor (Eds.), Self-care theory in nursing: Selected papers of Dorothea Orem (pp. 339–354). New York: Springer.

Harré, R. (1970). The Principles of Scientific Thinking. Chicago: University of Chicago Press.

Hartnett-Rauckhorst, L. (1968). Development of a theoretical model for the identification of nursing requirements in a selected aspect of self-care. Unpublished master's thesis. Washington, DC: Catholic University of America.

Henderson, V. (1955). Textbook of the principles and practice of nursing (5th ed.). New York: Macmillan.

Hooten, S.L. (1992). Education of staff nurses to practice within a conceptual framework. Nursing Administration Quarterly, 16(3), 34–35.

International Orem Society for Nursing Science and Scholarship (1994, March). Orem-based schools of nursing in the United States (National League for Nursing Accredited). Columbia, MO: The Society for Nursing Science and Scholarship.

Isenberg, M.A. (2001). Self-care deficit nursing theory: Directions for advancing nursing science and professional practice. In M.E. Parker (Ed.), Nursing Theories and Nursing Practice (pp. 179–191). Philadelphia: F.A. Davis.

Kotarbinski, T. (1965). Praxiology: An introduction to the sciences of efficient action [Trans. O. Wojtasiewicz]. New York: Pergamon Press.

Kyle, B.A.S., & Pitzer, S.A. (1990). A self-care approach to today's challenges. Nursing Management, 21(3), 37–39.

Lonergan, B.J.F. (1958). Insight: A study of human understanding. New York: Philosophical Library.

Marriner-Tomey, A. (Ed.). (1989). Nursing theorists and their work (2nd ed). St. Louis: Mosby.

Mason, T., & Chandley, M. (1990). Nursing models in a special hospital: A critical analysis of efficacy. Journal of Advanced Nursing, 15, 667–673.

McLaughlin, K., Taylor, S., Bliss-Holtz, J., Sayers, P., & Nickle, L. (1990). Shaping the future: The marriage of nursing theory and informatics. Computers in Nursing, 8, 174–179.

McQuiston, C.M., & Campbell, J.C. (1997). Theoretical substruction: A guide for theory testing. Nursing Science Quarterly, 10, 117–123.

Meleis, A.I. (1997). Theoretical nursing. Development and progress (3rd ed.). Philadelphia: Lippincott.

Moore, J.B. (1993). Predictors of children's self-care performance: Testing the theory of self-care deficit. Scholarly Inquiry for Nursing Practice, 7, 199–212.

Moore, J.B., & Mosher, R.B. (1997). Adjustment responses of children and their mothers to cancer: Self-care and anxiety. Oncology Nursing Forum, 24, 519–525.

Moore, J.B., & Pichler, V.H. (2000). Measurement of Orem's basic conditioning factors: A review of published research. Nursing Science Quarterly, 13, 137–142.

Mosher, R.R., & Moore, J.B. (1998). The relationship of self-concept and self-care in children with cancer. Nursing Science Quarterly, 11, 116–122.

Mullin, V.I., & Weed, F. (1980, October). Orem's self-care concept as a conceptual framework for a nursing curriculum. Paper presented at the Virginia State Nurses' Association Convention.

Munley, M.J., & Sayers, P.A. (1984). Self-care deficit theory of nursing: A primer for application of the concepts. North Brunswick, NJ: Personal and Family Health Associates.

Nunn, D., & Marriner-Tomey, A. (1989). Applying Orem's model in nursing administration. In B. Henry, C. Arndt, M. DiVincenti, & A. Marriner-Tomey (Eds.), Dimensions of nursing administration: Theory, research, education, practice (pp. 63–67). Boston: Blackwell Scientific.

Nursing Development Conference Group. (1973). Concept formalization in nursing: Process and product. Boston: Little, Brown.

Nursing Development Conference Group. (1979). Concept formalization in nursing: Process and Product (2nd ed.). Boston: Little, Brown.

Orem, D.E. (1956). Hospital nursing service: An analysis. Indianapolis: Indiana State Board of Health, Division of Hospital and Institutional Services.

Orem, D.E. (1959). Guides for developing curricula for the education of practical nurses. Washington, DC: US Government Printing Office.

Orem, D.E. (1971). Nursing: Concepts of practice. New York: McGraw-Hill.

Orem, D.E. (1978, December). A general theory of nursing. Paper presented at the Second Annual Nurse Educator Conference, New York. [Audiotape.]

Orem, D.E. (1980). Nursing: Concepts of practice (2nd ed.). New York: McGraw-Hill.

Orem, D.E. (1985). Nursing: Concepts of practice (3rd ed.). New York: McGraw-Hill.

Orem, D.E. (1989). Theories and hypotheses for nursing administration. In B. Henry, M. DiVincenti, C. Arndt, & A. Marriner (Eds.), Dimensions of nursing administration. Theory, research, education and practice (pp. 55–62). Boston: Blackwell Scientific.

Orem, D.E. (1990). A nursing practice theory in three parts, 1956–1989. In M.E. Parker (Ed.), Nursing theories in practice (pp. 47–60). New York: National League for Nursing.

Orem, D.E. (1991). Nursing: Concepts of practice (4th ed.). St. Louis: Mosby.

Orem, D.E. (1993). The Nurse Theorists: Excellence in Action—Dorothea Orem. Athens, OH: Fuld Institute for Technology in Nursing Education. [Videotape.]

Orem, D.E. (1995). Nursing: Concepts of practice (5th ed.). St. Louis: Mosby.

Orem, D.E. (1997). Views of human beings specific to nursing. Nursing Science Quarterly, 10, 26–31.

Orem, D.E. (2001). Nursing: Concepts of practice (6th ed.). St. Louis: Mosby.

Orem, D.E., & Taylor, S.G. (1986). Orem's general theory of nursing. In P. Winstead-Fry (Ed.), Case studies in nursing theory (pp. 37–71). New York: National League for Nursing.

Orem, D.E., & Vardiman, E.M. (1995). Orem's nursing theory and positive mental health: Practical considerations. Nursing Science Quarterly, 8, 165–173.

Parsons, T. (1937). The structure of social action. New York: McGraw-Hill.

Parsons, T. (1951). The social system. New York: The Free Press.

Paternostro, I. (1992). Developing theory-based software for nurses, by nurses. Nursing Administration Quarterly, 16(3), 33–34.

Phillips, J.R. (1977). Nursing systems and nursing models. Image: Journal of Nursing Scholarship, 9, 4–7.

Riehl, J.P., & Roy, C. (Eds.). (1980). Conceptual models for nursing practice (2nd ed.). New York: Appleton-Century-Crofts.

Riehl-Sisca, J. (1985a). Determining criteria for graduate and undergraduate self-care curriculums. In J. Riehl-Sisca (Ed.), The science and art of self-care (pp. 20–24). Norwalk, CT: Appleton-Century-Crofts.

Riehl-Sisca, J. (1985b). Epilogue: Future implications for the science and art of self-care. In J. Riehl-Sisca (Ed.), The science and art of self-care (pp. 307–309). Norwalk, CT: Appleton-Century-Crofts.

Riehl-Sisca, J. (1985c). The science and art of self-care. Norwalk, CT: Appleton-Century-Crofts.

Riehl-Sisca, J.P. (Ed.). (1989). Conceptual models for nursing practice (3rd ed.). Norwalk, CT: Appleton & Lange.

Roach, K.G., & Woods, H.B. (1993). Implementing cooperative care on an acute care medical unit. Clinical Nurse Specialist, 7, 26–29.

Rosenthal, R. (1991). Meta-analytic procedures for social research (Rev. ed.). Newbury Park, CA: Sage.

Rossow-Sebring, J., Carrieri, V., & Seward, H. (1992). Effect of Orem's model on nurse attitudes and charting behavior. Journal of Nursing Staff Development, 8, 207–212.

Scherer, P. (1988). Hospitals that attract (and keep) nurses. American Journal of Nursing, 88, 34–40.

Shanks, K.M. (2001). Prevalence of herbal therapy use in active duty Air Force women. Unpublished master's thesis, Uniformed Services University of the Health Sciences.

Smith, M.C. (1979). Proposed metaparadigm for nursing research and theory development. An analysis of Orem's self-care theory. Image, 11, 75–79.

Smith, M.J. (1987). A critique of Orem's theory. In R.R. Parse (Ed.), Nursing science: Major paradigms, theories, and critiques (pp. 91–105). Philadelphia: W.B. Saunders.

Taylor, S.G. (1985a). Curriculum development for preservice programs using Orem's theory of nursing. In J. Riehl-Sisca (Ed.), The science and art of self-care (pp. 25–32). Norwalk, CT: Appleton-Century-Crofts.

Taylor, S.G. (1985b). Teaching self-care deficit theory to generic students. In J. Riehl-Sisca (Ed.), The science and art of self-care (pp. 41–46). Norwalk, CT: Appleton-Century-Crofts.

Taylor, S.G. (1990). Practical applications of Orem's self-care deficit nursing theory. In M.E. Parker (Ed.), Nursing theories in practice (pp. 61–70). New York: National League for Nursing.

Taylor, S.G. (1991). The structure of nursing diagnoses from Orem's theory. Nursing Science Quarterly, 4, 24–32.

Taylor, S.G., Geden, E., Isaramalai, S., & Wongvatunyu, S. (2000). Orem's self-care deficit nursing theory: Its philosophic foundation and the state of the science. Nursing Science Quarterly, 13, 104–110.

Taylor, S.G., & McLaughlin, K. (1991). Orem's general theory of nursing and community nursing. Nursing Science Quarterly, 4, 153–160.

Taylor, S.G., & Renpenning, K.M. (1995). The practice of nursing in multiperson situations, family and community. In D.E. Orem (Ed.), Nursing: Concepts of practice (5th ed., pp. 348–380). St. Louis: Mosby.

Taylor, S.G., & Renpenning, K.M. (2001). The practice of nursing in multiperson situations, family and community. In D.E. Orem (Ed.), Nursing: Concepts of practice (6th ed., pp. 394–433). St. Louis: Mosby.

Taylor, S.G., Renpenning, K.E., Geden, E.Z., Neuman, B.M., & Hart, M.A. (2001). A theory of dependent-care: A corollary theory to Orem's theory of self-care. Nursing Science Quarterly, 14, 39–47.

Wagnild, G., Rodriguez, W., & Pritchett, P. (1987). Orem's self-care theory: A tool for education and practice. Journal of Nursing Education, 26, 343–343.

Wallace, W.A. (1983). From a realist point of view: Essays on the philosophy of science. Washington, DC: Catholic University of America Press.

Wallace, W.A. (1996). The modeling of nature. Washington, DC: Catholic University of America Press.

Weiss, P. (1980). You, I, and the others. Carbondale, IL: Southern Illinois University Press.

Young, A., Taylor, S.G., & McLaughlin-Renpenning, K. (2001). Connections: Nursing research, theory, and practice. St. Louis: Mosby.

RESEARCH

Ailinger, R.L., & Dear, M.R. (1993). Self-care agency in persons with rheumatoid arthritis. Arthritis Care and Research, 6, 134–140.

Ailinger, R.L., & Dear, M.R. (1997). An examination of the self-care needs of clients with rheumatoid arthritis. Rehabilitation Nursing, 22, 135–140.

Ailinger, R.L., & Dear, M.R. (1998). Adherence to tuberculosis preventive therapy among Latino immigrants. Public Health Nursing, 15, 19–24.

Aish, A. (1996). A comparison of female and male cardiac patients' responses to nursing care promoting nutritional self-care. Canadian Journal of Cardiovascular Nursing, 7(3), 4–13.

Aish, A.E., & Isenberg, M. (1996). Effects of Orem-based nursing intervention on nutritional self-care of myocardial infarction patients. International Journal of Nursing Studies, 33, 259–270.

Alexander, J., Divin-Cosgrove, C., Faner, M.L., & O'Connell, M. (2000). Increasing the knowledge base of asthmatics and their families through asthma clubs along the Southwest border. Journal of the American Academy of Nurse Practitioners, 17, 260–266.

Alexander, J.S., Younger, R.E., Cohen, R.M., & Crawford, L.V. (1988). Effectiveness of a nurse-managed program for children with chronic asthma. Journal of Pediatric Nursing, 3, 312–317.

Allen, J.D. (1988). Knowing what to weigh: Women's self-care activities related to weight. Advances in Nursing Science, 11(1), 47–60.

Allison, S.E. (1971). The meaning of rest: An exploratory nursing study. In ANA Clinical Sessions (pp. 191–205). New York: Appleton-Century-Crofts.

Allison, S.E. (2003). A posthumous reconstruction of an unpublished study by Joan E. Backscheider on self-care capabilities and nursing required to manage diabetes mellitus. Self-Care, Dependent-Care, and Nursing, 11(2), 5–14.

Anastasio, C., McMahan, T., Daniels, A., Nicholas, P.K., & Paul-Simon, A. (1995). Self-care burden in women with human immunodeficiency virus. Journal of the Association of Nurses in AIDS Care, 6(3), 31–42.

Anderson, J.A. (2001). Understanding homeless adults by testing the theory of self-care. Nursing Science Quarterly, 14, 59–67.

Anderson, K.J., & Campbell, I.G. (1993). Comparison of frail elders' satisfaction and their caregivers' burden in community-based and nursing home systems of long-term care. Nursing Scan in Research, 6(6), 9–10.

Arneson, S.W., & Triplett, J.L. (1990). Riding with Bucklebear: An automobile safety program for preschoolers. Journal of Pediatric Nursing, 5, 115–122.

Artinian, N.T., Magnan, M., Sloan, M., & Lange, M.P. (2002). Self-care behaviors among patients with heart failure. Heart and Lung, 31, 161–172.

Aukamp, V. (1989). Defining characteristics of knowledge deficit in the third trimester. In R.M. Carroll-Johnston (Ed.), Classification of nursing diagnoses: Proceedings of the Eighth Conference: North American Nursing Diagnosis Association (pp. 299–306). Philadelphia: Lippincott.

Baird, K.K., & Pierce, L.L. (2001). Adherence to cardiac therapy for men with coronary artery disease. Rehabilitation Nursing, 26, 233–237, 243, 251.

Baker, S. (1997). The relationships of self-care agency and self-care actions to caregiver strain as perceived by female family caregivers of elderly patients. Journal of the New York State Nurses Association, 28(1), 7–11.

Baker, T.J. (1996). Factors related to the initiation of prenatal care in the adolescent nullipara. Nurse Practitioner: American Journal of Primary Health Care, 21(2), 26, 29–32, 42.

Barron, M.L., Ganong, L.H., & Brown, M. (1987). An examination of preconception health teaching by nurse practitioners. Journal of Advanced Nursing, 12, 605–610.

Baulch, Y.S., Larson, P.J., Dodd, M.J., & Deitrich, C. (1992). The relationship of visual acuity, tactile sensitivity, and mobility of the upper extremities to proficient breast self-examination in women 65 and older. Oncology Nursing Forum, 19, 1367–1372.

Baxley, S.G., Brown, S.T., Pokorny, M.E., & Swanson, M.S. (1997). Perceived competence and actual level of knowledge of diabetes mellitus among nurses. Journal of Nursing Staff Development, 12, 93–98.

Beach, E.K, Smith, A., Luthringer, L., Utz, S.K., Ahrens, S., & Whitmire, V. (1996). Self-care limitations of persons after acute myocardial infarction. Applied Nursing Research, 9, 24–28.

Beauchesne, M.A. (1997). Social support and self-care agency of mothers of children with developmental disabilities. Clinical Excellence for Nurse Practitioners, 1, 449–455.

Behm, L.K., & Frank, D.I. (1992). The relationship between self-care agency and job satisfaction in public health nurses. Applied Nursing Research, 5, 28–29.

Belcher, D. (1992). The effect of a career awareness program on the success rate of the practical nursing student [Abstract]. Kentucky Nurse, 40(3), 18.

Bennett, J.A., DeMayo, M., & Saint Germain, M. (1993). Caring in the time of AIDS: The importance of empathy. Nursing Administration Quarterly, 17(2), 46–60.

Bidigare, S.A., & Oermann, M.H. (1991). Attitudes and knowledge of nurses regarding organ procurement. Heart and Lung, 20, 20–24.

Blazek, B., & McClellan, M. (1983). The effects of self-care instruction on locus of control in children. Journal of School Health, 53, 554–556.

Bliss-Holtz, J. (1988). Primiparas' prenatal concern for learning infant care. Nursing Research, 37, 20–24.

Bliss-Holtz, J. (1991). Developmental tasks of pregnancy and parental education. International Journal of Childbirth Education, 6(1), 29–31.

Brillhart, B. (2002). Quality of life and life satisfaction associated with urinary management. Communicating Nursing Research, 35, 375.

Brillhart, B., Heard, L., & Kruse, B. (2001). Rehabilitation nursing in home care. Rehabilitation Nursing, 26, 177–181, 191, 202.

Brock, A.M., & O'Sullivan, P. (1985). A study to determine what variables predict institutionalization of elderly people. Journal of Advanced Nursing, 10, 533–537.

Brodtkorb, K. (2001). Nursing and self-mutilation. Vard I Norden, 21(2), 11–15.

Buckley, H.B. (1990). Nurse practitioner intervention to improve postpartum appointment keeping in an outpatient family planning clinic. Journal of the American Academy of Nurse Practitioners, 2(1), 29–32.

Callaghan, D.M. (2003). Health-promoting self-care behaviors, self-care self-efficacy, and self-care agency. Nursing Science Quarterly, 16, 247–254.

Campbell, J.C. (1989). A test of two explanatory models of women's responses to battering. Nursing Research, 38, 18–24.

Campbell, J.C., & Soeken, K.L. (1999). Women's responses to battering: A test of the model. Research in Nursing and Health, 22, 49–58.

Campbell, J.C., & Weber, N. (2000). An empirical test of a self-care model of women's responses to battering. Nursing Science Quarterly, 13, 45–53.

Carlisle, J.B., Corser, N., Cull, V., DiMicco, W., Luther, L., McCaleb, A., Robuck, J., & Powell, K. (1993). Cardiovascular risk factors in young children. Journal of Community Health Nursing, 10, 1–9.

Carroll, D.L. (1995). The importance of self-efficacy expectations in elderly patients recovering from coronary artery bypass surgery. Heart and Lung, 24, 50–59.

Chang, B., Uman, G., Linn, L., Ware, J., & Kane, R. (1984). The effect of systematically varying components of nursing care on satisfaction in elderly ambulatory women. Western Journal of Nursing Research, 6, 367–386.

Chang, B., Uman, G., Linn, L., Ware, J., & Kane, R. (1985). Adherence to health care regimens among elderly women. Nursing Research, 34, 27–31.

Clark, C.C. (1998). Wellness self-care by healthy older adults. Image: Journal of Nursing Scholarship, 30, 351–355.

Clark, M.D. (1986). Application of Orem's theory of self-care: A case study. Journal of Community Health Nursing, 3, 127–135.

Closson, B.L., Mattingly, L.J., Finne, K.M., & Larson, J.A. (1994). Telephone follow-up program evaluation: Application of Orem's self-care model. Rehabilitation Nursing, 19, 287–292.

Conn, V. (1991). Self-care actions taken by older adults for influenza and colds. Nursing Research, 40, 176–181.

Conn, V.S., Taylor, S.G., & Kelley, S. (1991). Medication regimen complexity and adherence among older adults. Image: Journal of Nursing Scholarship, 23, 231–235.

Conn, V.S., Taylor, S.G., & Wienke, J.A. (1995). Managing medications: Older adults and caregivers. Journal of Nursing Science, 1(1/2), 40–50.

Conner-Warren, R.L. (1996). Pain intensity and home pain management of children with sickle cell disease. Issues in Comprehensive Pediatric Nursing, 19, 183–195.

Cook, D.L., & Barber, K.P. (1997). Relationship between social support, self-esteem and codependency in the African American female. Journal of Cultural Diversity, 4, 32–34.

Corrarino, J.E., Walsh, P.J., & Nadel, E. (2001). Does teaching scald burn prevention to families of young children make a difference? A pilot study. Journal of Pediatric Nursing: Nursing Care of Children and Families, 16, 256–262.

Craddock, R.B., Adams, P.F., Usui, W.M., & Mitchell, L. (1999). An intervention to increase use and effectiveness of self-care measures for breast cancer chemotherapy patients. Cancer Nursing, 22, 312–319.

Crockett, M.S. (1982). Self-reported coping histories of adult psychiatric and nonpsychiatric subjects and controls (Abstract). Nursing Research, 31, 122.

Cutler, C.G. (2001). Self-care agency and symptom management in patients treated for mood disorder. Archives of Psychiatric Nursing, 15, 24–31.

Dahlen, A. (1997). Health status of elderly—67 years and older in a community—and their need of nursing care. Vard i Norden, 17(3), 36–42.

Dashiff, C.J. (1992). Self-care capabilities in black girls in anticipation of menarche. Health Care for Women International, 13, 67–76.

Degenhart-Leskosky, S.M. (1989). Health education needs of adolescent and nonadolescent mothers. Journal of Obstetric, Gynecologic, and Neonatal Nursing, 18, 238–244.

Denyes, M.J., Neuman, B.M., & Villarruel, A.M. (1991). Nursing actions to prevent and alleviate pain in hospitalized children. Issues in Comprehensive Pediatric Nursing, 14, 31–48.

Dodd, M.J. (1982). Assessing patient self-care for side effects of cancer chemotherapy—Part 1. Cancer Nursing, 5, 447–451.

Dodd, M.J. (1983). Self-care for side effects in cancer chemotherapy: An assessment of nursing interventions—Part 2. Cancer Nursing, 6, 63–67.

Dodd, M.J. (1984a). Measuring informational intervention for chemotherapy knowledge and self-care behavior. Research in Nursing and Health, 7, 43–50.

Dodd, M.J. (1984b). Patterns of self-care in cancer patients receiving radiation therapy. Oncology Nursing Forum, 11, 23–27.

Dodd, M.J. (1987). Efficacy of proactive information on self-care in radiation therapy patients. Heart and Lung, 16, 538–544.

Dodd, M.J. (1988a). Efficacy of proactive information on self-care in chemotherapy patients. Patient Education and Counseling, 11, 215–225.

Dodd, M.J. (1988b). Patterns of self-care in patients with breast cancer. Western Journal of Nursing Research, 10, 7–24.

Dodd, M.J., & Dibble, S.L. (1993). Predictors of self-care: A test of Orem's model. Oncology Nursing Forum, 20, 895–901.

Dodd, M.J., Larson, P.J., Dibble, S.L., et al. (1996). Randomized clinical trial of chlorhexidine versus placebo for prevention of oral mucositis in patients receiving chemotherapy. Oncology Nursing Forum, 23, 921–927.

Dowd, T.T. (1991). Discovering older women's experience of urinary incontinence. Research in Nursing and Health, 14, 179–186.

Edgar, L., Shamian, J., & Patterson, D. (1984). Factors affecting the nurse as a teacher and practitioner of breast self-examination. International Journal of Nursing Studies, 21, 255–265.

Evans, L.K. (1996). Knowing the patient: The route to individualized care. Journal of Gerontological Nursing, 22(3), 15–19, 47–53.

Evers, G., Viane, A., Sermeus, W., Simoens-De Smet, A., & Delesie, L. (2000). Frequency of and indications for wholly compensatory nursing care related to enteral food intake: A secondary analysis of the Belgium National Nursing Minimum Data Set. Journal of Advanced Nursing, 32, 194–201.

Ewing, G. (1989). The nursing preparation of stoma patients for self-care. Journal of Advanced Nursing, 14, 411–420.

Farias, M.C.A., & Nóbrega, M.M.L. (2000). Nursing diagnoses in high-risk pregnant women based on Orem's self-care theory: A case study. Revista Latino-Americana de Enfermagem, 8(6), 59–67. [Portuguese; English abstract]

Faucett, J., Ellis, V., Underwood, P., Naqvi, A., & Wilson, D. (1990).

The effect of Orem's self-care model on nursing care in a nursing home setting. Journal of Advanced Nursing, 15, 659–666.

Fetzer, S.J., & Hand, M.C. (2001). A profile of perianesthesia nursing patient outcome research, 1994–1999. Journal of PeriAnesthesia Nursing, 16, 315–324.

Folden, S.L. (1993). Effect of a supportive-educative nursing intervention on older adults' perceptions of self-care after a stroke. Rehabilitation Nursing, 18, 162–167, 207–208.

Foltz, A.T., Gaines, G., & Gullatte, M. (1996). Recalled side effects and self-care actions of patients receiving inpatient chemotherapy. Oncology Nursing Forum, 23, 679–683.

Forsberg, A. (2002). Liver transplant recipient's experienced meaning of health and quality of life one year after transplantation. Theoria: Journal of Nursing Theory, 11(3), 4–14.

Frank, D.I. (2003). Elderly clients' perceptions of communication with their health care provider and its relation to health deviation self care behaviors. Self-Care, Dependent-Care, and Nursing, 11(2), 15–30.

Frederick, J., & Cotanch, P. (1995). Self-help techniques for auditory hallucinations in schizophrenia. Issues in Mental Health Nursing, 16, 213–224.

Freston, M.S., Young, S., Calhoun, S., Fredericksen, T., Salinger, L., Malchodi, C., & Egan, J.F.X. (1997). Responses of pregnant women to potential preterm labor symptoms. Journal of Obstetric, Gynecologic, and Neonatal Nursing, 26, 35–41.

Frey, M.A., & Denyes, M.J. (1989). Health and illness self-care in adolescents with IDDM: A test of Orem's theory. Advances in Nursing Science, 12(1), 67–75.

Frey, M.A., & Fox, M.A. (1990). Assessing and teaching self-care to youths with diabetes mellitus. Pediatric Nursing, 16, 597–800.

Frieson, T.C., & Frieson, C.W. (1996). Relationship between hope and self-esteem in renal transplant recipients. Journal of Transplant Coordination, 6, 20–23.

Fujita, L.Y. & Dungan, J. (1994). High risk for ineffective management of therapeutic regimen: A protocol study. Rehabilitation Nursing, 19, 75–79, 126.

Furlong, S. (1996). Self-care: The application of a ward philosophy. Journal of Clinical Nursing, 5, 85–90.

Gaffney, K.F., & Moore, J.M. (1996). Testing Orem's theory of self-care deficit: Dependent care agent performance for children. Nursing Science Quarterly, 9, 160–164.

Gammon, J. (1991). Coping with cancer: The role of self-care. Nursing Practice, 4(3), 11–15.

Ganong, L.H., & Coleman, M. (1992). The effect of clients' family structure on nursing students' cognitive schemas and verbal behavior. Research in Nursing and Health, 15, 139–146.

Gardulf, A., Bjorvell, H., Andersen, V., et al. (1995). Lifelong treatment with gamma globulin for primary antibody deficiencies: The patient's experiences of subcutaneous self-infusions and home therapy. Journal of Advanced Nursing, 21, 917–927.

Geden, E.A. (1982). Effects of lifting techniques on energy expenditure: A preliminary investigation. Nursing Research, 31, 214–218.

Geden, E. Isaramalai, S., & Taylor, S. (2002). Influences of partners' views of asthma self-management and family environment on asthmatic adults' asthma quality of life. Applied Nursing Research, 15, 217–226.

Geden, E.A., & Taylor, S.G. (1999). Theoretical and empirical description of adult couples' collaborative self-care systems. Nursing Science Quarterly, 12, 329–334.

George, M. (2003). Preparing girls for menarche. Nursing Journal of India, 94(3), 54–56.

Germain, C.P., & Nemchik, R.M. (1988). Diabetes self-management and hospitalization. Image: Journal of Nursing Scholarship, 20, 74–78.

Getty, C., Perese, E., & Knab, S. (1998). Capacity for self-care of persons with mental illnesses living in community residences and the ability of their surrogate families to perform health care functions. Issues in Mental Health Nursing, 19, 53–70.

Glanz, D., Ganong, L., & Coleman, M. (1989). Client gender, diagnosis, and family structure. Western Journal of Nursing Research, 11, 726–735.

Goodwin, J.O. (1979). Programmed instruction for self-care following pulmonary surgery. International Journal of Nursing Studies, 16, 29–40.

Graling, P.R., & Grant, J.M. (1995). Demographics and patient treatment choice in stage I breast cancer. Association of Operating Room Nurses Journal, 62, 381–384.

Grant, M., & Hezekiah, J. (1996). Knowledge and beliefs about hypertension among Jamaican female clients. International Journal of Nursing Studies, 33, 58–66.

Green, C. (1996). Clinical: Study of moving and handling practices on two medical wards. British Journal of Nursing, 5, 303–304, 306–308, 310–311.

Griffiths, P. (1998). An investigation into the description of patients' problems by nurses using two different needs-based nursing models. Journal of Advanced Nursing, 28, 969–977.

Grov, E.K. (1999). Death at home—How can the nurse contribute in making death at home possible for people with terminal cancer? Vard I Norden, 19(4), 4–9. [English abstract]

Gulick, E.E. (1991). Self-assessed health and use of health services. Western Journal of Nursing Research, 13, 195–219.

Gulick, E.E., Yam, M., & Touw, M.M. (1989). Work performance by persons with multiple sclerosis: Conditions that impede or enable the performance of work. International Journal of Nursing Studies, 26, 301–311.

Guthrie, B.J., Billings, S., Martyn, K.K., Oakley, D., & Walker, D.S. (2001). Using cognitive theory to improve nurse practitioners' anticipatory guidance with contraceptive pill users. Journal of Community Health Nursing, 18, 223–234.

Hagopian, G.A. (1991). The effects of a weekly radiation therapy newsletter on patients. Oncology Nursing Forum, 18, 1199–1203.

Hagopian, G.A. (1996). The effects of informational audiotapes on knowledge and self-care behaviors of patients undergoing radiation therapy. Oncology Nursing Forum, 23, 697–700.

Hagopian, G.A., & Rubenstein, J.H. (1990). Effects of telephone call interventions on patients' well-being in a radiation therapy department. Cancer Nursing, 13, 339–344.

Hamera, E.K., Peterson, K.A., Young, L.M., & Schaumloffel, M.M. (1992). Symptom monitoring in schizophrenia: Potential for enhancing self-care. Archives of Psychiatric Nursing, 6, 324–330.

Hamilton, L.W., & Creason, N.S. (1992). Mental status and functional abilities: Change in institutionalized elderly women. Nursing Diagnosis, 3, 81–86.

Hanucharurnkul, S. (1989). Predictors of self-care in cancer patients receiving radiotherapy. Cancer Nursing, 12, 21–27.

Hanucharurnkul, S., & Vinya-nguag, P. (1991). Effects of promoting patients' participation in self-care on postoperative recovery and satisfaction with care. Nursing Science Quarterly, 4, 14–20.

Harper, D. (1984). Application of Orem's theoretical constructs to self-care medication behaviors in the elderly. Advances in Nursing Science, 6(3), 29–46.

Harris, J. (1990). Self-care actions of chronic schizophrenics associated with meeting solitude and social interaction requisites. Archives of Psychiatric Nursing, 4, 298–307.

Harris, J.L., & Williams, L.K. (1991). Universal self-care requisites as identified by homeless elderly men. Journal of Gerontological Nursing, 17(6), 39–43.

Harris, M.D., Rinehart, J.M., & Gerstman, J. (1993). Animal-assisted therapy for the homebound elderly. Holistic Nursing Practice, 8(1), 27–37.

Harrison, L.L., & Novak, D. (1988). Evaluation of a gerontological nursing continuing education programme: Effect on nurses' knowledge and attitudes and on patients' perceptions and satisfaction. Journal of Advanced Nursing, 13, 684–692.

Hart, M.A. (1995). Orem's self-care deficit theory: Research with pregnant women. Nursing Science Quarterly, 8, 120–126.

Hart, M.A. (1996). Nursing implications of self-care in pregnancy. American Journal of Maternal Child Nursing, 21, 137–143.

Hart, M.A., & Foster, S.N. (1998). Self-care agency in two groups of pregnant women. Nursing Science Quarterly, 11, 167–171.

Hartley, L.A. (1988). Congruence between teaching and learning self-care: A pilot study. Nursing Science Quarterly, 1, 161–167.

Hartweg, D. (1993). Self-care actions of healthy middle-aged women to promote well-being. Nursing Research, 42, 221–227.

Hartweg, D., & Metcalfe, S. (1986). Self-care attitude changes of nursing students enrolled in a self-care curriculum—A longitudinal study. Research in Nursing and Health, 9, 347–353.

Hautman, M.A. (1987). Self-care responses to respiratory illnesses among Vietnamese. Western Journal of Nursing Research, 9, 223–243.

Hinojosa, R.J. (1992). Nursing interventions to prevent or relieve postoperative nausea and vomiting. Journal of Post Anesthesia Nursing, 7, 3–14.

Horsburgh, M.E. (1999). Self-care of well adult Canadians and adult Canadians with end stage renal disease. International Journal of Nursing Studies, 36, 443–453.

Horsburgh, M.E., Beanlands, H., Locking-Cusolito, H., Howe, A., & Watson, D. (2000). Personality traits and self-care in adults awaiting renal transplant. Western Journal of Nursing Research, 22, 407–437.

Hubbard, H. (2001). Use of a CHF fluid volume management

journal as a home health intervention. Communicating Nursing Research, 34, 353.

Hubbard, H. (2002). What does the CHF home health admit know about CHF after hospitalization? Communicating Nursing Research, 35, 335.

Hudson, D.B., Elek, S.M., Westfall, J.R., Grabau, A., & Fleck, M.O. (1999). Young Parents Project: A 21st century nursing intervention. Issues in Comprehensive Pediatric Nursing, 22, 153–165.

Humphreys, J. (1991). Children of battered women: Worries about their mothers. Pediatric Nursing, 17, 342–345, 354.

Humphreys, J.C. (1995). Dependent-care by battered women: protecting their children. Health Care for Women International, 16, 9–20.

Huss, K., Salerno, M., & Huss, R.W. (1991). Computer-assisted reinforcement of instruction: Effects on adherence in adult atopic asthmatics. Research in Nursing and Health, 14, 259–267.

Ienatsch, G. (1999). Knowledge, attitudes, treatment practices, and health behaviors of nurses regarding blood cholesterol. Journal of Continuing Education in Nursing, 30, 13–19.

Ip, W., Chau, J., Leung, M., Leung, Y., Foo, Y., & Chang, A.M. (1996). Research forum: Relationship between self concept and perception of self care ability of elderly in a Hong Kong hostel. Hong Kong Nursing Journal, 72, 6–12.

Jaarsma, T., Halfens, R., Tan, F., Abu-Saad, H.H., Dracup, K., & Diederiks, J. (2000). Self-care and quality of life in patients with advanced heart failure: The effect of a supportive educational intervention. Heart and Lung, 29, 319–330.

Jaarsma, T., Philipsen, H., Kastermans, M.C., & Cassen, T. (1994). Information needs and problems of patients with myocardial infarct and coronary bypass. A study of information needs and problems from the viewpoint of Orem's theory [English abstract]. Verpleegkunde, 8, 233–242.

Jenny, J. (1991). Self-care deficit theory and nursing diagnosis: A test of conceptual fit. Journal of Nursing Education, 30, 227–232.

Jirovec, M.M., & Kasno, J. (1990). Self-care agency as a function of patient-environmental factors among nursing home residents. Research in Nursing and Health, 13, 303–309.

Jirovec, M.M., & Kasno, J. (1993). Predictors of self-care abilities among the institutionalized elderly. Western Journal of Nursing Research, 15, 314–326.

Jirovec, M.M., & Maxwell, B.A. (1993). Nursing home residents' functional ability and perceptions of choice. Journal of Gerontological Nursing, 19(9), 10–14.

Johnson, J., & Pearson, V. (2000). The effects of a structured education course on stroke survivors living in the community. Rehabilitation Nursing, 25, 59–65, 79–80.

Jopp, M., Carroll, M.C., & Waters, L. (1993). Using self-care theory to guide nursing management of the older adult after hospitalization. Rehabilitation Nursing, 18, 91–94.

Jose, T.T., Bhaduri, A., & Mathew, B. (2003). A study of factors associated with compliance or non-compliance to lithium therapy among the patients with bipolar affective disorder. Nursing Journal of India, 94(1), 9–11.

Kang, J.M. (2002). Using a self-learning module to teach nurses about caring for hospitalized children with tracheostomies. Journal of Nurses in Staff Development, 18, 28–35.

Kao, C., & Ku, N. (1997). A study on the self-care abilities and related factors of colostomy patients during pre-discharge period [English abstract]. Nursing Research (China), 5, 413–424.

Karl, C. (1982). The effect of an exercise program on self-care activities for the institutionalized elderly. Journal of Gerontological Nursing, 8, 282–285.

Kerkstra, A., Castelein, E., & Philipsen, H. (1991). Preventive home visits to elderly people by community nurses in the Netherlands. Journal of Advanced Nursing, 16, 631–637.

Kirkpatrick, M.K., Brewer, J.A., & Stocks, B. (1990). Efficacy of self-care measures for perimenstrual syndrome (PMS). Journal of Advanced Nursing, 15, 281–285.

Klemm, L.W., & Creason, N.S. (1991). Self-care practices of women with urinary incontinence—A preliminary study. Health Care for Women International, 12, 199–209.

Korniewicz, D.M., & O'Brien, M.E. (1994). Evaluation of a hemodialysis patient education and support program. American Nephrology Nurses Association Journal, 21, 33–39.

Krouse, H.J., & Roberts, S.J. (1989). Nurse-patient interactive styles. Power, control, and satisfaction. Western Journal of Nursing Research, 11, 717–725.

Kruger, S., Shawver, M., & Jones, L. (1980). Reactions of families to the child with cystic fibrosis. Image: Journal of Nursing Scholarship, 12, 67–72.

Kubricht, D. (1984). Therapeutic self-care demands expressed by outpatients receiving external radiation therapy. Cancer Nursing, 7, 43–52.

Lakin, J.A. (1988). Self-care, health locus of control, and health value among faculty women. Public Health Nursing, 5, 37–44.

Larson, P.J., Dodd, M.J., & Aksamit, I. (1998). A symptom-management program for patients undergoing cancer treatment: The Pro-Self Program. Journal of Cancer Education, 13, 248–252.

Lauder, W. (1999a). Constructions of self-neglect: A multiple case study design. Nursing Inquiry, 6, 48–57.

Lauder, W. (1999b). A survey of self-neglect in patients living in the community. Journal of Clinical Nursing, 8, 95–102.

Lauder, W., Scott, P.A., & Whyte, A. (2001). Nurses' judgments of self-neglect: A factorial survey. International Journal of Nursing Studies, 38, 601–608.

Lawrence, D.M., & Schank, M.J. (1995). Health care diaries of young women. Journal of Community Health Nursing, 12, 171–182.

Lee, M.B. (1999). Power, self-care and health in women living in urban squatter settlements in Karachi, Pakistan: A test of Orem's theory. Journal of Advanced Nursing, 30, 248–259.

Lev, E.L. (1995). Triangulation reveals theoretical linkages and outcomes in a nursing intervention study. Clinical Nurse Specialist, 9, 300–305.

Lev, E.L., & Owen, S.V. (2002). Association of cancer patients' quality of life, symptoms, moods, and self-care self-efficacy with family care givers' depression, reaction and health. Self-Care, Dependent-Care, and Nursing, 10(2), 3–12.

Lile, J.L., & Hoffman, R.(1991). Medication-taking by the frail elderly in two ethnic groups. Nursing Forum, 26(4), 19–24.

Lilley, M.D. (1997). Postprandial blood pressure changes in the elderly. Journal of Gerontological Nursing, 23(12), 17–25.

Loveland-Cherry, C., Whall, A., Griswold, E., Bronneville, R., & Page, G. (1985). A nursing protocol based on Orem's self-care model: Application with aftercare clients. In J. Riehl-Sisca (Ed.), The science and art of self-care (pp. 285–297). Norwalk, CT: Appleton-Century-Crofts.

Lowe, N.K., & Ryan-Wenger, N.A. (2000). A clinical test of women's self-diagnosis of genitourinary infections. Clinical Nursing Research, 9, 144–160.

Lucas, M.D., Morris, C.M., & Alexander, J.W. (1988). Exercise of self-care agency and patient satisfaction with nursing care. Nursing Administration Quarterly, 12(3), 23–30.

Lukkarinen, H., & Hentinen, M. (1997). Self-care agency and factors related to this agency among patients with coronary heart disease. International Journal of Nursing Studies, 34, 295–304.

MacVicar, M.G., Winningham, M.L., & Nickel, J.L. (1989). Effects of aerobic interval training on cancer patients' functional capacity. Nursing Research, 38, 348–351.

Maddox, M. (1999). Older women and the meaning of health. Journal of Gerontological Nursing, 25(12), 26–33.

Malik, U. (1992). Women's knowledge, beliefs and health practices about breast cancer and breast self-examination. Nursing Journal of India, 83, 186–190.

Malm, D., Karsson, J., & Fridlund, B. (1998). Quality of life in pacemaker patients from a nursing perspective. Coronary Health Care, 2, 17–27.

Mapanga, K.G., & Andrews, C.M. (1995). The influence of family and friends' basic conditioning factors and self-care agency on unmarried teenage primiparas' engagement in contraceptive practice. Journal of Community Health Nursing, 12, 89–100.

Marsigliese, A.M. (2001). Evaluation of comfort level and complication rates as determined by peripheral intravenous catheter sites. CINA: Official Journal of the Canadian Intravenous Nurses Association, 17, 26–27, 30–39.

Maunz, E.R., & Woods, N.F. (1988). Self-care practices among young adult women: Influence of symptoms, employment, and sex-role orientation. Health Care for Women International, 9, 29–41.

McCaleb, A., & Cull, V.V. (2000). Sociocultural influences and self-care practices of middle adolescents. Journal of Pediatric Nursing, 15, 30–35. Carlisle, J. (2000). Commentary. Journal of Child and Family Nursing, 3, 330–332.

McCaleb, A., & Edgil, A. (1994). Self-concept and self-care practices of healthy adolescents. Journal of Pediatric Nursing 9, 233–238.

McConnell, T. (2000). Military wives' recognition of alcoholism. Journal of Addictions Nursing, 12(2), 83–88.

McCord, A.S. (1990). Teaching for tonsillectomies. Details mean better compliance. Today's OR Nurse, 12(6), 11–14.

McDermott, M.A.N. (1993). Learned helplessness as an interacting variable with self-care agency: Testing a theoretical model. Nursing Science Quarterly, 6, 28–38.

McDonnell, M., Turner, J., & Weaver, M.T. (2001). Antecedents of adherence to antituberculosis therapy. Public Health Nursing, 18, 392–400.

McKeighen, R.J., Mehmert, P.A., & Dickel, C.A. (1991). Self-care deficit, bathing/hygiene: Defining characteristics and related factors utilized by staff nurses in an acute care setting. In R.M. Carroll-Johnson (Ed.), Classification of Nursing Diagnosis: Proceedings of the Ninth Conference: North American Nursing Diagnosis Association (pp. 247–248). Philadelphia: Lippincott.

McQuiston, C.M., & Campbell, J.C. (1997). Theoretical substruction: A guide for theory testing. Nursing Science Quarterly, 10, 117–123.

Meeker, B.J., Rodriguez, L., & Johnson, J.M. (1992). A comprehensive analysis of preoperative patient education. Today's OR Nurse, 14(3), 11–18, 33–34.

Mendias, E.P., Clark, M.C., & Guevara, E.B. (2001). Women's self-perception and self-care practice: Implications for health care delivery. Health Care for Women International, 22, 299–312.

Miller, J.F. (1982). Categories of self-care needs of ambulatory patients with diabetes. Journal of Advanced Nursing, 7, 25–31.

Min, A. (2002). The effects of an educational program for premenstrual syndrome on women of Korean industrial districts. Health Care for Women International, 23, 503–511.

Monsen, R.B. (1992). Autonomy, coping, and self-care agency in healthy adolescents and in adolescents with spina bifida. Journal of Pediatric Nursing, 7, 9–13.

Moore, J.B. (1987a). Determining the relationship of autonomy to self-care agency or locus of control in school-age children. Maternal-Child Nursing Journal, 16, 47–60.

Moore, J.B. (1987b). Effects of assertion training and first aid instruction on children's autonomy and self-care agency. Research in Nursing and Health, 10, 101–109.

Moore, J.B. (1993). Predictors of children's self-care performance: Testing the theory of self-care deficit. Scholarly Inquiry for Nursing Practice, 7, 199– 212. Denyes, M.J. (1993). Response to "Predictors of children's self-care performance: Testing the theory of self-care deficit." Scholarly Inquiry for Nursing Practice, 7, 213–217.

Moore, J.B., & Mosher, R.B. (1997). Adjustment responses of children and their mothers to cancer: Self-care and anxiety. Oncology Nursing Forum, 24, 519–525.

Mosher, R.R., & Moore, J.B. (1998). The relationship of self-concept and self-care in children with cancer. Nursing Science Quarterly, 11, 116–122.

Navuluri, R.B. (2000). Gender differences in the factors related to physical activity among adults with diabetes. Nursing and Health Sciences, 2, 191–199.

Neil, R.M. (1984). Self care agency and spouses/companions of alcoholics. Kansas Nurse, 59(10), 3–4. Grant, M. (1990). Study critique. Oncology Nursing Forum, 17(3, suppl), 36–38.

Oberst, M.T., Hughes, S.H., Chang, A.S., & McCubbin, M.A. (1991). Self-care burden, stress appraisal, and mood among persons receiving radiotherapy. Cancer Nursing, 14, 71–78.

Orem, D.E. (1995). Obstacles to and other factors that affect meeting universal self-care requisites. In D.E. Orem (Ed.), Nursing: Concepts of practice (5th ed., pp. 439–455). St. Louis: Mosby.

Orem, D.E., & Vardiman, E.M. (1995). Orem's nursing theory and positive mental health: Practical considerations. Nursing Science Quarterly, 8, 165–173.

Page, C., & Ricard, N. (1995). A comparative study on the requisites for self-care perceived by women being treated for depression. Canadian Journal of Nursing Research, 27, 87–109.

Pallikkathayil, L., & Morgan, S.A. (1988). Emergency department nurses' encounters with suicide attempters: A qualitative investigation. Scholarly Inquiry for Nursing Practice, 2, 237–253. Winstead-Fry, P. (1988). Response to "Emergency department nurses' encounters with suicide attempters: A qualitative investigation." Scholarly Inquiry for Nursing Practice, 2, 255–259.

Palmer, P., & Meyers, F.J. (1990). An outpatient approach to the delivery of intensive consolidation chemotherapy to adults with acute lymphoblastic leukemia. Oncology Nursing Forum, 17, 553–558.

Patterson, E., & Hale, E. (1985). Making sure: Integrating menstrual care practices into activities of daily living. Advances in Nursing Science, 7(3), 18–31.

Pickens, J.M. (1999). Living with serious mental illness: The desire for normalcy. Nursing Science Quarterly, 12, 233–239.

Porter, L., Youssef, M., Shaaban, I., & Ibrahim, W. (1992). Parenting enhancement among Egyptian mothers in a tertiary care setting. Pediatric Nursing, 18, 329–336, 386.

Pressly, K.B. (1995). Psychosocial characteristics of CAPD patients and the occurrence of infectious complications. American Nephrology Nurses Journal, 22, 563–574.

Reed, P.G. (1989). Mental health of older adults. Western Journal of Nursing Research, 11, 143–163.

Renker, P.R. (1999). Physical abuse, social support, self-care, and pregnancy outcomes of older adolescents. Journal of Obstetric, Gynecologic, and Neonatal Nursing, 28, 377–388.

Rew, L. (1987a). Children with asthma. The relationship between illness behaviors and health locus of control. Western Journal of Nursing Research, 9, 465–483.

Rew, L. (1987b). The relationship between self-care behaviors and selected psychosocial variables in children with asthma. Journal of Pediatric Nursing, 2, 333–341.

Rhodes, V.A., Watson, P.M., & Hanson, B.M. (1988). Patients' descriptions of the influence of tiredness and weakness on self-care abilities. Cancer Nursing, 11, 186–194.

Richardson, A., & Ream, E.K. (1997). Self-care behaviours initiated by chemotherapy patients in response to fatigue. International Journal of Nursing Studies, 34, 35–43.

Riesch, S.K. (1988). Changes in the exercise of self-care agency. Western Journal of Nursing Research, 10, 257–273.

Robinson, K.D., & Posner, J.D. (1992). Patterns of self-care needs and interventions related to biologic response modifier therapy: Fatigue as a model. Seminars in Oncology Nursing, 8(4, suppl 1), 17–22.

Rossow-Sebring, J., Carrieri, V., & Seward, H. (1992). Effect of Orem's model on nurse attitudes and charting behavior. Journal of Nursing Staff Development, 8, 207–212.

Rothert, M., Rovner, D., Holmes, M., Schmitt, N., Talarczyk, Kroll, J., & Gogate, J. (1990). Women's use of information regarding hormone replacement therapy. Research in Nursing and Health, 13, 355–366.

Rothlis, J. (1984). The effect of a self-help group on feelings of hopelessness and helplessness. Western Journal of Nursing Research, 6, 157–173.

Ruland, C.M. (1999). Decision support for patient preference-based care planning: Effects on nursing care and patient outcomes. Journal of the American Medical Informatics Association, 6, 304–312.

Sandman, P.O., Norberg, A., Adolfsson, R., Axelsson, K., & Hedly, V. (1986). Morning care of patients with Alzheimer-type dementia: A theoretical model based on direct observation. Journal of Advanced Nursing, 11, 369–378.

Saounatsou, M., Patsi, O., Fasoi, G., et al. (2001). The influence of the hypertensive patient's education in compliance with their medication. Public Health Nursing, 18, 436–442.

Saucier, C. (1984). Self concept and self-care management in school-age children with diabetes. Pediatric Nursing, 10, 135–138.

Schafer, S.L. (1989). An aggressive approach to promoting health responsibility. Journal of Gerontological Nursing, 15(4), 22–27.

Schneider, J.K., Hornberger, S., Booker, J., Davis, A., & Kralicek, R. (1993). A medication discharge planning program: Measuring the effect on readmissions. Clinical Nursing Research, 2, 41–53.

Schott-Baer, D. (1993). Dependent care, caregiver burden, and self-care agency of spouse caregivers. Cancer Nursing, 16, 230–236.

Schott-Baer, D., Fisher, L., & Gregory, C. (1995). Dependent care, caregiver burden, hardiness, and self-care agency of caregivers. Cancer Nursing, 18, 299–305.

Seidman, R.Y. (1990). Effects of a premenstrual syndrome education program on premenstrual symptomatology. Health Care for Women International, 11, 491–501.

Shuster, G., Clough, D.H., & Higgins, P.G. (2001). Diet related behaviors and beliefs among elderly Hispanic women. Communicating Nursing Research, 34, 380.

Siebert, K.D., Ganong, L.H., Hagemann, V., & Coleman, M. (1986). Nursing students' perceptions of a child: Influence of information on family structure. Journal of Advanced Nursing, 11, 333–337.

Singleton, J.K. (2000). Nurses' perspectives of encouraging clients' care-of-self in a short-term rehabilitation unit within a long-term care facility. Rehabilitation Nursing, 25, 23–30, 35, 39.

Sloman, R. (2002). Relaxation and imagery for anxiety and depression control in community patients with advanced cancer. Cancer Nursing, 25, 432–435.

Sloman, R., Brown, P., Aldana, E., & Chee, E. (1994). The use of relaxation for the promotion of comfort and pain relief in persons with advanced cancer. Contemporary Nurse, 3(1), 6–12. Gagne, J.A. (1996). Commentary on "The use of relaxation for the promotion of comfort and pain relief in persons with advanced cancer." AACN Nursing Scan in Critical Care, 6(3), 2.

Slusher, I.L. (1999). Self-care agency and self-care practice of adolescents. Issues in Comprehensive Pediatric Nursing, 22, 49–58.

Smits, J., & Kee, C.C. (1992). Correlates of self-care among the independent elderly: Self-concept affects well-being. Journal of Gerontological Nursing, 18(9), 13–18. Pardee, C. (1993). Commentary on "Correlates of self-care among the independent elderly: Self-concept affects well-being." ENA's Nursing Scan in Emergency Care, 3(2), 20.

Smolen, D.M., & Topp, R. (2001). Self-care agency and quality of life among adults diagnosed with inflammatory bowel disease. Quality of Life Research, 10, 379–387.

Söderhamn, O. (1998). Self-care ability in a group of elderly Swedish people: A phenomenological study. Journal of Advanced Nursing, 28, 745–753.

Söderhamm, O., & Cliffordson, C. (2001). The structure of self-care in a group of elderly people. Nursing Science Quarterly, 14, 55–58.

Söderhamn, O., Lindencrona, C., & Ek, A. (2000). Ability for self-care among home dwelling elderly people in a health district in Sweden. International Journal of Nursing Studies, 37, 361–368.

Spitzer, A., Bar-Tal, Y., & Ziv, L. (1996a). The moderating effect of age on self-care. Western Journal of Nursing Research, 18, 136–148.

Spitzer, A., Bar-Tal, Y., & Ziv, L. (1996b). The moderating effect of gender of benefits from self-and others' health care. Social Sciences in Health, 2, 162–173.

Spoelstra, S. (1996). Management update: Productivity of registered nurses in home care. Caring, 15(10), 76–78.

Steele, N.F., & Sterling, Y.M. (1992). Application of the case study design: Nursing interventions for discharge readiness. Clinical Nurse Specialist, 6, 79–84.

Stockdale-Woolley, R. (1984). The effects of education on self-care agency. Public Health Nursing, 1, 97–106.

Storm, D.S., & Baumgartner, R.G. (1987). Achieving self-care in the ventilator-dependent patient: A critical analysis of a case study. International Journal of Nursing Studies, 24, 95–106.

Taggert, H.M. (2001). Self-reported benefits of T'ai Chi practice by older women. Journal of Holistic Nursing, 19, 223–237.

Takahashi, J.J., & Bever, S.C. (1989). Preoperative nursing assessment. A research study. Association of Operating Room Nurses Journal, 50, 1022, 1024–1029, 1031–1032, 1034–1035.

Terakye, G., & Buldukoglu, K. (1997). Childhood enuresis: Application of Orem's self-care practice model to home visits in Turkey. Journal of Pediatric Nursing, 12, 193–197.

Torres, G.O.V., Davim, R.M.B., & da Nobrega, M.M.L. (1999). Application of the nursing process based in Orem's theory: A case study with a pregnant adolescent. Revista Latino-Americana de Enfermagem, 7, 47–53. [English abstract]

Toth, J.C. (1980). Effect of structured preparation for transfer on patient anxiety on leaving coronary care unit. Nursing Research, 29, 28–34.

Troesch, L.M., Rodehaver, C.B., Delaney, E.A., & Yanes, B. (1993).

The influence of guided imagery on chemotherapy-related nausea and vomiting. Oncology Nursing Forum, 20, 1179–1185.

Utz, S.W., Hammer, J., Whitmire, V.M., & Grass, S. (1990). Perceptions of body image and health status in persons with mitral valve prolapse. Image: Journal of Nursing Scholarship, 22, 18–22.

Utz, S.W., & Ramos, M.C. (1993). Mitral value prolapse and its effects: A programme of inquiry within Orem's self-care deficit theory of nursing. Journal of Advanced Nursing, 18, 742–751.

Utz, S.W., Shuster, G., Merwin, E., & Williams, B. (1994). A community-based smoking-cessation program: Self-care behaviors and success. Public Health Nursing, 11, 291–299.

Utz, S.W., Whitmire, V.M., & Grass, S. (1993). Perspectives of the person with mitral valve prolapse syndrome: A study of self-care needs derived from a health deviation. Progress in Cardiovascular Nursing, 8(1), 31–39.

Villarruel, A.M. (1995). Mexican-American cultural meanings, expressions, self-care and dependent-care actions associated with experiences of pain. Research in Nursing and Health, 18, 427–436.

Villarruel, A.M., & Denyes, M.J. (1997). Testing Orem's theory with Mexican Americans. Image: Journal of Nursing Scholarship, 29, 283–288.

Wagnild, G., Rodriguez, W., & Pritchett, P. (1987). Orem's self-care theory: A tool for education and practice. Journal of Nursing Education, 26, 343–343.

Walker, L.O., & Grobe, S.J. (1999). The construct of thriving in pregnancy and postpartum. Nursing Science Quarterly, 12, 151–157.

Wang, C. (1997). The cross-cultural applicability of Orem's conceptual framework. Journal of Cultural Diversity, 4, 44–48.

Wang, C., & Abbott, L.J. (1998). Development of a community-based diabetes and hypertension preventive program. Public Health Nursing, 15, 406–414.

Wang, C., & Fenske, M.M. (1996). Self-care of adults with non-insulin-dependent diabetes mellitus: Influence of family and friends. Diabetes Educator, 22, 465–470.

Wang, H. (2001). A comparison of two models of health-promoting lifestyle in rural elderly Taiwanese women. Public Health Nursing, 18, 204–211.

Wang, H., & Laffrey, S. (2001). A predictive model of well-being and self-care for rural elderly women in Taiwan. Research in Nursing and Health, 24, 122–132.

Wang, S, Ku, N., Lin, H., & Wei, J. (1998). The relationships of symptom distress, social support, and self-care behaviors in heart transplant recipients [English abstract]. Nursing Research (China), 6, 4–18.

Wanich, C.K., Sullivan-Marx, E.M., Gottlieb, G.L., & Johnson, J.C. (1992). Functional status outcomes of a nursing intervention in hospitalized elderly. Image: Journal of Nursing Scholarship, 24, 201–207.

Ward-Griffin, C., & Bramwell, L. (1990). The congruence of elderly client and nurse perceptions of the client's self-care agency. Journal of Advanced Nursing, 15, 1070–1077.

Warren, J.K. (1998). Perceived self-care capabilities of

abused/neglected and nonabused/non-neglected pregnant, low-socioeconomic adolescents. Journal of Child and Adolescent Psychiatric Nursing, 11, 30–37.

Watkins, G.R. (1995). Patient comprehension of gastroenterology (GI) educational materials. Gastroenterology Nursing, 18, 123–127.

Watson, M.K., McDaniel, J.L., & Gibson, M.H. (1996). An innovative approach to home health education: The critical path to self-care for adults with diabetes. Home Health Care Management and Practice, 8(6), 41–51.

Weinrich, S.P. (1990). Predictors of older adults' participation in fecal occult blood screening. Oncology Nursing Forum, 17, 715–720.

Weintraub, F.N., & Hagopian, G.A. (1990). The effect of nursing consultation on anxiety, side effects, and self-care of patients receiving radiation therapy. Oncology Nursing Forum, 17(3, suppl), 31–36.

Wengström, Y., Häggmark, C., Strander, H., & Forsberg, C. (2000). Perceived symptoms and quality of life in women with breast cancer receiving radiation therapy. European Journal of Oncology Nursing, 4, 78–90.

Whetstone, W.R. (1986). Social dramatics: Social skills development for the chronically mentally ill. Journal of Advanced Nursing, 11, 67–74.

Whetstone, W.R. (1987). Perceptions of self-care in East Germany: A cross-cultural empirical investigation. Journal of Advanced Nursing, 12, 167–176.

Whetstone, W.R., & Hansson, A.M.O. (1989). Perceptions of self-care in Sweden: A cross-cultural replication. Journal of Advanced Nursing, 14, 962–969.

Whetstone, W.R., & Reid, J.C. (1991). Health promotion of older adults: Perceived barriers. Journal of Advanced Nursing, 16, 1343–1349.

Williams, P.D., Valderrama, D.M., Gloria, M.D., et al. (1988). Effects of preparation for mastectomy/hysterectomy on women's post-operative self-care behaviors. International Journal of Nursing Studies, 25, 191–206.

Woods, N.F. (1985). Self-care practices among young adult married women. Research in Nursing and Health, 8, 227–233.

Woods, N.F., Taylor, D., Mitchell, E.S., & Lentz, M.J. (1992). Perimenstrual symptoms and health-seeking behavior. Western Journal of Nursing Research, 14, 418–443.

Young, J., O'Connell, B., & McGregor, S. (2000). Day surgery patient's convalescence at home; Does enhanced discharge education make a difference? Nursing and Health Sciences, 2(1), 29–39.

Youssef, F.A. (1987). Discharge planning for psychiatric patients: The effects of a family-patient teaching programme. Journal of Advanced Nursing, 12, 611–616.

Zadinsky, J.K., & Boyle, J.S. (1996). Experiences of women with chronic pelvic pain. Health Care for Women International, 17, 223–232.

Zhimin, L. (2003). Self-care in Chinese school–age children with nephrotic syndrome. American Journal of Maternal Child Nursing, 28, 81–85.

RESEARCH INSTRUMENTS AND PRACTICE TOOLS

Ailinger, R.L., Harper, D.C., & Lasus, H.A. (1998). Bone up on osteoporosis: Development of the Facts on Osteoporosis Quiz. Orthopaedic Nursing, 17(5), 66–73.

Ailinger, R.L., Lasus, H.A., & Braun, M.A. (2003). Revision of the Facts on Osteoporosis Quiz. Nursing Research, 52, 198–201.

Allison, S.E., & Renpenning, K. (1999a). Nursing administration in the 21st century (pp. 121–129). Thousand Oaks, CA: Sage.

Allison, S.E., & Renpenning, K. (1999b). Nursing administration in the 21st century (pp. 155–167). Thousand Oaks, CA: Sage.

Allison, S.E., & Renpenning, K. (1999c). Nursing administration in the 21st century (pp. 171–172). Thousand Oaks, CA: Sage.

Allison, S.E., & Renpenning, K. (1999d). Nursing administration in the 21st century (pp. 188–189). Thousand Oaks, CA: Sage.

Allison, S.E., & Renpenning, K. (1999e). Nursing administration in the 21st century (pp. 196–199). Thousand Oaks, CA: Sage.

Allison, S.E., & Renpenning, K. (1999f). Nursing administration in the 21st century (pp. 202–206). Thousand Oaks, CA: Sage.

Allison, S.E., & Renpenning, K. (1999g). Nursing administration in the 21st century (pp. 212). Thousand Oaks, CA: Sage.

Angeles, D.M. (1991). An Orem-based NICU orientation checklist. Neonatal Network, 9(7), 43–48.

Artinian, N.T., Magnan, M., Sloan, M., & Lange, M.P. (2002). Self-care behaviors among patients with heart failure. Heart and Lung, 31, 161–172.

Arts, S., Kersten, H., & Kerkstra, A. (1996). The daily practice in home help services in the Netherlands: Instrument development. Health and Social Care in the Community, 4, 280–289.

Baldwin, J., & Davis, L.L. (1989). Assessing parents as health educators. Pediatric Nursing, 15, 453–457.

Beech, E.K., Smith, A., Luthringer, L., Utz, S.K., Ahrens, S., & Whitmire, V. (1996). Self-care limitations of persons after myocardial infarction. Applied Nursing Research, 9, 24,28.

Bickel, L.S. (1982). A study to assess the factorial structure of the perception of self-care agency questionnaire. Master's Abstracts International, 21, 340.

Biggs, A.J. (1990). Family care-giver versus nursing assessments of elderly self-care abilities. Journal of Gerontological Nursing, 16(8), 11–16.

Bliss-Holtz, J. (1995). Computerized support for case management: ISAACC. Computers in Nursing, 13, 289–294.

Bliss-Holtz, J., & Riggs, J. (1996). Computerization of self-care deficit nursing theory in a medical center. In P. Hinton Walker & B. Neuman (Eds.), Blueprint for Use of Nursing Models (pp. 275–286). New York: NLN Press.

Bottorff, J.L. (1988). Assessing an instrument in a pilot project: The self-care agency questionnaire. Canadian Journal of Nursing Research, 20, 7–16.

Brennan, M., & Duffy, M. (1992). Utilizing theory in practice to empower nursing. Nursing Administration Quarterly, 16(3), 32–33.

Brundage, D.J., Swearengen, P., & Woody, J.W. (1993). Self-care instruction for patients with COPD. Rehabilitation Nursing, 18, 321–325.

Campbell, J.C. (1986). Nursing assessment for risk of homicide with battered women. Advances in Nursing Science, 8(4), 36–51.

Carlisle, J.B., Corser, N., Cull, V., DiMicco, W., Luther, L., McCaleb, A., Robuck, J., & Powell, K. (1993). Cardiovascular risk factors in young children. Journal of Community Health Nursing, 10, 1–9.

Cleveland, S.A. (1989). Re: Perceived self-care agency: A LISREL factor analysis of Bickel and Hanson's Questionnaire (Letter to the editor). Nursing Research, 38, 59. Weaver, M.T. (1989). Response (Letter to the editor). Nursing Research, 38, 59.

Clinton, J.F., Denyes, M.J., Goodwin, J.O., & Koto, E.M. (1977). Developing criterion measures of nursing care: Case study of a process. Journal of Nursing Administration, 7(7), 41–45.

Davidhizar, R., & Cosgray, R. (1990). The use of Orem's model in psychiatric rehabilitation assessment. Rehabilitation Nursing, 15(1), 39–41.

Dellasega, C. (1995). SCOPE: A practical method for assessing the self-care status of elderly persons. Rehabilitation Nursing Research, 4, 128–135.

Dennis, C.M. (1997). Self-care deficit theory of nursing: Concepts and applications (pp. 122–123). St. Louis: Mosby.

Denyes, M.J. (1980). Development of an instrument to measure self-care agency in adolescents. Dissertation Abstracts International, 41, 1716B.

Denyes, M.J. (1982). Measurement of self-care agency in adolescents (Abstract). Nursing Research, 31, 63.

Denyes, M.J. (1988). Orem's model used for health promotion: Directions from research. Advances in Nursing Science, 11(1), 13–21.

Dodd, M.J. (1982). Assessing patient self-care for side effects of cancer chemotherapy—Part 1. Cancer Nursing, 5, 447–451.

Dodd, M.J. (1984). Patterns of self-care in cancer patients receiving radiation therapy. Oncology Nursing Forum, 11, 23–27.

Eichelberger, K.M., Kaufman, D.N., Rundahl, M.E., & Schwartz, N.E. (1980). Self-care nursing plan: Helping children to help themselves. Pediatric Nursing, 6(3), 9–13.

Eith, C.A. (1983). The nursing assessment of readiness for instruction of breast self-examination instrument (NARIB): Instrument development. Dissertation Abstracts International, 44, 1780B.

Evers, G.C., Isenberg, M.A., Philipsen, H., Senten, M., & Brouns, G. (1993). Validity testing of the Dutch translation of the Appraisal of Self-Care Agency (A.S.A.) Scale. International Journal of Nursing Studies, 30, 331–342.

Fernandez, R., & Wheeler, J.I. (1990). Organizing a nursing system through theory-based practice. In G.G. Mayer, M.J. Madden, & E. Lawrenz (Eds.), Patient care delivery models (pp. 63–83). Rockville, MD: Aspen.

Fok, M.S.M., Alexander, M.F., Wong, T.K.S., & McFadyen, A.K. (2002). Contextualising the Appraisal of Self-Care Agency Scale in Hong Kong. Contemporary Nurse, 112, 124–134.

Fridgen, R., & Nelson, S. (1992). Teaching tool for renal transplant recipients using Orem's self-care model. Canadian Association of Nephrology Nurses and Technicians Journal, 2(3), 18–26.

Fukuda, N. (1990). Outcome standards for the client with chronic congestive heart failure. Journal of Cardiovascular Nursing, 4(3), 59–70.

Gallant, B.W., & McLane, A.M. (1979). Outcome criteria: A process for validation at the unit level. Journal of Nursing Administration, 9(1), 14–21.

Gast, H.L., Denyes, M.J., Campbell, J.C., Hartweg, D.L., Schott-Baer, D., & Isenberg, M. (1989). Self-care agency: Conceptualizations and operationalizations. Advances in Nursing Science, 12(1), 26–38.

Gaut, D.A., & Kieckhefer, G.M. (1988). Assessment of self-care agency in chronically ill adolescents. Journal of Adolescent Health Care, 9, 55–60.

Geden, E., & Taylor, S. (1991). Construct and empirical validity of the self-as-carer inventory. Nursing Research, 40, 47–50.

Graff, B.M., Thomas, J.S., Hollingsworth, A.D., Cohen, S.M., & Rubin, M.M. (1992). Development of a postoperative self-assessment form. Clinical Nurse Specialist, 6, 47–50.

Guerrero Gamboa, N.S. (2000). Use of self-care theory of Orem in the attention of the newborn. Investigacion y Educacion en Enfermeria, 18(1), 71–85.

Gulick, E.E. (1987). Parsimony and model confirmation of the ADL self-care scale for multiple sclerosis persons. Nursing Research, 36, 278–283.

Gulick, E.E. (1988). The self-administered ADL scale for persons with multiple sclerosis. In C.F. Waltz, & O.L. Strickland (Eds.), Measurement of nursing outcomes. Vol. 1. Measuring client outcomes (pp. 128–159). New York: Springer.

Gulick, E.E. (1989). Model confirmation of the MS-related symptom checklist. Nursing Research, 38, 147–153.

Hageman, P., & Ventura, M. (1981). Utilizing patient outcome criteria to measure the effects of a medication teaching regimen. Western Journal of Nursing Research, 3, 25–33.

Hagopian, G. (1990). The measurement of self-care strategies of patients in radiation therapy. In O.L. Strickland & C.F. Waltz (Eds.), Measurement of Nursing Outcomes. Vol. 4. Measuring Client Self-care and Coping Skills (pp. 45–57). New York: Springer.

Halfens, R.J.G., van Alphen, A., Hasman, A., & Philipsen, H. (1999). The effect of item observability, clarity and wording on patient/nurse ratings when using the ASA Scale. Scandinavian Journal of Caring Science, 13, 159–164.

Hanchett, E.S. (1988). Nursing frameworks and community as client: Bridging the gap. Norwalk, CT: Appleton & Lange.

Hanson, B. (1981). Development of a questionnaire measuring perception of self-care agency. Master's Abstracts International, 21, 68.

Hanson, B., & Bickel, L. (1985). Development and testing of the questionnaire on perception of self-care agency. In J. Riehl-Sisca (Ed.), The Science and Art of Self-care (pp. 271–278). Norwalk, CT: Appleton-Century-Crofts.

Hanucharurnkul, S. (1989). Predictors of self-care in cancer patients receiving radiotherapy. Cancer Nursing, 12, 21–27.

Hayward, M.B., Kish, J.P., Jr., Frey, G.M., Kirchner, J.M., Carr, L.S., & Wolfe, C.M. (1989). An instrument to identify stressors in renal transplant recipients. Journal of the American Nephrology Nurses Association, 16, 81–84.

Hedahl, K. (1983). Assisting the adolescent with physical disabilities through a college health program. Nursing Clinics of North America, 18, 257–274.

Herrington, J., & Houston, S. (1984). Using Orem's theory: A plan for all seasons. Nursing and Health Care, 5(1), 45–47.

Hiromoto, B.M., & Dungan, J. (1991). Contract learning for self-care activities. A protocol study among chemotherapy outpatients. Cancer Nursing, 14, 148–154.

Horn, B. (1978). Development of criterion measures of nursing care (Abstract). In Communicating Nursing Research. Vol 11: New Approaches to Communicating Nursing Research (pp. 87–89). Boulder, CO: Western Interstate Commission for Higher Education.

Horn, B.J., & Swain, M.A. (1976). An approach to development of criterion measures for quality patient care. In Issues in Evaluation Research (pp. 74–82). Kansas City: American Nurses' Association.

Horn, B.J., & Swain, M.A. (1977). Development of Criterion Measures of Nursing Care (Vols. 1–2, NTIS Nos. PB–267 004 and PB–267 005). Ann Arbor, MI: University of Michigan.

Jaarsma, T., Halfens, R., Tan, F., Abu-Saad, H.H., Dracup, K., & Diederiks, J. (2000). Self-care and quality of life in patients with advanced heart failure: The effect of a supportive educational intervention. Heart and Lung, 29, 319–330.

Johannsen, J.M. (1992). Self-care assessment: Key to teaching and discharge planning. Dimensions of Critical Care Nursing, 11, 48–56.

Kaufman, M.L., & Paulanka, B.J. (1994). Nursing information: Better outcomes, less costs. Seminars for Nurse Managers, 2, 102–109.

Kearney, B.Y., & Fleischer, B.J. (1979). Development of an instrument to measure exercise of self-care agency. Research in Nursing and Health, 2, 25–34.

Kitson, A.L. (1986). Indicators of quality in nursing care—An alternative approach. Journal of Advanced Nursing, 11, 133–144.

Kyle, B.A.S., & Pitzer, S.A. (1990). A self-care approach to today's challenges. Nursing Management, 21(3), 37–39.

Lantz, J.M., Fullerton, J., & Quayhagen, M.P. (1995). Perceptual and enactment measurement of self-care. Advanced Practice Nursing Quarterly, 1(3), 29–33.

Laschinger, H.S. (1990). Helping students apply a nursing conceptual framework in the clinical setting. Nurse Educator, 15(3), 20–24.

Leatt, P., Bay, K.S., & Stinson, S.M. (1981). An instrument for assessing and classifying patients by type of care. Nursing Research, 30, 145–150.

Lin, C., Lu, L., Wang, J., & Lai, Y. (1998). Developing and testing of a CAPD self-efficacy scale. Nursing Research (China), 6, 315–326.

Lisko, S.A. (1995). Development and use of videotaped instruction for preoperative education of the ambulatory gynecological patient. Journal of Post Anesthesia Nursing, 10, 324–328.

Lorensen, M. (1998). Psychometric properties of self-care management and life quality amongst elderly. Clinical Effectiveness in Nursing, 2, 78–85.

Lorensen, M., Holter, I.M., Evers, G.C., Isenberg, M.A., & van Achterberg, T. (1993). Cross-cultural testing of the appraisal of self-care agency: ASA scale in Norway. International Journal of Nursing Studies, 30, 15–23.

Lukkarinen, H., & Hentinen, M. (1994). The SCI (self-as-carer-inventory) tested by Finnish patients. Hoitotiede, 6, 147–154.

MacSweeney, J. (1992). A helpful assessment. Nursing Times, 88(29), 32–33.

Marvulli, C., Paternostro, I., & Trofino, J. (1992). On the cutting edge: Computer technology empowers nurses. Nursing Administration Quarterly, 16(3), 35–36.

Marvulli, C., & Trofino, J. (1992). Laptop computers. Nursing Administration Quarterly, 16(3), 36–37.

Massey, R., & Jedlicka, D. (2002). The Massey Bedside Swallowing Screen. Journal of Neuroscience Nursing, 34, 252–253, 257–260.

McBride, S. (1987). Validation of an instrument to measure exercise of self-care agency. Research in Nursing and Health, 10, 311–316.

McBride, S.H. (1991). Comparative analysis of three instruments designed to measure self-care agency. Nursing Research, 40, 12–16.

McFarland, S.M., Sasser, L., Boss, B.J., Dickerson, J.L., & Stelling, J.D. (1992). Self-Care Assessment Tool for spinal cord injured persons. Spinal Cord Injury Nursing, 9, 111–116.

Micek, W.T., Berry, L, Gilski, D., Kallenbach, A., Link, D., & Scharer, K. (1996). Patient outcomes: The link between nursing diagnoses and interventions. Journal of Nursing Administration, 26(11), 29–35.

Michaels, C. (1985). Clinical specialist consultation to assess self-care agency among hospitalized COPD patients. In J. Riehl-Sisca (Ed.), The science and art of self-care (pp. 279–284). Norwalk, CT: Appleton-Century-Crofts.

Michaels, C.L. (1986). Development of a self-care assessment tool for hospitalized chronic obstructive pulmonary disease patients: A methodological study. Dissertation Abstracts International, 46, 3783B.

Mitchell, P., & Irvin, N. (1977). Neurological examination: Nursing assessment for nursing purposes. Journal of Neurosurgical Nursing, 9(1), 23–28.

Moore, J.B. (1995). Measuring the self-care practice of children and adolescents: Instrument development. Maternal-Child Nursing Journal, 23, 101–108.

Moore, J.B., & Gaffney, K.F. (1989). Development of an instrument to measure mothers' performance of self-care activities for children. Advances in Nursing Science, 12(1), 76–83.

Moore, J.B., & Mosher, R.B. (1997). Adjustment responses of children and their mothers to cancer: Self-care and anxiety. Oncology Nursing Forum, 24, 519–525.

Mosher, R.R., & Moore, J.B. (1998). The relationship of self-concept and self-care in children with cancer. Nursing Science Quarterly, 11, 116–122.

Mulvey, K., Sowul, M.J., & Trofino, J. (1992). Staff nurses develop voice-activated computers for clinical areas. Nursing Administration Quarterly, 16(3), 37–38.

Nursing Development Conference Group. (1979). Concept formalization in nursing: Process and product. Boston: Little, Brown.

O'Connor, C.T. (1990). Patient education with a purpose. Journal of Nursing Staff Development, 6, 145–147.

O'Connor, N.A. (1995). Maieutic dimensions of self-care agency: Instrument development. Dissertation Abstracts International, 56, 2563B.

Orem, D.E. (1995). Elements of a nursing history. In D.E. Orem (Ed.), Nursing: Concepts of practice (5th ed., pp. 422–430). St. Louis: Mosby.

Page, C., & Ricard, N. (1996). Conceptual and theoretical foundations for an instrument designed to identify self-care requisites in women treated for depression [English abstract]. Canadian Journal of Nursing Research, 28, 95–112.

Paternostro, I. (1992). Developing theory-based software for nurses, by nurses. Nursing Administration Quarterly, 16(3), 33–34.

Rew, L. (1987). The relationship between self-care behaviors and selected psychosocial variables in children with asthma. Journal of Pediatric Nursing, 2, 333–341.

Riesch, S.K., & Hauck, M.R. (1988). The exercise of self-care agency: An analysis of construct and discriminant validity. Research in Nursing and Health, 11, 245–255.

Robichaud-Ekstrand, S., & Loiselle, C.G. (1998). French validation of the "Exercise of Self-Care Agency" scale in cardiac patients. Recherche en Soins Infirmiers, September(54), 77–86. [French; English abstract]

Rossow-Sebring, J., Carrieri, V., & Seward, H. (1992). Effect of Orem's model on nurse attitudes and charting behavior. Journal of Nursing Staff Development, 8, 207–212.

Snyder, M., Brugge-Wiger, P., Ahern, S., et al-. (1991). Complex health problems. Clinically assessing self-management abilities. Journal of Gerontological Nursing, 17(4), 23–27.

Söderhamn, O., & Cliffordson, C. (2001). The internal structure of the appraisal of self-care agency scale. Theoria: Journal of Nursing Theory, 10(4), 5–12.

Söderhamn, O., Ek, A., & Porn, I. (1996). The self-care ability scale for the elderly. Scandinavian Journal of Occupational Therapy, 3, 69–78.

Söderhamn, O., Evers, G., & Hamrin, E. (1996). A Swedish version of the appraisal of self-care agency (ASA) scale. Scandinavian Journal of Caring Sciences, 10, 3–9.

Söderhamn, O., Lindencrona, C., & Ek, A. (1996). Validity of two self-care instruments for the elderly. Scandinavian Journal of Occupational Therapy, 3, 172–179.

Sonninen, A.L. (1999). Testing reliability and validity of the Finnish version of the appraisal of self-care agency (ASA) scale with elderly Finns. Dissertation Abstracts International, 60, 604C.

Swindale, J.E. (1989). The nurse's role in giving preoperative information to reduce anxiety in patients admitted to hospital for elective minor surgery. Journal of Advanced Nursing, 14, 899–905.

Taira, F. (1991). Individualized medication sheets. Nursing Economics, 9, 56–58.

van Achterberg, T., Lorensen, M., Isenberg, M.A., Evers, G.C.M., Levin, E., & Philipsen, H. (1991). The Norwegian, Danish and Dutch version of the Appraisal of Self-Care Agency Scale: Comparing reliability aspects. Scandinavian Journal of Caring Sciences, 5, 101–108.

Villarruel, A.M., & Denyes, M.J. (1991). Pain assessment in children: Theoretical and empirical validity. Advances in Nursing Science, 14(2), 32–41.

Weaver, M.T. (1987). Perceived self-care agency: A LISREL factor analysis of Bickel and Hanson's questionnaire. Nursing Research, 36, 381–387.

West, P., & Isenberg, M. (1997). Instrument development: The Mental Health–Related Self-Care Agency Scale. Archives of Psychiatric Nursing, 11, 126–132.

Whetstone, W.R. (1987). Perceptions of self-care in East Germany: A cross-cultural empirical investigation. Journal of Advanced Nursing, 12, 167–176.

Whetstone, W.R., & Hansson, A.M.O. (1989). Perceptions of self-care in Sweden: A cross-cultural replication. Journal of Advanced Nursing, 14, 962–969.

Willard, G.A. (1990). Development of an instrument to measure the functional status of hospitalized patients. Dissertation Abstracts International, 51, 2823B.

Yamashita, M. (1998). The Exercise of Self-Care Agency Scale. Western Journal of Nursing Research, 20, 370–381.

Young, A., Taylor, S.G., & McLaughlin-Renpenning, K. (2001). Connections: Nursing research, theory, and practice. St. Louis: Mosby.

EDUCATION

deMontigny, F., Dumas, L., Bolduc, L., & Blais, S. (1997). Teaching family nursing based on conceptual models of nursing. Journal of Family Nursing, 3, 267–279.

Feldsine, F. (1982). Options for transition into practice: Nursing process orientation program. Journal of New York State Nurses Association, 13, 11–16.

Fenner, K. (1979). Developing a conceptual framework. Nursing Outlook, 27, 122–126.

Gordon, M.F., & Grundy, M. (1997). From apprenticeship to academia: An adult branch programme. Nurse Education Today, 17, 162–167.

Harman, L., Wabin, D., MacInnis, L., Baird, D., Mattiuzzi, D., & Savage, P. (1989). Developing clinical decision-making skills in staff nurses: An educational program. Journal of Continuing Education in Nursing, 20, 102–106.

Herrington, J., & Houston, S. (1984). Using Orem's theory: A plan for all seasons. Nursing and Health Care, 5(1), 45–47.

Hooten, S.L. (1992). Education of staff nurses to practice within a conceptual framework. Nursing Administration Quarterly, 16(3), 34–35.

Kurger, S.F. (1988). The application of the self-care concept of nursing in the Wichita State University baccalaureate program. Kansas Nurse, 63(12), 6–7.

Langland, R.M., & Farrah, S.J. (1990). Using a self-care framework for continuing education in gerontological nursing. Journal of Continuing Education in Nursing, 21, 267–270.

McCoy, S. (1989). Teaching self-care in a market-oriented world. Nursing Management, 20(5), 22, 26.

O'Brien, B., Koller, L., Mahoney, J., & Hooten, S.L. (1992). Management education empowers staff nurses. Nursing Administration Quarterly, 16(3), 24–25.

Piemme, J.A., & Trainor, M.A. (1977). A first-year nursing course in a baccalaureate program. Nursing Outlook, 25, 184–187.

Reid, B., Allen, A.F., Gauthier, T., & Campbell, H. (1989). Solving the Orem mystery: An educational strategy. Journal of Continuing Education in Nursing, 20, 108–110.

Richeson, M., & Huch, M. (1988). Self-care and comfort. A framework for nursing practice. New Zealand Nursing Journal, 81(6), 26–27.

Romine, S. (1986). Applying Orem's theory of self-care to staff development. Journal of Nursing Staff Development, 2(2), 77–79.

Story, E.L., & Ross, M.M. (1986). Family centered community health nursing and the Betty Neuman systems model. Nursing Papers, 18(2), 77–88.

Taylor, S.G. (1985). Curriculum development for preservice programs using Orem's theory of nursing. In J. Riehl-Sisca (Ed.), The Science and art of self-care (pp. 25–32). Norwalk, CT: Appleton-Century-Crofts.

Woolley, A.S., McLaughlin, J., & Durham, J.D. (1990). Linking diploma and bachelor's degree nursing education: An Illinois experiment. Journal of Professional Nursing, 6, 206–212.

ADMINISTRATION

Allison, S.E. (1973). A framework for nursing action in a nurse-conducted diabetic management clinic. Journal of Nursing Administration, 3(4), 53–60.

Allison, S.E. (1985). Structuring nursing practice based on Orem's theory of nursing: A nurse administrator's perspective. In J. Riehl-Sisca (Ed.), The science and art of self-care (pp. 225–235). Norwalk, CT: Appleton-Century-Crofts.

Angeles, D.M. (1991). An Orem-based NICU orientation checklist. Neonatal Network, 9(7), 43–48.

Avery, P. (1992). Self-care in the hospital setting. The Prince Henry Hospital experience. Lamp, 49(2), 26–28.

Bachscheider, J.E. (1974). Self-care requirements, self-care capabilities and nursing systems in the diabetic nurse management clinic. American Journal of Public Health, 64, 1138–1146.

Barnes, L.P. (1991). Teaching self-care to children. American Journal of Maternal Child Nursing, 16, 101.

Barth, D. (1992). Staff nurses design a closed unit concept and virtually eliminate floating. Nursing Administration Quarterly, 16(3), 26–27.

Brady, D., & Cadamuro, B. (1992). Collaborative practice: An element in nurse empowerment. Nursing Administration Quarterly, 16(3), 30–32.

Brennan, M., & Duffy, M. (1992). Utilizing theory in practice to empower nursing. Nursing Administration Quarterly, 16(3), 32–33.

Calhoun, J., & Casey, P. (2002). Redesigning case management in managed care—An eclectic approach: From city to ranch. Lippincott's Case Management, 7, 180–191.

Campbell, C. (1984). Orem's story. Nursing Mirror, 159(13), 28–30.

Clark, J., & Bishop, J. (1988). Model-making. Nursing Times, 84(27), 37–40.

Crews, J. (1972). Nurse-managed cardiac clinics. Cardiovascular Nursing, 8, 15–18.

Del Togno–Armanasco, V., Olivas, G.S., & Harter, S. (1989). Developing an integrated nursing case management model. Nursing Management, 20(10), 26–29.

Derstine, J.B. (1992). Theory-based advanced rehabilitation nursing: Is it a reality? Holistic Nursing Practice, 6(2), 1–6.

Dibner, L.A., & Murphy, J.S. (1991). Nurse entrepreneurs. Journal of Psychosocial Nursing and Mental Health Services, 29(5), 30–34.

Duffy, M. (1992). Staff nurses interview potential candidates. Nursing Administration Quarterly, 16(3), 28–29.

Duncan, S., & Murphy, F. (1988). Embracing a conceptual model. The Canadian Nurse, 84(4), 24–26.

Dyer, S. (1990). Team work for personal patient care. Nursing the Elderly, 3(7), 28–30.

Farwell, M., & Gossett, P. (1992). Staff nurses accountable for quality of patient care. Nursing Administration Quarterly, 16(3), 27–28.

Feldsine, F. (1982). Options for transition into practice: Nursing process orientation program. Journal of New York State Nurses Association, 13, 11–16.

Fernandez, R., Brennan, M.L., Alvarez, A.R., & Duffy, M.A. (1990). Theory-based practice: A model for nurse retention. Nursing Administration Quarterly, 14(4), 47–53.

Fernandez, R.D., Hebert, G.J., & Bliss-Holtz, J. (1996). Application of self-care deficit theory. In P. Hinton Walker & B. Neuman (Eds.), Blueprint for Use of Nursing Models (pp. 228–235). New York: NLN Press.

Fernandez, R., & Wheeler, J.I. (1990). Organizing a nursing system through theory-based practice. In G.G. Mayer, M.J. Madden, & E. Lawrenz (Eds.), Patient Care Delivery Models (pp. 63–83). Rockville, MD: Aspen.

Fitch, M., Rogers, M., Ross, E., Shea, H., Smith, I., & Tucker, D. (1991). Developing a plan to evaluate the use of nursing conceptual frameworks. Canadian Journal of Nursing Administration, 4(1), 22–28.

Gossett, P., & DeTata, J. (1992). Creating a clinical matrix environment. Nursing Administration Quarterly, 16(3), 39–41.

Hamm-Vida, D. (1990). Cost of non-nursing tasks. Nursing Management, 21(4), 46–52.

Harman, L., Wabin, D., MacInnis, L., Baird, D., Mattiuzzi, D., & Savage, P. (1989). Developing clinical decision-making skills in staff nurses: An educational program. Journal of Continuing Education in Nursing, 20, 102–106.

Hathaway, D., & Strong, M. (1988). Theory, practice, and research in transplant nursing. Journal of the American Nephrology Nurses Association, 15, 9–12.

Hunter, L. (1992). Applying Orem to skin. Nursing (London), 5(4), 16–18.

Husted, E., & Strzelecki, S. (1985). Orem: A foundation for nursing practice in a community hospital. In J. Riehl-Sisca (Ed.), The science and art of self-care (pp. 199–207). Norwalk, CT: Appleton-Century-Crofts.

Kane, E., & O'Brien, B. (1992). Empowered nurses eliminate non-nursing tasks. Nursing Administration Quarterly, 16(3), 38–39.

Kaufman, M.L., & Paulanka, B.J. (1994). Nursing information: Better outcomes, less costs. Seminars for Nurse Managers, 2, 102–109.

Lanigan, T.L. (2000). The Patient-Family Learning Centre. Canadian Nurse, 96(3), 18–21.

Lantz, C. (1992). Staff nurses practice self-scheduling. Nursing Administration Quarterly, 16(3), 25–26.

Laurie-Shaw, B., & Ives, S.M. (1988a). Implementing Orem's self-care deficit theory. Part I—Selecting a framework and planning for implementation. Canadian Journal of Nursing Administration, 1(1), 9–12.

Laurie-Shaw, B., & Ives, S.M. (1988b). Part II: Implementing Orem's self-care deficit theory. Adopting a conceptual framework of nursing. Canadian Journal of Nursing Administration, 1(2), 16–19.

Lott, T.F., Blazey, M.E., & West, M.G. (1992). Patient participation in health care: An underused resource. Nursing Clinics of North America, 27, 61–76.

MacLeod, J.A., & Sella, S. (1992). One year later: Using role theory to evaluate a new delivery system. Nursing Forum, 27(2), 20–28.

McCoy, S. (1989). Teaching self-care in a market-oriented world. Nursing Management, 20(5), 22, 26.

McVay, J. (1985). A beginning of service and caring. In J. Riehl-Sisca (Ed.), The science and art of self-care (pp. 245–252). Norwalk, CT: Appleton-Century-Crofts.

McWilliams, B., Murphy, F., & Sobiski, A. (1988). Why self-care theory works for us. The Canadian Nurse, 84(9), 38–40.

Murphy, P.P. (1981). A hospice model and self-care theory. Oncology Nursing Forum, 8(2), 19–21.

Nunn, D., & Marriner-Tomey, A. (1989). Applying Orem's model in nursing administration. In B. Henry, C. Arndt, M. DiVincenti, & A. Marriner-Tomey (Eds.), Dimensions of Nursing Administration: Theory, Research, Education, Practice (pp. 63–67). Boston: Blackwell Scientific.

O'Connor, C.T. (1990). Patient education with a purpose. Journal of Nursing Staff Development, 6, 145–147.

Porter, D., & Shamian, J. (1983). Self-care in theory and practice. The Canadian Nurse, 79(8), 21–23.

Reid, B., Allen, A.F., Gauthier, T., & Campbell, H. (1989). Solving

the Orem mystery: An educational strategy. Journal of Continuing Education in Nursing, 20, 108–110.

Roach, K.G., & Woods, H.B. (1993). Implementing cooperative care on an acute care medical unit. Clinical Nurse Specialist, 7, 26–29.

Romine, S. (1986). Applying Orem's theory of self-care to staff development. Journal of Nursing Staff Development, 2(2), 77–79.

Rossow-Sebring, J., Carrieri, V., & Seward, H. (1992). Effect of Orem's model on nurse attitudes and charting behavior. Journal of Nursing Staff Development, 8, 207–212.

Scherer, P. (1988). Hospitals that attract (and keep) nurses. American Journal of Nursing, 88, 34–40.

Sella, S., & MacLeod, J.A. (1991). One year later: Evaluating a changing delivery system. Nursing Forum, 26(2), 5–11.

Smith, J.M., & Sorrell, V. (1989). Developing wellness programs: A nurse-managed stay well center for senior citizens. Clinical Nurse Specialist, 3, 198–202.

Snyder, M., Brugge-Wiger, P., Ahern, S.- et al. (1991). Complex health problems. Clinically assessing self-management abilities. Journal of Gerontological Nursing, 17(4), 23–27.

Strickland, R., Muller, K., & Croce, C. (1992). Empowerment through the professional practice committee. Nursing Administration Quarterly, 16(3), 29–30.

Trofino, J. (1992). Historical overview: Riverview Medical Center. Nursing Administration Quarterly, 16(3), 20–24.

Turner, K. (1989). Orem's model and patient teaching. Nursing Standard, 3(50), 32–33.

Van Eron, M. (1985). Clinical application of self-care deficit theory. In J. Riehl-Sisca (Ed.), The science and art of self-care (pp. 208–224). Norwalk, CT: Appleton-Century-Crofts.

Walker, D.M. (1993). A nursing administration perspective on use of Orem's self-care deficit nursing theory. In M.E. Parker (Ed.), Patterns of nursing theories in practice (pp. 252–263). New York: National League for Nursing.

Weis, A. (1988). Cooperative care: An application of Orem's self-care theory. Patient Education and Counseling, 11, 141–146.

PRACTICE

Abraham, T., & Fallon, P.J. (1997). Caring for the community: Development of the advanced practice nurse role. Clinical Nurse Specialist, 11, 224–230.

Alford, D.M. (1985). Self-care practices in ambulatory nursing clinics for older adults. In J. Riehl-Sisca (Ed.), The science and art of self-care (pp. 253–261). Norwalk, CT: Appleton-Century-Crofts.

Anderson, S.B. (1992). Guillain-Barre syndrome: Giving the patient control. Journal of Neuroscience Nursing, 24, 158–162.

Anna, D.J., Christensen, D.G., Hohon, S.A., Ord, L., & Wells, S.R. (1978). Implementing Orem's conceptual framework. Journal of Nursing Administration, 8(11), 8–11.

Atkins, F.D. (1992). An uncertain future: Children of mentally ill parents. Journal of Psychosocial Nursing and Mental Health Services, 30(8), 13–16.

Barajas Román, J., Doñoro Álvaro, M.A., Fernández Manzano, M., et al. (2002). Care's plan for the geriatric patients with urgency's urinary incontinence. Gerokomos, 13, 32–36. [Spanish; English abstract]

Batra, C. (1996). Nursing theory and nursing process in the community. In J.M. Cookfair (Ed.), Nursing care in the community (2nd ed., pp. 85–124). St. Louis: Mosby.

Beed, P. (1991). Sight restored. Nursing Times, 87(30). 46–48.

Berbiglia, V.A. (1997). Orem's self-care deficit theory in nursing practice. In M.R. Alligood & A. Marriner-Tomey (Eds.), Nursing theory: Utilization and application (pp. 129–152). St. Louis: Mosby.

Berbiglia, V.A. (2002). Orem's self-care deficit nursing theory in nursing practice. In M.R. Alligood & A. Marriner Tomey (Eds.), Nursing theory: Utilization and application (2nd ed., pp. 239–266). St. Louis: Mosby.

Bernier, F. (2002). Applying Orem's self-care deficit theory of nursing to continence care. Part 2. Urologic Nursing, 22, 384–391.

Best, C. (1998). Caring for the individual. Elderly Care, 10(5), 20–24.

Blaylock, B. (1991). Enhancing self-care of the elderly client: Practical teaching tips for ostomy care. Journal Enterostomal Therapy Nursing, 18, 118–121.

Boon, E., & Graham, L. (1992). Hip arthroplasty for osteoarthritis. British Journal of Nursing, 1, 562–566.

Boulter, P. (1995). Increasing independence: Training in toileting skills for people with a learning disability. Nursing Standard, 10(4), 18–20.

Bracher, E. (1989). A model approach. Nursing Times, 85(43), 42–43.

Bromley, B. (1980). Applying Orem's self-care theory in enterostomal therapy. American Journal of Nursing, 80, 245–249.

Cade, N.V. (2001). Orem's self-care deficit theory applied to hypertensive people. Revista Latino-Americana de Enfermagem, 9(3), 43–50. [Portuguese; English abstract]

Calley, J.M., Dirksen, M., Engalla, M., & Hennrich, M.L. (1980). The Orem self-care nursing model. In J.P. Riehl & C. Roy (Eds.), Conceptual models for nursing practice (2nd ed., pp. 302–314). New York: Appleton-Century-Crofts.

Cámara González, L., Domínguez Martínez, J.R., Herranz Márquez, N., et al. (2002). Care's plan of geriatric patient with acute confusional syndrome as hospital. Gerokomos, 13, 75–79. [Spanish; English abstract]

Campuzano, M. (1982). Self-care following coronary artery bypass surgery. Focus on Critical Care, 9(2), 55–56.

Catanese, M.L. (1987). Vaginal birth after cesarean: Recommendations, risks, realities, and the client's right to know. Holistic Nursing Practice, 2(1), 35–43.

Cheung, J., (2002). Applying Orem's self-care framework to the nursing care of a patient with hepatocellular carcinoma after extended right hepatectomy. Hong Kong Nursing Journal, 38, 20–26.

Chin, S. (1985). Can self-care theory be applied to families? In J. Riehl-Sisca (Ed.), The science and art of self-care (pp. 56–62). Norwalk, CT: Appleton-Century-Crofts.

Clang, E.D. (1985). Nursing system design for a young married diabetic. In J. Riehl-Sisca (Ed.), The science and art of self-care (pp. 113–125). Norwalk, CT: Appleton-Century-Crofts.

Clark, A.P. (1985). Self-care by the person with diabetes mellitus. In J. Riehl-Sisca (Ed.), The science and art of self-care (pp. 126–131). Norwalk, CT: Appleton-Century-Crofts.

Cohen, R. (1985). Sexual and self-care practices of adults. In J. Riehl-Sisca (Ed.), The science and art of self-care (pp. 298–306). Norwalk, CT: Appleton-Century-Crofts.

Compton, P. (1989). Drug abuse: A self-care deficit. Journal of Psychosocial Nursing and Mental Health Services, 27(3), 22–26.

Craig, C. (1989). Mr. Simpson's hip replacement. Nursing (London), 3(44), 12–19.

Dear, M.R., & Keen, M.F. (1982). Promotion of self-care in the employee with rheumatoid arthritis. Occupational Health Nursing, 30(1), 32–34.

Dennis, C.M., & Jesek-Hale, S. (2003). Calculating therapeutic self-care demand for a nursing population of normal newborns. Self-Care and Dependent-Care Nursing, 11(1), 3–10.

Doll-Speck, L., Miller, B., & Rohrs, K. (1993). Sibling education: Implementing a program for the NICU. Neonatal Network, 12(4), 49–52.

Dornik, E. (2001). Quality of life of a tetraplegic: Case study. Obzornik Zdravstvene Nege, 35, 205–211. [Slovenian; English abstract]

Dropkin, M.J. (1981). Development of a self-care teaching program for postoperative head and neck patients. Cancer Nursing, 4, 103–106.

Duffey, J., Miller, M.P., & Parlocha, P. (1993). Psychiatric home care: A framework for assessment and intervention. Home Healthcare Nurse, 11(2), 22–28.

Dumas, L. (1992). Nursing care based Orem's theory [English abstract]. The Canadian Nurse, 88(6), 36–39.

Dunn, B. (1990). Alcohol dependency: Health promotion and Orem's model. Nursing Standard, 4(40), 34.

Dunphy, J., & Jackson, E. (1985). Planing nursing care for the postpartum mother and her newborn. In J. Riehl-Sisca (Ed.), The science and art of self-care (pp. 63–90). Norwalk, CT: Appleton-Century-Crofts.

Eagan, D.E. (1998). The survival basket: Use of data sources to improve patient care. Pennsylvania Nurse, 53(1), 16–18.

Eagle, M. (1996). Involving the patient in care: Leg ulcers. Nursing Times, 92(3 Wound Care), 59–60, 64.

Eichelberger, K.M., Kaufman, D.N., Rundahl, M.E., & Schwartz, N.E. (1980). Self-care nursing plan: Helping children to help themselves. Pediatric Nursing, 6(3), 9–13.

Eliopoulos, C. (1984). A self care model for gerontological nursing. Geriatric Nursing, 4, 366–369.

Engle, M. (1996). Involving the patient in care: Leg ulcers. Nursing Times, 92(3 Wound Care), 59–60.

Facteau, L.M. (1980). Self-care concepts and the care of the hospitalized child. Nursing Clinics of North America, 15, 145–155.

Fawcett, J., Archer, C.L., Becker, D., Brown, K.K., Gann, S., Wong, M.J., & Wurster, A.B. (1992). Guidelines for selecting a conceptual model of nursing: Focus on the individual patient. Dimensions of Critical Care Nursing, 11, 268–277.

Fawcett, J., Cariello, F.P., Davis, D.A., Farley, J., Zimmaro, D.M., & Watts, R.J. (1987). Conceptual models of nursing: Application to critical care nursing practice. Dimensions of Critical Care Nursing, 6, 202–213.

Fialho, A.V.M., Pagliuca, L.M.F., & Soares, E. (2002). The self-care deficit theory adjustment in home-care in the light of Barnum's model. Revista Latino-Americana de Enfermagen, 10, 715–720. [Portuguese; English abstract]

Fields, L.M. (1987). A clinical application of the Orem nursing model in labor and delivery. Emphasis: Nursing, 2, 102–108.

Finnegan, T. (1986). Self-care and the elderly. New Zealand Nursing Journal, 79(4), 10–13.

Fitzgerald, S. (1980). Utilizing Orem's self-care nursing model in designing an educational program for the diabetic. Topics in Clinical Nursing, 2(2), 57–65.

Flanagan, M. (1991). Self-care for a leg ulcer. Nursing Times, 87(23), 67–68, 70, 72.

Foote, A., Holcombe, J., Piazza, D., & Wright, P. (1993). Orem's theory used as a guide for the nursing care of an eight-year-old child with leukemia. Journal of Pediatric Oncology Nursing, 10(1), 26–32.

Gantz, S.B. (1980). A fourth-grade adventure in self-directed learning. Topics in Clinical Nursing, 2(2), 29–38.

García Velázquez, M.C. (2002). A healthy old man: Plan of care based on D. Orem's theory. Gerokomos, 13, 17–26. [Spanish; English abstract]

Garrett, A.P. (1985). A nursing system design for a patient with myocardial infarction. In J. Riehl-Sisca (Ed.), The science and art of self-care (pp. 142–160). Norwalk, CT: Appleton-Century-Crofts.

Garvan, P., Lee, M., Lloyd K., & Sullivan, T.J. (1980). Self-care applied to the aged. New Jersey Nurse, 10(1), 3–5.

Gast, H.I. (1992). Nursing intervention focuses on enhancing the self-concept in children and adolescents. In P. West & C.L. Evans (Eds.), Psychiatric mental health nursing with children and adolescents (pp. 286–302). Gaithersburg, MD: Aspen.

Gibson, K.T. (1980). The type A personality: Implications for nursing practice. Cardiovascular Nursing, 16(5), 25–28.

Hanchett, E.S. (1988). Nursing frameworks and community as client: Bridging the gap. Norwalk, CT: Appleton & Lange.

Harris, F. (1996). A new way of life: Renal failure—Transplantation. Nursing Times, 92(8), 52, 54.

Harris, J.K. (1980). Self-care is possible after cesarean delivery. Nursing Clinics of North America, 15, 191–204.

Hedahl, K. (1983). Assisting the adolescent with physical disabilities through a college health program. Nursing Clinics of North America, 18, 257–274.

Hewes, C.J., & Hannigan, E.P. (1985). Self-care model and the geriatric patient. In J. Riehl-Sisca (Ed.), The science and art of self-care (pp. 161–167). Norwalk, CT: Appleton-Century-Crofts.

Hitejc, Z. (2000). Application of the theory of [Dorothea] Orem in the process of nursing care of mentally and physically handicapped children. Obzornik Zdravstvene Nege, 34(3/4), 121–125. [Slovenian; English abstract]

Jaarsma, T., Halfens, R., Senten, M., Abu Saad, H.H., & Dracup, K. (1998). Developing a supportive-educative program for patients with advanced heart failure within Orem's general theory of nursing. Nursing Science Quarterly, 11, 79–85.

James, L.A. (1992). Nursing theory made practical. Journal of Nursing Education. 31, 42–44.

Jewell, J.A., & Sullivan, E.A. (1996). Application of nursing theories in health education. Journal of the American Psychiatric Nurses Association, 2, 79–85.

Jones, A. (1996). Education: Orem's self-care model and clinical supervision. International Journal of Palliative Nursing, 2, 77–83.

Kelly, G. (1995). A self-care approach: Parkinson's disease. Nursing Times, 91(2), 40–41.

Keohane, N.S., & Lacey, L.A. (1991). Preparing the woman with gestational diabetes for self-care. Use of a structured teaching plan by nursing staff. Journal of Obstetric, Gynecologic, and Neonatal Nursing, 20, 189–193.

Kerr, J.A.C. (1985). A case of adolescent turmoil: Use of the self-care model. In J. Riehl-Sisca (Ed.), The science and art of self-care (pp. 105–112). Norwalk, CT: Appleton-Century-Crofts.

Knigge-Demal, B. (1998). The child experiencing pain and coping with pain in situations of invasive diagnostics, therapy and nursing care. Pflege, 11, 324–329. [German, English abstract]

Laferriere, R.H. (1995). Orem's theory of practice: Hospice nursing care. Home Healthcare Nurse, 13(5), 50–54.

Langley, T. (1989). Please, deliver more incontinence pads. Nursing Times, 85(15), 73–75.

LeRoy, L., (1998). Facial rejuvenation: Use of a teaching model in care planning. Dermatology Nursing, 10, 269–272.

Logue, G.A. (1997). An application of Orem's theory to the nursing management of pertussis. Journal of School Nursing, 13(4), 20–25.

MacDonald, G. (1991). Plans for a better future. Nursing Times, 87(31), 42–43.

Mack, C.H. (1992). Assessment of the autologous bone marrow transplant patient according to Orem's self-care model. Cancer Nursing, 15, 429–436.

MacLellan, M. (1989). Community care of a patient with multiple sclerosis. Nursing (London), 3(33), 28–32.

Mann, R. (1994). Imbalance of power. Nursing Times, 90(49 Learning Disabilities), 54–56.

Marten, L. (1978). Self-care nursing model for patients experiencing radical change in body image. Journal of Obstetric, Gynecologic and Neonatal Nursing, 7(6), 9–13.

McCracken, M.J. (1985). A self-care approach to pediatric chronic illness. In J. Riehl-Sisca (Ed.), The science and art of self-care (pp. 91–104). Norwalk, CT: Appleton-Century-Crofts.

Mehta, S.M. (1993). Applying Orem's self-care framework. Geriatric Nursing, 14, 182–185.

Meriney, D.K. (1990). Application of Orem's conceptual framework to patients with hypercalcemia related to breast cancer. Cancer Nursing, 13, 316–323.

Michael, M.M., & Sewall, K.S. (1980). Use of the adolescent peer group to increase the self-care agency of adolescent alcohol abusers. Nursing Clinics of North America, 15, 157–176.

Miller, J. (1989). DIY health care. Nursing Standard, 3(43), 35–37.

Monteiro, E.M.L., Nóbrega, M.M.L., & Lima, L.S. (2002). Self-care and the adult with asthma: The sistemization [sic] of nursing assistance. Revista Brasileira de Enfermagem, 55, 134–139. [Portuguese; English abstract]

Moore, R. (1989). Diogenes syndrome. Nursing Times, 85(30), 46–48.

Morse, W., & Werner, J.S. (1988). Individualization of patient care using Orem's theory. Cancer Nursing, 11, 195–202.

Mulkeen, H. (1989). Diabetes: Teaching the teaching of self-care. Nursing Times, 85(3), 63–65.

Noone, J. (1995). Acute pancreatitis: An Orem approach to nursing assessment and care. Critical Care Nurse, 15(4), 27–37.

Norris, M.K.G. (1991). Applying Orem's theory to the long-term care of adolescent transplant recipients. American Nephrology Nurses' Association Journal, 18, 45–47, 53.

Nowakowski, L. (1980). Health promotion/self-care programs for the community. Topics in Clinical Nursing, 2(2), 21–27.

Oakley, D., Denyes, M.J., & O'Connor, N. (1989). Expanded nursing care for contraceptive use. Applied Nursing Research, 2, 121–127.

O'Donovan, S. (1990a). Nursing models: More of Orem. Nursing the Elderly, 2(3), 22–23.

O'Donovan, S. (1990b). Nursing models: More of Orem—Part 2. Nursing the Elderly, 2(4), 20–22.

O'Donovan, S. (1992). Simon's nursing assessment. Nursing Times, 88(2), 30–33.

Ogden, V. (1996). Complex conditions: Hidradenitis suppurativa. Nursing Times, 92(46), 82–83, 85–86.

Oliver, C.J. (2003). Triage of the autistic spectrum child utilizing the congruence of case management concepts and Orem's nursing theories. Lippincott's Case Management, 8, 66–82.

Orem, D.E. (1983a). The family coping with a medical illness. Analysis and application of Orem's theory. In I.W. Clements & F.B. Roberts (Eds.), Family health: A theoretical approach to nursing care (pp. 385–386). New York: Wiley.

Orem, D.E. (1983b). The family experiencing emotional crisis. Analysis and application of Orem's self-care deficit theory. In I.W. Clements & F.B. Roberts (Eds.), Family Health: A Theoretical Approach to Nursing Care (pp. 367–368). New York: Wiley.

Park, P.B. (1989). Health care for the homeless: A self-care approach. Clinical Nurse Specialist, 3, 171–175.

Payne, A. (1987). Caring with Orem. Journal of District Nursing, 5(11), 5–6.

Perras, S., & Zappacosta, A. (1982). The application of Orem's theory in promoting self-care in a peritoneal dialysis facility. American Association of Nephrology Nurses and Technicians Journal, 9(3), 37–39.

Petrlik, J. C. (1976). Diabetic peripheral neuropathy. American Journal of Nursing, 76, 1794–1797.

Phillips, K.D., & Morrow, J.H. (1998). Nursing management of anxiety in HIV infection. Issues in Mental Health Nursing, 19, 375–393.

Priddy, J. (1989). Surgical care of the elderly: Home help. Nursing Times, 85(29), 30–32.

Raven, M. (1988–1989). Application of Orem's self-care model to nursing practice in developmental disability. Australian Journal of Advanced Nursing, 6(2), 16–23.

Raven, M. (1989). A conceptual model for care in developmental disability services. Australian Journal of Advanced Nursing, 6(4), 10–17.

Redfern, S. (1990). Care after a stroke. Nursing (London), 4(4), 7–11.

Rice, B.R. (1994). Self-care deficit nursing theory and the care of persons with developmental disabilities. In S.P. Roth & J.S. Morse (Eds.), A life-span approach to nursing care for individuals with developmental disabilities (pp. 105–117). Baltimore: Paul H. Brookes.

Robichaud-Ekstrand, S. (1990). Orem in medical-surgical nursing [English abstract]. The Canadian Nurse, 86(5), 42–47.

Roper, J.M., Shapira, J., & Chang, B. (1991). Agitation in the demented patient: A framework for management. Journal of Gerontological Nursing, 17(3), 17–21.

Roy, O., & Collin, F. (1994). Behavioral problems in elders with dementia. Canadian Nurse, 90(1), 39–41, 43.

Ruddick-Bracken, H., & Mackie, N. (1989). Helping the workers help themselves. Nursing Times, 85(24), 75–76.

Runtz, S.E., & Urtel, J.G. (1983). Evaluating your practice via a nursing model. Nurse Practitioner, 8(3), 30,32,37–40.

Sandman, P.O., Norberg, A., Adolfsson, R., Axelsson, K., & Hedly, V. (1986). Morning care of patients with Alzheimer-type dementia: A theoretical model based on direct observation. Journal of Advanced Nursing, 11, 369–378.

Shebel, N.D. (2002). An early intervention plan for identification and control of chronic lower extremity edema. Journal of Vascular Nursing, 20(2), 45–52.

Smith, C. (1996). Care of the older hypothermic patient using a self-care model. Nursing Times, 92(3), 29–31.

Smith, M.C. (1989). An application of Orem's theory in nursing practice. Nursing Science Quarterly, 2, 159–161.

Steele, S., Russell, F., Hansen, B., & Mills, B. (1989). Home management of URI in children with Down syndrome. Pediatric Nursing, 15, 484–488.

Stein, L.M.L. (1993). Health care delivery to farm workers in the Southwest: An innovative nursing clinic. Journal of the American Academy of Nurse Practitioners, 5, 119–124.

Stevens, J. (1994). Treating keratoconus. Nursing Times, 90(26), 36–39.

Stewart, M., & Basset, P. (1992). Using models in practice. Journal of Community Nursing, 6(6), 16, 18–20, 22.

Strong, M., Catindig, C., Cheney, A.M., Delim, M., Divina, C., Flynn, B., & Santellano, P. (1995). The nurse's role in fracture rehabilitation. Physical Medicine and Rehabilitation: State of the Art Reviews, 9, 227–249.

Sullivan, T., & Monroe, D. (1986). A self-care practice theory of nursing the elderly. Educational Gerontology, 12, 13–26.

Sullivan, T., & Monroe, D. (1987). Self-care model for long term care. California Nurse, 83(6), 6–7.

Summerton, H. (1995). End-stage renal failure: The challenge to the nurse. Nursing Times, 91(6), 27–29.

Swindale, J.E. (1989). The nurse's role in giving pre-operative information to reduce anxiety in patients admitted to hospital for elective minor surgery. Journal of Advanced Nursing, 14, 899–905.

Taylor, S.G. (1988). Nursing theory and nursing process: Orem's theory in practice. Nursing Science Quarterly, 1, 111–119.

Taylor, S.G. (1990). Practical applications of Orem's self-care deficit nursing theory. In M.E. Parker (Ed.), Nursing theories in practice (pp. 61–70). New York: National League for Nursing.

Thomas, J.S., Graff, B.M., Hollingsworth, A.O., Cohen, S.M., & Rubin, M.M. (1992). Home visiting for a posthysterectomy population. Home Healthcare Nurse, 10(3), 47–52.

Titus, S., & Porter, P. (1989). Orem's theory applied to pediatric residential treatment. Pediatric Nursing, 15, 465–468, 556.

Tolentino, M.B. (1990). The use of Orem's self-care model in the neonatal intensive care unit. Journal of Obstetric, Gynecologic, and Neonatal Nursing, 19, 496–500.

Underwood, P.R. (1980). Facilitating self-care. In P. Pothier (Ed.). Psychiatric nursing: A basic text (pp. 115–132). Boston: Little, Brown.

van der Weyden, R.S. (1994). Caring for a patient with Huntington's disease. Nursing Times, 90(49), 33–35.

Walborn, K.A. (1980). A nursing model for the hospice: Primary and self-care nursing. Nursing Clinics of North America, 15, 205–217.

Walsh, M. (1989). Asthma: The Orem self-care nursing model approach. Nursing (London), 3(38), 19–21.

Walsh, M., & Judd, M. (1989). Long term immobility and self care: The Orem nursing approach. Nursing Standard, 3(41), 34–36.

Whall, A.L. (1994). What is the nursing treatment for depression? Journal of Gerontological Nursing, 20, 42, 45.

Whelan, E.G. (1984). Analysis and application of Dorothea Orem's self-care practice model. Journal of Nursing Education, 23, 342–345.

Whenery-Tedder, M. (1991). Teaching acceptance. Nursing Times, 87(12), 36–39.

Woolery, L. (1983). Self-care for the obstetrical patient. Journal of Obstetric, Gynecologic, and Neonatal Nursing, 12, 33–37.

Wright, J. (1988). Trolley full of trouble. Nursing Times, 84(9), 24–26.

Wright, P.S., Piazza, D., Holcombe, J., & Foote, A. (1994). A comparison of three theories of nursing used as a guide for the nursing care of an 8-year-old child with leukemia. Journal of Pediatric Oncology Nursing, 11, 14–19.

Zach, P. (1982). Self-care agency in diabetic ocular sequelae. Journal of Ophthalmic Nursing Techniques, 1(2), 21–31.

Zinn, A. (1986). A self-care program for hemodialysis patients based on Dorothea Orem's concepts. Journal of Nephrology Nursing, 3, 65–77.

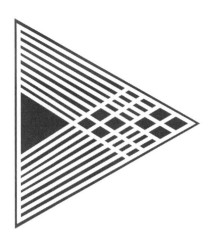

Chapter **9**

Rogers' Science of Unitary Human Beings

Martha E. Rogers' conceptual model of nursing is referred to as the Science of Unitary Human Beings. Rogers first presented her conceptual model, known then as the Life Process Model, in her 1970 book, *An Introduction to the Theoretical Basis of Nursing*. Further development and refinement of the conceptual model was presented by Rogers (1978a) at the Second Annual Nurse Educator Conference. That presentation, with additional refinements, was later published in Riehl and Roy's (1980) book *Conceptual Models for Nursing Practice* (Rogers, 1980a). The latter two papers also introduced theoretical formulations derived from the conceptual model. Rogers (1980b–g) presented an expanded explanation of the conceptual model, as well as a comprehensive discussion of the theories derived from it, in a series of videotapes and audiotapes in 1980. Further refinements in the conceptual model were published in a chapter in Malinski's (1986a) book *Explorations on Martha Rogers' Science of Unitary Human Beings* (Rogers, 1986). Still further refinements were published in a chapter in Barrett's (1990d) book *Visions of Rogers' Science-Based Nursing* (Rogers, 1990a), and in Rogers' 1992b journal article. Martha Rogers died on March 13, 1994.

Overview

Rogers' work focuses on unitary, irreducible human beings and their environments. Rogers (personal communication, June 17, 1987) regarded her work as an abstract conceptual system that "is not of the same order as the other conceptual models, nor does it derive from the same world view. Rather, it derives from a different world view and deals with a different phenomenon." The Science of Unitary Human Beings does, however, fit the definition of a conceptual model used in this book.

The concepts of the Science of Unitary Human Beings and their dimensions are listed here, along with the components of the associated practice methodol-

ogy. Each concept and its dimensions and the components of the practice methodology are defined and described, and the goal of nursing is discussed in detail, later in this chapter.

Key Terms

HUMAN BEINGS AND ENVIRONMENT
ENERGY FIELD
    Human Energy Field
    Environmental Energy Field
OPENNESS
PATTERN
PANDIMENSIONALITY
HOMEODYNAMICS

ANALYSIS OF ROGERS' SCIENCE OF UNITARY HUMAN BEINGS

This section presents an analysis of the Science of Unitary Human Beings. The analysis draws from several of Rogers' publications, including her 1970 book *An Introduction to the Theoretical Basis of Nursing*; her 1989 book chapter "Nursing: A Science of Unitary Man"; her 1990a book chapter "Nursing: Science of Unitary, Irreducible Human Beings: Update 1990"; her 1992b journal article "Nursing Science and the Space Age"; and her last two publications, the 1994a book chapter "Nursing Science Evolves" and the 1994b journal article "The Science of Unitary Human Beings: Current Perspectives."

ORIGINS OF THE NURSING MODEL

Historical Evolution and Motivation.

Rogers was a pioneer in the development of unique nursing knowledge. She was one of the first modern nurse scholars to explicitly identify man as the central phenomenon of interest to the discipline of nursing (Newman, 1972). Moreover, she focused attention on the environment as an equally important phenomenon for study. Rogers (1978a, 1992a) traced the dual concern with people and their environments to Nightingale. She explained, "Rogerian science of irreducible human beings provides a framework rooted in a new reality and directed toward moving us from what might be called a prescientific era to a scientific era. Certainly Nightingale laid a firm foundation for this kind of an approach to nursing knowledge and its use" (Rogers, 1992a, p. 61).

Rogers (1978a) stated that she directed her efforts "to evolve a conceptual system that would give identity to nursing as a knowledgeable endeavor." She added that she deliberately set out to develop a conceptual model when she realized that "there had to be a body of knowledge that was specific to and unique to nursing, or there was no need for higher education in nursing at all" (Rogers, 1978b). Rogers' recognition of the need for an organized body of unique nursing knowledge was evident in her early

316

writings on nursing education, especially in the books *Educational Revolution in Nursing* (Rogers, 1961) and *Reveille in Nursing* (Rogers, 1964).

Several changes have been made in the conceptual model as it evolved from the Life Process Model to the Science of Unitary Human Beings. The term for human beings evolved from man (Rogers, 1970) to unitary man (Rogers, 1980a) and later to unitary human beings (Rogers, 1986). The concepts or basic building blocks of the Rogerian conceptual system evolved from energy field, wholeness, openness, unidirectional, pattern and organization, and sentience and thought (Rogers, 1970) to energy field, openness, pattern, and four-dimensional (Rogers, 1980a) to energy field, openness, pattern, and multidimensional (Rogers, 1990a), and finally to energy field, openness, pattern, and pandimensional (Rogers, 1992b).

Rogers eliminated the term unidirectional because it led to the false interpretation of human development as linear. Multidimensional replaced four-dimensional in an effort "to select words best suited to portray one's thought.... Multidimensional provides for an infinite domain without limit" (Rogers, 1990a, p. 7). Pandimensional replaced multidimensional for the same reason. Rogers (1992b) explained that despite the changes in the actual word used, the definition has remained the same.

The principles of homeodynamics evolved from reciprocy, synchrony, helicy, and resonancy (Rogers, 1970) to helicy, resonancy, and complementarity (Rogers, 1980a) to helicy, resonancy, and integrality (Rogers, 1986). Reciprocy and synchrony were eliminated and complementarity was replaced by integrality because the terms reciprocy, synchrony, and complementarity led to the false interpretation of separation between the human and environmental energy fields. Furthermore, the notion of mutual and simultaneous interaction (Rogers, 1970), with its false connotation of separate human and environmental fields, evolved into complementarity and then to integrality. A change also was made in the definition of helicy. Here, the term probabilistic used in the definition was replaced by the term unpredictable because "the literature now points up that unpredictability transcends probability" (Rogers, 1990a, p. 7).

The many revisions and refinements in the Science of

Unitary Human Beings reflect Rogers' concern with language and the insights she gained over the years from new knowledge. She commented:

> The development of a science of unitary human beings is a never-ending process. This abstract system first presented some years ago has continued to gain substance. Concomitantly, early errors have undergone correction, definitions have been revised for greater clarity and accuracy, and updating of content is ongoing (Rogers, 1992b, p. 28).

Philosophical Claims

Rogers presented the philosophical claims undergirding the Science of Unitary Human Beings in the form of beliefs about human beings, beliefs about energy fields, a belief about the world, assumptions about causality, assumptions about nursing, assumptions about human beings and nursing, and a belief about licensure for professional nursing practice. Those philosophical claims are listed here.

Beliefs About Human Beings

- People have the capacity to participate knowingly and probabilistically in the process of change (Rogers, 1970, 1978a, 1978b, 1980a, 1986, 1992b).
- [A belief] in a humane and optimistic view of life's potentials [that] grows as a new reality appears (Rogers, 1992b, p. 28).

Beliefs About Energy Fields

- [Energy fields] constitute the fundamental unit of both the living and the nonliving (Rogers, 1992b, p. 30).
- [Energy fields] are not biological fields, physical fields, social fields, or psychological fields. Nor are human and environmental fields a summation of biological, physical, social, and psychological fields (Rogers, 1992b, p. 30).

Belief About the World

- [A belief in a] new vision of a world encompassing far more than planet earth ... [and a future] of growing diversity, of accelerating evolution, and of nonrepeating rhythmicities (Rogers, 1992b, p. 33).

Assumptions About Causality

- The appearance of causality is an illusion, a mirage (Rogers, 1980a, p. 334).
- In a universe of open systems, causality is not an option (Rogers, 1992b, p. 30).

Assumptions About Nursing

- Nursing ... is ... an independent discipline with its own unique phenomena, unique in terms of any other field (Rogers, 1994b, p. 34).

- The uniqueness of nursing lies in its focus on unitary, irreducible human beings and their environments (Rogers, 1994a, p. 3).
- If ... we believe that there is a body of knowledge unique to nursing, we start out with a phenomenon that is unique, and nursing is certainly unique in focusing on the irreducible human being and its environment, both defined as energy fields (Rogers, 1994b, p. 33).
- Nursing knowledge is rooted in the new reality [of new age science] and emerges as a synthesis of this new science and metaphysics (Rogers, 1994a, p. 3).
- Nursing is a learned profession (Rogers, 1970, 1978a, 1978b, 1980a, 1986, 1992b).
- The explication of an organized body of abstract knowledge specific to nursing is indispensable to nursing's transition from pre-science to science (Rogers, 1970, 1978a, 1978b, 1980a, 1986, 1992b).
- Nursing is ... an independent science (Rogers, 1994b, p. 34).
- [Nursing is a basic, open-ended science that builds and refines as] new knowledge brings new insights (Rogers, 1992b, p. 28).
- [Nursing] science provides a unique view of people and their world (Rogers, 1994a, p. 3).
- The focus of [nursing] science is different from that of any other field's phenomenon of concern (Rogers, 1994a, p. 3).
- A science of unitary or irreducible human beings is unique to nursing (Rogers, 1994a, p. 3).
- Nursing is both an empirical science and an art (Rogers, 1970, 1978a, 1978b, 1980a, 1986, 1992b).
- The descriptive, explanatory, and predictive principles that direct nursing practice are derived from a conceptual system (Rogers, 1970, 1978a, 1978b, 1980a, 1986, 1992b).
- Nursing is an organized abstract system that uses its knowledge in practice (Rogers, 1994a, p. 5).
- [Nursing] practice is not nursing; rather, it is the way in which we use nursing knowledge. ... Practice is the use of nursing knowledge (Rogers, 1994a, p. 5).

Assumptions About Human Beings and Nursing

- Nursing exists to serve people. Its direct and over-riding responsibility is to society ... the safe practice of nursing depends on the nature and amount of scientific nursing knowledge the individual brings to practice and the imaginative, intellectual judgment with which such knowledge is made explicit in service to mankind (Rogers, 1970, p. 122).
- Nursing's abstract system is the outgrowth of concern for human health and welfare. The science of nursing aims to provide a growing body of theoretical knowledge

whereby nursing practice can achieve new levels of meaningful service to man (Rogers, 1970, p. 88).

- Nursing's story is a magnificent epic of service to mankind. It is about people: how they are born, and live and die; in health and in sickness; in joy and in sorrow. Its mission is the translation of knowledge into human service. ... [Nursing is] a field long dedicated to serving the health needs of people (Rogers, 1992c, p. 1339).
- Nursing's long-established concern is with people and their worlds (Rogers, 1970, 1978a, 1978b, 1980a, 1986, 1992b).
- People need knowledgeable nursing (Rogers, 1970, 1978a, 1978b, 1980a, 1986, 1992b).
- The practice of nursing is the use of nursing knowledge in human service (Rogers, 1970, 1978a, 1978b, 1980a, 1986, 1992b).
- In [nursing's] creative use of its knowledge, manifested in the art of practice, nursing begins to achieve its recognition as a truly important human service (Rogers, 1994a, p. 5).
- The art of nursing is the utilization of scientific nursing knowledge for the betterment of people (Rogers, 1970, 1978a, 1978b, 1980a, 1986, 1992b).

Belief About Licensure for Professional Nursing Practice

- Licensure for professional practice in nursing is long overdue. In its absence, human health is jeopardized, fraudulence in recruitment practices continues, and placement of a high value on ignorance is pervasive. Licensing laws for professional practice must be written and professional examinations must be developed. People are at stake (Rogers, 1985b, p. 384).

Strategies for Knowledge Development

Rogers used a primarily deductive approach to develop the Science of Unitary Human Beings but also engaged in inductive thinking. She explained that the deductive approach yielded "a creative synthesis of facts and ideas ... an emergent, a new product" (Rogers, 1992b, p. 28). Elaborating, she stated that the Science of Unitary Human Beings

> has not derived from one or more of the basic sciences. Neither has it come out of a vacuum. It flows instead in novel ways from a multiplicity of knowledge, from many sources, to create a kaleidoscope of potentialities. In turn, fundamental concepts are identified and significant terms are defined congruent with the evolving system.... Neither does it derive from ... applied sciences, nor is it a summation of knowledge drawn from other fields. Nursing, instead, consists of its own unique irreducible mix (Rogers, 1992b, p. 28).

Rogers' (1994a) description of the thinking she engaged in to select the term pandimensional reflects an inductive approach. She stated, "One of the most significant updates was the replacement of the term four-dimensional with pandimensional.... Suddenly, one morning about 3:00 a.m., I knew that pandimensional was the right word" (p. 4).

Influences from Other Scholars

Rogers always emphasized the uniqueness of nursing knowledge in general and the Science of Unitary Human Beings in particular. However, she clearly stated that the new product that is her conceptual system was synthesized from the work of many scholars in adjunctive disciplines. Indeed, Rogers cited many notable philosophers and scientists, including Bohm (1980), Burr and Northrop (1935), Capra (1982), de Chardin (1961), Einstein (1961), Fuller (1981), Goldstein (1939), Herrick (1956), Lewin (1964), Polanyi (1958), Russell (1953), Sheldrake (1981), Stewart (1989), and von Bertalanffy (1960), among others.

Rogers (1985c) implied that system theory and knowledge gleaned from the exploration of space have been especially influential in the development and refinement of the Science of Unitary Human Beings when she stated:

> The introduction of systems theories several decades ago set in motion new ways of perceiving people and their world. Science and technology escalated. Space exploration revised old views. New knowledge merged with new ways of thinking. The second industrial revolution was born—far more dramatic in its implications and potentials than the first. A pressing need to study people in ways that would enhance their humanness coordinate with accelerating technological advances forced a search for new models (p. 16).

World View

The Science of Unitary Human Beings clearly reflects the *simultaneous action* world view. That classification is supported by analyses of Rogers' philosophical positions. Sellers (1991) maintained that the Science of Unitary Human Beings "is an eclectic synthesis of idealism, progressivism, and humanism that moves away from rationalism and scientific realism" (p. 147). Sarter (1988) pointed out that the major philosophical threads of the Science of Unitary Human Beings are "holism, process, [pan]dimensionality, evolution, energy fields, openness, noncausality, and pattern" (p. 54). Hanchett (1992) pointed out the similarities between certain concepts of the Science of Unitary Human Beings and the Madhyamika-Prasangika school of Tibetan Buddhism. She commented, "The activity and awareness of the energy field of Rogers' science bear relationships to the Buddhist concept[s] of karma ... [and] direct perception. Rogers' denial of parts as constituting the person is similar to the Buddhist argument that the aggregates do not constitute the person" (p. 170). In addition, Hanchett (1992) noted that the Rogerian notion of unique pattern within the integral human and environmental energy fields "is similar to the functioning of recognizable, conventional persons and phenomena within the interconnected web of dependent arising in the middle way consequence school of Tibetan Buddhist philosophy" (p. 170).

Although the Science of Unitary Human Beings reflects a holistic view of the world, Rogers (1992b) did not initially use the term holistic because of its ambiguous and varied meanings. She pointed out, "The use of the term unitary human beings is not to be confused with current popular usage of the term holistic, generally signifying a summation of parts, whether few or many. The unitary nature of environment is equally irreducible. The concept of field provides a means of perceiving people and their respective environments as irreducible wholes' (p. 29).

Rogers (1970) explicitly rejected the reaction world view tenet of reductionism, with its focus on parts, stating, "Reductionism, representative of an atomistic world view in which complex things are built up of simple elements, is contrary to a perception of wholeness" (p. 87). She also stated that her conceptual system "is humanistic, not mechanistic. Moreover, this is an optimistic model though not a utopian one" (Rogers, 1987d, p. 141). She also explicitly rejected mechanistic causality, stating, "In a universe of open systems, causality is not an option. Acausality had come in with quantum theory.... Causality is invalid" (Rogers, 1986, p. 5). Furthermore, Rogers (1970) rejected the reaction world view of human beings as reacting to environmental stimuli. She commented, "The all-too-common perception of man predominantly subjected to multiple negative environmental influences with pathological outcomes denies man's unity with nature and his evolutionary becoming" (p. 85).

The features of the simultaneous action world view that are evident in Rogers' Science of Unitary Human Beings are:

- The Science of Unitary Human Beings clearly reflects a holistic view of human beings and environment. Human beings and the environment are clearly conceptualized as irreducible, indivisible wholes (Rogers, 1970, 1978a, 1978b, 1980a, 1986, 1990b, 1992b).
- My own work focuses on developing a holistic world view by proposing a science of unitary, irreducible beings that is coordinate with a world view that includes outer space. ... A holistically oriented space-age paradigm is the substance of nursing's science of unitary, irreducible human beings (Rogers, 1990b, pp. 106–107).
- [We are on] the threshold of a new reality, a new world-

view. ... This new reality, whether called new age science or a similar expression, represents the foundation on which the science of nursing is built. This new reality is one of synthesis and holism and gives a broadened perspective of science in the future (Rogers, 1994a, p. 3).
- [A new world view,] compatible with the most progressive knowledge available ... has become a necessary prelude to studying human health and to determining modalities for its promotion both on this planet and in outer space. The [Science of Unitary Human Beings] is rooted in this new world view, a pandimensional view of people and their world (Rogers, 1992b, pp. 27–28).
- The human energy field is regarded as an active organism who is integral with the environmental energy field (Rogers, 1986, 1990b, 1992b).
- Human and environmental energy fields change continuously. Change, therefore, is regarded as natural and desirable.
- Change just is (Rogers et al., 1990, p. 377).
- Change is creative and innovative, always in the direction of increasing diversity. Thus human beings always are progressing, always reaching toward their potential.
- Change is continuous, relative, and innovative. The increasing diversity of field patterning characterizes this process of change. Individual differences serve only to point up the significance of this relative diversity (Rogers, 1992b, p. 31).
- People's capacity to participate knowingly in the process of change is postulated (Rogers, 1992b, p. 28).

UNIQUE FOCUS OF THE NURSING MODEL

The unique focus of the Science of Unitary Human Beings is "people and their worlds in a pandimensional universe" (Rogers, 1992b, p. 29). The distinction between nursing and other disciplines and the uniqueness of nursing lie in the phenomenon of central interest to each, in what is known rather than what is done in practice (Rogers, 1990b). The phenomenon of central concern to nursing is "the study of unitary, irreducible human beings and their respective environments" (Rogers, 1990b, p. 108).

The uniqueness of nursing, like that of other sciences, lies in the phenomenon central to its focus. For nurses, that focus consists of a long-established concern with people and the world they live in. It is the natural forerunner of an organized, abstract system encompassing people and their environments. The irreducible nature of individuals is different from the sum of their parts. Furthermore, the integrality of people and their environments coordinates with a pandimensional universe of open systems, points to a new paradigm, and initiates the identity of nursing as a science (Rogers, 1992b, p. 28).

The Science of Unitary Human Beings is concerned with those patterns of the human and environmental energy fields that are associated with maximum well-being, as well-being is defined by the society in which the human being is located (Rogers, 1970, 1986, 1992a). The Science of Unitary Human Beings does not deal with health problems, but rather is concerned with the evolution of change in the direction of wherever human beings think they are going (Rogers, 1987c).

Categories of Knowledge

Riehl and Roy (1974, 1980) classified the Science of Unitary Human Beings as a systems model. Riehl-Sisca (1989) classified it as a developmental model. Meleis (1997) regarded the Science of Unitary Human Beings as a prominent example of the outcomes category of models and also classified it within her human being–environment interaction category. Marriner-Tomey (1989) placed Rogers' work in the energy fields category. Barnum (1998) relegated Rogers' work to her enhancement category. Careful review of the content of the Science of Unitary Human Beings indicates that it reflects characteristics of both the systems category and the developmental category of knowledge. Although Rogers addressed the characteristics of systems models, she placed major emphasis on human development in the form of evolutionary changes in human field pattern. Rogers (as cited in Malinski, 1986b), however, stopped using the term human development "because development implies certain kinds of linearity" (p. 11). The appropriateness of the systems and development category classifications is evident in the comparison of the Science of Unitary Human Beings content with the characteristics of the systems and developmental categories of knowledge, as can be seen here.

Systems Category of Knowledge

- System and Open System: The human energy field and the environmental energy field are open systems (Rogers, 1970). [Energy fields are always open—] not a little bit or sometimes, but continuously (Rogers, 1992b, p. 30).
- Integration of Parts: [Unitary human beings and their environments are irreducible and indivisible energy fields that] have their own identity and are not to be confused with parts (Rogers, 1992b, p. 30). [Unitary human beings are regarded as] irreducible wholes [and] a whole cannot be understood when it is reduced to its particulars (Rogers, 1992b, p. 29). The irreducible nature of individuals is different from the sum of their parts (Rogers, 1992b, p. 28).

- Environment: A pandimensional energy field that is integral with the human pandimensional energy field (Rogers, 1992b).
- Boundary: Not addressed explicitly in the recent versions of the Science of Unitary Human Beings. The lack of boundaries is evident in the statement that the "human and environmental fields are infinite and integral with one another" (Rogers, 1986, p. 5).
- Tension, Stress, Strain, and Conflict: Not addressed in the Science of Unitary Human Beings. Rogers clearly rejected the idea that any external force impinges on the human field. Rather, the human and environmental fields are integral.
- Equilibrium and Steady State and Feedback: These are obsolete ideas for Rogers. The relationship between human beings and their environments goes beyond general system thinking. There is no fixed equilibrium point or even a dynamic equilibrium, nor is there any feedback process of input and output. Rather, the principle of integrality postulates that the human and environmental energy fields engage in the continuous, mutual process of change. "The continuous change emerges out of nonequilibrium and exhibits punctualism not gradualism. In addition, change is accelerating" (Rogers, 1992b, p. 32).

Developmental Category of Knowledge

- Growth, Development, and Maturation; Change; and Direction of Change: Addressed by the principles of helicy and resonancy. These principles postulate that field pattern is characterized by continuous change that is innovative, unpredictable, and increasing in diversity. The direction of change always is toward increasing diversity, from lower frequency to higher frequency wave patterns (Rogers, 1992b).
- Identifiable State: Addressed by the concept of pattern, which is "the distinguishing characteristic of an energy field perceived as a single wave. … it gives identity to the field" (Rogers, 1992b, p. 30).
- Form of Progression: The principle of helicy postulates that human and environmental field patterns increase in diversity and are characterized by nonrepeating rhythmicities. Although the term helicy might imply a spiral, Chin's (1980) definition of that form as returning to former problems, but dealing with them at a higher level, is at odds with Rogers' (1980a) contention that "there is no going back, no repetition" (p. 333).
- Forces: Rogers rejected the idea of forces. Rather, she posited that the nature of the energy field is to evolve. No special forces are required for evolution.
- Potentiality: The potentiality for development is overt.

CONTENT OF THE NURSING MODEL

Concepts

The metaparadigm concepts of human beings, environment, health, and nursing are reflected in the concepts of the Science of Unitary Human Beings. Each conceptual model concept is classified here according to its metaparadigm forerunner.

The metaparadigm concepts of human beings and environment are represented by the Science of Unitary Human Beings concepts of ENERGY FIELD, OPENNESS, PATTERN, PANDIMENSIONALITY, and HOMEODYNAMICS. The concept of ENERGY FIELD has two dimensions—**Human Energy Field** and **Environmental Energy Field**. The concept of HOMEODYNAMICS has three dimensions—**Resonancy, Helicy,** and **Integrality.** The remaining concepts are unidimensional.

The metaparadigm concept of health is represented by the Science of Unitary Human Beings concept of WELL-BEING. That concept is unidimensional.

The metaparadigm concept of nursing is represented by the Science of Unitary Human Beings concepts of INDEPENDENT SCIENCE OF NURSING and ART OF NURSING PRACTICE. Both of those concepts are unidimensional.

Nonrelational Propositions

The definitions of the concepts of the Science of Unitary Human Beings are given here. These constitutive definitions are the nonrelational propositions of this nursing model.

ENERGY FIELD

- A means of perceiving people and their respective environments as irreducible wholes (Rogers, 1992b, p. 29).
- Field … is a unifying concept and energy signifies the dynamic nature of the field. Energy fields are infinite and pandimensional; they are in continuous motion (Rogers, 1992b, p. 30).

The concept of **Energy Field** encompasses two dimensions—Human Energy Field and Environmental Energy Field. Rogers (1992b) pointed out that "human beings and the environment are energy fields; they do not have energy fields" (p. 30). Consequently, the possessive cannot be used when referring to a human energy field or an environmental energy field.

- **Human Energy Field:** [The unitary human being is] an irreducible, indivisible, pandimensional energy field identified by pattern and manifesting characteristics that are specific to the whole and which cannot be predicted from knowledge of the parts (Rogers, 1992b, p. 29).

Rogers (1992b) extended the notion of the Human Energy Field to groups. She commented that the Science of Unitary Human Beings "is equally as applicable to groups as it is to individuals. The group energy field to be considered is identified. It may be a family, a social group, or a community, a crowd or some other combination" (p. 30). Group energy fields have the same characteristics as individual energy fields—they are continuously open and integral with their own environmental fields, they are pandimensional, and they have pattern that changes continuously.

- **Environmental Energy Field:** [The environment is] an irreducible, [indivisible] pandimensional energy field identified by pattern and integral with the human [energy] field (Rogers, 1992b, p. 29).

OPENNESS

- Energy fields are open, not a little bit or sometimes, but continuously (Rogers, 1992b, p. 30).
- Openness is nonvariant (Rogers, 1992b).

PATTERN

- [Pattern is] the distinguishing characteristic of an energy field perceived as a single wave (Rogers, 1992b, p. 30).
- Pattern is an abstraction, its nature changes continuously, and it gives identity to the field. … Each human field pattern is unique and is integral with its own unique environmental field pattern (Rogers, 1992b, p. 30).
- Energy field patterns are not directly observable (Rogers, 1992b).
- Manifestations of field patterning are observable events in the real world. They are postulated to emerge out of the human-environmental field mutual process (Rogers, 1992b, p. 31).
- Manifestations of energy field pattern range from the physical body to such rhythmical phenomena as diversity in the experiences of time passing, the speed of motion, and sleep-wake cycles (Rogers, 1986, 1992b).
- Rogers has stated that she considers "physical bodies to be manifestations of field [pattern]" (Rogers et al., 1990, p. 377).
- The evolution of life and non-life is a dynamic, irreducible, nonlinear process characterized by increasing complexification of energy field patterning. The nature of change is unpredictable and increasingly diverse (Rogers, 1990a, p. 8) (see Table 9–1).

The **Pattern** of an **Energy Field** is conceptualized as a wave phenomenon. Rogers (1970) noted, "A multiplicity of waves characterizes the universe. Light waves, sound waves, thermal waves, atomic waves, and gravity waves flow in rhythmic patterns" (p. 101).

Pattern changes continuously. The change, according to Rogers (1992b), is continuous, relative, innovative, increasingly diverse, and unpredictable. This means that there is no repetition in human life, no regression to former states or stages. Rather, the human and environmental field patterns change constantly, always evolving into other novel, innovative forms (Rogers, 1970). Although the direction of changes is invariant, the rate of change may vary for an individual over the course of life. Change also varies among individuals. Indeed, "individual differences … point up the significance of this relative diversity" (Rogers, 1992b, p. 31). The diversity of rhythmical patterns is summarized in Table 9–1.

PANDIMENSIONALITY

- [Pandimensionality is] a nonlinear domain without spatial or temporal attributes (Rogers, 1992b, p. 29).
- [Pandimensional] best expresses the idea of a unitary whole (Rogers, 1992b, p. 31).
- One does not move into or become pandimensional. Rather, this is a way of perceiving reality (Rogers, 1992b, p. 31).
- [All reality is pandimensional, and in such a pandimensional world,] the relative nature of change becomes explicit (Rogers, 1992b, p. 31).

HOMEODYNAMICS

The concept of **Homeodynamics** encompasses three dimensions—Resonancy, Helicy, and Integrality. The definitions of the dimensions Resonancy, Helicy, and Integrality are considered principles (Rogers, 1990a).

The three dimensions of the concept of **Homeodynamics**, or the principles of homeodynamics, concisely explicate Rogers' ideas about human and environmental energy field patterns. The three mutually exclusive principles are equally applicable to individual energy fields and group energy fields, as well as environmental energy fields.

- **Resonancy:** [Resonancy is the] continuous change from lower to higher frequency wave patterns in human and environmental fields (Rogers, 1990a, p. 8). Resonancy delineates the direction of evolutionary change in energy field pattern (Rogers, 1990a).
- **Helicy:** [Helicy is the] continuous, innovative, unpredictable, increasing diversity of human and environmental field patterns (Rogers, 1990a, p. 8). Helicy addresses the continuous change that characterizes human and environmental field patterns (Rogers, 1990a).
- **Integrality:** [Integrality is the] continuous mutual human field and environmental field process (Rogers, 1990a, p. 8). Integrality emphasizes the nature of the relationship between the human and environmental fields (Rogers, 1990a).

WELL-BEING

- An expression of the life process (Rogers, 1970, 1994b).
- Well-being is a value, it is not an absolute (Rogers et al., 1990, p. 378).

Rogers (1994b) maintained that **Well-Being** "is a much better term [than health] because the term health is very ambiguous" (p. 34). Earlier, Rogers (1970) had referred to health and illness, ease and dis-ease, normal and pathological processes, and maximum well-being and sickness. Such dichotomous notions, Rogers (1970) maintained, "are ar-

---

TABLE 9–1
MANIFESTATIONS OF RELATIVE DIVERSITY IN ENERGY FIELD PATTERNING

Less Diverse	More Diverse	Most Diverse
Longer rhythms	Shorter rhythms	Seem continuous
Slower motion	Faster motion	Seem continuous
Lower frequency	Higher frequency	Seem continuous
Time experienced as slower	Time experienced as faster	Timelessness
Pragmatic	Imaginative	Visionary
Sleeping	Waking	Beyond waking

Adapted from Rogers, M.E. (1990). Nursing: Science of unitary, irreducible, human beings: Update 1990. In E.A.M. Barrett (Ed.), Visions of Rogers' science-based nursing (p. 9). New York: National League for Nursing, with permission.

bitrarily defined, culturally infused, and value laden" (p. 85). She went on to explain:

> Health and sickness, however defined, are expressions of the process of life. Whatever meaning they may have is derived out of an understanding of the life process in its totality. Life's deviant course demands that it be viewed in all of its dimensions if valid explanations of its varied manifestations are to emerge (p. 85).

Wellness and illness, then, are not differentiated within the context of the Science of Unitary Human Beings. Rather, they are considered value terms imposed by society. As such, "manifestations of human and environmental field pattern deemed to have high value are labeled wellness by the society, and those deemed to have low value are labeled illness" (Rogers, 1980f). Similarly, "Disease and pathology are value terms applied when the human field manifests characteristics that may be deemed undesirable" (Rogers, 1992b, p. 33). More specifically, within the Science of Unitary Human Beings, "There are no absolute norms for health. There are patterns that emerge from the human process that may be experienced as pain, happiness, illness, or any behavior. Society labels some of these behaviors 'sick.' What behaviors a society accepts as sick or well varies with culture and history. Families also have their own definitions of sick or well. … So there are no absolutes about what constitutes sickness or wellness" (Madrid & Winstead-Fry, 1986, p. 91).

In keeping with the Science of Unitary Human Beings, Madrid and Winstead-Fry (1986) then defined health as "participation in the life process by choosing and executing behaviors that lead to the maximum fulfillment of a person's potential" (p. 91).

Despite her lack of differentiation of wellness and illness, Rogers (1970) viewed those health states in the form of a continuum. She explained, "Health and illness are part of the same continuum. They are not dichotomous conditions. The multiple events taking place along life's axis denote the extent to which man is achieving his maximum health potential and vary in their expressions from greatest health to those conditions which are incompatible with maintaining life processes" (p. 125). However, Rogers (1970) indicated that she thought that society views wellness and illness as dichotomous, discrete entities.

NURSING

The concept of **Nursing** encompasses two dimensions—Independent Science of Nursing and Art of Nursing Practice.

- **Independent Science of Nursing**: An organized body of abstract knowledge arrived at by scientific research and logical analysis (Rogers, 1992b, p. 28; 1994b). A body of knowledge specific to nursing (Rogers, 1994a, p. 5).

- **Art of Nursing Practice**: The creative use of the science of nursing for human betterment (Rogers, 1992b, p. 28). [Nursing's] creative use of its knowledge [is] the art of practice (Rogers, 1994a, p. 5).

Nursing, for Rogers (1994b), is "a learned field of endeavor" (p. 34). Earlier, Rogers (1992b) referred to nursing as "a learned profession" (p. 28).

Rogers (1992b) noted that "historically, the term 'nursing' most often has been used as a verb signifying 'to do,' rather than as a noun meaning 'to know.' When nursing is identified as a science the term 'nursing' becomes a noun signifying 'a body of abstract knowledge'" (pp. 28–29). The combination of the concepts of **Independent Science of Nursing** and **Art of Nursing Practice** is evident in Rogers' (1992c) description of nursing as "compassionate concern for human beings. It is the heart that understands and the hand that soothes. It is the intellect that synthesizes many learnings into meaningful ministrations" (p. 1339).

The **GOAL OF NURSING** is "to promote human betterment wherever people are, on planet earth or in outer space" (Rogers, 1992b, p. 33). Although Rogers mentioned prevention of disease as a nursing goal in her 1970 book, she later pointed out that prevention is a negative concept that is contradicted by the philosophical and conceptual tenets of the Science of Unitary Human Beings (Rogers, 1980g). She also pointed out that the term promotion reflects a more positive, optimistic approach and therefore is consistent with the Science of Unitary Human Beings.

The nursing process, according to Rogers (1970), follows from the **Independent Science of Nursing**. She explained:

> Broad principles are put together in novel ways to help explain a wide range of events and multiplicity of individual differences. Action, based on predictions arising out of intellectual skill in the merging of scientific principles, becomes underwritten by intellectual judgments (pp. 87–88).

Rogers (1978b) regarded the nursing process as a modality for application of nursing knowledge but lacking in any substance of its own. She did not specify a particular nursing process format but did mention assessment, diagnosis, goal setting, intervention, and evaluation in her 1970 book. Although Rogers' later publications and presentations did not explicitly address a nursing process, components of a **PRACTICE METHODOLOGY** can be extracted from those and related works, especially Barrett's (1988, 1990c, 1998) and Cowling's (1990) descriptions of health patterning and Cowling's (1997) description of pattern appreciation. The Science of Unitary Human Beings **PRACTICE METHODOLOGY, THE HEALTH PATTERNING PRACTICE METHOD**, is outlined in Table 9–2.

PATTERN MANIFESTATION KNOWING AND APPRECIATION—ASSESSMENT

The continuous process of apprehending and identifying manifestations of the human energy field and environmental energy field patterns that relate to current health events.

The nurse uses one or more Science of Unitary Human Beings–based research instruments or practice tools to guide application and documentation of the practice methodology (see Table 9–3).

The nurse acts with pandimensional authenticity, that is, with a demeanor of genuineness, trustworthiness, and knowledgeable caring.

The nurse approaches each situation with gratefulness, enjoyment, understanding, unconditional love, compassion, and empathy.

The nurse makes the cherished values of Rogerian ethics intentional, including reverence, human betterment, generosity, commitment, diversity, responsibility, compassion, wisdom, justice-creating openness, courage, optimism, humor, unity, transformation, and celebration.

The nurse expresses intentionality by approaching the nursing situation with the intent to facilitate human betterment.

The nurse focuses on the client as a unified whole, a unitary human being.

The nurse appreciates the uniqueness of each client.

The nurse participates in individualized nursing by looking at each client and determining the range of behaviors that are normal for him or her.

The nurse always takes diversity among clients into account, because that diversity has distinct implications for what will be done and how it will be done.

The nurse comes to know human energy field pattern and environmental energy field pattern through manifestations of that pattern in the form of the client's experiences, perceptions, and expressions.

The nurse attends to expressions of experiences and perceptions in such forms as the client's verbal responses, responses to questionnaires, and personal ways of living and relating.

The nurse uses multiple forms of knowing, including intuition, meditative insights, and tacit knowing.

The nurse collects such relevant pattern information as the client's sensations, thoughts, feelings, awareness, imagination, memory, introspective insights, intuitive apprehensions, recurring themes and issues that pervade the client's life, metaphors, visualizations, images, nutrition, work and play, exercise, substance use, sleep/wake cycles, safety, decelerated/accelerated field rhythms, space-time shifts, interpersonal networks, and professional health-care access and use.

The nurse synthesizes all pattern information into a narrative pattern profile that describes the essence of the human/environment health situation. The pattern profile may include diagrams, poems, metaphors, and interpretations of any practice tools that were administered.

VOLUNTARY MUTUAL PATTERNING

The continuous process whereby the nurse, with the client, patterns the environmental energy field to promote harmony related to the health events.

Voluntary mutual patterning may begin with discussion of the pattern profile.

The nurse facilitates the client's actualization of potentials for health, well-being, and betterment.

The nurse makes the cherished values of Rogerian ethics intentional, including reverence, human betterment, generosity, commitment, diversity, responsibility, compassion, wisdom, justice-creating openness, courage, optimism, humor, unity, transformation, and celebration.

The nurse has no investment in the client's changing in a particular way.

The nurse does not attempt to change anyone to conform to arbitrary health ideals. Rather, the nurse enhances the client's efforts to actualize health potentials from his or her point of view.

The nurse helps create an environment where healing conditions are optimal and invites the client to heal himself or herself as the nurse and the client participate in various health patterning modalities.

The nurse uses many different modes of health patterning, including such noninvasive modalities as therapeutic touch; imagery; meditation; relaxation; balancing activity and rest; unconditional love; attitudes of hope, humor, and upbeat moods; the use of sound, including music; use of color; use of motion, such as movement, dance, and exercise; health education; wellness counseling; nutrition counseling; meaningful presence; meaningful dialogue; affirmations (expressions of intentionality); bibliotherapy; journal keeping; esthetic experiences of art, poetry, and nature; collaborative advocacy; and computer-based virtual reality.

The nurse recognizes that both noninvasive modalities and technology are simply tools used to apply knowledge in practice.

PATTERN MANIFESTATION KNOWING AND APPRECIATION—EVALUATION

The nurse evaluates voluntary mutual patterning by means of pattern manifestation knowing.

The nurse makes the cherished values of Rogerian ethics intentional, including reverence, human betterment, generosity, commitment, diversity, responsibility, compassion, wisdom, justice-creating openness, courage, optimism, humor, unity, transformation, and celebration.

The nurse monitors and collects additional pattern information as it unfolds during voluntary mutual patterning.

The nurse considers the pattern information within the context of continually emerging health patterning goals affirmed by the client.

Constructed from Barrett, 1988, 1990b, 1990c, 1993, 1998; Boguslawski, 1990; Butcher, 2001; Cowling, 1990, 1997; Rogers, 1970, 1980f, 1980g, 1985c, 1987b, 1990a, 1992b, 1994a; Rogers et al., 1990.

With regard to nursing practice, Rogers (1992b) noted that as the diversity of the **Pattern** of the Human Energy Field and the Environmental Energy Field increases, "so too will individualization of [nursing] services" (p. 33). She maintained that the individualization of nursing services is necessary to help people achieve their maximum potential in a positive fashion.

The diversity of human and environment energy field pattern manifestations is apprehended through what Rogers (1990a, 1992b) referred to as synthesis and pattern seeing. Elaborating, Barrett (1988) identified pattern manifestation appraisal, which she later renamed Pattern Manifestation Knowing (Barrett, 1998), as the first component of the Science of Unitary Human Beings HEALTH PATTERNING PRACTICE METHOD. The **Pattern Manifestation Knowing and Appreciation—Assessment** component encompasses what typically is regarded as the assessment, diagnosis, and goal-setting phases of the nursing process. Knowing refers to apprehending pattern manifestations (Barrett, 1988), and appreciation refers to perception of the pattern (Cowling, 1997). Drawing from Cowling (1997), Butcher (2001) explained that "Appreciation requires sensitivity [and] recognition of the excellence of the meaning of energy field patterning .... Appreciation is reaching for the essence of pattern and has the potential to deepen understanding [of] ... the client's process of knowing participation in change and transformation" (p. 209).

The second component of the **HEALTH PATTERNING PRACTICE METHOD** originally was called deliberative mutual patterning (Barrett, 1988) but has been renamed **Voluntary Mutual Patterning** (Barrett, 1998). That component refers to what typically is regarded as the intervention phase of the nursing process.

Rogers (1970) explained that the diversity of field pattern manifestations within an individual and between individuals mandates novel nursing interventions. She stated:

> Judicious and wise identification of interventive measures consonant with the diagnostic pattern and the purposes to be achieved in any given situation requires the imaginative pulling together of nursing knowledges in new ways according to the particular needs of the individual or group (p. 125).

Rogers (1970) acknowledged the importance of technological tools and personal procedural activities as nursing interventions, but pointed out that "it must be thoroughly understood that tools and procedures are adjuncts to practice and are safe and meaningful only to the extent that knowledgeable nursing judgments underwrite their selection and the ways in which they may be used" (p. 126). The Science of Unitary Human Beings, Rogers (1990a) pointed out, "sparks new interventive modalities— that evolve as life evolves from earth to space and beyond" (p. 10). Many of the new modalities are noninvasive (see Table 9–2). Indeed, Rogers (1994b) maintained that "in practice, non-invasive modalities will characterize the next century" (p. 34). She went on to point out that noninvasive alternative modalities "have been around in the literature for some 20 or 30 years, not necessarily in nursing, although there are nurses who have more and more recognized this. The public, interestingly enough, wants alternatives. Things are changing in the delivery of health care" (p. 34).

Voluntary Mutual Patterning is voluntary in that the nurse and the client engage in the process with an understanding of freedom of choice and act without external compulsion (Barrett, 1988). Voluntary Mutual Patterning is a mutual process, whereby "Both the nurse and the client are changed with each encounter, each patterning one another and coevolving together" (Butcher, 2001, p. 210). In addition, Voluntary Mutual Patterning is an intentional process, "in that the nurse approaches each nursing situation with the intention of promoting well-being and human betterment" (Butcher, 2001, p. 210).

The third component of the Science of Unitary Human Beings **HEALTH PATTERNING PRACTICE METHOD** is **Pattern Manifestation Knowing and Appreciation— Evaluation**. This component refers to what typically is regarded as the evaluation phase of the nursing process. "Evaluation," Butcher (2001) explained, "is continuous and is integral to both pattern manifestation knowing and appreciation[-assessment] and to voluntary mutual patterning. The nurse is continuously evaluating changes in patterning emerging from the human/environmental field mutual process" (p. 211).

Relational Propositions

The relational propositions of the Science of Unitary Human Beings are listed here. The metaparadigm concepts of human beings, environment, and health are linked in relational propositions A and B. Relational proposition C links the metaparadigm concepts of health and nursing. The metaparadigm concepts of human beings, health, and nursing are linked in relational propositions D and E. All four metaparadigm concepts—human beings, environment, health, nursing—are linked in relational propositions F and G.

A. For nurses, [the] focus consists of a long-established concern with people and the world they live in. It is the natural forerunner of an organized, abstract system encompassing people and their environments (Rogers, 1992b, p. 28).
B. [The nurse is] an environmental component for the individual receiving services (Rogers, 1970, pp. 124–125).
C. The primary focus of nursing is to promote health (Rogers, 1992a, p. 61).
D. The purpose of nurses is to promote ... well-being for all persons wherever they are (Rogers, 1992b, p. 28).
E. Nurses participate in the process of change, to help people move toward what is deemed better health (Rogers, 1980g).
F. The purpose of nurses is to promote health and well-being for all persons wherever they are (Rogers, 1992b, p. 28).
G. The purpose of nursing is to promote human betterment wherever people are, on planet earth or in outer space (Rogers, 1992b, p. 33).

 ## EVALUATION OF ROGERS' SCIENCE OF UNITARY HUMAN BEINGS

This section presents an evaluation of the Science of Unitary Human Beings. The evaluation is based on the results of the analysis, as well as on publications by Rogers and by others who have used or commented on the Science of Unitary Human Beings.

EXPLICATION OF ORIGINS

The origins of the Science of Unitary Human Beings are evident. Rogers explained why she decided to develop a conceptual model, identified various refinements in her conceptual system, and explained the reasons for changes in terminology. She also explicitly identified many of the assumptions undergirding the Science of Unitary Human

Beings. Other philosophical claims, in the form of Rogers' beliefs, were easily extracted from her publications. Those assumptions and beliefs indicate that Rogers viewed nursing as a legitimate science and an art that must base its practice on a body of empirically adequate knowledge. The assumptions also indicate that Rogers valued a unitary view of human beings and the environment. Rogers pointed out that this perspective of human beings identifies nursing as a unique discipline.

Rogers repeatedly emphasized her view that health is socially defined, which suggests that she expected specific goals for nursing intervention to be based on the values of society, not those of the nurse or nursing alone. Moreover, Rogers' discussion of nursing intervention indicates that she valued individualized nursing for each person. Indeed, individualized nursing is mandated by the Science of Unitary Human Beings because of the uniqueness and diversity of each human energy field.

Rogers explained how she drew from the knowledge of various sciences in developing the Science of Unitary Human Beings, and she cited the works of several scholars from adjunctive disciplines. Refinements in the Science of Unitary Human Beings can clearly be traced to new knowledge in nursing and adjunctive disciplines. For example, in explaining the change in the definition of helicy from the term probabilistic to the term unpredictable, Rogers (1990a, 1992b) cited publications about chaos theory. Interestingly, however, Rogers (as cited in Huch, 1995) seemed to reject chaos theory when she noted that "chaos is from an old worldview" (p. 43). Elaborating, she stated:

> There is nothing new about the idea of chaos theory; it had been proposed 30 to 40 years ago and had been worked on then. But what they were saying was, since the human being is not very knowledgeable and he can't possibly know everything, then of course he can't predict everything. Then there was a great big but; but if the human being did know everything, it would all be laid out and he could predict everything. In other words, the some old absolutist philosophy that was supposedly pushed out of the way around the turn of the century when Einstein and some of the others came along (Rogers, as cited in Huch, 1995, p. 43).

COMPREHENSIVENESS OF CONTENT

The Science of Unitary Human Beings is sufficiently comprehensive with regard to depth of content. The many revisions and refinements in the conceptual system attest to Rogers' concern for precision in language. Rogers defined and described the four metaparadigm concepts—human beings, environment, health, nursing—sufficiently for a conceptual model. Human beings and environment are clearly defined, and the relationship between unitary human beings and their environments is explicitly identi-

fied. Health is designated as well-being and is defined through its relation to the life process. Furthermore, designation of health conditions as wellness or illness is considered a social value.

Moreover, nursing is described, and emphasis is placed on its characteristics as a noun. The goal of nursing is clearly delineated. A nursing process, in the form of the **Health Patterning Practice Method**, was extracted from Rogers' publications and from publications by main proponents of the Science of Unitary Human Beings.

The Science of Unitary Human Beings is consistent with scientific findings. That is particularly evident in Rogers' insistence that nursing actions—the **Art of Nursing Practice**—must stem from an organized and empirically adequate knowledge base—the **Independent Science of Nursing**. Indeed, Rogers repeatedly emphasized that nursing is an empirical science, such that any and all judgments must be based on scientific knowledge. She commented, "The education of nurses gains its identity by the transmission of nursing's body of theoretical knowledge. The practice of nurses, therefore, is the creative use of this knowledge in human service" (Rogers, 1992b, p. 29).

Rogers always maintained that nursing practice must be theory-based. More specifically, she declared, "Nursing practice must be flexible and creative, individualized and socially oriented, compassionate and skillful. Professional practitioners in nursing must be continuously translating theoretical knowledge into human service.... Nursing's conceptual system provides the foundation for nursing practice" (Rogers, 1970, p. 128).

Rogers (1987a) also declared, "For nurses to fulfill their social and professional responsibilities in the days ahead demands that their practice be based upon a substantive theoretical base specific to nursing. The practice of nurses is the use of this knowledge in service to people" (pp. 121–122). Furthermore, Rogers (1980a) stated, "Broad principles to guide practice must replace rule-of-thumb" (p. 337).

The dynamic nature of nursing is evident in Rogers' (1970) statement that "the dynamic nature of life signifies continuous revision of the nature and meaning of diagnostic data and concomitant revision of interventional measures" (p. 125). In addition, the dynamic nature of the **Health Patterning Practice Method** is evident in Voluntary Mutual Patterning as nurse and participants in nursing are in continuous mutual process and also is evident in the use of Pattern Manifestation Knowing and Appreciation for evaluation of pattern manifestations following the application of nursing modalities.

The Science of Unitary Human Beings is compatible with ethical standards for nursing practice. Rogers (1992b) commented, "Continued emphasis on human rights, client decision-making, and noncompliance with the traditional rules of thumb are … necessary dimensions of the new science and art of nursing" (p. 33).

Rogers linked the metaparadigm concepts of human beings, environment, and nursing; health and nursing; and human beings, health, and nursing in various statements. The linkage of all four metaparadigm concepts is stated concisely in two statements about the purpose of nurses and nursing (see Relational Propositions F and G, above).

The Science of Unitary Human Beings is comprehensive in breadth of content. The Rogerian conceptual system can be used in diverse settings, ranging from community-based health services to hospitals to the "human advent into outer space" (Rogers, 1992b, p. 27), and with people experiencing virtually any health-related condition from birth through death, "in health and in sickness, in joy and in sorrow" (Rogers, 1992c, p. 1339). Furthermore, the Science of Human Beings is equally applicable to individuals and groups, including families, social groups, communities, and crowds (Rogers, 1992b).

The breadth of the Science of Unitary Human Beings is further supported by the direction it provides for nursing research, education, administration, and practice. The guidelines for nursing research, which continue to be developed by proponents of the Science of Unitary Human Beings, as well as the guidelines for nursing education, administration of nursing services, and nursing practice are listed below.

Nursing Research Guidelines

The guidelines for nursing research based on the Science of Unitary Human Beings, which were constructed from Alligood and Fawcett (1999), Barrett (1996), Barrett et al. (1997), Bultemeier (1997b), Butcher (1994, 1998, 2001), Carboni (1995), Cowling (1986, 1997, 1998), Fawcett (1994), Fawcett and Downs (1986), Phillips (1989, 1991), Reeder (1984, 1986), Rogers (1987a, 1990b, 1992b, 1994a, 1994b), Rogers et al. (1990), and Sherman (1997), are:

• Purpose of the research
  • The Science of Unitary Human Beings requires both basic research and applied research.
  • The purpose of Science of Unitary Human Beings–based basic research is to develop new theoretical knowledge about unitary human energy fields in mutual process with environmental energy fields. The goal of basic nursing research is pattern seeing.
  • The purpose of Science of Unitary Human Beings–based applied research is to test already available knowledge in practice situations.
  • The term applied research is used instead of the term clinical research because "clinical" refers to investiga-

tion of a disease in the living subject by observation, as distinguished from controlled study, or it refers to something done at the bedside. The term clinical research, therefore, is inappropriate and inadequate for the scope and purposes of nursing research.

• Phenomena of interest
  • The phenomena to be studied are those that are central to nursing—irreducible unitary human beings and their environments. More specifically, the phenomena to be studied are manifestations of human and environmental energy field mutual process.
  • Nursing research does not focus on other fields of study or theories derived from other fields, nor does it focus on nurses and what they do.

• Problems to be studied
  • The problems to be studied are the manifestations of human energy field patterns and environmental energy field patterns, especially pattern profiles, which are clusters of related pattern manifestations.

• Study participants
  • Inasmuch as nursing is a service to all people, wherever they may be, virtually any human being or group in its natural setting would be appropriate for study, with the proviso that both human being or group and environment are taken into account.

• Research methods
  • A variety of qualitative and quantitative research methods currently are regarded as appropriate designs for Science of Unitary Human Beings–based research, although qualitative methods are more congruent with the Science of Unitary Human Beings than quantitative methods.
  • Although descriptive and correlational designs are regarded as consistent with the Science of Unitary Human Beings, strict experimental designs are of questionable value because of Rogers' rejection of the notion of causality.
  • Specific existing methodologies that are used across disciplines but currently are regarded as appropriate include Husserlian phenomenology; existentialism; rational interpretive hermeneutics; interpretive evaluation methods, such as Fourth Generation Evaluation; participatory action and cooperative inquiry; focus groups; ecological thinking; dialectical thinking; and historical inquiries, as well as methods that focus on the uniqueness of each human being, such as imagery, direct questioning, personal structural analysis, and the Q-sort.
  • New Science of Unitary Human Beings–specific methodologies include the unitary pattern appreciation case method, the Rogerian process of inquiry

method, the unitary field pattern portrait research method, and the photo-disclosure methodology.

- Case studies and longitudinal research designs that focus on the identification of manifestations of human and environmental energy field patterns are more appropriate than cross-sectional designs, given the emphasis in the Science of Unitary Human Beings on the uniqueness of the unitary human being.
- Hypotheses should not be stated in causal language, in recognition of the unitary nature of the problem to be studied and Rogers' rejection of the notion of causality.
- Purposive sampling is appropriate, so that study participants who manifest the phenomenon of interest may be included.
- Research instruments that are directly derived from the Science of Unitary Human Beings should be used (see Table 9–3).
- Researchers are the primary pattern-apprehending instrument, as they are the only instrument sensitive to and able to interpret and understand pandimensional potentialialities in manifestations of human and environmental energy field patterns. The researcher may use tacit and mystical intuition and all forms of sensory knowing to apprehend pattern manifestations.
- Inclusion of study participants in the process of inquiry enhances mutual exploration, discovery, and knowing participation in change.
- Research design may change and evolve during a study; any changes should be documented.

- Data analysis
  - Synthesis rather than an analysis that separates parts is the goal of data analysis.
  - Data analysis techniques must take the unitary nature of human beings and the integrality of the human and environmental energy fields into account. Consequently, the use of standard data analysis techniques that employ the components of variance model of statistics is precluded, because this statistical model is logically inconsistent with the assumption of holism stating that the whole is greater than the sum of parts.
  - Multivariate analysis procedures, particularly canonical correlation, are useful techniques for generating a constellation of variables representing human field pattern properties. However, canonical correlation is a component of variance procedure, as are all parametric correlational techniques.
  - New data analysis techniques that permit examination of the integrality of human and environmental energy fields must be developed so that the ongoing testing of the Science of Unitary Human Beings does not have to be done through the logical empiricist criterion of

meaning, testing the hypodeductive system for consistency, and then testing correspondence to the world.
  - Data should be interpreted within the context of the concepts and propositions of the Science of Unitary Human Beings.
  - Bracketing and objectivity are not possible given the integral nature of the researcher and the study participants as energy fields in mutual process.

- Contributions
  - Science of Unitary Human Beings–based research enhances understanding of the continuous mutual process of human and environmental energy fields and manifestations of changes in energy field patterns. Ultimately, Science of Unitary Human Beings–based research will yield a body of nursing-specific knowledge.

Nursing Education Guidelines

The guidelines for nursing research based on the Science of Unitary Human Begins, which were constructed from Barrett (1990a), Gueldner et al. (1994), Mathwig et al. (1990), Rogers (1961, 1970, 1985a, 1987a, 1990b, 1994a), Rogers (as cited in Takahashi, 1992), and Young (1985), are:

- Focus of the curriculum
  - Nursing education can be for professional nursing or for technical nursing. The type of practice depends on the nature and amount of knowledge that underwrites the two separate career paths.
  - Although Rogers acknowledged the importance of both professional and technical nursing education as entry levels to practice, the focus of the guidelines for Science of Unitary Human Beings–based nursing education is on preparation for professional nursing.
  - The purpose of professional education is to provide knowledge and the tools to use that knowledge in practice.
  - The focus of Science of Unitary Human Beings–based professional nursing education programs is the transmission of a body of scholarly nursing knowledge.

- Nature and sequence of content
  - The content of a Science of Unitary Human Beings–based curriculum encompasses a body of scientific knowledge specific to nursing. That body of knowledge determines the safety and scope of nursing practice. The imaginative and creative use of knowledge for the betterment of humankind finds expression in the art of nursing.

- Courses in the adjunctive disciplines that are appropriate as a background for the study of the Science of Unitary Human Beings include written and spoken English, foreign languages, communication skills, logic, mathematics, economics, literature, history, political science, cultural anthropology, the world's religions, Eastern philosophy, ethics, astronomy, modern physics, a one-semester course in anatomy and physiology, computer science, and the creative arts.
- Nursing courses focus on the study of humankind and the Science of Unitary Human Beings.
- Baccalaureate degree program nursing courses provide knowledge of the beginning tools of inquiry and the application of knowledge for the improvement of practice.
- Master's degree program nursing courses provide knowledge of more sophisticated tools of inquiry and more complex practice problems, and knowledge of the design and utilization of applied research.
- Doctoral degree program nursing courses provide knowledge of basic research and strategies for pushing back the frontiers of nursing knowledge.
- The principles of resonancy, helicy, and integrality can serve as the major integrating concepts of the curriculum.
- The stages of the human life process, from conception through aging and in stages of terminal illness and dying, can provide the organizational theme for the sequence of didactic content and practicum experiences. The principles of resonancy, helicy, and integrality are introduced in the first course in the nursing major and are then considered at more advanced levels of understanding and application in subsequent courses.
- Settings for nursing education
  - Education for professional nursing occurs at the baccalaureate, master's, and doctoral levels in senior college and university settings.
  - Baccalaureate nursing education requires 5 years of study.
  - The faculties of nursing education programs situated in senior colleges and universities must be prepared at the doctoral level.
- Characteristics of students
  - Students must meet the requirements for matriculation in the particular professional nursing program of interest.
- Teaching-learning strategies
  - Teaching and learning are regarded as complex, interactive processes of growth and development and emphasize how to learn; how to think critically; and how to see patterns, find meanings, and gain scholarly insights.
  - Teaching-learning strategies also emphasize development of the student's awareness of self as an aspect of the client's environmental energy field and the dynamic role the nurse's pattern manifestations have on the client.
  - Teaching-learning strategies include didactic content and laboratory experiences encompassing maintenance and promotion of health, as well as care and rehabilitation of the sick and disabled. Laboratory study, which is directed toward the well and the sick of all ages and conditions, is a necessary adjunct to didactic content and provides students with the opportunity to demonstrate their capacity to translate theory into practice. Laboratory settings include homes, schools, industrial settings, clinics, hospitals, and other places where people may be.
  - A collection of the most important readings and other resources about the Science of Unitary Human Beings is made available to students in each course.
  - Attention is given to environmental attributes that legitimize and promote Science of Unitary Human Beings–based thinking.
  - Media that promote freedom and opportunity for expression are used.
  - Assignments include a combination of traditional written papers and such creative expressions as poetry writing and reading and expressive movement, which can be videotaped.
  - Time is allotted for nonjudgmental dialogue and independent reflection.
  - Faculty and students continue to develop new insights and creative applications for nursing practice as they explore the meaning of the content of the Science of Unitary Human Beings.

Administration of Nursing Services Guidelines

Guidelines for the administration of nursing services based on the Science of Unitary Human Beings, which were constructed from Alligood (1989), Caroselli-Dervan (1990), Gueldner (1989), Rizzo (1990), and Rogers (1985b, 1990a, 1990b, 1992b, 1994b), are:

- Focus of nursing in the health-care organization
  - The distinctive focus of Science of Unitary Human Beings–based nursing services is the creative use of nursing knowledge.

- Purpose of nursing services
  - Nursing services are at the center of any health-care system.
  - The purpose of nursing services is promotion of well-being.

- Characteristics of nursing personnel
  - Nursing services are regarded as energy fields that are seen as more than employees and staffing schedules or a count of functionaries required to staff a shift. Rather, all personnel on all shifts are viewed as interdependent.
  - The practitioners of professional nursing should hold valid baccalaureate or higher degrees in nursing and should be licensed as such.
  - Leaders of nursing services must be visionary and willing to embrace innovative and creative change.
  - The nurse administrator must have the ability to identify ways of patterning energy fields to ensure integrated behaviors for clients and employees.

- Settings for nursing services
  - Nursing services are located in all areas where there are people: at home, at school, at work, at play; in hospitals, nursing homes, and clinics; on this planet and in outer space.
  - Community-based health services, which eventually will extend to extraterrestrial centers, provide the umbrella for and should take precedence over hospital- and nursing home–based illness services. Hospitals and nursing homes are regarded as supplemental or satellite services that are pathology and disease oriented.

- Management strategies and administrative policies
  - Management strategies and administrative policies reflect the understanding that administrative systems consist of all human and environmental energy fields integral to the delivery of nursing services.
  - The strategy of participatory management, in the form of power sharing, is consistent with the Science of Unitary Human Beings. This strategy is operationalized as the situation in which primary nurses are able to make autonomous decisions and involve clients and their significant others in nursing.
  - Administrative policies foster an open and supportive administrative climate that enhances staff members' self-esteem, actualization, confidence, available options, and freedom of choice and provides opportunities for staff development and continuing education.
  - The ultimate goal of all management strategies and administrative policies is the client's well-being. This goal is attained by increasing the capacity of each individual involved in the delivery of nursing services to participate knowingly in change. The nurse administrator's energy, therefore, is directed toward facilitating changes in the environment that will enhance systems of communication and harmonious human-environmental energy field mutual process.

Nursing Practice Guidelines

Guidelines for nursing practice based on the Science of Unitary Human Beings, which were constructed from Malinski (1986c) and Rogers (1992b), are:

- Purpose of nursing practice
  - The primary purpose of Science of Unitary Human Beings–based nursing practice is to promote well-being for all human beings, wherever they are.
  - Another purpose of Science of Unitary Human Beings–based nursing practice is to assist both client and nurse to increase their awareness of their own rhythms and to make choices among a range of options congruent with their perceptions of well-being.

- Practice problems of interest
  - Practice problems of interest are those manifestations of human and environmental field patterns that nursing as a discipline and society as a whole deem relevant for nursing.

- Settings for nursing practice
  - Nursing may be practiced in any setting in which nurses encounter people, ranging from the community to hospitals to outer space.

- Characteristics of legitimate participants in nursing practice
  - Legitimate participants in nursing practice encompass all people of all ages, both as individual human energy fields and as group energy fields.

- Nursing process
  - The nursing process for the Science of Unitary Human Beings is the **Health Patterning Practice Method**. The components of the method are pattern manifestation knowing and appreciation—assessment, voluntary mutual patterning, and pattern manifestation knowing and appreciation—evaluation (see Table 9–2).

- Contributions of nursing practice to participants' well-being
  - Science of Unitary Human Beings–based nursing practice contributes to human betterment, however that might be defined by a society.

• Science of Unitary Human Beings–based nursing practice leads to acceptance of diversity as the norm and of the integral connectedness of human beings and their environments, as well as to viewing change as positive.

LOGICAL CONGRUENCE

There is no evidence of logical incompatibility in the content of the Science of Unitary Human Beings. The content of the Rogerian conceptual system flows directly from Rogers' philosophical claims, and the distinctive view of human beings and the environment is carried throughout all components of the Rogerian conceptual system. Furthermore, the characteristics of systems and developmental models that are reflected in the content of the Science of Unitary Human Beings are addressed in a logically congruent manner.

GENERATION OF THEORY

Several grand theories and middle-range theories have been derived from the Science of Unitary Human Beings. The grand theories are:

• Theory of Accelerating Evolution (Rogers, 1980a, 1986, 1992b)
• Theory of Rhythmical Correlates of Change (Rogers, 1980a, 1986, 1992b)
• Theory of Paranormal Phenomena (Rogers, 1980a, 1986, 1992b)
• Theory of Health as Expanding Consciousness (Newman, 1986, 1994)
• Theory of Human Becoming (Parse, 1981, 1992, 1998)
• Life Perspective Rhythm Model (Fitzpatrick, 1983, 1989)

Rogers derived the rudimentary grand theories of Accelerating Evolution, Rhythmical Correlates of Change, and Paranormal Phenomena from the Science of Unitary Human Beings. The **Theory of Accelerating Evolution** posits that evolutionary change is speeding up and that the range of diversity of life processes is widening. The theory postulates that change proceeds "in the direction of higher wave frequency field pattern … characterized by growing diversity" (Rogers, 1980a, p. 334). Accordingly, "the higher frequency wave patterns manifesting growing diversity portend new norms to coordinate with this accelerating change" (Rogers, 1992b, p. 32). Examples of new norms offered by Rogers are higher blood pressure readings in all age groups compared with readings from a few decades ago and increased length of the average waking period. Moreover, the theory provides a novel explanation for hy-

peractivity in children, regarding that pattern manifestation as accelerating evolution of the human energy field. Rogers (1992b) commented, "interestingly, gifted children and the so-called hyperactive [children] not uncommonly manifest similar behaviors. It would seem more reasonable, then, to hypothesize that hyperactivity was accelerating evolution, rather than to denigrate rhythmicities that diverge from outdated norms and erroneous expectations" (p. 32).

The **Theory of Rhythmical Correlates of Change** focuses on human and environmental energy field rhythms, which "are not to be confused with biologic rhythms or psychologic rhythms or similar particulate phenomena" (Rogers, 1980a, p. 335). The theory proposes that the accelerating evolution and increasing diversity of human energy field patterns are integral with accelerating evolution and increasing diversity in environmental energy field patterns. The theory postulates that "manifestations of the speeding up of human field rhythms are coordinate with higher frequency environmental field patterns. Humans and their environments evolve and change together" (Rogers, 1992b, p. 32). Evidence in support of the theory cited by Rogers includes the population explosion and increased longevity along with quickened environmental motion, growing atmospheric and cosmological complexity, escalating levels of science and technology, and development of space communities.

The **Theory of Paranormal Phenomena** provides explanations for precognition, deja vu, clairvoyance, and telepathy. Rogers (1980a) pointed out that within the Science of Unitary Human Beings "such occurrences become 'normal' rather than 'paranormal'" (p. 335). This is because in a pandimensional world, there is no linear time or any separation of human and environmental fields, so that the present is relative to each human being. The theory also provides an explanation for the efficacy of such alternative methods of healing as meditation, imagery, and therapeutic touch. Rogers (1992b) commented, "Meditative modalities, for example, bespeak 'beyond waking' [pattern] manifestations" (p. 32).

Rogers (1980a, 1986) cited several examples of changes in human life that she claimed as support for her theories. For example, she noted that Toffler's (1970, 1980) work provides evidence of the increasing rate of change in many aspects of life. She also noted that sleep/wake patterns are changing, such that people of all ages sleep less now. More definitive empirical evidence supporting her theory of rhythmic correlates comes from research by Johnston, Fitzpatrick, and Donovan (1982), who found that developmental stage is related to past and future time orientation.

Other grand theories also have been derived from the Science of Unitary Human Beings. Newman (1986, 1994) proposed a grand theory of health titled the Theory of

Health as Expanding Consciousness. The central thesis of the theory is that health is the expansion of consciousness. According to Newman (1986, 1994), the meanings of life and health are found in the evolving process of expanding consciousness. More specifically, the theory asserts that "every person in every situation, no matter how disordered and hopeless it may seem, is part of the universal process of expanding consciousness" (Newman, 1992, p. 650).

Parse (1981, 1992, 1998) formulated a grand theory, now called the Theory of Human Becoming, that "synthesizes Martha E. Rogers' principles and concepts about man with major tenets and concepts from existential-phenomenological thought" (Parse, 1981, p. 4). In particular, Parse based her theory on Rogers' principles of helicy, complementarity (now integrality), and resonancy; Rogers' concepts of energy field, openness, pattern and organization, and four- dimensionality (now pandimensionality); and the existential phenomenological tenets of human subjectivity and intentionality and the concepts of coconstitution, coexistence, and situated freedom. The central thesis of the Theory of Human Becoming is that "humans participate with the universe in the cocreation of health" (Parse, 1992, p. 37). Parse (as cited in Takahashi, 1992) explained that "human becoming refers to the human being structuring meaning multidimensionally while cocreating rhythmical patterns of relating and cotranscending with possibles" (p. 86).

Fitzpatrick (1983, 1989) derived the Life Perspective Rhythm Model, which can be considered a grand theory, from the Science of Unitary Human Beings and from the findings of research by Fitzpatrick (1980), Fitzpatrick and Donovan (1978), and Fitzpatrick, Donovan, and Johnston (1980). The life perspective rhythm model, according to Fitzpatrick (1989), "is a developmental model which proposes that the process of human development is characterized by rhythms. Human development occurs within the context of continuous person-environment interaction. Basic human rhythms that describe the development of persons include the identified indices of holistic human functioning, that is, temporal patterns, motion patterns, consciousness patterns, and perceptual patterns. The rhythmic correlates developed by Rogers are consistent with this life perspective rhythm model" (p. 405).

The middle-range theories that have been derived from the Science of Unitary Human Beings are:

- Power as Knowing Participation in Change (Barrett, 1986; Caroselli & Barrett, 1998)
- Theory of Human Field Motion (Ference, 1986b, 1989)
- Theory of Sentience Evolution (Parker, 1989)
- Theory of Creativity, Actualization, and Empathy (Alligood, 1991)
- Theory of Self-Transcendence (Reed, 1991, 1997)

- Theory of Kaleidoscoping in Life's Turbulence (Butcher, (1993)
- Theory of Enfolding Health-as-Wholeness-and-Harmony (Barrett et al., 1997)
- Theory of Healthiness (Leddy & Fawcett, 1997)
- Theory of Perceived Dissonance (Bultemeier, 1997a)
- Theory of Aging (Alligood & McGuire, 2000)
- Theory of Enlightenment (Hills & Hanchett, 2001)
- Theory of the Art of Professional Nursing (Alligood, 2002b)

Barrett (1986; Caroselli & Barrett, 1998) derived a middle-range theory of power—the Theory of Knowing Participation in Change—from the principle of helicy. Power is defined as "the capacity to participate knowingly in the nature of change characterizing the continuous repatterning of the human and environmental fields" (p. 174). Elaborating, Barrett (1986) explained that knowing participation "is being aware of what one is choosing to do, feeling free to do it, and doing it intentionally. Awareness and freedom to act intentionally guide participation in choices and involvement in creating changes" (p. 175).

Ference (1986b, 1989) derived a middle-range theory from the principle of resonancy. The Theory of Human Field Motion proposes that "as a human field engages in ever-higher levels of human field motion, the pattern evolves toward greater complexity, diversity, and differentiation" (Ference, 1989, p. 123). Ference (1989) cited empirical evidence of the correlates of human field motion, stating that "human field motion expands with increased physical motion, with meditation, with risk-taking, and with higher levels of participation in change" (p. 123).

Parker (1989) derived the Theory of Sentience Evolution from the concept of sentience, which Rogers (1970) included as a concept in an early version of her conceptual system. The theory focuses on sleeping, waking, and beyond waking, which are regarded as manifestations of relative diversity in energy field patterning (see Table 9–1). "Sentience evolution," according to Parker (1989), "is thinking, feeling, and perceiving in the sleeping, waking, and beyond waking states" (p. 5). Accordingly, beyond waking is "sentience experienced as a higher frequency phenomenon" (p. 5).

Alligood (1991) derived her middle-range theory—the Theory of Creativity, Actualization, and Empathy—from Rogers' Theory of Accelerating Evolution, which is a grand theory. Alligood's theory proposes that creativity and actualization are related to empathy. The conceptual-theoretical-empirical structure for Alligood's work was presented by Fawcett (1994). Empirical research supported the empirical adequacy of Alligood's (1991) theory for men and women 18 to 60 years of age, but not for men and women 61 to 92 years of age.

Reed (1991, 1997) reformulated knowledge about self-transcendence from various life span theories within the context of the Science of Unitary Human Beings. "Self transcendence," she explained, "was identified as a particular pattern of expansion of conceptual boundaries" (Reed, 1991, p. 72). The reformulated Theory of Self Transcendence proposes that "expansion of conceptual boundaries through intrapersonal, interpersonal, and temporal experiences [is] developmentally appropriate in individuals confronted with end-of-own-life issues [and that] expansion of self-boundaries [is] positively related to indicators of well-being in these individuals" (Reed, 1991, p. 72). Later, Reed (1997) explained, "Rogers' principles of homeodynamics taken as a whole reflect the basic capacity of unitary human beings, as individuals or groups, to self-organize for well-being. Transcendence represents one example of this capacity of self-organizing for well-being" (p. 192).

Butcher's (1993) Theory of Kaleidoscoping in Life's Turbulence encompasses the concept of kaleidoscoping and its three dimensions—turbulence, patterning, and flow. Butcher (1993) defined kaleidoscoping as "flowing with turbulent manifestations of patterning" (p. 186). The dimension of turbulence was derived from the Science of Unitary Human Beings concept of pandimensionality; patterning, from the concept of pattern; and flow, from the concept of openness. Butcher (1993) pointed out that "Nurses are in frequent contact with persons experiencing turbulent life events. Turbulent disruptions in harmonious human/environmental field patterning are present in persons experiencing illness" (p. 191). He went on the explain, "Kaleidoscoping is concerned with the flowing of a client's human field with a turbulent environmental energy field associated with a turbulent health event. When caring for a client who is experiencing turbulent life change, the nurse also kaleidoscopes with the client's chaotic field pattern" (p. 191).

Carboni (Barrett et al., 1997) developed a middle-range theory of Rogerian nursing practice titled Enfolding Health-as-Wholeness-and-Harmony. The theory "provide[s] an evolutionary understanding of Rogerian nursing practice and provide[s] the conceptual understanding necessary for the identification and testing of theoretical statements" (p. 556).

Leddy (1993) reconceptualized the principle of integrality through an extensive review of the literature from many adjunctive disciplines. Her work led to the development of the Human Energy Systems (HES) Model and an explanatory theory—the Theory of Healthiness. The Theory of Healthiness "proposes that greater perceived ease and expansiveness of human-environment mutual process (participation) is associated with less perceived change. Greater participation and less change are associated with greater perceived energy, which in turn, contributes to higher healthiness. Greater participation, less change, greater energy, and greater healthiness are all associated with greater mental health, current health status, and satisfaction with life, and less symptom distress" (Leddy & Fawcett, 1997, p. 76). Research yielded a more parsimonious version of the theory, with little evidence of relations of participation, change, energy, and healthiness to mental health, current health status, and symptom distress.

Bultemeier (1997a) proposed the Theory of Perceived Dissonance, which was derived from the Science of Unitary Human Beings homeodynamic principles of resonancy and integrality. The theory, which "delineates a human/environmental field process that is perceived as illness within the healthcare system, … proposes that resonancy is altered periodically and rhythmically during the evolution of energy fields" (Bultemeier, 1993, p. 158). According to the theory, perceptions of dissonance occur as the human and environmental energy fields evolve rhythmically.

Alligood (1997, 2002a) identified a theory of aging that she claimed was "derived by Rogers" (1997, p. 38) but provided no information about the theory. Close examination of Rogers' many publications revealed no evidence of a specific theory of aging. Alligood and McGuire (2000) derived a Theory of Aging (a middle-range theory) from Rogers' Theory of Accelerating Change (a grand theory). They explained, "Rogers viewed aging as a normal process of changes which emerge as manifestations of the evolving pattern of a human being's life. Rogers theorized that aging was a developmental process and that accelerating change manifested in the aged as they sleep less, have more varied sleep-wake frequencies, and experience time as racing" (p. 8). Alligood and McGuire identified sleep patterns and time perceptions as the two concepts of the Theory of Aging and asserted that the two concepts are related. Their study, which was designed to test the theory in a sample of elderly persons, yielded no evidence to support the assertion that sleep patterns and time perception are related. Consequently, the empirical adequacy of the theory must be questioned.

The four concepts of Hills and Hanchett's (2001) Theory of Enlightenment—awareness, wakefulness, human field motion, and well-being—also were derived from the homeodynamic principles of helicy, resonancy, and integrality. Awareness and wakefulness were derived from the principle of helicy; human field motion, from the principle of resonancy; and well-being, from the principle of integrality. The propositions of the theory assert that awareness is positively related to wakefulness, human field motion, and well-being; wakefulness is positively related to human field motion and well-being; human field motion is positively related to well-being; and awareness, wakefulness, and human field motion together explain more variance in well-being than any one concept alone. Hills and

Hanchett (2001) reported that their research findings supported all but the last proposition. They explained, "The finding that awareness and human field motion were each associated with as much variance in well-being as all three [concepts, i.e., awareness, wakefulness, and human field motion] together suggest the theory of enlightening needs further development" (p. 16).

Alligood (2002b) formalized a Theory of the Art of Professional Nursing from Rogers' publications through use of an interpretive hermeneutic research approach. The three concepts of the theory—respect, responsibility, and empathy—were derived from the homeodynamic principles of the Science of Unitary Human Beings. Respect was derived from the principle of resonancy; responsibility, from the principle of helicy; and integrality, from the principle of integrality. The theory proposes that the art of professional nursing is the nurse's ability to balance respect for human freedom and individual rights with responsibility for the welfare of others through empathy.

Butcher (2001) considers the Personalized Nursing LIGHT Model (Anderson & Smereck, 1989a, 1989b, 1992) to be a middle-range practice theory. Close examination of the publications about that model, however, indicate that is it a derivative of the Science of Unitary Human Beings but has not been formalized as a set of relatively concrete and specific concepts and propositions.

CREDIBILITY OF THE NURSING MODEL

Social Utility

The social utility of the Science of Unitary Human Beings is well documented by its use as a guide for nursing research, education, administration, and practice. Rogerian conferences have been held in New York City every 2 to 4 years since 1983, and the Society of Rogerian Scholars sponsors conferences every 1 or 2 years. Malinski's (1986a) edited book, *Explorations on Martha Rogers' Science of Unitary Human Beings*, Barrett's (1990d) edited book, *Visions of Rogers' Science-Based Nursing*, Madrid and Barrett's (1994) edited book, *Rogers' Scientific Art of Nursing Practice*, and Madrid's (1997) edited book, *Patterns of Rogerian Knowing* are devoted exclusively to reports of and issues related to research and practice derived from the Science of Unitary Human Beings. Two other books, *Martha E. Rogers: Eighty Years of Excellence* and *Martha E. Rogers: Her Life and Her Work*, both edited by Barrett and Malinski, were published in 1994. In addition, the official journal of the Society of Rogerian Scholars, *Visions: The Journal of Rogerian Nursing Science*, premiered in 1993.

The use of the Science of Unitary Human Beings requires considerable background and ongoing study. Rogers (1990b) maintained that the implementation of nursing practice based on the Science of Unitary Human Beings requires a commitment to lifelong learning and the use of what nurses know as well as what they can imagine. Implementation also requires creativity and compassion. The new reality represented by the Science of Unitary Human Beings requires "new ways of thinking, new questions, new interpretations" (Rogers, 1990b, p. 111). In particular, nurses "should learn to think through what it is they are dealing with and then practice will always be new and innovative" (Rogers, as cited in Takahashi, 1992, p. 89). Gueldner and colleagues (1994) emphasized the importance of experiential learning when initially introduced to the Science of Unitary Human Beings. They recommended such strategies as a week-long retreat, mentoring by Science of Unitary Human Beings nurse experts, opportunities for free-flowing dialogue and reflection, and attendance at the Rogerian conferences.

Rogers' conception of human beings as unitary and the presentation of the Science of Unitary Human Beings in just a few concepts and propositions might be considered elegant in its simplicity. Yet as Newman (1972) noted, "Many a graduate student will attest to the difficulty of reorganizing one's thinking about [each human being] in order to consider [him or her] a unified being and not as a composite of organs and systems and various psychosocial components" (pp. 451–452). Although the same might be said about any conceptual model that puts forth a holistic view of human beings, some nurses find it especially difficult when studying the Science of Unitary Human Beings.

Perhaps the difficulty is associated with a view of the world that "requires a new synthesis, a creative leap and inculcation of new attitudes and values" (Rogers, 1989, p. 188). Or it may be due to Rogers' use of ideas and associated terms that are unfamiliar to some people. Rogers (1970, 1978a, 1980b, 1986, 1990a, 1992b) has, however, repeatedly defended her terminology, pointing out that she selected terms that are in the general language and initially defined those terms according to the dictionary. As the Science of Unitary Human Beings evolved, Rogers recognized the need for more specific definitions to facilitate uniformity of usage and precision. She noted that this procedure is common in all sciences. Nevertheless, use of the Science of Unitary Human Beings must be preceded by mastery of a vocabulary that may be new to many nurses. This task can be facilitated by use of the glossary of terms that is included in Rogers' (1986, 1990a, 1992b) publications.

The application of the Science of Unitary Human Beings in nursing practice is feasible. Comprehensive plans for introducing the Science of Unitary Human Beings into a nursing service setting have been described by Ference (1989), Heggie and colleagues (1989, 1994), and Caroselli (1994). The three plans are presented in an integrated manner here.

- Pre-Project Planning
  - The Chief Nurse Executive (CNE) takes on the role of leader-as-teacher and provides a standard for what is possible and powerful in a nursing department.
  - The CNE works with other nursing administrators, staff development educators, and staff nurses to review various conceptual models of nursing, the nursing department philosophy and mission statement, governance structure, and organizational structure. The Science of Unitary Human Beings is selected as the conceptual model to guide nursing practice.
  - A Project Director, who is an expert in Science of Unitary Human Beings–based nursing practice, is selected and serves as an internal consultant. Throughout the implementation project, the Project Director facilitates values clarification, acts as a liaison for the staff nurses and the various committees, and communicates current progress and future initiatives to the entire health-care organization.
  - A Research Advisor and a Nursing Financial Advisor are selected. The research and financial advisors collaborate on collection and analysis of data, including costs, throughout the project.
  - The CNE markets the Science of Unitary Human Beings–based nursing department in staff recruitment initiatives and when negotiating student placements with affiliating nursing education programs.

- Level One: Staff Development
  - The Science of Unitary Human Beings is formally introduced to the administrators and staff in a series of planned learning activities facilitated by the Project Director.
  - Phase One: Awareness
    - Planned discussions are held between the Project Director and the nursing staff and are supplemented with readings and annotated references.
  - Phase Two: Testing
    - The staff nurses become acclimated to the Science of Unitary Human Beings through such activities as Project Director-guided patient care conferences that focus on integrating the Science of Unitary Human Beings into everyday practice situations.
  - Phase Three: Readiness
    - The staff nurses begin to write care plans, which they use to explain the Science of Unitary Human Beings to their peers. The staff nurses also begin to implement the care plans and share the new modalities of nursing with one another as they begin to integrate the Science of Unitary Human Beings into their traditional practice.
  - Phase Four: Expert Reinforcement
    - Feedback is provided to the staff from the Project Director, who also acts as a role model for staff nurses who may be skeptical, or those who have difficulty understanding the content of and nursing modalities associated with the Science of Unitary Human Beings.
  - Phase Five: Peer Reinforcement
    - The staff nurses become more proficient with implementation. The Research Advisor facilitates development of a nursing process audit tool that can be used by staff nurses to critique the adherence of their nursing practice to the Science of Unitary Human Beings.

- Level Two: Tool Development
  - The CNE works with other nursing administrators, staff development educators, and staff nurses to revise the nursing department philosophy and mission statement, governance structure, organizational structure, nursing standards, nursing documentation system, and the quality assurance/quality improvement program so that they are congruent with the Science of Unitary Human Beings.

- Level Three: Implementation
  - The Science of Unitary Human Beings is implemented in the nursing department. Implementation may begin on a pilot unit or on all units simultaneously.
  - The Research Advisor collects the data required for evaluation of the project.

- Level Four: Evaluation
  - The Research Advisor and the Nursing Financial Advisor present reports of the outcomes of the project.

The time required for full implementation and evaluation of Science of Unitary Human Beings nursing practice in a health-care organization varies. Ference's (1989) plan, which focuses on the staff tool development components of an implementation project, spans 12 months. Caroselli (1994) noted that 3 to 5 years may be required, and Heggie and colleagues (1994) described an ongoing implementation project that had lasted 11 years at the time they prepared their paper.

Mason and Patterson (1990) noted that although Science of Unitary Human Beings–based nursing practice is feasible and is associated with beneficial patient outcomes, its proper use may be limited "in the secure environment of a special hospital" for mentally handicapped people (p. 141). In addition, Mason and Chandley (1990) commented that the application of the Science of Unitary Human Beings in special hospitals for the criminally insane "remains unsuccessful, not least of all because of its highly complex philosophical nature, but also because it cannot influence the politico-legal components" (p. 671).

Nursing Research. The utility of the Science of Unitary Human Beings for nursing research is very well documented. In recent years, Science of Unitary Human Beings-specific research methodologies have been developed. Those methodologies are:

- Unitary Pattern Appreciation Case Method (Cowling, 1997, 1998, 2001)
- Rogerian Process of Inquiry (Carboni, 1995)
- Unitary Field Pattern Portrait Research Method (Butcher, 1994, 1998, 2001)
- Photo-Disclosure Methodology (Bultemeier, 1997a)

Furthermore, several research instruments have been derived directly from the Science of Unitary Human Beings (Table 9–3). The research methodologies and instruments reflect the investigators' creative attempts to devise strategies for the study of energy field pattern manifestations. As Parse (2001) pointed out, the Science of Unitary Human Beings-specific research methodologies are qualitative approaches. In contrast, the research instruments are quantitative in nature, with the exception of Carboni's Mutual Exploration of the Healing Human-Environmental Field Relationship instrument, which employs a qualitative approach (see Table 9–3).

Garon (2002) listed the Time Metaphor Test as a tool developed for the Science of Unitary Human Beings. That research instrument was not, however, directly derived from the Science of Unitary Human Beings, although it has been used in studies based on the Science. The results of Watson, Sloyan, and Robalino's (2000) psychometric test of the Time Metaphor Test indicated that modifications are needed for use in Science of Unitary Human Beings-based research.

TABLE 9–3
RESEARCH INSTRUMENTS AND PRACTICE TOOLS DERIVED FROM THE SCIENCE OF UNITARY HUMAN BEINGS

Instrument or Tool and Citation*	Description
RESEARCH INSTRUMENTS	
Human Field Motion Test (HFMT) (Ference, 1980, 1986; Young et al., 2001)	Measures human field motion by means of semantic differential ratings of the concepts My Motor Is Running and My Field Expansion.
Perceived Field Motion Scale (PFM) (Yarcheski & Mahon, 1991; Young et al., 2001)	Measures the perceived experience of motion by means of semantic differential ratings of the concept My Field Motion.
Human Field Rhythms (HFR) (Yarcheski & Mahon, 1991; Young et al., 2001)	Measures the frequency of rhythms in human-environmental energy field mutual process by means of a one-item visual analogue scale.
Index of Field Energy (IFE) (Gueldner, as cited in Watson et al., 1997; Young et al., 2001)	Measures human field dynamics by means of semantic differential ratings of 18 pairs of simple black-and-white line drawings.
Power as Knowing Participation in Change Tool (PKPCT) (Barrett, 1984, 1986, 1990; Watson et al., 1997; Young et al., 2001)	Measures the person's capacity to participate knowingly in change by means of semantic differential ratings of the concepts Awareness, Choices, Freedom to Act Intentionally, and Involvement in Creating Changes.
Diversity of Human Field Pattern Scale (DHFPS) (Hastings-Tolsma, 1993; Watson et al., 1997; Young et al., 2001)	Measures diversity of human field pattern, or the degree of change in the evolution of human potential throughout the life process, by means of Likert scale ratings of 16 items.
Human Field Image Metaphor Scale (HFIMS) (Johnston, 1993a, 1993b, 1994; Young et al., 2001)	Measures the individual's awareness of the infinite wholeness of the human field by means of Likert scale ratings of 14 metaphors that represent perceived potential and 11 metaphors that represent perceived field integrality.
Temporal Experiences Scale (TES) (Paletta, 1988, 1990; Young et al., 2001)	Measures subjective experience of temporal awareness by means of Likert scale ratings of 24 metaphors representing the factors of time dragging, time racing, and timelessness.

*See the Research Instruments and Practice Tools section of the chapter references for complete citations.   *(continued)*

Instrument or Tool and Citation*	Description
Assessment of Dream Experience (ADE) (Watson, 1994, 1999; Watson et al., 1997; Young et al., 2001)	Measures dreaming as a beyond waking experience by means of Likert scale ratings of the extent to which 20 items describe what the individual's dreams have been like during the past 2 weeks.
Person-Environment Participation Scale (PEPS) (Leddy, 1995, 1999; Young et al., 2001)	Measures the person's experience of continuous human-environment mutual process by means of semantic differential ratings of 15 bipolar adjectives representing the content areas of comfort, influence, continuity, ease, and energy.
Leddy Healthiness Scale (LHS) (Leddy, 1996; Young et al., 2001)	Measures the person's perceived purpose and power to achieve goals by means of Likert scale ratings of 26 items representing meaningfulness, ends, choice, challenge, confidence, control, capacity, capability to function, and connections.
McCanse Readiness for Death Instrument (MRDI) (McCanse, 1988, 1995)	Measures physiological, psychological, sociological, and spiritual aspects of healthy field pattern as death is developmentally approached by means of a 26-item structured interview questionnaire.
Mutual Exploration of the Healing Human-Environmental Field Relationship (Carboni, 1992; Young et al., 2001)	Measures nurses' and clients' experiences and expressions of changing configurations of energy field patterns of the healing human-environmental field relationship using semi-structured and open-ended items. Forms for a nurse and a single client and a nurse and two or more clients are available.

PRACTICE TOOLS

Nursing Process Format (Falco & Lobo, 1995)	Guides use of a Rogerian nursing process, including nursing assessment, nursing diagnosis, nursing planning for implementation, and nursing evaluation according to the homeodynamic principles of integrality, resonancy, and helicy.
Assessment Tool (Smith et al., 1991)	Guides use of a Rogerian nursing process, including assessment, diagnosis, implementation, and evaluation according to the homeodynamic principles of complementarity (i.e., integrality), resonancy, and helicy, for patients hospitalized in a critical care unit and their family members, using open-ended questions.
Critical Thinking for Pattern Appraisal, Mutual Patterning, and Evaluation Tool (Bultemeier, 2002)	Provides guidance for the nurse's application of pattern appraisal, mutual patterning, and evaluation, as well as areas for the client's self-reflection, patterning activities, and personal appraisal.
Nursing Assessment of Patterns Indicative of Health (Madrid & Winstead-Fry, 1986)	Guides assessment of pattern, including relative present, communication, sense of rhythm, connection to environment, personal myth, and system integrity.
Assessment Tool for Postpartum Mothers (Tettero et al., 1993)	Guides assessment of mothers experiencing the challenges of their first child during the postpartum period.
Assessment Criteria for Nursing Evaluation of the Older Adult (Decker, 1989)	Guides assessment of the functional status of older adults living in their own homes, including demographic data, client prioritization of problems, sequential patterning (e.g., family of origin, culture, past illnesses), rhythmic patterning (e.g., health-care usage, medication usage, social contacts, acute illnesses), and cross-sectional patterning (e.g., current living arrangements and health concerns, cognitive and emotional status).

Holistic Assessment of the Chronic Pain Client (Garon, 1991)	Guides holistic assessment of clients living in their own homes and experiencing chronic pain, including the environmental field, the community, and all systems in contact with the client; the home environment; client needs and expectations; client and family strengths; the client's pain experience—location, intensity, cause, meaning, effects on activities, life, and relationships, relief measures, and goals; and client and family feelings about illness and pain.
Human Energy Field Assessment Form (Wright, 1989, 1991)	Used to record findings related to human energy field assessment as practiced in therapeutic touch, including location of field disturbance on body diagram and strength of the overall field and intensity of the field disturbance on visual analogue scales.
Family Assessment Tool (Whall, 1981)	Guides assessment of families in terms of individual subsystem considerations, interactional patterns, unique characteristics of the whole family system, and environmental interface synchrony.
An Assessment Guideline for Work with Families (Johnston, 1986)	Guides assessment of the family unit, in terms of definition of family, family organization, belief system, family developmental needs, economic factors, family field and environmental field complementarity, communication patterns, and supplemental data, including health assessment of individual family members, developmental factors, member interactions, and relationships.
Nursing Process Format for Families (Reed, 1986)	Guides the use of a developmentally oriented nursing process for families.
A Conceptual Tool Kit For Community Health Assessment (Hanchett, 1979)	Tools used to guide the assessment of the energy, individuality, and pattern and organization of a community.
Community Health Assessment (Hanchett, 1988)	Guides assessment of a community in the areas of diversity; rhythms, including frequencies of colors, rhythms of light, and patterns of sound; motion; experience of time; pragmatic-imaginative-visionary world views; and sleep—wake-beyond waking rhythms.

As can be seen in the Doctoral Dissertations and Master's Theses sections of the chapter bibliography on the CD-ROM, a great many dissertations and theses have been guided by the Science of Unitary Human Beings. Ference (1986a), who traced the evolution of research that was guided by the Science of Unitary Human Beings from the late 1960s through the mid-1980s, noted that the early studies were conducted as doctoral dissertations at New York University. She explained that all of those studies "were based upon some guiding assumptions and a philosophy that the nurse cares for the whole person" (p. 37). Her retrospective analysis of those studies yielded groupings of research. In the mid-1960s, studies focused on human development, such as Porter's (1968) research, and on man-environment interaction, exemplified by Mathwig's (1968) research. Research conducted from the late 1960s to the late 1970s focused on body image, exemplified by Fawcett's (1977) and Chodil's (1979) studies. Several studies completed in the early to mid-1970s focused on the variable of time, such as the research by Newman (1971) and Fitzpatrick (1976). Studies conducted during the early

1970s also focused on locus of control, field independence, and differentiation, exemplified by research conducted by Barnard (1973), Miller (1974), and Swanson (1976).

Ference (1986a) pointed out that much of the early research only mentioned Rogers' work and used theories borrowed from other disciplines as a basis for hypotheses. Research conducted during the late 1970s and into the 1980s used the Science of Unitary Human Beings in a more comprehensive manner, often identifying a particular principle of homeodynamics as the focus of study. One of the first studies that reflected that focus was conducted by Ference (1980) herself.

Review of published reports of Science of Unitary Human Beings–based research revealed a growing number of descriptive studies, many correlational studies, and several experimental studies. This research is listed in Table 9–4.

Much of the published research focuses on the individual human energy field, although some investigators have explored family-related phenomena in childbearing couples or mother-daughter dyads (see Table 9–4).

Furthermore, much of the research is limited to a single study on a single topic, although some programmatic research is evident. Fawcett (1989) summarized the findings from a program of descriptive and correlational research designed to examine similarities in wives' and husbands' pregnancy-related experiences, including body image changes and physical and psychological symptoms (see Table 9–4). In addition, the collective work of several investigators represents a broad program of experimental research focused on the effects of such noninvasive modalities as therapeutic touch, guided imagery, relaxation, movement therapy, and auditory input (see Table 9–4).

Nursing Education. The utility of the Science of Unitary Human Beings for nursing education is documented. Rogers (as cited in Safier, 1977) commented, "I know that many schools are using my book [*An Introduction to the Theoretical Basis of Nursing*], and also that many students are being oriented to this sort of thinking" (p. 328). Riehl's (1980) survey finding that Rogers' model was "being taught, practiced by students, and implemented by faculty" (p. 398) provided empirical evidence to support that statement. Riehl did not, however, provide the names of schools using the Rogerian conceptual system. Science of Unitary Human Beings-based nursing education programs and a medical center nursing orientation program that have been described in the literature are listed here.

- Associate Degree Program
  - University of Medicine and Dentistry, Newark, New Jersey, and Middlesex County College, Edison, New Jersey (Hellwig & Ferrante, 1993)
- Baccalaureate Programs
  - New York University, New York City, New York (Mathwig et al., 1990)
  - Mercy College, Dobbs Ferry, New York (Mathwig et al., 1990)
  - University of Medicine and Dentistry, Newark, New Jersey, and Ramapo College, Mahwah, New Jersey (Hellwig & Ferrante, 1993)
  - Washburn University, Topeka, Kansas (Mathwig et al., 1990; Young, 1985)
- Master's Program
  - University of Medicine and Dentistry, Newark, New Jersey (Hellwig & Ferrante, 1993)
- Doctoral Program
  - Medical College of Georgia, Augusta, Georgia, Doctoral Program Course—Rogerian Conceptual System of Nursing (Gueldner et al., 1994)
- Staff Orientation Program
  - Veterans Affairs Medical Center, San Diego, California (Woodward & Heggie, 1997)

Nursing Administration. The utility of the Science of Unitary Human Beings for nursing administration is documented. The health-care organizations and private nursing practice in which Science of Unitary Human Beings–based nursing practice has been implemented, as described in the available literature, are listed here.

- Health-Care Organizations
  - Children's Hospital Medical Center, Cincinnati, Ohio (Tudor et al., 1994)
  - University of Michigan Surgical Intensive Care Unit, Ann Arbor, Michigan (Smith et al., 1991)
  - Health Patterning Clinic, Arizona State University, Tempe, Arizona (Matas, 1997)
  - Veterans Affairs Medical Center, San Diego, California (Garon, 1991; Heggie et al., 1994; Heggie et al., 1989; Kodiath, 1991)

- Private Nursing Practices
  - Health patterning for individuals and families (Malinski, 1994)
  - Private practice in health patterning (Barrett, 1990b, 1992)
  - Private practice in therapeutic touch (Hill & Oliver, 1993)
  - Private practice with polio survivors (Smith, 1994)
  - Personalized Nursing Corporation, Plymouth, Michigan (Andersen & Smereck, 1989a, 1989b, 1992, 1994; Andersen et al., 1993)

In addition, Decker (1989) devised a Science of Unitary Human Beings–based nursing practice model for use at an unnamed outpatient geriatric assessment center. The model encompasses observation of behavior, assessment of the person and environment, diagnosis of total person function, establishment of congruent goals, implementation of interventions, guidance of patterning, and evaluation of total person function. She pointed out that "the role of the clinical nurse specialist as a member of the geriatric assessment team is clarified when nursing actions are based [on the principles of helicy, resonancy, and integrality]" (p. 28). And, Joseph (1990) described the use of the Science of Unitary Human Beings in an inpatient and outpatient pain management clinic located within an unnamed acute care hospital.

Nursing Practice. Rogers (1987a) maintained that "the practical implications [of the Science of Unitary Human Beings] for human health and well-being are already demonstrable" (p. 123). Indeed, the utility of the Science of Unitary Human Beings for creative nursing of individuals across the life span with diverse medical diagnoses and in various settings is well documented (Table 9–5).

(Text continues on page 349)

Research Topic	Study Participants	Citation*
	DESCRIPTIVE STUDIES	
Evaluation of the Time Metaphor Test	Adults living in the mid-Atlantic region of the United States	Watson et al., 2000
Perception of the human energy field	Children 3–9 years of age	France, 1993
Physical and psychological symptoms during pregnancy and the postpartum	Childbearing women and their husbands residing in Canada	Drake, Verhulst, & Fawcett, 1988
Essence of the lived experience of an ecospiritual consciousness	Registrants of the American Holistic Nurses' Association Certificate Program in Holistic Nursing	Lincoln, 2000
The lived experience of recovering from addiction	Recovering addicts	Banonis, 1989
Description of self-attributes	Elderly persons residing in a retirement home	Donahue & Alligood, 1995
Factors associated with patterns of hope	Older adults who experienced a stroke	Bays, 2001
Description of dispiritedness	Adults 52–92 years of age who identified themselves as having experienced dispiritedness	Butcher, 1996
Physical, social, and emotional obstacles to and self-strategies to enhance taking prescribed HIV antiretroviral medications	Gay men, heterosexual men, and women taking highly active antiretroviral therapy	Halkitis & Kirton, 1999
The process of extraordinary healing	Individuals who experienced spontaneous remissions or healing that could not be explained by medical treatment received	Schneider, 1995
Description of patterns of symptoms and activities of daily living	Adults with multiple sclerosis	Gulick & Bugg, 1992
Description of nursing practice with addicted clients	Case study of a nurse expert in addictions nursing practice	Conti-O'Hare, 1998
Experiences of giving and receiving therapeutic touch	Case study of a woman suffering from migraine headache and a nurse	Green, 1996
	Case study of a client experiencing pain and associated anxiety and a nurse	Green, 1998
Description of the experience of therapeutic touch	Adults who received therapeutic touch	Samarel, 1992
	Adults who received therapeutic touch and the nurses who gave the therapeutic touch	Heidt, 1990
Description of the experience of meditation	Individuals who work with the meditations of Lazaris	Gibson, 1996
Mental health status	Older adults	Reed, 1989
The meaning of laughing at oneself	Senior citizens	Reeder, 1991

*See the Research section of the chapter references for complete citations.

(continued)

Research Topic	Study Participants	Citation
The experience of laughing at one-self	Older couples	Malinski, 1991
The lived experience of traumatic brain injury	An individual who had suffered a traumatic brain injury and the individual's parents and siblings	Johnson, 1995
Description of effects of critical care hospitalization on family roles and responsibilities	Adult family members of individuals in intensive care units	Johnson et al., 1995
The experience of power	Adults with schizophrenia	Dzurec, 1994
Comparison of death anxiety and self-esteem	African-American and Latino children 4–6 years of age diagnosed with AIDS and those who were well	Ireland, 1997, 1997–1998
Perceived preferences for sounds to be included in study participants' own hypothetical dying environments	Healthy men and women 18–82 years of age	Johnson, 2001
Comparison of patterns of person-environment process	Ambulatory, mentally alert nursing home residents and community-dwelling, independently living older adults	Gueldner, 1994
Comparison of human field motion and power	Adults in chronic pain management programs and community-dwelling adults without chronic pain	Matas, 1997
Comparison of health perceptions and locus of control	Parents who did and did not follow through on school nurse referrals for their school-age children	Bush, 1997
Comparison of injury-associated behaviors and life events	Parents of injured, ill, and well preschool children	Bernardo, 1996
Themes associated with parent satisfaction	Parents of hospitalized children	Schaffer et al., 2000
Comparison of perceptions of family needs as met during critical care experiences of an adult family member	Registered nurses Family members	Kosco & Warren, 2000
Comparison of sleep-wakefulness patterns	Rotating and nonrotating shift workers	Floyd, 1983
Comparison of use of self-healing and psychosocial techniques before and after 1987	Secondary analysis of the Cancer Survivorship Questionnaire from the 1992 National Health Interview Survey	Abu-Realh et al., 1996
Mutuality	Literature: Selected journal articles and book chapters	Curley, 1997
Philosophic inquiry regarding idea of energy	Literature	Todaro-Franceschi, 1999
Description of unit culture and work characteristics	Nursing department staff members	Rizzo et al., 1994

Awareness of and attitude toward use of research findings	Members of the Midwives' Association of Sweden	Berggren, 1996
Comparison of power	University administrators Faculty Staff	Mahoney, 2001
Description of perceptions of participating in an experimental therapeutic touch and dialogue and control quiet time and dialogue study	Women with breast cancer	Kelly et al., 2004

CORRELATIONAL STUDIES

Relation of creativity and actualization to empathy	Well adult males and females	Alligood, 1986, 1991
Relations among perception of time, sleep patterns, and activity	Men and women 55–94 years of age	Alligood & McGuire, 2000
Relation of mystical experience and differentiation to creativity	Male and female college students	Cowling, 1986
Relation of the experience of dying to the experience of paranormal events and creativity	Adults with a medical diagnosis of cancer who were dying and adults free of life-threatening illness	McEvoy, 1990
Relation between temporal experience and human time	Female graduate nursing students	Paletta, 1990
Relation between perception of the speed of time and the process of dying	Male and female hospitalized cancer patients	Rawnsley, 1986
Relation of time experience, creativity, and differentiation to human field motion	Well adult males and females	Ference, 1986
Relations among human field motion, human field rhythms, creativity, diversity of sensory phenomena, perception of time moving fast, and waking periods	Well adolescents	Yarcheski & Mahon, 1991
Relation of human field motion, human field rhythms, creativity, and sentience to perceived health status	Well adolescents	Yarcheski & Mahon, 1995
Relation between imposed motion and human field motion	Elderly adults residing in nursing homes	Gueldner, 1986
Relation between human field motion and power	Well adult males and females	Barrett, 1986
Relation of sleep-wake rhythm and dream experience to human field motion and time experience	Women 60–83 years of age	Watson, 1997
Relation between human field motion and preferred visible wavelengths	College students and faculty	Benedict & Burge, 1990
Relations among awareness, wakefulness, human field motion, and well-being	Breastfeeding mothers of 6-month-old infants	Hills & Hanchett, 2001

(continued)

Research Topic	Study Participants	Citation
Relation between humor and health, as mediated by perceived human field motion	Adolescents	Yarcheski et al. 2002
Relation between visible light and the experience of pain	Adult females with the medical diagnosis of rheumatoid arthritis	McDonald, 1986
Relation between degree of hyperactivity and perception of short-wavelength light	Hyperactive male and female school-age children	Malinski, 1986
Interactions between sleep-wakefulness rhythms and a hospital rest-activity schedule	Patients in a psychiatric hospital	Floyd, 1984
Relation of contextual factors (age, income, years of education, number of children, years married) and interpersonal factors (social support, professional support) to health empowerment (power as knowing participation in change, health-promoting lifestyle behaviors)	Adult females	Shearer, 2001
Relation between power and self-perceived health	Blind Swedish individuals with and without diabetes Nonblind, nondiabetic Swedish individuals, matched with the blind individuals on age and gender	Leksell et al., 2001
Relations among temporal experience, power, and depression	Depressed and nondepressed women	Malinski, 1997
Relation of hope and power to perception of self	Individuals recovering from schizophrenia and participating in community-based psychiatric rehabilitation programs	Salerno, 2002
Relations among power, perceived health, and life satisfaction	Adults with long-term care needs residing in a long-term care facility and employees of the long-term care facility	McNiff, 1997
Relation between power and spirituality	Adult polio survivors and adults who never had polio	Smith, 1994
Relations among spirituality, perceived social support, death anxiety, and nurses' willingness to care for AIDS patients	Female nurses who care for patients with AIDS	Sherman, 1996
Relation of spirituality, personal resources, and willingness to care for AIDS patients to death anxiety	Nurses who care for persons with AIDS	Sherman, 1996
Relation between power and feminism	Female nurse executives	Caroselli, 1995
Relations among gender role identity, femininity, self-concept, and perception of comfort in the mothering role	Women during late pregnancy and the early postpartum	Brouse, 1985

Relations among father-fetus attachment, mother-fetus attachment, and couvade	Expectant mothers and fathers	Schodt, 1989
Relation between spouses' strength of identification and similarities in their pregnancy-related experiences (body image, physical and psychological symptoms)	Childbearing couples during pregnancy and the postpartum residing in the United States	Fawcett, 1977, 1978, 1989a, 1989b; Fawcett et al., 1986; Fawcett & York, 1986, 1987
Changes in body image during and after pregnancy	Childbearing women and their husbands residing in Canada	Drake, Verhulst, Fawcett, & Barger, 1988
Relations among attachment, conflict, and mother-daughter identities	Mother-daughter dyads	Boyd, 1990
Relations among empathy, diversity, and telepathy	Mother-daughter dyads	Sanchez, 1989
Relation of body temperature and activation circadian rhythms to well-being	Well women 65–80 years of age	Mason, 1988
Relation of self-actualization to health conception and health behavior choice	Adult men and women	Laffrey, 1985
Relation of early risk indicators, sensation-seeking behaviors, and parental drug or alcohol history to substance abuse impairment	Substance-impaired registered nurses in recovery Nonimpaired registered nurses	West, 2002

EXPERIMENTAL STUDIES

Effect of experimental therapeutic touch (TT) and control mimic TT on anxiety	Adult males and females hospitalized in a cardiovascular unit	Quinn, 1984
	Adult males and females scheduled for open heart surgery	Quinn, 1989
Effects of therapeutic touch (TT) on anxiety, mood, time perception, perception of TT effectiveness, and immune function	Recently bereaved individuals	Quinn & Strelkauskas, 1993
Effect of TT on time distortion	Recently bereaved individuals	Quinn, 1992
Effect of experimental TT and control mimic TT on tension headache pain	Males and females experiencing tension headaches	Keller & Bzdek, 1986
Effect of experimental TT, control mimic TT, and narcotic analgesia on postoperative pain	Adult postoperative patients	Meehan, 1993
Effects of experimental therapeutic touch and dialogue and control quiet time and dialogue on anxiety, mood, and postoperative pain	Women with breast cancer before and after surgery	Samarel et al., 1998
Effect of experimental TT, control progressive muscle relaxation, and control routine treatment on functional ability	Older adult males and females with a medical diagnosis of degenerative arthritis	Peck, 1998
Effect of an educational intervention on willingness to receive TT	Nursing students Women belonging to a professional business women's group	Lowry, 2002
Effects of experimental therapeutic massage and control nurse interaction on pain intensity, pain distress, sleep quality, symptom distress, and anxiety	Hospitalized male and female cancer patients receiving chemotherapy or radiation treatment	Smith et al., 2002

(continued)

Research Topic	Study Participants	Citation
Effects of experimental guided imagery and control educational information on the experience of time and human field motion	Community hospital staff members	Butcher & Parker, 1988, 1990
Effects of guided imagery and relaxation on anxiety and movement	Adults undergoing magnetic resonance imaging	Thompson & Coppens, 1994
Effects of experimental relaxation plus music or ocean sounds and control relaxation alone and biofeedback modalities	Lamaze-trained primigravida women	Wiand, 1997
Effects of music on anxiety and dyspnea	People with chronic obstructive pulmonary disease	McBride et al., 1999
Effect of reminiscence on power	Well elderly persons	Bramlett & Gueldner, 1993
Effect of movement therapy on morale and self-esteem	Nursing home residents	Goldberg & Fitzpatrick, 1980
Effects of a preoperative exercise program on hope and power	People with lung cancer	Wall, 2002
Effects of magnet, placebo, and standard treatments on pain and power	Individuals with chronic primary headache	Kim, 2001
Effect of epidermal growth factor on wound healing	Porcine skin	Gill & Atwood, 1981
Effect of budgetary knowledge on attitudes toward administration and cost containment	Staff nurses	Meehan, 1992
Effects of petting one's own dog, petting an unknown dog, and reading quietly on heart rate and blood pressure	Adult males and females who owned a dog	Gaydos & Farnham, 1988
Effects of varied harmonious auditory input and quiet ambience on temporal experience and perception of restfulness	Well adults confined to bed for the purposes of the study	Smith, 1975, 1979, 1984, 1986
Effect of lower and higher frequency light waves and standard nursery lighting on sleep-wakefulness frequency	Well, full-term Hispanic infants	Girardin, 1992
Effects of passive cycling exercises on growth and development	Infants	Porter, 1972a, 1972b
Effects of experimental Personalized LIGHT nursing practice and a control standard education and counseling program on HIV risk behaviors	Adults self-identified as injecting drug users or crack cocaine users	Andersen & Hockman, 1997

Practice Situation	Population	Citation*
	INDIVIDUALS	
Application of the Science of Unitary Human Beings	Clients in an ambulatory primary care practice	Thomas, 1990
	A 51-year-old woman with chronic low back pain	Kodiath, 1991
	Patients with decreased cardiac output	Whelton, 1979
	A 35-year-old man with a cerebral aneurysm	Madrid & Winstead-Fry, 1986
	An 82-year-old man admitted to the hospital with the medical diagnoses of sepsis, atrial fibrillation, and pemphigus	J. Gold, 1997
	An 89-year-old woman admitted to the hospital with the medical diagnosis of severe cerebrovascular accident	J. Gold, 1997
	A 74-year-old woman who had experienced a stroke and was admitted to an acute elderly care/assessment ward	Webb, 1992
	A man, admitted to an intensive care unit with multiple injuries after being hit by a car, and his family, including two Rogerian-educated nurses, who shared his care with the unit staff	Chapman et al., 1994
	Patients with impaired neurological function	Whelton, 1979
	A 15-year-old girl with borderline personality disorder admitted to an inpatient psychiatric unit	Thompson, 1990
	An adolescent with a behavioral disturbance admitted to a children's mental health outpatient department	Sheu et al., 1997
	A 36-year-old woman hospitalized repeatedly for self-mutilative behavior	Horvath, 1994
	A young male musician who experienced pervasive anxiety, fits of anger, and destructive relationships	Horvath, 1994
	A 52-year-old man who was afraid to leave his apartment	Horvath, 1994
	Clients seeking brief, solution-oriented therapy	Tuyn, 1992, 1994
	A male nurse who was a pain medication abuser	Johnson, 1996
	An elderly man with metastatic cancer who is terminally ill	Buczny et al., 1989
	Persons who are dying	Ference, 1989 Talley, 1994
Assessing pattern	Women with hyperthyroidism	Sayre-Adams & Wright, 1995
Pattern manifestation appraisal and deliberative mutual patterning	Clients of a private nursing practice	Malinski, 1994
	A 29-year-old woman who underwent a radical hysterectomy for cervical cancer	Bultemeier, 1997, 2002
	A 33-year-old woman with a medical diagnosis of leukemia who was dying	Madrid, 1994
	A 42-year-old woman with metastatic breast cancer	Bultemeier, 1997, 2002
	A woman who underwent a bilateral mastectomy	Biley, 1993
	A 76-year-old man with advanced lung cancer	Barrett, 1988
	Groups of people living with AIDS	Sargent, 1994
	Elderly persons experiencing confusion, depression, incontinence, or sleeplessness	Cowling, 1990
Use of Rogerian Health Patterning Practice Methodology	A young woman who had been treated for an arteriovenous malformation in the brain	Barrett, 2000

*See the Practice section of the chapter references for complete citations.

(continued)

Practice Situation	Population	Citation
Application of the Unitary Pattern Appreciation Practice Methodology	A woman in her early 50s who was experiencing ongoing despair	Cowling, 2000
A patient's perspective of the application of the Science of Unitary Human Beings	A woman admitted to an emergency department and then to the inpatient service	Mandl, 1997
Use of health patterning	Clients of a private nursing practice	Barrett, 1990
Use of innovative imagery	A 29-year-old female client of a private nursing practice who experienced depression and felt "nervous"	Barrett, 1992
Use of music	Psychiatric inpatients	Covington, 2001
Use of centering	Women who had been raped and later had a gynecologic examination	Dole, 1996
Use of therapeutic touch	Clients of a pain management center associated with an acute care hospital	Joseph, 1990
	A patient experiencing pain from metastatic cancer	Meehan, 1990
	A 29-year-old man with AIDS who was experiencing respiratory and gastrointestinal symptoms, fever, pain, and anxiety	Newshan, 1989
	A man who fell from a ladder and injured his elbow	Herdtner, 2000
	A 66-year-old woman with multiple sclerosis admitted to a rehabilitation center	Payne, 1989
	A 62-year-old woman who underwent a below-the-knee amputation and was admitted to a rehabilitation center	Payne, 1989
Use of therapeutic touch and imagery	A 30-year-old man with AIDS hospitalized for gastrointestinal bleeding	Madrid, 1990, 1994
	Male and female clients of a private nursing practice who experienced mental health problems	Hill & Oliver, 1993
Use of energy healing	A 20-year-old mother and her 2-year-old son	Starn, 1998
	A 43-year-old single mother	Starn, 1998
	A woman with metastatic cancer	Starn, 1998
Medical practice guided by a unitary perspective	Patients in private medical practices	Field, 1997 J.L. Gold, 1997
GROUPS		
Application of the Science of Unitary Human Beings	Elderly Black adults participating in a clinical group encounter in the community	Forker & Billings, 1989
FAMILIES		
Application of the Science of Unitary Human Beings	A woman who underwent a mastectomy and her family	Rogers, 1983
	A family experiencing an argument between members	Johnston, 1986
	A 13-year-old girl who ran away from home and her family	Reed, 1986
Pattern manifestation appraisal and deliberative mutual patterning	Children with heart variations and their families	Morwessel, 1994
COMMUNITIES		
Community health assessment	The midwestern city of Kalamazoo	Hanchett, 1988

(Text continued from page 340)

As is evident from the published reports listed in Table 9–5 and the publications listed in the Commentary: Practice section of the chapter bibliography on the CD-ROM, the Science of Unitary Human Beings has been used to guide nursing practice in both inpatient and outpatient settings, including large medical centers, rehabilitation centers, ambulatory clinics, and private nursing practices. More specifically, the Science of Unitary Human Beings has been used to guide practice with children and adults, and with persons experiencing diverse medical diagnoses such as hyperactivity, chronic low back pain, decreased cardiac output, cerebral aneurysm, sepsis, atrial fibrillation, pemphigus, trauma, impaired neurological function, psychiatric illness, self-mutilative behavior, anxiety, depression, medication abuse, metastatic cancer, acquired immunodeficiency syndrome (AIDS), and multiple sclerosis.

Science of Unitary Human Beings-based nursing practice extends to the family (Fawcett, 1975; Rogers, 1983), including applications to a woman who had a mastectomy and her family, a family experiencing an argument, a family dealing with a teenage member who ran away, and children with cardiac arrhythmias and their families (see Table 9–5). In addition, Hanchett (1990) explained how the Science of Unitary Human Beings can be extended for use in the community, with the community as the client.

Furthermore, several practice tools have been developed to guide Science of Unitary Human Beings–based nursing practice and to facilitate documentation of that practice. The tools are identified and described in Table 9–3.

Social Congruence

Implementation of the Science of Unitary Human Beings carries with it the understanding that "nursing, as a learned profession, has no dependent functions. Like all other professions, nursing has many collaborative functions, which are indispensable to providing society with a higher order of service than any one profession can offer. Moreover, no profession has the knowledge, competence, or prerogative to delegate anything to another profession. Each profession is responsible for determining its own boundaries within the context of social need" (Rogers, 1985a, p. 381). Consequently, "professionally educated nurses are independent practitioners prepared to knowledgeably provide health services to individuals, families, groups, and communities. They are accountable for their own acts and liable to the public they serve. They are peer participants in collaborative judgments made with professional personnel in other fields" (Rogers 1985a, p. 382).

Rogers' view of professional practice, coupled with her focus on promotion of well-being and noninvasive modalities of nursing intervention directed to all human beings, wherever they are, may exceed the expectations of some consumers of health care, some nurses, and some other health-care team members. Clearly, the Science of Unitary Human Beings reflects a view of human beings and their environments that requires a new way of thinking that not all people are willing or able to undertake. Indeed, the Science of Unitary Human Beings "will not be accepted if a nurse cannot perceive [energy] fields and resonating waves as the 'real world' of nursing" (Barnum, 1990, p. 43).

However, as more consumers increasingly recognize the value, cost-effectiveness, and benefits of promotion of well-being and noninvasive modalities, and as continued health-care reform requires new views of what constitutes appropriate care, the nursing activities guided by the Science of Unitary Human Beings should be more fully accepted and even anticipated. As Mandl (1997), a self-described "intelligent, professional [woman], living a full life crammed with activities, family, and culture" (p. 236) who became a patient and experienced Science of Unitary Human Beings–based nursing practice, recommended:

> Let's take Martha Rogers' thinking beyond the realm of health-care practitioners and "mainstream" her. She is so "of today." Let's educate the general public, whether ill or well, about the possibilities of a change in healthcare by explaining Rogers' beliefs. Let those people who are hungry for alternative ways to look at health and illness know about the Science of Unitary Human Beings. Let's watch as people discover their power to change their expectations about healthcare and let's help people find different ways to approach health issues for themselves and their loved ones (pp. 237–238).

The Science of Unitary Human Beings is congruent with societal expectations that individuals should participate actively in decisions about their health care. Indeed, Rogers (as cited in Randell, 1992) took the position that "our job is better health, and people do better making their own choices. The best prognosis is for the individual who is non-compliant" (p. 181). Bramlett, Gueldner, and Sowell (1990) pointed out that Rogers' position reflects consumer-centric advocacy.

Proponents, of course, find Science of Unitary Human Beings–based nursing practice congruent with their views of nursing. Indeed, for many of its proponents, the Rogerian conceptual system and its related theories and research constitute *the* nursing science. For example, as early as 1979, Blair commented, "Nursing science as conceptualized by Rogers provides a sound basis for achieving the goal of nursing—to serve man throughout the life process" (p. 302). Almost 20 years later, J. Gold (1997) declared, "Rogers' new worldview of irreducible wholeness and a unitary nursing model will best serve nurses as we move toward the 21st century" (p. 255). Moreover, Gold noted that Rogers' clarification of the unique focus of nursing has served not only "to guide the vision, purpose, and practice of nursing, it is also integral to nurses finding meaning, value, and satisfaction in their work" (p. 255).

Rogers (1987c) pointed out that her perspective of nursing is humanistic and optimistic but not utopian. Barber (1987), a physician, cited Rogers' humanistic and scholarly approach to nursing as "a model for emulation" (p. 12). He pointed out that "the new orientation of the nursing profession is achieving in a more sophisticated manner what physicians have been striving to achieve. However, while nursing is drawing closer to this goal, physicians seem to be slowly moving in the opposite direction" (p. 15). Ten years later, two physicians identified the value of the Rogerian perspective to their practice of medicine. Field (1997) commented, "Rogerian science has much to teach physicians and nurses about healthcare and healing" (p. 283). And J.L. Gold (1997) commented, "As a physician, practicing medicine from a unitary perspective is a way of being that … urges me to go beyond what our present system offers in order to deliver care in a manner that acknowledges and addresses the wholeness of human beings" (p. 265).

Social Significance

Rogers (1992b) maintained that the purpose of Science of Unitary Human Beings–based nursing practice is "to promote health and well-being for all persons wherever they are" (p. 28). Whelton (1979) speculated that use of the Rogerian conceptual system could make differences in clients' health status. She stated, "By entering into a scientifically based therapeutic relationship with the patient, the nurse can make the difference between the patient continuing a life of inadvertent self-destruction or reaching for his optimum health potential" (p. 19). Miller (1979) added, "If Rogers' [conceptual system] is followed, then perhaps nursing approaches would take into account a wider range of behavioral variability among individuals" (p. 286).

The evidence supporting the social significance of Science of Unitary Human Beings–based nursing practice is mixed, with evaluation continuing to focus primarily on the effects of the use of therapeutic touch. Anecdotal evidence comes from practitioners, who claim that therapeutic touch elicits a profound relaxation response; promotes a positive mood state; and reduces anxiety, pain, and the need for pain medication (Jurgens, Meehan, & Wilson, 1987; Madrid, 1990; Newshan, 1989).

Empirical evidence provides some support for these anecdotal claims. Qualitative and quantitative studies have systematically documented the beneficial effects of therapeutic touch, including increased relaxation, reduced pain and anxiety, and increased positive mood (Heidt, 1990; Meehan, 1993; Samarel, 1992). Experimental research has, however, yielded mixed results. In one study, for example,

Quinn (1984) found that therapeutic touch resulted in a reduction in state anxiety, but that finding was not replicated in her later investigation (Quinn, 1989). The findings of Peters' (1999) meta-analysis indicated that therapeutic touch has had a positive, medium size effect on physiological and psychological variables within study participants who received therapeutic touch in pretest-posttest studies. Although a similar effect was found for physiological variables (pain, wound healing, immune status) when therapeutic touch was compared with control treatments, Peters concluded that an insufficient number of studies have been done to support the claim that therapeutic touch is more effective than control treatments for psychological variables (various measures of anxiety). She went on to declare, "More rigorous research still needs to be done to establish a solid body of evidence" (p. 59) for the efficacy of therapeutic touch. Samarel and colleagues (1998) reported a medium effect size for preoperative state anxiety in their study of the effects of an experimental therapeutic touch and dialogue nursing intervention and a control quiet time and dialogue nursing intervention; the women who received the experimental intervention before breast cancer surgery had lower state anxiety, controlling for trait anxiety, than did their counterparts who received the control intervention. There was, however, no evidence of an effect of the interventions on preoperative or postoperative mood, postoperative state anxiety, or postoperative pain. Additional, carefully controlled research is required to determine the efficacy of therapeutic touch and other noninvasive modalities (see Table 9–2) that are consistent with the Science of Unitary Human Beings.

 ## CONTRIBUTIONS TO THE DISCIPLINE OF NURSING

Rogers was one of the first nurse scholars to explicitly identify the human being as the central phenomenon of nursing's concern. Summarizing the significance of that contribution to nursing knowledge, Newman (1972) stated, "Much of the confusion about what we should be studying was eliminated, in my opinion, when Rogers identified the phenomenon which is the center of nursing's purpose: MAN.… The clear-cut delineation of man as the focus of nursing gave direction for the development of theory that is not just relevant to nursing, but basic to nursing" (pp. 451–452).

Although other conceptual models consider human beings in a holistic manner, Rogers' view of human beings as unitary is distinctive in that no parts or components or subsystems of the human being are delineated—each human being is a unified whole. Furthermore, although other conceptual models consider the environment and its relationship with human beings, Rogers' view of human beings and environment as integral energy fields is unique and visionary.

Commenting on the contributions of her model, Rogers (as cited in Safier, 1977) stated, "The conceptual system ... provides for a substantive body of knowledge in nursing that will have relevance for all workers concerned with people, but with special relevance for nurses, not because it matters to nurses per se, but because it matters to human beings, and consequently to nurses" (p. 320). Moreover, Rogers (1986) pointed out that "the Science of Unitary Human Beings identifies nursing's uniqueness and signifies the potential of nurses to fulfill their social responsibility in human service" (p. 8).

Whall (1987) noted that the Science of Unitary Human Beings has advanced the discipline of nursing through the many debates it has sparked. She pointed out that Rogers' conceptual model "has generated lively debates and seems to have raised more questions than it answers. It has explained disparate views while engendering debate regarding techniques that may be used to measure concepts and relationships. The debates engendered by [Rogers'] model have in a sense forced nursing to move on. In a sense, it forced nurse scholars to question and seek answers again and again. If this ... is in essence the value of a [conceptual model], Rogers' framework will stand as a milestone" (p. 158).

Rogers continued to refine her conceptual system until shortly before her death. Speaking to the need for continued evolution of her model, Rogers (1970) declared, "The emergence of a science of nursing demands a clear, unequivocal conceptual frame of reference. This is not to propose that nursing's conceptual system is either static or inflexible. Quite the contrary. In its evolution it is properly subject to reformulation and change as empirical knowledge grows, as conceptual data achieve greater clarity, and as the interconnectedness between ideas takes on new dimensions" (p. 84).

Later, Rogers (1987a) noted that nursing research is crucial for the continued refinement of the Science of Unitary Human Beings. She stated, "The future of research in nursing is based on a commitment to nursing as a science in its own right. The science of nursing is identified as the science of unitary human beings" (p. 123). For Rogers, then, "science is never finished. It is always open ended" (Rogers et al., 1990, p. 380). Stated in other words, "science is open-ended; it will never stop" (Rogers, 1994b, p. 34).

Rogers was largely successful in her commitment to advancing the discipline of nursing through development of a unique and substantive body of knowledge. She commented, "The future of nursing is based on a commitment to nursing as a science in its own right. The [independent] science of nursing is identified as the science of unitary human beings. The research potentials of nursing's abstract system are multiple. It is logically and scientifically tenable, it is flexible and open-ended. The practice implications for human health and well-being are already demonstrable" (Rogers, 1987a, p. 123).

Potential users of the Science of Unitary Human Beings are urged to consider its strengths and its limitations and work to systematically evaluate its credibility as a guide for the plethora of nursing activities for which it was developed. The advancement, continued refinement, and evaluation of the credibility of the Science of Unitary Human Beings should be ensured by the work of the members of the Society of Rogerian Scholars, which was founded in 1986. The mission of the Society is "to advance nursing science through an emphasis on the Science of Unitary Human Beings. The focus of the Society is education, research, and practice in service to humankind" (Mission Statement, Society of Rogerian Scholars, 1996). The Society published a newsletter, *Rogerian Nursing Science News*, for many years, and continues to publish the journal, *Visions: The Journal of Rogerian Nursing Science*.

The advancement, continued refinement, and evaluation of the credibility of the Science of Unitary Human Beings also should be ensured by the establishment of the Martha E. Rogers Center for the Study of Nursing Science. The Center was established in 1995 at New York University "to honor Martha Rogers and to provide a structure through which her work could be continued. The Center has helped to focus national and international scholarly activity relating to the Science of Unitary Human Beings; disseminate relevant information through conferences and publication; provide an interactive mechanism for sharing ideas and knowledge; generate support for further research and scholarship; and provide for a collection of writings and other works related to the science of unitary human beings" (Mission Statement, Martha E. Rogers Center for the Study of Nursing Science, 1995). The Center has sponsored a visiting scholar program and published a newsletter, and is a cosponsor of periodic dialogues among Rogerian scholars and the Rogerian Conference held at New York University.

In conclusion, Martha Rogers made a substantial contribution to the discipline of nursing by proposing a visionary conceptual model that may be an appropriate guide for nursing activities as human beings continue to evolve and as we move farther into the space age. As Rogers (1990b) stated:

> As a holistic reality revolutionizes our thinking and as space exploration and space living provide spin-off from space that can be helpful on planet Earth, nursing will change, as will other fields. We are on the threshold of a fantastic and unimagined future. Our potential for human service is greater than it has ever been (p. 112).

Finally, in her last two publications Rogers declared, "New frontiers continue to open as nurses move into the future. Their responsibility for knowledgeable nursing and human services also grows. The opportunity is there for nurses to use their infinite potential" (Rogers, 1994a, p. 9), and "The science of unitary human beings provides the knowledge for imaginative and creative promotion of the well-being of all people" (Rogers, 1994b, p. 35).

 ## REFERENCES

Alligood, M.R. (1989). Applying Rogers' model to nursing administration: Emphasis on environment, health. In B. Henry, C. Arndt, M. DiVincenti, & A. Marriner-Tomey (Eds.), Dimensions of nursing administration. Theory, research, education, and practice (pp. 105–111). Boston: Blackwell Scientific.

Alligood, M.R. (1991). Testing Rogers' theory of accelerating change. The relationships among creativity, actualization, and empathy in persons 18 to 92 years of age. Western Journal of Nursing Research, 13, 84–96.

Alligood, M.R. (1997). Models and theories: Critical thinking structures. In M.R. Alligood & A. Marriner Tomey (Eds.), Nursing theory: Utilization and application (pp. 31–45). St. Louis: Mosby.

Alligood, M.R. (2002a). Philosophies, models, and theories: Critical thinking structures. In M.R. Alligood & A. Marriner Tomey (Eds.), Nursing theory: Utilization and application (2nd ed., pp. 41–61). St. Louis: Mosby.

Alligood, M.R. (2002b). A theory of the art of nursing discovered in Rogers' science of unitary human beings. International Journal for Human Caring, 6(2), 55–60.

Alligood, M.R., & Fawcett, J. (1999). Acceptance of the invitation to dialogue: Examination of an interpretive approach for the science of unitary human beings. Visions: The Journal of Rogerian Nursing Science, 7, 5–13.

Alligood, M.R., & McGuire, S.L. (2000). Perception of time, sleep patterns, and activity in senior citizens: A test of Rogerian theory of aging. Visions: The Journal of Rogerian Nursing Science, 8, 6–14.

Anderson, M.D., & Smereck, G.A.D. (1989a). Personalized LIGHT model. Nursing Science Quarterly, 2, 120–130.

Anderson, M.D., & Smereck, G.A.D. (1989b). Personalized nursing: A science-based model of the art of nursing. In M. Madrid & E.A.M. Barrett (Eds.), Rogers' scientific art of nursing practice (pp. 261–283). New York: National League for Nursing.

Anderson, M.D., & Smereck, G.A.D. (1992). The consciousness rainbow: An explication of Rogerian field pattern manifestation. Nursing Science Quarterly, 5, 72–79.

Andersen, M.D., & Smereck, G.A.D. (1994). Personalized nursing: A science-based model of the art of nursing. In M. Madrid & E.A.M. Barrett (Eds.), Rogers' scientific art of nursing practice (pp. 261–283). New York: National League for Nursing Press.

Andersen, M.D., Smereck, G.A., & Braunstein, M.S. (1993). LIGHT model: An effective intervention model to change high-risk AIDS behaviors among hard-to-reach urban drug users. American Journal of Drug and Alcohol Abuse, 19, 309–325.

Barber, H.R.K. (1987). Editorial: Trends in nursing: A model for emulation. The Female Patient 12(3), 12, 14.

Barnard, R.M. (1973). Field independence-dependence and selected motor abilities. Dissertation Abstracts International, 34, 2737B.

Barnum, B.J.S. (1990). Nursing theory. Analysis, application, evaluation (3rd ed). Glenview, IL: Scott, Foresman/Little, Brown Higher Education.

Barnum, B.J.S. (1998). Nursing theory. Analysis, application, evaluation (5th ed). Philadelphia: Lippincott.

Barrett, E.A.M. (1986). Investigation of the principle of helicy: The relationship of human field motion and power. In V.M. Malinski (Ed.), Explorations on Martha Rogers' science of unitary human beings (pp. 173–188). Norwalk, CT: Appleton-Century-Crofts.

Barrett, E.A.M. (1988). Using Rogers' science of unitary human beings in nursing practice. Nursing Science Quarterly, 1, 50–51.

Barrett, E.A.M. (1990a). The continuing revolution of Rogers' science-based nursing education. In E.A.M. Barrett (Ed.), Visions of Rogers' science-based nursing (pp. 303–317). New York: National League for Nursing.

Barrett, E.A.M. (1990b). Health patterning with clients in a private practice environment. In E.A.M. Barrett (Ed.), Visions of Rogers' science-based nursing (pp. 105–115). New York: National League for Nursing.

Barrett, E.A.M. (1990c). Rogers' science-based nursing practice. In E.A.M. Barrett (Ed.), Visions of Rogers' science-based nursing (pp. 31–44). New York: National League for Nursing.

Barrett, E.A.M. (Ed.). (1990d). Visions of Rogers' science-based nursing. New York: National League for Nursing.

Barrett, E.A.M. (1992). Innovative imagery: A health-patterning modality for nursing practice. Journal of Holistic Nursing, 10, 154–166.

Barrett, E.A.M. (1993). Virtual reality: A health patterning modality for nursing in space. Visions: The Journal of Rogerian Nursing Science, 1, 10–21.

Barrett, E.A.M. (1996). Canonical correlation analysis and its use in Rogerian research. Nursing Science Quarterly, 9, 50–52.

Barrett, E.A.M. (1998). A Rogerian practice methodology for health patterning. Nursing Science Quarterly, 11, 136–138.

Barrett, E.A.M., Cowling, W.R., III, Carboni, J.T., & Butcher, H.K. (1997). Unitary perspectives on methodological practices. In M. Madrid (Ed.), Patterns of Rogerian knowing (pp. 47–62). New York: National League for Nursing Press.

Barrett, E.A.M., & Malinski, V.M. (Eds.). (1994a). Martha E. Rogers: Eighty years of excellence. New York: Society of Rogerian Scholars.

Barrett, E.A.M., & Malinski, V.M. (Eds.). (1994b). Martha E. Rogers: Her life and her work. Philadelphia: F.A. Davis.

Blair, C. (1979). Hyperactivity in children: Viewed within the framework of synergistic man. Nursing Forum, 18, 293–303.

Bohm, D. (1980). Wholeness and the implicate order. Boston: Routledge & Kegan Paul.

Boguslawski, M. (1990). Unitary human field practice modalities. In E.A.M. Barrett (Ed.), Visions of Rogers' science-based nursing (pp. 83–92). New York: National League for Nursing.

Bramlett, M.H., Gueldner, S.H., & Sowell, R.L. (1990). Consumer-centric advocacy: Its connection to nursing frameworks. Nursing Science Quarterly, 3, 156–161.

Bultemeier, K. (1997a). Photo-disclosure: A research methodology for investigating unitary human beings. In M. Madrid (Ed.), Patterns of Rogerian knowing (pp. 63–74). New York: National League for Nursing Press.

Bultemeier, K. (1997b). Rogers' science of unitary human beings in nursing practice. In M.R. Alligood & A. Marriner-Tomey (Eds.). Nursing theory: Utilization and practice (pp. 153–174). St. Louis: Mosby.

Burr, H.S., & Northrop, F.S.C. (1935). The electro-dynamic theory of life. Quarterly Review of Biology, 10, 322–333.

Butcher, H.K. (1993). Kaleidoscoping in life's turbulence: From Seurat's art to Rogers' nursing science. In M.E. Parker (Ed.), Patterns of nursing theories in practice (pp. 183–198). New York: National League for Nursing.

Butcher, H.K. (1994). The unitary human field pattern portrait method: Development of a research method for Rogers' science of unitary human beings. In M. Madrid & E.A.M. Barrett (Eds.), Rogers' scientific art of nursing practice (pp. 397–429). New York: National League for Nursing Press.

Butcher, H.K. (1998). Crystallizing the process of the unitary field pattern portrait research method. Visions: Journal of Rogerian Nursing Science, 6, 13–26.

Butcher, H.K. (2001). Nursing science in the new millennium: Practice and research within Rogers' science of unitary human beings. In M.E. Parker (Ed.), Nursing theories and nursing practice (pp. 205–226). Philadelphia: F.A. Davis.

Capra, F. (1982). The turning point. New York: Simon & Schuster.

Carboni, J.T. (1995). A Rogerian process of inquiry. Nursing Science Quarterly, 8, 22–37.

Caroselli, C. (1994). Opportunities for knowing participation: A new design for the nursing service organization. In M. Madrid & E.A.M. Barrett (Eds.), Rogers' scientific art of nursing practice (pp. 243–259). New York: National League for Nursing Press.

Caroselli, C., & Barrett, E.A.M. (1998). A review of the power as knowing participation in change literature. Nursing Science Quarterly, 11, 9–16.

Caroselli-Dervan, C. (1990). Visionary opportunities for knowledge development in nursing administration. In E.A.M. Barrett (Ed.), Visions of Rogers' science-based nursing (pp. 151–158). New York: National League for Nursing.

Chin, R. (1980). The utility of systems models and developmental models for practitioners. In J.P. Riehl & C. Roy (Eds.), Conceptual models for nursing practice (2nd ed., pp. 21–37). New York: Appleton-Century-Crofts.

Chodil, J.J. (1979). An investigation of the relation between per-

ceived body space, actual body space, body image boundary, and self-esteem. Dissertation Abstracts International, 39, 3760B.

Cowling, W.R., III. (1986). The science of unitary human beings: Theoretical issues, methodological challenges, and research realities. In V.M. Malinski (Ed.), Explorations on Martha Rogers' science of unitary human beings (pp. 65–77). Norwalk, CT: Appleton-Century-Crofts.

Cowling, W.R., III (1990). A template for unitary pattern-based nursing practice. In E.A.M. Barrett (Ed.), Visions of Rogers' science-based nursing (pp. 45–65). New York: National League for Nursing.

Cowling, W.R., III. (1997). Pattern appreciation: The unitary science/practice of reaching for essence. In M. Madrid (Ed.), Patterns of Rogerian knowing (pp. 129–142). New York: National League for Nursing Press.

Cowling, W.R., III. (1998). Unitary case inquiry. Nursing Science Quarterly, 11, 139–141.

Cowling, W.R. (2001). Unitary appreciative inquiry. Advances in Nursing Science, 23(4), 32–48.

de Chardin, P.T. (1961). The phenomenon of man. New York: Harper Torchbooks.

Decker, K. (1989). Theory in action: The geriatric assessment team. Journal of Gerontological Nursing, 15(10), 25–28.

Einstein, A. (1961). Relativity. New York: Crown.

Fawcett, J. (1975). The family as a living open system: An emerging conceptual framework for nursing. International Nursing Review, 22, 113–116.

Fawcett, J. (1977). The relationship between spouses' strength of identification and their patterns of change in perceived body space and articulation of body concept during and after pregnancy. Dissertation Abstracts International, 37, 4396B.

Fawcett, J. (1989). Spouses' experiences during pregnancy and the postpartum: A program of research and theory development. Image: Journal of Nursing Scholarship, 21, 149–152.

Fawcett, J. (1994). Theory development using quantitative methods within the science of unitary human beings. In M. Madrid & E.A.M. Barrett (Eds.), Rogers' scientific art of nursing practice (pp. 369–379). New York: National League for Nursing Press.

Fawcett, J., & Downs, F.S. (1986). The relationship of theory and research. Norwalk, CT: Appleton-Century-Crofts.

Ference, H.M. (1980). The relationship of time experience, creativity traits, differentiation and human field motion. An empirical investigation of Rogers' correlates of synergistic human development. Dissertation Abstracts International, 40, 5206B.

Ference, H.M. (1986a). Foundations of a nursing science and its evolution: A perspective. In V.M. Malinski (Ed.), Explorations on Martha Rogers' science of unitary human beings (pp. 25–32). Norwalk, CT: Appleton-Century-Crofts.

Ference, H.M. (1986b). The relationship of time experience, creativity traits, differentiation, and human field motion. In V.M. Malinski (Ed.), Explorations on Martha Rogers' science of unitary human beings (pp. 95–106). Norwalk, CT: Appleton-Century-Crofts.

Ference, H.M. (1989). Nursing science theories and administration. In B. Henry, C. Arndt, M. DiVincenti, & A. Marriner-Tomey (Eds.), Dimensions of nursing administration. Theory, research, education, and practice. (pp. 121–131). Boston: Blackwell Scientific.

Field, S. (1997). The scientific art of medical practice. In M. Madrid (Ed.), Patterns of Rogerian knowing (pp. 267–284). New York: National League for Nursing Press.

Fitzpatrick, J.J. (1976). An investigation of the relationship between temporal orientation, temporal extension, and time perception. Dissertation Abstracts International, 36, 3310B.

Fitzpatrick, J.J. (1980). Patients' perceptions of time: Current research. International Nursing Review, 27, 148–153, 160.

Fitzpatrick, J.J. (1983). Life perspective rhythm model. In J.J. Fitzpatrick & A.L. Whall (Eds.), Conceptual models of nursing: Analysis and application (pp. 295–302). Bowie, MD: Brady.

Fitzpatrick, J.J. (1989). A life perspective rhythm model. In J.J. Fitzpatrick & A.L. Whall (Eds.), Conceptual models of nursing: Analysis and application (2nd ed., pp. 401–407). Norwalk, CT: Appleton & Lange.

Fitzpatrick, J.J., & Donovan, M.J. (1978). Temporal experience and motor behavior among the aging. Research in Nursing and Health, 1, 60–68.

Fitzpatrick, J.J., Donovan, M.J., & Johnston, R.L. (1980). Experience of time during the crisis of cancer. Cancer Nursing, 3, 191–194.

Fuller, R.B. (1981). Critical path. New York: St. Martin's Press.

Garon, M. (1991). Assessment and management of pain in the home care setting: Application of Rogers' science of unitary human beings. Holistic Nursing Practice, 6(1), 47–57.

Garon, M. (2002). Science of unitary human beings: Martha E. Rogers. In J. B. George (Ed.), Nursing theories: The base for professional nursing practice (5th ed., pp. 269–294). Upper Saddle River, NJ: Prentice Hall.

Gold, J. (1997). The practice of nursing from a unitary perspective. In M. Madrid (Ed.), Patterns of Rogerian knowing (pp. 249–256). New York: National League for Nursing Press.

Gold, J.L. (1997). Practicing medicine in the nineties with an emphasis on the unitary perspective of patient care. In M. Madrid (Ed.), Patterns of Rogerian knowing (pp. 257–266). New York: National League for Nursing Press.

Goldstein, K. (1939). The organism. New York: American Book Company.

Gueldner, S.H. (1989). Applying Rogers' model to nursing administration: Emphasis on client and nursing. In B. Henry, C. Arndt, M. DiVincenti, & A. Marriner-Tomey (Eds.), Dimensions of nursing administration. Theory, research, education, and practice (pp. 113–119). Boston: Blackwell Scientific.

Gueldner, S.H., Daniels, W., Sauter, M., Johnson, M., Talley, B., & Bramlett, M.H. (1994). Learning Rogerian science: An experiential process. In M. Madrid & E.A.M. Barrett (Eds.), Rogers' scientific art of nursing practice (pp. 355–368). New York: National League for Nursing Press.

Hanchett, E.S. (1990). Nursing models and community as client. Nursing Science Quarterly, 3, 67–72.

Hanchett, E.S. (1992). Concepts from eastern philosophy and

Rogers' science of unitary human beings. Nursing Science Quarterly, 5, 164–170.

Heggie, J., Garon, M., Kodiath, M., & Kelly, A. (1994). Implementing the science of unitary human beings at the San Diego Veterans Affairs Medical Center. In M. Madrid & E.A.M. Barrett (Eds.), Rogers' scientific art of nursing practice (pp. 285–304). New York: National League for Nursing Press.

Heggie, J.R., Schoemenhl, P.A., Chang, M.K., & Grieco, C. (1989). Selection and implementation of Dr. Martha Rogers' nursing conceptual model in an acute care setting. Clinical Nurse Specialist, 3, 143–147.

Heidt, P.R. (1990). Openness: A qualitative analysis of nurses' and patients' experiences of therapeutic touch. Image: Journal of Nursing Scholarship, 22, 180–186.

Hellwig, S.D., & Ferrante, S. (1993). Martha Rogers' model in associate degree education. Nurse Educator, 18(5), 25–27.

Herrick, J. (1956). The evolution of human nature. Austin: University of Texas Press.

Hill, L., & Oliver, N. (1993). Technique integration: Therapeutic touch and theory-based mental health nursing. Journal of Psychosocial Nursing and Mental Health Services, 31(2), 19–22.

Hills, R.G.S., & Hanchett, E. (2001). Human change and individuation in pivotal life situations: Development and testing the theory of enlightenment. Visions: The Journal of Rogerian Nursing Science, 9, 6–19.

Huch, M.H. (1995). Nursing and the next millennium. Nursing Science Quarterly, 8, 38–44.

Johnston, R.L., Fitzpatrick, J.J., & Donovan, M.J. (1982). Developmental stage: Relationship to temporal dimensions (Abstract). Nursing Research, 31, 120.

Joseph, L. (1990). Practical application of Rogers' theoretical framework for nursing. In M.E. Parker (Ed.), Nursing theories in practice (pp. 115–125). New York: National League for Nursing.

Jurgens, A., Meehan, T.C., Wilson, H.L. (1987). Therapeutic touch as a nursing intervention. Holistic Nursing Practice, 2(1), 1–13.

Kodiath, M.F. (1991). A new view of the chronic pain client. Holistic Nursing Practice, 6(1), 41–46.

Leddy, S.K. (1993). Controversies column: Commentary and critique [Human Energy Systems Model]. Visions: Journal of Rogerian Nursing Science, 1, 56–57.

Leddy, S.K., & Fawcett, J. (1997). Testing the theory of healthiness: Conceptual and methodological issues. In M. Madrid (Ed.), Patterns of Rogerian knowing (pp. 75–86). New York: National League for Nursing Press.

Lewin, K. (1964). Field theory in the social sciences (D. Cartwright, Ed.). New York: Harper Torchbooks.

Madrid, M. (1990). The participating process of human field patterning in an acute-care environment. In E.A.M. Barrett (Ed.), Visions of Rogers' science-based nursing (pp. 93–104). New York: National League for Nursing.

Madrid, M. (Ed.). (1997). Patterns of Rogerian knowing. New York: National League for Nursing Press.

Madrid, M., & Barrett, E.A.M. (Eds.) (1994). Rogers' scientific art of nursing practice. New York: National League for Nursing Press.

Madrid, M., & Winstead-Fry, P. (1986). Rogers' conceptual model.

In P. Winstead-Fry (Ed.), Case studies in nursing theory (pp. 73–102). New York: National League for Nursing.

Malinski, V.M. (Ed.). (1986a). Explorations on Martha Rogers' science of unitary human beings. Norwalk, CT: Appleton-Century-Crofts.

Malinski, V.M. (1986b). Further ideas from Martha Rogers. In V.M. Malinski (Ed.), Explorations on Martha Rogers' science of unitary human beings (pp. 9–14). Norwalk, CT: Appleton-Century-Crofts.

Malinski, V.M. (1986c). Nursing practice within the science of unitary human beings. In V.M. Malinski (Ed.), Explorations on Martha Rogers' science of unitary human beings (pp. 25–32). Norwalk, CT: Appleton-Century-Crofts.

Malinski, V. (1994). Health patterning for individuals and families. In M. Madrid & E.A.M. Barrett (Eds.), Rogers' scientific art of nursing practice (pp. 105–117). New York: National League for Nursing Press.

Mandl, A. (1997). A plea to educate the public about Martha Rogers' science of unitary human beings. In M. Madrid (Ed.), Patterns of Rogerian knowing (pp. 236–238). New York: National League for Nursing Press.

Marriner-Tomey, A. (1989). Nursing theorists and their work (2nd ed.). St. Louis: Mosby.

Mason, T., & Chandley, M. (1990). Nursing models in a special hospital: A critical analysis of efficacity. Journal of Advanced Nursing, 15, 667–673.

Mason, T., & Patterson, R. (1990). A critical review of the use of Rogers' model within a special hospital: A single case study. Journal of Advanced Nursing, 15, 130–141.

Matas, K.E. (1997). Therapeutic touch: A model for community-based health promotion. In M. Madrid (Ed.), Patterns of Rogerian knowing (pp. 218–229). New York: National League for Nursing Press.

Mathwig, G.M. (1968). Living open systems, reciprocal adaptations and the life process. Dissertation Abstracts International, 29, 666B.

Mathwig, G.M., Young, A.A., & Pepper, J.M. (1990). Using Rogerian science in undergraduate and graduate nursing education. In E.A.M. Barrett (Ed.), Visions of Rogers' science-based nursing (pp. 319–334). New York: National League for Nursing.

Meehan, T.C. (1993). Therapeutic touch and postoperative pain: A Rogerian research study. Nursing Science Quarterly, 6, 69–78.

Meleis, A.I. (1997). Theoretical nursing: Development and progress (2nd ed.). Philadelphia: Lippincott.

Miller, L.A. (1979). An explanation of therapeutic touch using the science of unitary man. Nursing Forum, 18, 278–287.

Miller, S.R. (1974). An investigation of the relationship between mothers' general fearfulness, their daughters' locus of control, and general fearfulness in the daughter. Dissertation Abstracts International, 35, 2281B.

Newman, M.A. (1971). An investigation of the relationship between gait tempo and time perception. Dissertation Abstracts International, 32, 2821B.

Newman, M.A. (1972). Nursing's theoretical evolution. Nursing Outlook, 20, 449–453.

Newman, M.A. (1986). Health as expanding consciousness. St. Louis: Mosby.

Newman, M.A. (1992). Window on health as expanding consciousness. In M. O'Toole (Ed.), Miller-Keane encyclopedia and dictionary of medicine, nursing, and allied health (5th ed., p. 650). Philadelphia: Saunders.

Newman, M.A. (1994). Health as expanding consciousness (2nd ed.). New York: National League for Nursing.

Newshan, G. (1989). Therapeutic touch for symptom control in persons with AIDS. Holistic Nursing Practice, 3(4), 45–51.

Parker, K.P. (1989). The theory of sentience evolution: A practice-level theory of sleeping, waking, and beyond waking patterns based on the science of unitary human beings. Rogerian Nursing Science News, 2(1), 4–6. [See also Malinski, V.M. (2001). Martha E. Rogers: Science of unitary human beings. In M.E. Parker (Ed.), Nursing theories and nursing practice (p. 199). Philadelphia: F.A. Davis.]

Parse, R.R. (1981). Man-Living-Health. A theory of nursing. New York: Wiley. [Reprinted 1989. Albany, NY: Delmar.]

Parse, R.R. (1992). Human becoming: Parse's theory of nursing. Nursing Science Quarterly, 5, 35–42.

Parse, R.R. (1998). The human becoming school of thought: A perspective for nurses and other health professionals. Thousand Oaks, CA: Sage.

Parse, R.R. (2001). Emerging qualitative methods of the science of unitary human beings. In R.R. Parse, Qualitative inquiry: The path of sciencing (pp. 237–242). Boston: Jones and Bartlett.

Peters, R. (1999). The effectiveness of therapeutic touch: A meta-analytic review. Nursing Science Quarterly, 12, 52–61.

Phillips, J.R. (1989). Science of Unitary Human Beings: Changing research perspectives. Nursing Science Quarterly, 2, 57–60.

Phillips, J.R. (1991). Human field research. Nursing Science Quarterly, 4, 142–143.

Polanyi, M. (1958). Personal knowledge. Chicago: University of Chicago Press.

Porter, L. (1968). Physical-physiological activity and infants' growth and development. Dissertation Abstracts International, 28, 4829B.

Quinn, J.F. (1984). Therapeutic touch as energy exchange: Testing the theory. Advances in Nursing Science, 6(2), 42–49.

Quinn, J.F. (1989). Therapeutic touch as energy exchange: Replication and extension. Nursing Science Quarterly, 2, 79–87.

Randell, B.P. (1992). Nursing theory: The 21st century. Nursing Science Quarterly, 5, 176–184.

Reed, P.G. (1991). Toward a nursing theory of self-transcendence: Deductive reformulation using developmental theories. Advances in Nursing Science, 13(4), 64–77.

Reed, P.G. (1997). The place of transcendence in nursing's science of unitary human beings: Theory and research. In M. Madrid (Ed.), Patterns of Rogerian knowing (pp. 187–196). New York: National League for Nursing Press.

Reeder, F. (1984). Philosophical issues in the Rogerian science of unitary human beings. Advances in Nursing Science, 6(2), 14–23.

Reeder, F. (1986). Basic theoretical research in the conceptual system of unitary human beings. In V.M. Malinski (Ed), Explorations on Martha Rogers' science of unitary human beings (pp. 45–64). Norwalk, CT: Appleton-Century-Crofts.

Riehl, J.P. (1980). Nursing models in current use. In J.P Riehl & C. Roy (Eds.), Conceptual models for nursing practice (2nd ed., pp. 393–398). New York: Appleton-Century-Crofts.

Riehl, J.P., & Roy, C. (1974). Conceptual models for nursing practice. New York: Appleton-Century-Crofts.

Riehl, J.P., & Roy, C. (1980). Conceptual models for nursing practice (2nd ed). New York: Appleton-Century-Crofts.

Riehl-Sisca, J.P. (1989). Conceptual models for nursing practice (3rd ed.). Norwalk, CT: Appleton & Lange.

Rizzo, J.A. (1990). Nursing service as an energy field: A response to "Visionary opportunities for knowledge development in nursing administration." In E.A.M. Barrett (Ed.), Visions of Rogers' science-based nursing (pp. 159–164). New York: National League for Nursing.

Rogers, M.E. (1961). Educational revolution in nursing. New York: Macmillan.

Rogers, M.E. (1964). Reveille in nursing. Philadelphia: F.A. Davis.

Rogers, M.E. (1970). An introduction to the theoretical basis of nursing. Philadelphia: F.A. Davis.

Rogers, M.E. (1978a, December). Nursing science: A science of unitary man. Paper presented at Second Annual Nurse Educator Conference, New York. [Audiotape.]

Rogers, M.E. (1978b, December). Application of theory in education and service. Paper presented at Second Annual Nurse Educator Conference, New York. [Audiotape.]

Rogers, M.E. (1980a). Nursing: A science of unitary man. In J.P. Riehl & C. Roy (Eds.), Conceptual models for nursing practice (2nd ed., pp. 329–337). New York: Appleton-Century-Crofts.

Rogers, M.E. (1980b). Science of unitary man. Tape I. Unitary man and his world: A paradigm for nursing. New York: Media for Nursing. [Videotape and audiotape.]

Rogers, M.E. (1980c). Science of unitary man. Tape II. Developing an organized abstract system: Synthesis of facts and ideas for a new product. New York: Media for Nursing. [Videotape and audiotape.]

Rogers, M.E. (1980d). Science of unitary man. Tape III. Principles and theories: Directions for description, explanation and prediction. New York: Media for Nursing. [Videotape and audiotape.]

Rogers, M.E. (1980e). Science of unitary man. Tape IV. Theories of accelerating evolution, paranormal phenomena and other events. New York: Media for Nursing. [Videotape and audiotape.]

Rogers, M.E. (1980f). Science of unitary man. Tape V. Health and illness: New perspectives. New York: Media for Nursing. [Videotape and audiotape.]

Rogers, M.E. (1980g). Science of unitary man. Tape VI. Interventive modalities: Translating theories into practice. New York: Media for Nursing. [Videotape and audiotape.]

Rogers, M.E. (1983). Science of unitary human beings: A paradigm for nursing. In I.W. Clements and F.B. Roberts (Eds.), Family health: A theoretical approach to nursing care (pp. 219–227). New York: Wiley.

Rogers, M.E. (1985a). The nature and characteristics of professional education for nursing. Journal of Professional Nursing, 1, 381–383.

Rogers, M.E. (1985b). The need for legislation for licensure to practice professional nursing. Journal of Professional Nursing, 1, 384.

Rogers, M.E. (1985c). A paradigm for nursing. In R. Wood & J. Kekahbah (Eds.), Examining the cultural implications of Martha E. Rogers' science of unitary human beings (pp. 13–23). Lecompton, KS: Wood-Kekahbah Associates.

Rogers, M.E. (1986). Science of unitary human beings. In V.M. Malinski (Ed.), Explorations on Martha Rogers' science of unitary human beings (pp. 3–8). Norwalk, CT: Appleton-Century-Crofts.

Rogers, M.E. (1987a). Nursing research in the future. In J. Roode (Ed.), Changing patterns in nursing education (pp. 121–123). New York: National League for Nursing.

Rogers, M.E. (1987b, May). Rogers' framework. Paper presented at Nurse Theorist Conference, Pittsburgh, PA. [Audiotape.]

Rogers, M.E. (1987c, May). Small group D. Discussion at Nurse Theorist Conference, Pittsburgh PA. [Audiotape.]

Rogers, M.E. (1987d). Rogers' science of unitary human beings. In R.R. Parse (Ed.), Nursing science. Major paradigms, theories, and critiques (pp. 139–146). Philadelphia: Saunders.

Rogers, M.E. (1989). Nursing: A science of unitary human beings. In J.P. Riehl-Sisca (Ed.), Conceptual models for nursing practice (3rd ed., pp. 181–188). Norwalk, CT: Appleton & Lange.

Rogers, M.E. (1990a). Nursing: Science of unitary, irreducible, human beings: Update 1990. In E.A.M. Barrett (Ed.), Visions of Rogers' science-based nursing (pp. 5–11). New York: National League for Nursing.

Rogers, M.E. (1990b). Space-age paradigm for new frontiers in nursing. In M.E. Parker (Ed.), Nursing theories in practice (pp. 105–113). New York: National League for Nursing.

Rogers, M.E. (1992a). Nightingale's notes on nursing: Prelude to the 21st century. In F.N. Nightingale, Notes on nursing: What it is, and what it is not (Commemorative edition, pp. 58–62). Philadelphia: Lippincott.

Rogers, M.E. (1992b). Nursing science and the space age. Nursing Science Quarterly, 5, 27–34.

Rogers, M.E. (1992c). Window on science of unitary human beings. In M. O'Toole (Ed.), Miller-Keane encyclopedia and dictionary of medicine, nursing, and allied health (p. 1339). Philadelphia: Saunders.

Rogers, M.E. (1994a). Nursing science evolves. In M. Madrid & E.A.M. Barrett (Eds.), Rogers' scientific art of nursing practice (pp. 3–9). New York: National League for Nursing Press.

Rogers, M.E. (1994b). The science of unitary human beings: Current perspectives. Nursing Science Quarterly, 7, 33–35.

Rogers, M.E., Doyle, M.B., Racolin, A., & Walsh, P.C. (1990). A conversation with Martha Rogers on nursing in space. In E.A.M. Barrett (Ed.), Visions of Rogers' science-based nursing (pp. 375–386). New York: National League for Nursing.

Russell, B. (1953). On the notion of cause, with applications to the free-will problem. In H. Feigl & M. Brodbeck (Eds.), Readings in the philosophy of science (pp. 387–407). New York: Appleton-Century-Crofts.

Safier, G. (1977). Contemporary American leaders: An oral history. New York: McGraw-Hill.

Samarel, N. (1992). The experience of receiving therapeutic touch. Journal of Advanced Nursing, 17, 651–657.

Samarel, N., Fawcett, J., Davis, M. M., & Ryan, F. M. (1998). Effects of dialogue and therapeutic touch on preoperative and postoperative experiences of breast cancer surgery: An exploratory study. Oncology Nursing Forum, 25, 1369–1376.

Sarter, B. (1988). Philosophical sources of nursing theory. Nursing Science Quarterly, 1, 52–59.

Sellers, S.C. (1991). A philosophical analysis of conceptual models of nursing. Dissertation Abstracts International, 52, 1937B.

Sheldrake, R. (1981). A new science of life. Los Angeles: Jeremy Tarcher.

Sherman, D.W. (1997). Rogerian science: Opening new frontiers of nursing knowledge through its application in quantitative research. Nursing Science Quarterly, 10, 131–135.

Smith, D.W. (1994). Viewing polio survivors through violet-tinted glasses. In M. Madrid & E.A.M. Barrett (Eds.), Rogers' scientific art of nursing practice (pp. 141–145). New York: National League for Nursing Press.

Smith, K., Kupferschmid, B.J., Dawson, C., & Briones, T.L. (1991). A family-centered critical care unit. AACN Clinical Issues, 2, 258–268.

Stewart, I. (1989). Does God play dice? The mathematics of chaos. Cambridge, MA: Brasil Blackwell.

Swanson, A. (1976). An investigation of the relationship between a child's general fearfulness and the child's mother's anxiety, self differentiation, and accuracy of perception of her child's general fearfulness. Dissertation Abstracts International, 36, 3313B.

Takahashi, T. (1992). Perspectives on nursing knowledge. Nursing Science Quarterly, 5, 86–91.

Toffler, A. (1970). Future shock. New York: Random House.

Toffler, A. (1980). The third wave. New York: William Morrow.

Tudor, C.A., Keegan-Jones, L., & Bens, E.M. (1994). Implementing Rogers' science-based nursing practice in a pediatric nursing service setting. In M. Madrid & E.A.M. Barrett (Eds.), Rogers' scientific art of nursing practice (pp. 305–322). New York: National League for Nursing Press.

von Bertalanffy, L. (1960). Problems of life. New York: Harper Torchbooks.

Watson, J., Sloyan, C.M., & Robalino, J.E. (2000). The time metaphor test re-visited: Implications for Rogerian research. Visions: The Journal of Rogerian Nursing Science, 8, 32–45.

Whall, A.L. (1987). A critique of Rogers' framework. In R.R. Parse (Ed.), Nursing science. Major paradigms, theories, and critiques (pp. 147–158). Philadelphia: Saunders.

Whelton, B.J. (1979). An operationalization of Martha Rogers' theory throughout the nursing process. International Journal of Nursing Studies, 16, 7–20.

Woodward, T.A., & Heggie, J. (1997). Rogers in reality: Staff nurse

application of the science of unitary human beings in the clinical setting following changes in an orientation program. In M. Madrid (Ed.), Patterns of Rogerian knowing (pp. 239–248). New York: National League for Nursing Press.

Young, A.A. (1985). The Rogerian conceptual system: A framework for nursing education and service. In R. Wood & J. Kekahbah (Eds.), Examining the cultural implications of Martha E. Rogers' science of unitary human beings (pp. 53–69). Lecompton, KS: Wood-Kekahbah Associates.

RESEARCH

Abu-Realh, M.H, Magwood, G., Narayan, M.C., Rupprecht, C., & Suraci, M. (1996). The use of complementary therapies by cancer patients. NursingConnections, 9(4), 3–12.

Alligood, M.R. (1986). The relationship of creativity, actualization, and empathy in unitary human development. In V.M. Malinski (Ed.), Explorations on Martha Rogers' science of unitary human beings (pp. 145–160). Norwalk, CT: Appleton-Century-Crofts.

Alligood, M.R. (1991). Testing Rogers' theory of accelerating change. The relationships among creativity, actualization, and empathy in persons 18 to 92 years of age. Western Journal of Nursing Research, 13, 84–96.

Alligood, M.R., & McGuire, S.L. (2000). Perception of time, sleep patterns, and activity in senior citizens: A test of Rogerian theory of aging. Visions: The Journal of Rogerian Nursing Science, 8, 6–14.

Andersen, M., & Hockman, E.M. (1997). Well-being and high-risk drug use among active drug users. In M. Madrid (Ed.), Patterns of Rogerian knowing (pp. 152–166). New York: National League for Nursing Press.

Banonis, B.C. (1989). The lived experience of recovering from addiction: A phenomenological study. Nursing Science Quarterly, 2, 37–43.

Barrett, E.A.M. (1986). Investigation of the principle of helicy: The relationship of human field motion and power. In V.M. Malinski (Ed.), Explorations on Martha Rogers' science of unitary human beings (pp. 173–188). Norwalk, CT: Appleton-Century-Crofts.

Bays, C.L. (2001). Older adults' descriptions of hope after a stroke. Rehabilitation Nursing, 26, 18–20, 23–27.

Benedict, S.C., & Burge, J.M. (1990). The relationship between human field motion and preferred visible wavelengths. Nursing Science Quarterly, 3, 73–80.

Berggen, A. (1996). Swedish midwives' awareness of, attitudes to and use of selected research findings. Journal of Advanced Nursing, 23, 462–470.

Bernardo, L.M. (1996). Parent-reported injury-associated behaviors and life events among injured, ill, and well preschool children. Journal of Pediatric Nursing, 11, 100–110.

Boyd, C. (1990). Testing a model of mother-daughter identification. Western Journal of Nursing Research, 12, 448–468.

Bramlett, M.H., & Gueldner, S.H. (1993). Reminiscence: A viable option to enhance power in elders. Clinical Nurse Specialist, 7, 68–74.

Brouse, S.H. (1985). Effect of gender role identity on patterns of feminine and self-concept scores from late pregnancy to early postpartum. Advances in Nursing Science, 7(3), 32–40.

Bush, M.R. (1997). Influence of health locus of control and parental health perceptions on follow-through with school nurse referral. Issues in Comprehensive Pediatric Nursing, 20, 175–182.

Butcher, H.K. (1996). A unitary field pattern portrait of dispiritedness in later life. Visions: Journal of Rogerian Nursing Science, 4(1), 41–58.

Butcher, H.K., & Parker, N.I. (1988). Guided imagery within Rogers' science of unitary human beings. An experimental study. Nursing Science Quarterly, 1, 103–110.

Butcher, H.K., & Parker, N.I. (1990). Guided imagery within Rogers' science of unitary human beings: An experimental study. In E.A.M. Barrett (Ed.), Visions of Rogers' science-based nursing (pp. 269–286). New York: National League for Nursing. Rapacz, K.E. (1990). The patterning of time experience and human field motion during the experience of pleasant guided imagery: A discussion. In E.A.M. Barrett (Ed.), Visions of Rogers' science-based nursing (pp. 287–294). New York: National League for Nursing. Butcher, H.K., & Parker, N.I. (1990). Response to "Discussion of a study of pleasant guided imagery." In E.A.M. Barrett (Ed.), Visions of Rogers' science-based nursing (pp. 295–297). New York: National League for Nursing.

Caroselli, C. (1995). Power and feminism: A nursing science perspective. Nursing Science Quarterly, 8, 115–119.

Conti-O'Hare, M. (1998). Examining the wounded healer archetype: A case study in expert addictions nursing practice. Journal of the American Psychiatric Nurses Association, 4(3), 71–76.

Cowling, W.R., III. (1986). The relationship of mystical experience, differentiation, and creativity in college students. In V.M. Malinski (Ed.), Explorations on Martha Rogers' science of unitary human beings (pp. 131–143). Norwalk, CT: Appleton-Century-Crofts.

Curley, M.A.Q. (1997). Mutuality—An expression of nursing practice. Journal of Pediatric Nursing, 12, 208–213.

Donahue, L., & Alligood, M.R. (1995). A description of the elderly from self-selected attributes. Visions: Journal of Rogerian Nursing Science, 3(1), 12–19.

Drake, M. L., Verhulst, D., & Fawcett, J. (1988). Physical and psychological symptoms experienced by Canadian women and their husbands during pregnancy and the postpartum. Journal of Advanced Nursing, 13, 436–440.

Drake, M.L., Verhulst, D., Fawcett, J., & Barger, D.F. (1988). Spouses' body image changes during and after pregnancy: A replication in Canada. Image: Journal of Nursing Scholarship, 20, 88–92.

Dzurec, L.C. (1994). Schizophrenic clients' experiences of power: Using hermeneutic analysis. Image: Journal of Nursing Scholarship, 26, 155–159.

Fawcett, J. (1977). The relationship between identification and patterns of change in spouses' body images during and after pregnancy. International Journal of Nursing Studies, 14, 199–213.

Fawcett, J. (1978). Body image and the pregnant couple. American Journal of Maternal Child Nursing, 3, 227–233.

Fawcett, J. (1989a). Spouses' experiences during pregnancy and the postpartum (Brief report). Applied Nursing Research, 2, 49–50.

Fawcett, J. (1989b). Spouses' experiences during pregnancy and the postpartum: A program of research and theory development. Image: Journal of Nursing Scholarship, 21, 149–152. Eberhard, S.H. (1990). Letter to the editor. Image: Journal of Nursing Scholarship, 22, 197. Fawcett, J. (1990). Response to "Letter to the editor." Image: Journal of Nursing Scholarship, 22, 197.

Fawcett, J., Bliss-Holtz, V.J., Haas, M.B., Leventhal, M., & Rubin, M. (1986). Spouses body image changes during and after pregnancy: A replication and extension. Nursing Research, 35, 220–223.

Fawcett, J., & York, R. (1986). Spouses' physical and psychological symptoms during pregnancy and the postpartum. Nursing Research, 35, 144–148.

Fawcett, J., & York, R. (1987). Spouses' strength of identification and reports of symptoms during pregnancy and the postpartum. Florida Nursing Review, 2(2), 1–10.

Ference, H.M. (1986). The relationship of time experience, creativity traits, differentiation, and human field motion. In V.M. Malinski (Ed.), Explorations on Martha Rogers' science of unitary human beings (pp. 95–106). Norwalk, CT: Appleton-Century-Crofts.

Floyd, J.A. (1983). Research using Rogers' conceptual system: Development of a testable theorem. Advances in Nursing Science, 5(2), 37–48.

Floyd, J.A. (1984). Interaction between personal sleep-wake rhythms and psychiatric hospital rest-activity schedule. Nursing Research, 33, 255–259.

France, N.E. (1993). The child's perception of the human energy field using therapeutic touch. Journal of Holistic Nursing, 11, 319–331.

Gaydos, L.S., & Farnham, R. (1988). Human-animal relationships within the context of Rogers' principle of integrality. Advances in Nursing Science, 10(4), 72–80.

Gibson, A. (1996). Personal experiences of individuals using meditations from a metaphysical source. Visions: Journal of Rogerian Nursing Science, 4(1), 12–23.

Gill, B.P., & Atwood, J.R. (1981). Reciprocy and helicy used to relate mEFG and wound healing. Nursing Research, 30, 68–72. Kim, H.S. (1983). Use of Rogers' conceptual system in research: Comments. Nursing Research, 32, 89–91. Atwood, J.R., & Gill-Rogers, B. (1984). Metatheory, methodology and practicality: Issues in research uses of Rogers' science of unitary man. Nursing Research, 33, 88–91.

Girardin, B.W. (1992). Lightwave frequency and sleep wake frequency in well, full-term neonates. Holistic Nursing Practice, 6(4), 57–66.

Goldberg, W.G., & Fitzpatrick, J.J. (1980). Movement therapy with the aged. Nursing Research, 29, 339–346.

Green, C.A. (1996). A reflection of a therapeutic touch experience: Case study 1. Complementary Therapies in Nursing and Midwifery, 2, 122–125.

Green, C.A. (1998). Reflections of a therapeutic touch experience: Case study 2. Complementary Therapies in Nursing and Midwifery, 4, 17–21.

Gueldner, S.H. (1986). The relationship between imposed motion and human field motion in elderly individuals living in nursing homes. In V.M. Malinski (Ed.), Explorations on Martha Rogers' science of unitary human beings (pp. 161–172). Norwalk, CT: Appleton-Century-Crofts.

Gueldner, S.H. (1994). Pattern diversity and community presence in the human-environmental process: Implications for Rogerian-based practice with nursing home residents. In M. Madrid & E.A.M. Barrett (Eds.), Rogers' scientific art of nursing practice (pp. 131–140). New York: National League for Nursing Press.

Gulick, E.E., & Bugg, A. (1992). Holistic health patterning in multiple sclerosis. Research in Nursing and Health, 15, 175–185.

Halkitis, P.N., & Kirton, C. (1999). Self-strategies as means of enhancing adherence to HIV antiretroviral therapies: A Rogerian approach. Journal of the New York State Nurses Association, 30(2), 22–27.

Heidt, P.R. (1990). Openness: A qualitative analysis of nurses' and patients' experiences of therapeutic touch. Image: Journal of Nursing Scholarship, 22, 180–186.

Hills, R.G.S., & Hanchett, E. (2001). Human change and individuation in pivotal life situations: Development and testing the theory of enlightenment. Visions: The Journal of Rogerian Nursing Science, 9, 6–19.

Ireland, M. (1997). Pediatric acquired immunodeficiency syndrome (AIDS) as studied from a Rogerian perspective: A sense of hope. In M. Madrid (Ed.), Patterns of Rogerian knowing (pp. 143–151). New York: National League for Nursing Press.

Ireland, M. (1997–1998). Death anxiety and self-esteem in your children with AIDS: A sense of hope. Omega: Journal of Death and Dying, 36, 131–145.

Johnson, B.P. (1995). One family's experience with head injury: A phenomenological study. Journal of Neuroscience Nursing, 27, 113–118.

Johnson, L.W. (2001). An exploration of individual preferences for audio enhancement of the dying environment. Visions: The Journal of Rogerian Nursing Science, 9, 20–26.

Johnson, S.K., Craft, M., Titler, M., Halm, M., Kleiber, C., Montgomery, L.A., Megivern, K., Nicholson, A., & Buckwalter, K. (1995). Perceived changes in adult family members' roles and responsibilities during critical illness. Image: Journal of Nursing Scholarship, 27, 238–243.

Keller, E., & Bzdek, V.M. (1986). Effects of therapeutic touch on tension headache pain. Nursing Research, 35, 101–106.

Kelly, A.E., Sullivan, P., Fawcett, J., & Samarel, N. (2004) Therapeutic touch, quiet time, and dialogue: Perceptions of women with breast cancer. Oncology Nursing Forum 31, 625–631.

Kim, T.S. (2001). Relation of magnetic field therapy to pain and power over time in persons with chronic primary headache: A pilot study. Visions: The Journal of Rogerian Nursing Science, 9, 27–42.

Kosco, M., & Warren, N.A. (2000). Critical care nurses' perceptions of family needs as met. Critical Care Nursing Quarterly, 23 (2), 60–72.

Laffrey, S.C. (1985). Health behavior choice as related to self-actualization and health conception. Western Journal of Nursing Research, 7, 279–295.

Leksell, J.K., Johansson, I., Wibell, L.B., & Wikblad, K.F. (2001). Power and self-perceived health in blind diabetics and nondiabetic individuals. Journal of Advanced Nursing, 34, 511–519.

Lincoln, V. (2000). Ecospirituality; A pattern that connects. Journal of Holistic Nursing, 18, 227–244.

Lowry, R.C. (2002). The effect of an educational intervention on willingness to receive therapeutic touch. Journal of Holistic Nursing, 20, 48–60.

Mahoney, J. (2001). The comparison of university staff employees, faculty, and administrators on power as knowing participation in change. Visions: The Journal of Rogerian Nursing Science, 9, 43–51.

Malinski, V.M. (1986). The relationship between hyperactivity in children and perception of short wavelength light. In V.M. Malinski (Ed.), Explorations on Martha Rogers' science of unitary human beings (pp. 107–118). Norwalk, CT: Appleton-Century-Crofts.

Malinski, V.M. (1991). The experience of laughing at oneself in older couples. Nursing Science Quarterly, 4, 69–75.

Malinski, V.M. (1997). The relationship of temporal experience and power as knowing participation in change in depressed and nondepressed women. In M. Madrid (Ed.), Patterns of Rogerian knowing (pp. 197–208). New York: National League for Nursing Press.

Mason, D.J. (1988). Circadian rhythms of body temperature and activation and the well-being of older women. Nursing Research, 37, 276–281.

Matas, K.E. (1997). Human patterning and chronic pain. Nursing Science Quarterly, 10, 88–96.

McBride, S., Graydon, J., Sidani, S., & Hall, L. (1999). The therapeutic use of music for dyspnea and anxiety in patients with COPD who live at home. Journal of Holistic Nursing, 17, 229–250.

McDonald, S.F. (1986). The relationship between visible lightwaves and the experience of pain. In V.M. Malinski (Ed.), Explorations on Martha Rogers' science of unitary human beings (pp. 119–130). Norwalk, CT: Appleton-Century-Crofts.

McEvoy, M.D. (1990). The relationships among the experience of dying, the experience of paranormal events, and creativity in adults. In E.A.M. Barrett (Ed.), Visions of Rogers' science-based nursing (pp. 209–228). New York: National League for Nursing.

Winstead-Fry, P. (1990). Reflections on death as a process: A response to a study of the experience of dying. In E.A.M. Barrett (Ed.), Visions of Rogers' science-based nursing (pp. 229–236). New York: National League for Nursing. McEvoy, M.D. (1990). Response to "Reflections on death as a process." In E.A.M. Barrett (Ed.), Visions of Rogers' science-based nursing (pp. 237–238). New York: National League for Nursing.

McNiff, M.A. (1997). Power, perceived health, and life satisfaction in adults with long-term care needs. In M. Madrid (Ed.), Patterns of Rogerian knowing (pp. 177–186). New York: National League for Nursing Press.

Meehan, D.B. (1992). Effects of budgetary knowledge on staff nurses attitudes toward administration and cost containment [Abstract]. Kentucky Nurse, 40(2), 12.

Meehan, T.C. (1993). Therapeutic touch and postoperative pain: A Rogerian research study. Nursing Science Quarterly, 6, 69–78.

Paletta, J.R. (1990). The relationship of temporal experience to human time. In E.A.M. Barrett (Ed.), Visions of Rogers' science-based nursing (pp. 239–254). New York: National League for Nursing. Rawnsley, M.M. (1990). What time is it? A response to a study of temporal experience. In E.A.M. Barrett (Ed.), Visions of Rogers' science-based nursing (pp. 255–264). New York: National League for Nursing. Paletta, J.R. (1990). Response to "What time is it?" In E.A.M. Barrett (Ed.), Visions of Rogers' science-based nursing (pp. 265–268). New York: National League for Nursing.

Peck, S.D. (Eckes). (1998). The efficacy of therapeutic touch for improving functional ability in elders with degenerative arthritis. Nursing Science Quarterly, 11, 123–132.

Porter, L.S. (1972a). The impact of physical-physiological activity on infants' growth and development. Nursing Research, 21, 210–219.

Porter, L.S. (1972b). Physical-physiological activity and infants' growth and development. In American Nurses' Association, Seventh Nursing Research Conference (pp. 1–43). New York: American Nurses' Association.

Quinn, J.F. (1984). Therapeutic touch as energy exchange: Testing the theory. Advances in Nursing Science, 6(2), 42–49.

Quinn, J.F. (1989). Therapeutic touch as energy exchange: Replication and extension. Nursing Science Quarterly, 2, 79–87.

Quinn, J.F. (1992). Holding sacred space: The nurse as healing environment. Holistic Nursing Practice, 6(4), 26–36.

Quinn, J.F., & Strelkauskas, A.J. (1993). Psychoimmunologic effects of Therapeutic Touch on practitioners and recently bereaved recipients: A pilot study. Advances in Nursing Science, 15(4), 13–26.

Rawnsley, M.M. (1986). The relationship between the perception of the speed of time and the process of dying. In V.M. Malinski (Ed), Explorations on Martha Rogers' science of unitary human beings (pp. 79–93). Norwalk, CT: Appleton-Century-Crofts.

Reed, P. G. (1989). Mental health of older adults. Western Journal of Nursing Research, 11, 143–163.

Reeder, F. (1991). The importance of knowing what to care about: A phenomenological inquiry using laughing at oneself as a clue. In P.L. Chinn (Ed.), Anthology on caring (pp. 259–279). New York: National League for Nursing.

Rizzo, J.A., Gilman, M.P., & Mersmann, C.A. (1994). Facilitating care delivery redesign using measures of unit culture and work characteristics. Journal of Nursing Administration, 24(5), 32–37.

Salerno, E.M. (2002). Hope, power and perception of self in individuals recovering from schizophrenia: A Rogerian perspective. Visions: The Journal of Rogerian Science, 10, 23–36.

Samarel, N. (1992). The experience of receiving therapeutic touch. Journal of Advanced Nursing, 17, 651–657.

Samarel, N., Fawcett, J., Davis, M.M., & Ryan, F.M. (1998). Effects of dialogue and therapeutic touch on preoperative and postoperative experiences of breast cancer surgery: An exploratory study. Oncology Nursing Forum, 25, 1369–1376.

Sanchez, R. (1989). Empathy, diversity, and telepathy in mother-daughter dyads: An empirical investigation utilizing Rogers' conceptual framework. Scholarly Inquiry for Nursing Practice, 3, 29–44. Rawnsley, M.M. (1989). Response to "Empathy, diversity, and telepathy in mother-daughter dyads: An empirical investigation utilizing Rogers' conceptual framework." Scholarly Inquiry for Nursing Practice, 3, 45–51.

Schaffer, P., Vaughn, G., Kenner, C., Donohue, F., & Longo, A. (2000). Revision of a parent satisfaction survey based on the parent perspective. Journal of Pediatric Nursing, 15, 373–377.

Schneider, P.E. (1995). Focusing awareness: The process of extraordinary healing from a Rogerian perspective. Visions: Journal of Rogerian Nursing Science, 3(1), 32–43.

Schodt, C.M. (1989). Parental-fetal attachment and couvade: A study of patterns of human-environment integrality. Nursing Science Quarterly, 2, 88–97.

Shearer, N.B.C. (2001). Process of health empowerment in women. Communicating Nursing Research, 34(9), 379.

Sherman, D.W. (1996). Nurses' willingness to care for AIDS patients and spirituality, social support, and death anxiety. Image: Journal of Nursing Scholarship, 28, 205–213.

Sherman, D.W. (1996). Correlates of death anxiety in nurses who provide AIDS care. Omega; Journal of Death and Dying, 34, 117–137.

Smith, D.W. (1994). Toward developing a theory of spirituality. Visions: Journal of Rogerian Nursing Science, 2, 35–43.

Smith, D.W. (1995). Power and spirituality in polio survivors: A study based on Rogers' science. Nursing Science Quarterly, 8, 133–139.

Smith, M.C., Kemp, J., Hemphill, L., & Vojir, C.P. (2002). Outcomes of therapeutic massage for hospitalized cancer patients. Journal of Nursing Scholarship, 34, 257–262.

Smith, M.J. (1975). Changes in judgment of duration with different patterns of auditory information for individuals confined to bed. Nursing Research, 24, 93–98.

Smith, M.J. (1979). Duration experience for bed-confined subjects: A replication and refinement. Nursing Research, 28, 139–144.

Smith, M.J. (1984). Temporal experience and bed rest: Replication and refinement. Nursing Research, 33, 298–302.

Smith, M.J. (1986). Human-environment process: A test of Rogers' principle of integrality. Advances in Nursing Science, 9(1), 21–28.

Thompson, M.B., & Coppens, N.M. (1994). The effects of guided imagery on anxiety levels and movement of clients undergoing magnetic resonance imaging. Holistic Nursing Practice, 8(2), 59–69.

Todaro-Franceschi, V. (1999). The idea of energy as phenomenon and Rogerian nursing science: Are they congruent? Visions: The Journal of Rogerian Nursing Science, 7, 30–41.

Wall, L.M. (2000). Changes in hope and power in lung cancer patients who exercise. Nursing Science Quarterly, 13, 234–242.

Watson, J. (1997). Using Rogers' model to study sleep-wake pattern changes in older women. In M. Madrid (Ed.), Patterns of Rogerian knowing (pp. 167–176). New York: National League for Nursing Press.

Watson, J., Sloyan, C.M., & Robalino, J.E. (2000). The time metaphor test re-visited: Implications for Rogerian research. Visions: The Journal of Rogerian Nursing Science, 8, 32–45.

West, M.M. (2002). Early risk indicators of substance abuse among nurses. Journal of Nursing Scholarship, 34, 187–193.

Wiand, N.E. (1997). Relaxation levels achieved by Lamaze-trained pregnant women listening to music and ocean sound tapes. Journal of Perinatal Education, 6(4), 1–8.

Yarcheski, A., & Mahon, N. E. (1991). An empirical test of Rogers' original and revised theory of correlates in adolescents. Research in Nursing and Health, 14, 447–455.

Yarcheski, A., & Mahon, N.E. (1995). Roger's pattern manifestations and health in adolescents. Western Journal of Nursing Research, 17, 383–397.

Yarcheski, A., Mahon, N.E., & Yarcheski, T.J. (2002). Human and health in early adolescents; Perceived field motion as a mediating variable. Nursing Science Quarterly, 15, 1150–1155.

RESEARCH INSTRUMENTS AND PRACTICE TOOLS

Barrett, E.A.M. (1984). An empirical investigation of Martha E. Rogers' principle of helicy: The relationship of human field motion and power. Dissertation Abstracts International, 45, 615A.

Barrett, E.A.M. (1986). Investigation of the principle of helicy: The relationship of human field motion and power. In V.M. Malinski (Ed.), Explorations on Martha Rogers' science of unitary human beings (pp. 173–188). Norwalk, CT: Appleton-Century-Crofts.

Barrett, E.A.M. (1990). An instrument to measure power as Knowing-Participation-in-Change. In O. Strickland & C. Waltz (Eds.), The measurement of nursing outcomes. Vol. 4. Measuring client self-care and coping skills (pp. 159–180). New York: Springer.

Bultemeier, K. (2002). Rogers' science of unitary human beings in nursing practice. In M.R. Alligood & A. Marriner Tomey (Eds.), Nursing theory: Utilization and application (2nd ed., pp. 267–288). St. Louis: Mosby.

Carboni, J.T. (1992). Instrument development and the measurement of unitary constructs. Nursing Science Quarterly, 5, 134–142.

Decker, K. (1989). Theory in action: The geriatric assessment team. Journal of Gerontological Nursing, 15(10), 25–28.

Falco, S.M., & Lobo, M.L. (1995). Martha E. Rogers. In J.B. George (Ed.), Nursing theories. The base for professional nursing practice (4th ed., pp. 229–248). Norwalk, CT: Appleton & Lange.

Ference, H.M. (1980). The relationship of time experience, creativity traits, differentiation and human field motion. An empirical investigation of Rogers' correlates of synergistic human development. Dissertation Abstracts International, 40, 5206B.

Ference, H.M. (1986). The relationship of time experience, creativity traits, differentiation, and human field motion. In V.M. Malinski (Ed.), Explorations on Martha Rogers' science of unitary human beings (pp. 95–106). Norwalk, CT: Appleton-Century-Crofts.

Garon, M. (1991). Assessment and management of pain in the home care setting: Application of Rogers' science of unitary human beings. Holistic Nursing Practice, 6(1), 47–57.

Hanchett, E.S. (1979). Community health assessment: A conceptual tool kit. New York: Wiley.

Hanchett, E.S. (1988). Nursing frameworks and community as client: Bridging the gap. Norwalk, CT: Appleton & Lange.

Hastings-Tolsma, M.T. (1993). The relationship of diversity of human field pattern to risk-taking and time experience: An investigation of Rogers' principles of homeodynamics. Dissertation Abstracts International, 53, 4029B.

Johnston, L.W. (1993a). The development of the human field image metaphor scale. Dissertation Abstracts International, 54, 1890B.

Johnston, L.W. (1993b). The development of the human field image metaphor scale. Visions: Journal of Rogerian Nursing Science, 1, 55–56.

Johnston, L.W. (1994). Psychometric nalysis of Johnston's human field image metaphor scale. Visions: Journal of Rogerian Nursing Science, 2, 7–11.

Johnston, R.L. (1986). Approaching family intervention through Rogers' conceptual model. In A.L. Whall (Ed.), Family therapy theory for nursing. Four approaches (pp. 11–32). Norwalk, CT: Appleton-Century-Crofts.

Leddy, S.K. (1995). Measuring mutual process: Development and psychometric testing of the person-environment participation scale. Visions: Journal of Rogerian Nursing Science, 3(1), 20–31.

Leddy, S.K. (1996). Development and psychometric testing of the Leddy Healthiness Scale. Research in Nursing and Health, 19, 431–440.

Leddy, S.K. (1999). Further exploration of the psychometric properties of the Person-Environment Participation Scale: Differentiating instrument reliability and construct stability. Visions: The Journal of Rogerian Nursing Science, 7, 55–57.

Madrid, M., & Winstead-Fry, P. (1986). Rogers' conceptual model. In P. Winstead-Fry (Ed.), Case studies in nursing theory (pp. 73–102). New York: National League for Nursing.

McCanse, R.L. (1988). Healthy death readiness: Development of a measurement instrument. Dissertation Abstracts International, 48, 2606B.

McCanse, R.P. (1995). The McCanse Readiness for Death Instrument (MRDI): A reliable and valid measure for hospice care. Hospice Journal: Physical, Psychosocial, and Pastoral Care of the Dying, 10(1), 15–26.

Paletta, J.L. (1988). The relationship of temporal experience to human time. Dissertation Abstracts International, 49, 1621B–1622B.

Paletta, J.R. (1990). The relationship of temporal experience to human time. In E.A.M. Barrett (Ed.), Visions of Rogers' science-based nursing (pp. 239–254). New York: National League for Nursing.

Reed, P.G. (1986). The developmental conceptual framework: Nursing reformulations and applications for family therapy. In A.L. Whall (Ed.), Family therapy for nursing. Four approaches (pp. 69–91). Norwalk, CT: Appleton-Century-Crofts.

Smith, K., Kupferschmid, B.J., Dawson, C., & Briones, T.L. (1991). A family-centered critical care unit. AACN Clinical Issues, 2, 258–268.

Tettero, I., Jackson, S., & Wilson, S. (1993). Theory to practice: Developing a Rogerian-based assessment tool. Journal of Advanced Nursing, 18, 776–782.

Watson, J. (1994). The relationships of sleep-wake rhythm, dream experience, human field motion, and time experience in older women. Dissertation Abstracts International, 54, 6137B.

Watson, J. (1999). Measuring dreaming as a beyond waking experience in Rogers' conceptual model. Nursing Science Quarterly, 12, 245–250.

Watson, J., Barrett, E.A.M., Hastings-Tolsma, M., Johnston, L., & Gueldner, S. (1997). Measurement in Rogerian science: A review of selected instruments. In M. Madrid (Ed.), Patterns of Rogerian knowing (pp. 87–99). New York: National League for Nursing Press.

Whell, A.L. (1981). Nursing theory and the assessment of families. Journal of Psychiatric Nursing and Mental Health Services, 19(1), 30–36.

Wright, S.M. (1989). Development and construct validity of the energy field assessment form. Dissertation Abstracts International, 49, 3113B.

Wright, S.M. (1991). Validity of the human energy field assessment form. Western Journal of Nursing Research, 13, 635–647.

Yarcheski, A., & Mahon, N.E. (1991). An empirical test of Rogers' original and revised theory of correlates in adolescents. Research in Nursing and Health, 14, 447–455.

Young, A., Taylor, S.G., & McLauglin-Renpenning, K. (2001). Connections: Nursing research, theory, and practice. St. Louis: Mosby.

PRACTICE

Barrett, E.A.M. (1988). Using Rogers' science of unitary human beings in nursing practice. Nursing Science Quarterly, 1, 50–51.

Barrett, E.A.M. (1990). Health patterning in clients in a private practice. In E.A.M. Barrett (Ed.), Visions of Rogers' science-based nursing (pp. 105–116). New York: National League for Nursing.

Barrett, E.A.M. (1992). Innovative imagery: A health-patterning modality for nursing practice. Journal of Holistic Nursing, 10, 154–166.

Barrett, E.A.M. (2000). The theoretical matrix for a Rogerian nursing practice. Theoria: Journal of Nursing Theory, 9(4), 3–7.

Biley, F.C. (1993). Energy fields nursing: A brief encounter of a unitary kind. International Journal of Nursing Studies, 30, 519–525.

Buczny, B., Speirs, J., & Howard, J.R. (1989). Nursing care of a terminally ill client. Applying Martha Rogers' conceptual framework. Home Healthcare Nurse, 7(4), 13–18.

Bultemeier, K. (1997). Rogers' science of unitary human beings in nursing practice. In M.R. Alligood & A. Marriner-Tomey (Eds.), Nursing theory: Utilization and application (pp. 153–174). St. Louis: Mosby.

Bultemeier, K. (2002). Rogers' science of unitary human beings in nursing practice. In M.R. Alligood & A. Marriner Tomey (Eds.), Nursing theory: Utilization and application (2nd ed., pp. 267–288). St. Louis: Mosby.

Chapman, J.S., Mitchell, G.J., & Forchuk, C. (1994). A glimpse of nursing theory-based practice in Canada. [Chapman, J.S. Rogerian theory-based practice and research.] Nursing Science Quarterly, 7, 104–112.

Covington, H. (2001). Therapeutic music for patients with psychiatric disorders. Holistic Nursing Practice, 15, 59–69.

Cowling, W.R. III. (1990). Chronological age as an anomaly of evolution. In E.A.M. Barrett (Ed.), Visions of Rogers' science-based nursing (pp. 143–150). New York: National League for Nursing.

Cowling, W.R, III. (2000). Healing as appreciating wholeness. Advances in Nursing Science, 22(3), 16–32.

Dole, P.J. (1996). Centering: Reducing rape trauma syndrome anxiety during a gynecologic examination. Journal of Psychosocial Nursing and Mental Health Services, 34(10), 32–37, 52–53.

Ference, H.M. (1989). Comforting the dying. Nursing practice according to the Rogerian model. In J.P. Riehl-Sisca (Ed.), Conceptual models for nursing practice (3rd ed., pp. 197–205). Norwalk, CT: Appleton & Lange.

Field, S. (1997). The scientific art of medical practice. In M. Madrid (Ed.), Patterns of Rogerian knowing (pp. 267–284). New York: National League for Nursing Press.

Forker, J.E., & Billings, C.V. (1989). Nursing therapeutics in a group encounter. Archives of Psychiatric Nursing, 3, 108–112.

Gold, J. (1997). The practice of nursing from a unitary perspective. In M. Madrid (Ed.), Patterns of Rogerian knowing (pp. 249–256). New York: National League for Nursing Press.

Gold, J.L. (1997). Practicing medicine in the nineties with an emphasis on the unitary perspective of patient care. In M. Madrid (Ed.), Patterns of Rogerian knowing (pp. 257–266). New York: National League for Nursing Press.

Hanchett, E.S. (1988). Nursing frameworks and community as client: Bridging the gap. Norwalk, CT: Appleton & Lange.

Herdtner, S. (2000). Using therapeutic touch in nursing practice. Orthopaedic Nursing, 19(5), 77–82.

Hill, L., & Oliver, N. (1993). Technique integration: Therapeutic touch and theory-based mental health nursing. Journal of Psychosocial Nursing and Mental Health Services, 31(2), 19–22.

Horvath, B. (1994). The science of unitary human beings as a foundation for nursing practice with persons experiencing life patterning difficulties: Transforming theory into motion. In M. Madrid & E.A.M. Barrett (Eds.), Rogers' scientific art of nursing practice (pp. 163–176). New York: National League for Nursing Press.

Johnson, M.O. (1996). A mutual field manifestation: Substance abuse and nursing. Visions: Journal of Rogerian Nursing Science, 4(1), 24–30.

Johnston, R.L. (1986). Approaching family intervention through Rogers' conceptual model. In A.L. Whall (Ed.), Family therapy theory for nursing. Four approaches (pp. 11–32). Norwalk, CT: Appleton-Century-Crofts.

Joseph, L. (1990). Practical application of Rogers' theoretical framework for nursing. In M.E. Parker (Ed.), Nursing theories in practice (pp. 115–125). New York: National League for Nursing.

Kodiath, M.F. (1991). A new view of the chronic pain client. Holistic Nursing Practice, 6(1), 41–46.

Madrid, M. (1990). The participating process of human field patterning in an acute-care environment. In E.A.M. Barrett (Ed.), Visions of Rogers' science-based nursing (pp. 93–104). New York: National League for Nursing. Madrid, M. (1996). The participating process of human field patterning in an acute care environment [English abstract]. Pflege, 9, 246–254.

Madrid, M. (1994). Participating in the process of dying. In M. Madrid & E.A.M. Barrett (Eds.), Rogers' scientific art of nursing practice (pp. 91–100). New York: National League for Nursing Press. Griffin, J. (1994). Storytelling as a scientific art form. In M. Madrid & E.A.M. Barrett (Eds.), Rogers' scientific art of nursing practice (pp. 101–104). New York: National League for Nursing Press.

Madrid, M., & Winstead-Fry, P. (1986). Rogers' conceptual model. In P. Winstead-Fry (Ed.), Case studies in nursing theory (pp. 73–102). New York: National League for Nursing.

Malinski, V. (1994). Health patterning for individuals and families. In M. Madrid & E.A.M. Barrett (Eds.), Rogers' scientific art of nursing practice (pp. 105–117). New York: National League for Nursing Press.

Mandl, A. (1997). A plea to educate the public about Martha Rogers' science of unitary human beings. In M. Madrid (Ed.), Patterns of Rogerian knowing (pp. 236–238). New York: National League for Nursing Press.

Meehan, T.C. (1990). The science of unitary human beings and theory-based practice: Therapeutic touch. In E.A.M. Barrett (Ed.), Visions of Rogers' science-based nursing (pp. 67–82). New York: National League for Nursing.

Morwessel, N.J. (1994). Developing an effective pattern appraisal to guide nursing care of children with heart variations and their families. In M. Madrid & E.A.M. Barrett (Eds.), Rogers' scientific

art of nursing practice (pp. 147–161). New York: National League for Nursing Press.

Newshan, G. (1989). Therapeutic touch for symptom control in persons with AIDS. Holistic Nursing Practice, 3(4), 45–51.

Payne, M.B. (1989). The use of therapeutic touch with rehabilitation clients. Rehabilitation Nursing, 14(2), 69–72.

Reed, P.G. (1986). The developmental conceptual framework: Nursing reformulations and applications for family therapy. In A.L. Whall (Ed.), Family therapy for nursing. Four approaches (pp. 69–91). Norwalk, CT: Appleton-Century-Crofts.

Rogers, M.E. (1983). The family coping with a surgical crisis. Analysis and application of Rogers' theory of nursing. In I.W. Clements & F.B. Roberts (Eds.), Family health: A theoretical approach to nursing care (pp. 390–391). New York: Wiley.

Sargent, S. (1994). Healing groups: Awareness of a group field. In M. Madrid & E.A.M. Barrett (Eds.), Rogers' scientific art of nursing practice (pp. 119–129). New York: National League for Nursing Press.

Sayre-Adams, J., & Wright, S. (1995). Change in consciousness. Nursing Times, 91(41), 44–45.

Sheu, S.L., Shiau, S.J., & Hung, C.H. (1997). The application of Rogers' science of unitary human beings to an adolescent with mental illness [English abstract]. Journal of Nursing (China), 44, 51–57.

Starn, J.R. (1998). Energy healing with women and children. Journal of Obstetric, Gynecologic, and Neonatal Nursing, 27, 576–584.

Talley, B. (1994). Dying. In M. Madrid & E.A.M. Barrett (Eds.), Rogers' scientific art of nursing practice (pp. 239–240). New York: National League for Nursing Press.

Thomas, S.D. (1990). Intentionality in the human-environment encounter in an ambulatory care environment. In E.A.M. Barrett (Ed.), Visions of Rogers' science-based nursing (pp. 117–128). New York: National League for Nursing.

Thompson, J.E. (1990). Finding the borderline's border: Can Martha Rogers help? Perspectives in Psychiatric Care, 26(4), 7–10.

Tuyn, L.K. (1992). Solution-oriented therapy and Rogerian nursing science: An integrated approach. Archives of Psychiatric Nursing, 6, 83–89.

Tuyn, L.K. (1994). Rhythms of living: A Rogerian approach to counseling. In M. Madrid & E.A.M. Barrett (Eds.), Rogers' scientific art of nursing practice (pp. 207–221). New York: National League for Nursing Press.

Webb, J. (1992). A new lease on life. Nursing Times, 88(11), 30–32.

Whelton, B.J. (1979). An operationalization of Martha Rogers' theory throughout the nursing process. International Journal of Nursing Studies, 16, 7–20.

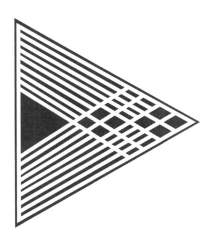

Chapter **10**

Roy's Adaptation Model

Sister Callista Roy first published the basic ideas that make up her conceptual model in 1970 in an article titled "Adaptation: A Conceptual Framework for Nursing." She went on to publish additional elements of the model and implications for practice and education in journal articles that were published 1971 and 1973. The model was explicated more fully in a chapter of the 1974 edition of Riehl and Roy's book *Conceptual Models for Nursing Practice* (Roy, 1974). A major expansion of the model was presented in Roy's (1976b) text *Introduction to Nursing: An Adaptation Model*. Refinements of the model then were presented in Roy's 1978 speech at the Second Annual Nurse Educator Conference, in the 1980 edition of Riehl and Roy's book (Roy, 1980), and in Roy and Roberts' (1981) text *Theory Construction in Nursing: An Adaptation Model*. Further refinements of the model were published in the second edition of Roy's (1984a) text *Introduction to Nursing: An Adaptation Model*, in Andrews and Roy's (1986) book *Essentials of the Roy Adaptation Model*, and in a chapter (Roy, 1989) of the third edition of *Conceptual Models for Nursing Practice* (Riehl-Sisca, 1989).

Roy articulated her philosophical assumptions in the 1988b journal article "An Explication of the Philosophical Assumptions of the Roy Adaptation Model," and she elaborated on her definitions of adaptation and health in the 1990 journal article "Strengthening the Roy Adaptation Model through Conceptual Clarification: Commentary and Response" (Artinian & Roy, 1990). The 1991 text *The Roy Adaptation Model: The Definitive Statement* (Roy & Andrews, 1991) contained further refinements in the model. The authors explicitly stated that the purpose of that book was "to assume the role of the definitive text on the model" (Roy & Andrews, 1991, p. xvii). A 1993 book chapter, "The Roy Adaptation Model: Theoretical Update and Knowledge for Practice" (Roy & Corliss, 1993), presented additional refinements and a restatement of so-called scientific assumptions, presented earlier in Roy's 1989 book chapter and the 1991 book, in the form of philosophical claims. Roy presented a new definition of adaptation and refined and restated her scientific assumptions and philosophical assumptions in the 1997 journal article "Future of the Roy Model: Challenge to Redefine Adaptation." Some rewording of the scientific assumptions and philosophical assumptions and considerable refinement in the content of the conceptual model are evident in the second edition of the Roy and Andrews (1999) book, now titled *The Roy Adaptation Model*. The purpose of the second edition, which Roy and Andrews (1999) still regard as "the definitive text" (p. xvii), is "to provide an update that (1) maintains the essential concepts of the model while reflecting new developments and enhanced integration of the model elements; (2) focuses on contemporary issues of health care delivery with social and

Overview

Roy's work focuses on human adaptive system responses and environmental stimuli, which are constantly changing. Roy's work clearly fits the definition of conceptual model used in this book, and Roy always has referred to her work as a conceptual model. The concepts of the Roy Adaptation Model and their dimensions and subdimensions are listed here, along with the components of Roy's practice methodology. Each concept and its dimensions and subdimensions and the practice methodology components are defined and described, and the goal of nursing is discussed in detail, later in this chapter.

Key Terms

HUMAN BEINGS
HUMAN ADAPTIVE SYSTEM
    Individual Persons
    Groups or Relational Persons
COPING PROCESSES
    Individuals: Regulator Coping Subsystem
    Individuals: Cognator Coping Subsystem
    Groups: Stabilizer Subsystem Control Process
    Groups: Innovator Subsystem Control Process
BEHAVIOR
    Individuals and Groups: Adaptive Response
    Individuals and Groups: Ineffective Response
ADAPTIVE MODES
    Individuals: Physiological Mode
      Oxygenation
      Nutrition
      Elimination
      Activity and Rest
      Protection
      Senses
      Fluid, Electrolyte, and Acid-Base Balance
      Neurological Function
      Endocrine Function
    Groups: Physical Mode
    Individuals: Self-Concept Mode
      Physical Self (Body Sensation, Body Image)
      Personal Self (Self-Consistency, Self-Ideal, Moral-Ethical-Spiritual Self)
    Groups: Group Identity Mode
      Interpersonal Relationships
      Group Self-Image
      Social Milieu
      Group Culture

    Individuals and Groups: Role Function Mode
      Primary Role
      Secondary Role
      Tertiary Role
      Instrumental Behavior
      Expressive Behavior
      Role-Taking
      Integrating Roles
    Individuals and Groups: Interdependence Mode
      Affectional Adequacy (Individuals and Groups)
      Developmental Adequacy (Individuals and Groups)
      Resource Adequacy (Individuals and Groups)
      Significant Others (Individuals)
      Support Systems (Individuals)
      Context (Groups)
      Infrastructure (Groups)
      Resources (Groups)
ENVIRONMENT
STIMULI
    Focal Stimulus
    Contextual Stimuli
    Residual Stimuli
HUMAN BEINGS AND ENVIRONMENT
ADAPTATION
    Survival
    Growth
    Reproduction
    Mastery
    Person and Environment Transformations
ADAPTATION LEVEL
    Integrated Life Process
    Compensatory Life Process
    Compromised Life Process
HEALTH
HEALTH
NURSING
SCIENCE
    Basic Nursing Science
    Clinical Nursing Science
ART
GOAL OF NURSING
    To Promote Adaptation for Individuals and Groups in the Four Adaptive Modes, Thus Contributing to Health, Quality of Life, and Dying with Dignity by Assessing Behavior and Factors That Influence Adaptive Abilities and by Intervening to Expand Those Abilities and to Enhance Environmental Interactions

PRACTICE METHODOLOGY: THE ROY ADAPTATION MODEL NURSING PROCESS	THEORY OF THE PERSON AS AN ADAPTIVE SYSTEM
Assessment of Behavior	THEORY OF THE PHYSIOLOGICAL MODE
Assessment of Stimuli	THEORY OF THE SELF-CONCEPT MODE
Nursing Diagnosis	THEORY OF THE ROLE FUNCTION MODE
Goal Setting	THEORY OF THE INTERDEPENDENCE MODE
Intervention	NURSING MODEL OF COGNITIVE PROCESSING
Evaluation	

 ## ANALYSIS OF ROY'S ADAPTATION MODEL

This section presents an analysis of the Roy Adaptation Model. The analysis draws heavily from the second edition of Roy and Andrews' (1999) book, *The Roy Adaptation Model*.

ORIGINS OF THE NURSING MODEL

Historical Evolution and Motivation

In tracing the historical development of her conceptual model, Roy (1989) explained:

> The Roy model had its beginning in 1964 when the author was challenged to develop a conceptual model for nursing in a seminar with Dorothy E. Johnson, at the University of California, Los Angeles. The adaptation concept, presented in a psychology class, had impressed [me] as an appropriate conceptual framework for nursing. The work on adaptation by the physiologic psychologist, Harry Helson, was added to the beginning concept and the model's present form began to take shape. In subsequent years the model was developed as a framework for nursing practice, research, and education. In 1968 work began on operationalizing the model in the baccalaureate nursing curriculum at Mount Saint Mary's College in Los Angeles. The first class of students to study with the model began their nursing major in the spring of 1970 and were graduated in June, 1972. Use of the model in nursing practice led to further clarification and refinement. In the summer of 1971 a pilot research study was conducted and in 1976 to 1977 a survey research study was done that led to some tentative confirmations of the model (p. 105).

Development of the model continued during the 1970s, according to Roy and Andrews (1999), as "more than 1,500 faculty and students at Mount St. Mary's College in Los Angeles helped to clarify, refine, and develop the basic concepts of the Roy Adaptation Model for nursing" (p. 29).

Continued refinement of the content of the Roy Adaptation Model and the scientific and philosophical assumptions on which it is based continued throughout the 1980s and the 1990s and into the 2000s. During much of the 1980s and continuing into the 1990s, Roy engaged in postdoctoral research in neuroscience nursing, which contributed to the further development of Roy Adaptation Model content. Throughout the 1990s and early 2000s, as a faculty member at Boston College, a participant in religious retreats, and a member of the Boston Theological Institute Faith and Science Exchange advisory board, Roy has refined the scientific and philosophical assumptions and turned her attention to contemporary movements in nursing knowledge development and spirituality (Roy, 1997, 2003; Roy & Andrews, 1999).

By accepting Johnson's challenge to develop a conceptual model when she was a student, Roy joined the group of nurse scholars who recognized the need to explicate a body of nursing knowledge. Indeed, she stated that "as nursing education moves more and more into institutions of higher learning, the nurse educator needs a basis for developing a body of nursing knowledge. And as the general public becomes more sophisticated in knowing the meaning of good health, it expects the nurse to provide care based on scientific knowledge. It is from the theoretical conceptual framework of any discipline that its area of practice, its body of knowledge, and its scientific basis are developed" (Roy, 1970, p. 42).

Philosophical Claims

Roy (1987c, 1988b, 1992b, 1989, 1997, Roy & Andrews, 1999) presented the philosophical claims undergirding the Roy Adaptation Model in the form of a claim about human beings and the environment, a claim about adaptation, scientific assumptions and philosophical assumptions about human beings and the environment, values about nursing, and claims about nursing and nurse scholars/nurse theorists. All of the philosophical claims are listed here.

Philosophical Claim About Human Beings and Environment

- Persons are seen as coextensive with their physical and social environments (Roy & Andrews, 1999, p. 539).

Philosophical Claim About Adaptation

- [The Roy Adaptation Model] assumes the universal importance of promoting adaptation in states of health and illness (Roy, 1992b, p. 66).

Scientific Assumptions

- Systems of matter and energy progress to higher levels of complex self-organization (Roy & Andrews, 1999, p. 35).
- Consciousness and meaning are constitutive of person and environment integration (Roy & Andrews, 1999, p. 35).
- Awareness of self and environment is rooted in thinking and feeling (Roy & Andrews, 1999, p. 35).
- Humans by their decisions are accountable for the integration of creative processes (Roy & Andrews, 1999, p. 35).
- Thinking and feeling mediate human action (Roy & Andrews, 1999, p. 35).
- System relationships include acceptance, protection, and fostering of interdependence (Roy & Andrews, 1999, p. 35).
- Persons and the earth have common patterns and integral relationships (Roy & Andrews, 1999, p. 35).
- Person and environment transformations are created in human consciousness (Roy & Andrews, 1999, p. 35).
- Integration of human and environment meanings results in adaptation (Roy & Andrews, 1999, p. 35).

Philosophical Assumptions

- Persons have mutual relationships with the world and God (Roy & Andrews, 1999, p. 35).
- Human meaning is rooted in an omega point convergence [with] the universe (Roy & Andrews, 1999, p. 35).
- God is intimately revealed in the diversity of creation and is the common destiny of creation (Roy & Andrews, 1999, p. 35).
- Persons use human creative abilities of awareness, enlightenment, and faith (Roy & Andrews, 1999, p. 35).
- Persons are accountable for the processes of deriving, sustaining, and transforming the universe (Roy & Andrews, 1999, p. 35).

Values About Nursing

- Nursing's concern with the person as a total being in the areas of health and illness is a socially significant activity (Roy, 1989, p. 109).
- The nursing goal of supporting and promoting patient adaptation is important for patient welfare (Roy, 1989, p. 109).
- Promoting the process of adaptation is assumed to conserve patient energy; thus nursing makes an important contribution to the overall goal of the health team by making energy available for the healing process (Roy, 1989, p. 109).
- Nursing is unique because it focuses on the patient as a person adapting to those stimuli present as a result of his

or her position on the health-illness continuum (Roy, 1989, p. 109).
- The nurse takes a values-based stance, focusing on awareness, enlightenment, and faith (Roy & Andrews, 1999, p. 539).

Philosophical Claims About Nursing and Nurse Scholars/Nurse Theorists

- Nurse scholars take a value-based stance. Rooted in beliefs and hopes about the human person, they fashion a discipline that participates in the well-being of persons (Roy, 1997, p. 42).
- Nurse scholars are accountable for consciously guiding the future eras of humankind.... The mission of the future well-being of humankind in environmental interactions approaches as the defining moment for nursing and the major challenge of nurse theorists (Roy, 1997, p. 42).

Roy (1997) regarded the most recent statement of her scientific assumptions and philosophical assumptions as appropriate for the twenty-first century. The scientific assumptions undergirding the Roy Adaptation Model "combine expanded notions of systems and adaptation theory" drawn from von Bertalanffy's (1968) and Helson's (1964) work (Roy, 1997, p. 45). The scientific and philosophical assumptions reflect the principles of cosmic unity and common purposefulness. The principle of cosmic unity asserts that "persons and earth have common patterns and mutuality of relations and meaning" (Roy, 2003). The principle of comic unity further asserts that "Persons, through thinking and feeling capacities, rooted in consciousness and meaning, are accountable for deriving, sustaining, and transforming the universe" (Roy, 2003). The principle of common purposefulness asserts that "All persons and earth have both unity and diversity; are united in a common destiny; [and] find meaning in mutual relations with each other, the treated world, and a God-figure" (Roy, 2003).

The philosophical assumptions encompass several values and beliefs associated with the general principles of humanism, veritivity, and creation spirituality. Humanism, according to Roy (1988b), is "a broad movement in philosophy and psychology that recognizes the person and subjective dimensions of human experience as central to knowing and valuing" (p. 29). Humanism includes such schools of thought as secular, atheistic, and Christian humanism (Roy, 2003).

Veritivity is a philosophical premise asserting that "there is an absolute truth" (Roy, 1988b, p. 29). Veritivity focuses attention on "the richness of rootedness in absolute truth" (Roy, 2003). As a principle of human nature, veritivity "affirms a common purposefulness of human existence" (Roy,

1988b, p. 30). Components of veritivity include "(a) purposefulness of human existence, (b) unity of purpose in humankind, (c) activity and creativity for the common good, and (d) value and meaning of life" (Hanna & Roy, 2001, p. 10; Roy, 2003)

Creation spirituality, according to Roy's (1997) interpretation of Fox's (1983) work, declares that "Persons and the earth are one, and that they are in God and of God" (p. 46). Citing Swimme and Berry (1994), Roy and Andrews (1999) noted that creation spirituality focuses attention on "awareness and the notion of eliminating false consciousness; enlightenment to reach self-control, balance, and quietude; and the reclamation of early creation as the core of faith" (p. 35).

Roy and Andrews (1999) pointed out that the scientific assumptions and philosophical assumptions "have constituted the basis for and are evident in the specific description of the following major concepts of the Roy Adaptation Model—humans as adaptive systems as both individuals and groups, the environment, health, and the goal of nursing" (p. 35).

Strategies for Knowledge Development

The Roy Adaptation Model evolved from a combination of inductive and deductive thinking. Roy (1992b) explained, "As a young staff nurse I was immediately impressed with the resilience of children in the recovery process, both from disease and from the many changes of hospitalization, with even a small amount of well-timed nursing care. Thus, my original insights into viewing the person as having innate and acquired abilities to deal with a changing environment were developed. Later I articulated this belief by using the concept of adaptation" (p. 64).

Deduction clearly was the approach used by Roy to develop her conceptualization of adaptation and the factors that influence the level of adaptation. Initially, she drew heavily from Helson's (1964) work on adaptation of the retina of the eye to environmental changes. Later, she drew from more contemporary views of science and the relationship of person and environment. Moreover, her conceptualization of the human being as an adaptive system was deduced from general system theory.

Roy used an inductive approach to identify the four modes of adaptation. That was accomplished through classification of "about 500 samples of behavior of patients collected by nursing students over a period of several months in all clinical settings" (Roy, 1971, p. 255). The classification was based in part on Strickler and LaSor's (1970) work on threats in crisis situations. The modes were then compared with the typologies developed by Abdellah and colleagues (1960) and McCain (1965).

Influences from Other Scholars

Roy (1988c) noted that her personal and professional life has been shaped by "my family, my religious commitment, my teachers, and my mentors" (p. 292). She is the second child and first daughter in a large nuclear family. She joined the religious community of the Sisters of Saint Joseph of Carondelet when she completed high school. She completed her undergraduate nursing studies at Mount St. Mary's College in Los Angeles and went on to graduate study at the University of California, Los Angeles.

Andrews and Roy (1991a) explained that "the roots of the [Roy Adaptation] Model lie in Roy's own personal and professional background.... Under the mentorship of Dorothy E. Johnson, Roy became convinced of the importance of defining nursing. She was influenced also by studies in the social sciences, and clinical practice in pediatric nursing provided experience with the resiliency of the human body and spirit" (p. 4).

In addition to acknowledging the contributions to her thinking made by her mentor, Dorothy Johnson, Roy (1978) acknowledged her colleagues at Mount St. Mary's College, nursing students across the country, and other nurse theorists. In particular, she cited the influences of Dorothy Johnson's focus on behavior, Martha Rogers' concern with holistic man, and Dorothea Orem's notion of self-care. Roy (1988c) also acknowledged the contributions of Dr. Burton Meyer, who "gave me a firm grounding in both inductive and deductive processes for developing a framework, as well as in the meticulous steps of design, data collection, and analysis" during her graduate study at the University of California, Los Angeles (p. 293); and Dr. Connie Robinson, who provided mentorship in "the world of basic and clinical neurosciences" during her Robert Wood Johnson Clinical Nurse Scholars postdoctoral fellowship at the University of California, San Francisco (p. 296).

Roy (1997) explained that her experiences in the mid-1980s as a Clinical Nurse Scholar and subsequent research with patients who had neurological deficits, along with her experiences as the recipient of a 1989 Fulbright Senior Scholar Award from the Australian-American Educational Foundation, influenced her thinking about adaptation and broadened her insights to an international level. She explained, "Two relevant influences from this work were, first, a sensitivity to the immense potential of the human body and spirit to adapt to major neurologic injury, and secondly, entree to scholars and literature in the neurosciences that provide insights into current study of brain and mind functions, including human consciousness" (pp. 42–43).

Roy (1970; Andrews & Roy, 1991a; Roy & Corliss, 1993) stated that the scientific foundation for the Roy Adaptation

Model initially came from the work of Helson (1964) and von Bertalanffy (1968). Later, Roy (1997) explained that Helson's work "remains the parent theory for the origin of the Roy adaptation concept. However, given a broad view of person and environment interactions that is the focus of nursing practice now and in the future, the time has come to be free of the limitation of [Helson's] particular definition of adaptation. The notion from Helson that will remain useful in nursing assessment is that adaptation is a pooled effect of multiple influences, which he called focal, contextual, and residual stimuli" (p. 45).

In addition, Roy (1997) cited Gould (1983) and Zohar (1990) in the discussion of her revised definition of adaptation. In discussing the revisions in her scientific assumptions, Roy (1997) also cited Davies (1988), Gendreau and Caranfa (1984), Maloney (1991), and Swimme and Berry (1992).

Roy's notions of coping are tied to the work of Coelho, Hamburg, and Adams (1974) and Lazarus, Averill, and Opton (1974). She also drew from Levine (1966) and compared the concepts of her model with ideas put forth by Henderson (1960), Nightingale (1859), and Peplau (1952). Elaborating on influences from Nightingale, Roy (1992b) noted that her own work is congruent with Nightingale's beliefs about "how to promote 'health existences' and the proper use of the environment to aid the natural reparative processes" (p. 64).

Moreover, Roy (1988b, 1997, 2002) acknowledged the influence of several philosophers on the development of her philosophical assumptions. Among those whose works were cited are Chaisson (1981), de Chardin (1956, 1959, 1964, 1965, 1969), Ewing (1951), Fox (1983), Haught (1993), Helminiak (1998), Kant (Boas, 1957), O'Murchu (1995, 1997), Pinckaers (1995), Popper (Popper & Eccles, 1981), Rush (1981), Wilbur (1997), and Young (1993). Roy and Corliss (1993) explained that the philosophical assumptions "stem from Roy's lifelong study, conviction, and living of a theologically based religious faith. In addition, Roy built upon both undergraduate and graduate studies in philosophy, especially related to the nature of person and the place of persons in a cosmos set in motion by a loving Creator. Early on, she studied the philosophies of Aristotle and Thomas Aquinas, as well as the philosophical roots and historical methods of hermeneutical exegesis of biblical texts. Later the works of Freud, Jung, Adler, de Chardin, Kant, Hegel, Marx, and Freire were added. A strong basis in sociology, social psychology, and anthropology opened doors into structural analysis, empirical deductive knowledge strategies, interactionist theory, and phenomenology. Current teaching of the epistemology of nursing has allowed Roy to study the philosophy of science movements affecting nursing over the past few decades and the thinking of current nurse philosophers" (p. 218).

World View

The Roy Adaptation Model reflects the *reciprocal interaction* world view. Human beings and groups, for Roy (1997; Roy & Andrews, 1999), are holistic, adaptive systems that are constantly changing in concert with a constantly changing environment. The features of the reciprocal interaction world view that are evident in the Roy Adaptation Model are:

* The Roy Adaptation Model reflects a holistic view of the person.
* [Individuals and groups are holistic adaptive systems] that function as wholes in one unified expression of meaningful human behavior. They are, then, more than the sum of their parts (Roy & Andrews, 1999, p. 35).
* Persons represent unity in diversity. Similarly, there is diversity among persons and their earth, yet all are united in a common destiny (Roy & Andrews, 1999, pp. 35–36).
* The adaptive system is regarded as active.
* The notion of adaptation level conveys that the human system is not passive in relation to the environment (Roy & Andrews, 1999, p. 41).
* Human systems have thinking and feelings capacities, rooted in consciousness and meaning, by which they adjust effectively to changes in the environment and, in turn, affect the environment (Roy & Andrews, 1999, p. 36).
* According to this nursing model, the person is to be respected as an active participant in his care. It is the information that the patient shares with the nurse that forms the assessment. The goal arrived at is one of mutual agreement between nurse and patient. Interventions are the options that the nurse provides for the patient (Roy & Roberts, 1981, p. 47).
* Humans and environment are constantly in the process of change (Roy & Andrews, 1999, p. 37).
* For human beings, life is never the same. It is constantly changing and presenting new challenges (Roy & Andrews, 1999, p. 51).

UNIQUE FOCUS OF THE NURSING MODEL

The unique focus of the Roy Adaptation Model is changes that occur in the human adaptive system and the environment (Roy & Andrews, 1999). Adaptation is the central feature and a core concept of the Roy Adaptation Model. Problems in adaptation arise when the human adaptive system is unable to cope with or respond to stimuli from the internal and external environments in a manner that maintains the integrity of the system (Roy, 1989; Roy & Andrews, 1999).

Category of Knowledge

Roy (1989) maintained that the Roy Adaptation Model "can be viewed primarily as a systems model, although it also contains interactionist levels of analysis" (p. 105). Meleis (1997) regarded the Roy Adaptation Model as an example of the outcomes school of thought and also categorized it as client focused. Marriner-Tomey (1989) placed the model in the systems category. Barnum (1998) regarded the model as an example of her intervention category. Examination of the content of the model revealed that it reflects the characteristics of the systems category of knowledge, and some characteristics of the interaction category, as can be seen here.

Systems Category of Knowledge

- System and Integration of Parts: Living systems … are … nonlinear, multifaceted, and complex phenomena (Roy & Andrews, 1999, p. 33). Living systems, particularly human adaptive systems, involve complex processes of interaction (Roy & Andrews, 1999, p. 33). A system is a set of parts connected to function as a whole for some purpose and it does so by virtue of the interdependence of its parts (Roy & Andrews, 1999, p. 36). [A system is a] whole with parts that function as a unity for some purpose (Roy & Andrews, 1999, p. 31). Two subsystems are the regulator and cognator coping processes, which are linked through the process of perception (Roy & Roberts, 1981). Two other subsystems are the stabilizer and innovator control processes (Roy & Andrews, 1999).
- Environment: All conditions, circumstances, and influences that surround and affect the development and behavior of individuals and groups as adaptive systems, with particular consideration of mutuality of person and earth resources (Roy & Andrews, 1999, pp. 13, 31). Environment is both physical and social (Roy & Andrews, 1999, p. 38). The environment is more specifically classified as stimuli: focal, contextual, and residual (Roy & Andrews, 1999, p. 38). Human systems are affected by and, in turn, affect the world around and within. In the broadest sense, this world is called the environment (external and internal) (Roy & Andrews, 1999, p. 38). The nurse soon learns that persons never act in isolation, but are influenced by the environment and in turn affect the environment (Roy & Andrews, 1999, p. 38).
- Boundary: Not addressed explicitly in the Roy Adaptation Model.
- Tension, Stress, Strain, and Conflict: Increased force, or tension, comes from strains within the [adaptive] system or from the environment that impinges on the system (Roy, 1989, p. 105). The tension is created by the focal, contextual, and residual stimuli from the internal and external environments (Roy, 1989).

- Equilibrium: Helson's work points to adaptation as a dynamic state of equilibrium involving both heightened and lowered responses brought about by autonomic and cognitive processes triggered by internal and external stimuli (Roy & Roberts, 1981, p. 54).
- Feedback: Input for humans has been termed stimuli…. Behavior as the output of human systems takes the form of adaptive responses and ineffective responses. These responses act as feedback or further input to the systems, allowing people to decide whether to increase or decrease efforts to cope with the stimuli (Roy & Andrews, 1999, pp. 36–37). The human system and the environment are in constant interaction with each other (Roy & Andrews, 1999, p. 41).

Interaction Category of Knowledge

- Social Acts and Relationships: The Role Function Mode addresses social integrity (Roy & Andrews, 1999). The Interdependence Mode addresses relational integrity and relationships between significant others (Roy & Andrews, 1999). The group identity component of the Self-Concept/Group Identity Mode addresses interpersonal relationships (Roy & Andrews, 1999).
- Perception: Perception is addressed within the cognator coping process and the senses component of the Physiologic/Physical Mode (Roy & Andrews, 1999). [Perception is] the interpretation of a sensory stimulus and the conscious appreciation of it (Roy & Andrews, 1999, p. 259). Inputs to the regulator are transformed into perceptions. Perception is a process of the cognator [coping process]. The responses following perception are feedback into both the cognator and regulator (Roy & Roberts, 1981, p. 67).
- Communication: Communication is addressed within the context of the Interdependence Mode (Roy & Andrews, 1999).
- Role: Role is explicitly addressed through the Role Function Mode, which was deliberately developed within the context of the interactionist viewpoint (Roy, 1989).
- Self-Concept: Self-concept is explicitly addressed through the Self-Concept/Group Identity Mode, which was deliberately developed within the context of the interactionist viewpoint (Roy, 1989).

CONTENT OF THE NURSING MODEL

Concepts

The metaparadigm concepts of human beings, environment, health, and nursing are reflected in the concepts of the Roy Adaptation Model. Each conceptual model concept is classified here according to its metaparadigm forerunner.

The metaparadigm concept of human beings is represented by the Roy Adaptation Model concepts of **HUMAN ADAPTIVE SYSTEM, COPING PROCESSES, BEHAVIOR,** and **ADAPTIVE MODES.** The concept of **HUMAN ADAPTIVE SYSTEM** is has two dimensions—**Individual Persons** and **Groups or Relational Persons.** The concept of COPING PROCESSES has four dimensions—**Regulator Coping Subsystem, Cognator Coping Subsysteml, Stabilizer Subsystem Control Process,** and **Innovator Subsystem Control Process.** The concept of **BEHAVIOR** has two dimensions—**Adaptive Response** and **Ineffective Response.** The concept of **ADAPTIVE MODES** has four dimensions—**Physiological/Physical Mode, Self-Concept/Group Identity Mode, Role Function Mode,** and **Interdependence Mode.** The Physiological Mode component of the dimension **Physiological/Physical Mode** has nine subdimensions—Oxygenation; Nutrition; Elimination; Activity and Rest; Protection; Senses; Fluid, Electrolyte, and Acid-Base Balance; Neurological Function; and Endocrine Function.

The Self-Concept component of the dimension **Self-Concept/Group Identity Mode** encompasses two subdimensions—Physical Self (Body Sensation, Body Image) and Personal Self (Self-Consistency, Self-Ideal, Moral-Ethical-Spiritual Self). The Group Identity Mode component of the dimension **Self-Concept/Group Identity Mode** encompasses four subdimensions—Interpersonal Relationships, Group Self-Image, Social Milieu, and Group Culture.

The dimension **Role Function** encompasses seven subdimensions—Primary Role, Secondary Role, Tertiary Role, Instrumental Behavior, Expressive Behavior, Role-Taking, and Integrating Roles. The dimension **Interdependence Mode** encompasses three subdimensions for individuals and groups—Affectional Adequacy, Developmental Adequacy, and Resource Adequacy; two subdimensions for individuals—Significant Others and Support Systems; and three subdimensions for groups—Context, Infrastructure, and Resources.

The metaparadigm concept of environment is represented by the Roy Adaptation Model concept of **STIMULI.** That concept has three dimensions—**Focal Stimulus, Contextual Stimuli,** and **Residual Stimuli.**

The metaparadigm concepts of human beings and environment are represented by the Roy Adaptation Model concepts of **ADAPTATION** and **ADAPTATION LEVEL.** The concept of **ADAPTATION** has five dimensions—**Survival, Growth, Reproduction, Mastery,** and **Person and Environment Transformations.** The concept of ADAPTATION LEVEL has three dimensions—**Integrated Life Process, Compensatory Life Process,** and **Compromised**

Life Process. The metaparadigm concept of health is represented by the Roy Adaptation Model concept of **HEALTH,** which is unidimensional.

The metaparadigm concept ofnursing is represented by the Roy Adaptation Model concepts of **SCIENCE** and **ART.** The concept of **SCIENCE** has two dimensions—**Basic Nursing Science** and **Clinical Nursing Science.** The concept of **ART** is unidimensional.

Nonrelational Propositions

The definitions of the concepts of the Roy Adaptation Model are given listed here. Those constitutive definitions are the nonrelational propositions of this nursing model.

HUMAN ADAPTIVE SYSTEM

- A whole with parts that function as a unity for some purpose (Roy & Andrews, 1999, p. 31).
- Human systems function as wholes in one unified expression of meaningful human behavior. They are, then, more than the sum of their parts (Roy & Andrews, 1991, p. 35).
- Human systems have thinking and feeling capacities rooted in consciousness and meaning, by which they adjust effectively to changes in the environment and, in turn, affect the environment (Roy & Andrews, 1999, p. 36).
- Human systems include people as individuals or in groups including families, organizations, communities, and society as a whole (Roy & Andrews, 1999, p. 31).

The concept of **Human Adaptive System** has two dimensions—Individual Persons and Groups or Relational Persons.

- **Individual Persons:** Refers to a single person as the human adaptive system.
- **Groups or Relational Persons:** Groups refer to the human adaptive system as a collective or aggregate (Roy & Andrews, 1999). Relational Persons refers to the human adaptive system as individuals relating in groups such as families, organizations, communities, nations, and society as a whole (Hanna & Roy, 2001; Roy, 2003), or groups of persons in relationships (Hanna & Roy, 2001, p. 9).

COPING PROCESSES

- Innate or acquired ways of interacting with (responding to and influencing) the changing environment (Roy & Andrews, 1999, p. 46).
- Innate coping processes are genetically determined or common to the species and are generally viewed as

automatic process; humans do not have to think about them (Roy & Andrews, 1999, p. 46).

- Acquired coping processes are developed through strategies such as learning. The experiences encountered throughout life contribute to customary responses to particular stimuli (Roy & Andrews, 1999, p. 46).

Roy and Andrews (1999) identified dimensions for the concept of **Coping Processes** that pertain to individuals and dimensions that pertain to groups. The dimension Regulator Coping Subsystem pertains to the individual; its group counterpart is the dimension Stabilizer Subsystem Control Process. Similarly, the dimension Cognator Coping Subsystem pertains to the individual; its group counterpart is the dimension Innovator Subsystem Control Process. Roy and Andrews (1999) explained, "Just as the adaptive individual has neural-chemical-endocrine activities and engages in processes that act to maintain homeostasis, equilibrium, and growth potential, so the group, as an adaptive system, has strategies and engages in processes that act to stabilize. … [And] just as the cognator for the person involves cognitive and emotional channels for responding to a changing environment, the aggregate has parallel information and human processes for innovation and change. The innovator dynamism involves cognitive and emotional [short-term and long-term] strategies for change to higher levels of potential' (pp. 47–48).

Consequently, the concept of **Coping Processes** encompasses four dimensions—Regulator Coping Subsystem, Cognator Coping Subsystem, Stabilizer Subsystem Control Process, and Innovator Subsystem Control Process.

- **Regulator Coping Subsystem**: For individuals, a major coping process involving the neural, chemical, and endocrine systems (Roy & Andrews, 1999, p. 32). A basic type of adaptive process … [that] responds automatically through neural, chemical, and endocrine coping channels (Roy & Andrews, 1999, p. 46).
- **Cognator Coping Subsystem**: For individuals, a major coping process involving four cognitive-emotive channels: perceptual and information processing, learning, judgment, and emotion (Roy & Andrews, 1999, p. 31). Perceptual and information processing includes the activities of selective attention, coding, and memory (Roy & Andrews, 1999, pp. 46–47). Learning involves imitation, reinforcement, and insight (Roy & Andrews, 1999, p. 47). The judgment process encompasses such activities as problem solving and decision making (Roy & Andrews, 1999, p. 47). Through the person's emotions, defenses are used to seek relief from anxiety to make affective appraisal and attachments (Roy & Andrews, 1999, p. 47).

Roy (1984a) explained that for the Regulator Coping Subsystem, "the internal and external stimuli are basically chemical or neural and act as inputs to the central nervous system and may be transduced into neural inputs. The spinal cord, brain stem, and autonomic reflexes act through effectors to produce automatic, unconscious effects on the body responses. The chemical stimuli in the circulation influence the endocrine glands to produce the appropriate hormone. The responsiveness of target organs or tissues then [a]ffects body responses. By some unknown process, the neural inputs are transformed into conscious perceptions in the brain. Eventually, this perception leads to psychomotor choices of response which activate a body response. These bodily responses, brought about through the chemical-neural-endocrine channels, are fed back as additional stimuli to the regulator" (p. 31). For the Cognator Coping Subsystem, information is processed through the perceptual and information processing, learning, judgment, and emotion channels, and responses are produced (Roy & Andrews, 1999).

Elaborating on the differences between the Regulator Coping Subsystem and the Cognator Coping Subsystem, Roy and Corliss (1993) noted that "the cognitive-emotional processes of the cognator act within varying levels of consciousness as the person deals with internal and external states. [In contrast,] the neuro-chemical-endocrine processes of the regulator may be outside of consciousness, but provide the substrates of human conscious processes and actions" (p. 219).

- **Stabilizer Subsystem Control Process**: For groups, the subsystem associated with system maintenance and involving established structures, values, and daily activities whereby participants accomplish the purpose of the social system (Roy & Andrews, 1999, p. 32). Act[s] to stabilize [and] involves the established structures, values, and daily activities whereby participants accomplish the primary purpose of the group and contribute to common purposes of society (Roy & Andrews, 1999, p. 47).
- **Innovator Subsystem Control Process**: Pertaining to humans in a group, the internal subsystem that involves structures and processes for change and growth (Roy & Andrews, 1999, p. 31). [The] subsystem [that] involves the structures and processes for change and growth in human social systems (Roy & Andrews, 1999, p. 48).

BEHAVIOR

- Internal or external actions and reactions under specified circumstances (Roy & Andrews, 1999, p. 30).
- All responses of the human adaptive system including capacities, assets, knowledge, skills, abilities, and commitments (Roy & Andrews, 1999, p. 63).

Behavior, Roy and Andrews (1999) explained, pertains to both individuals and groups, and can be "observed, sometimes measured, or subjectively reported" (p. 43).

The concept of **Behavior** encompasses two dimensions—Adaptive Responses and Ineffective Responses.

- **Adaptive Responses:** Behaviors that promote integrity in terms of the goals of human systems (Roy & Andrews, 1999, pp. 30, 67). Responses that promote the integrity of the human system in terms of the goals of adaptation: survival, growth, reproduction, mastery, and person and environment transformations (Roy & Andrews, 1999, p. 44).

Adaptive Responses refers to those behaviors that appropriately meet the goals of adaptation. Although one goal is survival, "in some situations and at some developmental stages, the appropriate response may be discontinuation of the system [i.e., the group], or death, as it relates to the individual" (Roy & Andrews, 1999, p. 44).

- **Ineffective Responses:** Behaviors that do not contribute to integrity in terms of the goals of the human system (Roy & Andrews, 1999, pp. 31, 67). Responses ... that neither promote integrity nor contribute to the goals of adaptation and the integration of persons with the earth (Roy & Andrews, 1999, p. 44). [Responses that] can, in the immediate situation or if continued over a long time, threaten the human system's survival, growth, reproduction, mastery, or person and environment transformations (Roy & Andrews, 1999, p. 44).

ADAPTIVE MODES

- Ways of behaving (Roy & Andrews, 1999, p. 99).
- Ways of manifesting adaptive processes (Roy, 2003)
- Four categories or modes in which behaviors of both individuals and [groups] that result from coping activity can be observed (Roy & Andrews, 1999).

The concept of **Adaptive Modes** encompasses four dimensions—Physiological/Physical Mode, Self-Concept/Group Identity Mode, Role Function Mode, and Interdependence Mode. Although the four dimensions of the concept of **Adaptive Modes** are discussed separately, they are interrelated. In particular, "behavior in [one] mode may have an effect on or act as a stimulus for one or all of the other modes" (Roy & Andrews, 1999, p. 51).

Adaptive Modes pertain to both individual and group **Human Adaptive Systems**, with certain components of the four dimensions (Physiological/Physical Mode, Self-Concept/Group Identity Mode, Role Function Mode, Interdependence Mode) encompassing subdimensions relevant for the individual and others for the group.

- **Physiological/Physical Mode:** The Physiological/Physical Mode is made up of two components—the Physiological Mode and the Physical Mode. [The Physiological Mode component pertains to the individual. It is the mode] in which a person manifests the physical and chemical processes involved in the function and activities of a living organism (Roy & Andrews, 1999, p. 101). [The Physiological Mode component] is associated with the way humans as individuals interact as physical beings with the environment. Behavior in this mode is the manifestation of the physiologic activities of all the cells, tissues, organs, and systems comprising the human body. ... The underlying need ... is physiologic integrity (Roy & Andrews, 1999, pp. 48–49). [The Physical Mode component pertains to groups. It is the] manner in which the collective human adaptive system manifests adaptation relative to needs associated with basic operating resources (Roy & Andrews, 1999, p. 100). The Physical Mode component focuses on physical operating resources (Roy, 2003). [The Physical Mode component] pertains to the manner in which the collective human adaptive system manifests adaptation relative to basic operating resources, that is, participants, physical facilities, and fiscal resources. The basic need ... for the group is resource adequacy, or wholeness achieved by adapting to change in physical resource needs (Roy & Andrews, 1999, p. 49).

The Physiological Mode component of the dimension Physiological/Physical Mode encompasses nine subdimensions—*Oxygenation*; *Nutrition*; *Elimination*; *Activity and Rest*; *Protection*; *Senses*; *Fluid, Electrolyte, and Acid-Base Balance*; *Neurological Function*; and *Endocrine Function*.

- *Oxygenation*: One of five basic needs (Roy & Andrews, 1999). The processes (ventilation, gas exchange, and transport of gases [to and from the tissues]) by which cellular oxygen supply is maintained in the body (Roy & Andrews, 1999, p. 126).
- *Nutrition*: One of five basic needs (Roy & Andrews, 1999). The series of processes by which a person takes in nutrients and assimilates and uses them to maintain body tissue, promote growth, and provide energy (Roy & Andrews, 1999, p. 149). Concerns the food people eat and how their bodies use it (Roy & Andrews, 1999, p. 149).
- *Elimination*: One of five basic needs (Roy & Andrews, 1999). A life process that concerns elimination of waste products from the body, including intestinal elimination and urinary elimination (Roy & Andrews, 1999). Intestinal elimination is the expulsion from the body of undigested substances via the anus in the form of feces (Roy & Andrews, 1999, p. 171). Urinary elimination pertains to the elimination of fluid wastes

and excess ions as a result of the filtering process in which the kidneys maintain the purity and constancy of internal fluids (Roy & Andrews, 1999, p. 171).

- *Activity and Rest*: One of five basic needs (Roy & Andrews, 1999). Activity refers to body movement and serves various purposes such as carrying out daily living chores and protecting self or others from bodily injuries. Mobility is the basic life process for activity (Roy & Andrews, 1999, p. 193). Rest … involves changes in activity in which energy requirements are minimal.… Sleep is the basic life process for rest (Roy & Andrews, 1999, p. 193). [Rest] more generally [refers to] refreshing relaxation (Roy & Andrews, 1999, p. 193).
- *Protection*: One of five basic needs (Roy & Andrews, 1999). Consists of two basic life processes: nonspecific defense processes and specific defense processes. Together these two functional defense systems work to protect the body from "foreign" substances such as bacteria, viruses, transplanted tissues, and abnormal body cells (Roy & Andrews, 1999, p. 233). Nonspecific defenses processes [are] surface membrane barriers and cellular and chemical defenses which function to hinder pathogen entry, prevent the spread of disease-causing microorganisms, and strengthen the immune response (Roy & Andrews, 1999, p. 233). Specific defense processes [are those] that are targeted against specific antigens (Roy & Andrews, 1999, p. 233).
- *Senses*: One of four complex processes (Roy & Andrews, 1999). Channels of input necessary for the person to interact with the changing environment … [including] seeing [vision], hearing, and feeling (Roy & Andrews, 1999, p. 257). Vision is a complex process involving the peripheral structure of the eye, visual neural pathways, and the visual area of the cerebral cortex in the occipital lobe of the brain (Roy & Andrews, 1999, p. 260). Hearing [is] a complex process involving the peripheral structure of the ear, auditory neural pathways, and the auditory areas of the brain whereby sound waves are detected, transmitted, and interpreted (Roy & Andrews, 1999, p. 258). Feeling [is] a complex process involving the somatosensory system whereby touch and pressure, position sense, heat and cold, and pain are detected, transmitted, and interpreted (Roy & Andrews, 1999, p. 258).
- *Fluid, Electrolyte, and Acid-Base Balance*: One of four complex processes (Roy & Andrews, 1999). Fluid Balance [refers to the balance of fluids] between intracellular and extracellular compartments (Roy & Andrews, 1999, p. 296). [Fluids are] internal body fluids located within (intracellular) and outside (extracellular) body cells, [or] in various parts of the body not available for general body use, for example, joint fluid

or pericardial fluid (third space fluids) (Roy & Andrews, 1999, p. 294). Electrolyte Balance addresses concentrations of salts within the body (Roy & Andrews, 1999, p. 297). [Electrolytes are] substances [salts] that break down into ions when in solution (Roy & Andrews, 1999, p. 294). [Acid-Base Balance refers to the] status of body fluids [with regard to] the concentration of hydrogen ions and is described in terms of pH (Roy & Andrews, 1999, p. 298).

- *Neurological Function*: One of four complex processes (Roy & Andrews, 1999). Refers to the components of the central nervous system (brain and spinal cord) and peripheral nervous system (cranial and spinal nerves); the peripheral nervous system has afferent and efferent components; the efferent component includes the autonomic nervous system (Roy & Andrews, 1999) Two basic life processes that are key to neurologic function are cognition and consciousness (Roy & Andrews, 1999, p. 313). Cognition [is] a broad term encompassing the human abilities to think, feel, and act (Roy & Andrews, 1999, p. 314). Consciousness [is] the level of arousal and awareness, including orientation to the environment and self-awareness (Roy & Andrews, 1999, p. 314).
- *Endocrine Function*: One of four complex processes (Roy & Andrews, 1999). In close association with the autonomic nervous system, integrates and maintains all the body's physiologic processes to promote normal growth, development, and maintenance of structure and function (Roy & Andrews, 1999, p. 355).

- **Self-Concept/Group Identity Mode:** [Behavior] pertaining to the personal aspects of human systems (Roy & Andrews, 1999, p. 49). The Self-Concept/Group Identity Mode is made up of two components—the Self-Concept Mode and the Group Identity Mode. [The Self-Concept Mode component pertains to the individual. It addresses] the composite of beliefs and feelings that a person holds about him- or herself at a given time. … The basic [underlying] need … [is] psychic and spiritual integrity, the need to know who one is so that one can be or exist with a sense of unity, meaning, and purposefulness in the universe (Roy & Andrews, 1999, pp. 49, 382). [The Self-Concept Mode component addresses] the composite of beliefs and feelings that is held about oneself at a given time, formed from internal perceptions and perceptions of others' reactions (Roy, 2003). [The Group Identity Mode component pertains to groups. It addresses] shared relations, goals, and values, which create a social milieu and culture, a group self-image, and coresponsibility for goal achievement. Identity integrity is the [underlying] need, [which] implies the honesty, soundness, and completeness of the group members' identification with the group [and] involves [the] process of sharing identity and goals (Roy & Andrews, 1999, pp. 49, 381).

The Self-Concept component of the dimension Self-Concept/Group Identity Mode encompasses two subdimensions—*Physical Self* (Body Sensation, Body Image) and *Personal Self* (Self-Consistency, Self-Ideal, Moral-Ethical-Spiritual Self).

- *Physical Self*: A component of the Self-Concept Mode (Roy & Andrews, 1999, p. 49). The person's appraisal of one's own physical being, including physical attributes, functioning, sexuality, health and illness states, and appearance; includes the components of body sensation and body image (Roy & Andrews, 1999, p. 383). Body sensation [refers to] how one feels and experiences the self as a physical being (Roy & Andrews, 1999, p. 381). Body image [refers to] how one views oneself physically and one's view of personal appearance (Roy & Andrews, 1999, p. 381).
- *Personal Self*: A component of the Self-Concept Mode (Roy & Andrews, 1999, p. 49). The individual's appraisal of one's own characteristics, expectations, values, and worth, including self-consistency, self-ideal, and the moral-ethical-spiritual self (Roy & Andrews, 1999, p. 381). Self-Consistency [refers to] that part of the personal self ... which strives to maintain a consistent self-organization and to avoid disequilibrium; an organized system of ideas about self (Roy & Andrews, 1999, p. 382). Self-Ideal [refers to] that aspect of the personal self ... which relates to what the person would like to be or is capable of doing (Roy & Andrews, 1999, p. 382). Moral-Ethical-Spiritual Self [refers to] that aspect of the personal self which includes a belief system and an evaluation of who one is in relation to the universe (Roy & Andrews, 1999, p. 381).

The Group Identity Mode component of the dimension Self-Concept/Group Identity Mode encompasses four subdimensions—*Interpersonal Relationships, Group Self-Image, Social Milieu*, and *Group Culture*.

- *Interpersonal Relationships*: A component of the Group Identity Mode (Roy & Andrews, 1999, p. 49).
- *Group Self-Image*: A component of the Group Identity Mode (Roy & Andrews, 1999, p. 49).
- *Social Milieu*: A component of the Group Identity Mode (Roy & Andrews, 1999, p. 49).
- *Group Culture*: A component of the Group Identity Mode (Roy & Andrews, 1999, p. 49). The group's agreed upon expectations, including values, goals, and norms for relating (Roy & Andrews, 1999, p. 381).

- **Role Function Mode**: Behavior pertaining to roles in human systems (Roy & Andrews, 1999, p. 49). [The Role Function Mode for the individual] focuses on the roles that the individual occupies in society. Role [refers to] the functioning unit of society [and] is defined as a set of expectations about how a person occupying one position behaves toward a person occupying another position. The basic [underlying] need is social integrity, the need to know who one is in relation to others so that one can act (Roy & Andrews, 1999, pp. 49–50). [The Role Function Mode for the group focuses on] the action components associated with group infrastructure [that] are designed to contribute to the accomplishment of the group's mission, or the tasks or functions associated with the group. ...The basic [underlying] need is ... role clarity, the need to understand and commit to fulfill expected tasks, so that the group can achieve common goals (Roy & Andrews, 1999, p. 50).

The dimension Role Function Mode encompasses seven subdimensions—*Primary Role, Secondary Role, Tertiary Role, Instrumental Behavior, Expressive Behavior, Role-Taking*, and *Integrating Roles*.

- *Primary Role*: An ascribed role based on age, sex, and developmental stage; it determines the majority of behaviors engaged in by a person during a particular growth period of life (Roy & Andrews, 1999, p. 431).
- *Secondary Role*: A role that a person assumes to complete the tasks associated with a developmental stage and primary role (Roy & Andrews, 1999, p. 432).
- *Tertiary Role*: A role that is freely chosen by a person, temporary in nature, and often associated with the accomplishment of a minor task in a person's current development (Roy & Andrews, 1999, p. 432).
- *Instrumental Behavior*: Goal-oriented behavior; role activities the person performs (Roy & Andrews, 1999, p. 430).
- *Expressive Behavior*: The feelings and attitudes held by the person about role performance (Roy & Andrews, 1999, p. 430).
- *Role-Taking*: A process of looking at or anticipating another person's behavior by viewing it within a role attributed to the other; basing one's interaction on the judgment about the other's role; focuses on the meaning that the acts have to both persons in a role interaction (Roy & Andrews, 1999, p. 431).
- *Integrating Roles*: The process of managing different roles and their expectations (Roy & Andrews, 1999, p. 431).

- **Interdependence Mode:** Behavior pertaining to interdependent relationships of individuals and groups. ... The basic [underlying] need is ... relational integrity, the feeling of security in nurturing relationships (Roy & Andrews, 1999, p. 50). The close relationships of people aimed at satisfying needs for affection, development and resources to achieve relational integrity (Roy, 2003). [The Interdependence Mode for the individual] focuses on interactions related to the giving and receiving of love, respect, and value (Roy & Andrews, 1999, p. 50). [The Interdependence Mode for the group] pertains to the social context in which the group operates [including] both private and public contacts both within the group and with those outside the group (Roy & Andrews, 1999, p. 50).

The dimension Interdependence Mode encompasses three subdimensions for individuals and groups—*Affectional Adequacy, Developmental Adequacy*, and *Resource Adequacy*; two subdimensions for individuals—*Significant Others* and *Support Systems*; and three subdimensions for groups—*Context, Infrastructure*, and *Resources*.

- *Affectional Adequacy* (*Individuals and Groups*): The need to give and receive love, respect, and value satisfied through effective relations and communication (Roy & Andrews, 1999, p. 474).
- *Developmental Adequacy* (*Individuals and Groups*): [Refers to] learning and maturation in relationships achieved through developmental processes (Roy & Andrews, 1999, p. 474).
- *Resource Adequacy* (*Individuals and Groups*): The need for food, clothing, shelter, health, and security achieved through interdependent processes (Roy & Andrews, 1999, p. 475).
- *Significant Others* (*Individuals*): The individuals to whom the most meaning or importance is given [by a person] (Roy & Andrews, 1999, p. 475).
- *Support Systems* (*Individuals*): Persons, groups, [and] organizations with whom one associates in order to achieve affectional, developmental, and resources requirements (Roy & Andrews, 1999, p. 475).
- *Context* (*Groups*): External (economic, social, political, cultural, belief, family systems) and internal (mission, vision, values, principles, goals, plans) influences within relationships (Roy & Andrews, 1999, p. 474).
- *Infrastructure* (*Groups*): The affectional, resource, and developmental processes that exist within a relationship (Roy & Andrews, 1999, p. 474).
- *Resources* (*Groups*): Refers to food, clothing, shelter, meeting places, physical facilities for organizations, supplies, equipment, technology, and finances (Roy & Andrews, 1999).

Roy and Andrews (1999) include the notion of integrity in their definitions of the dimensions of the concepts of **Behavior** and **Adaptive Modes**. In particular, they speak to **Behavior** that promotes (Adaptive Responses) or does not contribute to (Ineffective Responses) integrity, and to the need for physiological integrity (Physiological Mode component of the Physiological/Physical Mode), psychic and spiritual integrity (Self-Concept component of the Self-Concept/Group Identity Mode), identity integrity (Group Identity component of the Self-Concept/Group Identity Mode), social integrity (Role Function Mode), and relational integrity (Interdependence Mode). They explained that they use the term integrity "to mean soundness or an unimpaired condition leading to wholeness" (p. 54).

STIMULI

- [A stimulus is] that which provokes a response, or more generally, the point of interaction of the human system and the environment (Roy & Andrews, 1999, p. 32).
- A stimulus is a factor in the internal environment (internal stimulus) or external environment (external stimulus) that provokes a response (Roy & Andrews, 1999).
- Common stimuli are culture, including socioeconomic status, ethnicity, and belief system; the structure and tasks of a family or aggregate; developmental stage, including the individual's age, sex, tasks, heredity, and genetic factors, or the longevity and vision of an aggregate; the integrity of the adaptive modes; the adaptation level; the perception, knowledge, and skill aspects of cognator or innovator effectiveness; and environmental considerations, including changes in the internal or external environment, medical management, use of drugs, alcohol, and tobacco, and political or economic stability (Roy & Andrews, 1999, p. 72).

The concept of **Stimuli** encompasses three dimensions—**Focal Stimulus, Contextual Stimuli,** and **Residual Stimuli.**

- **Focal Stimulus:** The internal or external [environmental] stimulus most immediately in the awareness of the human system; the object or event most present in consciousness (Roy & Andrews, 1999, p. 38). The internal or external stimulus most immediately confronting the human adaptive system (Roy & Andrews, 1999, p. 66).
- **Contextual Stimuli:** All other stimuli present in the situation that contribute to the effect of the focal stimulus.... All the environmental factors that present to the human system from within or without but which are not the center of attention or energy. These factors will influence how the human system can deal with the focal stimulus (Roy & Andrews, 1999, p. 39). All internal and external stimuli evident in the situation other than the focal stimulus (Roy & Andrews, 1999, p. 66).

- **Residual Stimuli:** Environmental factors within or without human systems, the effects of which are unclear in the current situation. There may not be awareness of the influence of these factors, or it may not be clear to the observer that they are having an effect (Roy & Andrews, 1999, p. 39). Those stimuli having an undetermined effect on the behavior of the human adaptive system (Roy & Andrews, 1999, p. 66).

The classification of any stimulus as a Focal Stimulus, a Contextual Stimulus, or a Residual Stimulus depends on its influence on adaptation in a particular situation. Moreover, the classification of a particular stimulus as focal, contextual, or residual changes rapidly as the situation changes. "What is focal at one time soon becomes contextual and what is contextual may slip far enough into the background to become residual, that is, just a possible influence" (Roy & Andrews, 1999, p. 40).

Roy and Corliss (1993) pointed out that the dimension Residual Stimuli of the concept of Stimuli "is particularly compatible with [Roy's] philosophical assumptions about the person. ... [A]lways being aware of a category for residual stimuli allows for the mystery in each person since each is unique within the common destiny and the nurse may not expect to know the other as the other knows self or is known by the Creator" (pp. 220–221). Residual stimuli become contextual stimuli or the focal stimulus when their effects on the person are validated (Andrews & Roy, 1991b).

ADAPTATION

- The process and outcome whereby thinking and feeling persons, as individuals or in groups, use conscious awareness and choice to create human and environmental integration (Roy & Andrews, 1999, p. 30).

The concept of **Adaption** encompasses five dimensions—Survival, Growth, Reproduction, Mastery, and Person and Environment Transformations.

- **Survival:** A goal of adaptation (Roy & Andrews, 1999, p. 44). A goal of human systems (Roy & Andrews, 1999, p. 30).
- **Growth:** A goal of adaptation (Roy & Andrews, 1999, p. 44). A goal of human systems (Roy & Andrews, 1999, p. 30).
- **Reproduction:** A goal of adaptation (Roy & Andrews, 1999, p. 44). A goal of human systems (Roy & Andrews, 1999, p. 30). Not limited to a physiologic bringing forth of off-spring, but also is seen as generativity of other kinds, e.g., mentoring, producing works of art, and generating other accomplishments that actualize oneself (Artinian & Roy, 1990, p. 65). Includes the continuation of the human species by having children, but it also in-

volves the many ways that people extend themselves in time and space by creative works and moral presence (Roy & Andrews, 1999, p. 44).
- **Mastery:** A goal of adaptation (Roy & Andrews, 1999, p. 44). A goal of human systems (Roy & Andrews, 1999, p. 30).
- **Person and Environment Transformations:** A goal of adaptation (Roy & Andrews, 1999, p. 44). A goal of human systems (Roy & Andrews, 1999, p. 30).

ADAPTATION LEVEL

- A key factor of the internal environment (Roy & Andrews, 1999, p. 42).
- A significant internal stimulus (Roy & Andrews, 1999, p. 38).
- The condition of the life processes as a significant focal, contextual, or residual stimulus in a situation (Roy & Andrews, 1999, p. 42).
- The pooled defect of focal, contextual, and residual stimuli determines the adaptation level (Roy & Andrews, 1999, p. 547).
- A changing point influenced by the demands of the situation and the internal resources [of the human adaptive system, including] capabilities, hopes, dreams, aspirations, motivations, and all that makes humans constantly move toward mastery (Roy & Andrews, 1999, p. 33).

The concept of **Adaptation Level** encompasses three dimensions—Integrated Life Process, Compensatory Life Process, and Compromised Life Process.

- **Integrated Life Process:** Adaptation level at which the structures and functions of a life process are working as a whole to meet human needs (Roy & Andrews, 1999, p. 31).
- **Compensatory Life Process:** Adaptation level at which the cognator and regulator [or stabilizer and innovator] have been activated by a challenge to the integrated life processes (Roy, 2003; Roy & Andrews, 1999, p. 31).
- **Compromised Life Process:** Adaptation level resulting from inadequate integrated and compensatory life process; an adaptation problem (Roy & Andrews, 1999, p. 31).

The definitions for Integrated Life Process, Compensatory Life Process, and Compromised Life Process suggest that they are hierarchical. That inference is supported by Roy and Andrews' (1999) statement that "an integrated life process may change to a compensatory process which evokes attempts to reestablish adaptation. If the compensatory processes are not adequate, compromised processes result" (p. 37).

HEALTH

- A state and process of being and becoming integrated and whole that reflects person and environment mutuality (Roy & Andrews, 1999, p. 13).
- Being integrated is a state at any given point in time and may be described as such at that point in time. This state is reflective of the adaptation process. It is manifested by the wholeness and integration of physiologic components, self concept, role function, and interdependence (Artinian & Roy, 1990, p. 65).
- Becoming is a process that is continuous and made up of the systematic series of actions directed toward some end. … This end [is] related to both individual goals and the purposefulness of human existence (Artinian & Roy, 1990, p. 65).
- A whole person is one with the highest possible fulfillment of human potential (Andrews & Roy, 1986, p. 8).

The definition of **Health** is linked to the interaction between human beings and the environment, that is, to **Adaptation**. Andrews and Roy (1991a) explained, "[The] person [is] described as an adaptive system constantly growing and developing within a changing environment. A person's health can be described as a reflection of this interaction or adaptation. … Health can be viewed in light of individual goals and the purposefulness of human existence. The fulfillment of one's purpose in life is reflected in becoming an integrated and whole person" (p. 19).

Roy and Corliss (1993) regard **Adaptation** and **Health** as "on-going processes" (p. 221). They went on to explain that **Adaptation** "is a process of promoting integrity, or one may also say that adaptation means interacting positively with the environment and thereby promoting health. One's health does not depend on the absence or presence of disease, rather it relates to use of the processes that lead to patterns of integrity of the person and the ability to move toward effective unity of the adaptive modes" (p. 221). "A lack of integration [is] a lack of health" (Andrews & Roy, 1991a, p. 8).

Roy (1987c; Artinian & Roy, 1990) rejected her earlier conceptualization of health as a continuum from maximum wellness to maximum illness. Indeed, she maintained that her view of health is not consistent with the notion of the health-illness continuum, because it "is a limited view and reflects a given point in time on a continuum" (Roy, 1987c, p. 42). She noted that being and becoming integrated and whole may occur throughout life. Even "dying individuals are going through that process of final being and becoming where they are integrating themselves" (Roy, 1987c, pp. 42–43). Thus "it is more consistent with the model's scientific and philosophical assumptions to continue conceptual explication of the notion of health without reference to illness" (Artinian & Roy, 1990, p. 65). However, Roy and Andrews (1999) referred to both health

and illness in their statement that "it is the nurse's role to promote adaptation in situations of health and illness" (p. 55).

It may be inferred that health is viewed as a dichotomy of Adaptive Responses and Ineffective Responses to changing environmental **Stimuli**. This interpretation is supported by the definition of Adaptive Responses as those promoting integrity of the person and the definition of Ineffective Responses as those not contributing to integrity.

SCIENCE

- Deals with understanding both the how and the why questions (Roy & Andrews, 1999, p. 536).

The concept of Science encompasses two dimensions—Basic Nursing Science and Clinical Nursing Science.

- **Basic Nursing Science:** The basic science of nursing focuses on human life processes [which are mutually interactive with the total ecology] as the core of knowledge to be developed (Roy, 1988b, p. 27). Understanding of the basic life processes that promote health (Roy & Andrews, 1999, p. 536).
- **Clinical Nursing Science:** The clinical science of nursing is based on the basic science of nursing as well as on the history and philosophy of nursing, which includes a strong ethical heritage. It [is directed toward the development of] substantive knowledge related to the diagnosis and treatment of the patterning of the life processes in wellness and traditional life situations, in chronic and acute illness, and particularly in life situations when the positive [adaptive] processes are threatened by health technologies and behaviorally induced health problems (Roy, 1988b, p. 28). Understanding how human systems cope with health and illness and what can be done to promote adaptive coping (Roy & Andrews, 1999, p. 536).

ART

- Deals with understanding and expressing the realities of life (Roy & Andrews, 1999, p. 536).

Roy (1976a) described nursing as "a theoretical system of knowledge which prescribes a process of analysis and action related to the care of the ill or potentially ill person" (p. 3). Furthermore, nursing is "a scientific discipline that is practice oriented" (Andrews & Roy, 1991b, p. 27). The Roy Adaptation Model stipulates that a nurse is needed "when unusual stresses or weakened coping mechanisms make the person's usual attempts to cope ineffective" (Roy & Roberts, 1981, p. 45).

Roy (1970; Roy & Roberts, 1981) distinguished nursing from medicine by noting that medicine focuses on biological systems and the person's disease, whereas nursing focuses on the person as a total being who responds to internal and external environmental stimuli. This distinction is elaborated further by a comparison of the goals of medicine and nursing. The physician's goal is "to move the patient along the continuum from illness to health" (Roy, 1970, p. 43).

In contrast, the **GOAL OF NURSING** is:

> To promote adaptation for individuals and groups in the four adaptive modes, thus contributing to health, quality of life, and dying with dignity by assessing behavior and factors that influence adaptive abilities and by intervening to expand those abilities and to enhance environmental interactions (Roy & Andrews, 1999, p. 13).

Roy and Roberts (1981) placed the **Goal of Nursing** within the context of the overall goal of the health team when they stated, "The projected outcome [of nursing] is an adapted state in the patient which frees him to respond to other stimuli. This freeing of energy makes it possible for the goal of nursing to contribute to the overall goal of the health team, high-level wellness. When energy is freed from inadequate coping attempts, then it can promote healing and wellness" (p. 45).

Roy and Andrews (1999) pointed out that it is not possible for every human system to experience optimal health, in the commonly recognized form of complete physical, mental, and social well-being. It is therefore the nurse's role "to increase the person's adaptive response[s] and to decrease ineffective responses" (Roy, 1984a, p. 37). It also is the nurse's role "to promote adaptation in situations of health and illness and to enhance the interaction of human systems with the environment ... through acceptance, protection, and fostering of interdependence and to promote personal and environmental transformations" (Roy & Andrews, 1999, p. 55).

The Roy Adaptation Model includes a detailed **PRACTICE METHODOLOGY**, in the form of the **ROY ADAPTATION MODEL NURSING PROCESS**. Roy and Andrews (1999) regard the **ROY ADAPTATION MODEL NURSING PROCESS** as "a problem-solving approach for gathering data, identifying capacities and needs, establishing goals, selecting and implementing approaches for nursing care, and evaluating the outcomes of care provided" (pp. 63–64). The components of the **ROY ADAPTATION MODEL NURSING PROCESS** are outlined in Table 10–1.

▶ **TABLE 10–1**
PRACTICE METHODOLOGY: THE ROY ADAPTATION MODEL NURSING PROCESS

ASSESSMENT OF BEHAVIOR

The nurse systematically gathers data about the behavior of the human adaptive system and judges the current state of adaptation in each adaptive mode.

The nurse uses one or more of the Roy Adaptation Model–based research instruments or practice tools to guide application and documentation of the practice methodology (see Table 10–2).

Gathering Behavioral Data
The nurse systematically gathers data about observable and nonobservable behaviors for each dimension and subdimension of the four adaptive modes, focusing on the individual or the group of interest.

The nurse gathers behavioral data by means of observation, using the senses of sight, sound, touch, taste, and smell; objective measurement, using paper and pencil instruments and measures of physiological parameters; and purposeful interviews.

Tentative Judgment of Behavior
The nurse, in collaboration with the human adaptive system of interest, makes a tentative judgment about behaviors in each adaptive mode.

Behaviors are tentatively judged as adaptive or ineffective responses, using the criteria of the human adaptive system's individualized goals and comparison of the behaviors with norms signifying adaptation. If norms are not available, the nurse considers adaptation difficulty as pronounced regulator activity with cognator ineffectiveness for individuals, or pronounced stabilizer activity with innovator ineffectiveness for groups.

The nurse sets priorities for further assessment, taking the dimensions (goals) of adaptation into account.

(continued)

> **TABLE 10–1**
> **PRACTICE METHODOLOGY: THE ROY ADAPTATION MODEL NURSING PROCESS** *(continued)*

- The first priority is behaviors that threaten the survival of the individual, family, group, or community.
- The second priority is behaviors that affect the growth of the individual, family, group, or community.
- The third priority is behaviors that affect the continuation of the human race or of society.
- The fourth priority is behaviors that affect the attainment of full potential for the individual or group.

ASSESSMENT OF STIMULI

The nurse recognizes that stimuli must be amenable to independent nurse functions. Consequently, factors such as medical diagnoses and medical treatments are not considered stimuli because those factors cannot be independently managed by nurses.

The nurse identifies the internal and external focal and contextual stimuli that are influencing the behaviors of particular interest, in the order of priority established at the end of the Assessment of Behavior component of the Roy Adaptation Model Nursing Process.

The nurse recognizes that residual stimuli typically are present and attempts to confirm the presence of those stimuli by asking the human adaptive system about other stimuli or by recourse to theoretical or experiential knowledge. When residual stimuli are identified, they are classified as contextual or focal stimuli.

The nurse identifies the internal stimulus of the adaptation level and determines whether it reflects integrated, compensatory, or compromised life processes.

Stimuli associated with ineffective responses are of interest because the nurse wants to change them to adaptive behaviors, and adaptive responses are of interest because the nurse wants to maintain or enhance them.

In situations where all behaviors are judged as adaptive responses, assessment of stimuli focuses on identifying potential threats to adaptation.

The nurse identifies stimuli by means of observation, using the senses of sight, sound, touch, taste, and smell; objective measurement, using paper and pencil instruments and measures of physiological parameters; and purposeful interviews.

The nurse validates perceptions and thoughts about relevant stimuli with the human adaptive system of interest, using Orlando's (1961) deliberative nursing process (see Chapter 14, Table 14–4):

- The nurse shares perceptions and thoughts about relevant stimuli with the human adaptive system.
- The nurse asks if those are the relevant stimuli.
- The human adaptive system confirms or does not confirm the identified stimuli as relevant.
- If the stimuli are not confirmed as relevant, the nurse and the human adaptive system discuss their perceptions of the situation until agreement about relevant stimuli is reached.

NURSING DIAGNOSIS

The nurse uses a process of judgment to make a statement conveying the adaptation status of the human adaptive system of interest.

The nursing diagnosis is a statement that identifies the behaviors of interest together with the most relevant influencing stimuli.

The nurse uses one of three different approaches to state the nursing diagnosis:

- Behaviors are stated within each adaptive mode and with their most relevant influencing stimuli.
- A summary label for behaviors in each adaptive mode with relevant stimuli is used.
- A label that summarizes a behavioral pattern across adaptive modes that is affected by the same stimuli is used.

The nurse may link the Roy Adaptation Model-based nursing diagnosis with a relevant diagnosis from the taxonomy of the North American Nursing Diagnosis Association (NANDA).

The nurse assigns a priority to each nursing diagnosis. The first priority is behaviors that threaten the survival of the individual, family, group, or community; the second priority is behaviors that affect the growth of the individual, family, group, or community; the third priority is behaviors that affect the continuation of the human race or of society; the fourth priority is behaviors that affect the attainment of full potential for the individual or group.

GOAL SETTING

The nurse articulates a clear statement of the behavioral outcomes in response to nursing provided to the human adaptive system.

The nurse actively involves the human adaptive system in the formation of behavioral goals if possible, recognizing that that involvement provides an opportunity to explore the rationale behind certain goals and gives the adaptive system a chance to suggest goals and evaluate whether others are realistic.

The nurse states goals as specific short-term and long-term behavioral outcomes of nursing intervention.

The goal statement designates the behavior of interest, the way in which the behavior will change, and the time frame for attainment of the goal.

Goals may be stated for ineffective behaviors that are to be changed to adaptive behaviors and also for adaptive behaviors that should be maintained or enhanced.

INTERVENTION

The nurse selects and implements nursing approaches that have a high probability of changing stimuli or strengthening adaptive processes.

Nursing intervention is the management of stimuli. The nurse may alter stimuli, increase stimuli, decrease stimuli, remove stimuli, or maintain stimuli.

The nurse manages the focal stimulus first if possible, and then manages the contextual stimuli.

Identification and Analysis of Possible Nursing Interventions
The nurse uses the McDonald and Harms (1966) nursing judgment method, in collaboration with the human adaptive system, to select a nursing intervention:

- Alternative approaches to management of stimuli are listed, along with the consequences of management of each stimulus.
- The probability (high, moderate, low) for each consequence is determined.
- The value of the outcomes of each approach is designated as desirable or undesirable.
- The options are shared with the human adaptive system.
- The nursing intervention with the highest probability of reaching the valued goal is selected.

Implementation

- The nurse determines and implements the steps that will manage the stimulus appropriately.

EVALUATION

The nurse judges the effectiveness of nursing interventions in relation to the behaviors of the human adaptive system.

The nurse systematically reassesses observable and nonobservable behaviors for each dimension and subdimension of the four adaptive modes.

The nurse gathers the behavioral data by means of observation, using the senses of sight, sound, touch, taste, and smell; objective measurement, using paper and pencil instruments and measures of physiological parameters; and purposeful interviews.

The nurse uses the following criteria to judge the effectiveness of nursing intervention:

- The goal was attained.

(continued)

> **TABLE 10-1**
> **PRACTICE METHODOLOGY: THE ROY ADAPTATION MODEL NURSING PROCESS** *(continued)*

- The human adaptive system manifests behavior stated in the goals.
- The human adaptive system demonstrates a positive response to the stimuli that frees energy for responses to other stimuli.

If the criteria for nursing intervention effectiveness are met, and if there is no threat that the behavior will become ineffective again, that behavior may be deleted from nursing concern.

If, however, the criteria are not met, the nurse must determine what went wrong. Possibilities include:

- The goals were unrealistic or unacceptable to the human adaptive system.
- The assessment data were inaccurate or incomplete.
- The selected nursing intervention approaches were not implemented properly.
- The nurse then returns to Assessment of Behaviors to closely examine behaviors that continue to be ineffective and to try to further understand the situation.

The end result of the Roy Adaptation Model Nursing Process is an update of the nursing care plan.

Constructed from Andrews & Roy, 1991b, pp. 29–47; Logan, 1990; Roy, 1984a; Roy, 1989, p. 109; Roy & Andrews, 1999, pp. 63–96.

Relational Propositions

Within the context of the **Human Adaptive System** and **Adaptation**, the relation of the concept of **Stimuli** to the concepts of **Coping Processes, Adaptive Modes**, and **Behavior** is depicted in Figure 10–1. The diagram illustrates that **Stimuli** (Focal, Contextual, Residual) act as inputs to the **Human Adaptive System** and are processed by the **Coping Processes** (Cognator and Regulator for the individual, Stabilizer and Innovator for groups). The output is **Behavior**, in the form Adaptive Responses and Ineffective Responses for each component of each of the four interrelated **Adaptive Modes**. Adaptive Responses, which promote the integrity of the **Human Adaptive System**, are depicted by the arrow that remains within the **Adaptation** circle. Ineffective Responses, which do not contribute to the integrity of the **Human Adaptive System**, are depicted by the arrow that extends beyond the **Adaptation** circle. In a cyclical manner, the responses then act as feedback, which is further input for the **Human Adaptive System**.

The specific relational propositions of the Roy Adaptation Model are listed here. The metaparadigm concepts of human beings and environment are linked in relational propositions A, B, C, D, E, F, G, and H. The metaparadigm concepts of human beings, environment, and health are linked in relational proposition I. Relational propositions J and K specify the linkage of the metaparadigm concepts of human beings, health, and nursing. The

linkage of all four metaparadigm concepts—human beings, environment, health, nursing—is evident in relational proposition L.

A. Stimuli from the internal and external environment (through the senses) act as inputs to the nervous system

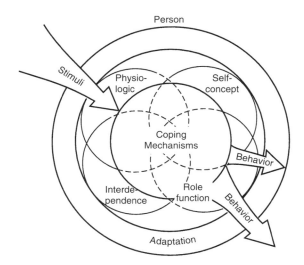

FIG. 10–1. Diagram of the human adaptive system. (From Roy, C., & Andrews, H.A. (1999). The Roy adaptation model (2nd ed., p. 50). Stamford, CT: Appleton and Lange, with permission from Prentice-Hall, Inc.)

and affect the fluid and electrolyte, and acid-base balance, and the endocrine system. The information is channeled automatically in the appropriate manner and an automatic, unconscious response is produced (Roy & Andrews, 1999, p. 46) [Explanation of the action of the Regulator Coping Subsystem].

B. Internal and external stimuli including psychological, social, physical, and physiological factors act as inputs to the cognator subsystem (Roy & Andrews, 1999, p. 47).

C. Stimuli and adaptation level serve as input to human adaptive systems. ... Processing of this input through control processes [i.e., regulator and cognator coping subsystems or stabilizer and innovator subsystem control processes] results in behavioral responses (Roy & Andrews, 1999, p. 43).

D. Human systems, as individuals, families, groups, organizations, or communities, must sense changes in the environment and make adaptations in the way they function to accommodate new environmental requirements (Roy & Andrews, 1999, p. 44).

E. Adaptation level affects the human system's ability to respond positively in a situation (Roy & Andrews, 1999, p. 36).

F. The changing environment stimulates the person to make adaptive responses. For human beings, life is never the same. It is constantly changing and presenting new challenges. The person has the ability to make new responses to these changing conditions. As the environment changes, the person has the opportunity to continue to grow, to develop, and to enhance the meaning of life for everyone (Andrews & Roy, 1991a, p. 18).

G. The characteristics of the internal and external stimuli influence the adequacy of cognitive and emotional processes [i.e., cognator coping subsystem] (Roy & Andrews, 1999, p. 547).

H. The characteristics of the internal and external stimuli influence [behavioral] responses (Roy & Andrews, 1999, p. 547).

I. Human beings [are] described as adaptive systems constantly growing and developing within changing environments. Health for human adaptive systems can be described as a reflection of this interaction or adaptation (Roy & Andrews, 1999, pp. 53–54).

J. The goal of nursing [is] the promotion of adaptation in each of the four [adaptive] modes, thereby contributing to health, quality of life, or dying with dignity (Roy & Andrews, 1999, p. 55).

K. The general goal of nursing intervention ... is to maintain and enhance adaptive behavior and to change ineffective behavior to adaptive (Roy & Andrews, 1999, p. 81).

L. It is the nurse's role to promote adaptation in situations

of health and illness and to enhance the interaction of human systems with the environment, thereby promoting health (Roy & Andrews, 1999, p. 55).

EVALUATION OF ROY'S ADAPTATION MODEL

This section presents an evaluation of the Roy Adaptation Model. The evaluation is based on the results of the analysis of the conceptual model, as well as on publications by Roy and by others who have used or commented on Roy's work.

EXPLICATION OF ORIGINS

Roy has explicated the origins of the Roy Adaptation Model clearly and concisely. She chronicled the development of the model over time and identified her motivation to formulate a conceptual model of nursing. Furthermore, she explicitly stated her philosophical claims in the form of a claim about the person and the environment, a claim about adaptation, scientific assumptions and philosophical assumptions about the person and the environment, values about nursing, and claims about nursing and nurse scholars/nurse theorists.

Roy's (1997; Roy & Andrews, 1999) refinement of her philosophical assumptions made explicit her beliefs about God. Inasmuch as adoption of a conceptual model as a guide for nursing activities is predicated on the nurse's acceptance of the underlying philosophical claims, Roy's explication of her spiritual beliefs in the form of God, rather than in a broader spirituality, may limit the adoption of the Roy Adaptation Model by nurses who do not believe in God and may limit the applicability of the model to those human adaptive systems who do believe in God.

Roy assumes that people are integrated wholes capable of action, and she values the active participation of human adaptive systems in the **Roy Adaptation Model Nursing Process** (see Table 10–1). Roy noted that although active participation may not always be possible, as in the case of infants and unconscious or suicidal patients, the nurse "is constantly aware of the active responsibility of the patient to participate in his own care when he is able to do so" (Roy & Roberts, 1981, p. 47).

Roy acknowledged the nurses and other scholars whose works influenced her thinking. Moreover, she provided bibliographic citations to the works that were especially relevant and explained how each one contributed to the development of the Roy Adaptation Model.

COMPREHENSIVENESS OF CONTENT

Roy addressed each of the metaparadigm concepts explicitly and adequately for the level of abstraction of a conceptual model. At least rudimentary definitions are provided for each concept and for most dimensions and subdimensions of the Roy Adaptation Model. It should be noted, however, that Roy and Andrews (1999) provided slightly different versions of definitions for the same concept in various places throughout their book.

The Roy Adaptation Model concepts representing the metaparadigm concept of human beings are, for the most part, adequately defined and described. Although some difficulty had been reported in distinguishing the adaptive mode to which a particular behavior belongs, especially in the self-concept, role function, and interdependence modes (Wagner, 1976), the continuing refinements in the Roy Adaptation Model have clarified the focus of each adaptive mode. Roy (1987c) explained, "Through many revisions with input from educators, clinicians, and theory critics, the physiological mode has been reorganized, and can now be used for nursing assessment and the organization of curriculum content" (p. 39). She went on to say, "The content changes in the interdependence mode have been significant over the last couple of years. This allows interdependence to be distinguished from self-concept and role function" (p. 41). Moreover, the distinctions between individual and group adaptive systems in terms of the adaptive modes are evident in Roy and Andrews (1999). However, definitions still are needed for the subdimensions of the Group Identity component of the Self-Concept/Group Identity Mode.

The Roy Adaptation Model concepts representing the metaparadigm concept of environment are generally defined in a sufficient manner for a conceptual model. The distinction between the internal and external environments, however, is not always clear. Acknowledging this, Roy and Roberts (1981) commented, "Further clarification of environment as distinct from internal stimuli awaits additional theoretical work on the model" (p. 43). Additional work also is needed to describe the nature of environmental change. Further development of the concept of environment was undertaken by Randell, Poush Tedrow, and Van Landingham (1982). Roy (1982) acknowledged that the introduction of the ideas of transaction and perception in their treatment of environment has expanded the conceptual model.

The dimensions of the Roy Adaptation Model concept of Adaptation, which represents the metaparadigm concepts of human beings and environment, are stated as the goals of adaptation or the goals of the human adaptive system. Close examination of many of Roy's publications about the model failed to reveal a definition for any of the goals with the exception of reproduction. Especially troubling is the lack of a definition for the goal of person and environment transformations, which was introduced by Roy and Andrews in their 1999 book.

Health is clearly defined. Given that Roy (1987c) regarded the health-illness continuum as a limited viewpoint, it is not surprising that she gave no explicit definitions of wellness or illness. Although it is tempting to interpret Adaptive Responses as signifying wellness and Ineffective Responses as signifying illness, it is unclear whether Roy would agree with such an interpretation. Consequently, the exact meanings of the two types of responses with regard to health state must be clarified to avoid confusion and misinterpretations.

Clarification also is required with regard to the use of the term "illness" in the vocabulary of the Roy Adaptation Model. A lack of consistency is noted between Artinian and Roy's 1990 journal article and Roy and Andrews' 1999 book. In the 1990 article, Roy stated that further explication of health should be "without reference to illness" (p. 65). Yet at least one reference to "situations of health and illness" (p. 55) appears in the 1999 text, which is regarded as "the definitive statement" about the model (p. xvii).

Another point about health requiring clarification is the connection between needs and responses. Roy (1987b) pointed out that the notion of needs was omitted from her 1984a discussion of the person as an adaptive system; yet she discussed and diagrammed the source of difficulty for the person as originating with a need excess or deficit in her 1989 book chapter. Furthermore, "identifying the capacities and needs of the human adaptive system" (pp. 64, 66) is part of the definition of the **Roy Adaptation Model Nursing Process** given in the 1999 Roy and Andrews text. Furthermore, Roy and Andrews (1999) systematically identified the underlying basic need for each of the adaptive modes.

The metaparadigm concept of nursing is defined and described clearly. Slightly different versions of the goal of nursing are articulated, and the nursing process is described in considerable detail. The **Roy Adaptation Model Nursing Process** is consistent with scientific findings about human behavior. A major concern in relation to the scientific basis of earlier versions of the Roy Adaptation Model was the heavy reliance on Helson's (1964) work on adaptation, which was limited to investigation of the responses of the retina of the eye to environmental stimuli. The concern centered around the question of the generalizability of Helson's findings to the whole person, which has never been established. That concern was eliminated with the publication of Roy's 1997 journal article, in which she put forth a new definition of adaptation and explained that she now limits reliance on Helson's theory to his notion of focal, contextual, and residual stimuli.

Roy has consistently maintained that nursing science should provide the basis for the selection of behaviors to observe when assessing the adaptive system. Furthermore, judgments about the behaviors should be based on explicit criteria drawn from existing scientific knowledge, and interventions with the highest probability of empirically documented success should be selected.

The **Roy Adaptation Model Nursing Process** is dynamic in that the components, or steps, are "ongoing and simultaneous" (Roy & Andrews, 1999, p. 64). Moreover, the results of the last step, Evaluation, lead back to the first step, Assessment of Behaviors, and subsequent updating of the nursing care plan.

Roy's insistence that the human adaptive system be an active participant in the decision-making aspects of the nursing process attests to her concern for ethical standards of nursing practice. Indeed, "collaboration with the person in each step of the nursing process is important. Individuals must be involved in observation of and decisions relative to their state of adaptation. They provide valuable insight that may assist the nurse in attempts to promote adaptation" (Andrews & Roy, 1991b, p. 28).

Roy's concern with ethical standards is especially evident in the statement that "In fulfilling nursing activities, nurses hold a profound regard for human and environmental consciousness, meaning, and common destiny. These beliefs are held with respect to individuals and groups receiving care, other participants in the provision of the care, and nurses themselves. As such, nurses promote the rights of individuals to define their own health-related goals and seek out health care that reflects their values" (Roy & Andrews, 1999, p. 64).

Roy linked the metaparadigm concepts of human beings and environment; human beings, environment, and health; and human beings, health, and nursing in various relational propositions. The linkage of all four metaparadigm concepts is stated concisely in one statement regarding the nurse's role (see Relational Proposition L).

The Roy Adaptation Model is sufficiently comprehensive with regard to breadth of content. The model is equally applicable to individuals, families, groups, communities, or society as a whole, in diverse health situations.

The comprehensiveness of the breadth of content of the Roy Adaptation Model is further supported by the direction it provides for nursing research, education, administration, and practice. Guidelines for each area continue to be formulated. The current guidelines for nursing research, nursing education, nursing administration, and nursing practice are listed below.

Nursing Research Guidelines

The guidelines for nursing research based on the Roy Adap-tation Model, which were constructed from Fawcett (1999), Roy (1988b, 2003), and Roy and Andrews (1999), are:

- Purpose of the research
  - Study of the phenomena encompassed by the Roy Adaptation Model requires both basic nursing research and clinical nursing research.
  - The purpose of Roy Adaptation Model-based basic nursing research is to understand and explain people adapting within their life situations, including descriptions of individual and group coping processes and adaptation to environmental stimuli and explanations of the relation between adaptation and health.
  - The purpose of Roy Adaptation Model-based clinical nursing research is to develop and test interventions and other strategies designed to enhance positive life processes and patterns.

- Phenomena of interest
  - The phenomena to be studied include basic life processes and how nursing maintains or enhances adaptive responses or changes ineffective responses to adaptive responses. The particular foci of inquiry are focal, contextual, and residual stimuli; adaptation level; regulator and cognator coping processes in individuals and stabilizer and innovator coping processes in groups; and responses in the physiological/physical, self-concept/group identity, role function, and interdependence adaptive modes.
  - Within the context of basic nursing science, phenomena of particular interest are the person or group as an adaptive system, including coping processes (cognator and regulator processes for individuals, stabilizer and innovator processes for groups); stability of adaptive patterns; dynamics of evolving adaptive patterns; cultural and other influences on the development and interrelatedness of the adaptive modes; and adaptation related to health, including person and environment interaction and integration of the adaptive modes.
  - Within the context of clinical nursing science, the phenomena of particular interest are changes in the effectiveness of coping processes; changes within and among the adaptive modes; and nursing interventions that promote adaptive behavioral responses, in times of transition, during changes in the environment, and during acute and chronic illness, injury, treatment, and threats from use of health technology.

- Problems to be studied
  - The problems to be studied are those stemming from the attempts made by the human adaptive system to meet needs for physiological integrity (individuals), resource adequacy (groups), psychic and spiritual integrity (individuals), identity integrity (groups), social integrity (individuals), role clarity (groups), and relational integrity (individuals and groups). Particular interest is in situations in which adaptive behavioral responses are threatened by health technologies and behaviorally induced health problems.

- Study participants
  - Research participants may be individuals or groups who are well or who have acute or chronic medical conditions.

- Research methods
  - Descriptive, correlational, and experimental research designs are required to study the phenomena encompassed by the Roy Adaptation Model.
  - Both qualitative and quantitative methods of data collection are appropriate.
  - Data can be gathered in any health-care setting in which human adaptive systems are found.
  - Research instruments should reflect the unique focus and intent of the Roy Adaptation Model and may include the instruments that have been directly derived from the Roy Adaptation Model (see Table 10–2).
  - The process of knowledge development when employing experimental designs is:
    - Select a relevant population
    - Identify a life process of interest
    - Develop a middle-range theory of the life process of interest from the Roy Adaptation Model and related literature
    - Derive an intervention strategy to enhance the life process for a given sample
    - State an hypothesis addressing the effects of the intervention
    - Conduct an experimental study with the selected sample

- Data analysis
  - Data analysis techniques encompass qualitative content analysis and nonparametric and parametric statistical procedures, with an emphasis on statistical techniques that facilitate analysis of nonlinear and reciprocal relations.

- Contributions
  - Roy Adaptation Model-based research enhances understanding of the human adaptive system and the role of nursing intervention in the promotion of adaptation.

Nursing Education Guidelines

The guidelines for nursing research based on the Roy Adaptation Model, which were constructed from Baldwin and Schaffer (1990), Camooso et al. (1981), Morales-Mann and Logan (1990), Porth (1977), and Roy (1979), are:

- Focus of the curriculum
  - The distinctive focus of a Roy Adaptation Model-based curriculum is understanding factors that influence the ability of human adaptive systems to adjust effectively to changes in the environment and also to create changes in the environment.
  - The purpose of nursing education is to prepare adaptation nurses by providing opportunities for students to develop knowledge of basic and clinical nursing sciences and nursing practice skills.

- Nature and sequence of content
  - The content of the curriculum is guided by the concepts and propositions of the Roy Adaptation Model. The vertical strands of the curriculum focus on theory and practice. The theory strand encompasses content on the adapting person, health/illness, and stress/disruption. The practice strand emphasizes nursing management of environmental stimuli. The horizontal strands include the Roy Adaptation Model Nursing Process and student adaptation and leadership.
  - Nonnursing courses include anatomy, physiology, pathophysiology, chemistry, psychology, sociology, human growth and development, anthropology, family studies, community studies, organizational behavior, economics, ecology and cosmology, religious studies, and the humanities.
  - The curricular sequence for a baccalaureate nursing program could begin with a sophomore year course that introduces the student to the content of the Roy Adaptation Model and the role of the nurse. The nursing process emphasizes identification of behaviors. Junior year courses would then focus on nursing science and medical science. The nursing process progresses to an emphasis on assessment of behavior and common stimuli and intervention using known approaches to the management of stimuli. Senior year courses would focus on nursing theory, nursing application, and issues in health care. The nursing process progresses to assessment of behavior and complex stimuli and creative approaches to the management of stimuli.

- Settings for nursing education
  - The Roy Adaptation Model is an appropriate curriculum guide for nursing programs offered by hospital-based schools of nursing, community colleges, and

universities. Thus the model may be used to guide curricula for diploma, associate degree, and baccalaureate and higher degree programs.

- Characteristics of students
  - Students have to meet the requirements for admission to the relevant nursing program.
  - Students must have the ability to adapt to a variety of stimuli in the educational environment, which is facilitated by faculty and peer support and personal awareness of relevant influencing factors.

- Teaching-learning strategies
  - An introductory course could include such teaching strategies as exposing students to the views of experts in adjunctive disciplines and to the notions of systems theory before presenting the content of the Roy Adaptation Model, contracting with an adult client in the community to develop a nursing care plan that includes interventions to maintain health or correct existing problems, small group (15 or fewer students) seminars, group discussions, individual faculty-student consultations, and pen-and-paper tests.
  - Another teaching strategy is the use of a continuing case study dealing with a fictional extended family throughout the academic year.
  - Physiological mode content can be taught effectively by asking students to consider why the body exhibits a particular set of physiological behaviors.
  - Practicum courses focus on helping students learn how to use practice tools directly derived from the Roy Adaptation Model (see Table 10–3). The hospital record can be used as a source of information rather than a guide for nursing practice when practice at the health-care organization is not based on the Roy Adaptation Model.

Administration of Nursing Services Guidelines

Guidelines for the administration of nursing services based on the Adaptation Model, which were constructed from DiIorio (1989), Fawcett et al. (1989), Roy (1991), and Roy and Anway (1989), are:

- Focus of nursing in the health-care organization
  - The distinctive focus of Roy Adaptation Model-based nursing in a health-care organization is provision of nursing services designed to promote the adaptation of individuals and groups in the physiological/physical, self-concept/group identity, role function, and interdependence modes.

- Purpose of nursing services
  - The specific goal of nursing service management is to ensure the most effective delivery of nursing services to

clients by means of organizational nursing systems and associated resources.

- Characteristics of nursing personnel
  - The collective nursing staff is viewed as an adaptive system in an environment of constantly changing internal and external conditions. The department of nursing or the entire health-care institution also may be viewed as an adaptive system. Consequently, the nursing personnel, the department, and the institution must possess individual and collective abilities to adapt to the changing environmental conditions.
  - Nursing personnel are differentiated on the basis of knowledge of the Roy Adaptation Model, rather than by educational level or institutional definitions.
  - The two levels of personnel are the general health-care aide and the professional nurse.
    - The aide possesses public information, common sense, and basic instruction about persons and their needs related to the adaptive mode that is used in assisting professionals in providing care based on individual pattern maintenance.
    - Professional nurses are differentiated from aides and each other on the basis of their knowledge.
      - The first-level professional nurse deals more specifically than the aide with developing patterns of the human adaptive system, such as growth and development, eating, and sleeping.
      - The second-level professional nurse is prepared to deal with complex changes in patterns of the human adaptive system and specializes in understanding particular processes for particular patient populations.
      - The third-level professional nurse conducts basic and clinical nursing research.

- Settings for nursing services
  - The settings for nursing services encompass most types of health-care organizations and most specialty practice areas.

- Management strategies and administrative policies
  - Management strategies emphasize promotion of staff, departmental, and institutional adaptation to constantly changing environmental stimuli.
  - The goal of the nurse manager is to manage stimuli so that the staff's adaptive behavioral responses are enhanced. Thus the nurse manager strives to maintain or enhance the health of the organization.
  - The managerial process emphasizes planning, organizing, staffing, leading, controlling, and especially goal setting, which is recognized as a key managerial activity.
  - The nurse manager assesses behaviors related to planning, organizing, staffing, leading, and controlling;

identifies relevant focal, contextual, and residual stimuli; develops an administratively oriented nursing diagnosis; sets goals; intervenes by changing the focal stimulus, managing the contextual stimuli, and broadening the adaptation level; and evaluates the outcomes of intervention.

Nursing Practice Guidelines

Guidelines for nursing practice based on the Roy Adaptation Model, which were constructed from Roy (1987a, 1989), Roy and Andrews (1999), and Roy and Anway (1989, p. 78), are:

- Purpose of nursing practice
  - The broad purpose of Roy Adaptation Model-based nursing practice is to promote the ability of human adaptive systems to adjust effectively to changes in the environment and also to create changes in the environment.
  - The more specific purpose of Roy Adaptation Model-based nursing practice is to promote the human adaptive system's adaptation in the physiological/physical, self-concept/group identity, role function, and interdependence modes.

- Practice problems of interest
  - Practice problems of interest encompass adaptive and ineffective behavioral responses of human adaptive systems in the physiological/physical, self-concept/group identity, role function, and interdependence adaptive modes.

- Settings for nursing practice
  - Nursing may be practiced in any setting in which nurses encounter individuals and groups, ranging from virtually every type of health-care institution to people's homes and the community at large.

- Characteristics of legitimate participants in nursing practice
  - Legitimate participants in nursing practice are human adaptive systems, including individuals, families and other groups, communities, and society, that are considered sick or well. Those adaptive systems may or may not manifest specific adaptation problems and ineffective behavioral responses.

- Nursing process
  - The practice methodology is the **Roy Adaptation Model Nursing Process**. The components of the process are assessment of behavior, assessment of stimuli, nursing diagnosis, goal setting, intervention, and evaluation (see Table 10–1).

- Contributions of nursing practice to participants' well-being
  - Roy Adaptation Model-based nursing practice contributes to the well-being of human adaptive systems by maintaining or enhancing the adaptation level and adaptive behavioral responses.

LOGICAL CONGRUENCE

The Roy Adaptation Model is generally logically congruent. Roy and Roberts (1981) began to translate the essentially reaction world view idea of adaptation to a view that is more in keeping with the reciprocal interaction world view. They stated, "This notion of adaptation does not negate the fact that humans do not merely respond to stimuli in the environment, but can take the initiative to change the environment" (p. 45). Elaborating, Roy and Corliss (1993) explained, "The use of the term stimuli sometimes has been misinterpreted as related to the framework of behaviorism. The language of behaviorism was in wide use during early stages of the Roy model development[;] however, it was clear from the beginning that Roy used the classes of stimuli to describe the complexity of the environment taken in by the person, and never referred to stimulus-response effects" (p. 220).

Moreover, Roy and Corliss (1993) pointed out that the scientific assumptions of the Roy Adaptation Model "established belief in holism and in the person as the initiator of adaptive processes. The patterning of these processes in exchange with the environment allows one's adaptive abilities to provide the dynamic energy for health and effective living" (p. 217). Roy (1997) initiated a complete break from any notion of stimulus and response in the articulation of her twenty-first century scientific assumptions, philosophical assumptions, definition of adaptation, and use of such terminology as "mutual complex person and environment self-organization" (p. 44).

Sellers (1991) maintained that the Roy Adaptation Model "proposes a nursing philosophy of scientific realism and behaviorism" (p. 150). She went on to say that the model puts forth a conceptualization of the person that reflects "the mechanistic, deterministic, persistence world view … and a view of person as a passive, reactive participant in the human-environment relationship" (pp. 150–151). Her conclusions are in sharp contrast to those reached in this chapter. Furthermore, Roy (1988b) dismissed the charge that the conceptual model reflects a mechanistic view of the person and the environment. She explained that "the complexities and subtleties of the process whereby the person takes in and responds to the environment preclude such a behavioristic interpretation" of her use of the terms stimuli and behavior (p. 32). Moreover, adaptation "is far from being a passive process, because the adaptation level includes all the person's capabilities, hopes, dreams, aspirations, and motivations, in other words, all that makes the person constantly move toward greater mastery" (Artinian & Roy, 1990, p. 64).

Work remains to be done, however, in the full translation of the twenty-first century scientific assumptions and philosophical assumptions into the concepts and propositions of the Roy Adaptation Model. For example, the scientific assumption addressing person and environment transformations is mentioned as an additional goal of adaptation in Roy and Andrews' 1999 book, but that goal is not defined or described in any detail. Furthermore, the philosophical assumption addressing the human being's relationships with the world and God is not yet fully integrated into the discussion of the moral-ethical-spiritual self aspect of the Personal Self component of the Self-Concept/Group Identity Mode.

GENERATION OF THEORY

The Roy Adaptation Model has led to the generation of a general **Theory of the Person as an Adaptive System** and separate theories of the four adaptive modes—the **Theory of the Physiological Mode**, the **Theory of the Self-Concept Mode**, the **Theory of the Role Function Mode**, and the **Theory of the Interdependence Mode** (Roy & Roberts, 1981). Roy (1984a, 1987a) pointed out that her distinctions between conceptual models and theories are based on form and function rather than on levels of abstraction, as is the case in this book. Alligood (2001) classified the Theory of the Person as an Adaptive System as a grand theory and the other theories as middle-range theories.

The **Theory of the Person as an Adaptive System** considers the person holistically. The major concepts of the theory are System Adaptation, Regulator Subsystem, and Cognator Subsystem. The propositions of this theory, which were constructed from Roy (personal communication, September 22, 1982) and Roy and Roberts (1981, pp. 62, 65), are:

- Basic Regulator Subsystem Propositions
  1.1. Internal and external stimuli are basically chemical or neural; chemical stimuli may be transduced into neural inputs to the central nervous system.
  1.2. Neural pathways to and from the central nervous system must be intact and functional if neural stimuli are to influence body responses.
  2.1. Spinal cord, brainstem, and autonomic reflexes act through effectors to produce automatic, unconscious effects on the body responses.
  3.1. The circulation must be intact for chemical stimuli to influence endocrine glands to produce the appropriate hormone.

3.2. Target organs and tissues must be able to respond to hormone levels to effect body responses.
4.1. Neural inputs are transformed into conscious perceptions in the brain (process unknown).
4.2. Increase in short-term or long-term memory will positively influence the effective choice of psychomotor response to neural input.
4.3. Effective choice of response, retained in long-term memory, will facilitate future effective choice of response.
4.4. The psychomotor response chosen will determine the effectors activated and the ultimate body response.
5.1. The body response resulting from regulator processes is fed back into the system.

- Propositions That Link the Basic Regulator Subsystem Propositions
  - The magnitude of the internal and external stimuli will positively influence the magnitude of the physiological response of an intact system (1.1 through 2.1, 3.2, 4.4).
  - Intact neural pathways will positively influence neural output to effectors (2.1 through 3.1, 4.4).
  - Chemical and neural inputs will influence normally responsive endocrine glands to hormonally influence target organs in a positive manner to maintain a state of dynamic equilibrium (1.1 through 3.2).
  - The body's response to external and internal stimuli will alter those external and internal stimuli (1.1 through 5.1).
  - The magnitude of the external and internal stimuli may be so great that the adaptive systems cannot return the body to a state of dynamic equilibrium (1.1 through 5.1).

- Cognator Subsystem Propositions
  1.1. The optimum amount and clarity of input of internal and external stimuli positively influences the adequacy of selective attention, coding, and memory.
  1.2. The optimum amount and clarity of input of internal and external stimuli positively influences the adequacy of imitation, reinforcement, and insight.
  1.3. The optimum amount and clarity of input of internal and external stimuli positively influences the adequacy of problem solving and decision making.
  1.4. The optimum amount and clarity of input of internal and external stimuli positively influences the adequacy of defenses to seek relief, and affective appraisal and attachment.
  2.1. Intact pathways and perceptual/information-processing apparatus positively influences the adequacy of selective attention, coding, and memory.

2.2. Intact pathways and learning apparatus positively influences imitation, reinforcement, and insight.

2.3. Intact pathways and judgment apparatus positively influences problem solving and decision making.

2.4. Intact pathways and emotional apparatus positively influences defenses to seek relief, and affective appraisal and attachment.

3.1. The higher level of adequacy of all the cognator processes, the more effective the psychomotor choice of response.

4.1. The psychomotor response chosen will be activated through intact effectors.

5.1. Effector activity produces the response that is at an adaptive level determined by the total functioning of the cognator subsystem.

6.1. The level of adaptive responses to internal and external stimuli will alter those internal and external stimuli.

The **Theory of the Physiological Mode** applies the propositions from the regulator subsystem to physiological needs. The theory encompasses adaptive and ineffective regulatory responses related to exercise and rest, nutrition, elimination, fluid and electrolytes, oxygen and circulation, temperature, the senses, and the endocrine system. Roy and Roberts (1981) pointed out that by considering regulator activity, they avoided exploration of biological systems, which they viewed as the focus of medicine. Roy and Roberts (1981) formulated one or more sample hypotheses for each component of the physiological mode. Each hypothesis was based on a deductive line of reasoning that proceeds from a general proposition (axiom) to a more specific proposition (theorem) to the hypothesis. The deductive proposition sets for components of the physiological mode are presented here.

• Exercise
    Axiom: The magnitude of the internal and external stimuli will positively influence the magnitude of the physiological response of an intact system.
    Theorem: The amount of mobility in the form of exercising positively influences the level of muscle integrity.
    Hypothesis: If the nurse helps the patient maintain muscle tone through proper exercising, the patient will experience fewer problems associated with immobility. (Roy & Roberts, 1981, p. 90)

• Rest
    Axiom: The magnitude of the internal and external stimuli will positively influence the magnitude of the physiological response of an intact system.
    Theorem: The quality of uninterrupted [rapid eye movement (REM)] sleep positively influences the patient's avoidance of REM sleep deprivation and dream deprivation.
    Hypothesis: If the nurse provides the patient with uninterrupted sleep where REM can be achieved, the patient will not experience sleep deprivation (Roy & Roberts, 1981, pp. 90–91).

• Nutrition
    Axiom: The magnitude of the internal and external stimuli will positively influence the magnitude of the physiological response of an intact system.
    Theorem$_1$: The diet that is based on both biological needs and patient preference will positively influence the amount of dietary intake.
    Hypothesis$_1$: If the nurse assesses the patient's dietary needs in relation to his dietary preference, the patient will achieve an optimal level of nutritional intake (Roy & Roberts, 1981, pp. 109–110).
    Axiom: The magnitude of the internal and external stimuli will positively influence the magnitude of the physiological response of an intact system.
    Theorem$_2$: An environment conducive for eating will positively influence the level of anorexia or nausea.
    Hypothesis$_2$: If the nurse establishes an environment conducive for dietary intake, the patient will be less likely to experience anorexia or nausea (Roy & Roberts, 1981, p. 110).

• Elimination
    Axiom: The magnitude of the internal and external stimuli will positively influence the magnitude of the physiological response of an intact system.
    Theorem: The magnitude of internal and external stimuli will positively influence the level of urinary and intestinal elimination.
    Hypothesis: If the nurse helps the patient achieve an optimal level of urinary and intestinal elimination, the patient's eliminatory system will perform at a higher level (Roy & Roberts, 1981, p. 129).

• Fluids and Electrolytes
    Axiom: The magnitude of the internal and external stimuli will positively influence the magnitude of the physiological response of an intact system.
    Theorem: The level of hydration achieved will positively influence the level of fluid and electrolyte balance.
    Hypothesis: If the nurse helps the patient maintain an optimal level of hydration, the patient will perform at a higher cellular level (Roy & Roberts, 1981, p. 156).

• Oxygen and Circulation
    Axiom: The magnitude of the internal and external stimuli will positively influence the magnitude of the physiological response of an intact system.

Theorem: The level of alveolar-capillary exchange and perfusion will positively influence the level of oxygenation and circulatory balance.

Hypothesis: If the nurse helps the patient achieve an optimal level of oxygenation and circulation, the patient's alveolar-capillary system will perform at a higher level (Roy & Roberts, 1981, p. 181).

- Temperature

  Axiom: The magnitude of the internal and external stimuli will positively influence the magnitude of the physiological response of an intact system.

  Theorem: The amount of input in the form of heat will positively influence the temperature regulatory system.

  Hypothesis: If the nurse helps the patient maintain a temperature level for normal physiological functioning, the patient's cellular activity and body metabolism will perform at a more optimal level (Roy & Roberts, 1981, p. 199).

- The Senses

  Axiom: The magnitude of the internal and external stimuli will positively influence the magnitude of the physiological response of an intact system.

  Theorem: The amount of sensory input via each sensory modality will positively influence the level of cortical arousal.

  Hypothesis: If the nurse provides optimal sensory input, the patient will achieve an optimal level of cortical arousal (Roy & Roberts, 1981, p. 218).

- Endocrine System

  Axiom: Chemical and neural inputs will influence normally responsive endocrine glands to hormonally influence target organs in a positive manner to maintain a state of dynamic equilibrium.

  Theorem: The amount of hormonal input and control will positively influence hormonal balance.

  Hypothesis: If the nurse helps the patient maintain an optimal level of hormonal secretion, the patient will achieve a higher level of hormonal or endocrine balance (Roy & Roberts, 1981, p. 243).

The **Theory of the Self-Concept Mode**, the **Theory of the Role Function Mode**, and the **Theory of the Interdependence Mode** consider those modes as systems "through which the regulator and cognator subsystems act to promote adaptation" (Roy & Roberts, 1981, p. 248). Each theory describes the relevant system in terms of its wholeness, subsystems, relation of parts, inputs, outputs, and self-regulation and control. The propositions and a deductive set of propositions for each theory are presented here.

- Theory of the Self-Concept Mode
  - Propositions
    1.1. The positive quality of social experience in the form of others' appraisals positively influences the level of feelings of adequacy.
    1.2. Adequacy of role taking positively influences the quality of input in the form of social experience.
    1.3. The number of social rewards positively influences the quality of social experience.
    1.4. Negative feedback in the form of performance compared with ideals leads to corrections in levels of feelings of adequacy.
    1.5. Conflicts in input in the form of varying appraisals positively influences the amount of self-concept confusion experienced.
    1.6. Confused self-concept leads to activation of mechanisms to reduce dissonance and maintain consistency.
    1.7. Activity of mechanisms for reducing dissonance and maintaining consistency (e.g., choice) tends to lead to feelings of adequacy.
    1.8. The level of feelings of adequacy positively influences the quality of presentation of self (Roy & Roberts, 1981, p. 255).
  - Deductive Proposition Set

    Axiom$_1$: Adequacy of role taking positively influences the quality of input in the form of social experience.

    Axiom$_2$: The positive quality of social experience positively influences the level of feelings of adequacy.

    Theorem: Adequacy of role taking positively influences the level of feelings of adequacy.

    Hypothesis: If the nurse helps the new mother to practice role taking, the mother will develop a higher level of feelings of adequacy. (Roy & Roberts, 1981, p. 258).

- Theory of the Role Function Mode
  - Propositions
    1.1. The amount of clarity of input in the form of role cues and cultural norms positively influences the adequacy of role taking.
    1.2. Accuracy of perception positively influences the clarity of input in the form of role cues and cultural norms.
    1.3. Adequacy of social learning positively influences the clarity of input in the form of role cues and cultural norms.
    1.4. Negative feedback in the form of internal and external validations leads to corrections in adequacy of role taking.
    1.5. Conflicts in input in the form of conflicting role

sets positively influences the amount of role strain experienced.

1.6. Role strain leads to activation of mechanisms for reducing role strain and for articulating role sets.

1.7. Activity of mechanisms for reducing role strain and for articulating role sets (e.g., choice) leads to adequacy of role taking.

1.8. The level of adequacy of role taking positively influences the level of role mastery (Roy & Roberts, 1981, p. 267).

- Deductive Proposition Set

    Axiom$_1$: The amount of clarity of input in the form of role cues positively influences the adequacy of role taking.

    Axiom$_2$: The level of adequacy of role taking positively influences the level of role mastery.

    Theorem: The amount of clarity of input in the form of role cues positively influences the level of role mastery.

    Hypothesis: If the nurse orients the patient to the sick role, the patient will perform at a higher level of role mastery in the sick role (Roy & Roberts, 1981, p. 270).

- Theory of the Interdependence Mode
  - Propositions
    1.1. The balance and flexibility of coping style positively influences the adequacy of seeking nurturance and nurturing.

    1.2. The optimum amount of environmental changes positively influences the adequacy of seeking nurturance and nurturing.

    1.3. Clarity of feedback about self positively influences the balance and flexibility of coping style.

    1.4. Clarity of validation regarding others positively influences the balance and flexibility of coping style.

    1.5. Commonality and freedom of communication patterns positively influences the adequacy of seeking nurturance and nurturing.

    1.6. The balance of dependency and aggressive drives positively influences the adequacy of seeking nurturance and nurturing.

    1.7. Adequacy of seeking nurturance and nurturing positively influences interdependence (Roy & Roberts, 1981, p. 277).

  - Deductive Proposition Set

    Axiom$_1$: The optimum amount of environmental changes positively influences the adequacy of seeking nurturance and nurturing.

    Axiom$_2$: Adequacy of seeking nurturance and nurturing positively influences interdependence.

Theorem: The optimum amount of environmental changes positively influences interdependence.

Hypothesis: If the nurse provides time and space for private family visits, the patient will demonstrate more appropriate attention-seeking behavior (Roy & Roberts, 1981, p. 280).

The hypotheses derived from the propositions of each theory still have not been tested empirically. However, Roy and Roberts (1981) recognized the need for a systematic program of research to test the sample hypotheses, as well as other hypotheses that could be derived from the theories. They also recognized the need to further develop and test the Theory of the Person as an Adaptive System. They commented, "We must look at the theory of the adaptive person to further explain the interrelatedness of the adaptive modes. In this process we must also search for multivariable and nonlinear relationships. Cognator and regulator processes must be studied to discover the proposed hierarchy of processes" (p. 289).

Furthermore, as Roy and Roberts (1981) pointed out, nursing practice theory, or what Roy (1988b) later called clinical nursing science, must be developed within the context of the Roy Adaptation Model. That is, theories must be formulated to explain and predict the effects of specific nursing interventions on the responses of individuals and groups.

Recently, Roy (2003) introduced the notion of theories of processes, which apparently extend the Theory of the Self-Concept Mode, the Theory of the Role Function Mode, and the Theory of the Interdependence Mode. She proposed that within the Self-Concept Mode, theories about the physical self and personal self address processes of developing self; theories about self consistency address processes of focusing self, theories about self ideal address processes of choosing self, and theories about the moral-ethical-spiritual self address processes of valuing self. Theories about the Group Identity Mode addres processes of sharing identity. Within the Role Function Mode, theories about primary, secondary, and tertiary roles address processes of developing roles; theories about role transition address processes of role taking; and theories about role set address processes of integrating roles. Within the Interdependence Mode, theories about significant others address processes of giving and receiving, as well as processes of learning and maturing in relationships; and theories about support systems address processes of securing resources.

The **Nursing Model of Cognitive Processing** also was developed within the context of the Roy Adaptation Model (Roy, 1988a, 2001). The cognitive processing model, which actually is a rudimentary middle-range theory of information processing, focuses attention on the basic cognitive processes of arousal and attention, sensation and perception, coding, concept formation, memory, language, planning, and motor responses. The model proposes that the basic cognitive processes, which occur within the field of consciousness, are dependent on neurological and neurochemical functions. The model further proposes that cognitive processes are directed toward dealing with the focal stimulus of the immediate sensory experience, within the reference frame of contextual and residual stimuli in the form of the person's education and experience.

In recent years, other explicit middle-range theories have been derived from the Roy Adaptation Model. Those theories are:

- Theory of caregiver stress (Tsai, 1999, 2003)
- Theory of adapting to diabetes (Whittemore & Roy, 2002)
- Theory of psychosocial adaptation to termination of pregnancy for fetal anomaly (Kruszewski, 1999)
- Theory of adaptation during childbearing (Tulman & Fawcett, 2003)

Additional theory development work stemming from the Roy Adaptation Model includes the construction of explicit conceptual-theoretical-empirical structures for several studies, including preparation for cesarean childbirth (Fawcett, 1990); correlates of functional status in normal life situations and serious illness (Fawcett & Tulman, 1990; Samarel & Fawcett, 1992; Tulman & Fawcett, 1990a, 1990b); adaptation to chronic illness (Pollock, 1993); cross-cultural responses to pain (Calvillo & Flaskerud, 1993); stress experiences of spouses of coronary artery bypass graft patients (Artinian, 1991, 1992); correlates of physiological and psychosocial adaptation in spinal cord–injured persons (Barone & Roy, 1996); correlates of psychological distress and life satisfaction in diverse caregiver populations (Ducharme et al., 1998; Levesque et al., 1998); and the effects of walking exercise for women with breast cancer (Mock et al., 1994, 1997).

CREDIBILITY OF THE NURSING MODEL

Social Utility

The utility of the Roy Adaptation Model for nursing research, education, administration, and practice is well documented. The conceptual model is being used by nurses throughout the United States and in other countries, including Canada, Colombia, Switzerland, and Japan (Fawcett, 2003a; Roy, personal communication, May 15, 1982). In addition to Roy's own texts (Andrews & Roy, 1986; Roy, 1976b, 1984a; Roy & Andrews, 1991, 1999; Roy & Roberts, 1981), books related to the Roy Adaptation

Model have been published by Randell, Poush Tedrow, and Van Landingham (1982), Rambo (1984), and Welsh and Clochesy (1990).

The Roy Adaptation Model encompasses an extensive vocabulary with several new words. Furthermore, even familiar words, such as adaptation, have been given new meanings in Roy's attempt to translate notions that reflect the reaction world view into ideas that reflect the reciprocal interaction world view. Consequently, considerable study is required to fully understand the unique focus and content of the Roy Adaptation Model. Roy (1991) emphasized the need to study "development, interrelatedness, cultural, and other influences" on adaptive mode responses (p. 35). Andrews (1989) pointed out that "conceptual clarity relative to the understanding of the essential elements of a nursing model is a particular challenge and of great importance if the conceptualization is to be effective in its application" (p. 139). She recommended detailed study of the content of the four adaptive modes and highlighted the importance of diagrams (such as Fig. 10–1) to facilitate understanding of the various components of the Roy Adaptation Model.

Implementation of Roy Adaptation Model-based nursing practice is feasible. The human and material resources needed for implementation of the model at the health-care organization level are evident in the following descriptions of implementation projects.

Gray (1991) presented a comprehensive report of the strategies used for implementation of the Roy Adaptation Model at five Southern California hospitals. The hospitals ranged from a 100-bed proprietary hospital to a 248-bed nonprofit, community-owned hospital. Drawing from the Ingalls (1972) System of Management, Gray (1991) described the processes of climate setting, mutual planning, assessing needs, forming objectives, designing, implementing, and evaluating. Climate setting focuses on assessment of the physical, psychological, and organizational climate. She pointed out that "if a hospital waits for the perfect time to begin a change project, no change projects would ever be started" (p. 433). Planning should be carried out by all levels of nursing staff, along with the hospital personnel responsible for medical records, purchasing, central supply, social services, laboratories, x-ray, and respiratory therapy. Needs assessment encompasses the individual staff nurse, the nursing department, and the health-care system as a whole. Gray (1991) underscored the importance of marketing the model-based nursing services to consumers as a method of contributing to the fiscal needs of the health-care organization.

Gray (1991) went on to point out that the overall objective of an implementation project dealing with the Roy Adaptation Model is "to improve the quality of patient care through the use of written care plans" (p. 437). More specific objectives should be developed for each nursing unit and individual staff nurses. Designing is a time-consuming but "exciting and professionally exhilarating" phase of implementation and is best accomplished through a committee structure (p. 439). Gray (1991) recommended establishment of a Standards of Practice Steering Committee and working committees on quality assurance, procedures and protocol, nursing process, professional development, and patient education.

Implementing, according to Gray (1991), is "the easiest step" if the previous phases were accomplished in an effective manner and if hospital personnel were adequately oriented to the model (p. 440). Evaluation is carried out continuously, from climate setting through implementation.

Mastal, Hammond, and Roberts (1982) cited the importance of a thorough analysis of the model, the heuristic value of a diagram to depict the relations between the components of the model, and the pragmatic necessity of support from the agency administrators. They noted that funds for the necessary staff education can be allocated from the agency's continuing education budget. They added that if funds are not available, it may be possible to recruit one or more volunteers from the health-care organization and local schools of nursing to serve as implementation project staff.

Mastal and associates (1982) also noted the importance of the appointment of a project change team, as well as an introductory meeting of all personnel who would be involved in the change to model-based practice, including "float" staff. They commented that shared power, which involves group decision making and group problem solving, was especially effective as the implementation project progressed.

Connerley and colleagues (1999) reported that they used the Roy Adaptation Model Nursing Process as a guide for their implementation project at St. Joseph Regional Medical Center in Lewiston, Idaho. They stated that "successful model implementation requires the presence of multiple positive conditions and the use of a variety of strategies and processes to support change. Paramount among these is support and recognition of the value of defining the role of nursing in the organization" (p. 517). They went on to identify other strategies, including articulating the value of model-based nursing practice in general and Roy Adaptation Model-based nursing practice in particular, staff nurse involvement in selection of the nursing model, educational programs designed to help nurses understand the focus and content of the Roy Adaptation Model, the enthusiastic commitment and support of the nursing leaders in the organization, communication of the nursing leader's vision for nursing practice, carefully

planned changes in nursing practice that actively involve all members of the organization, consideration of the rapid environmental changes in health-care organizations, and a systems perspective of the implementation project.

Dorsey and Purcell (1987) reported that remodeling a unit by removing the nursing station walls, which promoted increased nursing home resident–staff interaction, was a particularly important aspect of the implementation of Roy Adaptation Model-based nursing practice. They highlighted the importance of comprehensive orientation and inservice programs for staff.

The importance of revising nursing documents so that they are consistent with the Roy Adaptation Model has been underscored by various authors (Jakocko & Sowden, 1986; Mastal et al., 1982; Rogers et al., 1991). Relevant documents include the health-care organization's philosophy of nursing, mission statement, standards of practice, nursing history and assessment forms, nursing care plans, patient classification systems, computer information systems, job descriptions, performance appraisals, and quality monitoring tools. Many such tools already have been developed and can be modified for use in particular health-care organizations (Table 10–2).

Weiss and colleagues' (1994) study of the implementation of the Roy Adaptation Model at Sharp Memorial Hospital in San Diego, California, revealed both facilitators and inhibitors to the integration of the model into nursing practice. Facilitators included experience with the model in an educational program, participation in the implementation project through shared governance councils, participation in career advancement programs, and ongoing continuing education. Inhibitors were resistance to change, the language of the model, increased time required for documentation, and lack of continuing education about nursing models.

The application of the Roy Adaptation Model is feasible in many different practice settings. However, Mason and Chandley (1990) noted that the lack of success in applying the model in special hospitals for the criminally insane "is due firstly to the limitation of adaptive responses in terms of the patient's goal due to the secure environment, and secondly, it creates a level of frustration when the 'treatment' values conflict with the social, political and legal values" (p. 671). Conversely, although she noted certain limitations in its use, Miller (1991) presented a largely successful application of the Roy Adaptation Model in the special hospital with which Mason was affiliated.

Ingram (1995) noted that the time required for comprehensive assessment of psychosocial behaviors makes the use of the Roy Adaptation Model difficult in the rapid-paced emergency department setting. She also pointed to the difficulty of involving gravely injured patients in decision making as a drawback. Ingram (1995) weighed those limitations with the advantages of the nursing diagnosis and goal-setting components of the Roy Adaptation Model Nursing Process and suggested that the model be modified so that it could be used effectively in emergency departments.

Echoing Ingram's (1995) concerns, Galbreath (2002) commented, "In a practice arena that is increasingly challenged with time constraints, the amount of time required to fully implement the two areas of [Roy Adaptation Model] assessment [assessment of behaviors, assessment of stimuli] may be viewed as insurmountable. This is particularly true as one begins to use the [model]; a nurse more experienced in the use of the [model] may find the time constraints less compelling" (p. 330). It could be argued that conversely, a less systematic assessment or an ad hoc assessment could take more time in the long run, as nurses have to add crucial information to the patient data base as they realize that aspects of the initial assessment were not completed.

Nursing Research. The Roy Adaptation Model has proved very useful as a guide for nursing research. Several research instruments have been derived directly from the Roy Adaptation Model (see Table 10–2). Moreover, as can be seen in the Doctoral Dissertations and Master's Theses sections of the chapter bibliography on the CD-ROM, many dissertations and theses have been guided by the model. Published reports of research based on the Roy Adaptation Model include descriptive studies of patients' responses to diverse environmental stimuli, correlational studies of the relation of focal and contextual stimuli to diverse manifestations of physiological and psychosocial adaptation, and experimental studies of the effects of Roy Adaptation Model-based nursing interventions on adaptation. These reports are listed in Table 10–3.

In 1999, Roy and her colleagues in the Boston Based Adaptation Research Nursing Society (BBARNS) published the results of their integrative review of Roy Adaptation Model-based research from 1970 through 1994 (Boston Based Adaptation Research Nursing Society, 1999). They classified 163 reports of empirical nursing research, including 51 doctoral dissertations, 25 master's theses, and 87 published research articles, into categories of studies focusing on stimuli ($n = 19$), coping processes ($n = 36$), the physiological mode ($n = 21$), the self-concept mode ($n = 18$), the role function mode ($n = 21$), the interdependence mode ($n = 20$), and effects of nursing interventions ($n = 28$). They found that 116 of the studies were explicitly designed to test propositions of the Roy Adaptation Model.

More recently, Roy (2003) presented the results of a review of 54 Roy Adaptation Model-based studies published between 1995 and 2001, including 28 journal articles, 25 doctoral dissertations, and 1 master's thesis. Twenty-two studies focused on adaptive modes and processes; seven, on the physiological mode; seven, on the self-concept mode; five, on the role function mode; three, on the interdependence mode; five, on stimuli; and five, on the effects of interventions.

The authors of the Boston Based Adaptation Research Nursing Society (1999) book noted that although some programs of research were evident, many more research programs are needed. Fawcett and Newman (2003) reviewed the publications listed in Table 10–3 and identified several programs of research, some of which have become evident since the Boston Based Adaptation Research Nursing Society book (1999) was completed (see, for example, research by Cottrell and Shannahan; Fawcett and colleagues; Ducharme and Levesque and colleagues; Lutjens; Mock and colleagues; Modrcin and colleagues; Niska; Pollock and colleagues; and Tulman and colleagues). In addition, Fawcett (2003b) presented a brief overview of the research on functional status that she and her colleagues and doctoral students have been conducting for several years. And, Tulman and Fawcett (2003) published a book-length report of their study of correlates of women's functional status during and after pregnancy, which is one of several of the studies in their program of research (see Table 10–3).

Nursing Education. The utility of the Roy Adaptation Model for nursing education is well documented. The early and widespread interest in using the model in educational programs is attested to by three conferences that were held for faculty members who planned to use or were already using the model as a basis for curriculum development in their schools. The first and second conferences were held at Alverno College in Milwaukee, Wisconsin, in 1978 and 1979. The third conference was held at Mount St. Mary's College in Los Angeles, California, in 1981. Annual conferences have been held at Mount St. Mary's College to recognize the leadership role of the College in the initial development of the Roy Adaptation Model and to provide a forum for Roy Adaptation Model-based issues in education and practice (Wallace, 1993). In addition, Mount St. Mary's College initiated a lecture and seminar series in honor of Sr. Callista Roy in 1991.

Roy (personal communication, May 15, 1982) provided a list of schools of nursing where she or a faculty member from Mount St. Mary's College had made consultant visits and there was "some evidence of follow-through with curriculum development." The nursing programs named are listed on page 414.

(Text continues on page 414)

Instrument and Citation*	Description
RESEARCH INSTRUMENTS	
Health-Illness (Powerlessness) Questionnaire (Roy, 1979)	Measures hospitalized patients' perception of powerlessness in illness.
Hospitalized Patient Decision Making (Roy, 1979)	Measures hospitalized patients' perceptions of decisions they actually make while in a hospital and the decisions they would prefer to make.
Cognitive Adaptation Processing Scale (CAPS) (Roy & Andrews, 1999f; Roy & Zhan, 2001; Zhan, 1994)	Measures five dimensions of cognitive adaptation strategies— cognitive processing of self-perception, clear focus and method, knowing awareness, sensory regulation, and selective focus; a measure of ways of coping.
Self-Consistency Scale (Roy & Zhan, 2001; Young et al., 2001; Zhan, 1994; Zhan & Shen, 1994)	Measures self-consistency in older adults, including self-esteem, private consciousness, social anxiety, and stability of self-concept.
Inventory of Functional Status—Antepartum Period (IFSAP) (Tulman, Higgins et al., 1991; Young et al., 2001)	Measures the extent to which women continue to perform their usual household, social and community, personal care, child care, occupational, and educational activities during pregnancy.
Inventory of Functional Status—Fathers (IFS-F) (Tulman et al., 1993; Young et al., 2001)	Measures the extent to which expectant and new fathers continue to perform their usual household, social and community, personal care, child care, occupational, and educational activities.
Parental Roles Questionnaire (Varnell, 1990)	Measures parentization, operationalized as expectant parents' own and spouse's perceptions of parental role behaviors, including mothering behaviors, fathering behaviors, incorporating of norms, and childhood background.
Interdependence Questionnaire (Short, 1994)	Measures Roy's interdependence adaptive mode giving and receiving behaviors, in the categories of significant other, support systems (friendships and extended family), and the experience of feeling alone in newly delivered mothers.
Inventory of Functional Status After Childbirth (IFSAC) (Fawcett et al., 1988; Young et al., 2001)	Measures the extent to which women resume performance of their usual household, social and community, personal care, and occupational activities and assume infant care responsibilities following childbirth.
Inventory of Functional Status— Caregiver of a Child in a Body Cast (Newman, 1997; Young et al., 2001)	Measures the extent to which parental caregivers or their surrogates continue their usual household, social and community, child care, personal care, and occupational activities while caring for a child in a body cast.
Self-Perceived Adaptation Level (SPAL) (Ide, 1978)	Measures the perceived ability of well elderly persons to manage or cope with changes in their internal or external environment within the context of Roy's role function and interdependence adaptive modes.
Inventory of Functional Status in the Elderly (DiMattio, 2001; DiMattio & Tulman, 2003; Paier, 1994)	Measures the extent to which independent, community-dwelling older adults perform personal care, household, social and community, volunteer/ work, care of another, and leisure activities.
Sleep/Activity Behavior Log (O'Leary, 1991)	Used to record sleep and activity patterns of persons with Alzheimer's disease.

*See the Research Instruments and Practice Tools section of the chapter references for complete citations.

Inventory of Functional Status—Cancer (IFSCA) (Tulman et al., 1991; Fawcett et al., 1991; Fawcett & Tulman, 1996; Young et al., 2001)	Measures the extent to which women continue their usual household, social and community, personal care, and occupational activities following diagnosis of cancer.
Adaptation After Surviving Cancer Profile (Dow, 1993)	Measures transcendence after cancer, uncertainty over future, mastery of cancer, family relationships, work disclosure, and risk-taking in women who are survivors of breast cancer.
Health Outcomes Questionnaire (Lewis et al., 1978, 1979)	Measures health outcomes of nursing care for adult cancer patients receiving chemotherapy, in the areas of nausea and vomiting, body regard, anxiety, and functional effectiveness.
Varricchio-Wright Impact of Cancer Questionnaire—Parents (VWICS-P) (Wright, 1993)	Measures perceptions of quality of life of parents of children with cancer in Roy's physiological, self-concept, role function, and interdependence adaptive modes.
Inventory of Functional Status—Dialysis (Thomas-Hawkins et al., 1998)	Measures the extent to which men and women receiving hemodialysis continue their usual household, social and community, and personal care activities.
Structured Interview Guide (LeMone, 1995)	Used to collect data regarding psychosexual concerns of individuals with diabetes mellitus, within the context of Roy's physiological, self-concept, role function, and interdependence adaptive modes.
Prosthetic Problem Inventory Scale (Huber et al., 1988)	Used to identify problem areas in the use of prostheses by lower extremity amputees, in the areas of activities of daily living, social participation, sexual activity, and athletic participation.

PRACTICE TOOLS

Nursing Process Manual (Seo-Cho, 1999)	Guides detailed assessment of the physiological, self-concept, role function, and interdependence modes of adaptation, along with a discussion of and form for the Roy Adaptation Model Nursing Process Format.
Questions for Nursing Assessment of Sensory Impairment (Roy & Andrews, 1999c)	Provides a list of questions to ask when assessing the senses aspect of the physiological/physical adaptive mode.
Adaptation Assessment Form (Rambo, 1984)	Guides assessment within the context of Roy's physiological adaptive mode and the growth and developmental tasks associated with the person's primary role within the context of the role function adaptive mode.
Admission History and Assessment Form (Jakocko & Sowden, 1986)	Guides assessment of hospitalized children within the context of Roy's physiological, self-concept, role function, and interdependence adaptive modes.
Admission Nursing Assessment (Galbreath, 2002)	A form developed by nurses at Upper Valley Medical Centers in Troy, Ohio. Questions guide assessment of each adaptive mode and reflect the age or acuity of the relevant client population. Subjective, objective, and measurement data are collected.
Family Development/ Nursing Intervention Identifier (Hinman, 1983)	Guides Roy Adaptation Model-based assessment of school-age children and their families.
Admission Assessment Form (Hamner, 1989)	Guides assessment of adults hospitalized in a coronary care unit, within the context of Roy's physiological, self-concept, role function, and interdependence adaptive modes.
Nursing History Tool (Robitaille-Tremblay, 1984)	Guides assessment of hospitalized psychiatric patients within the context of Roy's physiological, self-concept, role function, and interdependence adaptive modes.

(continued)

Instrument and Citation	Description
PACU [Postanesthesia Care Unit] Preoperative Assessment Tool (Jackson, 1990)	Guides preoperative assessment of surgical patients within the context of Roy's physiological, self-concept, role function, and interdependence adaptive modes.
Comprehensive Sexual Assault Assessment Tool (CSAAT) (Burgess & Fawcett, 1996)	Guides documentation of the assessment of sexual assault victims by Sexual Assault Nurse Examiners; items tap Roy Adaptation Model stimuli, coping processes, and adaptive modes. CSAAT data can be used for clinical agency statistical analyses.
Joseph Continence Assessment Tool (JCAT) (Joseph & Lantz, 1996)	Permits assessment of factors that may affect success or failure of incontinence treatment, within the context of Roy's physiological, self-concept, role function, and interdependence adaptive modes; particularly useful for providers in ambulatory care or community settings.
Osteoporosis Assessment (Doyle & Rajacich, 1991)	Guides assessment of individuals with osteoporosis within the context of Roy's self-concept, role function, interdependence, and physiological adaptive modes.
Questions for Assessing Emotional and Social Adaptation to Dialysis (Frank, 1988)	Guides assessment of the renal dialysis patient within the context of Roy's self-concept, role function, interdependence, and physiological adaptive modes.
Community Health Assessment (Hanchett, 1988)	Guides assessment of a community in the areas of survival, continuity, growth, transactional patterns, and member control.
Typology of Indicators of Positive Adaptation (Roy & Andrews, 1999a)	A list of the indicators of positive adaptation for individuals and groups in the physiological/physical, self-concept/group identity, role function, and interdependent adaptive modes.
Typology of Commonly Recurring Adaptation Problems (Roy & Andrews, 1999b)	A list of the common adaptation problems for individuals and groups in the physiological/physical, self-concept/group identity, role function, and interdependence adaptive modes.
Nursing Diagnostic Categories (Roy & Andrews, 1999d)	A list of generic nursing diagnoses within the context of indicators of positive adaptation, common adaptation problems, and NANDA nursing diagnoses for all aspects of the physiological/physical adaptive mode, and the self-concept/group identity, role function, and interdependence adaptive modes.
Potential Nursing Diagnoses (Frank, 1988)	A list of potential nursing diagnoses within Roy's self-concept, role function, interdependence, and physiological adaptive modes that are relevant for patients receiving renal dialysis.
Nursing Diagnoses for MI Patients (Hamner, 1989)	A list of nursing diagnoses and associated focal and contextual stimuli that are relevant for patients who have had a myocardial infarction.
A Parent's Guide to Cesarean Birth (Fawcett & Burritt, 1985; Fawcett & Henklein, 1987)	A pamphlet to prepare expectant parents for unplanned or planned cesarean birth. Provides procedural, sensory, and coping strategies information about the labor (in the case of unplanned cesarean birth), delivery, and postpartum periods, organized according to the four Roy Adaptation Model adaptive modes.
The Patient's Guide to Preterm Labor (Taylor, 1993)	A pamphlet to help women deal with preterm labor. Provides procedural, sensory, and coping strategies information about home- and hospital-based treatment of preterm labor, organized according to the four Roy Adaptation Model adaptive modes.

Standards of Nursing Practice (Rogers et al., 1991)	Provides descriptions of performance expectations for provision of high-quality nursing that reflect the Roy Adaptation Model, in the areas of nursing assessment, nursing care planning, implementation of nursing care, evaluation of nursing, and professional development and accountability.
Perinatal Standards of Care (Weiss & Teplick, 1993, 1995)	Provides separate guidelines and expectations for nursing practice and desired patient outcomes for antepartal patients, intrapartum laboring patients, postpartum patients, neonates, and neonatal intensive care unit patients. Standards are made up of adaptation goals, outcome criteria, and relevant nursing interventions.
Nursing Judgment Method (Roy & Andrews, 1999e)	Provides a format for use of the McDonald and Harms method of judging the probability of attaining goals and value of alternative nursing interventions.
COPD Outcome Criteria (Laros, 1977)	Provides outcome criteria for patients with chronic obstructive pulmonary disease. Criteria are listed for each adaptive mode in a progressive sequence of days following hospital admission.
MCN Developmental/Diagnostic Model Nursing Care Plan Format (Starn & Niederhauser, 1990)	Provides a nursing care plan format for childbearing and child-rearing families.
Nursing Process Format for Families (Whall, 1986)	Guides the use of a Roy Adaptation Model–oriented nursing process for families.
Documentation System (Weiss & Teplick, 1993, 1995)	Facilitates recording of nursing assessments, interventions, and progress toward patient outcomes. Flow sheets provide consistency between desired patient outcomes and nursing interventions included in the relevant patient standard of care.
Nursing Care Plan (Rambo, 1984)	Provides a general form for documentation of Roy Adaptation Model-based nursing practice, including medical problems, medical treatment, and associated nursing actions; and nursing problems and associated focal and contextual stimuli, goals, and nursing interventions; and evaluation.
Nursing Care Plan Form (Fawcett, 1992)	Provides a general form for documentation of Roy Adaptation Model-based nursing assessment, intervention, and evaluation of outcomes.
Kardex Form, Flow Sheet, Care Plan, Charting Form (Peters, 1993)	Provide organized worksheets and documentation forms for Roy Adaptation Model-based assessment, goal setting, interventions, and evaluation for use on a general medical unit.
Nursing Care Plan Form (Hamner, 1980)	Permits documentation of Roy Adaptation Model-based assessment of behaviors and stimuli, nursing diagnoses and goals, intervention, and evaluation for use on a coronary care unit.
STRESS Tool (Modrcin-McCarthy et al., 1997)	Permits documentation of signs of stress, touch interventions, reduction of pain, environmental considerations, state, and stability in medically fragile preterm infants.
Nursing Job Descriptions (Rogers et al., 1991)	Provides Roy Adaptation Model-based job descriptions for nurse administrators (director of nursing department, unit managers), registered nurses, registered nursing assistants, and technicians.
Quality Assessment Tools (Weiss & Teplick, 1993, 1995)	Provides a Roy Adaptation Model-based method for quality assessment and monitoring. Separate tools are available for particular patient populations.
Performance Appraisal System (Rogers et al., 1991)	Provides a Roy Adaptation Model-based system for appraisal of nurses' performance of their responsibilities.
Intershift Report Format (Riegel, 1985)	Provides guidelines for presenting intershift reports organized according to the Roy Adaptation Model nursing diagnosis, stimuli, and adaptive mode responses.

Research Topic	Study Participants	Citation*
	DESCRIPTIVE STUDIES	
Quality of nursing services	Women undergoing termination of pregnancy (TOP) and TOP unit staff nurses	Blain, 1993
Experiences of pregnancy	Pregnant women who had spinal cord injuries	Craig, 1990
Incidence of couvade symptoms	Thai expectant fathers	Khanobdee et al., 1993
Comparison of reactions to vaginal birth after cesarean (VBAC) with reactions to the previous cesarean birth, description of factors that influenced the decision to attempt VBAC, and causes ascribed to the outcome of the birth experience	Women who had experienced a VBAC	Fawcett et al., 1994
Responses to cesarean birth	Mothers and fathers who experienced cesarean birth of their infant	Fawcett, 1981
	White, Hispanic, and Asian mothers who experienced cesarean birth of their infant	Fawcett & Weiss, 1993
Needs of cesarean birth mothers	Women who experienced cesarean birth of their infant	Eakes & Brown, 1998; Kehoe, 1981
Attitudes toward cesarean birth	Women who experienced cesarean birth of their infant	Reichert et al., 1993
Differences in perceptions of women's needs during preterm labor	Registered nurses and postpartum mothers	Lynam & Miller, 1992
Postpartum functional status	Women who had experienced vaginal or cesarean delivery	Tulman & Fawcett, 1988
Interdependence needs	Newly delivered mothers	Short, 1994
Comparison of perceptions of maternal and infant stressors	Mothers of infants in a neonatal intensive care unit (NICU) and NICU nurses	Raeside, 1997
Advice to nurses and other mothers regarding breastfeeding	Swedish mothers of full-term infants in a neonatal intensive care unit	Nyqvist & Sjoden, 1993
Kinds of touch used during resuscitation immediately after delivery	Videotapes of premature infants who required resuscitation immediately after delivery	Kitchin & Hutchinson, 1996
Time required to measure stable axillary temperature	Newborn infants	Hunter, 1991
Experience of adapting to problems of caring for a very-low-birth-weight infant	Parents of very-low-birth-weight infants interviewed at 1, 3, and 5 months after hospital discharge	Vasquez, 1995

*See the Research section of the chapter references for complete citations.

400

Parents' needs	Mothers and fathers of children in a pediatric intensive care unit	Fisher, 1994
Differences in parental perception of stress and coping experiences	Parents of children in a neonatal or pediatric intensive care unit	Seideman et al., 1997
Perceptions and coping mechanisms	Neonatal nurses who care for dying babies	Raeside, 2000
Perceptions of pediatric intensive care unit stressors	Nurses working in a pediatric intensive care unit	Munn & Tichey, 1987
Sleep-wake patterns and environmental stressors	1- and 2-year-old children in an intensive care unit	Corser, 1996
Components of nursing care	Nurses caring for Finnish preschool children with minimal brain dysfunction	Kiikkala & Peitsi, 1991
Family support and child adjustment	Single-parent families	Friedemann & Andrews, 1990
Adaptation to a child with developmental disabilities	Foster parents of children with developmental disabilities	Rodriguez & Jones, 1996
Common health problems	Abused women and their children residing in a shelter	Germain, 1984
Process of adaptation to cancer	Taiwanese children with cancer	Yeh, 2001
Perceptions of isolation	Children who had been hospitalized in isolation for infectious diseases or immunodeficiency disorders	Broeder, 1985
Knowledge of internal anatomy and physiology	Deaf adults	Leyva et al., 2000
Family experiences	Members of families with a child with Duchenne muscular dystrophy	Gagliardi, 1991
Gender differences in reported stressors	Male and female high school freshmen	Thomas et al., 1988
Experience of transferring to adult health-care services	Adolescents with cystic fibrosis	Russell et al., 1996
Differences in depression according to age, gender, smoking, and alcohol use	Adolescents	Pullen et al., 2000
Experiences of living with ulcerative colitis	Swedish adolescents and young adults with ulcerative colitis	Brydolf & Segesten, 1996
Description of experience of integrating type 2 diabetes treatment recommendations into an existing lifestyle while participating in a nurse-coaching intervention	Women with type 2 diabetes	Whittemore et al., 2002
Long-term physical health status	Swedish adolescents and young adults who had surgery for ulcerative colitis	Brydolf & Segesten, 1994
Description of adaptive behaviors	Thai school-aged children with a sibling who has cancer	Phuphaibul & Muensa, 1999
Adaptive strengths	Parents of children with cancer	Smith et al., 1983

(continued)

Research Topic	Study Participants	Citation
Parental quality of life	Parents of children with cancer	Wright, 1993
Description of effects of interleukin-2 (IL-2) therapy on severity of illness, symptom distress, emotional distress, long-term quality of life, and hospital charges	Male and female cancer patients receiving IL-2 therapy	Jackson et al., 1991
Reports of adaptation to breast cancer and participation in support groups	Women with breast cancer who participated in cancer support groups	Samarel et al., 1998
Description of and report of content validity of educational materials used in a study of the effects of individual and group support on adaptation to breast cancer	Women with breast cancer who received individual and/or group support	Samarel et al., 1999
Differences in sexual functioning	Women with breast cancer treated with or without chemotherapy or endocrine therapy	Young-McCaughan, 1996
Sexual role performance of chronic alcoholics	Literature review	Frank & Lang, 1990
Description of responses to a music intervention	Case study of a 76-year-old man hospitalized for gastrointestinal bleeding due to alcohol consumption	Janelli et al., 1995
Characteristics of preoperative nursing assessments	Staff nurses	Takahashi & Bever, 1989
Concerns about surgery	Patients scheduled for open heart surgery and their significant others	Bradley & Williams, 1990
Differences in diuresis	Women who had a hysterectomy that could or could not potentially cause obstruction of the urinary tract	Sheppard & Cunnie, 1996
Spouses' needs	Spouses of surgical patients	Silva, 1987
Spouses' life stressors, supports, perception of illness severity, role strain, stress symptoms, and marital quality	Spouses of patients having coronary artery bypass surgery	Artinian, 1991, 1992
Changes in direction and degree of simultaneous and successive modes of information processing	Patients recovering from mild and moderate closed-head injuries	Roy & Andrews, 1999
Profile of nursing diagnoses related to oxygenation in trauma victims	Trauma victims admitted to an intensive care unit	Gomes de Arruda & Garcia, 2000
Functional and psychosocial adaptation to trauma	Adolescent and adult survivors of multiple trauma, at home 6 months after hospital discharge	Strohmyer et al., 1993

Quality of life	Men and women who had total hip replacement surgery 12 to 24 months before study	Selman, 1989
Perception of quality of life	Patients with non-small cell lung cancer who receive radiation therapy	John, 2001
Differences in prosthesis use problems	Men and women who had undergone above-the-knee or below-the-knee amputation	Medhat et al., 1990
Parental concerns	Mexican-American first-time mothers and fathers	Niska et al., 1997
Ethnographic study of intergenerational family rituals of Mexican-American families that facilitate adaptation to parenthood	Mexican-American families residing in Hidalgo County, Texas, experiencing transition to parenthood	Niska et al., 1998
Ethnographic study of the meaning of family health of Mexican-American first-time mothers and fathers	Mexican-American families residing in Hidalgo County, Texas, experiencing transition to parenthood	Niska et al., 1999
Ethnographic study of similarities and receptivity of nursing interventions to existing ways families were nurtured, supported, and socialized	Mexican-American families residing in Hidalgo County, Texas, experiencing transition to parenthood	Niska, 1999a
Ethnographic study of characteristics of Mexican-American family processes of nurturing, support, and socialization	Mexican-American families residing in Hidalgo County, Texas, experiencing transition to parenthood	Niska, 1999b
Description of family goals of survival, continuity, and growth	Mexican-American parents residing in Hidalgo County, Texas	Niska, 2001a
Field test of a methodology using parental stories to enhance family socialization when a firstborn child enters the community school system	Mexican-American parents residing in Hidalgo County, Texas	Niska, 2001b
Development of a conceptual framework to explain the interaction between caregiver and care receiver during discharge transition from hospital to home	Taiwanese care receivers and caregivers	Shyu, 2000
Family coping and family functioning	Caregivers of ventilator-dependent adults living at home	Smith et al., 1991
Caregiving responsibilities and reactions	Family caregivers of relatives who require total parenteral nutrition at home	Smith et al., 1993
Differences in anxiety, depression, and psychosocial adjustment	Male patients on home hemodialysis, in-center hemodialysis, or peritoneal dialysis	Courts & Boyette, 1998
Immune status and nutritional status	Women with HIV disease receiving therapy at the United States National Institutes of Health	Orsi et al., 1997

(continued)

Research Topic	Study Participants	Citation
Semantic structure of the term "person" related to women with HIV	Text of research report by Orsi et al., 1997	Neto & Pagliuca, 2002
Experiences and adaptation	Swedish women heterosexually infected with HIV	Florence et al., 1994
Differences in body image	Spinal cord–injured adults with and without pressure ulcers	Harding-Okimoto, 1997
Meaning of suffering	Adults with multiple sclerosis	Pollock & Sands, 1997
Description of making sense of the experience of living with multiple sclerosis	Individuals with multiple sclerosis	Gagliardi et al., 2002
Psychosexual concerns	Men and women hospitalized for diabetes mellitus	LeMone, 1995
Coping strategies	Older people with hypertension	Oliverira & Araujo, 2002
Physiological and psychosocial adaptation to chronic illness	Adults with hypertension, diabetes, rheumatoid arthritis, or multiple sclerosis	Pollock, 1986, 1989, 1993; Pollock et al., 1990
Physical and psychological adjustment	Women who had a mastectomy	Chen et al., 1999
Description of Roy Adaptation Model nursing process	Case studies of two adults with schizophrenia exhibiting withdrawal behavior	Schmidt, 1981
Attitudes toward nursing interventions	Hospitalized psychiatric patients	Leonard, 1975
Experiences of daily living	Blind adults living in a rural community in KwaZulu, South Africa	Zungu, 1993
Comparison of the importance and availability of expected and received types of assistance during convalescence, from an informal social support network	Older persons who had cardiac surgery	Paul & Rochichaud-Ekstrand, 2002
Perceived unmet needs, biopsychosocial problems, and coping strategies following termination of home care services	Elderly persons who had a stroke	Brandriet et al., 1994
Readiness to exercise and time devoted to the wife, household, grandmother, personal care, and recreational roles	Elderly Mexican women	Salazar-Gonzalez & Jirovec, 2001
Elements of holistic nursing	Case study of a 79-year-old woman who had a stroke	McIllmurray, 1997
Use of traditional and complementary therapies	Patients with chronic sinusitis	Krouse & Krouse, 1999

Differences in perceived life stressors	Elderly Chinese immigrants and other elderly Americans	Lee & Ellenbecker, 1998
Problems in adaptation	Elderly persons and their significant others	Farkas, 1981
Description of the pattern of the becoming-self	Home hospice patients	Dobratz, 2002
Comparison of perceptions of needs	Patients at different phases of organ transplant and nurses who work on transplant units	Baert et al., 2000
Incidence and impact of verbal abuse from physicians	Perioperative nurses	Cook et al., 2001
Description of effects of strikes by nursing personnel	Nurse managers and various categories of nursing personnel working in the KwaZulu-Natal Province of South Africa	Kunene & Nzimande, 1996
Nurses' perspectives of the use of the Roy Adaptation Model in practice	Registered nurses employed for more than 2 years at the hospital where the Roy Adaptation Model was used to guide nursing practice	Weiss et al., 1994

CORRELATIONAL STUDIES

Relation of pre-pregnant weight gain and weight gain during pregnancy to functional status, physical symptoms, and physical energy	Pregnant women	Tulman et al., 1998
Relation of expectations about the possibility of cesarean birth to type of delivery (vaginal or cesarean) and perception of the birth experience	Women who attended childbirth education classes and expected to have a vaginal delivery, who later had either a vaginal or an unplanned cesarean delivery	Fawcett et al., 1994
Relations of health, individual psychosocial, and family variables to functional status	Women interviewed at 3 weeks, 6 weeks, 3 months, and 6 months postpartum	Tulman et al., 1990; Tulman & Fawcett, 1990b
Relation of physical health, psychosocial health, and family relationships variables to functional status	Childbearing women interviewed during the first, second, and third trimesters of pregnancy and at 3 weeks, 6 weeks, 3 months, and 6 months postpartum	Tulman & Fawcett, 2003
Relation of fraction of inspired oxygen levels and number of hand ventilations to transcutaneous oxygen pressure	Intubated very-low-birth-weight infants receiving chest physiotherapy	Cheng & Williams, 1989
Relations among social support, parenting stress, coping style, and psychological distress	Parents caring for children with cancer	Yeh, 2003
Relation of age, gender, past painful experiences, temperament, general and medical fears, and child-rearing practices to pain-related responses	School-aged children having a venipuncture and their female caregivers	Bournaki, 1997

(continued)

Research Topic	Study Participants	Citation
Relation of self-esteem to age, gender, smoking, exercise, depression, anger, and parental alcohol use	Adolescents aged 12–19 years being treated in an outpatient mental health setting	Modrcin-Talbott, Pullen, Ehrenberger et al., 1998
Relation of self-esteem to age group, gender, exercise participation, smoking, parental alcohol use, depression, and anger	Healthy adolescents aged 12–19 years	Modrcin-Talbott, Pullen, Zandstra et al., 1998
Relation between religiosity and tobacco use	Male and female adolescents aged 12–19 years who were clients of a mental health agency or members of a church youth group	Pullen, Modricin-Talbott, West, Fenske et al., 1999
Relation of alcohol and drug abuse to frequency of religious service attendance	Adolescents living in the southeast United States	Pullen, Modrcin-Talbott, West, & Muenchen, 1999
Relations among appraisal of vaso-occlusive events, coping behavior during the event, and adjustment	Adolescents with sickle cell disease	Fletcher, 2000
Relation of physical abuse, emotional abuse, risk of homicide to post-traumatic stress disorder, as mediated by physiological stress response, self-esteem, functional status, and interpersonal relationships	Currently abused, post-abused, and non-abused women	Woods & Isenberg, 2001
Relation of symptoms of endometriosis to severity of pain and self-esteem	Women with a diagnosis of endometriosis	Christian, 1993
Relation of circadian type, work environment, and coping style to adaptation to shift work	Paper mill workers who rotate shifts	Phillips & Brown, 1992
Relation of conflicts, social support, perceived stress, and coping strategies to psychological distress and life satisfaction	Informal caregivers of demented relatives at home, informal caregivers of psychiatrically ill relatives at home, professional caregivers of elderly institutionalized patients, and elderly spouses in the community	Ducharme et al., 1998
Relation of gender, conflicts, social support, perceived stress, and coping strategies to psychological distress	Informal caregivers of demented relatives at home, informal caregivers of psychiatrically ill relatives at home, professional caregivers of elderly institutionalized patients, and elderly spouses in the community	Levesque et al., 1998
Relation between adaptation to focal stimuli and emotional distress	Hospitalized adult patients	Roy, 1978

Factors contributing to postoperative adjustment	Patients who had colostomy surgery	Piwonka & Merino, 1999
Relation of anxiety, sociodemographic variables, and acculturation to vital signs, nurse and patient ratings of pain, amount of pain medication, adaptation, self-esteem, sense of coherence, activities of daily living, length of hospital stay, and social support	Anglo-American and Mexican-American patients who had undergone cholecystectomy	Calvillo & Flaskerud, 1993
Relation of severity of illness, perceived control over visitation, hardiness, and state anxiety to length of stay in an intensive care unit	General medical-surgical intensive care unit patients	Hamner, 1996
Relation of length of stay in intensive care unit and number of hours after surgery when ambulation occurred to overall postoperative length of hospital stay	Patients who had coronary artery bypass graft surgery	Anderson et al., 1999
Relation between life satisfaction and physical functioning	Spinal cord–injured persons who had completed a rehabilitation program	Dunnum, 1990
Relation of age, gender, marital status, educational level, time postinjury, level and grade of injury, time in rehabilitation, hardiness, and ways of coping to physiological and psychosocial adaptation	Adults with spinal cord injuries resulting in quadriplegia or paraplegia	Barone & Roy, 1996
Relation of gender, partner's previous health, length of time of diagnosis, number of years married, and general state of the marital relationship to psychosocial adjustment to the partner's illness	Male and female spouses of persons who had undergone open heart surgery	Gardner, 1996
Relation between personal values and psychosocial adjustment to surgery	Adults who had coronary artery bypass surgery at 1 day before and 6 months after surgery	Flanagan, 1998
Relation of immune status, depression, and interpersonal relations to functional status	Women with breast cancer	Tulman & Fawcett, 1990a, 1996a, 1996b
Relation of social support, personal resources, coping styles, and household structure to psychosocial adjustment	Women with diabetes mellitus	Willoughby et al., 2000
Relation of symptom distress to functional status	Chronic in-center hemodialysis patients]	Thomas-Hawkins, 2000
Relations among severity of illness, symptom distress, and psychosocial adaptation	Male and female cancer patients receiving IL-2 therapy	Frederickson et al., 1991

(continued)

Research Topic	Study Participants	Citation
Test of a Roy model-based theory of health-related quality of life—relation of severity of illness, age, gender, communication with others, and understanding of the illness with physical function, psychologic function, peer/school function, treatment/disease symptoms, and cognition functions	Taiwanese children with cancer	Yeh, 2002
Test of a Roy model-based theory of health-related quality of life-symptom distress, emotional distress, functional status, and social support	Secondary analysis of data from newly diagnosed postsurgical cancer patients, 60–92 years of age	Nuamah et al., 1999
Relations among alternative therapies, functional status, and symptom severity	Men and women with multiple sclerosis	Fawcett et al., 1996
Relation of comorbidity, household composition, fatigue, and surgical pain to functional status	Women who had coronary bypass graft surgery	DiMattio & Tulman, 2003
Relation between physical health and hope	Elderly persons with and without cancer	McGill, 1992; McGill & Paul, 1993
Relation between marital status (married/ unmarried/widowed) and level of functioning	Stroke patients who had completed a rehabilitation program	Baker, 1993
Relations among functional health status, social support, and morale	Older women living alone in Appalachia	Collins, 1993
Relation of marital status and gender to health status and vulnerability to stress	Elderly married and unmarried men and women	Preston & Dellasega, 1990
Relations among loneliness, social support, depression, and cognitive functioning	Adults living in senior housing	Ryan, 1996
Relation of hearing loss to loneliness and self-esteem	Elderly men and women	Chen, 1994
Relation between cognitive adaptation processes and self-consistency	Older persons with hearing loss	Zhan, 2000; Roy & Zhan, 2001
Relation of age, sex, length of illness, social support, pain, and physical function to psychological adaptation	Adults in a home hospice program	Dobratz, 1993
Relation of social support, social network, income/education, spiritual beliefs, and coping processes to grief responses	Widows during the second year of bereavement	Robinson, 1995

Relation of medical condition, nursing condition, nursing intensity, and medical severity to length of hospital stay	Retrospective record review	Lutjens, 1991, 1992
Relation between payment source (DRG or per diem) and hospital length of stay	Retrospective record review	Lutjens, 1994
Relation of length of time after surgery and ventilator status on pain medication decisions	Critical care unit nurses	Gujol, 1994
Codependency issues	Hospital nursing staff	Chappelle & Sorrentino, 1993
Magnitude of interrelationships between the four Roy Adaptation Model modes	Reports of nine studies	Chiou, 2000

EXPERIMENTAL STUDIES

Effect of written birth plans or no birth plans on anxiety	Nulliparous pregnant women	Springer, 1996
Effect of an antenatal cesarean birth information program on responses to cesarean birth	Expectant parents attending childbirth education classes who later experienced a cesarean birth	Fawcett & Burritt, 1985; Fawcett & Henklein, 1987
Effects of an experimental antenatal cesarean birth information program and control usual cesarean birth information on perception of the birth experience, pain intensity, distress, self-esteem, functional status, feelings about the baby, and changes in the quality of the relationship with the spouse	Expectant parents attending childbirth education classes who later experienced an unplanned cesarean birth	Fawcett, 1990; Fawcett et al., 1993
Effects of a birthing chair and the traditional delivery table position on duration of second-stage labor, maternal blood loss, and infant outcomes	Women in labor and their infants	Cottrell & Shannahan,1986, 1987; Shannahan & Cottrell, 1985
Effects of suctioning, repositioning, and performing a heel stick on transcutaneous oxygen tension	Premature infants	Norris et al., 1982
Effects of environmental illumination level on oxygen saturation	Preterm infants	Shogan & Schumann, 1993
Effects of experimental taste, smell, and oral tactile stimulation and control traditional tactile stimulation on reinitiation of respiratory effort	Preterm infants experiencing an apneic episode	Garcia & White-Traut, 1993
Effects of early parent touch on heart rate and arterial oxygen saturation	Preterm infants	Harrison et al., 1990

(continued)

Research Topic	Study Participants	Citation
Effects of experimental gentle human touch intervention and control routine neonatal intensive care unit nursing care on inactivity, motor activity, behavioral distress cues, quiet sleep time, active sleep time, heart rate, oxygen saturation, length of hospitalization, and weight gain	Medically fragile preterm infants	Modrcin-Talbott et al., 2003
Effects of conventional system versus managed care clinical system on feeding behaviors, length of stay, severity of illness, readmissions, and cost of care	High-risk neonates	Jones & Smyth, 1999
Effects of structured home nursing visits on anxiety and retention of cardiopulmonary resuscitation knowledge	Parents of home apnea-monitored infants	Komelasky, 1990
Effects of type of thermometer and site on accuracy and reliability of temperature measurement	Children admitted to an emergency department	Pontious, Kennedy, Chang, et al., 1994; Pontious, Kennedy, Shelly, et al., 1994
Effects of a home ventilator care program on child and family psychosocial adjustment, parental and family preparation for home care, follow-up care, use of support services, child and family unmet needs, costs of home care, and changes in financial status or employment associated with the child's home care	Children with home ventilator assistance and their mothers	Hazlett, 1989
Effect of the Frame Model of Preadolescent Empowerment on perception of self-worth	Preadolescent children with attention-deficit hyperactivity disorder	Frame, 2003
Effects of an experimental school-based, nurse-facilitated support group and a control substantial attention group on perceptions of scholastic competence, social acceptance, behavioral conduct, perceived athletic competence, perceived physical appearance, and perceived global self-worth	Preadolescents diagnosed with attention deficit disorder or attention deficit hyperactivity disorder	Frame et al., 2003
Effect of a psychotherapy group, a self-help group, or no group on depression	College-age adult children of alcoholics	Kuhns, 1997
Effects of a safer sex educational module on AIDS-related beliefs and safer sex practices	College students	Vicenzi & Thiel, 1992

Effect of Roy Adaptation Model pre-operative nursing assessments or routine preoperative assessments on knowledge of patients' physiological and psychosocial needs	Circulating operating room nurses	Leuze & McKenzie, 1987
Effects of experimental Tellington touch and control social conversation with a friendly medic on blood pressure, heart rate, state anxiety, and procedural pain	Healthy members of the National Guard in the Midwest receiving a routine physical examination	Wendler, 2003
Effect of experimental music therapy and control no music on anxiety	Ambulatory patients undergoing colonoscopy	Smolen et al., 2002
Effect of humorous audiotapes, tranquil music audiotapes, or no audiotapes on preoperative anxiety	Men and women scheduled for same-day, elective, nondiagnostic surgery	Gaberson, 1991, 1995
Effects of an experimental structured preoperative teaching program and control usual teaching on postoperative atelectasis incidence and patient satisfaction	Men and women scheduled for surgery	Meeker, 1994
Effects of a preoperative experimental structured or control unstructured education program on postoperative vital signs, use of analgesics, nausea and vomiting, length of postanesthesia care unit stay, and patient satisfaction	Women scheduled for laparoscopic tubal ligation	Coslow & Eddy, 1998
Effects of an experimental nursing assessment and supportive intervention and a control routine nursing intervention on postoperative recall of perceptions in relation to the environment, feelings, events, and people during the immediate preanesthesia preoperative period	Sedated surgical patients awaiting general anesthesia induction	Nolan, 1977
Effect of family member visitation, familiar nurse visitation, or no visitation on anxiety	Women surgical patients in a postanesthesia care unit	Vogelsang & Ragiel, 1987
Effects of a substance abuse clinical pathway on co-morbidity, number of re-admissions, provider satisfaction, patient satisfaction, length of stay, hospital discharge statistics, and number of referrals to outpatient substance abuse treatment	Hospitalized medical patients at risk for substance abuse	Lopez-Bushnell & Fassler, 2002
Effect of an experimental care conference and a control no care conference on anxiety	Family members of patients being transferred from a neurological intensive care unit to a general care unit	Bokinskie, 1992

(continued)

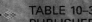
Research Topic	Study Participants	Citation
Effects of attachment of invasive (intravenous) or noninvasive (telemetry) technology on comfort, self-esteem, patient role, and social relationships	Medical-surgical patients	Campbell-Heider, 1993; Campbell-Heider & Knapp, 1993
Effects of placement of nitroglycerin ointment on severity of headache and flushing	Patients with cardiac disease	Riegel et al., 1988
Effects of a structured exercise program on exercise tolerance, activity and sleep patterns, and quality of life	Men and women diagnosed with cancer	Young-McCaughan et al., 2003
Effects of timing of an experimental cardiac teaching program on psychological anxiety, physiological anxiety, and knowledge of illness and related health-care issues	Male hospitalized myocardial infarction patients	Guzzetta, 1979
Effect of an experimental information-processing practice protocol or no protocol on changes in information processing	Patients recovering from mild and moderate head injuries	Roy & Andrews, 1999
Effect of an experimental stroke club and a control no stroke club on caregiver burden	Caregivers of stroke survivors	Printz-Fedderson, 1990
Effects of cancer support groups with and without coaching and no support group on symptom distress, emotional distress, functional status, and quality of relationship with significant other	Women with newly diagnosed early-stage breast cancer	Samarel & Fawcett, 1992; Samarel et al., 1993, 1997
Effects of an experimental structured walking exercise program and support groups and control usual care on performance status, physical functioning, psychosocial adjustment, self-concept, body image, and symptom intensity	Women with breast cancer receiving adjuvant chemotherapy	Mock et al., 1994
Effects of an experimental walking exercise program and control usual care on physical functioning, exercise level, emotional distress, and symptom experience (fatigue)	Women with breast cancer receiving radiation therapy	Mock et al., 1997
Effects of an experimental humor intervention and control no humor on mood and pain	Cancer patients	Dant, 1993

Effect of an experimental nursing intervention aimed at reinforcing positive-input thought patterns, control craft classes, and a no-intervention control on depressive symptoms	Community-dwelling, low-income, well elderly persons	Campbell, 1992
Effect of rocking in a rocking chair on relaxation (heart rate, systolic and diastolic blood pressure, skin temperature)	Community-residing women and men	Houston, 1993
Effects of a Roy Adaptation Model-based treatment protocol, a Neuman Systems Model-based treatment protocol, and a treatment protocol not based on an explicit conceptual model on depression and life satisfaction	Retired persons attending a senior citizen center	Hoch, 1987
Effect of home environment-based nursing intervention on urine control	Incontinent memory-impaired elders and their caregivers	Jirovec et al., 1999
Effects of an individualized scheduled toileting program	Incontinent, memory-impaired elders being cared for at home	Jirovec & Templin, 2001
Effect of experimental domestic animal visitation and control no animal visitation on social interaction, psychosocial function, life satisfaction, mental function, depression, social competence, psychological well-being, personal neatness, and health self-concept	Male and female nursing home residents	Francis et al., 1985
Effect of level of human-pet interaction during resident and visitation pet programs on loneliness	Male and female nursing home residents	Calvert, 1989
Effect of an experimental wheelchair bike riding intervention and control standard care on depression	Elderly long-term care residents	Fitzsimmons, 2001
Effect of an experimental formal invitation to have greater involvement in care of relative and control usual involvement in care on satisfaction with care given	Former caregivers of relatives newly admitted to a nursing home	Toye et al., 1996
Effect of experimental slow-stroke back massage on relaxation (blood pressure, heart rate, skin temperature)	Hospice clients	Meek, 1993
Effects of bereavement group postvention and social group postvention on depression, psychological distress, grief resolution, and social adjustment	Bereaved widows and widowers who survived the suicide of a spouse	Constantino, 1993
Effect of use of Roy Adaptation Model first-level (behaviors) and second-level assessment (stimuli) data or use of first-level assessment data only on accuracy of nursing diagnoses	Registered nurses familiar with the Roy Adaptation Model	Hammond et al., 1983

(Text continued from page 395)

- Cerritos Community College, Cerritos, California
- Golden West College, Huntington Park, California
- Mount St. Mary's College, Los Angeles, California
- Point Loma College, San Diego, California
- Harbor Community College, San Pedro, California
- Wesley Passavant School of Nursing, Chicago, Illinois
- Kansas State College, Pittsburg, Kansas
- Maryland General Hospital, Baltimore, Maryland
- Graceland College, Independence, Missouri
- Northwest Missouri State University, Kirksville, Missouri
- William Paterson College, Wayne, New Jersey
- Central State College, Edmond, Oklahoma
- University of Tulsa, Tulsa, Oklahoma
- University of Portland, Portland, Oregon
- Widener University, Chester, Pennsylvania
- Edinboro State College, Edinboro, Pennsylvania
- Villa Maria College, Erie, Pennsylvania
- Community College of Philadelphia, Philadelphia, Pennsylvania
- University of Texas at Arlington and at Austin
- Alverno College, Milwaukee, Wisconsin
- Columbia Hospital, Milwaukee, Wisconsin
- Royal Alexander Hospital, Edmonton, Alberta, Canada
- University of Calgary, Calgary, Alberta, Canada
- Health Sciences Centre, Winnipeg, Manitoba, Canada
- Vanier College, Montreal, Quebec, Canada
- Ecole Génévoise d'Infirmière, Le Bon Secours, Geneva, Switzerland

Some reports of nursing education programs based on the Roy Adaptation Model have been published. The names of the schools in which those programs are located are listed here. The complete citations for the publications are given in the Education section of the chapter references. The Roy Adaptation Model also has been used as a guide for a professional nursing staff competency-based orientation program at Our Lady of Bellefonte Hospital in Ashland, Kentucky (Runyon, 1994).

- Associate Degree Nursing Programs
  - Community College of Philadelphia, Philadelphia, Pennsylvania (Mengel et al., 1989)
  - North Central Technical College, Wausau, Wisconsin (Flood & Schneider, 1993)
  - Mount St. Mary's College, Los Angeles, California (Rambo, 1984)
- Baccalaureate Programs
  - University of Hartford, Hartford, Connecticut (Heinrich, 1989)
  - The Catholic University of America, Washington, DC (Knowlton et al., 1983)
  - University of Miami, Geriatric Nurse Practitioner Program, Coral Gables, Florida (Brower & Baker, 1976)

- Saginaw Valley State University, University Center, Michigan (Claus et al., 1991)
- University of Wisconsin–Green Bay, Green Bay, Wisconsin—Computer Applications in Nursing course (Curl et al., 1988)
- Mount St. Mary's College, Los Angeles, California (Rambo, 1984; Roy, 1973, 1974, 1979, 1980, 1989)
- University of Quebec in Hull, Hull, Quebec, Canada—Family nursing theory and practice courses (deMontigny et al., 1997)
- University of Ottawa, Ottawa, Ontario, Canada—First-, second-, and third-year nursing courses (Morales-Mann & Logan, 1990; Story & Ross, 1986)
- La Sabana University, Bogotá, Colombia (Fawcett, 2003)
- Robert Gordon University, Foresterhill Campus, Aberdeen, Scotland—Adult Branch Program of a Diploma in Higher Education Course (Gordon & Grundy, 1997)

An interesting application of the model in nursing education was presented by Camooso, Greene, and Reilly (1981). The authors, who were graduate nursing students, described their adjustment to graduate school within the context of the four adaptive modes of Roy's model, citing adaptive and ineffective behaviors they exhibited throughout the master's degree program.

Another interesting and innovative application of the Roy Adaptation Model was described by Dobratz (2003). She reported that undergraduate students who were enrolled in a nursing research course that was guided by the Roy Adaptation Model indicated that they were able to successfully put the pieces of the research puzzle together by working in groups, being supported by the instructor, and learning from diverse teaching methods. Dobratz (2003) concluded, "[I]nformation on conceptual models of nursing at the undergraduate level provides a powerful tool by which students learn nursing's distinct knowledge base, and gain skill in differentiating the separate knowledge found within the context of medicine" (p. 389).

Nursing Administration. Roy (1987a) commented, "Implementing the [Roy Adaptation] model of nursing care in whole health care systems will require … expertise both in implementation and in evaluation of the outcomes. Some of the outcomes are important in relation to what the model does for nursing, such as increasing autonomy, accountability, and professionalism in general, and in changing relationships with other disciplines" (p. 44).

The utility of the Roy Adaptation Model for nursing service administration is documented. The published reports listed in the Administration section of the chapter references indicate that the Roy Adaptation Model has been used to guide the administration of nursing services in hospitals and medical centers across the United States and in Canada, England, and Sweden. Moreover, practice tools that are particularly relevant to the administration of nursing services, including standards of nursing practice, nursing job descriptions, quality assessment tools, a performance appraisal system, and a format for intershift report, have been developed within the context of the Roy Adaptation Model (see Table 10–2). The health-care organizations in which Roy Adaptation Model-based nursing practice has been implemented, as described in the available literature, are listed here. The complete citations for the publications are given in the Administration section of the chapter references.

- Montefiore Medical Center, Henry and Lucy Moses Division Neurosurgical Nursing Unit, New York City, New York (Frederickson, 1991, 1993; Frederickson & Williams, 1997; Parse, 1990; Roy, 1992)
- Hospital of the University of Pennsylvania, Day Gynecologic Chemotherapy Unit, Philadelphia, Pennsylvania (Torosian et al., 1985)
- National Hospital for Orthopaedics and Rehabilitation, Arlington, Virginia (Mastel et al, 1982; Silva & Sorrell, 1992)
- St. Joseph Regional Medical Center, Lewiston, Idaho (Connerley et al., 1999)
- Veterans Administration Medical Center, Nursing Home Care Unit, Roseburg, Oregon (Dorsey & Purcell, 1987)
- Providence Hospital, Oakland, California (Laros, 1977)
- South Coast Medical Center, Laguna Beach, California (Gray, 1991)
- Anaheim Memorial Hospital, Anaheim, California (Gray, 1991)
- Children's Hospital of Orange County, Orange, California (Jakocko & Sowden, 1986)
- Sharp Memorial Hospital, Mary Birch Hospital for Women, San Diego, California (Weiss & Teplick, 1993, 1995)
- Centre Hospitalier Pierre Janet, Hull, Quebec, Canada (Robitaille-Tremblay, 1984)
- Mount Sinai Hospital, Toronto, Ontario, Canada (Fitch et al., 1991)
- Orthopedic and Arthritic Hospital, Toronto, Ontario, Canada (Rogers et al., 1991)
- La Sanbana University Hospital, Bogotá, Colombia (Fawcett, 2003)
- Fundación Cardio Infantil-Istituto de Cardiologia, Pediatric Critical Care and Neonatal Units, Bogotá, Colombia (Fawcett, 2003)
- Brighton General Hospital, Acute Surgery Ward, Brighton, England (Lewis, 1988)
- University Children's Hospital, Neonatal Intensive Care Unit, Uppsala, Sweden (Nyqvist & Karlsson, 1997)

Furthermore, Roy and Anway (1989) presented an adaptation of the Roy Adaptation Model for nursing administration (RAMA). The organizational modes of adaptation are the physical system, the role system, the interpersonal system, and the interdependence system. Those systems adapt to internal and external environmental conditions through stabilizer and innovator central mechanisms. The notions of the physical system and the stabilizer and innovator mechanisms presented in Roy and Anway's (1989) description of the RAMA have been incorporated into the most recent version of the Roy Adaptation Model, as presented in Roy and Andrews' (1999) book.

DiIorio (1989) also described the application of the conceptual model to nursing administration. Furthermore, Roy and Martinez (1983) presented a conceptual framework for clinical specialist nursing practice based on the Roy Adaptation Model and systems notions. In addition, Zarle (1987) described a Roy Adaptation Model-based model for planning continuing care following hospitalization.

Nursing Practice. The Roy Adaptation Model has documented utility for nursing practice with patients across the lifespan who have various health conditions and are in various settings. Phillips (2002) agreed that "Roy's model is generalizable to all settings in nursing practice" (p. 287) but criticized the model for the limitations in its scope, "because it primarily addresses the concept of person-environment adaptation and focuses primarily on the patient. Information on the nurse is implied" (p. 287). Published reports of the application of the Roy Adaptation Model in practice are listed in Table 10–4.

Galbreath (2002) pointed to the broad applicability of the Roy Adaptation Model. She stated:

> The concepts of the model have application for individuals across the life span and for families, groups, and other collective human adaptive systems. No age or situation is particularly outside the scope of the model [although] portions of the model may be of greater concern to the nurse at different times. … The model helps the nurse organize and apply the vast body of knowledge of nursing science and related sciences and arts to promote adaptation of individuals and groups (p. 324).

More specifically, a review of the published reports listed in Table 10–4 and the publications listed in the Commentary: Practice section of the chapter bibliography on the CD-ROM reveals that the Roy Adaptation Model has been used to guide nursing practice with children and adolescents with chronic and acute medical conditions, such as Kawasaki disease, juvenile dermatomyositis, diabetes, acute lymphocytic leukemia, and cancer. The model also has guided nursing practice with well adults, including childbearing women and new fathers, and with men and women with such chronic or acute medical conditions as emotional problems or psychiatric illness; spinal cord, burn, or other injuries; cardiac surgery; cardiac disease; respiratory disease; Hodgkin's disease; cancer; human immunodeficiency virus (HIV) disease; acquired immunodeficiency syndrome (AIDS); substance abuse; diabetes; end-stage renal disease; psoriasis; scleroderma; neurofibromatosis; osteoporosis; Parkinson's disease; and Alzheimer's disease. In addition, the model has been used to guide nursing with dying persons and the family caregivers of terminally ill persons. Moreover, the model has been used in acute care settings, operating rooms, critical care and coronary care units, psychiatric units, emergency departments, and outpatient settings, including clinics and people's homes.

Roy (1983) and Hanna and Roy (2001) expanded the Roy Adaptation Model to encompass nursing care of the family. Roy (1984b) and Hanchett (1990) extended the model for use in community health nursing.

In addition, several generic and health condition–specific practice tools have been developed to guide Roy Adaptation Model-based nursing practice and to facilitate documentation of that practice. Those tools are identified and described in Table 10–2.

Social Congruence

The Roy Adaptation Model is generally congruent with societal expectations for nursing practice. Individuals and groups who expect to have input into nursing should find this model to be consistent with their views. Moreover, the model's emphasis on adaptation within a constantly changing environment is congruent with many people's perspective of the world today as a place of turmoil and rapid change. Indeed, Mastal and colleagues (1982) reported enhanced patient satisfaction and health outcomes as a result of the initial implementation of the Roy Adaptation Model at the National Hospital for Orthopaedics and Rehabilitation in Arlington, Virginia. In addition, Robitaille-Tremblay (1984; personal communication, August 4, 1982) reported that use of a Roy Adaptation Model-based nursing history tool for psychiatric patients (see Table 10–2) at a Canadian hospital enhanced the patients' satisfaction with care, quoting them as saying, "It is the first time a professional has evaluated me so fully"; "I realize that most of my problems interrelate"; and "I have learned to know myself better than I have during any previous hospitalization" (Robitaille-Tremblay, 1984, p. 28).

Frederickson and Williams (1997) reported a very positive response by patients and their families to the use of Roy Adaptation Model-based nursing practice on the neurosurgical unit of the Moses Division of Montefiore Medical Center in New York. The patients' and family members' responses indicated much satisfaction in the areas of caring, holistic nursing care, communication, professional fulfillment of nurses, and interdisciplinary collegiality among nurses and other health professionals. In addition, Frederickson and Williams (1997) reported that a survey comparing the responses of patient/family satisfaction before and after implementation of the Roy Adaptation Model on the unit revealed increases in the 10 areas on the survey questionnaire, with the greatest improvement in the areas of "The nursing staff really cared about you as a person," "The nursing staff included your family in decision making and your care," and "The nursing staff was interested in all aspects of your life not just your current medical problems" (p. 54).

However, as with other conceptual models that include a focus on the well person, the Roy Adaptation Model may not be entirely congruent with some people's expectations of nursing. This would be especially so when the nurse's action is directed toward reinforcement of already adaptive behaviors.

The Roy Adaptation Model is congruent with nurses', physicians', and hospital administrators' expectations for nursing. Robitaille-Tremblay (1984) reported increased nurse satisfaction as the result of using a Roy Adaptation Model-based nursing history tool for psychiatric patients (see Table 10–2) at Centre Hospitalier Pierre Janet. She noted that the tool "helped [nurses] get to know the patient more fully and to broaden their perspective in establishing priorities on the basis of identified stimuli. Some felt closer to the patient with whom the tool was used. One nurse stated, 'I have acquired more confidence in my independent role and I'm proud, very proud'" (p. 28). Nurses have also indicated their satisfaction with Roy Adaptation Model-based nursing practice by means of reduced turnover; Montefiore Medical Center in New York City realized a savings of approximately $300,000 in staff orientation costs due to the lack of resignations following the implementation of the model on the neurosurgical unit (K. Frederickson, cited in Roy, 1992a).

Furthermore, Mastal and her colleagues (1982) noted that the initial use of the model at the National Hospital for Orthopaedics and Rehabilitation led to enhanced professional nursing practice. Elaborating, they explained, "The staff has contributed to developing a tool that provides a way to assess the biopsychosocial status of patients. In planning for patient care, the nurses are not only meticulous about writing complete plans, but phrase existing patient problems in terms of nursing diagnoses, consistent with the concepts of the Adaptation Model" (p. 14).

Weiss and colleagues (1994) found that many nurses at Sharp Memorial Hospital in San Diego, California experienced positive outcomes of the implementation of Roy Adaptation Model-based nursing practice. The nurses

(Text continues on page 419)

Nursing Situation	Population	Citation*
	INDIVIDUALS	
Application of Roy's Adaptation Model	Young children who are hospitalized	Galligan, 1979
	10-month-old child with tracheomalacia	Lankester & Sheldon, 1999
	Children with Kawasaki disease	Nash, 1987
	An 8-year-old boy with leukemia	Wright et al., 1993
	A 9-year-old girl with juvenile dermatomyositis	Hartley & Campion-Fuller, 1994
	Adolescents with cancer	Ellis, 1991
	Adolescents with asthma	Hennessy-Harstad, 1999
	A teenager with diabetes mellitus	Roy, 1971
	A 19-year-old college student	Barnfather et al., 1989
	A pregnant woman	Sato, 1986
	Women undergoing genetic testing during pregnancy	Stringer et al., 1991
	Women experiencing preterm labor	Eganhouse, 1994
	A 22-year-old multipara who did not want the baby, in active labor	Wagner, 1976
	Postpartum cesarean-delivered mothers	Kehoe, 1981
	Fathers whose infants were born by cesarean	Fawcett, 1981
	A 27-year-old woman who delivered an infant in respiratory distress	Downey, 1974
	Women experiencing cardiomyopathy during the peripartum period	Sirignano, 1987
	A 25-year-old new mother experiencing emotional problems	Fawcett, 1997
	A 23-year-old man who was severely injured in a farm accident	Giger et al., 1987
	Adults experiencing multiple trauma	DiMaria, 1989
	Adults who suffered severe burns	Summers, 1991
	A 25-year-old woman with Hodgkin's disease	Gerrish, 1989
	A 29-year-old woman recovering from surgery for cervical cancer	Phillips, 1997, 2002
	A woman scheduled for excision of bilateral breast lumps	Fox, 1990
	A 37-year-old woman who had a benign chest mass	West, 1992
	A woman who had gynecologic surgery	Roy, 1971
	A 38-year-old woman with metastatic breast cancer	Piazza et al., 1992
	Adults with HIV disease	Griffiths-Jones & Walker, 1993
	A 27-year-old man with AIDS	Phillips, 1997, 2002
	A hospitalized 34-year-old woman and a 39-year-old man experiencing anxiety due to surgical or medical problems	Frederickson, 1993
	A 30-year-old woman alcoholic admitted to a detoxification unit	McIver, 1987
	Adult cocaine abusers recovering from anesthesia for surgery	Rogers, 1991
	A 44-year-old man who had a heart transplant	Cardiff, 1989
	A 47-year-old man recovering from surgery for a cerebral aneurysm	Fawcett et al., 1992
	Adults who had stomal surgery	Hughes, 1991
	Women experiencing changes associated with menopause	Cunningham, 2002
	Women experiencing depression during the climacteric	Coleman, 1993
	Adults experiencing depression	Lambert, 1994

*See the Practice section of the chapter references for complete citations.

(continued)

Nursing Situation	Population	Citation
	Individuals with schizophrenia experiencing withdrawal behavior	Schmidt, 1981
	Individuals diagnosed with organic brain damage, mild to moderate mental retardation, or schizoaffective disorder	Hamer, 1991
	A 22-year-old man hospitalized for criminal behavior	Miller, 1991
	Adults with respiratory problems	Innes, 1992
	Adults with diabetes mellitus	Miller & Hellenbrand, 1981; O'Reilly, 1989
	A man with end-stage renal disease undergoing hemodialysis	Keen et al., 1998
	Adults with renal disorders	Frank, 1988
	A woman with psoriasis	Forsdyke, 1993
	Adults with scleroderma	Crossfield, 1990
	Individuals who have neurofibromatosis	Messner & Smith, 1986
	A 60-year-old man admitted to a rehabilitation center with a spinal cord injury	Piazza & Foote, 1990
	Adults with osteoporosis	Doyle & Rajacich, 1991
	Adults with Parkinson's disease undergoing stereotactic posteroventral pallidotomy	Bonnema, 1997
	A 69-year-old man undergoing a below-the-knee amputation	Dawson, 1998
	A man admitted to an emergency department with chest pain	Ingram, 1995
	An individual who had an acute myocardial infarction	Hernández, 2002
	An individual with cardiac disease	Araich, 2001
	A 70-year-old man who had a myocardial infarction	Gordon, 1974
	A 65-year-old woman admitted to a psychiatric hospital with a diagnosis of manic depression and recovering in a nursing home from partial gastrectomy surgery	Janelli, 1980
	Elderly persons with hypernatremia	Aaronson & Seaman, 1989
	An elderly women with rheumatoid arthritis	Madina Lizarralde, 2001
	Community-dwelling elderly individuals	Smith, 1988
	Elderly persons with Alzheimer's disease	Thornbury & King, 1992
	Individuals who are dying	Logan, 1986; Starr, 1980
	Individuals caring for their terminally ill relatives	Jay, 1990
Application of Roy's Adaptation Model and Orem's Self-Care Framework	An individual with tetraplegia	Dornik, 2002

FAMILIES

Nursing Situation	Population	Citation
Application of Roy's Adaptation Model	An older couple expecting their first child	Roy, 1983a
	A family with an infant	deMontigny, 1992a, 1992b
	A family made up of a 23-year-old mother, her three young children, and the children's grandmother	Schmitz, 1980
	A family with an adolescent member with diabetes	Roy, 1983b
	A mother and her children, all of whom have hypophosphatemic rickets	Dudek, 1989
	A family with a mentally retarded child	Hitejc, 2001
	A 32-year-old mother and her children dealing with the sudden death of the 42-year-old father from a heart attack	Whall, 1986
	A family made up of an elderly couple, their daughter and her husband, and their two children	Donnelly, 1993
	A family experiencing the terminal illness of a member	Logan, 1988

GROUPS

Application of Roy's Adaptation Model	Mothers of developmentally delayed children in a psychoeducational group	Bawden et al., 1991
	Inpatient psychiatric patients in group therapy	Kurek-Ovshinsky, 1991

COMMUNITIES

Application of Roy's Adaptation Model	A community	Batra, 1996
	A county in need of a shelter for the victims of domestic violence	Hanchett, 1988

(Text continued from page 416)

reported that the model provided "a structure for thinking about patient care, direction for organizing nursing work, and a focus on comprehensive, holistic care for patient and family ... [and] on the development of nursing skills" (p. 82). The nurses also reported a positive impact on the quality of patient care, due to the model's comprehensive approach. In addition, the nurses reported a positive impact on "their personal sense of professionalism as well as the image of nursing as a whole ... and the uniqueness of the nursing role" (p. 84).

Connerley and her colleagues (1999) reported positive nurse-focused outcomes of the implementation of Roy Adaptation Model-based nursing practice in the areas of practice, management, and staff education at St. Joseph's Regional Medical Center. They explained, "Model-based nursing has influenced patient care, the documentation system, and communication, while empowering nurses. ... Nurses are now able to identify and describe their practice and the influence they have on patient outcomes. ... Education focuses on patient care and model-based nursing practice. Skills fairs have become nursing practice fairs" (pp. 530–531).

Another indicator of enhanced professional practice at the National Hospital for Orthopaedics and Rehabilitation is the finding that an increased number of staff members received baccalaureate and master's degrees after implementation of the Roy Adaptation Model (Silva & Sorrell, 1992). Moreover, physicians and hospital administrators have expressed their acceptance of the Roy Adaptation Model as an appropriate guide for nursing practice (Roy, 1992a).

Social Significance

The social significance of the Roy Adaptation Model continues to be established. Anecdotal evidence regarding the impact of Roy Adaptation Model-based nursing care comes from Starn and Niederhauser (1990). They reported that several practicing nurses who used their Roy-based MCN Developmental/Diagnostic Model (see Table 10–2) "were better able to identify problems [and] determine interventions more effectively" (p. 182).

Additional anecdotal evidence comes from Robitaille-Tremblay (personal communication, August 4, 1982), who commented, "Interestingly, patients stayed longer in the hospital" after a Roy Adaptation Model-based nursing history tool for psychiatric patients (see Table 10–2) was implemented. She indicated that use of the tool led to more comprehensive assessments and nursing care plans. She went on to say that research was planned to determine whether there is a relation between use of the tool and length of hospital stay. To date, no reports of that research have been located.

Empirical evidence comes from the findings of many studies. Hoch (1987), for example, studied the effects of a treatment protocol derived from the Roy Adaptation Model on depression and life satisfaction in a sample of retired persons. She found that the Roy protocol group had lower depression scores and higher life satisfaction scores than a control group who received a nursing intervention that was not based on an explicit conceptual model. Although the logical connection between depression and life satisfaction and the adaptive modes of the Roy Adaptation Model might be questioned, Hoch's study represents the beginning of the empirical work that is needed to determine the credibility of conceptual models of nursing.

Additional evidence, albeit mixed, comes from research that was based explicitly on propositions of the Roy Adaptation Model addressing relations between the adaptive modes. Calvillo and Flaskerud (1993), for example, carefully constructed a conceptual-theoretical-empirical structure to test the empirical adequacy of the Roy Adaptation Model. Their mixed findings for relation between the adaptive modes revealed that "the empirical adequacy of the model as a whole could not be established" (p. 127).

In contrast, Chiou (2000) and Tulman and Fawcett (2003) presented impressive empirical evidence supporting the credibility of the Roy Adaptation Model with regard to the interrelationships among the four adaptive modes. Collectively, the evidence they presented revealed that "The magnitude of statistically significant correlations between variables representing the four [adaptive] modes indicated that the modes are interrelated but also independent components of adaptation to environmental stimuli" (Tulman & Fawcett, 2003, p. 160). In addition, Tulman and Fawcett (2003) and DiMattio and Tulman (2003) reported substantial evidence of relations between variables representing focal and contextual stimuli and those representing one or more of the adaptive modes.

Some experimental studies have revealed the expected adaptive responses to Roy Adaptation Model-based nursing interventions, others have yielded mixed findings, and still others have revealed no differences between the experimental and control conditions. Findings from some experimental studies support the effectiveness of Roy Adaptation Model-based nursing interventions. For example, Sparks (1998) found that children who received Roy Adaptation Model-based nursing interventions of distraction (bubble-blowing) or cutaneous stimulation (touch) reported less pain during a Diphtheria-Tetanus-Pertussis injection than did children who received standard care. Smolen, Topp, and Singer (2002) reported that music therapy decreased heart rate, blood pressure, and the amount of sedation required during colonoscopy. Young-McCaughan and colleagues (2003) found that cancer patients who completed a Roy Adaptation Model-based exercise program experienced significant improvements in exercise tolerance, activity and sleep patterns, and quality of life, compared to patients who did not complete the exercise program. Fitzsimmons (2001) reported that long-term care residents who were depressed and who participated in a Roy Adaptation Model-based wheelchair bike intervention experienced a statistically significant improvement in depression scores than did depressed residents who did not participate in the intervention. And, Banks (1998) found that long-term care residents who participated in an animal-assisted therapy intervention experienced a reduction in loneliness when compared to their counterparts who did not participate in the animal-assisted therapy intervention.

Mixed findings come, for example, from Wendler's (2003) study. She found that Tellington touch, which she regarded as management of a contextual stimulus, was effective in reducing blood pressure and heart rate in response to the noxious focal stimulus of venipuncture. The Tellington touch intervention did not, however, have any effect on state anxiety and perceived pain.

An example of findings of no differences is Fawcett and associates' (1993) study. They concluded that their findings of no differences in outcomes between the experimental and control conditions of antenatal information about cesarean birth raised questions about the credibility of the Roy Adaptation Model. However, they pointed out that then recent changes in childbirth education with regard to provision of cesarean birth information may have prevented an adequate test of the effects of increasing the contextual stimulus of information.

On the basis of an integrative review of 163 Roy Adaptation Model-based studies, the Boston Based Adaptation Research Nursing Society (1999) concluded that the research as a whole provides theoretical and empirical support for the Roy Adaptation Model concepts and propositions. The results of many studies confirmed the role of stimuli in adaptation, although the relative importance of such common stimuli as single demographic variables (e.g., age, gender) is doubtful. Instead, the role of research variables representing stimuli in adaptation may be better understood if future research focuses on pooled effects of stimuli and on adaptation level. Furthermore, the findings of several studies revealed a reciprocal relation between coping processes and responses in the adaptive modes, indicating the need to employ multivariate and structural equation model statistical techniques in future research. Moreover, several studies supported the Roy Adaptation Model contention that the four adaptive modes are interrelated. Lacking, however, is a sufficient number of longitudinal and cross-sectional studies of adaptive mode responses across the life span. In addition, although some studies documented the importance of patients' perceptions, and some ways to measure those perceptions have been identified, research is needed to better understand patient and family perceptions in diverse practice situations. Research also is needed that focuses on the identification of the appropriate timing of interventions and measurement of subsequent outcomes.

A meta-analytic study that extends Ayers (1991) early work and Chiou's (2000) more recent work is the next step in integrating the Roy Adaptation Model-based research. Such a study would be especially helpful in determining the magnitude of effects of interventions and identifying design and other factors that might be contributing to the mixed findings (Rosenthal, 1991).

 ## CONTRIBUTIONS TO THE DISCIPLINE OF NURSING

The Roy Adaptation Model makes a significant contribution to nursing knowledge by focusing attention on the nature of the changes in a person's or a group's adaptation. Roy's perspective of adaptation goes beyond that presented by other disciplines by placing it within the context of the person or group as a holistic adaptive system. Thus, the Roy Adaptation Model presents a distinctive view of the person and the group, one that developed within the discipline of nursing.

Roy and others (e.g., Randell, Poush Tedrow, & Van Landingham, 1982) have continued to develop the various concepts of the conceptual model, so that only a few gaps and omissions remain. Roy and Roberts' (1981) work to develop the Theory of the Person as an Adaptive System and the theories of the adaptive modes and Roy's (2003) more recent work is especially noteworthy. That work resulted in construction of the beginning of logically congruent conceptual-theoretical-empirical structures that can be used for nursing activities. The importance of the Theory of the Person as an Adaptive System to nursing was summarized by Roy and Roberts (1981). They stated, "Investigation of adaptive systems is evident in the literature of a number of fields including genetics, biology, physiology, physics, psychology, anthropology, and sociology. All of these approaches can be helpful in conceptualizing the adaptive system. Yet each approach views the person or the group from the perspective of that discipline. The nursing model directs that the nurse view the patient holistically. We need a theory of the holistic person as an adaptive system. Since the basic sciences do not provide nurses with a single working theory, the nurse using the adaptation model must create one for herself. This ... is a beginning effort to do this—to create a theory of the holistic person as an adaptive system" (p. 49). Given the importance of that work, it is unfortunate more programs of research designed to systematically test propositions still have not been developed.

With regard to middle-range theory development, Phillips (2002) explained that "Roy has explicated a great number of propositions, theorems, and axioms that serve well in the development of middle-range theory. The holistic nature of the model serves well for nurse researchers who are interested in the complex reaction between physiological and psychosocial adaptive processes" (p. 287). He went on to point out, researchers need to "continue to build middle-range theory based on the [Roy Adaptation Model] and to develop empirical referents [that is, research instruments] specifically designated to measure concepts proposed in the derived theory" (p. 287).

Additional work is needed to fully establish the credibility of conceptual-theoretical-empirical structures derived from the Roy Adaptation Model. Gerrish's (1989) thoughtful evaluation of her use of the model in nursing practice represents a prototype case study for credibility determination. Hoch's (1987) clinical study comparing the use of an explicit conceptual model of nursing with an implicit model is a prototype for more systematic credibility

determination. More comprehensive case studies and clinical research that draw definitive conclusions regarding the credibility of the Roy Adaptation Model are needed.

In conclusion, "few can fail to be excited by the explosive use of the Roy Adaptation Model in [nursing] practice, nursing administration, nursing education, and scholarly research" (Galbreath, 2002, p. 329). The Roy Adaptation Model has been adopted enthusiastically by many nurse educators, nurse researchers, and practicing nurses. Although such enthusiasm about the model could result in its uncritical application, Roy has attempted to guard against that by pointing out areas of the model needing further clarification and development. She commented:

> As models and frameworks continue to make their contribution to nursing, conceptual clarification and other theoretical development will be done by the theorists and others. ... A number of issues related to the concepts of the Roy adaptation model [have been raised]. Although major changes in the model do not seem to be called for, a rethinking of some basic definitions and distinctions among the key concepts provides the stimulus for further theoretical and empirical growth (Artinian & Roy, 1990, p. 66).

> Some assumptions about the model should be validated—for example, the assumption that the person has four modes of adaptation. Assumed values, particularly the value concerning the uniqueness of nursing, need to be made more explicit, and perhaps should also be supported. The model's goal, patiency, source of difficulty, and intervention in terms of focus and mode are all replete with possibilities for further clarification. A particularly fruitful field for study is the patient's use of adaptive mechanisms and the nurse's support of these in each adaptive mode (Roy, 1989, p. 113).

Further clarification and development of the Roy Adaptation Model may be spearheaded by the Roy Adaptation Association (RAA; formerly known as the Boston Based Adaptation Research Nursing Society). The purposes of the RAA are to advance nursing practice by developing basic and clinical nursing knowledge based on the Roy Adaptation Model and its philosophical perspective, provide forums for special interest in Roy Adaptation Model based research, education and practice all focused on creative social change, and enhance networks of dissemination of knowledge for practice and education. Continued development of the Roy Adaptation Model should progress as RAA members and other nurses continue their work. The RAA has held annual conferences each year since 2000. Practicing nurses, faculty, and researchers have opportunities to present their Roy Adaptation Model-based practice and education innovations and the findings of their Roy Adaptation Model-based studies at those conferences. The RAA also publishes a bi-annual newsletter, the *Roy Adaptation Association Review*.

Roy is confident that the Roy Adaptation Model "is compatible with futurists' views of the universe as progressing in structure, organization, and complexity" (Roy & Andrews, 1999, p. 34). Moreover, Roy's (1997) redefinition of the concept of Adaptation serves "the development of knowledge for practice in the future. In this way the discipline of nursing can meet a defining moment in accepting social accountability. The problem of the universe has been placed in a cosmic perspective. The solution has been offered to nurses using the Roy adaptation model" (p. 47).

 ## REFERENCES

Abdellah, F.G., Beland, I., Martin, A., & Matheney, R. (1960). Patient-centered approaches to nursing. New York: Macmillan.

Alligood, M.R. (2001). Philosophies, models, and theories: Critical thinking structures. In M.R. Alligood & A. Marriner Tomey (Eds.), Nursing theory: Utilization and application (2nd ed., pp. 41–61). St. Louis: Mosby.

Andrews, H.A. (1989). Implementation of the Roy adaptation model: An application of educational change research. In J.P. Riehl-Sisca (Ed.), Conceptual models for nursing practice (3rd ed., pp. 133–148). Norwalk, CT: Appleton & Lange.

Andrews, H.A., & Roy, C. (1986). Essentials of the Roy Adaptation Model. Norwalk, CT: Appleton-Century-Crofts.

Andrews, H.A., & Roy, C. (1991a). Essentials of the Roy adaptation model. In C. Roy & H.A. Andrews, The Roy adaptation model: The definitive statement (pp. 3–25). Norwalk, CT: Appleton & Lange.

Andrews, H.A., & Roy, C. (1991b). The nursing process according to the Roy adaptation model. In C. Roy and H.C. Andrews, The Roy adaptation model: The definitive statement (pp. 27–54). Norwalk, CT: Appleton & Lange.

Artinian, N.T. (1991). Stress experience of spouses of patients having coronary artery bypass during hospitalization and 6 weeks after discharge. Heart and Lung, 20, 52–59.

Artinian, N.T. (1992). Spouse adaptation to mate's CABG surgery: 1-year follow-up. American Journal of Critical Care, 1(2), 36–42.

Artinian, N.T., & Roy, C. (1990). Strengthening the Roy adaptation model through conceptual clarification. Commentary [Artinian] and response [Roy]. Nursing Science Quarterly, 3, 60–66.

Ayers, C.J. (1991). A meta-analysis of the effects of social support on adaptation in Roy's four modes. Dissertation Abstracts International, 51, 4773B.

Baldwin, J., & Schaffer, S. (1990). The continuing case study. Nurse Educator, 15(5), 6–9.

Banks, M.R. (1998). The effects of animal-assisted therapy on loneliness in an elderly population in long-term care facilities. Dissertation Abstracts International, 59, 1043B.

Barnum, B.J.S. (1998). Nursing theory. Analysis, application, evaluation (5th ed.). Philadelphia: Lippincott.

Barone, S.H., & Roy, C. (1996). The Roy adaptation model in research: Rehabilitation nursing. In P. Hinton Walker & B. Neuman (Eds.), Blueprint for use of nursing models (pp. 64–87). New York: NLN Press.

Boas, G. (1957). Dominant themes of modern philosophy. New York: Ronald Press.

Boston Based Adaptation Research Nursing Society. (1999). Roy adaptation model-based research: 25 years of contributions to nursing science. Indianapolis: Sigma Theta Tau International Center Nursing Press.

Calvillo, E.R., & Flaskerud, J.H. (1993). The adequacy and scope of Roy's adaptation model to guide cross-cultural pain research. Nursing Science Quarterly, 6, 118–129.

Camooso, C., Greene, M., & Reilly, P. (1981). Students' adaptation according to Roy. Nursing Outlook, 29, 108–109.

Chaisson, E. (1981). Cosmic dawn: The origins of matter and life. New York: Norton.

Coelho, G., Hamburg, D., & Adams, J. (Eds.). (1974). Coping and adaptation. New York: Basic Books.

Chiou, C-P. (2000). A meta-analysis of the interrelationships between the modes in Roy's adaptation model. Nursing Science Quarterly, 13, 252–258.

Connerley, K., Ristau, S., Lindberg, C., & McFarland, M. (1999). The Roy model in practice. In C. Roy & H.A. Andrews, The Roy adaptation model (2nd ed., pp. 515–534). Stamford, CT: Appleton & Lange.

Davies, P. (1988). The cosmic blueprint. New York: Simon & Schuster.

de Chardin, P.T. (1956). Man's place in nature. New York: Harper & Row.

de Chardin, P.T (1959). The phenomenon of man. New York: Harper & Row.

de Chardin, P.T. (1964). Human energy. New York: Harcourt Brace Jovanovich.

de Chardin, P.T. (1965). Hymn of the universe. [S. Bartholomew, Trans.]. New York: Harper & Row.

de Chardin, P.T. (1969). The future of man. New York: Harper & Row.

DiIorio, C. (1989). Applying Roy's model to nursing administration. In B. Henry, M. DiVincenti, C. Arndt, & A. Marriner (Eds.), Dimensions of nursing administration. Theory, research, education, and practice (pp. 89–104). Boston: Blackwell Scientific.

DiMattio, M.J.K., & Tulman, L. (2003). A longitudinal study of functional status and correlates following coronary artery bypass graft surgery in women. Nursing Research, 52, 98–107.

Dobratz, M.C. (2003). Putting the pieces together: Teaching undergraduate research from a theoretical perspective. Journal of Advanced Nursing, 41, 383–392.

Dorsey, K., & Purcell, S. (1987). Translating a nursing theory into a nursing system. Geriatric Nursing, 8, 167–137.

Ducharme, F., Ricard, N., Duquette, A., Levesque, L., & Lachance, L. (1998). Empirical testing of a longitudinal model derived from the Roy adaptation model. Nursing Science Quarterly, 11, 149–159.

Ewing, A.C. (1951). The fundamental questions of philosophy. London: Routledge & Kegan Paul.

Fawcett, J. (1990). Preparation for caesarean childbirth: Derivation of a nursing intervention from the Roy adaptation model. Journal of Advanced Nursing, 15, 1418–1425.

Fawcett, J. (1999). The relationship of theory and research (3rd ed.). Philadelphia: F.A. Davis.

Fawcett, J. (2003a). Conceptual models of nursing: International in scope and substance? The case of the Roy Adaptation Model. Nursing Science Quarterly, 16, 315–318.

Fawcett, J. (2003b). The Roy Adaptation Model: A program of nursing research. Japanese Journal of Nursing Research, 36(1), 67–73.

Fawcett, J., Botter, M.L., Burritt, J., Crossley, J.D., & Frink, B.B. (1989). Conceptual models of nursing and organization theories. In B. Henry, M. DiVincenti, C. Arndt, & A. Marriner (Eds.), Dimensions of nursing administration. Theory, research, education, and practice (pp. 143–154). Boston: Blackwell Scientific.

Fawcett, J., Pollio, N., Tully, A., Baron, M., Henklein, J.C., & Jones, R.C. (1993). Effects of information on adaptation to cesarean birth. Nursing Research, 42, 49–53.

Fawcett, J., & Newman, D.M.L. (2003, May). The Roy adaptation model: Identification and categorization of programs of research. Paper presented at the 4th Annual Conference of the Roy Adaptation Association, Kennebunkport, ME.

Fawcett, J., & Tulman, L. (1990). Building a programme of research from the Roy adaptation model of Nursing. Journal of Advanced Nursing, 15, 720–725.

Fitzsimmons, S. (2001). Interdisciplinary care. Easy Rider wheelchair biking: A nursing-recreation clinical trial for the treatment of depression. Journal of Gerontological Nursing, 27(5), 14–23.

Fox, M. (1983). Original blessing: A primer in creation spirituality. Santa Fe: Bear & Co.

Frederickson, K., & Williams, J.K. (1997). Nursing theory–guided practice: The Roy adaptation model and patient/family experiences. Nursing Science Quarterly, 10, 53–54.

Galbreath, J.G. (2002). Roy adaptation model: Sister Callista Roy. In J. B. George (Ed.), Nursing theories: The base for professional nursing practice (5th ed., pp. 295–338). Upper Saddle River, NJ: Prentice Hall.

Gendreau, F.R., & Caranfa, A. (1984). Western heritage: Man's encounter with himself and the world. Lanham, MD: University Press of America.

Gerrish, C. (1989). From theory to practice. Nursing Times, 85(35), 42–45.

Gould, S.J. (1983). The hardening of the synthesis. In M. Grene (Ed.), Dimensions of Darwinism (pp. 346–360). Cambridge: Cambridge University Press.

Gray, J. (1991). The Roy adaptation model in nursing practice. In C. Roy & H.A. Andrews, The Roy adaptation model: The definitive statement (pp. 429–443). Norwalk, CT: Appleton & Lange.

Hanchett, E.S. (1990). Nursing models and community as client. Nursing Science Quarterly, 3, 67–72.

Hanna, D.R., & Roy, C. (2001). Roy adaptation model and perspectives on the family. Nursing Science Quarterly, 14, 9–13.

Haught, J. (1993). The promise of nature: Ecology and cosmic purpose. New York: Paulist Press.

Helminiak, D.A. (1998). Religion and the human sciences. Albany: State University of New York Press.

Helson, H. (1964). Adaptation-level theory. New York: Harper & Row.

Henderson, V. (1960). Basic principles of nursing care. London: International Council of Nurses.

Hoch, C.C. (1987). Assessing delivery of nursing care. Journal of Gerontological Nursing, 13(1), 10–17.

Ingalls, J.D. (Ed.). (1972). A trainer's guide to androgogy (rev. ed.). Waltham, MA: Data Education, Inc.

Ingram, L. (1995). Roy's adaptation model and accident and emergency nursing. Accident and Emergency Nursing, 3, 150–153.

Jakocko, M.T., & Sowden, L.A. (1986). The Roy adaptation model in nursing practice. In H.A. Andrews & C. Roy, Essentials of the Roy adaptation model (pp. 165–177). Norwalk, CT: Appleton & Lange.

Kruszewski, A.Z. (1999). Psychosocial adaptation to termination of pregnancy for fetal anomaly. Dissertation Abstracts International, 61, 194B.

Lazarus, R.S., Averill, J.R., & Opton, E.M., Jr. (1974). The psychology of coping: Issues of research and assessment (pp. 249–315). In G.V. Coelho, D.A. Hamburg, & J.E. Adams (Eds.), Coping and adaptation. New York: Basic Books.

Levesque, L., Ricard, N., Ducharme, F., Duquette, A., & Bonin, J.P. (1998). Empirical verification of a theoretical model derived from the Roy adaptation model: Findings from five studies. Nursing Science Quarterly, 11, 23–30.

Levine, M.E. (1966). Adaptation and assessment: A rationale for nursing intervention. American Journal of Nursing, 66, 2450–2453.

Logan, M. (1990). The Roy adaptation model: Are nursing diagnoses amenable to independent nurse functions? Journal of Advanced Nursing, 15, 468–470.

Maloney, G.A. (1991). Mysticism and the new age. New York: Alba House.

Marriner-Tomey, A. (Ed.). (1989). Nursing theorists and their work (2nd ed.). St. Louis: Mosby.

Mason, T., & Chandley, M. (1990). Nursing models in a special hospital: A critical analysis of efficacy. Journal of Advanced Nursing, 15, 667–673.

Mastal, M.F., Hammond, H., & Roberts, M.P. (1982). Theory into hospital practice: A pilot implementation. Journal of Nursing Administration, 12(6), 9–15.

McCain, R.F. (1965). Nursing by assessment—not intuition. American Journal of Nursing, 65(4), 82–84.

McDonald, F.J., & Harms, M. (1966). Theoretical model for an experimental curriculum. Nursing Outlook, 14(8), 48–51.

Meleis, A.I. (1997). Theoretical nursing: Development and progress (3rd ed.). Philadelphia: Lippincott.

Miller, F. (1991). Using Roy's model in a special hospital. Nursing Standard, 5(27), 29–32.

Mock, V., Burke, M.B., Sheehan, P., Creaton, E.M., Winningham, M.L., McKenney-Tedder, S., Schwager, L.P., & Liebman, M. (1994). A nursing rehabilitation program for women with breast cancer receiving adjuvant chemotherapy. Oncology Nursing Forum, 21, 899–908.

Mock, V., Dow, K.H., Meares, C.J., Grimm, P.M., Dienemann, J.A., Haisfield-Wolfe, M.E., Quitasol, W., Mitchell, S., Chakravarthy, A., & Gage, I. (1997). Effects of exercise on fatigue, physical functioning, and emotional distress during radiation therapy for breast cancer. Oncology Nursing Forum, 24, 991–1000.

Morales-Mann, E.T., & Logan, M. (1990). Implementing the Roy model: Challenges for nurse educators. Journal of Advanced Nursing, 15, 142–147.

Nightingale, F. (1859). Notes on nursing: What it is and what it is not. London: Harrison. [Reprinted 1946. Phildelphia: Lippincott.]

O'Murchu, D. (1995). Our world in transition: Making sense of a changing world. Sussex, England: The Book Guild, Ltd.

O'Murchu, D. (1997). Quantum theology. New York: Crossroad Publishing.

Orlando, I.J. (1961). The dynamic nurse-patient relationship. New York: G.P. Putnam's Sons.

Peplau, H. (1952). Interpersonal relations in nursing. New York: G.P. Putnam's Sons.

Phillips, K.D. (2002). Sister Callista Roy: Adaptation model. In A. Marriner Tomey & M.R. Alligood (Eds.), Nursing theorists and their work (5th ed., pp. 269–298). St. Louis: Mosby.

Pinckaers, S. (1995). The sources of Christian ethics (3rd ed., Trans. Sr. M.T. Noble). Washington, D.C.: Catholic University of American Press.

Pollock, S.E. (1993). Adaptation to chronic illness: A program of research for testing nursing theory. Nursing Science Quarterly, 6, 86–92.

Popper, K.R., & Eccles, J.C. (1981). The self and its brain. New York: Springer.

Porth, C.M. (1977). Physiological coping: A model for teaching pathophysiology. Nursing Outlook, 25, 781–784.

Rambo, B. (1984). Adaptation nursing: Assessment and intervention. Philadelphia: Saunders.

Randell, B., Poush Tedrow, M., & Van Landingham, J. (1982). Adaptation nursing: The Roy conceptual model applied. St. Louis: Mosby.

Riehl, J.P., & Roy, C. (Eds.). (1974). Conceptual models for nursing practice. New York: Appleton-Century-Crofts.

Riehl, J.P., & Roy, C. (Eds.). (1980). Conceptual models for nursing practice (2nd ed.). New York: Appleton-Century-Crofts.

Riehl-Sisca, J.P. (Ed.). (1989). Conceptual models for nursing practice (3rd ed.). Norwalk, CT: Appleton & Lange.

Robitaille-Tremblay, M. (1984). A data collection tool for the psychiatric nurse. Canadian Nurse, 80(7), 26–28.

Rogers, M., Paul, L.J., Clarke, J., Mackay, C., Potter, M., & Ward, W. (1991). The use of the Roy adaptation model in nursing administration. Canadian Journal of Nursing Administration, 4(2), 21–26.

Rosenthal, R. (1991). Meta-analytic procedures for social research (rev. ed.). Newbury Park, CA: Sage.

Roy, C. (1970). Adaptation: A conceptual framework for nursing. Nursing Outlook, 18(3), 42–45.

Roy, C. (1971). Adaptation: A basis for nursing practice. Nursing Outlook, 19, 254–257.

Roy, C. (1973). Adaptation: Implications for curriculum change. Nursing Outlook, 21, 163–168.

Roy, C. (1974). The Roy Adaptation Model. In J.P. Riehl & C. Roy (Eds.), Conceptual models for nursing practice (pp. 135–144). New York: Appleton-Century-Crofts.

Roy, C. (1976a). Comment. Nursing Outlook, 24, 690–691.

Roy, C. (1976b). Introduction to nursing: An adaptation model. Englewood Cliffs, NJ: Prentice-Hall.

Roy, C. (1978, December). Adaptation model. Paper presented at Second Annual Nurse Educator Conference, New York. [Audiotape.]

Roy, C. (1979). Relating nursing theory to education: A new era. Nurse Educator, 4(2), 16–21.

Roy, C. (1980). The Roy adaptation model. In J.P. Riehl & C. Roy (Eds.), Conceptual models for nursing practice (2nd ed., pp. 179–188). New York: Appleton-Century-Crofts.

Roy, C. (1982). Foreword. In B. Randell, M. Poush Tedrow, & J. Van Landingham, Adaptation nursing: The Roy conceptual model applied (pp. vii–viii). St. Louis: Mosby.

Roy, C. (1983). The expectant family. Analysis and application of the Roy Adaptation Model. In I.W. Clements & F.B. Roberts (Eds.), Family health: A theoretical approach to nursing care (pp. 298–303). New York: Wiley.

Roy, C. (1984a). Introduction to nursing: An adaptation model (2nd ed.). Englewood Cliffs, NJ: Prentice-Hall.

Roy, C. (1984b). The Roy Adaptation Model: Applications in community health. In M.K. Asay & C.C. Ossler (Eds.), Conceptual models of nursing. Applications in community health nursing. Proceedings of the Eighth Annual Community Health Nursing Conference (pp. 51–73). Chapel Hill: Department of Public Health Nursing, School of Public Health, University of North Carolina.

Roy, C. (1987a). The influence of nursing models on clinical decision making II. In K.J. Hannah, M. Reimer, W.C. Mills, & S. Letourneau (Eds.), Clinical judgment and decision making: The future with nursing diagnosis (pp. 42–47). New York: Wiley.

Roy, C. (1987b). Response to "Needs of spouses of surgical patients: A conceptualization within the Roy adaptation model." Scholarly Inquiry for Nursing Practice, 1, 45–50.

Roy, C. (1987c). Roy's adaptation model. In R.R. Parse (Ed.), Nursing science. Major paradigms, theories, and critiques (pp. 35–45). Philadelphia: Saunders.

Roy, C. (1988a). Altered cognition: An information processing approach. In P.H. Mitchell, L.C. Hodges, M. Muwaswes, & C.A. Walleck (Eds.), AANN's neuroscience nursing: Phenomenon and practice: Human responses to neurological health problems (pp. 185–211). Norwalk, CT: Appleton & Lange.

Roy, C. (1988b). An explication of the philosophical assumptions of the Roy Adaptation Model. Nursing Science Quarterly, 1, 26–34.

Roy, C. (1988c). Sister Callista Roy. In T.M. Schorr & A. Zimmerman (Eds.), Making choices. Taking chances. Nurse leaders tell their stories (pp. 291–298). St. Louis: Mosby.

Roy, C. (1989). The Roy adaptation model. In J.P. Riehl-Sisca (Ed.), Conceptual models for nursing practice (3rd ed., pp. 105–114). Norwalk, CT: Appleton & Lange.

Roy, C. (1991). Structure of knowledge: Paradigm, model, and research specifications for differentiated practice. In I.E. Goertzen (Ed.), Differentiating nursing practice. Into the twenty-first century (pp. 31–39). Kansas City, MO: American Academy of Nursing.

Roy, C. (1992a). The Nurse Theorists: Excellence in Action— Callista Roy. Athens, OH: Fuld Institute of Technology in Nursing Education. [Videotape.]

Roy, C. (1992b). Vigor, variables, and vision: Commentary on Florence Nightingale. In F.N. Nightingale, Notes on nursing: What it is, and what it is not (Commemorative ed., pp. 63–71). Philadelphia: Lippincott.

Roy, C. (1997). Future of the Roy model: Challenge to redefine adaptation. Nursing Science Quarterly, 10, 42–48.

Roy, C. (2001). Alterations in cognitive processing. In C. Stewart-Amidei & J.A. Kunkel (Eds.), AANN's neuroscience nursing: Human responses to neurologic dysfunction (2nd ed., pp. 275–323). Philadelphia: Saunders.

Roy, C. (2002, May). Expanding on the Roy adaptation model for the 21st century. Paper presented at the 3rd Annual Conference of the Roy Adaptation Association. Kennebunkport, ME.

Roy, C. (2003, May). Implications of the 21st century developments of the Roy adaptation model. Paper presented at the 4th Annual Conference of the Roy Adaptation Association. Kennebunkport, ME.

Roy, C., & Andrews, H.A. (1991). The Roy adaptation model: The definitive statement. Norwalk, CT: Appleton & Lange.

Roy, C., & Andrews, H.A. (1999). The Roy adaptation model (2nd ed.). Stamford, CT: Appleton & Lange.

Roy, C., & Anway, J. (1989). Theories and hypotheses for nursing administration. In B. Henry, M. DiVincenti, C. Arndt, & A. Marriner-Tomey (Eds.), Dimensions of nursing administration. Theory, research, education, and practice (pp. 75–88). Boston: Blackwell Scientific.

Roy, C., & Corliss, C.P. (1993). The Roy adaptation model: Theoretical update and knowledge for practice. In M.E. Parker (Ed.), Patterns of nursing theories in practice (pp. 215–229). New York: National League for Nursing.

Roy, C., & Martinez, C. (1983). A conceptual framework for CNS practice. In A. Hamric & J. Spross (Eds.), The clinical nurse spe-

cialist in theory and practice (pp. 3–20). New York: Grune & Stratton.

Roy, C., & Roberts, S.L. (1981). Theory construction in nursing. An adaptation model. Englewood Cliffs, NJ: Prentice-Hall.

Runyon, C.A.H. (1994). Competency-based orientation for the professional nursing staff. Kentucky Nurse, 42(4), 23.

Rush, J.E. (1981). Towards a general theory of healing. Washington, DC: University Press of America.

Samarel, N., & Fawcett, J. (1992). Enhancing adaptation to breast cancer: The addition of coaching to support groups. Oncology Nursing Forum, 19, 591–596.

Sellers, S.C. (1991). A philosophical analysis of conceptual models of nursing. Dissertation Abstracts International, 52, 1937B.

Silva, M.C., & Sorrell, J.M. (1992). Testing of nursing theory: Critique and philosophical expansion. Advances in Nursing Science, 14(4), 12–23.

Smolen, D., Topp, R., & Singer, L. (2002). The effect of self-selected music during colonoscopy on anxiety, heart rate, and blood pressure. Applied Nursing Research, 15, 126–136.

Sparks, L.G. (1998). A comparison of the effects of cutaneous stimulation and distraction on children's perceptions of injection pain. Dissertation Abstracts International, 60, 1536B.

Starn, J., & Niederhauser, V. (1990). An MCN model for nursing diagnosis to focus intervention. MCN: American Journal of Maternal/Child Nursing, 15, 180–183.

Strickler, M., & LaSor, B. (1970). Concept of loss in crisis intervention. Mental Hygiene, 54, 301–305.

Swimme, B., & Berry, T. (1994). The universe story. San Francisco: Harper.

Tsai, P-F. (1999). Development of a middle-range theory of caregiver stress from the Roy adaptation model. Dissertation Abstracts International, 60, 133B.

Tsai, P-F. (2003) A middle-range theory of caregiver stress. Nursing Science Quarterly, 16, 137–145.

Tulman, L., & Fawcett, J. (1990a). A framework for studying functional status after diagnosis of breast cancer. Cancer Nursing, 13, 95–99.

Tulman, L., & Fawcett, J. (1990b). Functional status during pregnancy and the postpartum: A framework for research. Image: Journal of Nursing Scholarship, 22, 191–194.

Tulman, L., & Fawcett, J. (2003). Women's health during and after pregnancy: A theory-based study of adaptation to change. New York: Springer.

von Bertalanffy, L. (1968). General system theory. New York: George Braziller.

Wagner, P. (1976). Testing the adaptation model in practice. Nursing Outlook, 24, 682–685.

Wallace, C.L. (1993). Resources for nursing theories in practice. In M.E. Parker (Ed.), Patterns of nursing theories in practice (pp. 301–311). New York: National League for Nursing.

Weiss, M.E., Hastings, W.J., Holly, D.C., & Craig, D.I. (1994).

Using Roy's adaptation model in practice: Nurses' perspectives. Nursing Science Quarterly, 7, 80–86.

Welsh, M.D., & Clochesy, J.M. (Eds.). (1990). Case studies in cardiovascular critical care nursing. Rockville, MD: Aspen.

Wendler, M.C. (2003). Effects of Tellington touch in healthy adults awaiting venipuncture. Research in Nursing and Health, 26, 40–52.

Whittemore, R., & Roy, C. (2002). Adapting to diabetes mellitus: A theory synthesis. Nursing Science Quarterly, 15, 311–317.

Wilbur, K. (1997). The eye of the spirit: An integral vision for a world gone slightly mad. Boston: Shambhala Publications.

Young, L.B. (1993). The unfinished universe. New York: Oxford University Press.

Young-McCaughan, S., Mays, M.Z., Arzola, S.M., Yoder, L.H., Dramiga, S.A., Leclerc, K.M., Caton, J.R. Jr., Sheffler, R.L., & Nowlin, M.U. (2003). Changes in exercise tolerance, activity and sleep patterns, and quality of life in patients with cancer participating in a structured exercise program. Oncology Nursing Forum, 30, 441–454.

Zarle, N.C. (1987). Continuing care: The process and practice of discharge planning. Rockville, MD: Aspen.

Zohar, D. (1990). The quantum self: Human nature and consciousness defined by the new physics. New York: Quill/William Morrow.

RESEARCH

Anderson, B., Higgins, L., & Rozmus, C. (1999). Critical pathways: Application to selected patient outcomes following coronary artery bypass graft. Applied Nursing Research, 12, 168–174.

Artinian, N.T. (1991). Stress experience of spouses of patients having coronary artery bypass during hospitalization and 6 weeks after discharge. Heart and Lung, 20, 52–59.

Artinian, N.T. (1992). Spouse adaptation to mate's CBG surgery: 1-year follow-up. American Journal of Critical Care, 1(2), 36–42.

Baert, C., Cocula, N., Delran, J., Faubel, E., Foucaud, C., & Martins, V. (2000). Comparative study of transplant or pending patients' needs. Recherche En Soins Infirmiers, December (63), 26–51. [French; English abstract]

Baker, A.C. (1993). The spouse's positive effect on the stroke patient's recovery. Rehabilitation Nursing, 18, 30–33, 67–68.

Barone, S.H., & Roy, C. (1996). The Roy adaptation model in research: Rehabilitation nursing. In P. Hinton Walker & B. Neuman (Eds.), Blueprint for use of nursing models (pp. 64–87). New York: NLN Press.

Blain, S., (1993). Attitudes of women undergoing TOP [termination of pregnancy]. Nursing Standard, 7(37), 30–33.

Bokinskie, J.C. (1992). Family conferences: A method to diminish transfer anxiety. Journal of Neuroscience Nursing, 24, 129–133.

Bournaki, M.C. (1997). Correlates of pain-related responses to venipunctures in school-aged children. Nursing Research, 46, 147–153.

Bradley, K.M., & Williams, D.M. (1990). A comparison of the preoperative concerns of open heart surgery patients and their significant others. Journal of Cardiovascular Nursing, 5, 43–53.

Brandriet, L.M., Lyons, M., & Bentley, J. (1994). Perceived needs of poststroke elders following termination of home health services. Nursing and Health Care, 15, 514–520.

Broeder, J.L. (1985). School-age children's perceptions of isolation after hospital discharge. Maternal-Child Nursing Journal, 14, 153–174.

Brydolf, M., & Segesten, K. (1994). Physical health status in young subjects after colectomy: An application of the Roy model. Journal of Advanced Nursing, 20, 500–508.

Brydolf, M., & Segesten, K. (1996). Living with ulcerative colitis: Experiences of adolescents and young adults. Journal of Advanced Nursing, 23, 39–47.

Calvert, M.M. (1989). Human-pet interaction and loneliness: A test of concepts from Roy's adaptation model. Nursing Science Quarterly, 2, 194–202.

Calvillo, E.R., & Flaskerud, J.H. (1993). The adequacy and scope of Roy's adaptation model to guide cross-cultural pain research. Nursing Science Quarterly, 6, 118–129.

Campbell, J.M. (1992). Treating depression in well older adults: Use of diaries in cognitive therapy. Issues in Mental Health Nursing, 13, 19–29.

Campbell-Heider, N. (1993). Patient adaptation to technology: An application of the Roy model to nursing research. Journal of the New York State Nurses Association, 24(2), 22–27.

Campbell-Heider, N., & Knapp, T.R. (1993). Toward a hierarchy of adaptation to biomedical technology. Critical Care Nursing Quarterly, 16(3), 42–50.

Chappelle, L.S., & Sorrentino, E.A. (1993). Assessing codependency issues within a nursing environment. Nursing Management, 24(5), 40–42.

Chen, H. (1994). Hearing in the elderly: Relation of hearing loss, loneliness, and self-esteem. Journal of Gerontological Nursing, 20(6), 22–28.

Chen, H., Ma, F., Kuo, B., & Shyr, Y. (1999). Physical and psychological adjustment in women with mastectomy: Based on Roy's adaptation model. Nursing Research (China), 7, 321–332. [Chinese; English abstract]

Cheng, M., & Williams, P.D. (1989). Oxygenation during chest physiotherapy of very-low-birth-weight infants: Relations among fraction of inspired oxygen levels, number of hand ventilations, and transcutaneous oxygen pressure. Journal of Pediatric Nursing, 4, 411–418.

Chiou, C-P. (2000). A meta-analysis of the interrelationships between the modes in Roy's adaptation model. Nursing Science Quarterly, 13, 252–258.

Christian, A. (1993). The relationship between women's symptoms of endometriosis and self-esteem. Journal of Obstetric, Gynecologic, and Neonatal Nursing, 22, 370–376.

Collins, J.M. (1993). Functional health, social support, and morale of older women living alone in Appalachia. Kentucky Nurse, 41(3), 13.

Constantino, R. (1993). Nursing postvention for suicide survivors. Pennsylvania Nurse, 48(11), 19.

Cook, J.K., Green, M., & Topp, R.V. (2001). Exploring the impact of physician verbal abuse on perioperative nurses. Association of Operating Room Nurses Journal, 74, 317–331.

Corser, N.C. (1996). Sleep of 1- and 2-year-old children in intensive care. Issues in Comprehensive Pediatric Nursing, 19(1), 17–31.

Coslow, B.I.F., & Eddy, M.E. (1998). Effects of preoperative ambulatory gynecological education: Clinical outcomes and patient satisfaction. Journal of Perianesthesia Nursing, 13, 4–10.

Cottrell, B., & Shannahan, M. (1986). Effect of the birth chair on duration of second stage labor and maternal outcome. Nursing Research, 35, 364–367.

Cottrell, B., & Shannahan, M. (1987). A comparison of fetal outcome in birth chair and delivery table births. Research in Nursing and Health, 10, 239–243.

Courts, N.F., & Boyette, B.G. (1998). Psychosocial adjustment of males on three types of dialysis. Clinical Nursing Research, 7, 47–63.

Craig, D.I. (1990). The adaptation to pregnancy of spinal cord injured women. Rehabilitation Nursing, 15(1), 6–9.

Dant, D. (1993). The effects of humor on self-reported mood and pain levels in the oncology patient population. Kentucky Nurse, 41(4), 21.

DiMattio, M.J.K., & Tulman, L. (2003). A longitudinal study of functional status and correlates following coronary artery bypass graft surgery in women. Nursing Research, 52, 98–107.

Dobratz, M.C. (1993). Causal influences of psychological adaptation in dying. Western Journal of Nursing Research, 15, 708–729.

Dobratz, M.C. (2002). The pattern of the becoming-self in death and dying. Nursing Science Quarterly, 15, 137–142.

Ducharme, F., Ricard, N., Duquette, A., Levesque, L., & Lachance, L. (1998). Empirical testing of a longitudinal model derived from the Roy adaptation model. Nursing Science Quarterly, 11, 149–159.

Dunnum, L. (1990). Life satisfaction and spinal cord injury: The patient perspective. Journal of Neuroscience Nursing, 22, 43–47.

Eakes, M., & Brown, H. (1998). Home alone: Meeting the needs of mothers after cesarean birth. AWHONN Lifelines, 2(1), 36–40.

Farkas, L. (1981). Adaptation problems with nursing home application for elderly persons: An application of the Roy Adaptation Nursing Model. Journal of Advanced Nursing, 8, 363–368.

Fawcett, J. (1981). Needs of cesarean birth parents. Journal of Obstetric, Gynecologic, and Neonatal Nursing, 10, 371–376.

Fawcett, J. (1990). Preparation for caesarean childbirth: Derivation of a nursing intervention from the Roy adaptation model. Journal of Advanced Nursing, 15, 1418–1425.

Fawcett, J., & Burritt, J. (1985). An exploratory study of antenatal preparation for cesarean birth. Journal of Obstetric, Gynecologic, and Neonatal Nursing, 14, 224–230.

Fawcett, J., & Henklein, J. (1987). Antenatal education for cesarean birth: Extension of a field test. Journal of Obstetric, Gynecologic, and Neonatal Nursing, 16, 61–65.

Fawcett, J., Henklein, J.C., Pollio, N., Tully, A., & Baron, M. (1994). Expectations about cesarean birth and birth outcomes. International Journal of Childbirth Education, 9(4), 12–17.

Fawcett, J., Pollio, N., Tully, A., Baron, M., Henklein, J.C., & Jones, R.C. (1993). Effects of information on adaptation to cesarean birth. Nursing Research, 42, 49–53. Beal, J.A. (1993). Commentary on "Effects of information on adaptation to cesarean birth." Nursing Scan in Research, 6(4), 5.

Fawcett, J., Sidney, J.S., Riley-Lawless, K., & Hanson, M.J.S. (1996). An exploratory study of the relationship between alternative therapies, functional status, and symptom severity among people with multiple sclerosis. Journal of Holistic Nursing, 14, 115–129.

Fawcett, J., Tulman, L., & Spedden, J.P. (1994). Responses to vaginal birth after cesarean (VBAC). Journal of Obstetric, Gynecologic, and Neonatal Nursing, 23, 253–259.

Fawcett, J., & Weiss, M.E. (1993). Cross-cultural adaptation to cesarean birth. Western Journal of Nursing Research, 15, 282–297.

Fisher, M.D. (1994). Identified needs of parents in a pediatric intensive care unit. Critical Care Nurse, 14(3), 82–90.

Fitzsimmons, S. (2001). Interdisciplinary care. Easy Rider wheelchair biking: A nursing-recreation clinical trial for the treatment of depression. Journal of Gerontological Nursing, 27(5), 14–23.

Flanagan, N.A. (1998). An analysis of patients' psychosocial adjustment and values before and after coronary artery surgery. Rehabilitation Nursing, 23, 234–239.

Fletcher, C. (2000). Appraisal and coping with vaso-occlusive crisis in adolescents with sickle cell disease. Pediatric Nursing, 26, 319–324.

Florence, M.E., Lützen, K., & Alexius, B. (1994). Adaptation of heterosexually infected HIV-positive women: A Swedish pilot study. Health Care of Women International, 15, 265–273.

Frame, K. (2003). Empowering preadolescents with ADHD: Demons or delights. Advances in Nursing Science, 26, 131–139.

Frame, K., Kelly, L., & Bayley, E. (2003). Increasing perceptions of self-worth in preadolescents diagnosed with ADHD. Journal of Nursing Scholarship, 35, 225–229.

Francis, G., Turner, J.T., & Johnson, S.B. (1985). Domestic animal visitation as therapy with adult home residents. International Journal of Nursing Studies, 22, 201–206.

Frank, D.I., & Lang, A.R. (1990). Disturbances in sexual role performance of chronic alcoholics: An analysis using Roy's adaptation model. Issues in Mental Health Nursing, 11, 243–254.

Frederickson, K., Jackson, B.S., Strauman, T., & Strauman, J. (1991). Testing hypotheses derived from the Roy adaptation model. Nursing Science Quarterly, 4, 168–174.

Friedemann, M., & Andrews, M. (1990). Family support and child adjustment in single-parent families: Secondary analysis. Issues in Comprehensive Pediatric Nusing, 13, 289–301.

Gaberson, K.B. (1991). The effect of humorous distraction on preoperative anxiety. A pilot study. Association of Operating Room Nurses Journal, 54, 1258–1261, 1263–1264.

Gaberson, K.B. (1995). The effect of humorous and musical distraction of preoperative anxiety. Association of Operating Room Nurses Journal, 62, 784, 786–788, 790–791.

Gagliardi, B.A. (1991). The impact of Duchenne muscular dystrophy on families. Orthopaedic Nursing, 10(5), 41–49.

Gagliardi, B.A., Frederickson, K., & Shanley, D.A. (2002). Living with multiple sclerosis: A Roy adaptation model-based study. Nursing Science Quarterly, 15, 230–236.

Garcia, A.P., & White-Traut, R. (1993). Preterm infants' responses to taste/smell and tactile stimulation during an apneic episode. Journal of Pediatric Nursing, 8, 245–252.

Gardner, M.J. (1996). Do male and female spouses differ in their perceptions and adaptation to their partner's open heart surgery? Michigan Nurse, 69(8), 22–23.

Germain, C.P. (1984). Sheltering abused women: A nursing perspective. Journal of Psychosocial Nursing, 22(9), 24–31.

Gomes de Arruda, A.J.C., & Garcia, T.R. (2000). Nursing diagnoses related to oxygenation, attributed to trauma victims admitted to ICU. Revista Brasileira De Enfermagem, 53, 363–374. [Portuguese; English abstract]

Gujol, M.C. (1994). A survey of pain assessment and management practices among critical care nurses. American Journal of Critical Care, 3, 123–128.

Guzzetta, C. (1979). Relationship between stress and learning. Advances in Nursing Science, 1(4), 35–49.

Hammond, H., Roberts, M., & Silva, M. (1983, Spring). The effect of Roy's first level and second level assessment on nurses' determination of accurate nursing diagnoses. Virginia Nurse, 14–17.

Hamner, J.B. (1996). Preliminary testing of a proposition from the Roy adaptation model. Image: Journal of Nursing Scholarship, 28, 215–220.

Harding-Okimoto, M.B. (1997). Pressure ulcers, self-concept and body image in spinal cord injury patients. SCI [Spinal Cord Injury] Nursing, 14, 111–117.

Harrison, L.L., Leeper, J.D., & Yoon, M. (1990). Effects of early parent touch on preterm infants' heart rates and arterial oxygen saturation levels. Journal of Advanced Nursing, 15, 877–885.

Hartweg, D.L. (1993). Commentary on "Cross-cultural adaptation to cesarean birth." AWHONN's Women's Health Nursing Scan, 7(6), 12.

Hazlett, D.E. (1989). A study of pediatric home ventilator management: Medical, psychosocial, and financial aspects. Journal of Pediatric Nursing, 4, 284–294.

Hoch, C.C. (1987). Assessing delivery of nursing care. Journal of Gerontological Nursing, 13(1), 10–17.

Houston, K.A. (1993). An investigation of rocking as relaxation for the elderly. Geriatric Nursing, 14, 186–189.

Hunter, L.P. (1991). Measurement of axillary temperatures in neonates. Western Journal of Nursing Research, 13, 324–335.

Jackson, B.S., Strauman, J., Frederickson, K., & Strauman, T.J. (1991). Long-term biopsychosocial effects of interleukin-2 therapy. Oncology Nursing Forum, 18, 683–690.

Janelli, L.M., Kanski, G.W., Jones, H.M., & Kennedy, M.C. (1995). Exploring music intervention with restrained patients. Nursing Forum, 30(4), 12–18.

Jirovec, M.M., Jenkins, J., Isenberg, M., & Bairdi, J. (1999). Urine control theory derived from Roy's conceptual framework. Nursing Science Quarterly, 12, 251–255.

Jirovec, M.M., & Templin, T. (2001). Predicting success using individualized scheduled toileting for memory-impaired elders at home. Research in Nursing and Health, 24, 1–8.

John, L.D. (2001). Quality of life in patients receiving radiation therapy for non-small cell lung cancer. Oncology Nursing Forum, 28, 807–813.

Jones, M.L.H., & Smyth, K.A. (1999). Outcomes for high-risk neonates in a managed care clinical system. Nursing Case Management, 4, 71–76.

Kehoe, C.F. (1981). Identifying the nursing needs of the postpartum cesarean mother. In C.F. Kehoe (Ed.), The cesarean experience: Theoretical and clinical perspectives for nurses (pp. 85–141). New York: Appleton-Century-Crofts.

Khanobdee, C., Sukratanachaiyakul, V., & Gay, J.T. (1993). Couvade syndrome in expectant Thai fathers. International Journal of Nursing Studies, 30, 125–131.

Kiikkala, I., & Peitsi, T. (1991). The care of children with minimal brain dysfunction: A Roy Adaptation analysis. Journal of Pediatric Nursing, 6, 290–292.

Kitchin, L.W., & Hutchinson, S. (1996). Touch during preterm infant resuscitation. Neonatal Network: Journal of Neonatal Nursing, 15(7), 45–51.

Komelasky, A.L. (1990). The effect of home nursing visits on parental anxiety and CPR knowledge retention of parents of apnea-monitored infants. Journal of Pediatric Nursing, 5, 387–392.

Krouse, H.J., & Krouse, J.H. (1999). Complementary therapeutic practices in patients with chronic sinusitis. Clinical Excellence for Nurse Practitioners, 3, 346–352.

Kuhns, M.L. (1997). Treatment outcomes with adult children of alcoholics: Depression. Advanced Practice Nursing Quarterly, 3(2), 64–69.

Kunene, P.J., & Nzimande, P.N. (1996). Strikes by nursing personnel: A challenge for nurse managers in Kwazulu-Natal Province. Curationis: South African Journal of Nursing, 19(3), 41–46.

Lee, A.A., & Ellenbecker, C.H. (1998). The perceived life stressors among elderly Chinese immigrants: Are they different from those of other elderly Americans? Clinical Excellence for Nurse Practitioners, 2, 96–101.

LeMone, P. (1995). Assessing psychosexual concerns in adults with diabetes: Pilot project using Roy's modes of adaptation. Issues in Mental Health Nursing, 16, 67–78.

Leonard, C. (1975). Patient attitudes toward nursing interventions. Nursing Research, 24, 335–339.

Leuze, M., & McKenzie, J. (1987). Preoperative assessment using the Roy adaptation model. Association of Operating Room Nurses Journal, 46, 1122–1134.

Levesque, L., Ricard, N., Ducharme, F., Duquette, A., & Bonin, J.P. (1998). Empirical verification of a theoretical model derived from the Roy adaptation model: Findings from five studies. Nursing Science Quarterly, 11, 23–30.

Leyva, T.L., Whiteford, V.N., & Jones, E. (2000). Deaf adult's knowledge of internal anatomy and physiology. Journal for Undergraduate Nursing Scholarship, 2(1), 7.

Lopez-Bushnell, K., & Fassler, C. (2002). Risk reduction for hospitalized medical patients with substance abuse. Communicating Nursing Research, 35, 272.

Lutjens, L.R.J. (1991). Medical condition, nursing condition, nursing intensity, medical severity, and length of stay in hospitalized adults. Nursing Administration Quarterly, 15(2), 64–65.

Lutjens, L.R.J. (1992). Derivation and testing of tenets of a theory of social organizations as adaptive systems. Nursing Science Quarterly, 5, 62–71.

Lutjens, L.R.J. (1994). Hospital payment source and length-of-stay. Nursing Science Quarterly, 7, 174–179.

Lynam, L.E., & Miller, M.A. (1992). Mothers' and nurses' perceptions of the needs of women experiencing preterm labor. Journal of Obstetric, Gynecologic, and Neonatal Nursing, 21, 126–136.

McGill, J.S. (1992). Functional status as it relates to hope in elders with and without cancer (Abstract). Kentucky Nurse, 40(4), 6.

McGill, J.S., & Paul, P.B. (1993). Functional status and hope in elderly people with and without cancer. Oncology Nursing Forum, 20, 1207–1213.

McIllmurray, A. (1997). Adaptation to stroke. Assignment, 3(3), 9–21.

Medhat, A., Huber, P.M., & Medhat, M.A. (1990). Factors that influence the level of activities in persons with lower extremity amputation. Rehabilitation Nursing, 15, 13–18.

Meek, S.S. (1993). Effects of slow stroke back massage on relaxation in hospice clients. Image: Journal of Nursing Scholarship, 25, 17–21.

Meeker, B.J. (1994). Preoperative patient education: Evaluating postoperative patient outcomes. Patient Education and Counseling, 23, 41–47.

Mock, V., Burke, M.B., Sheehan, P., Creaton, E.M., Winningham, M.L., McKenney-Tedder, S., Schwager, L.P., & Liebman, M. (1994). A nursing rehabilitation program for women with breast cancer receiving adjuvant chemotherapy. Oncology Nursing Forum, 21, 899–908.

Mock, V., Dow, K.H., Meares, C.J., Grimm, P.M., Dienemann, J.A., Haisfield-Wolfe, M.E., Quitasol, W., Mitchell, S., Chakravarthy, A., & Gage, I. (1997). Effects of exercise on fatigue, physical functioning, and emotional distress during radiation therapy for breast cancer. Oncology Nursing Forum, 24, 991–1000.

Modrcin-Talbott, M.A., Harrison, L.L., Groer, M.W., & Younger, M.S. (2003). The biobehavioral effects of gentle human touch on preterm infants. Nursing Science Quarterly, 16, 60–67.

Modrcin-Talbott, M.A., Pullen, L., Ehrenberger, H., Zandstra, K., & Muenchen, B. (1998). Self-esteem in adolescents treated in an outpatient mental health setting. Issues in Comprehensive Pediatric Nursing, 21, 159–171.

Modrcin-Talbott, M.A., Pullen, L., Zandstra, K., Ehrenberger, H., & Muenchen, B. (1998). A study of self-esteem among well adolescents: Seeking a new direction. Issues in Comprehensive Pediatric Nursing, 21, 229–241.

Munn, V.A., & Tichy, A.M. (1987). Nurses' perceptions of stressors in pediatric intensive care. Journal of Pediatric Nursing, 2, 405–411.

Neto, D.L., & Pagliuca, L.M.F. (2002). Holistic approach of the term "person" in an empirical study: A critical analysis. Revista Latino Americana de Enfermagem, 10, 825–830. [Portuguese; English abstract]

Niska, K.J. (1999a). Family nursing interventions: Mexican American early family formation, Nursing Science Quarterly, 12, 335–340.

Niska, K.J. (1999b). Mexican American family processes: Nurturing, support, and socialization, Nursing Science Quarterly, 12, 138–142.

Niska, K.J. (2001a). Mexican American family survival, continuity, and growth: The parental perspective. Nursing Science Quarterly, 14, 322–329.

Niska, K.J. (2001b). Therapeutic use of parental stories to enhance Mexican American family socialization: Family transition to the community school system. Public Health Nursing, 18, 149–156.

Niska, K.J., Lia-Hoagberg, B., & Snyder, M. (1997). Parental concerns of Mexican American first-time mothers and fathers. Public Health Nursing, 14, 111–117.

Niska, K.J., Snyder, M., & Lia-Hoagberg, B. (1998). Family ritual facilitates adaptation to parenthood. Public Health Nursing, 15, 329–337.

Niska, K.J., Snyder, M., & Lia-Hoagberg, B. (1999). The meaning of family health among Mexican-American first-time mothers and fathers. Journal of Family Nursing, 5, 218–233.

Nolan, M. (1977). Effects of nursing intervention in the operating room as recalled on the third postoperative day. In M.V. Batey (Ed.), Communicating nursing research in the bicentennial year (Vol. 9, pp. 41–50). Boulder, CO: Western Interstate Commission for Higher Education.

Norris, S., Campbell, L., & Brenkert, S. (1982). Nursing procedures and alterations in transcutaneous oxygen tension in premature infants. Nursing Research, 31, 330–336. Holloway, E., & King, I. (1983). Re: "What's going on here?" (Letter to the editor). Nursing Research, 32, 319. Berkemeyer, S.N., & Campbell, L.A. (1983). To the editor (Letter to the editor). Nursing Research, 32, 319–329. Roy, C. (1983). To the editor (Letter to the editor). Nursing Research, 32, 320.

Nuamah, I.F., Cooley, M.E., Fawcett, J., & McCorkle, R. (1999). Testing a theory for health-related quality of life in cancer patients: A structural equation approach. Research in Nursing and Health, 22, 231–242.

Nyqvist, K.H., & Sjoden, P.O. (1993). Advice concerning breast-feeding from mothers of infants admitted to a neonatal intensive care unit: The Roy adaptation model as a conceptual structure. Journal of Advanced Nursing, 18, 54–63.

Oliverira, T.C., & Araujo, T.L. (2002). Mechanisms developed by old-aged people to face arterial hypertension. Revista da Escola de Enfermagen UPS (San Paulo), 36, 276–281.

Orsi, A.J., Grady, C., Tax, A., McCorkle, R. (1997). Nutritional adaptation of women living with human immunodeficiency virus: A pilot study. Holistic Nursing Practice, 12(1), 71–79.

Paul, R., & Rochichaud-Ekstrand, S. (2002). Expected and received assistance from the informal social support network by older persons undergoing heart surgery. Recherche Soins Infirmiers, 71, 38–55. [French; English abstract]

Phillips, J.A., & Brown, K.C. (1992). Industrial workers on a rotating shift pattern: Adaptation and injury status. American Association of Occupational Health Nurses Journal, 40, 468–476.

Phuphaibul, R., & Muensa, W. (1999). Negative and positive adaptive behaviors of Thai school-aged children who have a sibling with cancer. Journal of Pediatric Nursing, 14, 342–348.

Piwonka, M.A., & Merino, J.M. (1999). A multidimensional modeling of predictors influencing the adjustment to a colostomy. Journal of Wound, Ostomy, and Continence Nursing, 26, 298–305.

Pollock, S.E. (1986). Human responses to chronic illness: Physiologic and psychosocial adaptation. Nursing Research, 35, 90–95.

Pollock, S.E. (1989). Adaptive responses to diabetes mellitus. Western Journal of Nursing Research, 11, 265–280.

Pollock, S.E. (1993). Adaptation to chronic illness: A program of research for testing nursing theory. Nursing Science Quarterly, 6, 86–92.

Pollock, S.E., Christian, B.J., & Sands, D. (1990). Responses to chronic illness: Analysis of psychological and physiological adaptation. Nursing Research, 39, 300–304.

Pollock, S.E., & Sands, D. (1997). Adaptation to suffering. Clinical Nursing Research, 6, 171–185.

Pontious, S.L., Kennedy, A., Chung, K.L., Burroughs, T.E., Libby, L.J., & Vogel, D.W. (1994). Accuracy and reliability of temperature measurement in the emergency department by instrument and site in children. Pediatric Nursing, 20, 58–63.

Pontious, S.L., Kennedy, A.H., Shelley, S., Mittrucker, C. (1994). Accuracy and reliability of temperature measurement by instrument and site. Journal of Pediatric Nursing, 9, 114–123.

Preston, D.B., & Dellasega, C. (1990). Elderly women and stress. Does marriage make a difference? Journal of Gerontological Nursing, 16, 26–32.

Printz-Feddersen, V. (1990). Effect of group process on caregiver burden. (Abstract). Journal of Neuroscience Nursing, 22, 50–51.

Pullen, L.M., Modrcin-McCarthy, M.A., & Graf, E.V. (2000). Adolescent depression: Important facts that matter. Journal of Child and Adolescent Psychiatric Nursing, 13, 69–75.

Pullen, L., Modrcin-Talbott, M.A., West, W.R., Fenske, M.M., & Muenchen, B. (1999). Keeping the faith or just blowing smoke? Journal of Addictions Nursing, 11, 13–18.

Pullen, L., Modrcin-Talbott, M.A., West, W.R., & Muenchen, R. (1999). Spiritual high vs. high on spirits: Is religiosity related to adolescent alcohol and drug abuse? Journal of Psychiatric and Mental Health Nursing, 6, 3–8.

Raeside, L. (1997). Perceptions of environmental stressors in the neonatal unit. British Journal of Nursing, 6, 914–916, 918, 920–923.

Raeside, L. (2000). Caring for dying babies: Perceptions of neonatal nurses. Journal of Neonatal Nursing, 6, 93–99.

Reichert, J.A., Baron, M., & Fawcett, J. (1993). Changes in attitudes toward cesarean birth. Journal of Obstetric, Gynecologic, and Neonatal Nursing, 22, 159–167.

Riegel, B., Heywood, G., Jackson, W., & Kennedy, A. (1988). Effect of nitroglycerin ointment placement on the severity of headache and flushing in patients with cardiac disease. Heart and Lung, 17, 426–431.

Robinson, J.H. (1995). Grief responses, coping processes, and social support of widows: Research with Roy's model. Nursing Science Quarterly, 8, 158–164.

Rodriguez, J.A., & Jones, E.G. (1996). Foster parents' early adaptation to the placement of a child with developmental disabilities in their homes. Journal of Pediatric Nursing, 11, 111–118.

Roy, C. (1978). The stress of hospital events: Measuring changes in level of stress (Abstract). In Communicating nursing research. Vol. 11: New approaches to communicating nursing research (pp. 70–71). Boulder, CO: Western Interstate Commission for Higher Education.

Roy, C., & Andrews, H.A. (1999). The Roy adaptation model (2nd ed., pp. 542–546). Stamford, CT: Appleton & Lange.

Roy, C., & Zhan, L. (2001). Sister Callista Roy: The Roy adaptation model. In M.E. Parker (Ed.), Nursing theories and nursing practice (pp. 315–327). Philadelphia: F.A. Davis

Russell, M.T., Reinbold, J., & Maltby, H.J. (1996). International pediatric nursing: Transferring to adult health care: Experiences of adolescents with cystic fibrosis. Journal of Pediatric Nursing, 11, 262–268.

Ryan, M.C. (1996). Loneliness, social support and depression as interactive variables with cognitive status: Testing Roy's model. Nursing Science Quarterly, 9, 107–114.

Salazar-Gonzalez, B.C, & Jirovec, M.M. (2001). Elderly Mexican women's perceptions of exercise and conflicting role responsibilities. International Journal of Nursing Studies, 38, 45–49.

Samarel, N., & Fawcett, J. (1992). Enhancing adaptation to breast cancer: The addition of coaching to support groups. Oncology Nursing Forum, 19, 591–596.

Samarel, N., Fawcett, J., & Tulman, L. (1993). The effects of coaching in breast cancer support groups: A pilot study. Oncology Nursing Forum, 20, 795–798.

Samarel, N., Fawcett, J., & Tulman, L. (1997). Effect of support groups with coaching on adaptation to early stage breast cancer. Research in Nursing and Health, 20, 15–26.

Samarel, N., Fawcett, J., Krippendorf, K., et al. (1998). Women's perceptions of group support and adaptation to breast cancer. Journal of Advanced Nursing, 28, 1259–1268.

Samarel, N., Fawcett, J., Tulman, L., et al. (1999). A resource kit for women with breast cancer: Development and evaluation. Oncology Nursing Forum, 26, 611–618.

Schmidt, C.S. (1981). Withdrawal behavior of schizophrenics: Application of Roy's model. Journal of Psychosocial Nursing and Mental Health Services, 19(11), 26–33.

Seideman, R.Y., Watson, M.A., Corff, K.E., Odle, P., Haase, J., & Bowerman, J.L. (1997). Parent stress and coping in NICU and PICU. Journal of Pediatric Nursing, 12, 169–177.

Selman, S.W. (1989). Impact of total hip replacement on quality of life. Orthopaedic Nursing, 8(5), 43–49.

Shannahan, M., & Cottrell, B. (1985). Effect of the birth chair on duration of second stage labor, fetal outcome, and maternal blood loss. Nursing Research, 34, 89–92.

Sheppard, V.A., & Cunnie, K.L. (1996). Incidence of diuresis following hysterectomy. Journal of Post Anesthesia Nursing, 11, 20–28.

Shogan, M.G., & Schumann, L.L. (1993). The effect of environmental lighting on the oxygen saturation of preterm infants in the NICU. Neonatal Network, 12(5), 7–13.

Short, J.D. (1994). Interdependence needs and nursing care of the new family. Issues in Comprehensive Pediatric Nursing, 17, 1–14.

Shyu, Y.L. (2000). Role tuning between caregiver and care receiver during discharge transition: An illustration of role function mode in Roy's adaptation model. Nursing Science Quarterly, 13, 323–331.

Silva, M.C. (1987). Needs of spouses of surgical patients: A conceptualization within the Roy adaptation model. Scholarly Inquiry for Nursing Practice, 1, 29–44. Roy, C. (1987). Response to "Needs of spouses of surgical patients: A conceptualization within the Roy adaptation model." Scholarly Inquiry for Nursing Practice, 1, 45–50.

Smith, C., Garvis, M., & Martinson, I. (1983). Content analysis of interviews using nursing model: A look at parents adapting to the impact of childhood cancer. Cancer Nursing, 6, 269–275.

Smith, C.E., Mayer, L.S., Parkhurst, C., Perkins, S.B., & Pingleton, S.K. (1991). Adaptation in families with a member requiring mechanical ventilation at home. Heart and Lung, 20, 349–356.

Smith, C.E., Moushey, L., Ross, J.A., & Gieffer, C. (1993). Responsibilities and reactions of family caregivers of patients dependent on total parenteral nutrition at home. Public Health Nursing, 10, 122–128.

Smolen, D., Topp, R., & Singer, L. (2002). The effect of self-selected music during colonoscopy on anxiety, heart rate, and blood pressure. Applied Nursing Research, 15, 126–136.

Springer, D. (1996). Birth plans: The effect on anxiety in pregnant women. International Journal of Childbirth Education, 11(3), 20–25.

Strohmyer, L.L., Noroian, E.L., Patterson, L.M., & Carlin, B.P.

(1993). Adaptation six months after multiple trauma: A pilot study. Journal of Neuroscience Nursing, 25, 30–37.

Takahashi, J.J., & Bever, S.C. (1989). Preoperative nursing assessment. A research study. Association of Operating Room Nurses Journal, 50, 1022, 1024–1029, 1031–1032, 1034–1035.

Thomas, S.P., Shoffner, D.H., & Groer, M.W. (1988). Adolescent stress factors: Implications for the nurse practitioner. Nurse Practitioner, 13(6), 20, 22, 24.

Thomas-Hawkins, C. (2000). Symptom distress and day-to-day changes in functional status in chronic hemodialysis patients. Nephrology Nursing Journal, 27, 369–380.

Toye, C., Percival, P., & Blackmore, A. (1996). Satisfaction with nursing home care of a relative: Does inviting greater input make a difference? Collegian: Journal of the Royal College of Nursing, Australia, 3(2), 4–6.

Tulman, L., & Fawcett, J. (1988). Return of functional ability after childbirth. Nursing Research, 37, 77–81.

Tulman, L., & Fawcett, J. (1990a). A framework for studying functional status after diagnosis of breast cancer. Cancer Nursing, 13, 95–99.

Tulman, L., & Fawcett, J. (1990b). Maternal employment following childbirth. Research in Nursing and Health, 13, 181–188.

Tulman, L., & Fawcett, J. (1996a). Biobehavioral correlates of functional status following diagnosis of breast cancer: Report of a pilot study. Image: Journal of Nursing Scholarship, 28, 181.

Tulman, L., & Fawcett, J. (1996b). Lessons learned from a pilot study of biobehavioral correlates of functional status in women with breast cancer. Nursing Research, 45, 356–358.

Tulman, L., & Fawcett, J. (2003). Women's health during and after pregnancy: A theory-based study of adaptation to change. New York: Springer.

Tulman, L., Fawcett, J., Groblewski, L., & Silverman, L. (1990). Changes in functional status after childbirth. Nursing Research, 39, 70–75.

Tulman, L., Morin, K.H., & Fawcett, J. (1998). Prepregnant weight and weight gain during pregnancy: Relationship to functional status, symptoms, and energy. Journal of Obstetric, Gynecologic, and Neonatal Nursing, 27, 629–634.

Vasquez, E. (1995). Creating paths: Living with a very-low-birth-weight infant. Journal of Obstetric, Gynecologic, and Neonatal Nursing, 24, 619–624.

Vicenzi, A.E., & Thiel, R. (1992). AIDS education on the college campus: Roy's adaptation model directs inquiry. Public Health Nursing, 9, 270–276.

Vogelsang, J., & Ragiel, C. (1987). Anxiety levels in female surgical patients. Journal of Post Anesthesia Nursing, 2, 230–236.

Weiss, M.E., Hastings, W.J., Holly, D.C., & Craig, D.I. (1994). Using Roy's adaptation model in practice: Nurses' perspectives. Nursing Science Quarterly, 7, 80–86.

Wendler, M.C. (2003). Effects of Tellington touch in healthy adults awaiting venipuncture. Research in Nursing and Health, 26, 40–52.

Whittemore, R., Chase, S.K., Mandle, C.L., & Roy, C. (2002). Lifestyle changes in type 2 diabetes: A process model. Nursing Research, 51, 18–25.

Willoughby, D.F., Kee, C., & Demi, A. (2000). Women's psychosocial adjustment to diabetes. Journal of Advanced Nursing, 32, 1422–1430.

Woods, S.J., & Isenberg, M.A. (2001). Adaptation as a mediator of intimate abue and traumatic stress in battered women. Nursing Science Quarterly, 14, 215–221.

Wright, P.S. (1993). Parents' perception of their quality of life. Journal of Pediatric Oncology Nursing, 10, 139–145.

Yeh, C-H. (2001). Adaptation in children with cancer: Research with Roy's model. Nursing Science Quarterly, 14, 141–148.

Yeh, C-H. (2002). Health-related quality of life in pediatric patients with cancer: A structural equation approach with the Roy adaptation model. Cancer Nursing, 25, 74–80.

Yeh, C-H. (2003). Psychological distress: Testing hypotheses based on Roy's adaptation model. Nursing Science Quarterly, 16, 255–263.

Young-McCaughan, S. (1996). Sexual functioning in women with breast cancer after treatment with adjuvant therapy. Cancer Nursing, 19, 308–319.

Young-McCaughan, S., Mays, M.Z., Arzola, S.M., et al. (2003). Changes in exercise tolerance, activity and sleep patterns, and quality of life in patients with cancer participating in a structured exercise program. Oncology Nursing Forum, 30, 441–454.

Zhan, L. (2000). Cognitive adaptation and self-consistency in hearing impaired older persons: Testing Roy's adaptation model. Nursing Science Quarterly, 13, 158–165.

Zungu, B.M. (1993). Assessment of the life experiences of visually impaired adults in the Empangeni region of KwaZulu. Curationis, 16(4), 38–42.

RESEARCH INSTRUMENTS AND PRACTICE TOOLS

Burgess, A.W., & Fawcett, J. (1996). The Comprehensive Sexual Assault Assessment Tool. Nurse Practitioner, 21(4), 66, 71–72, 74–76, 78, 83, 86.

DiMattio, M.J.K. (2001). Women's home recovery from coronary artery bypass surgery: A longitudinal study of functional status and correlates. Dissertation Abstracts International, 62, 2254B.

DiMattio, M.J.K., & Tulman, L. (2003). A longitudinal study of functional status and correlates following coronary artery bypass graft surgery in women. Nursing Research, 52, 98–107.

Dow, K.H.M. (1993). An analysis of the experience of surviving and having children after breast cancer. Dissertation Abstracts International, 53, 5641B.

Doyle, R., & Rajacich, D. (1991). The Roy adaptation model. Health teaching about osteoporosis. American Association of Occupational Health Nursing Journal, 39, 508–512.

Fawcett, J. (1992). Documentation using a conceptual model of nursing. Nephrology Nursing Today, 2(5), 1–8.

Fawcett, J., & Burritt, J. (1985). An exploratory study of antenatal preparation for cesarean birth. Journal of Obstetric, Gynecologic, and Neonatal Nursing, 14, 224–230.

Fawcett, J., & Henklein, J. (1987). Antenatal education for cesarean birth: Extension of a field test. Journal of Obstetric, Gynecologic, and Neonatal Nursing, 16, 61–65.

Fawcett, J., & Tulman, L. (1996). Assessment of function. In R. McCorkle, M. Grant, M. Frank-Stromborg, & S.B. Baird (Eds.), Cancer nursing: A comprehensive textbook (2nd ed., pp. 66–73). Philadelphia: Saunders.

Fawcett, J., Tulman, L., & Myers, S. (1988). Development of the Inventory of Functional Status after Childbirth. Journal of Nurse-Midwifery, 33, 252–260.

Galbreath, J.G. (2002). Roy adaptation model: Sister Callista Roy. In J.B George (Ed.), Nursing theories: The base for professional nursing practice (5th ed., pp. 295–338). Upper Saddle River, NJ: Prentice Hall.

Frank, D.I. (1988). Psychosocial assessment of renal dialysis patients. American Nephrology Nurses Association Journal, 15, 207–232.

Hamner, J.B. (1989). Applying the Roy adaptation model to the CCU. Critical Care Nurse, 9(3), 51–61.

Hanchett, E.S. (1988). Nursing frameworks and community as client: Bridging the gap. Norwalk, CT: Appleton & Lange.

Hinman, L.M. (1983). Focus on the school-aged child in family intervention. Journal of School Health, 53, 499–502.

Huber, P.M., Medhat, A., & Carter, M.C. (1988). Prosthetic problem inventory scale. Rehabilitation Nursing, 13, 326–329.

Ide, B.A. (1978). SPAL: A tool for measuring self-perceived adaptation level appropriate for an elderly population. In E.E. Bauwens (Ed.), Clinical nursing research: Its strategies and findings (Monograph series 1978: Two, pp. 56–63). Indianapolis: Sigma Theta Tau.

Jackson, D.A. (1990). Roy in the postanesthesia care unit. Journal of Post Anesthesia Nursing, 5, 143–148.

Jakocko, M.T., & Sowden, L.A. (1986). The Roy adaptation model in nursing practice. In H.A. Andrews & C. Roy (Eds.), Essentials of the Roy adaptation model (pp. 165–177). Norwalk, CT: Appleton & Lange.

Joseph, A., & Lantz, J. (1996). A systematic tool to assess urinary incontinence parameters: A closer look at unfamiliar parameters. Urologic Nursing, 16, 93–98.

Laros, J. (1977). Deriving outcome criteria from a conceptual model. Nursing Outlook, 25, 333–336.

LeMone, P. (1995). Assessing psychosexual concerns in adults with diabetes: Pilot project using Roy's modes of adaptation. Issues in Mental Health Nursing, 16, 67–78.

Lewis, F.M., Firsich, S.C., & Parsell, S. (1978). Development of reliable measures of patient health outcomes related to quality nursing care for chemotherapy patients. In J.C. Krueger, A.H. Nelson, & M.O. Wolanin (Eds.), Nursing research: Development, collaboration, and utilization (pp. 225–228). Germantown, MD: Aspen.

Lewis, F.M., Firsich, S.C., & Parsell, S. (1979). Clinical tool development for adult chemotherapy patients: Process and content. Cancer Nursing, 2, 99–108.

Modrcin-McCarthy, M.A., McCue, S., & Walker, J. (1997). Preterm infants and STRESS: A tool for the neonatal nurse. Journal of Perinatal and Neonatal Nursing, 10(4), 62–71.

Newman, D.M.L. (1997). The Inventory of Functional Status—Caregiver of a Child in a Body Cast. Journal of Pediatric Nursing, 12, 142–147.

O'Leary, P.A. (1991). Family caregivers' log reports of sleep and activity behaviors of persons with Alzheimer's disease. Dissertation Abstracts International, 51, 4780B.

Paier, G.S. (1994). Development and testing of an instrument to assess functional status in the elderly. Dissertation Abstracts International, 55, 1806B.

Peters, V.J. (1993). Documentation using the Roy adaptation model. American Nephrology Nurses Association Journal, 20, 522.

Rambo, B. (1984). Adaptation nursing: Assessment and intervention (pp. 385–395). Philadelphia: Saunders.

Riegel, B. (1985). A method of giving intershift report based on a conceptual model. Focus on Critical Care, 12(4), 12–18.

Robitaille-Tremblay, M. (1984). A data collection tool for the psychiatric nurse. Canadian Nurse, 80(7), 26–28.

Rogers, M., Paul, L.J., Clarke, J., Mackay, C., Potter, M., & Ward, W. (1991). The use of the Roy adaptation model in nursing administration. Canadian Journal of Nursing Administration, 4(2), 21–26.

Roy, C. (1979). Health-illness (powerlessness) questionnaire and hospitalized patient decision making. In M.J. Ward & C.A. Lindeman (Eds.), Instruments for measuring nursing practice and other health care variables (Vol. 1, pp. 147–153). Hyattsville, MD: US Department of Health, Education, and Welfare.

Roy, C., & Andrews, H.A. (1999a). The Roy adaptation model (2nd ed., pp. 79–81). Stamford, CT: Appleton & Lange.

Roy, C., & Andrews, H.A. (1999b). The Roy adaptation model (2nd ed., pp. 82–84). Stamford, CT: Appleton & Lange.

Roy, C., & Andrews, H.A. (1999c). The Roy adaptation model (2nd ed., p. 263). Stamford, CT: Appleton & Lange.

Roy, C., & Andrews, H.A. (1999d). The Roy adaptation model (2nd ed., pp. 139, 161, 184, 214, 247, 279, 305, 340, 372, 417, 462, 503). Stamford, CT: Appleton & Lange.

Roy, C., & Andrews, H.A. (1999e). The Roy adaptation model (2nd ed., p. 91). Stamford, CT: Appleton & Lange.

Roy, C., & Andrews, H.A. (1999f). The Roy adaptation model (2nd ed., p. 546). Stamford, CT: Appleton & Lange.

Roy, C., & Zhan, L. (2001). Sister Callista Roy: The Roy adaptation model. In M.E. Parker (Ed.), Nursing theories and nursing practice (pp. 315–327). Philadelphia: F.A. Davis

Seo-Cho, J.M. (1999). Nursing process manual: Assessment tool for the Roy adaptation model. Glendale, CA: Polaris Publishing.

Short, J.D. (1994). Interdependence needs and nursing care of the new family. Issues in Comprehensive Pediatric Nursing, 17, 1–14.

Starn, J., & Niederhauser, V. (1990). An MCN model for nursing diagnosis to focus intervention. MCN: American Journal of Maternal/Child Nursing, 15, 180–183.

Taylor, C. (1993). The patient's guide to preterm labor. Woodbury, NJ: Underwood-Memorial Hospital.

Thomas-Hawkins, C., Fawcett, J., & Tulman, L. (1998). The Inventory of Functional Status—dialysis: Development and testing. American Association of Nephrology Nurses Journal, 25, 483–490.

Tulman, L., Fawcett, J., & McEvoy, M.D. (1991). Development of the Inventory of Functional Status—cancer. Cancer Nursing, 14, 254–260.

Tulman, L., Fawcett, J., & Weiss, M. (1993). The Inventory of Functional Status—fathers: Development and psychometric testing. Journal of Nurse-Midwifery, 38, 117–123.

Tulman, L., Higgins, K., Fawcett, J., Nunno, C., Vansickel, C., Haas, M.B., & Speca, M.M. (1991). The Inventory of Functional Status—antepartum period: Development and testing. Journal of Nurse-Midwifery, 36, 117–123.

Varnell, G.M.P. (1990). Parental role perceptions: Instrument development. Dissertation Abstracts International, 51, 1197B.

Weiss, M.E., & Teplick, F. (1993). Linking perinatal standards, documentation, and quality monitoring. Journal of Perinatal and Neonatal Nursing, 7(2), 18–27. [Reprinted in Neonatal Intensive Care, 8(1), 38–43, 58, 1995.]

Weiss, M.E., & Teplick, F. (1995). Linking perinatal standards, documentation, and quality monitoring. Neonatal Intensive Care, 8(1), 38–43, 58.

Whall, A.L. (1986). Strategic family therapy: Nursing reformulations and applications. In A.L. Whall, Family therapy theory for nursing: Four approaches (pp. 51–67). Norwalk, CT: Appleton-Century-Crofts.

Wright, P.S. (1993). Parents' perception of their quality of life. Journal of Pediatric Oncology Nursing, 10, 139–145.

Young, A., Taylor, S.G., & McLaughlin-Renpenning, K. (2001). Connections: Nursing research, theory, and practice. St. Louis: Mosby.

Zhan, L. (1994). Cognitive adaptation processing and self-consistency in the hearing impaired elderly. Dissertation Abstracts International, 54, 4086B.

Zhan, L., & Shen, C. (1994). The development of an instrument to measure self-consistency. Journal of Advanced Nursing, 20, 509–516.

EDUCATION

Brower, H.T.F., & Baker, B.J. (1976). Using the adaptation model in a practitioner curriculum. Nursing Outlook, 24, 686–689.

Claus, S., Graiver, M., Krawczyk, M., & Wallace, R., Sr. (1991). An outcome assessment of liberal education for the baccalaureate nursing major. In M. Garbin (Ed.), Assessing educational outcomes: Third National Conference on Measurement and Evaluation in Nursing (pp. 69–77). New York: National League for Nursing.

Curl, L., Hoehn, J., & Theile, J.R. (1988). Computer applications in nursing: A new course in the curriculum. Computers in Nursing, 6, 263–268.

deMontigny, F., Dumas, L., Bolduc, L., & Blais, S. (1997). Teaching family nursing based on conceptual models of nursing. Journal of Family Nursing, 3, 267–279.

Fawcett, J. (2003). Conceptual models of nursing: International in scope and substance? The case of the Roy Adaptation Model. Nursing Science Quarterly, 16, 315–318.

Flood, J., & Schneider, L. (1993). A unique approach to first semester. In J. Simmons (Ed.), Prospectives: Celebrating 40 years of associate degree nursing education (pp. 91–97). New York: National League for Nursing Press.

Gordon, M.F., & Grundy, M. (1997). From apprenticeship to academia: An adult branch programme. Nurse Education Today, 17, 162–167.

Heinrich, K. (1989). Growing pains: Faculty stages in adopting a nursing model. Nurse Educator, 14(1), 3–4, 29.

Knowlton, C., Goodwin, M., Moore, J., Alt-White, A., Guarino, S., & Pyne, H. (1983). Systems adaptation model for nursing for families, groups and communities. Journal of Nursing Education, 22, 128–131.

Mengel, A., Sherman, S., Nahigian, E., & Coleman, I. (1989). Adaptation of the Roy model in an educational setting. In J.P. Riehl-Sisca (Ed.), Conceptual models for nursing practice (3rd ed., pp. 125–131). Norwalk, CT: Appleton & Lange.

Morales-Mann, E.T., & Logan, M. (1990). Implementing the Roy model: Challenges for nurse educators. Journal of Advanced Nursing, 15, 142–147.

Rambo, B. (1984). Adaptation nursing: Assessment and intervention (p. v). Philadelphia: Saunders.

Roy, C. (1973). Adaptation: Implications for curriculum change. Nursing Outlook, 21, 163–168.

Roy, C. (1974). The Roy adaptation model. In J.P. Riehl & C. Roy (Eds.), Conceptual models for nursing practice (pp. 135–144). New York: Appleton-Century-Crofts.

Roy, C. (1979). Relating nursing theory to education: A new era. Nurse Educator, 4(2), 16–21.

Roy, C. (1980). The Roy adaptation model. In J.P. Riehl & C. Roy (Eds.), Conceptual models for nursing practice (2nd ed., pp. 179–188). New York: Appleton-Century-Crofts.

Roy, C. (1989). The Roy adaptation model. In J.P. Riehl-Sisca (Ed.), Conceptual models for nursing practice (3rd ed., pp. 105–114). Norwalk, CT: Appleton & Lange.

Story, E.L., & Ross, M.M. (1986). Family centered community health nursing and the Betty Neuman systems model. Nursing Papers, 18(2), 77–88.

ADMINISTRATION

Connerley, K., Ristau, S., Lindberg, C., & McFarland, M. (1999). The Roy model in practice. In C. Roy & H.A. Andrews (Eds.), The Roy adaptation model (2nd ed., pp. 515–534). Stamford, CT: Appleton & Lange.

Dorsey, K., & Purcell, S. (1987). Translating a nursing theory into a nursing system. Geriatric Nursing, 8, 167–137.

Fawcett, J. (2003). Conceptual models of nursing: International in scope and substance? The case of the Roy Adaptation Model. Nursing Science Quarterly, 16, 315–318.

Fitch, M., Rogers, M., Ross, E., Shea, H., Smith, I., & Tucker, D. (1991). Developing a plan to evaluate the use of nursing conceptual frameworks. Canadian Journal of Nursing Administration, 4(1), 22–28.

Frederickson, K. (1991). Nursing theories—A basis for differentiated practice: Application of the Roy adaptation model in nursing practice. In I.E. Goertzen (Ed.), Differentiating nursing practice: Into the twenty-first century (pp. 41–44). Kansas City, MO: American Academy of Nursing.

Frederickson, K. (1993). Translating the Roy Adaptation Model into practice and research. In M.E. Parker (Ed.), Patterns of nursing theories in practice (pp. 230–238). New York: National League for Nursing.

Frederickson, K., & Williams, J.K. (1997). Nursing theory–guided practice: The Roy adaptation model and patient/family experiences. Nursing Science Quarterly, 10, 53–54.

Gray, J. (1991). The Roy adaptation model in nursing practice. In C. Roy & H.A. Andrews (Eds.), The Roy adaptation model: The definitive statement (pp. 429–443). Norwalk, CT: Appleton & Lange.

Jakocko, M.T., & Sowden, L.A. (1986). The Roy adaptation model in nursing practice. In H.A. Andrews & C. Roy (Eds.), Essentials of the Roy adaptation model (pp. 165–177). Norwalk, CT: Appleton & Lange.

Laros, J. (1977). Deriving outcome criteria from a conceptual model. Nursing Outlook, 25, 333–336.

Lewis, T. (1988). Leaping the chasm between nursing theory and practice. Journal of Advanced Nursing, 13, 345–351.

Mastel, M.F., Hammond, H., & Roberts, M.P. (1982). Theory into hospital practice: A pilot implementation. Journal of Nursing Administration, 12(6), 9–15.

Nyqvist, K.H., & Karlsson, K.H. (1997). A philosophy of care for a neonatal intensive care unit: Operationalization of a nursing model. Scandinavian Journal of Caring Sciences, 11, 91–96.

Parse, R.R. (1990). Nursing theory-based practice: A challenge for the 90s (Editorial). Nursing Science Quarterly, 3, 53.

Robitaille-Tremblay, M. (1984). A data collection tool for the psychiatric nurse. Canadian Nurse, 80(7), 26–28.

Rogers, M., Paul, L.J., Clarke, J., Mackay, C., Potter, M., & Ward, W. (1991). The use of the Roy adaptation model in nursing administration. Canadian Journal of Nursing Administration, 4(2), 21–26.

Roy, C. (1992). The nurse theorists: Excellence in action—Callista Roy. Athens, OH: Fuld Institute of Technology in Nursing Education. [Videotape.]

Silva, M.C., & Sorrell, J.M. (1992). Testing of nursing theory: Critique and philosophical expansion. Advances in Nursing Science, 14(4), 12–23.

Torosian, L.C., DeStefano, M., & Dietrick-Gallagher, M. (1985). Day gynecologic chemotherapy unit: An innovative approach to changing health care systems. Cancer Nursing, 8, 221–227.

Weiss, M.E., & Teplick, F. (1993). Linking perinatal standards, documentation, and quality monitoring. Journal of Perinatal and

Neonatal Nursing, 7(2), 18–27. [Reprinted in Neonatal Intensive Care, 8(1), 38–43, 58, 1995.]

Weiss, M.E., & Teplick, F. (1995). Linking perinatal standards, documentation, and quality monitoring. Neonatal Intensive Care, 8(1), 38–43, 58.

PRACTICE

Aaronson, L., & Seaman, L.P. (1989). Managing hypernatremia in fluid deficient elderly. Journal of Gerontological Nursing, 15(7), 29–34.

Araich, M. (2001). Roy's adaptation model: Demonstration of theory integration into process of care in coronary care unit. ICUs and Nursing Web Journal, July-August (7), 12.

Barnfather, J.S., Swain, M.A.P., & Erickson, H.C. (1989). Evaluation of two assessment techniques for adaptation to stress. Nursing Science Quarterly, 2, 172–182.

Batra, C. (1996). Nursing theory and nursing process in the community. In J.M. Cookfair (Ed.), Nursing care in the community (2nd ed., pp. 85–124). St. Louis: Mosby.

Bawden, M., Ralph, J., & Herrick, C.A. (1991). Enhancing the coping skills of mothers with developmentally delayed children. Journal of Child and Adolescent Psychiatric Mental Health Nursing, 4, 25–28.

Bonnema, R. (1997). Steriotactic posteroventral pallidotomy. Seminars in Perioperative Nursing, 6(1), 49–58.

Cardiff, J. (1989). Heartfelt care. Nursing Times, 85(3), 42–45.

Coleman, P.M. (1993). Depression during the female climacteric period. Journal of Advanced Nursing, 18, 1540–1546.

Crossfield, T. (1990). Patients with scleroderma. Nursing (London), 4(10), 19–20.

Cunningham, D.A. (2002). Application of Roy's adaptation model when caring for a group of women coping with menopause. Journal of Community Health Nursing, 19, 49–60.

Dawson, S. (1998). Adult/elderly care nursing: Pre-amputation assessment using Roy's adaptation model. British Journal of Nursing, 7, 536, 538–542.

deMontigney, F. (1992a). L'Intervention familiale selon Roy [Family intervention according to Roy]: La famille Joly: Cueillette et analyse des donnees [English abstract]. Canadian Nurse, 88(8), 41–45.

deMontigney, F. (1992b). L'Intervention familiale selon Roy [Family intervention according to Roy]: Planification, execution et evaluation [English abstract]. Canadian Nurse, 88(9), 43–46.

DiMaria, R.A. (1989). Posttrauma responses: Potential for nursing. Journal of Advanced Medical-Surgical Nursing, 2(1), 41–48.

Donnelly, E. (1993). Family health assessment. Home Healthcare Nurse, 11(2), 30–37.

Dornik, E. (2001). Quality of life of a tetraplegic: Case study. Obzornik Zdravstvene Nege, 35, 205–211. [Slovenian; English abstract]

Downey, C. (1974). Adaptation nursing applied to an obstetric patient. In J.P. Riehl & C. Roy (Eds.), Conceptual models for nursing practice (pp. 151–159). New York: Appleton-Century-Crofts.

Doyle, R., & Rajacich, D. (1991). The Roy adaptation model. Health teaching about osteoporosis. American Association of Occupational Health Nursing Journal, 39, 508–512.

Dudek, G. (1989). Nursing update: Hypophosphatemic rickets. Pediatric Nursing, 15(1), 45–50.

Eganhouse, D.J. (1994). A nursing model for a community hospital preterm birth prevention program. Journal of Obstetric, Gynecologic, and Neonatal Nursing, 23, 756–766.

Ellis, J.A. (1991). Coping with adolescent cancer: It's a matter of adaptation. Journal of Pediatric Oncology Nursing, 8, 10–17.

Fawcett, J. (1981). Assessing and understanding the cesarean father. In C.F. Kehoe (Ed.), The cesarean experience. Theoretical and clinical perspectives for nurses (pp. 143–156). New York: Appleton-Century-Crofts.

Fawcett, J. (1997). Conceptual models as guides for psychiatric nursing practice. In A.W. Burgess (Ed.), Psychiatric nursing: Promoting mental health (pp. 627–642). Stamford, CT: Appleton & Lange.

Fawcett, J., Archer, C.L., Becker, D., Brown, K.K., Gann, S., Wong, M.J., & Wurster, A.B. (1992). Guidelines for selecting a conceptual model of nursing: Focus on the individual patient. Dimensions of Critical Care Nursing, 11, 268–277.

Forsdyke, H. (1993). Treatment for life. Nursing Times, 89(32), 34–36.

Fox, J.A. (1990). Bilateral breast lumps. A care plan in theatre using a stress adaptation model. NATNews: British Journal of Theatre Nursing, 27(11), 11–14.

Frank, D.I. (1988). Psychosocial assessment of renal dialysis patients. American Nephrology Nurses Association Journal, 15, 207–232.

Frederickson, K. (1993). Using a nursing model to manage symptoms: Anxiety and the Roy adaptation model. Holistic Nursing Practice, 7(2), 36–43.

Galligan, A.C. (1979). Using Roy's concept of adaptation to care for young children. MCN: American Journal of Maternal/Child Nursing, 4, 24–28.

Gerrish, C. (1989). From theory to practice. Nursing Times, 85(35), 42–45.

Giger, J.A., Bower, C.A., & Miller, S.W. (1987). Roy Adaptation Model: ICU application. Dimensions of Critical Care Nursing, 6, 215–224.

Gordon, J. (1974). Nursing assessment and care plan for a cardiac patient. In J.P. Riehl & C. Roy (Eds.), Conceptual models for nursing practice (pp. 144–151). New York: Appleton-Century-Crofts.

Griffiths-Jones, A., & Walker, G. (1993). A new way forward: How care can be planned for clients who are HIV positive, using Roy's adaptation model. Nursing Times, 89(19), 76, 78.

Hamer, B.A. (1991). Music therapy: Harmony for change.

Journal of Psychosocial Nursing and Mental Health Services, 29(12), 5–7.

Hanchett, E.S. (1988). Nursing frameworks and community as client: Bridging the gap. Norwalk, CT: Appleton & Lange.

Hartley, B., & Camion-Fuller, C. (1994). Juvenile dermatomyositis: A Roy nursing perspective. Journal of Pediatric Nursing, 9, 175–182.

Hennessy-Harstad, E.B. (1999). Empowering adolescents with asthma to take control through adaptation. Journal of Pediatric Health Care, 13, 273–277.

Hernández, G.E. (2002). The Callista Roy adaptation model: Caring for the patient with an acute myocardial infarction. Meta de Enfermeria, 5(44), 52–58. [Spanish; English abstract]

Hitejc, Z. (2001). Practical application of the theory of Callista Roy in the process of adaptation of the family to a mentally retarded child. Obzornik Zdravstvene Nege, 35, 185–191.

Hughes, A. (1991). Life with a stoma. Nursing Times, 87(25), 67–68.

Ingram, L. (1995). Roy's adaptation model and accident and emergency nursing. Accident and Emergency Nursing, 3, 150–153.

Innes, M.H. (1992). Management of an inadequately ventilated patient. British Journal of Nursing, 1, 780–784.

Janelli, L. (1980). Utilizing Roy's adaptation model from a gerontological perspective. Journal of Gerontological Nursing, 6, 140–150.

Jay, P. (1990). Relatives caring for the terminally ill. Nursing Standard, 5(5), 30–32.

Keen, M., Breckenridge, D., Frauman, A.C., et al. (1998). Nursing assessment and intervention for adult hemodialysis patients: Application of Roy's adaptation model. American Association of Nephrology Nurses Journal, 25, 311–319. [Erratum: American Association of Nephrology Nurses Journal, 25, 532, 1998.]

Kehoe, C.F. (1981). Identifying the nursing needs of the postpartum cesarean mother. In C.F. Kehoe (Ed.), The cesarean experience: Theoretical and clinical perspectives for nurses (pp. 85–141). New York: Appleton-Century-Crofts.

Kurek-Ovshinsky, C. (1991). Group psychotherapy in an acute inpatient setting: Techniques that nourish self-esteem. Issues in Mental Health Nursing, 12, 81–88.

Lambert, C. (1994). Depression: Nursing management, part 2. Nursing Standard, 8(48), 57–64.

Lankester, K., & Sheldon, L.M. (1999). Health visiting with Roy's model: A case study. Journal of Child Health Care, 3, 28–34.

Logan, M. (1986). Palliative care nursing: Applicability of the Roy model. Journal of Palliative Care, 1(2), 18–24.

Logan, M. (1988). Care of the terminally ill includes the family. Canadian Nurse, 84(5), 30–33.

Madina Lizarralde, E. (2001). A study of a case of homecare in accordance with Roy's adaptation model. Meta de Enfermeria, 4(33), 18–25. [Spanish; English abstract]

McIver, M. (1987). Putting theory into practice. Canadian Nurse, 83(10), 36–38.

Messner, R., & Smith, M.N. (1986). Neurofibromatosis: Relinquishing the masks; a quest for quality of life. Journal of Advanced Nursing, 11, 459–464.

Miller, F. (1991). Using Roy's model in a special hospital. Nursing Standard, 5(27), 29–32.

Miller, J.F., & Hellenbrand, D. (1981). An eclectic approach to practice. American Journal of Nursing, 81, 1339–1343.

Nash, D.J. (1987). Kawasaki disease: Application of the Roy adaptation model to determine interventions. Journal of Pediatric Nursing, 2, 308–315.

O'Reilly, M. (1989). Familiarity breeds acceptance. Nursing Times, 85(12), 29–30.

Phillips, K.D. (1997). Roy's adaptation model in nursing practice. In M.R. Alligood & A. Marriner-Tomey (Eds.), Nursing theory: Utilization and application (pp. 175–200). St. Louis: Mosby.

Phillips, K.D. (2002). Roy's adaptation model in nursing practice. In M.R. Alligood & A. Marriner Tomey (Eds.), Nursing theory: Utilization and application (2nd ed., pp. 289–314). St. Louis: Mosby.

Piazza, D., & Foote, A. (1990). Roy's adaptation model: A guide for rehabilitation nursing practice. Rehabilitation Nursing, 15, 254–259.

Piazza, D., Foote, A., Holcombe, J., Harris, M.G., & Wright, P. (1992). The use of Roy's adaptation model applied to a patient with breast cancer. European Journal of Cancer Care, 1(4), 17–22.

Rogers, E.J. (1991). Postanesthesia care of the cocaine abuser. Journal of Post Anesthesia Nursing, 6, 102–107.

Roy, C. (1971). Adaptation: A basis for nursing practice. Nursing Outlook, 19, 254–257.

Roy, C. (1983a). The expectant family. In I.W. Clements & F.B. Roberts (Eds.), Family health: A theoretical approach to nursing care (pp. 298–303). New York: Wiley.

Roy, C. (1983b). The family in primary care. In I.W. Clements & F.B. Roberts (Eds.), Family health: A theoretical approach to nursing care (pp. 375–378). New York: Wiley.

Sato, M.K. (1986). The Roy adaptation model. In P. Winstead-Fry (Ed.), Case studies in nursing theory (pp. 103–125). New York: National League for Nursing.

Schmidt, C.S. (1981). Withdrawal behavior of schizophrenics: Application of Roy's model. Journal of Psychosocial Nursing and Mental Health Services, 19(11), 26–33.

Schmitz, M. (1980). The Roy adaptation model: Application in a community setting. In J.P. Riehl & C. Roy (Eds.), Conceptual models for nursing practice (2nd ed., pp. 193–206). New York: Appleton-Century-Crofts.

Sirignano, R.G. (1987). Peripartum cardiomyopathy: An application of the Roy adaptation model. Journal of Cardiovascular Nursing, 2, 24–32.

Smith, M.C. (1988). Roy's adaptation model in practice. Nursing Science Quarterly, 1, 97–98.

Starr, S.L. (1980). Adaptation applied to the dying client. In J.P. Riehl & C. Roy (Eds.), Conceptual models for nursing practice (2nd ed., pp. 189–192). New York: Appleton-Century-Crofts.

Stringer, M., Librizzi, R., & Weiner, S. (1991). Establishing a prenatal genetic diagnosis: The nurse's role. MCN: American Journal of Maternal/Child Nursing, 16, 152–156.

Summers, T.M. (1991). Psychosocial support of the burned patient. Critical Care Nursing Clinics of North America, 3, 237–244.

Thornbury, J.M., & King, L.D. (1992). The Roy adaptation model and care of persons with Alzheimer's disease. Nursing Science Quarterly, 5, 129–133.

Wagner, P. (1976). Testing the adaptation model in practice. Nursing Outlook, 24, 682–685.

West, S. (1992). Number one priorities. Nursing Times, 88(17), 28–31.

Whall, A.L. (1986). Strategic family therapy: Nursing reformulations and applications. In A.L. Whall, Family therapy theory for nursing: Four approaches (pp. 51–67). Norwalk, CT: Appleton-Century-Crofts.

Wright, P.S., Holcombe, J., Foote, A., & Piazza, D. (1993). The Roy adaptation model used as a guide for the nursing care of an 8-year-old child with leukemia. Journal of Pediatric Oncology Nursing, 10, 68–74.

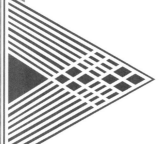

Part Three

ANALYSIS AND EVALUATION OF NURSING THEORIES

Part Three introduces the reader to nursing theories.

Chapter 11 presents a distinctive framework for the analysis and evaluation of nursing theories.

Chapters 12 through 16 illustrate the application of the analysis and evaluation framework. These chapters acquaint the reader with widely recognized and oft-cited nursing theories. In Chapters 12 and 13, the reader learns about two grand theories—Margaret Newman's Theory of Health as Expanding Consciousness and Rosemarie Parse's Theory of Human Becoming. In Chapters 14, 15, and 16, the reader learns about three middle-range theories—Ida Jean Orlando's Theory of the Deliberative Nursing Process, Hildegard Peplau's Theory of Interpersonal Relations, and Jean Watson's Theory of Human Caring.

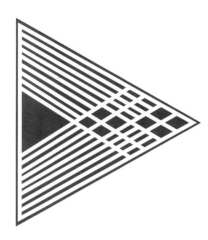

Chapter **11**

Framework for Analysis and Evaluation of Nursing Theories

This chapter presents a framework for analysis and evaluation of nursing theories. The framework emphasizes the most important features of grand theories and middle-range theories and is appropriate to the level of abstraction of these two types of nursing theories. The framework was first published several years ago (Fawcett, 1993) and was refined for the first edition of this book (Fawcett, 2000). The current version reflects attention to language that encompasses all nursing practice situations and settings, not just those situations and settings that connote nursing at the bedside of the sick, or clinical nursing (Parse, 2002).

This framework, like the framework for analysis and evaluation of nursing models presented in Chapter 3, reflects critical reasoning and, therefore, "highlights strengths and exposes problems inherent in a line of reasoning" (Silva & Sorrell, 1992, p. 17). Application of the framework yields a descriptive, analytical, and critical commentary that enhances understanding of the theory and can lead to refinements in its concepts and propositions (Meleis, 1997).

Overview

The framework for analysis and evaluation of nursing theories separates questions dealing with analysis from those more appropriate to evaluation. Analysis refers to an objective and nonjudgmental description of a nursing theory. In contrast, evaluation involves judgments about the extent to which a nursing theory satisfies certain criteria. The steps of the framework are listed here. Each step is discussed in detail in this chapter.

Key Terms

ANALYSIS
    Step 1: Theory Scope
    Step 2: Theory Context
    Step 3: Theory Content
EVALUATION
    Step 1: Significance
    Step 2: Internal Consistency
    Step 3: Parsimony
    Step 4: Testability
    Step 5: Empirical Adequacy
    Step 6: Pragmatic Adequacy

▶▶▶ ANALYSIS OF NURSING THEORIES

ANALYSIS of a nursing theory, using the framework presented in this chapter, is accomplished by a systematic examination of exactly what the author has written about the theory, rather than by relying on inferences about what might have been meant or by referring to other authors' interpretations of the theory. When the author of the theory has not been clear about a point or has not presented certain information, it may be necessary to make inferences or to turn to other reviews of the theory. That, however, must be noted explicitly, so that the distinction between the words of the theory author and those of others is clear. Theory analysis, therefore, involves a nonjudgmental, detailed examination of the theory, including **Theory Scope, Theory Context,** and **Theory Content.**

ANALYSIS STEP 1: THEORY SCOPE

The first step in theory analysis is to classify the **Theory Scope.** Recall, from Chapter 1, that grand theories are broad in scope and substantively nonspecific; their concepts and propositions are relatively abstract. Middle-range theories, in contrast, are more circumscribed and substantively specific; their concepts and propositions are relatively concrete. In addition, middle-range theories are classified as descriptive, explanatory, or predictive. The question that should be asked is:

• What is the scope of the theory?

ANALYSIS STEP 2: THEORY CONTEXT

The second step in theory analysis is examination of the **Theory Context.** Barnum (1998) regarded the context of a nursing theory to be "the environment in which nursing acts occur. It tells the nature of the world of nursing and, in most cases, this involves describing the salient characteristics of the patient's surroundings" (p. 19). Context, as used in this book, goes beyond Barnum's description to encompass identification of the concepts and propositions of the nursing metaparadigm addressed by the theory, the philosophical claims on which the theory is based, the conceptual model from which the theory was derived, and the contributions of knowledge from nursing and adjunctive disciplines to the theory development effort.

The metaparadigm of nursing, as explained in Chapter 1, is made up of four global concepts and four global propositions. The questions about the metaparadigm concepts and propositions are:

• Which metaparadigm concepts are addressed by the theory?
  • Does the theory deal with human beings?
  • Does the theory deal with the environment?
  • Does the theory deal with health?
  • Does the theory deal with nursing processes or goals?

• Which metaparadigm propositions are addressed by the theory?
  • Does the theory deal with human processes of living and dying?
  • Does the theory deal with patterning of human health experiences within the context of the environment.
  • Does the theory deal with nursing actions or processes that are beneficial to human beings?
  • Does the theory deal with human processes of living and dying, recognizing that human beings are in a continuous relationship with their environments?

Other questions about context focus on the philosophical claims on which the theory is based. Philosophical statements, as noted in Chapter 1, explicate values and beliefs about nursing, as well as the world view of the relationship between human beings and the environment. The questions are:

• On what philosophical claims is the theory based?
• What world view is reflected in the theory?

Another question dealing with the context of a theory focuses on the conceptual model from which the theory was derived. As explained in Chapter 1, a conceptual model is more abstract than a theory and serves as a guide for theory development. The question is:

• From what conceptual model was the theory derived?

The final question dealing with theory context highlights the knowledge from nursing and other disciplines used by the theorist. This question reflects recognition that "nursing theories do not spring forth fully formed" (Levine, 1988, p. 16). Instead, most nurse theorists draw on existing, or antecedent, knowledge from nursing and adjunctive disciplines as they construct and refine their theories. The question is:

• What antecedent knowledge from nursing and adjunctive disciplines was used in the development of the theory?

ANALYSIS STEP 3: THEORY CONTENT

The third step in theory analysis is examination of **Theory Content.** The content, or subject matter, of a theory is articulated through the theory's concepts and propositions.

The concepts of a theory are words or groups of words that express a mental image of some phenomenon. They represent the special vocabulary of a theory. Furthermore, the concepts give meaning to what can be imagined or observed through the senses. They enable the theorist to categorize, interpret, and structure the phenomena encompassed by the theory. Concepts can be unidimensional, or they can have more than one dimension.

The propositions of a theory are declarative statements about one or more concepts, statements that assert what is thought to be the case. As explained in Chapter 1, nonrelational propositions describe concepts by stating their constitutive definitions. Relational propositions express the associations or linkages between two or more concepts.

Analysis of the content of a theory requires systematic examination of all available descriptions of the theory by its author. The questions are:

- What are the concepts of the theory?
- What are the propositions of the theory?
  - Which propositions are nonrelational?
  - Which propositions are relational?

 ## EVALUATION OF NURSING THEORIES

EVALUATION of a theory requires judgments to be made about the extent to which a theory satisfies certain criteria. These criteria are **Significance, Internal Consistency, Parsimony, Testability, Empirical Adequacy,** and **Pragmatic Adequacy**. The evaluation is based on the results of the analysis, as well as on a review of previously published critiques, research reports, and reports of practical applications of the theory.

EVALUATION STEP 1: SIGNIFICANCE

The first step in theory evaluation focuses on the context of the theory. The criterion is **Significance**.

The criterion of significance requires justification of the importance of the theory to the discipline of nursing. That criterion is met when the metaparadigmatic, philosophical, and conceptual or paradigmatic origins of the theory are explicit, when the antecedent nursing and adjunctive knowledge is cited (Levine, 1995), and when the special contributions made by the theory are identified. The questions to be asked when evaluating the significance of the theory are:

- Are the metaparadigm concepts and propositions addressed by the theory explicit?
- Are the philosophical claims on which the theory is based explicit?

- Is the conceptual model from which the theory was derived explicit?
- Are the authors of antecedent knowledge from nursing and adjunctive disciplines acknowledged and are bibliographical citations given?

EVALUATION STEP 2: INTERNAL CONSISTENCY

The second step in theory evaluation focuses on both the context and the content of the theory. The criterion is **Internal Consistency**. This criterion requires all elements of the theorist's work, including the philosophical claims, conceptual model, and theory concepts and propositions, to be congruent.

Furthermore, the internal consistency criterion requires the theory concepts to reflect semantic clarity and semantic consistency. The semantic clarity requirement is more likely to be met when a constitutive definition is given for each concept than when no explicit definitions are given.

The semantic consistency requirement is met when the same term and the same definition are used for each concept in all of the author's discussions about the theory. Semantic inconsistency occurs when different terms are used for a concept or different meanings are attached to the same concept.

The internal consistency criterion also requires that propositions reflect structural consistency, which means that the linkages between concepts are specified and that no contradictions in relational propositions are evident.

The questions to be asked when evaluating the internal consistency of a theory are:

- Are the context (philosophical claims and conceptual model) and the content (concepts and propositions) of the theory congruent?
- Do the concepts reflect semantic clarity and semantic consistency?
- Do the propositions reflect structural consistency?

EVALUATION STEP 3: PARSIMONY

The third step in theory evaluation focuses only on the content of the theory. The criterion is **Parsimony**. This criterion requires a theory to be stated in the most economical way possible without oversimplifying the phenomena of interest. This means that the fewer the concepts and propositions needed to fully explicate the phenomena of interest, the better.

The parsimony criterion is met when the most parsimonious statements clarify rather than obscure the phenomena of interest. The question to be asked when evaluating the parsimony of a theory is:

- Is the theory content stated clearly and concisely?

EVALUATION STEP 4: TESTABILITY

The fourth step in theory evaluation again focuses on the content of the theory. The criterion is **Testability.**

Testability frequently is regarded as the major characteristic of a scientifically useful theory. Indeed, Marx (1976) maintained, "If there is no way of testing a theory it is scientifically worthless, no matter how plausible, imaginative, or innovative it may be" (p. 249). Elaborating, Marx and Cronan-Hillix (1987) explained that if the hypotheses derived from a theory do not assert testable expectations about one or more concepts, empirical observations cannot affect the theory. And "if empirical observations cannot affect it, then the theory fails the most critical test of all: it is not testable, and in that sense it is not a scientific theory at all" (p. 307).

The ultimate goal of theory development in such professional disciplines as nursing is the empirical testing of interventions that are specified in the form of predictive middle-range theories. It is, however, still important to be able to test theories that have not yet reached the precision of interventions. In other words, it is important to be able to test grand theories, middle-range descriptive theories, and middle-range explanatory theories, as well as middle-range predictive theories.

Testability of Grand Theories

The relatively abstract and general nature of grand theories means that their concepts lack operational definitions stating how the concepts are measured, and their propositions are not amenable to direct empirical testing. Consequently, an approach that Silva and Sorrell (1992) called description of personal experiences may be used to evaluate the testability of grand theories. The description of personal experiences approach requires specification of an inductive, qualitative research methodology that is in keeping with the philosophical claims and content of the grand theory and that has the capacity to generate middle-range theories. The product of the descriptions of personal experiences approach is "generalities that constitute the substance of [middle-range] nursing theories" (Silva & Sorrell, 1992, p. 19). In essence, then, evaluation of the testability of a grand theory involves determining the middle-range theory-generating capacity of a grand theory. The criterion of testability is met when the grand theory has led to the generation of one or more middle-range theories.

Three questions, which were adapted from requirements proposed by Silva and Sorrell (1992), are asked when evaluating the testability of a grand theory:

- Is the research methodology qualitative and inductive?
- Is the research methodology congruent with the philosophical claims and content of the grand theory?
- Will the data obtained from use of the research methodology represent sufficiently in-depth descriptions of one or more personal experience(s) to capture the essence of the grand theory?

Testability of Middle-Range Theories

The relatively concrete and specific nature of middle-range theories means that their concepts can have operational definitions and their propositions are amenable to direct empirical testing. Consequently, an approach called traditional empiricism is used to evaluate the testability of middle-range theories. That approach requires the concepts of a middle-range theory to be observable and the propositions to be measurable. Concepts are empirically observable when operational definitions identify the empirical indicators that are used to measure the concepts. Propositions are measurable when empirical indicators can be substituted for concept names in each proposition and when statistical procedures can provide evidence regarding the assertions made. The criterion of testability for middle-range theories, then, is met when specific instruments or experimental protocols have been developed to observe the theory concepts and statistical techniques are available to measure the assertions made by the propositions. The evaluation of testability for a middle-range theory is, therefore, facilitated by a thorough review of the research methodology literature associated with the theory, including descriptions of questionnaires and other instruments designed to measure the concepts, research designs that will elicit the required data, and statistical or other data management techniques that will yield evidence about the theory.

Three questions, which were adapted from requirements identified by Silva (1986) and Fawcett (1999), are asked when evaluating the testability of a middle-range theory:

- Does the research methodology reflect the middle-range theory?
- Are the middle-range theory concepts observable through instruments that are appropriate empirical indicators of those concepts?
- Do the data analysis techniques permit measurement of the middle-range theory propositions?

EVALUATION STEP 5: EMPIRICAL ADEQUACY

The fifth step in theory evaluation deals with an assessment of the theory's **Empirical Adequacy**. The empirical adequacy criterion requires the assertions made by the theory to be congruent with empirical evidence. The extent to which a theory meets the criterion of empirical adequacy is determined by means of a systematic review of the findings of all studies that have been guided by the theory.

The logic of scientific inference dictates that if the empirical data conform to the theoretical assertions, it may be appropriate to tentatively accept the assertions as reasonable or adequate. Conversely, if the empirical data do not conform to the assertions, it is appropriate to conclude that the assertions are false.

Evaluation of the empirical adequacy of a theory should take into consideration the potential for circular reasoning. More specifically, if data always are interpreted in light of a particular theory, it may be difficult to "see" results that are not in keeping with that theory. Indeed, if researchers constantly uncover, describe, and interpret data through the lens of a particular theory, the outcome may be limited to expansion of that theory and that theory alone (Ray, 1990). Therefore, unless alternative theories are considered when interpreting data or the data are critically examined for both their fit and nonfit with the theory, circular reasoning will occur and the theory will be uncritically perpetuated. Circular reasoning can be avoided if the data are carefully examined to determine the extent of their congruence with the concepts and propositions of the theory, as well as from the perspective of alternative theories (Platt, 1964).

In other words, evaluation of a theory always should take alternative theories into account when interpreting data collected within the context of the theory in question. Testability of a grand theory requires interpretations of descriptions of personal experiences within the context of the grand theory of interest, as well as within the context of one or more alternative grand theories. Testability of a middle-range theory requires interpretations of the empirical data within the context of the middle-range theory of interest, as well as within the context of one or more alternative middle-range theories.

It is unlikely that any one test of a theory will provide the definitive evidence needed to establish its empirical adequacy. Thus decisions about empirical adequacy should take the findings of all related studies into account. Meta-analysis, metasynthesis, metasummary, and other formal procedures can be used to integrate the results of related studies. Readers are referred to other texts for comprehensive discussions of those procedures (Cooper, 1989; Fawcett, 1999; Rosenthal, 1991, Sandelowski & Barnum, 2003; Sandelowski, Docherty, & Emden, 1997). Suffice it to

say here that the more tests of a theory that yield supporting evidence, the more empirically adequate the theory.

It is important to point out that a theory should not be regarded as the truth or an ideology that cannot be modified. Indeed, no theory should be considered final or absolute, because it is always possible that subsequent studies will yield different findings or that other theories will provide a better fit with the data. Thus the aim of evaluation of empirical adequacy is to determine the degree of confidence warranted by the best empirical evidence, rather than to determine the absolute truth of the theory. The outcome of evaluation of empirical adequacy is a judgment regarding the need to modify, refine, or discard one or more concepts or propositions of the theory.

Determining the Empirical Adequacy of Grand Theories

The extent to which a grand theory meets the criterion of empirical adequacy is determined by a continuation of the description of personal experiences approach discussed earlier in the section on testability of grand theories. The data used to determine the empirical adequacy of a grand theory may come from multiple personal experiences of an individual or similar personal experiences of several individuals. The question to be asked when evaluating the empirical adequacy of a grand theory is:

- Are the findings from studies of descriptions of personal experiences congruent with the concepts and propositions of the grand theory?

Determining the Empirical Adequacy of Middle-Range Theories

The extent to which a middle-range theory meets the criterion of empirical adequacy is determined by a continuation of the traditional empirical approach discussed earlier in the section on testability of middle-range theories. The question is:

- Are theoretical assertions congruent with empirical evidence?

EVALUATION STEP 6: PRAGMATIC ADEQUACY

The sixth step in evaluation of a theory focuses on the theory's utility for practice. The criterion is **Pragmatic Adequacy**. The extent to which a grand theory or a middle-range theory meets this criterion is determined by reviewing all descriptions of the use of the theory in practice.

The pragmatic adequacy criterion requires that nurses have a full understanding of the content of the theory, as well as the interpersonal and psychomotor skills necessary to apply it (Magee, 1994). Although that may seem obvious, it is important to acknowledge the need for education and special skill training before theory application.

The pragmatic adequacy criterion also requires that the theory actually is used in the real world of nursing practice (Chinn & Kramer, 1995). In addition, the pragmatic adequacy criterion requires that the application of the theory-based nursing actions is generally feasible (Magee, 1994). Feasibility is determined by an evaluation of the availability of the human and material resources needed to establish the theory-based nursing actions as customary practice, including the time needed to learn and implement the protocols for nursing actions; the number, type, and expertise of personnel required for their implementation; and the cost of in-service education, salaries, equipment, and protocol-testing procedures. Moreover, the willingness of those who control financial resources to pay for the theory-based nursing actions, such as health-care system administrators and third-party payors, must be determined. In sum, the nurse must be in a setting that is conducive to application of the theory and have the time and training necessary to apply it.

Furthermore, the pragmatic adequacy criterion requires the practitioner to have the legal ability to control the application and to measure the effectiveness of the theory-based nursing actions. Despite legal ability, such control may be problematic in that practitioners are not always able to carry out legally sanctioned responsibilities because of resistance from others. Sources of resistance against implementation of theory-based nursing actions include attempts by physicians and health-care system administrators to control nursing practice, financial barriers imposed by health-care institutions and third-party payors, and skepticism by other health professionals about the ability of nurses to carry out the proposed actions (Funk, Tornquist, & Champagne, 1995). The cooperation and collaboration of others may, therefore, have to be secured.

Moreover, the pragmatic adequacy criterion requires that theory-based nursing actions be compatible with expectations for practice (Magee, 1994). Compatibility should be evaluated in relation to expectations held by the public and the health-care system. If the actions do not meet existing expectations, they should be abandoned or people should be helped to develop new expectations. Johnson (1974) commented, "Current [nursing] practice is not entirely what it might become and [thus people] might come to expect a different form of practice, given the opportunity to experience it" (p. 376).

Finally, the pragmatic adequacy criterion requires the theory-based nursing actions to be socially meaningful by leading to favorable outcomes for those who participate in the actions. Examples of favorable outcomes include a re-duction in complications, improvement in health conditions, and increased satisfaction with the theory-based actions on the part of all who participate.

The questions to be asked when evaluating pragmatic adequacy are:

- Are education and special skill training required before application of the theory in nursing practice?
- Has the theory been applied in the real world of nursing practice?
- Is it generally feasible to implement practice derived from the theory?
- Does the practitioner have the legal ability to implement and measure the effectiveness of theory-based nursing actions?
- Are the theory-based nursing actions compatible with expectations for nursing practice?
- Do the theory-based nursing actions lead to favorable outcomes?

The outcomes of theory-based nursing actions are further judged by use of what Silva and Sorrell (1992) called the problem-solving approach. That approach emphasizes the problem-solving effectiveness of a theory and seeks to determine "whether what is purported or experienced accomplishes its purpose" (Silva & Sorrell, 1992, p. 19).

The problem-solving approach is based on the position that theories are developed "to solve human and technical problems and to improve practice" (Kerlinger, 1979, p. 280). It requires deliberative application of a theory. Chinn and Kramer (1995) explained that the application "involves using research methods to demonstrate how a theory affects nursing practice and places the theory within the context of practice to ensure that it serves the goals of the profession, … [and] provides evidence of the theory's usefulness in ensuring quality of care" (p. 164).

The problem-solving approach can be used with all types of theories but is most effective when applied to middle-range predictive theories. In that case, the application seeks to determine the effects of interventions specified in middle-range predictive theories on the health conditions of the human beings who participate in the interventions (Hegyvary, 1992).

Two questions, which were adapted from requirements identified by Silva and Sorrell (1992), are asked when evaluating the problem-solving effectiveness of nursing theories:

- Is the application of theory-based nursing actions designed so that comparisons can be made between outcomes of use of the theory and outcomes in the same situation when the theory was not used?
- Are outcomes measured in terms of the problem-solving effectiveness of the theory?

CONCLUSION

This chapter presents a framework for analysis and evaluation of grand and middle-range nursing theories. The framework, which is summarized in Table 11–1, will be applied in the next five chapters. Each of those chapters will present a comprehensive examination of a nursing theory.

The framework for analysis and evaluation of nursing theories presented in this chapter is *not* appropriate for examination of conceptual models of nursing. The framework for analysis and evaluation of nursing models is presented in Chapter 3.

TABLE 11–1
A FRAMEWORK FOR ANALYSIS AND EVALUATION OF NURSING THEORIES

QUESTIONS FOR ANALYSIS

Step 1: Theory Scope

- What is the scope of theory?

Step 2: Theory Context

- Which metaparadigm concepts are addressed by the theory?
  - Does the theory deal with human beings?
  - Does the theory deal with the environment?
  - Does the theory deal with health?
  - Does the theory deal with nursing processes or goals?
- Which metaparadigm propositions are addressed by the theory?
  - Does the theory deal with human processes of living and dying?
  - Does the theory deal with patterning of human health experiences within the context of the environment?
  - Does the theory deal with nursing actions or processes that are beneficial to human beings?
  - Does the theory deal with the human processes of living and dying, recognizing that human beings are in a continuous relationship with their environments?
- On what philosophical claims is the theory based?
- What world view is reflected in the theory?
- From what conceptual model was the theory derived?
- What antecedent knowledge from nursing and adjunctive disciplines was used in the development of the theory?

Step 3: Theory Content

- What are the concepts of the theory?
- What are the propositions of the theory?
  - Which propositions are nonrelational?
  - Which propositions are relational?

QUESTIONS FOR EVALUATION

Step 1: Significance

- Are the metaparadigm concepts and propositions addressed by the theory explicit?
- Are the philosophical claims on which the theory is based explicit?
- Is the conceptual model from which the theory was derived explicit?
- Are the authors of antecedent knowledge from nursing and adjunctive disciplines acknowledged and are bibliographical citations given?

Step 2: Internal Consistency

- Are the context (philosophical claims and conceptual model) and the content (concepts and propositions) of the theory congruent?
- Do the concepts reflect semantic clarity and semantic consistency?
- Do the propositions reflect structural consistency?

(continued)

> ▶️≪ **TABLE 11–1**
> **A FRAMEWORK FOR ANALYSIS AND EVALUATION OF NURSING THEORIES** *(continued)*

Step 3: Parsimony

- Is the theory content stated clearly and concisely?

Step 4: Testability

Grand Theories

- Is the research methodology qualitative and inductive?
- Is the research methodology congruent with the philosophical claims and content of the grand theory?
- Will the data obtained from use of the research methodology represent sufficiently in-depth descriptions of one or more personal experiences to capture the essence of the grand theory?

Middle-Range Theories

- Does the research methodology reflect the middle-range theory?
- Are the middle-range theory concepts observable through instruments that are appropriate empirical indicators of those concepts?
- Do the data analysis techniques permit measurement of the middle-range theory propositions?

Step 5: Empirical Adequacy

Grand Theories

- Are the findings from studies of descriptions of personal experiences congruent with the concepts and propositions of the grand theory?

Middle-Range Theories

- Are theoretical assertions congruent with empirical evidence?

Step 6: Pragmatic Adequacy

- Are education and special skill training required before application of the theory in practice?
- Has the theory been applied in the real world of nursing practice?
- Is it generally feasible to implement practice protocols derived from the theory?
- Does the practitioner have the legal ability to implement and measure the effectiveness of theory-based nursing actions?
- Are the theory-based nursing actions compatible with expectations for nursing practice?
- Do the theory-based nursing actions lead to favorable outcomes?
- Is the application of theory-based nursing actions designed so that comparisons can be made between outcomes of use of the theory and outcomes in the same situation when the theory was not used?
- Are outcomes measured in terms of the problem-solving effectiveness of the theory?

 REFERENCES

Barnum, B.J.S. (1998). Nursing theory: Analysis, application, evaluation (5th ed.). Philadelphia: Lippincott.

Chinn, P.L., & Kramer, M.K. (1995). Theory and nursing. A systematic approach (4th ed.). St. Louis: Mosby.

Cooper, H.M. (1989). Integrating research: A guide for literature reviews (2nd ed.). Newbury Park, CA: Sage.

Fawcett, J. (1993). Analysis and evaluation of nursing theories. Philadelphia: F.A. Davis.

Fawcett, J. (1999). The relationship of theory and research (3rd ed). Philadelphia: F.A. Davis.

Fawcett, J. (2000). Analysis and evaluation of contemporary nursing knowledge: Nursing models and theories. Philadelphia: F.A. Davis.

Funk, S.G., Tornquist, E.M., & Champagne, M.T. (1995). Barriers and facilitators of research utilization. Nursing Clinics of North America, 30, 395–407.

Hegyvary, S.T. (1992). From truth to relativism: Paradigms for doctoral education. In Proceedings of the 1992 Forum on Doctoral Education in Nursing (pp. 1–15). Baltimore: University of Maryland School of Nursing.

Johnson, D.E. (1974). Development of theory: A requisite for nursing as a primary health profession. Nursing Research, 23, 372–377.

Kerlinger, F.N. (1979). Behavioral research: A conceptual approach. New York: Holt, Rinehart & Winston.

Levine, M.E. (1988). Antecedents from adjunctive disciplines: Creation of nursing theory. Nursing Science Quarterly, 1, 16–21.

Levine, M.E. (1995). The rhetoric of nursing theory. Image: Journal of Nursing Scholarship, 27, 11–14.

Magee, M. (1994). Eclecticism in nursing philosophy: Problem or solution? In J.F. Kikuchi & H. Simmons (Eds.), Developing a philosophy of nursing (pp. 61–66). Thousand Oaks, CA: Sage.

Marx, M.H. (1976). Formal theory. In M.H. Marx & F.E. Goodson (Eds.), Theories in contemporary psychology (2nd ed., pp. 234–260). New York: Macmillan.

Marx, M.H., & Cronan-Hillix, W.A. (1987). Systems and theories in psychology (4th ed.). New York: McGraw-Hill.

Meleis, A.I. (1997). Theoretical nursing: Development and progress (3rd ed.). Philadelphia: Lippincott.

Parse, R.R. (2002). Words, words, words: Meanings, meanings, meanings! Nursing Science Quarterly, 15, 183.

Platt, J.R. (1964). Strong inference. Science, 146, 347–353.

Ray, M.A. (1990). Critical reflective analysis of Parse's and Newman's research methodologies. Nursing Science Quarterly, 3, 44–46.

Rosenthal, R. (1991). Meta-analytic procedures for social research (rev. ed.). Newbury Park, CA: Sage.

Sandelowski, M., & Barroso, J. (2003). Creating metasummaries of qualitative findings. Nursing Research, 52, 226–233.

Sandelowski, M., Docherty, S., & Emden, C. (1997). Qualitative metasynthesis: Issues and techniques. Research in Nursing and Health, 20, 365–371.

Silva, M.C. (1986). Research testing nursing theory: State of the art. Advances in Nursing Science, 9(1), 1–11.

Silva, M.C., & Sorrell, J.M. (1992). Testing of nursing theory: Critique and philosophical expansion. Advances in Nursing Science, 14(4), 12–23.

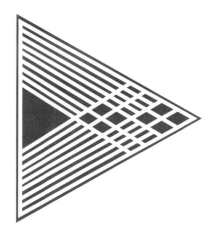

Chapter **12**

Newman's Theory of Health as Expanding Consciousness

Margaret Newman's ideas about health and the development of her Theory of Health as Expanding Consciousness were greatly influenced by her mother's struggle with amyotrophic lateral sclerosis and her experiences as an undergraduate and graduate nursing student (Newman, 1986, 1994a), as well as her concern "for those for whom health as the absence of disease is not a reality" (Newman, 1992, p. 650). Newman (1997a) explained, "My life experience prior to entering the profession of nursing, particularly as it related to the care of my mother, laid the foundation for this nursing theory" (p. 22).

Newman began to formalize her ideas in preparation for a paper delivered at the Nurse Educator Conference held in New York City in 1978, and she published the first version of the theory in her 1979 book, *Theory Development in Nursing*. The theory continued to evolve and became known as the Theory of Health as Expanding Consciousness with the publication of Newman's 1986 book, *Health as Expanding Consciousness*. Newman's continuing refinement of the theory and development of her ideas about a research/practice methodology culminated in the publication of the second edition of *Health as Expanding Consciousness* in 1994 (Newman, 1994a) and subsequent journal articles (Newman, 1994b, 1997a, 1997b).

Newman (1997b) noted that the Theory of Expanding Consciousness evolved in six stages as she thought about the theory and worked with nursing colleagues and students:

1. Identifying the underlying assumptions, key concepts, and axiomatic relations among movement, space, time, and consciousness as relevant to patterning of health
2. Seeing these concepts emerge from the implicit grasp of the total pattern of the person
3. Moving from identifying the pattern of person-environment at a point in time, as was done in the early days of nursing diagnosis, to seeing the pattern as sequential configurations evolving over time, like waves of explicit-implicit phenomena, unfolding-enfolding
4. Seeing the insights that occurred in the process as choice points of action potential

5. Realizing that both the client and the nurse mutually participate in a process of expanding consciousness
6. Experiencing the pattern unfolding

Newman (1994a) acknowledged that only as her ideas evolved did she realize "that the theory of health as expanding consciousness is a radical departure from traditional concepts of health … [that she] was calling for a revolution … [and that] the essence of the theory required an 180-degree turn [in thinking about health]" (p. xv). In reviewing what she had learned as a student and how she came to the understandings that have been formalized in the Theory of Health as Expanding Consciousness, Newman (1994a) commented:

> Basic among these learnings [from her undergraduate and graduate education] was that illness reflected the life pattern of the person and that what was needed was the recognition of that pattern and acceptance of it for what it meant to that person. Years later, I came to the conclusion that *health is the expansion of consciousness*. It frightens me to think I might have missed that revelation, it is so important to me now. But even my fear is unwarranted because the gist of all that I am saying is that one can trust the evolving pattern, that it is a pattern of evolving, expanding consciousness *regardless* of what form or direction it may take. This realization is such that illness and disease have lost their demoralizing power. (p. xxiii)

Overview

Newman's work is a grand theory that focuses on health as the expansion of consciousness. The concepts of the Theory of Health as Expanding Consciousness and dimensions are listed here, along with the components of Newman's research/practice methodology. Each concept and dimension and the methodology components are defined and described later in this chapter.

Key Terms

PATTERN
  Movement-Space-Time
  Rhythm
  Diversity

CONSCIOUSNESS
RESEARCH/PRACTICE METHODOLOGY
  Phenomenon of Interest
  The Interview
  Transcription
  Development of Narrative
    Pattern Recognition
  Diagram
    Pattern Recognition
  Follow-Up
    Pattern Recognition
  Application of the Theory of Health as
    Expanding Consciousness

ANALYSIS OF THE THEORY OF HEALTH AS EXPANDING CONSCIOUSNESS

This section presents an analysis of Newman's theory. The analysis is based on Newman's publications about her theory, drawing heavily from the first and second editions of her book, *Health as Expanding Consciousness* (Newman, 1986, 1994a), as well as from the journal articles "Newman's Theory of Health as Praxis" (Newman, 1990a) "Evolution of the Theory of Health as Expanding Consciousness" (Newman, 1997a), and "Experiencing the Whole" (Newman, 1997b) and a book chapter titled "Shifting to a Higher Consciousness" (Newman, 1990b).

SCOPE OF THE THEORY

The central thesis of the Theory of Health as Expanding Consciousness is that health is the expansion of consciousness. The meaning of life and health are, according to Newman (1986), found in the evolving process of expanding consciousness. More specifically, the theory "asserts that *every* person in *every* situation, no matter how disordered and hopeless it may seem, is part of the universal process of expanding consciousness" (Newman, 1992, p. 650). Newman's description of health, her definitions for the concepts of the theory, and the theory propositions all are at a relatively abstract level, which resulted in classification of Newman's work as a grand theory.

CONTEXT OF THE THEORY

Metaparadigm Concepts and Propositions

Newman alluded to the metaparadigm of nursing when she stated that "what we are concerned with is the health of persons in interaction with the environment" (Newman, 1986, p. 33). That statement indicates that the Theory of Health as Expanding Consciousness focuses on the metaparadigm concepts of *human beings, environment,* and *health.* The most relevant metaparadigm proposition is *the patterning of human health experiences within the context of the environment.*

Philosophical Claims

The analysis of Newman's published works resulted in identification of several statements that could be considered philosophical claims undergirding the Theory of Health as Expanding Consciousness. In addition, Newman has identified several assumptions that may be considered philosophical claims. The statements and assumptions address the universe; humans and the universe; consciousness; consciousness and the universe; pattern; pattern and the universe; pattern and consciousness; health, disease, and illness; the universe and disease; consciousness and disease; and pattern and disease. Those statements and assumptions are listed here.

Philosophical Claim About the Universe

- A universe of undivided wholeness (Newman, 1986, p. 68).

Philosophical Claim About Humans and the Universe

- The human being [is] unitary and continuous with the undivided wholeness of the universe (Newman, 1994a, p. 83).

Philosophical Claims About Consciousness

- Persons as individuals, and human beings as a species, are identified by their patterns of consciousness. The person does not *possess* consciousness—the person *is* consciousness (Newman, 1994a, p. 33).
- The process of life is toward higher levels of consciousness (Newman, 1994a, p. 23).
- Life is proceeding in the direction of higher consciousness (Newman, 1995, p. 168).
- The highest form of knowing is loving (Newman, 1986, p. 68).

Philosophical Claim About Consciousness and the Universe

- Consciousness is coextensive in the universe and is the essence of all matter (Newman, 1994a, p. 33).

Philosophical Claims About Pattern

- Pattern [identifies] the unique, evolving wholeness of the person (Newman & Moch, 1995, p. 153).
- Health [is the] pattern of the whole (Newman, 1994a, p. 10).
- An adequate understanding of patterns cannot be reduced to an understanding of the properties of the parts (Newman, 1994a, p. 73).
- Behavior [is] an indication of pattern (Newman, 1994a, p. 52).
- The task is not to try to change another person's pattern but to recognize it as information that depicts the whole and relate to it as it unfolds (Newman, 1994a, p. 13).

Philosophical Claim About Pattern and the Universe

- The whole of a person, or of a universe, is a pattern in which the parts cannot stand alone as separate (Newman, 1994a, p. 73).

Philosophical Claim About Pattern and Consciousness

- There is no basis for rejecting any experience as irrelevant. The important factor is to get in touch with one's own pattern of interaction and recognize that whatever it is, the process is in progress and the experience is one of expanding consciousness (Newman 1986, p. 67).

Philosophical Claims About Health, Disease, and Illness

- Health … is not a utopian state to be achieved, but the totality of the life process to be experienced (Newman, 1983, p. 168).
- Health and illness [are viewed] as a single process and, like rhythmic phenomena, becoming manifest in ups and downs, or peaks and troughs, moving through varying degrees of organization and disorganization, but all as one unitary process (Newman, 1986, p. 4).
- Ill or illness refers to a subjective sense of diminished health (Newman, 1983, p. 163).
- Health encompasses disease as a meaningful aspect of health, as a manifestation of the underlying pattern of person-environment interaction (Newman, 1990b, p. 133)
- Health encompasses conditions known as disease (Newman, 1997a, p. 22).

- Disease is a manifestation of health (Newman, 1994a, p. 5).
- Disease can be considered a manifestation of the underlying pattern of the person (Newman, 1997a, p. 22).
- Sometimes [the process of life] is smooth, pleasant, harmonious; other times it is difficult, disharmonious, as in disease (Newman, 1994a, p. 23).

Philosophical Claim About the Universe and Disease

- The physical manifestations of disease may be considered evidence of how one is interacting with the environment (Newman, 1986, p. 43).

Philosophic Claim About Consciousness and Disease

- It is possible to move to higher levels of consciousness without the necessity of disease (Newman, 1994a, p. 29).

Philosophical Claims About Pattern and Disease

- Disease conditions can be considered a manifestation of the unitary pattern of the person (Newman, 1983, p. 163).
- Disease, when present, is a manifestation of the evolving pattern of the whole and can provide insight into the human needs of the person (Newman, 1995, p. 159).
- The pattern of the person that eventually manifests itself as disease is part of a larger ongoing pattern (Newman, 1983, p. 164).
- The pattern of the person that manifests itself as disease is primary and exists prior to structural or functional changes (Newman, 1997a, p. 22).
- If developing a disease is the only way an individual['s pattern] can manifest itself, then that is health for that person (Newman, 1983, p. 164).
- Elimination of the disease condition in itself will not change the pattern of the person (Newman, 1983, p. 164).
- We are not separate people with separate diseases. ... The pattern manifested by a disease does not stop with one person but is part of the greater whole (Newman, 1994a, p. 25).

In addition, Newman offered several statements that represent the philosophical claims undergirding her research/practice methodology. These statements are listed here.

- [Research] involves *a priori* theory (Newman, 1994a, p. 93).
- The necessity of *a priori* theory renders a strictly interpretive, phenomenological approach inadequate (Newman, 1994a, p. 93).

- There is an interpenetration between the researcher's embodied theory and the researcher's understanding (Newman, 1994a, p. 93).
- Unbroken wholeness is what is real—not the fragments we devise with our way of describing things. And the wholeness is in the continual movement (Newman, 1997b, p. 37).
- The nature of wholeness is such that it cannot be addressed by the scientific method as currently conceived. It cannot be observed, named, or manipulated. The whole cannot be found in summation or integration of the parts. But the parts are manifestations of the whole. The whole is always present everywhere and ... is experienced by going to the parts (Newman, 1997b, pp. 37–38).
- [There is] uniqueness and wholeness of pattern in each client situation (Newman, 1997b, p. 35).
- Research in a paradigm characterized by pattern and process is participatory research (Newman, 1997b, p. 38).
- We come to the meaning of the whole not by viewing the pattern from the outside but by entering into the evolving pattern as it unfolds (Newman, 1997b, p. 38).
- [There is a] mutuality of interaction between nurse and client (Newman, 1997b, p. 35).
- If the way we know this reality is by experiencing it, then to study it we must engage in the process of practice (Newman, 1997b, p. 38).
- The researcher participates in the research to help the participants understand the meaning of their situations, with its potential for action (Newman, 1997b, p. 38).
- The knowledge of nursing is an immanent, transforming process of unfolding pattern (Newman, 1997b, p. 39).

Sarter (1988) maintained that Newman's theory is based on philosophical claims rooted in "relativity and quantum theory, mysticism, and early Greek and Eastern philosophy" (p. 55). But Yamashita and Tall (1998) countered that "Newman came to her insights not from Eastern thought but from modern physics as well as the work of Martha Rogers" (p. 66).

Newman's philosophical claims are consistent with holism (Sarter, 1988) and the unitary-transformative paradigm (Newman, 1994a). Indeed, Newman (1990a) maintained that her view of health "requires a nonfragmentary world view" (p. 39). More specifically, she noted that her theory of health reflects a "patterned, unpredictable, unitary, intuitive, and innovative" view of the world (Newman, personal communication, November 30, 1992). Clearly, then, the philosophical claims undergirding the Theory of Health as Expanding Consciousness reflect the *simultaneous action* world view.

Conceptual Model

The conceptual roots for the Theory of Health as Expanding Consciousness are, according to Newman (1990a), "a paradigm of evolving pattern of the whole" (p. 40). That paradigm, as Newman (1986, 1990a, 1990b, 1994a, 1997a) repeatedly pointed out, is Rogers' (1970) Life Process Model, which now is known as the Science of Unitary Human Beings (Rogers, 1990). Newman (1990a) explained that "Rogers' assumptions regarding the patterning of persons in interaction with the environment are basic to my view that consciousness is a manifestation of an evolving pattern of person-environment interaction. ... Rogers' insistence that health and illness are simply manifestations of the rhythmic fluctuations of the life process led me to view health and illness as a unitary process moving through variations in order-disorder" (p. 38).

Newman (1990b) identified two propositions about pattern from Rogers' conceptual model that are basic to the Theory of Health as Expanding Consciousness: (1) pattern identifies the wholeness of the person, and (2) pattern evolves unidirectionally. She then explained:

> If you can accept these two [propositions], then you can begin to think of disease as a manifestation of expanding consciousness. If you accept that pattern is a manifestation of the person, and that the process of life moves in the direction of increasing complexity, diversity, and higher consciousness, then when something appears or becomes manifest, it follows that it is a manifestation of the evolving pattern; it is not something separate to be gotten rid of or squelched, but something to be regarded as a clue to the underlying pattern. (p. 132)

In keeping with Rogers (1970, 1990), Newman regards the human being as unitary and as continuous with a unitary environment, which extends to the universe. Her view of the human-universe connection led Newman (1994a) to reject the view that nursing science is human science. She explained that this designation "admittedly emphasizes the human being as whole rather than a sum or integration of parts, but may serve to separate the human being from the flow within the larger dynamic context. It is important to see the human being as unitary and as continuous with the undivided wholeness of the universe" (p. 83). Nursing, for Newman (1994a), is caring. "Going through the motions of job responsibilities without caring is not nursing" (p. 141). The goal of nursing for Newman (1979) "is not to make people well, or to prevent their getting sick, but to assist people to utilize the power that is within them as they evolve toward higher levels of consciousness" (p. 67).

Newman (1994a) distinguished between nursing and medicine when she maintained that diagnosis and treatment of disease are the purview of medical science and practice, whereas recognition of the pattern of the whole is the responsibility of nursing science and practice. More specifically, the focus of the nursing discipline is "the unitary field that combines person-family-community all at once ... the pattern of the whole, health as pattern of the evolving whole, with caring as a moral imperative" (p. xix).

Antecedent Knowledge

Newman (1994a) noted that her ideas about nursing and the content of her theory were "stimulated by Martha Rogers' [1970] insistence on the unitary nature of a human being in interaction with the environment" (p. xxiv). Furthermore, Newman (1986) has acknowledged the contributions of several scholars from various adjunctive disciplines to the development and refinement of her ideas about health. She noted that de Chardin's (1959) belief "that a person's consciousness continues to develop beyond the physical life and becomes a part of a universal consciousness ... made sense to me" (p. 5). In addition, she cited Bohm's (1980) theory of the implicate order as a significant contribution to her notions about pattern manifestation and "the interconnectedness and omnipresence of all that there is" (p. 5). Newman (1987) also acknowledged Bateson's (1979) contributions to her understanding of pattern.

Moreover, Newman (1986) stated that Young's (1976a, 1976b) theory of human evolution "was the impetus for my efforts to integrate the basic concepts of my theory ... into a dynamic portrayal of life and health" (p. 6). She also noted that Moss' (1981) idea of "love as the highest level of consciousness provided affirmation and elaboration of my intuition regarding the nature of health" (p. 6). Furthermore, Newman commented that Bentov's (1978) work "provided logical explanations for many things I had taken on faith" (p. 5). Newman also commented that Prigogine's (1980) theory of change contributed to her understanding of the evolution of consciousness. In addition, Newman (1994a) cited Guba and Lincoln (1989), Moustakas (1990), Polkinghorne (1988), Lather (1986), and especially Heron (1981) as contributing to her thinking about ways to study health as expanding consciousness.

In an effort to clarify the place of antecedent knowledge in the development of her theory, Newman (1997a) commented that theories from adjunctive disciplines "provided substantiation and elaboration of the theory of health as expanding consciousness. *The theory is enriched by [those theories] but was not based on them.* The theory, like Rogers' [conceptual system], emerged from a new science of unitary human beings" (p. 23).

CONTENT OF THE THEORY

Concepts

An analysis of the first and second editions of Newman's books (Newman, 1986, 1994a) and other publications revealed that the concepts of the Theory of Health as Expanding Consciousness are **PATTERN** and **CONSCIOUSNESS**. The concept of **PATTERN** is multidimensional; the three dimensions are **Movement-Space-Time, Rhythm**, and **Diversity**. The concept of **CONSCIOUSNESS** is unidimensional.

Nonrelational Propositions

The definitions for the concepts of the Theory of Health as Expanding Consciousness are given here. Those constitutive definitions are the nonrelational propositions of the theory.

PATTERN

- A fundamental attribute of all there is and reveals unity in diversity (Newman, 1994a, p. 71).
- Information that depicts the whole, understanding of the meaning of all the relationships at once (Newman, 1994a, p. 71).
- A pattern possesses meaning. As meaning is discovered, the pattern becomes apparent (and vice versa) (Newman, 2002, p. 4).
- Pattern is relatedness and is self-organizing over time, i.e., it becomes more highly organized with more information (Newman, 1994a, p. 72).
- [Throughout life it is] a pattern that identifies us as a particular person (Newman, 1994a, p. 71).
- Pattern [is] an identification of the wholeness of the person (Newman, 1990b, p. 132).
- Pattern encompasses genetic pattern, voice pattern, movement pattern, and other types of patterns that are manifestations of the underlying pattern (Newman, 1994a).
- Exchanging, a manifestation of pattern, is defined as "interchanging matter and energy between person and environment and transforming energy from one form to another" (Newman, 1986, p. 74).
- Communicating, a manifestation of pattern, is defined as "interchanging information from one system to another" (Newman, 1986, p. 74).
- Relating, a manifestation of pattern, is defined as "connecting with other persons and the environment" (Newman, 1986, p. 74).
- Valuing, a manifestation of pattern, is defined as "assigning worth" (Newman, 1986, p. 74).

- Choosing, a manifestation of pattern, is defined as "selecting of one or more alternatives" (Newman, 1986, p. 74).
- Moving, a manifestation of pattern, is defined as "rhythmic alternating between activity and rest" (Newman, 1986, p. 74).
- Perceiving, a manifestation of pattern, is defined as "receiving and interpreting information" (Newman, 1986, p. 74).
- Feeling, a manifestation of pattern, is defined as "sensing physical and intuitive awareness" (Newman, 1986, p. 74).
- Knowing, a manifestation of pattern, is defined as "personal recognizing of self and world" (Newman, 1986, p. 74).

Newman drew from Rogers (1970) for her ideas about **Pattern**. Accordingly, she regards the **Pattern** of each person's life as that which gives identity, rather than the substance that makes up the pattern. But Newman (1987) has gone beyond Rogers in her assertion that pattern is "the essence of a holistic view of health" (p. 36). Also in keeping with Rogers, Newman regards **Pattern** as unitary but as manifested in various ways. Drawing from the work of the North American Nursing Diagnosis Association nurse theorist group (Roy et al., 1982), Newman (1986) defined the nine specific manifestations of unitary pattern listed above—exchanging, communicating, relating, valuing, choosing, moving, perceiving, feeling, and knowing.

The concept of **Pattern** encompasses three dimensions—Movement-Space-Time, Rhythm, and Diversity.

Newman (1994a) now refers to what she formerly (1979, 1986) treated as three separate concepts as the **Movement-Space-Time** dimension of the concept of **Pattern**. She explained, "The relevant task … is to see the concepts of movement-space-time in relation to each other, all at once, as patterns of evolving consciousness" (p. 52).

- **Movement-Space-Time:** Movement-space-time can be seen as dimensions [of] unitary evolving patterns (Newman, 1997a, p. 25). Movement is central to understanding the nature of reality (Newman, 1990a, p. 39). Movement is a characteristic of pattern (Newman, 1994a). Movement is the natural condition of life. When movement ceases, it is an indication that life has gone out of the organism (Newman, 1994a, pp. 56–57). [Movement is] an essential property of matter [and] a means of communicating (Newman, 1979, pp. 61, 62). [Movement is] the means whereby one perceives reality and, therefore, [the] means of becoming aware of self (Newman, 1983, p. 165). The pattern of movement reflects the overall organization of the thought and feeling processes of a person (Newman, 1994a, p. 57). It is through movement that the organism interacts with its environment and exercises control over its interactions (Newman, 1994a, p. 57). Movement is a means whereby space and time become a reality (Newman, 1979, p. 60). Through movement one discovers the world of time-space and establishes personal territory (Newman, 1990a, p. 39). Time is a function of movement (Newman, 1979, p. 60). The world contains time aspects and space aspects (Newman, 1979). Time and space have a complementary relationship (Newman, 1979, p. 60). Space is inextricably linked to ... time (Newman, 1979, p. 61). Matters of space-time are very much involved in one's struggles for self-determination and status (Newman, 1990a, p. 39). Subjective time is the amount of time perceived to be passing, and objective time is clock time (Newman, 1983). Subjective time, objective time, and use of time, and personal space, inner space, and life space, are all relevant for the individual. In contrast, private time, coordinated time, and shared time, and territoriality, shared space, and distancing, are relevant to the family (Newman, 1983).

- **Rhythm:** Rhythm is a characteristic of pattern (Newman, 1994a). Rhythm is basic to movement ... [and] the rhythm of movement is an integrating experience (Newman, 1994a, pp. 58–59). Rhythm as a powerful factor in interpersonal relations and an important aspect of communication between individuals (Newman, 1994a). When one cannot establish a mutually satisfying rhythm of relating, it is difficult if not impossible to communicate (Newman, 1994a, p. 58). The rhythm of talking—vocalizations and pauses, words and silence—influence interpersonal relations (Newman, 1994a).
- **Diversity:** Diversity is a characteristic of pattern (Newman, 1994a). Diversity is seen in the parts (Newman, 1994a).

The integral nature of all three dimensions of the concept of **Pattern—Movement-Space-Time, Rhythm,** and **Diversity**—is evident in the following statement: "The pattern is in constant movement or change; the parts are diverse and are changing in relation to each other; and movement is rhythmic" (Newman, 1994a, p. 72).

CONSCIOUSNESS

- The informational capacity of the ... human being, that is, the ability of the [person] to interact with the environment' (Newman, 1990a, p. 38).
- The information of the [human] system: the capacity of the [human] system to interact with the environment (Newman, 1994a, p. 33).
- The informational capacity of the human system encompasses interconnected cognitive (thinking) and affective (feeling) awareness, physiochemical maintenance

including the nervous and endocrine systems, growth processes, the immune system, and the genetic code (Newman, 1986, 1990a, 1994a).

Newman (1986, 1994a) maintained that the concept of **Consciousness** can be seen in the quantity and quality of the interaction between the information of the human system and the information of the environmental system. Moreover, Newman regards **Consciousness** as a process that continually expands rather than a static entity. Newman (1992) described the process of expanding consciousness as "a process of becoming more of oneself, of finding greater meaning in life, and of reaching new heights of connectedness with other people and the world in which one lives" (p. 650). She proposed that consciousness expands in a series of stages that are parallel to Young's (1976a, 1976b) stages of human evolution (Table 12–1).

Newman (1986, 1994a) explained that Young proposed that human beings evolve from a loss of potential freedom to real freedom through a process of interactions with each other and the social state. Freedom is lost as the person binds in with the larger network. Subsequently, identity, self-consciousness, and self-determination emerge through centering. When things that worked in the past no longer work, choice operates and the person evolves by decentering and unbinding, finally achieving real freedom. The stages of unbinding and real freedom are not physical but may manifest in such superhuman powers as healings and appearances in different forms.

Newman (1994a) described the evolution or progression of expanding consciousness that is parallel to Young's stages of human evolution as follows:

> Human beings come from a state of potential consciousness into the world of determinate matter and have the capacity for understanding that enables them to gain insight regarding their patterns. This insight represents a turning point in evolving consciousness with concomitant gains in freedom of action. (p. 43)

Newman (1994a) equated the process of expanding consciousness with the process of health: "The process of the evolution of consciousness is the process of health" (p. 43). She also equated absolute consciousness, the last stage of the process, with love. She explained:

> In [the last stage] all opposites are reconciled. This kind of love embraces all experience equally and unconditionally: pain as well as pleasure, failure as well as success, ugliness as well as beauty, disease as well as non-disease. (p. 48)

Relational Propositions

The relational propositions of the Theory of Health as Expanding Consciousness are listed here. Relational propositions A and B link the concepts of **Conscious-**

Stage	Young: Evolution of Human Beings	Newman: Expanding Consciousness
1	Potential freedom	Potential consciousness
2	Binding	Time
3	Centering	Space
4	Choice	Movement
5	Decentering	Infinite space or boundarylessness
6	Unbinding	Timelessness
7	Real freedom	Absolute consciousness

Adapted from Newman, M.A. (1990). Newman's theory of health as praxis. Nursing Science Quarterly, 3, 37–41, p. 39, with permission.

ness and **Pattern.** Relational propositions C, D, E, F, G, H, and I all provide linkages between the concept of **Consciousness** and the **Movement-Space-Time** dimension of the concept of **Pattern.** In addition, relational proposition I explains the integration of Young's (1976a, 1976b) theory of human evolution and Newman's theory. The concept of **Consciousness** is linked with the **Movement-Space-Time** and **Rhythm** dimensions of the concept of **Pattern** in relational proposition J.

A. Consciousness is a manifestation of an evolving pattern of person-environment interaction (Newman, 1990a, p. 38).
B. The evolving pattern of person-environment can be viewed as a process of expanding consciousness (Newman, 1994a, p. 33).
C. Movement is a pivotal choice point in the evolution of human consciousness (Newman, 1994a, p. 56).
D. When we reach the choice point when movement (both physical and social) is no longer an option, we learn to transcend the limitations of time-space-movement to higher levels of consciousness (Newman, 1994a, p. 57).
E. Movement is a reflection of consciousness (Newman, 1979, p. 60).
F. The consciousness that characterizes any form of life is expressed in its movement (Newman, 1994a, p. 57).
G. Time is a measure of consciousness (Newman, 1979, p. 60).
H. Manifestations of space-time-movement [are] indicators of consciousness (Newman, 1994a, p. 63).
I. A person comes into being from the ground of consciousness and loses freedom as one is bound in time

and finds one's identity in space. ... Through movement one discovers the world of time-space and establishes personal territory. It is also when movement is restricted that one becomes aware of personal limitations and the fact that the old rules don't work anymore. When one no longer has the power of movement (either physical or social), it is necessary to go beyond oneself. As one is able to recognize the boundarylessness and timelessness of human existence, one gains the freedom of returning to the ground of consciousness (Newman, 1990a, pp. 39–40).
J. The rhythm of living phenomena is a vivid portrayal of the embeddedness of matter (consciousness) in space-time (Newman, 1994a, p. 53).

EVALUATION OF THE THEORY OF HEALTH AS EXPANDING CONSCIOUSNESS

This section presents an evaluation of Newman's Theory of Health as Expanding Consciousness. The evaluation is based on the results of the analysis of the theory, as well as on publications by others who have used or commented on this nursing theory.

SIGNIFICANCE

The Theory of Health as Expanding Consciousness meets the criterion of significance. The metaparadigmatic origins of the theory are evident in Newman's publications. Furthermore, Newman explicitly identified some philosophical assumptions; other statements that can be

457

considered philosophical claims were extracted from her publications.

Newman explicitly identified the conceptual model from which the Theory of Health as Expanding Consciousness was derived. Rogers' (1970) model, especially the idea of pattern, clearly served as a starting point for development of the theory. Newman also explicitly acknowledged and cited the scholars from other disciplines whose works provided support for her ideas and contributed to their refinement. Of note is her comment that she used knowledge developed by other scholars to *enrich* her theory but that such knowledge did not serve as the *basis* for the theory (Newman, 1997a).

Noteworthy features of the theory are the focus on the evolution of expanding consciousness and the notion that consciousness expands in the presence of disease. But Newman (1994a) also pointed out that disease is not necessary for consciousness to expand.

The special significance of the Theory of Health as Expanding Consciousness lies in the theory's contributions to our understanding of wellness, illness, and disease as patterns of the whole person and as manifestations of health. Yamashita and Tall (1998) pointed out that "it is perhaps somewhat misleading to call Newman's theory a theory of health because of the usual connotations of that word. On the other hand, so doing challenges our values; which is more important, conventional health or expanding consciousness?" (p. 67).

INTERNAL CONSISTENCY

The Theory of Health as Expanding Consciousness meets the criterion of internal consistency in part. Sarter's (1988) philosophical analysis of the Theory of Health as Expanding Consciousness indicates congruence in philosophical viewpoints among the scholars from whose works Newman drew for her theory. For example, Sarter (1988) noted that the writings of Moss (1981), Young (1976a, 1976b), and de Chardin (1959) all reflect process philosophy and mysticism. In contrast, Mitchell and Cody (1992) pointed out that Newman's view of human beings as unitary seems to be inconsistent with her discussion of physiological structures and functions. In an attempt to reconcile the inconsistency, they offered the following interpretation of Newman's views:

> The unity of the human "system," for Newman, is predicated on the idea that "mind and matter are made of the same basic stuff" (1986, p. 37). It is apparently quite appropriate within Newman's model to discuss the physiological, psychological, and emotional processes of the "human system" in conventional terms, so long as one remembers that everything, from the atom to the human being and beyond, is a manifestation of the implicate order, or "absolute consciousness" (Newman, 1986, pp. 36–37) (p. 57).

Semantic clarity is evident in that Newman provided clear constitutive definitions for the concepts of **Consciousness** and **Pattern**. She did not, however, provide clear constitutive definitions for all three dimensions of the concept of **Pattern**. In particular, the Rhythm and Diversity dimensions are defined only in a rudimentary fashion, and the Space and Time components of the dimension Movement-Space-Time are not explicitly defined. More importantly, Movement-Space-Time as a single entity is not defined. Furthermore, repeated readings of several of Newman's publications were needed to locate the definitions that are available.

Semantic consistency is evident in the consistent use of terms and the consistent meaning attached to each term within each of Newman's publications. Any difference in terminology, such as the progression from movement, space, and time, to movement and space-time, to movement-space-time, reflects the evolution of Newman's thinking.

The analysis of Newman's theory revealed structural consistency, but only when relational propositions were extracted from different publications about the theory. No one publication contains all of the relational propositions, and some of the required propositions are not included in the most recent publications about the theory (Newman, 1994a, 1997a). Moreover, the Diversity dimension of the concept of **Pattern** was not included in any relational proposition.

PARSIMONY

The Theory of Health as Expanding Consciousness meets the criterion of parsimony. The analysis of the theory yielded two concepts, one of which is multidimensional, and several relational propositions.

The decision to include **Pattern** as a separate concept, rather than a dimension of the concept of **Consciousness**, was based on Newman's frequent reference to **Pattern** and the central role it plays in the theory. Indeed, she stated that "pattern … is basic to the theory" (Newman, 1990b, p. 132). The decision not to include health as a separate concept of the Theory of Health as Expanding Consciousness is supported by Newman's (1990a) statement that "health and the evolving pattern of consciousness are the same" (p. 38). Inasmuch as health and consciousness are equivalent, the inclusion of both would have created an unnecessary redundancy.

Furthermore, the decision to regard Movement-Space-Time, Rhythm, and Diversity as dimensions of the concept of **Pattern** is supported by Newman's own statements. In particular, she explicitly stated that "characteristics of patterning include movement, diversity, and rhythm" (Newman, 1994a, p. 72); and that "the original concepts of movement-space-time can be seen as dimensions in the unitary evolving patterns of consciousness" (Newman, 1997a, p. 25).

TESTABILITY

The Theory of Health as Expanding Consciousness meets the criterion of testability for grand theories. Newman has developed a specific yet fluid RESEARCH/PRACTICE METHODOLOGY for her theory that yields middle-range theories addressing the process of expanding conscious-

ness as expressed in life patterns (Newman, 1994a). The components of the Research/Practice Methodology are identified and described in Table 12–2.

Newman's Research/Practice Methodology was, as Barrett (1998) pointed out, designed to develop new discipline of nursing-specific knowledge. Newman (1997a) described the Research/Practice Methodology as "hermeneutic, to reflect the search for meaning and understanding and interpretation inherent in the researcher's embodiment of the theory; and dialectic because both the

---

► ◄ TABLE 12–2
NEWMAN'S RESEARCH AS PRAXIS PROTOCOL: A RESEARCH/PRACTICE METHODOLOGY

PHENOMENON OF INTEREST

The process of expanding consciousness.

THE INTERVIEW

The meeting of the nurse and the study participant/client occurs when there is a mutual attraction via congruent patterns, i.e., interpenetration of the two fields.

The nurse and study participant/client enter into a partnership, with the mutual goal of participating in an authentic relationship, trusting that in the process of its unfolding, both will emerge at a higher level of consciousness.

The nurse explains the study.

The study participant/client agrees to continue in the study and agrees to recording the interview on tape.

The nurse begins the initial interview with a simple, open-ended statement, such as "Tell me about the most meaningful persons and events in your life." This question may be modified to fit the focus of the study.

The nurse continues the interview in a nondirectional manner, although more direct questions can be used occasionally. Examples of additional questions are "Tell me what it has been like living with [a particular medical diagnosis, clinical condition, or life circumstance]." "What is meaningful to you?" "What do you think about what we have been talking about?"

The nurse may prompt the study participant/client to think of something from childhood that stands out in memory if he or she needs help in thinking of something considered important.

The nurse acts as an active listener and clarifies and reflects as necessary.

The nurse is fully present in the moment, is sensitive to intuitive hunches about what to say or ask, and waits for insight into the meaning of the pattern.

The nurse is free to disclose aspects of himself or herself that are deemed appropriate.

The initial interview lasts 45 to 60 minutes.

TRANSCRIPTION

The nurse listens carefully to and transcribes the tape of the interview soon after the interview is completed.

The nurse is sensitive to the relevance of the data and may omit comments made by the study participant/client that do not directly relate to his or her life pattern, with an appropriate note to the place on the tape where such comments occurred, in case those comments seem important later.

(continued)

► ≪ TABLE 12–2
NEWMAN'S RESEARCH AS PRAXIS PROTOCOL: A RESEARCH/PRACTICE METHODOLOGY *(continued)*

DEVELOPMENT OF THE NARRATIVE: *PATTERN RECOGNITION*

The nurse selects the statements deemed most important to the study participant/client and arranges the key segments of the data in chronological order to highlight the most significant events and persons.

The data remain the same except in the order of presentation. Natural breaks where a pattern shift occurs are noted and form the basis of the sequential patterns. Recogni-tion of the pattern of the whole, made up of segments of the study participant's/client's relationships over time, will emerge for the nurse.

DIAGRAM: *PATTERN RECOGNITION*

The nurse then transmutes the narrative into a simple diagram of the sequential pattern configurations.

FOLLOW-UP: *PATTERN RECOGNITION*

The nurse conducts a second interview with the study participant/client to share the diagram or other visual portrayal of the pattern.

The nurse does not interpret the diagram. Rather, it is used simply to illustrate the study participant's/client's story in graphic form, which tends to accentuate the contrasts and repetitions in relationships over time.

The mutual viewing of the graphic form is an opportunity for the study participant/client to confirm and clarify or revise the story being portrayed.

The mutual viewing also is an opportunity for the nurse to clarify any aspect of the story about which he or she has any doubt.

The nature of the pattern of person-environment interaction will begin to emerge in terms of energy flow, e.g., blocked, diffuse, disorganized, repetitive, or whatever descriptors and metaphors come to mind to describe the pattern.

The study participant/client may express signs that pattern recognition is occurring (or already has occurred in the interval following the first interview) as the nurse and study participant/client reflect together on the study participant's/client's life pattern.

If no signs of pattern recognition occur, the nurse and study participant/client may want to proceed with additional reflections in subsequent interviews until no further insight is reached.

Sometimes, no signs of pattern recognition emerge, and if so, that characterizes the pattern for that person. Pattern recognition is not to be forced.

APPLICATION OF THE THEORY OF HEALTH AS EXPANDING CONSCIOUSNESS

The nurse undertakes more intense analysis of the data in light of the Theory of Health as Expanding Consciousness after the interviews are completed.

The nurse evaluates the nature of the sequential patterns of interaction in terms of quality and complexity and interprets the patterns according to the study participant's/client's position on Young's spectrum of consciousness (see Table 12–1).

The sequential patterns represent presentational construing or relationships.

Any similarities of pattern among a group of study participants/clients having a similar experience may be designated by themes and stated in propositional form.

Constructed from Moch, 1990, p. 1429; Newman, 1994a, pp. 88–89, 93, 97, 109, 112, 147–149.

process and the content [are] dialectic. The process is the content. The content is the process" (p. 23). The methodology obviously is qualitative and inductive, and it is completely congruent with the philosophical claims undergirding the Theory of Health as Expanding Consciousness. Moreover, the particular philosophical claims on which the **Research/Practice Methodology** is based flow directly from the more general philosophical claims undergirding the theory.

The success of the **Interview** component of the

Research/Practice Methodology depends on establishing the mutuality of the process of inquiry. It requires the nurse to focus on the most meaningful persons and events in the study participant's/client's life. The nurse is precluded from viewing the person as an object and instead is required to participate in the evolving pattern of consciousness. Indeed, "the nurse-researcher cannot stand outside the person being researched in a subject-object fashion" (Newman, 1990a, p. 40). Rather, clients serve as partners or co-researchers in the search for health patterns (Newman, 1986, 1994a).

No specific instruments associated with the **Research/Practice Methodology** have been published, although the protocol for the **Interview** (see Table 12–2) includes relevant questions that can be asked to start and maintain the dialogue with the study participant/ client. In addition, Witucki (2002) identified elements of critical thinking that may be used with the **Interview, Development of the Narrative**, and **Follow-Up** components of the **Research/ Practice Methodology**. Boyd (1990) urged refinement of the interview method, as well as development of other data collection strategies that would be consistent with the Theory of Health as Expanding Consciousness. She stated:

> Explicit incorporation of nursing practice modalities of care in research methods need not be limited to interview, as ... Newman ... impl[ies], nor [do] data need to be limited to participants' verbal descriptions. Further development of these and other methods for nursing research will profit from the search for and admittance of a variety of data forms that include a fuller range of human expression. (p. 42)

Pattern Recognition is an important aspect of the **Development of Narrative, Diagram**, and **Follow-Up** components of the **Research/Practice Methodology**. Newman (1994a) explained that *Pattern Recognition* "comes from within the observer—which means that with any set of data or sequence of events, an infinite number of patterns are possible" (pp. 73–74). More specifically, *Pattern Recognition* occurs "by going into ourselves and getting in touch with our own pattern and through it in touch with the pattern of the person or persons with whom we are interacting" (p. 107). Newman (2002) explained that *Pattern Recognition* evolves

> from an authentic, mutual relationship [that] makes a meaningful difference in the experience of the participants. The dialogue of the encounter follows the lead of the client. The significant events described by the client are viewed as configurarions (patterns) of relatedness over time. In the process of this dialogue, insight regarding the client's evolving pattern occurs. The clients grasp greater understanding of themselves and their relationships. (p. 4)

Newman (1994a) pointed out that the pattern may not be seen all at once, that extending the time and distance from relevant events may facilitate recognition of the pattern,

and that it is paradoxical that the whole of the pattern can be seen in its component parts. The importance of *Pattern Recognition* is underscored by Newman's (1997a) claim that "pattern recognition, finding meaning and understanding, accelerates the evolution of consciousness" (p. 23).

The **Research/Practice Methodology** was designed to yield sufficiently in-depth descriptions of study participants'/clients' personal experiences to capture the essence of patterns that represent expanding consciousness. Indeed, the last component of the **Research/Practice Methodology, Application of the Theory of Health as Expanding Consciousness,** yields themes representing similarities of pattern among a group of study participants/clients having a similar experience. The themes then are summarized in middle-range theory-level propositions. For example, "experiences associated with coronary heart disease are the need to excel, the need to please others, and the feeling of being alone" (Newman, 1994a, p. 92) is the proposition that summarizes themes identified by Newman and Moch (1995) from transcriptions of interviews with seven men and four women who had a medical diagnosis of coronary heart disease and were clients in a cardiac rehabilitation program.

In summarizing her **Research/Practice Methodology**, Newman (2002) stated:

> This research takes on the form and purpose of practice (i.e., a shift form observation of "the other" to "we" knowledge) with the intent of assisting clients to get in touch with the meaning of their health experience and thereby get insight into the pattern of the process and its potential for action. The nurse comes to the situation with a theoretical perspective that then becomes a part of the process. Transformation occurs in the interpenetration of the client's and the nurse's patterns, which include the client's concept of health and the nurse's theoretical understanding. The theory illuminates the meaning of the experience and is in turn illuminated by the data of the experience. ... The process is directly, immediately applicable as nursing practice, and one that is illuminating to both the researched and the researcher. (p. 4)

EMPIRICAL ADEQUACY

The Theory of Health as Expanding Consciousness meets the criterion of empirical adequacy for grand theories. A review of the results of Theory of Health as Expanding Consciousness–based published research reports (Table 12–3), as well as the master's theses and doctoral dissertations listed in the chapter bibliography on the CD-ROM, reveals that some middle-range descriptive theories of patterns of expanding consciousness have been generated. These middle-range theories represent descriptions of the study participants'/clients' personal experiences that are congruent with the concepts and propositions of the grand theory.

Interestingly, Newman (1994b) pointed out that the evidence regarding the empirical adequacy of the Theory of Health as Expanding Consciousness "is not exclusive. [Indeed,] what one sees in the data depends on the theoretical perspective from which one views the data; therefore, the same data could be used to support other theories". (p. 156)

Some studies have employed Newman's **Research/Practice Methodology** (see Table 12–3). Many of the early studies, however, employed quantitative methods, and some more recent studies have used various qualitative methodologies. In tracing the evolution of her theory and associated research, Newman (1994b) stated:

> I was aware for a long time of a vague feeling of discontent, a feeling that things didn't quite fit, and yet I was determined to make them fit. I ignored the fact that I was deceiving myself: I was supporting a unitary theoretical framework on the one hand but conducting research based on assumptions contradictory to the theory. Finally I began to allow the assumptions of the theory to determine the methods of the research. I let go of the need to control and manipulate and shifted into a mode of being fully present, authentically myself—seeking to know and trusting that the knowledge inherent in the situation would emerge. One day I felt the relief and joy of method congruent with theory. (p. 156)

Elaborating, Newman (1997a) explained:

> The illumination of the theory of health as expanding consciousness has evolved in conjunction with the research, from the testing of discrete relationships of the concepts of movement, time and consciousness, to the identification of sequential patterns of person-environment, to recognition of the integrality of the nurse-client relationship (dialogue) in the client's evolving insight and potential action. (pp. 24–25)

The evolution of Newman's research and that of others who have used her work as a guide, from a focus on such concepts as time and movement to a focus on patterns, can be seen in the titles of the studies in the Research section of the chapter references, as well as in the Research, Doctoral Dissertations, and Master's Theses sections of the chapter bibliography on the CD-ROM. Much more research that employs Newman's **Research/Practice Methodology** is needed to better understand the process and patterns of health as expanding consciousness.

PRAGMATIC ADEQUACY

The Theory of Health as Expanding Consciousness meets the criterion of pragmatic adequacy. Newman has underscored the need for special education before use of the theory, and she has explained her view that research is practice.

Nursing Education

Within the context of the Theory of Health as Expanding Consciousness, research is regarded as praxis, or practice. Hence, teaching nursing students and clinicians to use Newman's **Research/Practice Methodology** teaches them a way to both study patterns of evolving consciousness and practice nursing within the context of the theory. Newman (1990b) commented, "I now see the theory, the research, and the practice as one process—not separate entities" (p. 131). Later, she declared, "Nursing praxis integrates theory, research, and practice. It is art, science, and practice" (Newman, 2002, p. 4).

Newman (1994a) maintained that the professional doctoral degree—the Doctor of Nursing (ND)—is required for professional nursing education. She explained that the ND degree "requires a strong arts and sciences background as pre-professional education, provides professional education comparable to that of the other major players in the health field, and brings to the program students with added personal maturity" (p. 127). She went on to point out that the ND curriculum is not the transference of a typical baccalaureate nursing program to the graduate level but rather a new curriculum based on the unitary-transformative (i.e., the simultaneous action) world view.

Specific education for use of the Theory of Health as Expanding Consciousness requires a curriculum that reflects a shift in thinking from the traditional view of health as a dichotomy of wellness and illness, or even a continuum from high-level wellness through disease to death, to a new, synthesized view of disease as a meaningful aspect of health. Furthermore, the nurse has to learn to let go of wanting to control the situation. The client's choices have to be respected and supported, even when those choices conflict with the nurse's personal values (Newman, 1990b; Newman, Lamb, & Michaels, 1991).

Moreover, use of the theory requires the ability to recognize patterns in such observable phenomena as body temperature, blood pressure, heart rate, neoplasms, biochemical variations, diet, exercise, and communication. Pattern, then, is substance, process, and method. Newman (1994a) recommended use of Gendlin's (1978) process of focusing as a starting point for Pattern Recognition. That process involves directed concentration on and naming of one's bodily feelings, which results in a feeling of relaxation that, in turn, releases energy for growth.

Students and practitioners who plan to use the Theory of Health as Expanding Consciousness have to be prepared for personal transformation. Indeed, "personal growth of the student/practitioner [is] paramount" (Newman, 1986, p. 89). Sensitive to that issue, Newman (1986) commented:

(Text continues on page 465)

Research Topic	Study Participants	Citation*
Patients' needs	Hospitalized patients	Newman, 1966
Time perspective and cerebral hemi-spheric dominance	People in Zaire	Butrin & Newman, 1986
Perceived duration of time, perceived situational control, age, and length of institutionalization	Aged women living in an extended care facility	Mentzer & Schorr, 1986
Subjective time and depression	Women older than 65 years of age	Newman & Guadiano, 1984
Temporal orientation, type A behavior, and death anxiety	Professionally employed men and women	Schorr & Schroeder, 1989
Time estimation and gait tempo	Healthy men	Newman, 1972
Perceived duration of time, preferred walking rate, and age	Healthy older men and women	Newman, 1982
Time estimation and movement tempo	Healthy individuals	Newman, 1976
Time perception and personal tempo	Residents of apartment complexes for the aged	Engle, 1984
Perceived duration of time, walking ca-dence, and functional health	Community-based older women	Engle, 1986
Perceived duration of time and level of physical exertion	University faculty, students and staff, and fitness center members who par-ticipated in regular aerobic exercise	Schorr & Schroeder, 1991
Frame of temporal reference, perceived impact of chronic illness, hope/hope-lessness, powerlessness, and death anxiety	Aging women	Schorr et al., 1991
Self-assessment of health, functional health, self-concept, and attitude	Female residents, older than 60 years of age, in apartment complexes for the aged	Engle & Graney, 1985–1986
Meanings of disabling events	Families who experienced altered mobility	Marchione, 1986
Experiences of breast cancer	Women with breast cancer	Moch, 1990
Description of inner strength	Women aged 35 to 72 years who were living with breast cancer	Roux et al., 2000, 2001
Description of inner strength	Women living with multiple sclerosis	Koob et al., 2002
Description of the interpreted reality of inner strength	Women aged 67 to 83 years recovering from coronary artery disease	Dingley et al., 2001
Life patterns†	Native American women who had had breast cancer	Kiser-Larson, 2002

*See the Research section of the chapter references for complete citations.

(continued)

Research Topic	Study Participants	Citation
Life patterns[†]	Men and women with coronary heart disease	Newman & Moch, 1991
Life patterns[†]	Icelandic men and women with chronic obstructive pulmonary disease	Jonsdottir, 1998
Evolving pattern[†]	Gay men with human immunodeficiency virus (HIV)/acquired immunodeficiency syndrome (AIDS)	Lamendola & Newman, 1994
Meaning of life pattern[†]	Men and women with cancer	Newman, 1995
Pattern recognition as a nursing intervention[†]	Japanese women with ovarian cancer	Endo, 1998
Health patterning	Persons with multiple sclerosis	Gulick & Bugg, 1992
Descriptions of health	Men and women with cancer or AIDS	Fryback, 1993
Transitions in life patterns[†]	Women living with rheumatoid arthritis or multiple sclerosis	Neill, 2002a
Transitions in life patterns[†]	Women living with rheumatoid arthritis	Neill, 2002b
Explication of the health experience	Men and women with rheumatoid arthritis	Schmidt et al., 2003
Description of common patterns of person-environment interaction	Men and women with rheumatoid arthritis	Brauer, 2001
Comparison of life patterns[†]	Adolescent males convicted of murder	Pharris, 2002
Patterns of interaction with family and environment[†]	Childhood cancer survivors	Karian et al., 1998
Pattern of nurse-parent interaction	Families with children who were medically fragile	Tommet, 2003
Family experience of health as expanding consciousness[†]	Family of a pre-school age child with asthma; Young families with complex health circumstances	Litchfield, 1999
Patterns and activities of expanding consciousness	Midlife women aged 40 to 65 years	Picard, 2000
Meaning of "staying healthy"	Rural African-American adult family members	Smith, 1995
Meaning of "staying healthy"	Immigrant Pakistani families living in the United States	Jan & Smith, 1998
Personal transformation[†]	Content analysis of literature from several disciplines	Wade, 1998

[†]Used Newman's research/practice methodology.

(continued)

Mutuality	Literature: Selected journal articles and book chapters	Curley, 1997
Experience of the time spent together	Dyads of nurses and clients who originated from different cultures	Butrin, 1992
Description of the meaning of advocacy	Hospital-based nurse case managers	Hellwig et al., 2003
Clients' views of nurse case management	Clients who had worked with or were working with a nurse case manager	Lamb & Stempel, 1994
Experience of being a primary family caregiver*	Primary family caregivers of Japanese people with schizophrenia	Yamashita, 1998
Patterns of caregiving in mental illness	Family members who were primary caregivers of a relative with schizophrenia	Yamashita, 1999
Process of a caring partnership	Japanese families of wife-mothers hospitalized with cancer	Endo et al., 2000
Secondary analysis of two studies of family members' reactions to a relative's mental illness	Family members of relatives with mental illness residing in the United States and Canada	Yamashita & Forsyth, 1998
Use of music to alter perception of chronic pain	Women with rheumatoid arthritis	Schorr, 1993

*Used Newman's research/practice methodology.

(Text continued from page 462)

The pathway is uncertain and the feeling is unsure. Those who have gone before us assure us that in letting go and experiencing the moment fully the transformation will take place, and through us others will find a new level of integration and growth. (p. 78)

Despite the potential difficulties of personal transformation, Newman (1992) claimed that nurses who practice within the context of the Theory of Health as Expanding Consciousness will "experience the joy of participating in the expanding process of others and find that their own lives are enhanced and expanded by the process" (p. 650). She also commented, "It is a matter of *the nurse's being transformed by the theory and thereby becoming a transforming partner in interaction with clients*" (Newman, 1994b, p. 156).

Nursing Practice

Newman's (1994a) view that research is praxis means that "the process of nursing practice is the content of nursing research. [Furthermore,] nursing research helps participants understand and act on their particular situations" (p. 92). More specifically, Newman (1995) explained that the results of use of the **Research/Practice Methodology** "provide retrospective illumination of the participants' patterns and guidance for the process of nursing practice

in facilitating clients' insight regarding their evolving patterns" (p. 164).

In keeping with her idea that research is praxis, Newman (1986) maintained that Pattern Recognition "is the essence of practice" (p. 18) and, therefore, "the task in intervention is pattern recognition" (p. 72). Pattern Recognition "illuminates the possibilities for action" (Newman, 1990a, p. 40). The objective of nursing practice, according to Newman (1986), is "an authentic involvement of [the nurse] with the patient in a mutual relationship of pattern recognition and augmentation" (p. 88).

The **Research/Practice Methodology** guides the nurse and study participant/client to meet, form shared consciousness, and move apart. Thus the nurse-client relationship has a beginning and an end. The end, the moving apart, comes when the client "is able to center without being connected to the nurse. This occurs gradually as the client and nurse move apart, then reconnect and move apart again, repeating the process until the client can see clearly" (Newman, 1994a, p. 112).

Nurses and clients become partners in Pattern Recognition and give up the traditional roles of nurse and patient. Instead, they are "participants in a greater whole … [and] are not separate persons. They are persons experiencing the pattern of consciousness formed by their interaction. Their relationship is based not only on problems and solutions … but is a manifestation of the evolving consciousness of the whole" (Newman, 1986, p. 89). Nurses also are partners with other nurses and other health care professionals and thereby form an integrated team (Newman, 1986; 1990b).

Published reports dealing with the application of the Theory of Health as Expanding Consciousness indicate that the theory has been used in the real world of nursing practice (Table 12–4) with diverse populations in various practice situations. Furthermore, Newman (1983) has discussed the implications of the use of the Theory of Health as Expanding Consciousness with families, explaining that when the family is considered as a whole, health is the expansion of consciousness of the family. In addition, Newman (1994a) briefly discussed the application of the theory to the community. She explained, "Health of the community is conceptualized in terms of changing patterns of energy in the evolution of the system. A pattern of disease endemic to a community can be considered a manifestation of the pattern of community health" (p. 29).

George (2002) added "Newman's Theory of Health as Expanding Consciousness is not limited by person or setting. It is generalizable to anybody, anywhere" (p. 530).

The feasibility of implementing practice protocols that reflect the Theory of Health as Expanding Con-sciousness is evident in implementation projects listed here, as well as in the applications of the theory cited in Table 12–4. The complete citations for the implementation projects are given in the Administration section of the chapter references.

- Carondelet St. Mary's Hospital and Health Center, Tucson, Arizona (Ethridge, 1991; Michaels, 1992; Newman et al., 1991)
- Healing Web Partners: North Valley Hospital and Salish Kootenai College in Montana; Sioux Valley Hospital, Augustana College, and University of South Dakota in South Dakota; LDS Hospital, Brigham Young University, and Salt Lake Community College, in Utah; Lutheran Hospital, Viterbo College, Western Wisconsin Technical

> **TABLE 12–4**
> **PUBLISHED REPORTS OF NURSING PRACTICE GUIDED BY THE THEORY OF HEALTH AS EXPANDING CONSCIOUSNESS**

Practice Situation	Population	Citation*
Substance abuse	Female recovering substance abusers in a residential treatment center in Edmonton, Alberta, Canada	Woods, 1993
Pattern recognition	Pregnant women experiencing preterm labor at Abbott Northwestern Hospital in Minneapolis, Minnesota	Kalb, 1990
	Various members of the Gloria Dei Lutheran Church in Duluth, Minnesota	Gustafson, 1990
Assessing pattern	Woman with hyperthyroidism	Sayre-Adams & Wright, 1995
Application of the Theory of Health as Expanding Consciousness	School-age children with insulin-dependent diabetes mellitus	Schlotzhauer & Farnham, 1997
	29-year-old woman with cervical cancer	Witucki, 2002
	An elderly woman at home	Capasso, 1998
	Family caregivers	Yamashita, 1997
	86-year-old woman with macular degeneration caring for her husband, who has Alzheimer's disease	Witucki, 2002
	A family with a child born with a developmental disability	Newman, 1994
	Baccalaureate psychiatric nursing students caring for elderly nursing home residents	Weingourt, 1998

*See the Practice section of the chapter references for complete citations.

College, and Winona State University in Wisconsin/ Minnesota (Fosbinder et al., 1997; Koener et al., 1989; Koerner & Bunkers, 1994)

The only resources required for application of the theory are the time and personnel needed to teach nurses to use the **Research/Practice Methodology**. Moreover, practitioners have the legal ability to implement the **Research/ Practice Methodology** and to measure the effectiveness of relevant theory-based outcomes.

The extent to which use of the **Research/Practice Methodology** is compatible with expectations for nursing practice and the actual effects of its use on health-care professionals and clients have begun to be explored. Evaluation of the use of the Theory of Health as Expanding Consciousness at Carondelet St. Mary's Health Center, which is a national and international exemplar for nursing theory-based nurse case management, has resulted in increased job satisfaction and decreased job stress for nurses, increased patient satisfaction with nursing services, and considerable savings of health-care dollars due to decreased incidence of hospitalization and decreased length of hospital stay (Ethridge, 1991). Controlled experimental studies are, however, necessary to determine the relative contributions of nurse case management and the use of the Theory of Health as Expanding Consciousness.

The teaching-learning-practice Healing Web project is an exceptional prototype for Theory of Health as Expanding Consciousness-based collaborative nursing education and practice. Nursing practice is differentiated on the basis of the nurse's educational preparation. Hence, nurses who hold the associate degree, those who hold the baccalaureate degree, and those who hold a graduate degree, such as the master's degree in nursing, take on different practice roles. Healing Web school of nursing partners educate students for the appropriate role, and health-care agency partners offer positions that allow nurses to practice in the role for which they were prepared. Faculty, student, administrator, and staff evaluations of the project have indicated positive outcomes (Fosbinder, Ashton, & Koerner, 1997). In particular, nursing faculty reported that they had become an active part of the unit staff, staff reported that they were actively involved in teaching students, students reported that they engaged in teaching staff and patients, and school of nursing and health-care organization administrators reported a high return on their investments in terms of satisfying and effective educational and practice environments. Students also reported that they were very confident of their practice and organizational skills, understood the value of a detailed care plan and its effects on the quality of patient care, actively participated in interdisciplinary planning and could see the importance of integrated planning, and understood the

importance of shared learning with staff, faculty, other students, other health-care professionals, and patients. Furthermore, all participants reported that they had a better understanding of the distinct roles of nurses prepared at the associate degree and baccalaureate degree levels. Again, controlled experimental studies are necessary, in this case to determine the relative contributions of differentiated nursing practice and the use of the Theory of Health as Expanding Consciousness.

Evaluation of the Carondelet St. Mary's Health Center nurse case management project provides an initial comparison of outcomes when the theory was used and when it was not used. Other comparisons that better control for use of the theory and use of a particular method of delivery of nursing services, such as case management, are needed.

The results of research projects (see table 12–3) practice applications (see Table 12–4), and formal implementation projects reveal that clients' problems are solved. Within the context of the Theory of Health as Expanding Consciousness, this means that patterns are recognized and used as a catalyst for action.

 ## CONCLUSION

Newman has made a meaningful contribution to nursing by explicating a theory of health that extends Rogers' (1970, 1990) concept of pattern in person-environment mutual process. Evidence of the empirical and pragmatic adequacy of the theory is accumulating. Evidence from implementation projects is especially impressive. Continued documentation of outcomes of the use of the Theory of Health as Expanding Consciousness is needed.

Exactly what outcomes should be considered may be difficult, for as George (2002) pointed out, "Since the focus is on process and not on fixing what is wrong, it is difficult to define favorable outcomes ... The theory is not intended to be measured by outcomes" (p. 531). Yet Newman provided some direction for the identification of outcomes when she declared, "The theory assets that every person in every situation, no matter how disordered and hopeless it may seem, is part of the universal process of expanding consciousness—a process of becoming more of oneself, of finding greater meaning in life, and of reaching new dimensions of connectedness with other people and the world" (Retrieved March 2, 2002 from *http:// www. healthasexpandingconsciousenss. org*).

The translation of the second edition of Newman's (1994a) book, *Health as Expanding Consciousness*, into Japanese and Korean indicates international interest in the theory (Retrieved March 2, 2002 from http://www.healthasexpandingconsciousenss.org/bibliography). In addition, two groups of nurses who are particularly interested in the Theory of Health as Expanding Consciousness meet periodically to study the theory and discuss its application in practice. One group, which has received funding from the Foundation of Cancer Research, meets at the Kanagawa Cancer Center in Japan. The other group meets in the Twin Cities (Minneapolis and St. Paul) area of Minnesota, in the United States (Retrieved July 14, 2003 from http://www. healthasexpandingconsciousenss.org/gatherings). The publication of a new book about the Theory of Health as Expanding Consciousness, which focuses on the linkage of the theory with the development of nursing knowledge, practice, and education, futher attests to Margaret Newman's many contributions to the discipline of nursing (Picard & Jones, 2005).

 ## REFERENCES

Barrett, E.A.M. (1998). Unique nursing research methods: The diversity chant of pioneers. Nursing Science Quarterly, 11, 94–96.

Bateson, G. (1979). Mind and nature: A necessary unity. Toronto: Bantam.

Bentov, I. (1978). Stalking the wild pendulum. New York: Dutton.

Bohm, D. (1980). Wholeness and the implicate order. London: Routledge & Kegan Paul.

Boyd, C.O. (1990). Critical appraisal of developing nursing research methods. Nursing Science Quarterly, 3, 42–43.

de Chardin, T. (1959). The phenomenon of man. New York: Harper & Brothers.

Ethridge, P. (1991). A nursing HMO: Carondelet St. Mary's experience. Nursing Management, 22(7), 22–27.

Fosbinder, D., Ashton, C.A., & Koerner, J.G. (1997). The national Healing Web partnership: An innovative model to improve health. Journal of Nursing Administration, 27(4), 37–41.

Gendlin, E.T. (1978). Focusing. New York: Everest.

George, J.B. (2002). Health as expanding consciousness: Margaret Newman. In J. B. George (Ed.), Nursing theories: The base for professional nursing practice (5th ed., pp. 519–538.). Upper Saddle River, NJ: Prentice Hall.

Guba, E.G., & Lincoln, Y.S. (1989). Fourth generation evaluation. Newbury Park, CA: Sage.

Heron, J. (1981). Philosophical basis for a new paradigm. In P. Reason & J. Rowan (Eds.), Human inquiry: A sourcebook of new paradigm research (pp. 19–35). New York: Wiley.

Lather, P. (1986). Research as praxis. Harvard Educational Review, 56, 257–277.

Mitchell, G.J., & Cody, W.K. (1992). Nursing knowledge and human science: Ontological and epistemological considerations. Nursing Science Quarterly, 5, 54–61.

Moch, S.D. (1990). Health within the experience of breast cancer. Journal of Advanced Nursing, 15, 1426–1435.

Moss, R. (1981). The I that is we. Millbrae, CA: Celestial Arts.

Moustakas, C. (1990). Heuristic research. Newbury Park, CA: Sage.

Newman, M.A. (1978, December). Toward a theory of health. Paper presented at the Second Annual Nurse Educator Conference, New York. [Audiotape.]

Newman, M.A. (1979). Theory development in nursing. Philadelphia: F.A. Davis.

Newman, M.A. (1983). Newman's health theory. In I. Clements & F. Roberts (Eds.), Family health: A theoretical approach to nursing care (pp. 161–175). New York: Wiley.

Newman, M.A. (1986). Health as expanding consciousness. St. Louis: Mosby.

Newman, M.A. (1987). Patterning. In M.E. Duffy & N.J. Pender (Eds.), Conceptual issues in health promotion: A report of proceedings of a Wingspread conference (pp. 36–50). Indianapolis: Sigma Theta Tau.

Newman, M.A. (1990a). Newman's theory of health as praxis. Nursing Science Quarterly, 3, 37–41.

Newman, M.A. (1990b). Shifting to higher consciousness. In M.E. Parker (Ed.), Nursing theories in practice (pp. 129–139). New York: National League for Nursing.

Newman, M.A. (1992). Window on health as expanding consciousness. In M. O'Toole (Ed.), Miller-Keane encyclopedia and dictionary of medicine, nursing, and allied health (5th ed., p. 650). Philadelphia: Saunders.

Newman, M.A. (1994a). Health as expanding consciousness (2nd ed.). New York: National League for Nursing.

Newman, M.A. (1994b). Theory for nursing practice. Nursing Science Quarterly, 7, 153–157.

Newman, M.A. (1995). A developing discipline: Selected works of Margaret Newman. New York: National League for Nursing Press.

Newman, M.A. (1997a). Evolution of the theory of health as expanding consciousness. Nursing Science Quarterly, 10, 22–25.

Newman, M.A. (1997b). Experiencing the whole. Advances in Nursing Science, 20(1), 34–39.

Newman, M.A. (2002). The pattern that connects. Advances in Nursing Science, 24(3), 1–7.

Newman, M.A., Lamb, G.S., & Michaels, C. (1991). Nurse case management: The coming together of theory and practice. Nursing and Health Care, 12, 404–408.

Newman, M.A., & Moch, S.D. (1995). Life patterns of persons with coronary heart disease. In M.A. Newman (Ed.), A developing discipline: Selected works of Margaret Newman (pp. 139–157). New York: National League for Nursing Press. [Originally published 1991.]

Picard, C., & Jones, D. (Eds.). (2005). Giving voice to what we know: Margaret Newman's theory of health as expanding consciousness in practice, research, and education. Sudbury, MA: Jones and Bartlett.

Polkinghorne, D.E. (1988). Narrative knowing and the human sciences. Albany: State University of New York Press.

Prigogine, I. (1980). From being to becoming. San Francisco: Freeman.

Rogers, M.E. (1970). An introduction to the theoretical basis of nursing. Philadelphia: F.A. Davis.

Rogers, M.E. (1990). Space-age paradigm for new frontiers in nursing. In M.E. Parker (Ed.), Nursing theories in practice (pp. 105–113). New York: National League for Nursing.

Roy, C., Rogers, M.E., Fitzpatrick, J.J., Newman, M.A., Orem, D., Field, L., Stafford, M.J., Weber, S., Rossi, L., & Krekeler, K. (1982). Nursing diagnosis and nursing theory. In M.J. Kim & D.A. Moritz (Eds.), Classification of nursing diagnosis (pp. 214–278). New York: McGraw-Hill.

Sarter, B. (1988). Philosophical sources of nursing theory. Nursing Science Quarterly, 1, 52–59.

Witucki, J.M. (2002). Newman's theory of health as expanding consciousness in nursing practice. In M.R. Alligood & A. Marriner Tomey (Eds.), Nursing theory: Utilization and application (2nd ed., pp. 429–449). St. Louis: Mosby.

Yamashita, M., & Tall, F.D. (1998). A commentary on Newman's theory of health as expanding consciousness. Advances in Nursing Science, 21(1), 65–75.

Young, A.M. (1976a). The geometry of meaning. San Francisco: Robert Briggs.

Young, A.M. (1976b). The reflexive universe: Evolution of consciousness. San Francisco: Robert Briggs.

RESEARCH

Brauer, D.J. (2001). Common patterns of person-environment interaction in persons with rheumatoid arthritis. Western Journal of Nursing Research, 23, 414–430.

Butrin, J. (1992). Cultural diversity in the nurse-client encounter. Clinical Nursing Research, 1, 238–251.

Butrin, J., & Newman, M.A. (1986). Health promotion in Zaire: Time perspective and cerebral hemispheric dominance as relevant factors. Public Health Nursing, 3, 183–191.

Curley, M.A.Q. (1997). Mutuality—An expression of nursing practice. Journal of Pediatric Nursing, 12, 208–213.

Dingley, C.E., Bush, H.A., & Roux, G. (2001). Inner strength in women recovering from coronary artery disease: A grounded theory. Journal of Theory Construction and Testing, 5(2), 45–52.

Endo, E. (1998). Pattern recognition as a nursing intervention with Japanese women with ovarian cancer. Advances in Nursing Science, 20(4), 49–61.

Endo, E., Nitta, N., Inayoshi, M., Saito, R., Takemura, K., Minegishi, H., Kubo, S., & Kondo, M. (2000). Pattern recognition as a caring partnership in families with cancer. Journal of Advanced Nursing, 32, 603–610.

Engle, V.F. (1984). Newman's conceptual framework and the measurement of older adults' health. Advances in Nursing Science, 7(1), 24–36.

Engle, V.F. (1986). The relationship of movement and time to older adults' functional health. Research in Nursing and Health, 9, 123–129.

Engle, V.F., & Graney, M.J. (1985–1986). Self-assessed and functional health of older women. International Journal of Aging and Human Development, 22, 301–313.

Fryback, P.B. (1993). Health for people with a terminal diagnosis. Nursing Science Quarterly, 6, 147–159.

Gulick, E.E., & Bugg, A. (1992). Holistic health patterning in multiple sclerosis. Research in Nursing and Health, 15, 175–185.

Hellwig, S.D., Yam, M., & DiGiulio, M. (2003). Nurse care managers' perceptions of advocacy: A phenomenological study. Lippicott's Case Mangement, 8(2), 53–65.

Jan, R., & Smith, C.A. (1998). Staying healthy in immigrant Pakistani families living in the United States. Image: Journal of Nursing Scholarship, 30, 157–159.

Jonsdottir, H. (1998). Life patterns of people with chronic obstructive pulmonary disease: Isolation and being closed in. Nursing Science Quarterly, 11, 160–166.

Karian, V.E., Jankowski, S.M., & Beal, J.A. (1998). Exploring the lived-experience of childhood cancer survivors. Journal of Pediatric Oncology Nursing, 15, 153–162.

Kiser-Larson, N. (2002). Life pattern of Native women experiencing breast cancer. International Journal for Human Caring, 6(2), 61–68.

Koob, P.B., Roux, G., & Bush, H.A. (2002). Inner strength in women dwelling in the world of multiple sclerosis. International Journal for Human Caring, 6(2), 20–28.

Lamb, G.S., & Stempel, J.E. (1994). Nurse case management from the client's view: Growing as insider-expert. Nursing Outlook, 42, 7–13.

Lamendola, F.P., & Newman, M.A. (1994). The paradox of HIV/AIDS as expanding consciousness. Advances in Nursing Science, 16(3), 13–21. [Reprinted in Newman, M.A. (1995). A developing discipline: Selected works of Margaret Newman. New York: National League for Nursing Press.]

Litchfield, M. (1999). Practice wisdom. Advances in Nursing Science, 22(2), 62–73.

Marchione, J.M. (1986). Pattern as methodology for assessing family health: Newman's theory of health. In P. Winstead-Fry (Ed.), Case studies in nursing theory (pp. 215–240). New York: National League for Nursing.

Mentzer, C.A., & Schorr, J.A. (1986). Perceived situational control and perceived duration of time: Expressions of life patterns. Advances in Nursing Science, 9(1), 12–20.

Moch, S.D. (1990). Health within the experience of breast cancer. Journal of Advanced Nursing, 15, 1426–1435.

Neill, J. (2002a). From practice to caring praxis through Newman's theory of health as expanding consciousness: A personal journey. International Journal for Human Caring, 6(2), 48–554.

Neill, J. (2002b). Transendence and transformation in the life patterns of women living with rheumatoid arthritis. Advances in Nursing Science, 24(4), 27–47.

Newman, M.A. (1966). Identifying and meeting patients' needs in short-span nurse-patient relationships. Nursing Forum, 5(1), 76–86.

Newman, M.A. (1972). Time estimation in relation to gait tempo. Perceptual and Motor Skills, 34, 359–366.

Newman, M.A. (1976). Movement tempo and the experience of time. Nursing Research, 25, 273–279.

Newman, M.A. (1982). Time as an index of expanding consciousness with age. Nursing Research, 31, 290–293.

Newman, M.A. (1995). Recognizing a pattern of expanding consciousness in persons with cancer. In M.A. Newman, A developing discipline: Selected works of Margaret Newman (pp. 159–171). New York: National League for Nursing Press.

Newman, M.A., & Gaudiano, J.K. (1984). Depression as an explanation for decreased subjective time in the elderly. Nursing Research, 33, 137–139.

Newman, M.A., & Moch, S.D. (1991). Life patterns of persons with coronary heart disease. Nursing Science Quarterly, 4, 161–167. [Reprinted in Newman, M.A. (1995). A developing discipline: Selected works of Margaret Newman. New York: National League for Nursing Press. Reprinted in Parse, R.R. (2001). Qualitative inquiry: The path to sciencing. Boston: Jones and Bartlett.]

Pharris, M.D. (2002). Coming to know ourselves as community through a nursing partnership with adolescents convicted of murder. Advances in Nursing Science, 24(3), 21–42.

Picard, C. (2000). Pattern of expanding consciousness in midlife women: Creative movement and the narrative as modes of expression. Nursing Science Quarterly, 13, 150–157.

Roux, G., Bush, H.A., & Dingley, C.E. (2000). Inner strength in women with breast cancer. Journal of Theory Construction and Testing, 4(2), 36–39.

Roux, G., Bush, H.A., & Dingley, C.E. (2001). Inner strength in women with breast cancer. Journal of Theory Construction and Testing, 5(1), 19–27.

Schmidt, B.J., Brauer, D.J., & Peden-McAlpine, C. (2003). Experiencing health in the context of rheumatoid arthritis. Nursing Science Quarterly, 16, 155–162.

Schorr, J.A. (1993). Music and pattern change in chronic pain. Advances in Nursing Science, 15(4), 27–36. Morse, L.K. (1993). Commentary on "Music and pattern change in chronic pain." ONS Nursing Scan in Oncology, 2(6), 10.

Schorr, J.A., Farnham, R.C., & Ervin, S.M. (1991). Health patterns in aging women as expanding consciousness. Advances in Nursing Science, 13(4), 52–63.

Schorr, J.A., & Schroeder, C.A. (1989). Consciousness as a dissipative structure: An extension of the Newman model. Nursing Science Quarterly, 2, 183–193.

Schorr, J.A., & Schroeder, C.A. (1991). Movement and time: Exertion and perceived duration. Nursing Science Quarterly, 4, 104–112.

Smith, C.A. (1995). The lived experience of staying healthy in rural African American families. Nursing Science Quarterly, 8, 17–21.

Tommet, P.A. (2003). Nurse-parent dialogue: Illuminating the evolving pattern of families with children who are medically fragile. Nursing Science Quarterly, 16, 239–246.

Wade, G.H. (1998). A concept analysis of personal transformation. Journal of Advanced Nursing, 28, 713–719.

Yamashita, M. (1998). Newman's theory of health as expanding consciousness: Research on family caregiving in mental illness in Japan. Nursing Science Quarterly, 11, 110–115.

Yamashita, M. (1999). Newman's theory of health applied in caregiving in Canada. Nursing Science Quarterly, 12, 73–79.

Yamashita, M., & Forsyth, D.M. (1998). Family coping with mental illness: An aggregate from two studies, Canada and United States. Journal of the American Psychiatric Nurses Association, 4, 1–8.

ADMINISTRATION

Ethridge, P. (1991). A nursing HMO: Carondelet St. Mary's experience. Nursing Management, 22(7), 22–27.

Fosbinder, D., Ashton, C.A.., & Koerner, J.G. (1997). The national healing web partnership: An innovative model to improve health. Journal of Nursing Administration, 27(4), 37–41.

Koerner, J.G., & Bunkers, S.S. (1994). The healing web: An expansion of consciousness. Journal of Holistic Nursing, 12(1), 51–63.

Koerner, J.G., Bunkers, S.S., Nelson, B., & Santema, K. (1989). Implementing differentiated practice: The Sioux Valley Hospital experience. Journal of Nursing Administration, 19(2), 13–22.

Michaels, C. (1992). Carondelet St. Mary's nursing enterprise. Nursing Clinics of North America, 27, 77–85.

Newman, M.A., Lamb, G.S., & Michaels, C. (1991). Nurse case management. The coming together of theory and practice. Nursing and Health Care, 12, 404–408. [Reprinted in Newman, M.A. (1995). A developing discipline: Selected works of Margaret Newman. New York: National League for Nursing Press.

PRACTICE

Capasso, V.A. (1998). The theory is the practice: An exemplar. Clinical Nurse Specialist, 12, 226–229.

Gustafson, W. (1990). Application of Newman's theory of health: Pattern recognition as nursing practice In M.E. Parker (Ed.), Nursing theories in practice (pp. 141–161). New York: National League for Nursing.

Kalb, K.A. (1990). The gift: Applying Newman's theory of health in nursing practice. In M.E. Parker (Ed.), Nursing theories in practice (pp. 163–186). New York: National League for Nursing.

Newman, M.A. (1994). Health as expanding consciousness (2nd ed., pp. 25–29). New York: National League for Nursing.

Sayre-Adams, J., & Wright, S. (1995). Change in consciousness. Nursing Times, 91(41), 44–45.

Schlotzhauer, M., & Farnham, R. (1997). Newman's theory and insulin dependent diabetes mellitus in adolescence. Journal of School Nursing, 13(3), 20–23.

Weingourt, R. (1998). Using Margaret A. Newman's theory of health with elderly nursing home residents. Perspectives in Psychiatric Care, 34(3), 25–30.

Witucki, J.M. (2002). Newman's theory of health as expanding consciousness in nursing practice. In M.R. Alligood & A. Marriner Tomey (Eds.), Nursing theory: Utilization and application (2nd ed., pp. 429–449). St. Louis: Mosby.

Woods, L. (1993). Substance abuse, existentialism, and anger. Addictions Nursing Network, 5(3), 78–83.

Yamashita, M. (1997). Family caregiving: Application of Newman's and Peplau's theories. Journal of Psychiatric and Mental Health Nursing, 4, 401–405.

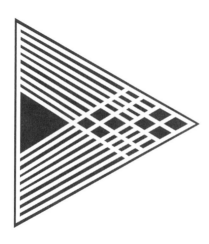

Chapter **13**

Parse's Theory of Human Becoming

Rosemarie Rizzo Parse set out to create a theory grounded in the human sciences that would enhance nursing knowledge. She explained:

> The idea to create such a theory began many years ago when I began to wonder and wander and ask why not? The theory itself … surfaced in me in Janusian fashion over the years in interrelationship with others primarily through my lived experience with nursing. The creation of it has been long and arduous, but with many moments of joy. (Parse, 1981, p. xiii)

Later, Parse (1997b) elaborated on the evolution of her theory:

> The was, is, and will be of the human becoming theory is a journey in the art of sciencing, a process of coming to know the world of human experience. The form and structure of the theory as written does not fully reflect the intuitive-rational process that birthed its creation. That process germinated multidimensionally throughout [my] life of being present to and conceptualizing the significance of the discipline's mission to humankind. The puzzle that surfaced a concern for the mission was related to early gnawing musing about whose desires were being served by the medical model practice of nursing and the keen and growing awareness in [me] that humans were mysteries emerging in living personal value priorities, not machines to be fixed. Once aware of such notions, there was a concentrated focus on moving with other possibilities for nursing. The theory was cast in written form, though not in stone, and thus it has been evolving ever since. (p. 32)

The initial result of Parse's intellectual effort was the Theory of Man-Living-Health, which was first published in her 1981 book, *Man-Living-Health: A Theory of Nursing*. Research and practice methodologies congruent with the theory were introduced in a chapter of Parse's 1987 edited book, *Nursing Science: Major Paradigms, Theories, and Critiques*. The theory was renamed the Theory of Human Becoming in 1990 because although the term man formerly referred to mankind, that term currently connotes the male gender (Parse, 1992). Refinements in the theory, focused primarily on wording, were published in Parse's 1992 journal article, "Human Becoming: Parse's Theory of Nursing." Refinements in wording continued, additional research methodologies were developed, and the research and practice methodologies were added to the second edition of Parse's 1981 book, newly titled *The Human Becoming School of Thought: A Perspective for Nurses and Other Health Professionals* (Parse, 1998). The 1998 book "is offered in the ongoing quest of defining unique nursing knowledge for the betterment of humankind" (Parse, 1998, p. xi). Most recently,

Parse (2003a) has offered a perspective of community change within the context of the Human Becoming School of Thought and has clarified the ontology of the theory by eliminating the term unitary (Parse, 2004).

Overview

Parse's work is a grand theory that focuses on the human-universe-health process, which Parse (1998) views as the phenomenon of concern for the discipline of nursing, as well as on cocreated human experiences (Parse, 2001b). The concepts and the propositions, which Parse calls principles, of the Theory of Human Becoming are listed here. In addition, the components of the research methodologies and the practice methodology are listed here. Each concept, proposition, and methodology component is defined and described later in this chapter.

Key Terms

HUMAN BECOMING
MEANING
RHYTHMICITY
TRANSCENDENCE
IMAGING
VALUING
LANGUAGING
REVEALING-CONCEALING
ENABLING-LIMITING
CONNECTING-SEPARATING
POWERING
ORIGINATING
TRANSFORMING
PRINCIPLE 1: Structuring meaning multidimensionally is cocreating reality through the languaging of valuing and imaging.
PRINCIPLE 2: Cocreating rhythmical patterns of relating is living the paradoxical unity of revealing-concealing and enabling-limiting while connecting-separating.
PRINCIPLE 3: Cotranscending with the possibles is powering unique ways of originating in the process of transforming.
HUMAN BECOMING AND COMMUNITY CHANGE CONCEPTS
MOVING-INITIATING
    Tunneling
    Driving
    Laddering
    Boating
    Swimming
    Submarining
    Ballooning
    Motorflying
    Swinging
ANCHORING-SHIFTING
    Savoring-Sacrificing
    Revering-Liberating

PONDERING-SHAPING
    Considering-Composing
    Dialoguing-Listening
THE PARSE METHOD OF BASIC RESEARCH
    Phenomena for Study
    Structure of the Phenomenon to Emerge
    Processes
    Participant Selection
    Dialogical Engagement
    Extraction-Synthesis
    Heuristic Interpretation
THE HUMAN BECOMING HERMENEUTIC METHOD OF BASIC RESEARCH
    Phenomena for Study
    Structure of the Phenomenon to Emerge
    Processes
    Participant Selection
    Discoursing
    Interpreting
    Understanding
    Disseminating Possibilities
PRACTICE METHODOLOGY
    Illuminating Meaning
    Explicating
    Synchronizing Rhythms
    Dwelling With
    Mobilizing Transcendence
    Moving Beyond
    Contexts for Nursing
    Goal of the Discipline of Nursing
    Goal of the Human Becoming Nurse
    True Presence
    Coming-to-be-Present
    Face-to-Face Discussions
    Silent Immersion
    Lingering Presence
    Ways of Changing Health Patterns in True Presence
    Creative Imagining
    Affirming Personal Becoming
    Glimpsing the Paradoxical
THE PREPROJECT-PROCESS-POSTPROJECT DESCRIPTIVE QUALITATIVE METHOD OF APPLIED RESEARCH
    Purpose
    Design
    Information Sources
    Teaching-Learning Process
    Nurses' Documentation
    Personal Health Descriptions
    Patterns of Becoming
    Nurse-Person Activities
    Plans, Goals, and Priorities for Change
    Analysis of Information Sources

ANALYSIS OF THE THEORY OF HUMAN BECOMING

This section presents an analysis of Parse's theory. The analysis is based on Parse's publications about her theory, drawing primarily from her 1998 book, *The Human Becoming School of Thought: A Perspective for Nurses and Other Health Professionals.*

SCOPE OF THE THEORY

The central thesis of the Theory of Human Becoming is that "humans in mutual process with the universe structure meaning multidimensionally, coauthor health, freely choose ways of becoming, and move beyond each moment with hopes and dreams" (Parse, 1998, pp. x–xi). Parse (1998) explained that her work has evolved from a theory of nursing to a school of thought, which she defined as "a theoretical point of view held by a community of scholars" (Parse, 1997c, p. 74). The school of thought encompasses the Theory of Human Becoming along with three research methodologies and a practice methodology (Parse, 2001b). Inasmuch as the theory concepts and propositions are written at a relatively abstract level of discourse, Parse's work is classified as a grand theory.

CONTEXT OF THE THEORY

Metaparadigm Concepts and Proposition

Parse's (1998) statement that her theory focuses on "the human-universe-health process" (p. x) indicates that the metaparadigm concepts of interest are *human beings, environment, and health.* Furthermore, her statement suggests that the metaparadigm proposition of particular interest is the *human processes of living and dying, recognizing that human beings are in a continuous relationship with their environments.*

Philosophical Claims

The philosophical foundation of the Theory of Human Becoming is the human sciences, as put forth by Dilthey (1988 [original work published 1883]). Parse (2001b) declared, "Human Becoming is a basic *human science* that has cocreated human experiences as its central focus" (p. 229). The human sciences "posit methodologies directed toward uncovering the meaning of phenomena as humanly experienced [and which] are used to study the ... human's participative experience with a situation" (Parse, 1998, p. 9).

More specifically, the philosophical foundation of the theory is existential-phenomenological thought. Drawing primarily from Heidegger (1962), Merleau-Ponty (1974), and Sartre (1966), Parse (1998) cited the concepts of co-constitution, coexistence, and situated freedom, along with the tenets of intentionality and human subjectivity. Parse has so linked the philosophical foundation of the Theory of Human Becoming with the conceptual model on which the theory was founded that specific assumptions cannot be fully articulated until after the conceptual model is discussed.

Parse's philosophical claims reflect the *simultaneous action* world view. Parse (1998) explicitly categorized her theory as grounded in the human sciences and an example of the simultaneity perspective. Moreover, she noted that "human becoming reflects the unity of the construct man-living-health [and that] there are no references to particular aspects of humans, such as biological, psychological, or spiritual" (Parse, 1992, p. 37). Even more to the point, Parse (1981) commented that her theory "is in contradistinction to a [philosophical perspective] that views man as the sum of parts, acted upon and delimited by such terms as disease and pathology" (p. 7).

Conceptual Model

In keeping with the simultaneous action world view, the conceptual foundation of the Theory of Human Becoming is Rogers' Science of Unitary Human Beings. In particular, Rogers' (1992) concepts of energy field, openness, pattern, and pandimensionality and her homeodynamic principles of helicy, integrality, and resonancy were used as the conceptual underpinnings of the Theory of Human Becoming.

Consistent with Rogers' (1970, 1992) conceptual system, Parse (1998) regards human beings as open, [indivisible] beings who mutually cocreate with the rhythmical patterns of the universe (the environment), who are recognized by patterns of relating, and who freely choose in situations. Health is defined as "a continuously changing process that the human cocreates in mutual process with the universe" (p. 33). Accordingly, disease "is not something a person contracts but, rather, a pattern of the human-universe mutual process" (p. 33). In addition, health is a cocreated process of becoming that is experienced and described by the person, family, and community. The goal of nursing is quality of life, which Parse (1998) defined as "the incarnation of lived experiences in the indivisible human's views on living moment to moment (becoming) as the changing patterns of shifting perspectives weave the fabric of life through the human-universe process" (p. 31).

Assumptions Arising from Philosophical Claims and Conceptual Model

Parse (1998) synthesized the concepts, tenets, and principles from existential-phenomenology and Rogers' Science of Unitary Human Beings into four assumptions about humans and five assumptions about becoming. All of these assumptions are listed here, along with their particular philosophical and conceptual roots (Parse, 1998, pp. 19–20, 27–28; Parse, 2004).

Assumptions About the Human

- The human is coexisting while coconstituting rhythmical patterns with the universe.
  - Philosophical concepts and tenets: Coexistence, Coconstitution
  - Conceptual model concept: Pattern

- The human is open, freely choosing meaning in situation, bearing responsibility for decisions.
  - Philosophical concept and tenet: Situated freedom
  - Conceptual model concepts: Openness, Energy field

- The human is [indivisible], continuously coconstituting patterns of relating.
  - Philosophical concept and tenet: Coconstitution
  - Conceptual model concepts: Energy field, Pattern

- The human is transcending multidimensionally with the possibles.
  - Philosophical concept and tenet: Situated freedom
  - Conceptual model concepts: Pandimensionality, Openness

Assumptions About Becoming

- Becoming is [indivisible], unpredictable, ever-changing human-living-health.
  - Philosophical concepts and tenets: Situated freedom, Coconstitution
  - Conceptual model concept: Openness

- Becoming is rhythmically coconstituting human-universe process.
  - Philosophical concept and tenet: Coconstitution
  - Conceptual model concepts: Pattern, Pandimensionality

- Becoming is the human's pattern of relating value priorities.
  - Philosophical concept and tenet: Situated freedom
  - Conceptual model concepts: Pattern, Openness

- Becoming is an intersubjective process of transcending with the possibles.
  - Philosophical concepts and tenets: Situated freedom, Coexistence
  - Conceptual model concept: Openness

- Becoming is [indivisible] human's emerging.
  - Philosophical concept and tenet: Coexistence
  - Conceptual model concepts: Energy field, Pandimensionality

Three other assumptions, which represent a synthesis of the assumptions about the human and becoming, address human becoming. These assumptions are listed here.

- Human becoming is freely choosing personal meaning in situations in the intersubjective process of living value priorities (Parse, 1998, p. 29).
- Human becoming is cocreating rhythmical patterns of relating in mutual process with the universe (Parse, 1998, p. 29).
- Human becoming is cotranscending multidimensionally with emerging possibles (Parse, 1998, p. 29).

Parse (2003a) also identified several tenets that undergird the human becoming view of community. Those tenets are:

- The individual is community (Parse, 2003a, p. 46).
- The group is community (Parse, 2003a, p. 46).
- Community bears witness-does not bear witness in unfolding meanings of the moment (Parse, 2003a, p. 46).
- Nurse-community process focuses on the hopes, dreams, desires, and intentions of community, one person or many (Parse, 2003a, p. 46).
- Nurse-community process is guided by community value priorities (Parse, 2003a, p. 46).
- Nurses are with community in digging, forging, climbing, steering, gliding, immersing, drifting, propelling, and soaring, as ways of moving-initiating community change (Parse, 2003a, p. 46).
- Nurses are with community in the persisting-diversifying of changing value priorities as the savoring-sacrificing and revering-liberating of anchoring-shifting community change unfolds with the changing patterns of preference.
- Nurses are with community in considering-composing and dialoguing-listening as ways of pondering-shaping community change.

Five assumptions, some of which are combinations or restatements of the assumptions about the human, becoming, and human becoming, are the basis for Parse's Basic Research Methodology. These assumptions are presented here.

- Humans are open beings in mutual process with the universe. The construct human becoming refers to the human-universe-health process (Parse, 1998, p. 63; 2001a, p. 172).
- Human becoming is uniquely lived by individuals and

groups. People make reflective-prereflective choices in connection with others and the universe that incarnate their health (Parse, 2001a, p. 170).

- Descriptions of lived experiences enhance knowledge of human becoming. Individuals and groups can describe their own experiences in ways that shed light on the meaning of health (Parse, 2001a, p. 170).
- Researcher-participant dialogical engagement discovers the meaning of phenomena as humanly lived. The researcher, in true presence with the participant, can elicit authentic information about lived experiences (Parse, 2001a, p. 170).
- The researcher, through inventing and abiding with logic while adhering to semantic consistency during the extraction-synthesis and heuristic interpretation processes, creates structures of lived experiences and weaves the structure with the theory in ways that enhance the knowledge base of nursing (Parse, 2001a, p. 170).

Parse (2001a) identified still other assumptions, which undergird the Human Becoming Hermeneutic Method of Basic Research. Those assumptions, which reflect "the He[i]deggerian [Heidegger, 1962]-Gadamerian [Gadamer, 1998 [original work published 1960], 1976] tradition to answer research questions such as *What does it mean to be human?*" (Parse, 2001a, p. 172), are:

- Human perspective is personal meaning cocreated with the human-universe mutual process (Parse, 2001a, p. 173).
- Human creations and interpretations of texts and artforms are perspectival (Parse, 2001a, p. 173).
- The rhythmical process of researcher-text and researcher-artform dialogue coconstructs meaning moments (Parse, 2001a, p. 173).
- New understandings of lived experiences arise with interpretations of texts and artforms (Parse, 2001a, p. 173).
- Understandings transfigure the researcher's life patterns (Parse, 2001a, p. 173).

Yet other assumptions undergird the Preproject-Process-Postproject Descriptive Qualitative Method of Applied Research. Those assumptions are:

- Value priorities are cherished beliefs that guide actions (Parse, 2001a, p. 174).
- New experiences shed light on the familiar-unfamiliar (Parse, 2001a, p. 174).
- New understandings are appropriated-disappropriated and woven with explicit-tacit knowings all-at-once (Parse, 2001a, p. 174).
- Fulfilling satisfaction arises with recognition and living cherished beliefs (Parse, 2001a, p. 174).

Antecedent Knowledge

Parse (1998) clearly and explicitly stated that her assumptions about the human and becoming of the Theory of Human Becoming emerged from Rogers' (1970, 1992) conceptual model of nursing and the existential-phenomenological thinking of Heidegger (1962), Merleau-Ponty (1974), and Sartre (1966). She also cited the contributions of Buber (1965), Marcel (1978), Tillich (1952, 1954), van den Berg (1971), van Kaam (1974), Camus (1946, 1995), and Simone de Beauvoir (1948, 1977). In addition, she mentioned Kafka but gave no citations to his works.

Parse cited numerous other scholars as she defined and discussed the concepts and propositions of her theory, including Ricoeur (1984, 1987, 1988, 1992); Toben (1975); Dilthey (1961); Whorf (1956); Polanyi (1959, 1969); Bruteau (1979); Schutz (1967); Greene (1978); Harman (1997); Raths, Harmin, and Simon (1978); B.P. Hall (1976); Bandler and Grinder (1975); Watzlawick (1978); Gadamer (1993); E.T. Hall (1976); Sapir (1966); von Bertalanffy (1959); Straus (1974); Dossey (1991); Grinder and Bandler (1976); Langer (1976); Leonard (1978); Jourard (1971); Kempler (1974); van Kaam, van Croonenburg, and Muto (1969); Weisskopf (1959); Frankl (1959); Nietzsche (1968); Watzlawick, Weakland, and Fisch (1974); and Laing, Phillipson, and Lee (1966).

CONTENT OF THE THEORY

Parse (1998) identified four essential ideas in her theory: the human-universe mutual process, the coconstitution of health, the multidimensional meanings the indivisible human gives to being and becoming, and the human's freedom in each situation to choose alternative ways of becoming. Those ideas are reflected in the concepts and propositions of the Theory of Human Becoming.

Concepts

Analysis of the Theory of Human Becoming yielded 13 unidimensional concepts. Parse (1998) explained that many of the concepts "are stated in verbal forms to express more clearly the idea of human becoming as an ongoing changing process" (p. 34). In other words, the use of the participle form—the "-ing" ending—for the name of a concept makes explicit the process orientation of the Theory of Human Becoming (Parse, 1992).

The central concept of the Theory of Human Becoming is **HUMAN BECOMING**. Three other concepts are **MEANING, RHYTHMICITY,** and **TRANSCENDENCE.** Although Parse (1998) viewed meaning, rhythmicity, and transcendence as major themes reflected in the philosophical assumptions about the human, becoming, and human becoming, analysis of the Theory of Human Becoming revealed that these themes can be considered concepts of the theory.

The concept of **MEANING** is further defined by three other concepts—**IMAGING, VALUING,** and **LANGUAGING.** The concept of **RHYTHMICITY** also is further defined by three other concepts—**REVEALING-CONCEALING, ENABLING-LIMITING,** and **CONNECTING-SEPARATING.** Similarly, the concept of **TRANSCENDENCE** is further defined by three other concepts—**POWERING, ORIGINATING,** and **TRANSFORMING.**

Nonrelational Propositions

The definitions for all of the concepts of the Theory of Human Becoming are given here. These constitutive definitions are the nonrelational propositions of the theory. The definitions of several of the concepts reflect paradoxes that Parse regards as fundamental to human becoming. She views a paradox as "one phenomenon with two dimensions" and explained that paradoxes "are not problems to be solved or eliminated, but are natural rhythms of life" (Parse, 1998, p. 34). Each paradox is a natural rhythm that is lived all-at-once.

HUMAN BECOMING

- A ... construct referring to the human being's living health (Parse, 1997b, p. 32).

Elaborating on the definition of **Human Becoming,** Parse (1998) stated that the human participates with the universe in creating health and quality of life by choosing imaged values in multidimensional experiences that are the human's paradoxical ways of relating. Ways of relating are rhythms lived as the human comes to know explicitly-tacitly, while confirming—not confirming cherished beliefs in speaking—being silent and moving—being still in the struggle of pushing-resisting with the conformity-nonconformity and certainty-uncertainty in inventing unique ways of viewing the familiar-unfamiliar (p. 55).

MEANING

- The linguistic and imagined content of something and the interpretation that one gives to something (Parse, 1998, p. 29).

Elaborating on the definition of **Meaning,** Parse (1998) noted that "meanings are the valued images of the is, was,

and will-be languaged in the now with and without words, with and without movement.... [Meaning] arises with the human-universe process and refers to ultimate meaning or purpose in life and the meaning moments of everyday living. Meaning moments change through the living of new experiences that shift imaged values, shedding a different light and thus changing ultimate meaning. Meaning, then, is not static but everchanging, and thus portends the unknown, the yet-to-be truths for the moment" (p. 29).

RHYTHMICITY

- The cadent, paradoxical patterning of the human-universe mutual process (Parse, 1998, p. 29).

When elaborating on the definition of **Rhythmicity,** Parse (1998) referred to rhythmical patterns, which she views as natural, paradoxical, unrepeatable, ever-shifting, recognizable configurations of human with universe. These patterns are "revealed and concealed all-at-once with a flowing process as cadences change with new experiences arising with diversity" (p. 30).

TRANSCENDENCE

- Reaching beyond with possibles—the hopes and dreams envisioned in multidimensional experiences [and] powering the originating of transforming (Parse, 1998, p. 30).

Parse (1998) explained that the notion of possibles that is part of the definition of **Transcendence** refers to "options from which to choose personal ways of becoming ... [that] arise with the human-universe process" (p. 30). She went on to note that "the human propels with the creation of new ventures, as struggling and leaping beyond shift the views of the now, expanding horizons and bringing to light other possibles" (p. 30).

IMAGING

- Reflective-prereflective coming to know the explicit-tacit all-at-once (Parse, 1998, p. 36).

Imaging contains the rhythmical paradox of explicit-tacit knowing. "Explicit knowing is that which is known reflectively and is utterable. Tacit knowing is prereflective unutterable knowing" (Parse, 1998, p. 34).

VALUING

- Confirming—not confirming cherished beliefs in light of a personal worldview (Parse, 1998, pp. 37–38).

Valuing contains the rhythmical paradox of confirming—not confirming. This paradox focuses on "the persistent living of what is cherished and not cherished" (Parse, 1998, p. 34).

LANGUAGING

- Signifying valued images through speaking—being silent and moving—being still (Parse, 1998, p. 39).

Languaging contains two rhythmical paradoxes: speaking—being silent and moving—being still. Parse (1998) views these paradoxes as the rhythms of languaging.

REVEALING-CONCEALING

- Disclosing—not disclosing all-at-once (Parse, 1998, p. 43).

ENABLING-LIMITING

- Living the opportunities-restrictions present in all choosings all-at-once (Parse, 1998, p. 44).

CONNECTING-SEPARATING

- Being with and apart from others, ideas, objects, and situations all-at-once (Parse, 1998, p. 45).

The concepts of **Revealing-Concealing, Enabling-Limiting**, and **Connecting-Separating** contain rhythmical paradoxes, which are evident in the actual labels for those concepts. Parse (1998) pointed out that one of the two aspects of each concept is in the foreground, and the other is in the background. She did not, however, indicate which aspect is foreground and which is background or whether which is foreground and which is background depends on the situation.

POWERING

- The pushing-resisting process of affirming—not affirming being in light of nonbeing (Parse, 1998, p. 47).

This concept encompasses three rhythmical paradoxes: pushing-resisting, affirming-not affirming, and being-nonbeing. "The pushing-resisting [paradox] is the mutually forging and holding that enlivens the ebb and flow of life, and [the] being-nonbeing [paradox] is all-at-once living the now and the unknown not-yet. The affirming–not affirming paradox is all-at-once living reverence and disregard" (Parse, 1998, p. 35).

ORIGINATING

- Inventing new ways of conforming-nonconforming in the certainty-uncertainty of living (Parse, 1998, p. 49).

This concept contains two paradoxes: conforming-nonconforming and certainty-uncertainty. The conform-

ing-nonconforming paradox "is the all-at-once movement to be like others and yet unique" and the certainty-uncertainty paradox "is all-at-once being sure and unsure in choosing among options" (Parse, 1998, p. 35).

TRANSFORMING

- Shifting the view of the familiar-unfamiliar, the changing of change in coconstituting anew in a deliberate way (Parse, 1998, p. 51).

This concept contains the paradox of familiar-unfamiliar. This paradox refers to "the all-at-once transfiguring of an unfamiliar perspective to the familiar, as others, ideas, objects, and situations are viewed in a new light" (Parse, 1998, p. 35).

PRINCIPLE 1

- Structuring meaning multidimensionally is cocreating reality through the languaging of valuing and imaging (Parse, 1998, p. 35).

This proposition focuses on the view that "humans are not given reality but have to construct it for themselves in their own way. ... [The proposition] means that human becoming is the ongoing constructing of reality through assigning significance to experiences at the many realms of the universe that are lived all-at-once" (Parse, 1998, p. 35). In other words, "humans construct what is real for them from choices made at many realms of the universe" (Parse, 1995, p. 6).

PRINCIPLE 2

- Cocreating rhythmical patterns of relating is living the paradoxical unity of revealing-concealing and enabling-limiting while connecting-separating (Parse, 1998, p. 42).

This proposition "means that human becoming is an emerging cadence of coconstituting ways of becoming with the universe. These ways of becoming (revealing-concealing, enabling-limiting, and connecting-separating) are paradoxical, lived rhythmically, and recognized in the human-universe process as patterns" (Parse, 1998, p. 42). In other words, "humans live in rhythm with the universe coconstituting patterns of relating" (Parse, 1995, p. 7). Rhythmical patterns of relating have the qualities of timing and flowing. Parse (1998) explained, "Timing refers to the cadence evident in a recurrent beat. It is sometimes fast, sometimes slow, but ever-emerging universally. Flowing refers to the continuity evident as the changing beats incarnate diverse patterns, like waves of the sea, moving with the alternating rise and fall, somewhat the same yet becoming different with each movement of wave with wave and wave with sea" (p. 43).

PRINCIPLE 3

- Cotranscending with the possibles is powering unique ways of originating in the process of transforming (Parse, 1998, 46).

This proposition "means that human becoming is moving beyond with intended hopes and dreams while pushing-resisting in creating new ways of viewing the familiar and unfamiliar" (Parse, 1998, p. 46). In other words, "humans forge unique paths with shifting perspectives as a different light is cast on the familiar" (Parse, 1995, p. 7). "The human exists with others," Parse (1998) explained, "and continues to cocreate new possibles that arise from the context of situations as opportunities from which alternatives are [freely] chosen" (p. 46).

Relational Propositions

The relational propositions of the Theory of Human Becoming are given here. Relational proposition A links the concept of **Human Becoming** with the concepts of **Meaning, Rhythmicity,** and **Transcendence.** Relational proposition B is a more elaborate statement of relations between concepts, and it links the concept of **Human Becoming** with three of the concepts that make up each of the three principles (**Languaging, Valuing, Imagining, Revealing-Concealing, Enabling-Limiting, Connecting-Separating, Powering, Originating, Transforming**).

Relational propositions C, D, and E are what Parse (1998) called theoretical structures. Each of these propositions links a concept from one of the three principles with a concept from each of the other principles. Relational proposition C links **Powering, Revealing-Concealing,** and **Imaging.** Relational proposition D links **Originating, Enabling-Limiting,** and **Valuing.** Relational proposition E links **Transforming, Connection-Separating,** and **Languaging.** All of the relational propositions are nondirectional and noncausal (Parse, 1992).

A. Human becoming is structuring meaning multidimensionally in cocreating paradoxical rhythmical patterns of relating while cotranscending with the possibles (Parse, 1998, p. 34).
B. Human becoming is the day-to-day creating of reality through the languaging of valuing and imaging as the paradoxical rhythmical patterns of revealing-concealing, enabling-limiting, and connecting-separating are powering ways of originating transforming (Parse, 1998, p. 55).

C. Powering emerges with the revealing-concealing of imaging (Parse, 1998, p. 55).
D. Originating emerges with the enabling-limiting of valuing (Parse, 1998, p. 55).
E. Transforming emerges with the languaging of connecting-separating (Parse, 1998, p. 55).

Human Becoming Community Change Concepts

Recently, Parse (2003a) presented a view of community from the perspective of the Theory of Human Becoming. She explained, "Community, from a human becoming perspective, is an [indivisible], unpredictable, and ever-changing phenomenon ... It is an incarnation of unique patterns of the coevolving life histories of diverse entities. Histories are cocreated multidimensionally with predecessors, contemporaries, successors, ideas, objects, and events" (p. 23). Three community change concepts, which "arise from the human becoming school of thought, ... are unitary paradoxical rhythms of change" (p. 23). The community change concepts are **MOVING-INITIATING, ANCHORING-SHIFTING,** and **PONDERING-SHAPING.** Each concept is made up of various processes, or dimensions. The definitions of each concept and its dimensions are given here.

MOVING-INITIATING

- A cocreated paradoxical rhythm of community change (Parse, 2003a, p. 23).
- [Moving-Initiating] is discarding and creating all-at-once, incarnating the value priorities of community, whether community is an individual or group (Parse, 2003a, p. 23).

Moving-Initiating has nine processes, or dimensions: Tunneling, Driving, Laddering, Boating, Swimming, Submarining, Ballooning, Motorflying, and Swinging.

- **Tunneling:** Digging under, piercing the depths in cocreating situations for deliberately earthing and unearthing ideas, objects, and events (Parse, 2003a, p. 24).
- **Driving:** Forging directly with intensity in cocreating shifting patterns of diversity (Parse, 2003a, p. 24).
- **Laddering:** Climbing multidirectionally in planning and executing strategies (Parse, 2003a, p. 24).
- **Boating:** Steering while navigating the calm-turbulence of shifting waves and winds, harnessing moments of buoyancy, yet always with ambiguity (Parse, 2003a, p. 24).
- **Swimming:** Gliding with diverse currents in keeping afloat with sureness-unsureness (Parse, 2003a, p. 24).
- **Submarining:** Immersing in a high pressure enveloping

at great depth with the shifting of what is known and not yet known explicitly (Parse, 2003a, p. 24).

- **Ballooning:** Drifting vigilantly with the pattern of the whole in a buoyant surgence-release, while shifting winds cocreate the unexpected (Parse, 2003a, p. 24).
- **Motorflying:** Propelling persistently with the gravity of weaving winds (Parse, 2003a, p. 24).
- **Swinging:** Soaring in undulating suspension with gusts of shifting winds in swingshifting to and fro in a bold leaping beyond (Parse, 2003a, p. 24).

ANCHORING-SHIFTING

- A cocreated paradoxical rhythm of community change (Parse, 2003a, p. 36).
- [Anchoring-Shifting] is the persisting-diversifying that pushes-resists as community (individual or group) invents new meanings, knowing that all that was and will be is inextricably woven into the now (Parse, 2003a, p. 36).

Anchoring-Shifting has two processes, or dimensions: Savoring-Sacrificing and Revering-Liberating.

- **Savoring-Sacrificing:** Delighting in and all-at-once foregoing something of value. Savoring is relishing ideas, objects, or events that are appealing to a community, and these arise as threads of constancy. Sacrificing is giving up something originally delighted in and all-at-once taking on something else, the view of which has changed with new experiences. (Parse, 2003a, p. 37)
- **Revering-Liberating:** Honoring while all-at-once freeing. Revering is respecting others, ideas, objects, and events. Liberating is a buoyant freeing. (Parse, 2003a, p. 37)

PONDERING-SHAPING

- A cocreated paradoxical rhythm of community change (Parse, 2003a, p. 36).
- [Pondering-Shaping] is contemplating while configuring (Parse, 2003a, p. 38).

Pondering-Shaping has two processes, or dimensions: Considering-Composing and Dialoguing-Listening.

- **Considering-Composing:** Deeply contemplating while all-at-once birthing anew. Considering is ruminating or deliberating about others, ideas, objects, or events that are important for the moment. Birthing anew is creating or carving out the possibles. Imaged possibles cocreate new meanings that are languaged in composing ways of connecting-separating that reveal-conceal value priorities. (Parse, 2003a, p. 39)
- **Dialoguing-Listening:** Unconditional witnessing with all-at-once speaking-being silent and moving-being still

(Parse, 2003a, p. 39). Dialoguing with community in pondering-shaping change arises with the discourse of the commingling of personal histories (Parse, 2003a, p. 40). Listening with pondering-shaping changes arises with the astringent regard integral with coming to know something in depth while gaining an understanding, yet knowing that no understanding is absolute or complete (Parse, 2003a, p. 40).

EVALUATION OF THE THEORY OF HUMAN BECOMING

This section presents an evaluation of Parse's Theory of Human Becoming. The evaluation is based on the results of the analysis of the theory, as well as on publications by others who have used or commented on this nursing theory.

SIGNIFICANCE

The Theory of Human Becoming meets the criterion of significance. Parse explicitly identified the focus of her theory as the human-universe-health process, which she views as the phenomenon of concern for the discipline of nursing. It is obvious, then, that the theory addresses the metaparadigm concepts of human beings, environment, and health and the metaparadigm proposition of human processes of living and dying, recognizing that human beings are in a continuous relationship with their environments.

Parse explicitly identified the philosophical and conceptual foundations of her theory. She has made clear that the human sciences, existential-phenomenological philosophy, and Rogers' conceptual model of nursing were the starting points for the assumptions on which her theory is based. Moreover, she clearly stated the assumptions, categorizing them into those about the human, becoming, and human becoming. Additional assumptions were easily extracted from her discussion about methodologies for Theory of Human Becoming–based research.

Parse acknowledged the scholars from nursing and adjunctive disciplines—especially philosophers—whose works undergird her theory. With the one exception of Kafka, she listed specific citations to the works that contributed to her thinking.

A noteworthy feature of the Theory of Human Becoming is its process orientation and the emphasis on paradoxical rhythmical patterns of relating between the human and the universe. Another feature is the focus on the human's participation and connectedness with the universe in cocreating health.

The special significance of the Theory of Human Becoming lies in its contributions to understanding how people experience health from a human science perspective. As Parse (1992) pointed out, her theory is consistent with human science because its essence "is embedded in meanings, patterns in relationships, and in hopes and dreams" (p. 37).

The special significance of the theory also lies in the recognition that values play a part in health. As Parse (1992) noted, "This theory takes into consideration that human beings live their health incarnating personal values which are each individual's unique connectedness with the universe" (p. 37).

INTERNAL CONSISTENCY

The Theory of Human Becoming meets the criterion of internal consistency. The content of the theory is completely consistent with its philosophical and conceptual origins. Indeed, Mitchell and Cody (1992) pointed out that Parse's philosophical claims and the content of the theory are consistent with "human science in Dilthey's traditional sense" (p. 59). Moreover, they claimed that the theory clarifies and expands the human science approach. Furthermore, as Sarter (1988) noted, Parse's synthesis of existentialism and Rogers' conceptual model is creative as well as logically constructed and organized.

The vocabulary of the Theory of Human Becoming is congruent with the philosophical and conceptual foundations of the theory. As Parse (1997b) explained, "This theory … created new language for the discipline in keeping with the notion that all disciplines must have unique expressions to specify the nature of their phenomena of concern" (p. 33). The terminology used by Parse may, however, limit understanding of her work. Holmes (1990) commented:

> Unfortunately, [Parse's] efforts have not had the impact on nursing that might have been hoped. Their accessibility is undermined by an obscure style, a penchant for the utterly novel use of familiar words, and a large crop of ill-explained neologisms. These problems are exacerbated if the reader is not familiar with the esoteric language and idiosyncratic conceptual tools of existential phenomenologists. (p. 193)

Adding to the discussion about terminology, Wimpenny (1993) stated:

> The complexity of the language for many nurses creates an immediate barrier to comprehension and also prevents any further critique. … Addressing this can prove difficult, especially when the level of abstraction in Parse's theory is unusual among nursing theorists and stems from a base within Rogers'

science of unitary [human beings] and existential phenomenology. For me, this complexity created difficulty, not only in my understanding but in transmitting these ideas to others as a teacher (p. 10).

Also, Edwards (2000) commented, "[T]he complex terminology of the [human becoming school of thought] does not render it easily accessible, and one wonders if anything important is gained by the employment of this terminology" (p. 196).

To her credit, Parse (1998) has done just about all that a theorist can to help readers understand the context and content of the Theory of Human Becoming. She provided an exceptionally clear explanation of the historical evolution and philosophical and conceptual foundations of the theory, clear and concise definitions for each theory concept, and informative descriptions of the three principles.

More specifically, semantic clarity is evident in the explicit constitutive definitions of all concepts of the Theory of Human Becoming. Semantic consistency also is evident. Parse has been consistent in her use of terms and has attached the same meaning to terms in her various publications. Furthermore, she provided a rationale for the change in the name of the theory and the subsequent rewording of propositions.

The analysis of the Theory of Human Becoming revealed structural consistency. Parse (personal communication, April 20, 1990) described the development of her theory as both inductive and deductive, as well as "intuitive-rational" (Parse, 1997b, p. 32). The analysis indicated that the derivation of relational propositions C, D, and E from the concepts contained in three of the nonrelational propositions (Parse's Principles) follows a logical line of deductive reasoning.

Parse's (2003a) recent work on community change would benefit from elaboration, despite the inclusion of examples from practice and research. In particular, Parse's rationale for regarding both an individual and a group as community is not clear. Furthermore, a clear definition of composing within the context of the considering-composing dimension of the community change concept of pondering-shaping is not evident.

PARSIMONY

The Theory of Human Becoming meets the criterion of parsimony. The analysis revealed that the theory encompasses 13 distinct concepts, three principles, and five relational propositions. Parse's description of her theory (as cited in Takahashi, 1992; Parse, 1998) led to identification of **Human Becoming** as a distinct concept of the theory. Moreover, the decision to consider **Meaning, Rhythmicity,** and, **Transcendence** as theory concepts rather than philosophical themes was based on their integral place in the three nonrelational propositions that Parse calls **Principles** and in relational proposition A. Overall, the concepts and propositions of the Theory of Human Becoming are stated clearly and concisely.

TESTABILITY

The Theory of Human Becoming meets the criterion of testability for grand theories. Parse (1997c, 1998) regards Theory of Human Becoming–based research as "sciencing human becoming," which she defined as "the process of coming to know and understand human experiences through creative conceptualization and formal inquiry" (1997c, p. 74; 1998, p. 60). The term sciencing "is used to reflect inquiry as an ongoing process" (1998, p. 60). Creative conceptualization "is a playful process of reflecting and contemplating phenomena to imaginatively construct ideas" (1997c, p. 74). Formal inquiry "is the process of coming to know through use of specific research methodologies" (1997c, p. 74).

"Sciencing," Parse (2001a) pointed out, "is in stark contrast to science, which specifies inquiry as pursuing and achieving the absolute truth, as if there are undisputable, unchanging truths. ... The term sciencing implies that knowing is ever-changing with new experiences" (p. 1).

Two basic research methodologies have been designed specifically for the Theory of Human Becoming. The **PARSE METHOD OF BASIC RESEARCH** was introduced by Parse in 1987, and the **HUMAN BECOMING HERMENEUTIC METHOD OF BASIC RESEARCH** was introduced by Cody in 1995.

The components of the **PARSE METHOD OF BASIC RESEARCH** are identified and described in Table 13–1. The method was, as Parse (1998) pointed out, "constructed to be in harmony with and evolve from the ontological beliefs of the research tradition" (p. 61). Furthermore, the method "is an overall design of precise processes that adhere to scientific rigor[, which] specifies the order within the processes appropriate for inquiry within the research tradition" (p. 61). In particular, the **Parse Method of Basic Research** is a "phenomenological-hermeneutic method in that the universal experiences described by participants who lived them provide the source of information, and participants' descriptions are interpreted in light of the human becoming theory' (Parse, 1998, p. 63). The findings of **Parse Method of Basic Research**–based research "contribute new knowledge and understanding of human experiences" (Parse, 1998, p. 65).

The components of the **HUMAN BECOMING**

HERMENEUTIC METHOD OF BASIC RESEARCH are identified and described in Table 13–2. This method permits interpretation of literary texts from the perspective of the Theory of Human Becoming. Cody (1995) explained that he drew primarily from Gadamer (1976, 1989 [original work published 1960]) for his understanding of hermeneutics. He proposed that "hermeneutic inquiry [with literary texts] surfaces truths of vital importance to the discipline of nursing" (p. 280).

Both basic research methods were, as Barrett (1998) pointed out, designed to develop new disciplines of nursing-specific knowledge. Both methods are qualitative and inductive and are completely congruent with the philosophical foundation of the theory. Parse (1998) explicitly identified assumptions that undergird the **Parse Method of Basic Research** and Cody (1995) explicated the connections between the hermeneutic study of literary text and Parse's Theory of Human Becoming.

Edwards (2000) challenged Parse's (1998, 2001a) claim that the **Parse Method of Basic Research** and the **Human Becoming Hermeneutic Method of Basic Research** focus on entities that are "universal lived experiences of health and quality of life, meaning that all persons experience the phenomenon" (2001a, p. 165). He pointed out that "the appeal to human universals may ... be threatened by the observation of cultural diversity .... [and that] the whole idea of universals has been called into question in both philosophical literature ... and in nursing literature" (p. 196).

The **Parse Method of Basic Research** yields sufficiently in-depth descriptions of personal experiences to capture the essence of the lived experience of interest. More specifically, the method yields the structure of a lived experience. Such structures may be considered middle-range theories, as middle-range theories are defined in this book. Parse, however, refers to the structures as findings, rather than theories. She declared, "The products of Theory of Human Becoming-guided research simply are the findings of the research, the emergent meanings and the structure of the universal lived experience that was studied" (Fawcett, 2001, p. 127). Two examples of structures of lived experiences are given here.

- [The lived experience of] hope is anticipating possibilities through envisioning the not-yet in harmoniously living the comfort-discomfort of everydayness while unfolding a different perspective of an expanding view (Parse, 1990b, p. 15).
- The lived experience of considering tomorrow is contemplating desired endeavors in longing for the cherished, while intimate alliances with isolating distance emerge, as resilient endurance surfaces amid disturbing unsureness (Bunkers, 1998, p. 60).

(Text continues on page 483)

PHENOMENA FOR STUDY

Universal human health lived experiences surfacing in the human-universe process reflecting being-becoming, value priorities, and quality of life.

Descriptions are from participants.

STRUCTURE OF THE PHENOMENON TO EMERGE

The answer to the research question.

The paradoxical living of the remembered, the now moment, and the not-yet, all-at-once.

PROCESSES

Participant Selection
Persons who can describe the meaning of the experience through words, symbols, music, metaphors, poetry, photographs, drawings, or movements. Participants can be of any age, but must be able to give an authentic accounting of the lived experience of interest. Two to 10 participants are sufficient for saturation or redundancy of the data. The criterion for saturation is a pattern in the engagements repeated by a number of participants.

Dialogical Engagement
A researcher-participant discussion that is not an interview in the traditional sense, but rather requires the researcher to be in true presence with the participant.

The researcher centers before the engagement with each participant.

The researcher obtains a signed consent for protection of participants.

The dialogue is audiotaped and, if possible, videotaped. Tapes are transcribed for later analysis.

The researcher opens the dialogue with a comment such as "Please tell me about your experience of …"

The researcher enters the flow with each participant and remains in true presence without interjecting questions. The researcher may, however, move the discussion by saying something such as "Go on" or "Please explain more about your experience of …"

Extraction-Synthesis
The researcher extracts and synthesizes essences from transcribed and recorded descriptions in the participant's language by dwelling with the transcribed audiotaped and videotaped dialogues in deep concentration.

The researcher synthesizes and extracts essences in his or her language to form a structure of the experience.

The researcher formulates a proposition from each participant's essences.

The researcher extracts and synthesizes core concepts from the formulated propositions of all participants.

The researcher synthesizes a structure of the lived experience from the core concepts. The result is movement of the descriptions of the lived experience from the language of the participants up the levels of abstraction to the language of science.

Heuristic Interpretation
The researcher weaves the structure of the lived experience with the Theory of Human Becoming and beyond through structural transposition and conceptual integration.

Structural transposition involves connecting the synthesized structure to the Theory of Human Becoming, which results in moving the structure of the lived experience up another level of abstraction.

Conceptual integration further specifies the structure of the lived experience by using concepts of the theory to create a unique theoretical structure that represents the meaning of the lived experience at the level of the theory.

Source: Constructed from Parse, 1987, p. 175; 1990b, pp. 10–11; 1997a, p. 33; 1998, pp. 64–65.

TABLE 13–2
THE HUMAN BECOMING HERMENEUTIC METHOD OF BASIC RESEARCH

PHENOMENA FOR STUDY

Universal human health lived experiences.

Descriptions are from published texts.

STRUCTURE OF THE PHENOMENON TO EMERGE

The answer to the research question.

Emergent meanings from literary texts.

PROCESSES

Participant Selection
A published literary work.

The sentences of a literary text are the fundamental unit of interpretation.

Each sentence consists essentially of an identifier (noun) and a predicate (verb).

Each sentence is understood in the context of its literal meaning and in the context of its figurative meaning.

Discoursing with Penetrating Engaging
A text, as something written and read, is a form of discourse. Author and reader are discoursing whenever the text is read.

The researcher engages in the interplay of shared and unshared meanings through which beliefs are appropriated and disappropriated.

The researcher fuses horizons when he or she assigns meaning to the text through appropriating and disappropriating beliefs.

The researcher identifies truths that emerge from the researcher-text dialectic.

Interpreting with Quiescent Beholding
The researcher expands the meaning moment through dwelling in situated openness with the disclosed and the hidden.

The researcher interprets the text by constructing meanings with the text through the rhythmical moment-to-moment movement between the language of the text and his or her own language. The process involves questioning and answering and questioning anew.

Understanding with Inspiring Envisaging
The researcher chooses from the possibles a unique way of moving beyond the meaning moment.

The researcher's understanding of a text is interweaving the meaning of the text with the pattern of his or her life in a chosen way.

Disseminating Possibilities
The researcher sets in text for publication his or her interpretation of the author's perspective, offering it as a possibility for the enhancement of nursing science.

Source: Constructed from Cody, 1995, pp. 275–281; Parse, 1998, p. 66; 2001a, p. 172.

(Text continued from page 481)

Still another approach to sciencing human becoming was mentioned by Parse (1987, 1992). She indicated that relational propositions C, D, and E of the Theory of Human Becoming, which she calls theoretical structures, can be used to guide research designed to generate what are referred to in this book as middle-range theories, and what Parse (1992) referred to as "lower level[s] of discourse to guide research or practice" (p. 39). That is accomplished by deriving propositions at a lower level of abstraction from the Theory of Human Becoming relational propositions and then selecting universal lived experiences for study. The three examples of middle-range theory propositions derived from the relational propositions of the Theory of Human Becoming that are listed here were constructed from examples given by Parse (1987, p. 170; 1992, p. 39; 1998, p. 55).

- Theory of Human Becoming proposition: Powering emerges with the revealing-concealing of imaging.
  - Derived middle-range theory proposition: Struggling toward goals discloses and hides the significance of situations.

- Theory of Human Becoming proposition: Originating emerges with the enabling-limiting of valuing.
  - Derived middle-range theory proposition: Creating anew shows one's cherished beliefs and leads in a directional movement.

- Theory of Human Becoming proposition: Transforming emerges with the languaging of connecting-separating.
  - Derived middle-range theory proposition: Changing views emerge in speaking and moving with others.

Concept inventing is yet another method of research that flows from the Theory of Human Becoming. Parse (1997a) defined concept inventing as "a multidimensional all-at-once process of analyzing-synthesizing, bringing to life novel unitary concepts" (p. 63). She explained:

> Concept inventing does not occur in a step-by-step linear fashion but, rather, entails the rational-intuitive origination of a unique synthetic definition of an idea surfacing from the beliefs and values of the scholar who is creating the concept. These beliefs and values shine through the process like luminaries leading the search through a labyrinth of ambiguity that is always present when moving with something new. (p. 63)

The idea for inventing a concept arises not from study participants' descriptions of their lived experiences but rather from the researcher's "interpretation of general and nursing literature, nursing practice situations, art, photography, architecture, rhythmic movements, metaphor, music, stories described in files, and other media" (Parse, 1997a, p. 63). Bournes (2000) explained that her ideas about the concept of having courage arose as she dwelled with "ideas, metaphors, and situations that arose with reviewing existing literature about the phenomenon courage, and by engaging in discussions with individuals who were willing to share their thoughts about the phenomenon" (p. 145). Wang (2000) used a Taiwanese folk song as the source of concept inventing for her interpretation of the concept of hope.

EMPIRICAL ADEQUACY

The Theory of Human Becoming meets the criterion of empirical adequacy for grand theories. The **Parse Method of Basic Research** has been used to guide many studies (Table 13–3), and the **Human Becoming Hermeneutic Method of Basic Research** has been employed for four

published studies to date (Table 13–3). Parse's (1997a) concept inventing method has been used to guide two published studies to date (Table 13–3). A translinguistic basic research project designed to identify the lived experience of hope by a total of 130 people in nine countries—Australia, Canada, Finland, Italy, Japan, Sweden, Taiwan, United Kingdom, United States—as expressed in the people's native languages, is worthy of special mention (see Table 13–3). An informative extension of that work is Parse's (2003b) interpretation of the study of hope as expressed by Native Americans (Kelley, 1999) within the context of her community change concepts.

In addition, various qualitative research methods borrowed from other disciplines, such as descriptive exploratory methods from the social sciences, phenomenological methods from existential phenomenological psychology, and ethnographic methods from anthropology were used initially and continue to be used to study universal lived experiences of health (see Table 13–3), which are the phenomena of particular interest for sciencing human becoming (Fawcett, 2001; Parse, 1998). A review of the results of all of these Theory of Human Becoming–based published studies (Table 13–3), as well as the master's theses and doctoral dissertations listed in the chapter bibliography on the CD-ROM, revealed that new middle-range descriptive theories of universal human health lived experiences were generated. These middle-range theories, or what Parse (Fawcett, 2001) calls findings, represent descriptions of personal experiences that are congruent with the concepts and propositions of the Theory of Human Becoming.

PRAGMATIC ADEQUACY

The Theory of Human Becoming meets the criterion of pragmatic adequacy. Parse has stated the need for special education before use of the theory in practice, and she has delineated a specific approach for practice.

Nursing Education

Use of the Theory of Human Becoming requires special education. This is because nursing practice based on the theory "is a different kind of nursing. It is not offering professional advice and opinions stemming from the personal value system of the nurse. It is not a canned approach to cure. It is a subject-to-subject interrelationship, a loving, true presence with the other to promote health and the quality of life" (Parse, 1987, p. 169).

Consequently, the nurse must learn to avoid making judgments about or labeling individuals' ways of being,

(Text continues on page 489)

Lived Experience	Participants	Citation*
[†]Lived experience of feeling loved	Women parolees residing in a shelter	Baumann, 2000
[†]Hope	Persons on hemodialysis	Parse, 1990
[†]Lived experience of hope	Women, 30 years old or older, from the Southern, Midwestern, or Eastern United States, who had children	Allchin-Petardi, 1999
	Sioux Indian Nation men and women 46–78 years old residing in South Dakota	Kelley, 1999b; Parse, 2003a
	Homeless men and women 25–50 years old in South Dakota and Illinois	Bunkers, 1999
	African-American and Caucasian women residing in a shelter in North Carolina	Cody & Filler, 1999
	African-American or Latina/Latino children 4–13 years old, living in a shelter or other supported facility in New York	Bauman, 1999
	Individuals of various ethnic backgrounds residing in a chronic care facility in Canada	Parse, 1999
	Individuals of various ethnic backgrounds living with coronary artery disease and relatives of individuals who had coronary artery disease, residing in Australia	Bunkers & Daly, 1999
	Men 59–80 years old living in a leprosarium in Taiwan	Wang, 1999
	Japanese men and women 20–70 years old	Takahashi, 1999
	Finnish men and women 18–83 years old	Toikkanen & Muurinen, 1999
	Swedish men and women 74–91 years old	Willman, 1999
	Italian men and women 21–60 years old	Zanotti & Bournes, 1999
	Welsh men and women 30–75 years old	Pilkington & Miller, 1999
Analysis of the concept of hope[#]	A Taiwanese folk song	Wang, 2000
Analysis of the concept of having courage[#]	Published literature Discussion with individuals	Bournes, 2000
[†]Lived experience of having courage	Individuals with spinal cord injuries	Bournes, 2002a, 2003
Laughter	Persons older than 65 years	Parse, 1993
Laughing and health[†]	Persons older than 65 years	Parse, 1994
Joy-sorrow[†]	Women older than 65 years	Parse, 1997
Lived experience of contentment[†]	Women older than 65 years who volunteer in community projects in a large metropolitan setting in North America	Parse, 2001a, 2001b

*See the Research section of the chapter references for complete citations.
[†]Used the Parse Method of Basic Research.
[#]Used Parse's method of concept inventing.

(continued)

Lived Experience	Participants	Citation*
Lived experience of feeling very tired[†]	Women older than 65 years who volunteer in community projects in a large metropolitan setting in North America	Parse, 2003b; Bunkers, 2003
	Men and women living in the southern region of the United States	Huch & Bournes, 2003; Bunkers, 2003
	Girls attending a suburban public high school in the northeast region of the United States	Baumann, 2003; Bunkers, 2003
Experience of living with the consequences of personal choices[†]	Persons diagnosed with diabetes	Mitchell & Lawton, 2000
Lived experience of the struggle of trying to change health patterns[†]	Women living in an abusive relationship	Pilkington, 2000a
Lived experience of bowel obstruction	Patients with bowel obstruction due to gynecological or gastric cancer	Gwilliam, & Bailey, 2001
Meaning of severe visual impairment	Older women diagnosed with macular degeneration	Moore, 2000
Health	Oldest-old persons living in the community	Wondolowski & Davis, 1991
Quality of life[†]	Persons with diabetes mellitus	Mitchell, 1998
	Men and women who had had a stroke	Pilkington, 2000b
	Men and women with Alzheimer's disease	Parse, 1996
Description of quality of life	Men and women living with stroke	Dawson, 2000
Quality of life[†]	Patients receiving acute psychiatric care	Fisher & Mitchell, 1998
Case study of changes in quality of life	Patients suffering from genital herpes	Kelley, 1999a
Meaning of serenity[†]	Survivors of cancer	Kruse, 1999
Rest	Young adults confined to bed for 2.5 hours	Smith, 1989
Choosing life goals	Married women nurse administrators	Costello-Nickitas, 1994
Wanting to help another[†]	Nurses whose practice incorporated nontraditional modalities	Mitchell & Heidt, 1994
Feeling understood[†]	A woman with cerebral palsy	Jonas-Simpson, 1997
Lived experience of being overweight	Overweight women and men	Overgaard, 2002
Perceptions of living with a chronic illness, using masterworks of art as a center point for dialogue	Nurses Students Chronically ill elderly individuals	Hodges et al., 2001

[†]Used the Parse Method of Basic Research.

Persistent pain	Persons living with persistent pain	Carson & Mitchell, 1998
Experiences with nurses	Hospitalized persons older than 65 years	Janes & Wells, 1997
Struggling through a difficult time[†]	Unemployed persons	Smith, 1990
Persevering through a difficult time[†]	Women with ovarian cancer	Allchin-Petardi, 1998
Struggling with going along in a situation you do not believe in[†]	Members of the American Academy of Nursing	Kelley, 1991
Meaning of fathering	Fathers of children with congenital anomalies	Baumann & Braddick, 1999
Feeling uncomfortable[†]	Children residing in shelters	Baumann, 1996
Having no place of their own	Mothers and children in emergency shelters	Baumann, 1994
Considering tomorrow[†]	Homeless women	Bunkers, 1998
Experience of waiting	Women hospitalized during pregnancy	Thornburg, 2002
Essences of the experience of waiting for persons who have family members or friends in a critical care unit[†]	Female and male family members of persons admitted to an adult medical-surgical critical care unit in a large teaching hospital in Canada	Bournes & Mitchell, 2002
Smoking cessation	Korean adolescents	Kim et al., 1998
Recovering from addiction	Recovering addicts	Banonis, 1989
Experience of coronary angiography	Individuals undergoing coronary angiography in Sweden	Stoltz & Willman, 2001
Relentless drive to be ever thinner	Young adult women	Santopinto, 1989
Meaning of time passing[†]	Men with HIV	Northrup, 2002
Living with acquired immunodeficiency syndrome (AIDS)	Persons with AIDS	Nokes & Carver, 1991
Suffering[†]	Persons in the general population	Daly, 1995
Grieving[†]	Persons grieving a personal loss (death, close relationship)	Cody, 1991
	Families living with AIDS	Cody, 1995b, 1995c
	Mothers who lost their babies at birth	Pilkington, 1993
Retirement	Italian communally living retired performing artists	Davis & Cannava, 1995
Aging	Scottish community-dwelling oldest-old persons	Futrell et al., 1993
	Spanish community-dwelling elders	Rendon et al., 1995
	Oldest-old persons living in the community in the United States	Wondolowski & Davis, 1988
Meaning of later life	Canadian persons 65 years or older	Mitchell, 1993
Phenomenon of feeling understood[†]	Women living with enduring health situations	Jonas-Simpson, 2001

[†]Used the Parse Method of Basic Research.

(continued)

Lived Experience	Participants	Citation
Structure of the lived experience of being listened to[†]	Older women receiving in-patient rehabilitation	Jonas-Simpson, 2003
Lived experience of autonomy	Elderly women who shared a household with a family member	Major & Pepin, 2001
Being a senior	Canadian persons 65 years or older	Mitchell, 1994
Taking life day by day[†]	Canadian persons older than 75 years	Mitchell, 1990
Being an elder	Nepalese persons 50 years or older	Jonas, 1992
Restriction of freedom in later life[†]	Persons 75 years or older	Mitchell, 1995b
Meaning of caring for an elderly relative	Middle-aged and older adults who cared for an older family member	Gates, 2000
Feeling restricted[†]	Institutionalized older adults	Heine, 1991
Spiritual perspectives	Mental heath nurses	Pullen et al., 1996
Description of the meaning of advocacy	Hospital-based nurse case managers	Hellwig et al., 2003
What it means to be human[‡]	Literary text: Walt Whitman's poems in *Leaves of Grass*	Cody, 1995a
Examination of bearing witness[‡]	Literary text: Script of the play, "Cat on a Hot Tin Roof"	Cody, 2001
Identification of meanings about human experiences[‡]	Literary text: Thomas Hegg's poem, "A Cup of Christmas Tea"	Baumann et al., 2001
Exploration of the meaning of lingering presence[‡]	Literary text: Letters in the book, *A Promise to Remember: The NAMES Project Book of Letters*	Ortiz, 2003
Mutuality	Literature: Selected journal articles and book chapters	Curley, 1997
A synthesis and discussion of six studies of use of the theory of human becoming in practice	Research reports	Bournes, 2002b
Relation of individual, dyadic, and family variables to perception of risk for sexually transmitted diseases	Sexually active, unmarried, heterosexual women, 17–26 years old	Hutchinson, 1999
Relation of social support and obtaining a mammogram	Women who had and had not undergone mammography screening	Fite et al., 1996; Fite & Frank, 1996
Effectiveness of therapeutic touch, healing touch, Reiki, and reflexology for reduction of stress and pain	Adult females having knee surgery	Scales, 2001

[†]Used the Parse Method of Basic Research.
[‡]Used the Human Becoming Hermeneutic Method of Basic Research.

(Text continued from page 484)

thinking, or feeling. "It is," according to Parse (1992), "essential to go with the person where the person is rather than attempting to judge, change, or control the person" (p. 40).

Moreover, nursing practice based on the Theory of Human Becoming requires considerable grounding in the basic tenets and vocabulary of existential phenomenology and the use of that vocabulary in the theory. Indeed, "one unfamiliar with existential phenomenology may initially have difficulty with Parse's terminology" (Phillips, 1987, p. 195). Bunkers (2000) provided a novel aid to comprehension of the vocabulary of the Theory of Human Becoming in her collection of poems, each of which was illustrated in a painting by her daughter.

In addition, students and practicing nurses must learn to interpret the content of the Theory of Human Becoming through the **PRACTICE METHODOLOGY** (see Table 13–4, later in this section). Furthermore, students and nurses who plan to use the Theory of Human Becoming to guide basic research must understand the **Parse Method of Basic Research** (see Table 13–1), the **Human Becoming Hermeneutic Method of Basic Research** (see Table 13–2), or both, as well as Parse's (1997a) method of concept inventing.

Parse (as cited in Bournes, 1997) noted that in her 1998 book, she did not specify "whether nursing education should begin at the baccalaureate or master's level but my learning these days is that perhaps nursing should be at the master's level—at least" (p. 2). Later, Parse (Fawcett, 2001) commented,

> I would like to see at least the master's level as the entry level. However, I think that is not going to be possible for a while; I don't know if it will ever be possible. But in order to be with people in a special way related to the human-universe-health process, no matter what theory or framework, our entry level should be the post-baccalaureate level, just as in medicine and law. Students then would come to nursing with a solid undergraduate liberal arts and sciences background, and we could teach them nursing, not medical science. At the master's level, then, for the Human Becoming theory, the students would learn the meaning of structuring meaning, cocreating rhythms, cotranscending the possibles—as the content of the courses, rather than diseases and other areas of the medical model. (p. 131)

Any nursing curriculum, according to Parse (as cited in Takahashi, 1992), should be based on educational theories of the teaching-learning process, and the substantive content of the curriculum should be nursing theories and frameworks. Elaborating, she explained, "Nursing theories and frameworks should not be the curriculum plan; the curriculum plan should be designed on an education theory since that comes from the science of education, but the substantive content to be taught is nursing science"

(p. 89). Several years later, Parse (Fawcett, 2001) declared that "nursing students at all levels of education should be taught the frameworks and theories of the discipline. The Human Becoming School of Thought could be the focus of nursing curricula where faculty espouses the beliefs congruent with the assumptions and principles" (p. 131).

Jacono and Jacono (1996) commented that use of the Theory of Human Becoming in a nursing curriculum can enhance both student and faculty creativity. They explained that the faculty "would help students see the many possible meanings which could be assigned to situations, and help them accept personal responsibility for assigning those meanings that they choose to situations" (p. 357). Moreover, they pointed out that as faculty members pause to contemplate the content and use of the Theory of Human Becoming, they will increase their own creativity in the teaching-learning process.

The Theory of Human Becoming has begun to be used as a guide for nursing education programs. Parse (1998) presented a detailed description of a master's degree program grounded in the Theory of Human Becoming. She specified the philosophy, program goals, program indicators, conceptual framework, themes, course content, instructional strategies, and evaluation strategies. That program was designed to prepare students for specialization in family health, with role concentrations in teaching nursing and administering nursing services. No published reports of the implementation of Parse's plan for a master's program were located. Bunkers (1999), however, described the Theory of Human Becoming as one central focus for the undergraduate and graduate nursing curricula at Augustana College in Sioux Falls, South Dakota. Furthermore, Milton (2001) described the Theory of Human Becoming-based master's program at Olivet Nazarene University in Bourbonnais, Illinois. And, Saltmarche, Kolodny, and Mitchell (1998) and Linscott, Spée, Flint, and Fisher (1999) described a Theory of Human Becoming-based continuing education course offered at Sunnybrook Health Sciences Center, in Toronto, Ontario, Canada.

Nursing Practice

Parse (1987) pointed out that "practice is the empirical life of [a] theory, which means that the practice of one theory would be very different from the practice of another" (p. 166). Accordingly, she developed a **PRACTICE METHODOLOGY** that is directly derived from and consistent with the Theory of Human Becoming (Table 13–4). The **Practice Methodology** encompasses three dimensions and three processes that are directly derived from the three principles of the Theory of Human Becoming. The dimensions are **Illuminating Meaning, Synchronizing Rhythms,** and **Mobilizing Transcendence.** The processes, which are empirical activities, are *Explicating, Dwelling With,* and *Moving Beyond.* Several reports of the application of the **Practice Methodology** for the Theory of Human Becoming have been published (Table 13–5).

The **Practice Methodology** dimension of **Illuminating Meaning,** which is derived from Principle 1, structuring meaning multidimensionally, occurs through the empirical activity of *Explicating.* **Illuminating Meaning** draws attention to the "unique ways in which generational and contemporary family interrelationships cocreate lived values. … [and focuses] on mobilizing family energies for structuring and languaging different meanings in light of family health possibilities" (Parse, 1981, p. 81). When using the empirical activity of *Explicating,* the nurse invites the person or family to relate the meaning of the situation by sharing thoughts and feelings with themselves, the nurse, and others in nurse-family-community situations. *Explicating,* according to Parse (1998), "sheds a new light on situations, and often the thoughts and feelings discussed have been lying dormant beneath the surface for some time. Articulation of such thoughts connected with the moment in the presence of the nurse may surface with *ah-has,* which are ways of viewing the familiar in a new light" (p. 70).

The dimension of **Synchronizing Rhythms,** which is derived from Principle 2, cocreating rhythmical patterns, happens through the empirical activity of *Dwelling With.* **Synchronizing Rhythms,** Parse (1987) explained, "happens in dwelling with the pitch, yaw, and roll of the interhuman cadence—the turning, spinning, and thrusting of human relationships. Pitch, yaw, and roll represent the ups and downs, the struggles, the moments of joy, the unevenness of day-to-day living" (p. 168).

When engaging in the empirical activity of *Dwelling With,* the nurse stays with the person or family as each person describes the rhythms of his or her life and the family's life. Through discussion, the nurse can lead the family "to recognize the harmony that exists within its own lived context. There is always a way to find the harmony in what appears to be the conflict in the spinning and turning of human relationships" (Parse, 1987, p. 168). "Awareness of patterns of relating," Parse (1981) claimed, "enhances opportunities for the changing of health patterns" (p. 82).

The dimension of **Mobilizing Transcendence,** which is derived from Principle 3, cotranscending with the possibles, is realized through the empirical activity of *Moving Beyond.* **Mobilizing Transcendence,** according to Parse (1987), happens "through moving beyond the meaning moment to what is not yet. It focuses on dreaming of the possibles and planning to reach for the dreams" (p. 169).

When engaged in the empirical activity of *Moving Beyond,* the nurse "guides individuals and families to plan for the changing of lived health patterns—these patterns uncovered in the illuminating of meaning, synchronizing of rhythms, and mobilizing of transcendence" (Parse, 1987, p. 169). Parse (1981) claimed that **Mobilizing Transcendence** through *Moving Beyond* results in "mobilizing family energies in reflectively choosing shifts in viewpoints relative to the possibilities available in the changing health process" (p. 82).

The use of the **Practice Methodology** requires the nurse to practice the interpersonal art of being truly present with a person or group. **True presence** is grounded in knowledge of the Theory of Human Becoming and in the belief that each person knows "the way" somewhere within himself or herself. Elaborating, Parse (1990a) stated, "The true presence of the nurse is a nonroutinized, nonmechanical way of 'being with' in which the nurse is authentic and attentive to moment-to-moment changes in meaning for the person or group" (p. 139).

Furthermore, "True presence is a powerful human-universe connection experienced at all realms of the universe. … [It] is a free-flowing attentiveness that does not arise from trying to attend to the other, because *trying to* is a distraction that demands a focus away from the other" (Parse, 1998, p. 71). Rather, what Parse (1998) calls *Coming-to-be-Present* requires preparation and attention. The nurse then enters the person's or group's world in **True Presence** through *Face-to-Face Discussions, Silent Immersion,* and *Lingering Presence.* When in **True Presence** with a nurse, people can change their health patterns through *Creative Imagining, Affirming Personal Becoming,* and *Glimpsing the Paradoxical* (see Table 13–4).

Parse (1987) pointed out that the middle-range theory propositions derived from the Theory of Human Become which are listed in the Testability section of this chapter, can serve as relatively concrete guides for nursing practice. The proposition, Struggling toward goals discloses and hides the significance of situations, guides practice by focusing on "illuminating the process of revealing-concealing unique ways a person and family can mobilize transcendence in considering new dreams, to image new possibles" (p. 170). Elaborating, she explained that, in a nurse-family process, members share their thoughts and feelings about a situation, which both tells and does not tell all they know in the continuous struggle to meet personal goals. In disclosing the significance of the situation, the meaning of it changes for the family members, thus for the family. (p. 170)

The proposition, Creating anew shows one's cherished beliefs and leads in a directional movement, guides practice by dealing with "illuminating ways of being alike and different from others in changing values" (Parse, 1987, p.

170). Here, "in a nurse-family process, by synchronizing rhythms, the members uncover the opportunities and limitations created by the decisions made in choosing irreplaceable ways of being together. The choices of new ways of being together mobilizes transcendence" (Parse, 1987, p. 170).

The proposition, Changing views emerge in speaking and moving with others, guides practice by focusing on "illuminating meaning of relating ways of being together as various changing perspectives shed different light on the familiar, which gives rise to new possibles" (Parse, 1987, p. 170). In this case, family members "relate their values through speech and movement; thus views change and through mobilizing transcendence ways of relating change. When changing views are talked about among family members new possibles are seen and thus the ways of relating among family members change" (Parse, 1987, p. 170).

In addition to the practice applications listed in Table 13–5, projects designed to implement the Theory of Human Becoming in health-care organizations have been evaluated using variations of Parse's PREPROJECT-PROCESS-POSTPROJECT DESCRIPTIVE QUALITATIVE METHOD OF APPLIED RESEARCH (Table 13–6), and the reports have been published (Table 13–7). The PREPROJECT-PROCESS-POSTPROJECT DESCRIPTIVE QUALITATIVE METHOD OF APPLIED RE-

(Text continues on page 494)

TABLE 13–4
THE PRACTICE METHODOLOGY FOR THE THEORY OF HUMAN BECOMING

PART 1

Theory of Human Becoming Principle	Practice Methodology Dimension	Practice Methodology Process (Empirical Activity)
PRINCIPLE 1: Structuring meaning multidimensionally	**Illuminating Meaning:** Explicating what was, is, and will be.	*Explicating:* Making clear what is appearing now through languaging.
PRINCIPLE 2: Cocreating rhythmical patterns	**Synchronizing Rhythms:** Dwelling with the pitch, yaw, and roll of the human-universe process.	*Dwelling With:* Immersing with the flow of connecting-separating.
PRINCIPLE 3: Mobilizing transcendence	**Mobilizing Transcendence:** Moving beyond the meaning moment with what is not-yet.	*Moving Beyond:* Propelling with envisioned possibles of transforming

PART 2

Contexts for Nursing
Nurse-person situations
Nurse-group situations
    Participants: Children, Adults
      Locations: Homes, shelters, health care centers, parish halls, all departments of hospitals and clinics, rehabilitation
        centers, offices, other milieus where nurses are with people

Goal of the Discipline of Nursing
Quality of life from the person's, family's, and community's perspective.

Goal of the Human Becoming Nurse
To be truly present with people as they enhance their quality of life.

True Presence
A special way of "being with" in which the nurse is attentive to moment-to-moment changes in meaning as she or he bears witness to the person's or group's own living of value priorities.

(continued)

▶ ◀   **TABLE 13–4**
THE PRACTICE METHODOLOGY FOR THE THEORY OF HUMAN BECOMING *(Continued)*

Coming-to-be-Present
An all-at-once gentling down and lifting up.
True presence begins in the coming-to-be-present moments of preparation and attention.
Preparation involves:
    An emptying to be available to bear witness to the other or others.
    Being flexible, not fixed but gracefully present from one's center.
    Dwelling with the universe at the moment, considering the attentive presence about to be.
Attention involves focusing on the moment at hand for immersion.

Face-to-Face Discussions
Nurse and person engage in dialogue.
The nurse tries to understand the person's perspective by initiating discussions using questions such as:
    How are you doing?
    How are things going?
    How was your day (or night)?
    What is life like for you?
    What is most important to you at this time?
    What do you need most right now?
Conversation may be through discussion in general or through interpretations of stories, films, drawings,
    photographs, music, metaphors, poetry, rhythmical movements, and other expressions.
The nurse really listens to the person, without interrupting.
The nurse may seek clarification through such statements as:
    Tell me more about that.
    What does … mean for you?
    What is it like for you to life with … ?
    What do you see yourself doing?
    What can you do to get help?
    What might help you to go on?
    What do you hope happens?

Silent Immersion
A process of the quiet that does not refrain from sending and receiving messages.

A chosen way of becoming in the human-universe process lived in the rhythm of speaking—being silent,
    moving—being still as valued images incarnate meaning.

True presence without words.

Lingering Presence
Recalling a moment through a lingering presence that arises after an immediate engagement.

A reflective-prereflective "abiding with" attended to through glimpses of the other person, idea, object, or situation.

Ways of Changing Health Patterns in True Presence

Creative Imagining
Picturing, by seeing, hearing, and feeling, what a situation might be like if lived in a different way.

Affirming Personal Becoming
Uncovering preferred personal health patterns by critically thinking about how or who one is.

Glimpsing the Paradoxical
Changing one's view of a situation by recognizing incongruities in that situation.

Source: Constructed from Parse, 1998, pp. 69–75; Pilkington, 1999, p. 5

TABLE 13–5
PUBLISHED REPORTS OF NURSING PRACTICE GUIDED BY THE THEORY OF HUMAN BECOMING

Practice Situation	Population	Citation*
Nurse-Person		
	Children in a school-based mental health program	Galligan, 2000
	Hospitalized adolescents	Arndt, 1995
	An adolescent male with cancer	Melnechenko, 1995
	A woman in her home, parish nursing	Bunkers, 1998
	A woman at a community center	Mitchell, 1993
	A 24-year-old woman grieving for her stillborn baby	Pilkington, 1997
	A 29-year-old woman with cervical cancer	G.J. Mitchell, 2002
	Persons with cancer considering treatment options	Plank, 1994
	A woman receiving dialysis	M.G. Mitchell, 2002
	An adult male with diabetes	G. J. Mitchell, 2002
	Adults, perioperative nursing	Andrus, 1995; Markovic, 1997; Mitchell & Copplestone, 1990
	Adults, orthopedic nursing	Balcombe et al., 1991
	A man with a heart transplant	Liehr, 1989
	A man at a rehabilitation center after a stroke	Mitchell, 1993
	A hospitalized elderly woman	Mitchell, 1986
	An elderly woman with terminal cancer	Mitchell, 1991
	A 45-year-old South Korean woman with rectal cancer, dying in a hospice	Lee & Pilkington, 1999
	Dying persons	Jonas, 1995; Jonas-Simpson, 1996
	Confused older adults	Mattice & Mitchell, 1991
	A woman with Alzheimer's disease	Mitchell, 1996a
	An elderly person in a home for the aged	Mitchell, 1988
	An elderly woman in a retirement home	Bunkers, 1996b
	A woman in a nursing home	Mitchell, 1996b
	Older adults in the community	Baumann, 1997
	Persons living with dementia	Jonas-Simpson, 2001
	Women in a drop-in center designed as a safe place for women and families to gather	Josephson, 2000
	Women living with violence	Smith, 2002
	A homeless woman	Bunkers, 1996a
	A homeless woman's personal report of her experience of nursing practice guided by the Human Becoming Theory	Williamson, 2000

*See the Practice section of the chapter references for complete citations.

(continued)

Practice Situation	Population	Citation*
Nurse-person		
	Homeless persons	Rasmusson, 1995; Rasmusson et al., 1991
	Persons living with human immunodeficiency virus (HIV) disease/acquired immunodeficiency syndrome (AIDS)	Relf, 1997
	Persons experiencing music	Jonas, 1994; Mavely & Mitchell, 1994
	A man who immigrated to the United States from Sudan	Letcher, 2000
Nurse-family		
as	A child and family	Cody et al., 1995
	Families living with HIV disease	Cody, 1995
	A family facing the death of a member	Butler, 1988
	A family living with unrest	Smith, 1989
	Abused women and their families	Butler & Snodgrass, 1991
Nurse-group		
	Persons with genital herpes in a community-based group	Kelley, 1995
Application of Human Becoming Community Change Concepts		
	A 24-year-old woman and her three children living in a shelter for homeless women and children	Cody, 2003

(continued from page 491)

SEARCH is distinctive in that the methodology is completely qualitative. Furthermore, the method is compatible with the concepts and propositions of the Theory of Human Becoming.

A review of the published reports reveals that the Theory of Human Becoming has been applied in many real world nursing practice situations with diverse populations. Although her claim may be too sweeping, Hickman (2002) declared, "Parse's theory of human becoming focuses on the lived experiences of ... human beings and therefore is applicable to all individuals, families, and communities, at all times, and in all contexts" (p. 444). In a more tempered summary, G.J. Mitchell (2002) commented, "Although not widely adopted, the theory is providing meaningful options for nursing in the twenty-first century. ... People are recognizing that the human becoming theory is a fitting guide for practitioners who want to create respectful partnerships with people seeking healthcare" (p. 539).

In addition to the situations listed in Table 13–5 and the

health-care organizations listed in Table 13–7, the Theory of Human Becoming also has been used to guide the delivery of the Rainbow PRISM Model of community health nursing services offered by the Nursing Center for Health Promotion, a nurse-managed free clinic serving the residents of a shelter for homeless women and children in Charlotte, North Carolina (Cody, 2003). Furthermore, The Health Action Model for Partnership in Community, which is in operation in Sioux Falls, South Dakota, is based on the Human Becoming School of Thought and reflects Parse's (2003a) ideas about community change (Bunkers, 2003; Bunkers, Nelson, Leuning, Crane, & Josephson, 1999).

Furthermore, M.G. Mitchell (2002) explained that the standards of nursing practice at Sunnybrook and Women's College Health Sciences Centre in Toronto, Canada, have been based on the Human Becoming School of Thought since 1995. The standards, which are based on the premise of patient-focused care, encourage "health care providers to respond to patients' wishes, needs and concerns ...

494

[and] have led the way for nurses and other health care professionals to begin the processes of listening and dialoguing in a new way" (p. 48).

Moreover, Spée (2000) and McLeod and Spée (2003) explained how nursing practice policies changed when the Human Becoming School of Thought was implemented in the Long Term and Veterans Care Directorate at Sunnybrook and Women's College Health Sciences Centre in Toronto, Ontario, Canada. McLeod and Spée (2003) explained that as nursing practice "moved from the traditional mechanistic model to a patient-focused model based on the values and beliefs of the human becoming school of thought ... we have participated in the struggles of professional nurses to identify what values they hold most dear, to choose how they will practice, who's definitions of *harm* they will listen to, and what actions they will take to support self-determination" (p. 119).

The feasibility of implementing practice protocols that reflect the Theory of Human Becoming by nurses who know the theory well is evident in these publications. Also, it is clear that nurses have the legal ability to implement those protocols and measure the effectiveness of theory-based nursing actions.

The reports of the implementation projects (see Table 13–7) indicate that several resources are required for successful implementation of Theory of Human Becoming–based practice in a health-care organization. These resources include "(a) the presence of a consistent, on-site, master's or doctorally prepared facilitator knowledgeable in the theory; (b) the allocation of resources necessary for learning; (c) the endorsement of Parse theory-based practice by management personnel; and (d) administrative support for continued educational opportunities related to Parse's theory of human becoming" (Northrup & Cody, 1998, p. 30).

Another resource is a coherent, easy-to-use set of documentation tools. Some such tools are available in a booklet published by the Nursing Council at Sunnybrook Health Science Centre, titled *Patient Focused Care: Sailing Beyond the Boundaries* (Bournes & Mitchell, 1997). Another documentation tool, the Human Becoming in Practice Sample Documentation Format, was devised by Parse (2001a, p. 178).

The extent to which nursing practice based on the Theory of Human Becoming is compatible with expectations for nursing practice and the actual results of its use have begun to be examined (see Table 13–7). Taken together, the findings of the implementation projects, all of which took place in the Canadian health-care organizations, revealed socially meaningful, favorable results that are compatible with expectations. In particular, nurses who gained knowledge of the Theory of Human Becoming and applied the theory in practice experienced personal trans-

formations in their thinking about nursing and themselves as nurses. Those personal transformations were reflected in "an enhanced respect for and concern with people as self-determining human beings [who] pursue and create their chosen way of being with the world" (Northrup & Cody, 1998, p. 29). Pilkington (1999) added,

> [N]urses ... report that [use of the Theory of Human Becoming] changes everything, not only for patients, but also, for them as care providers. People feel honored and respected, and they have chance to clarify the meaning of situations for themselves. In doing so, they also clarify their perspective for the nurse, which helps in better addressing person's needs and expectations. Clarifying the meaning of situations provides persons with opportunities to see things differently and to make choices about how to proceed. (p. 5)

Moreover, nurses have reported that they spent more time listening to and talking with persons and groups. In addition, persons and families reported enhanced satisfaction with nursing, and health-care professionals of other disciplines reported favorable changes in their opinions about nursing. Missing from these evaluation projects, however, are data regarding changes in health patterns or the quality of life of persons or groups.

Additional evidence of the extent to which the Theory of Human Becoming is compatible with expectations for nursing practice should come from the use of the South Dakota Board of Nursing regulatory decisioning model (Benedict, Bunkers, Damgaard, Duffy, Hohman, & Vander Woude, 2000; Damgaard & Bunkers, 1998; Vander Woude, 1998; Vander Woude & Hutcherson, 1999). That model, which reflects the values and principles of the Theory of Human Becoming, represents a new way of "exploring and honoring differing paradigms in nursing while grounding nursing regulatory decision-making in nursing science" (Damgaard & Bunkers, 1998, p. 144). Moreover, the presentation of the regulatory decisioning model at conferences served as a catalyst for development of nursing education, regulatory, and practice prototypes grounded in nursing science.

Use of Parse's **Preproject-Process-Postproject Descriptive Qualitative Method of Applied Research** permits comparisons of outcomes before and after the theory was used. The various reports published to date do not, however, fully address the problem-solving effectiveness of Theory of Human Becoming-based practice, in terms of the achievement of the disciplinary goal of enhanced quality of life for persons, families, and communities and the human becoming nurse's goal of being truly present with people as they enhance the quality of their lives.

Outcomes and problem-solving effectiveness may not be relevant criteria by which to evaluate the Theory of Human Becoming. Edwards (2000) commented, "One wonders what counts as being effective within the [human

(Text continues on page 498)

PURPOSE

To ascertain specific changes that emerge after initiation of a project to apply the Theory of Human Becoming in practice.

DESIGN

Information is gathered before the initiation of the project, midway, and at the end of the project.

An evaluator who is not engaged in the day-to-day activity of the setting makes a record of the responses from the information sources before the teaching-learning sessions begin, midway through the project, and at the end of the project.

INFORMATION SOURCES

Direct observation of nurses' documentation.

Written and tape-recorded interviews with nurses regarding their beliefs about human beings, health, and nursing.

Written and tape-recorded interviews with persons and their families regarding their experiences with nursing.

Tape-recorded interviews with nurse managers, physicians, and other multidisciplinary health professionals.

TEACHING-LEARNING PROCESS

Teaching-learning sessions are offered on a regular basis.

A human becoming nurse specialist instructs project participants (nurses and other health professionals) about the theory and guides them in consistent practice and documentation.

NURSES' DOCUMENTATION

Documentation is done in an easy-to-access format that is determined by nurses.

Personal Health Descriptions
Documentation of the meanings of the situation, the relationship with close others, and the hopes and wishes, as articulated by the person who is receiving nursing.

Patterns of Becoming
Documentation of themes surfacing in discussion, which are paradoxical and guide nurse-person activities.

Nurse-Person Activities
Documentation of activities in which the nurse participates, as decided by the person who is receiving nursing.

Plans, Goals, and Priorities for Change
Documentation of change in personal patterns of becoming, written from the perspective of the person who is receiving nursing, and written by that person or the nurse.

ANALYSIS OF INFORMATION SOURCES

All information sources are analyzed and synthesized to identify themes from each source.

Themes are further synthesized to determine what changes emerge in nurses' beliefs and practice, persons' and families' experiences of health care, and opinions of multidisciplinary health professionals.

Constructed from Parse, 1998, pp. 67–68.

Setting	Design Participants Data Sources	Citation*
28-bed medical unit in St. Michael's Hospital in Toronto, Ontario, Canada	Preproject-postproject descriptive evaluation Staff nurses Patients Unit manager Physicians Patient reports Unit manager's personal reflections Physician's anecdotal comments Staff nurse evaluations Quality assurance audits	Mattice, 1991
28-bed medical unit in St. Michael's Hospital in Toronto, Ontario, Canada	Preproject-postproject descriptive evaluation Staff nurses Patients Physicians Staff nurses' reports of changes in their thoughts and actions Patient reports Physician reports	Quiquero et al., 1991
28-bed medical unit in St. Michael's Hospital in Toronto, Ontario, Canada	Preproject-postproject descriptive evaluation Staff nurses Unit manager Patients Family members Written questionnaires Taped interviews Chart audits	Mitchell, 1991, 1995a
41-bed vascular and general surgery unit in Vancouver Hospital and Health Services Center, Vancouver, British Columbia, Canada	Preproject-process-postproject descriptive evaluation Patients Family members Staff nurses Unit manager Patients' and family members' perspectives Staff nurses' perspectives Unit manager's perspectives Researcher's documentation of experiences shared by nurses during teaching sessions, including stories about patients, changes happening on the unit, group process, and individual achievements	Legault & Ferguson-Paré, 1999
Family practice unit affiliated with an urban teaching hospital in Canada	Preproject-postproject descriptive evaluation Staff nurses Nurse manager Patients Written comments Taped interviews	Jonas, 1995

*See the Research section of the chapter references for complete citations.

(continued)

Setting	Design Participants Data Sources	Citation*
Two 20-bed pediatric units and one 42-bed medical-surgical unit in a 400-bed urban community teaching hospital in Canada	Preproject-postproject descriptive evaluation Staff nurses Adult clients Child clients Parents Nurse managers Physicians Child health workers Patient ombudsman Key representatives from other health professions Ethnographic interviews Written questionnaires Chart audits Photographs	Santopinto & Smith, 1995
One 16-bed forensic unit, one 9-bed neuropsychiatric unit, and one 24-bed geriatric psychiatry unit, all in a 200-bed acute care psychiatric hospital in Canada	Preproject-midproject-postproject descriptive evaluation Staff nurses Unit managers Hospital supervisors Patients Written questionnaires Taped interviews Chart audits	Northrup & Cody, 1998
Sunnybrook Health Science Centre in Toronto, Ontario, Canada	Time of information gathering not specified Patients' verbatim reports	Mitchell et al., 1997

(continued from page 495)

becoming school of thought]" (p. 194). Mitchell (1998) and Young, Taylor, and McLaughlin-Renpenning (2001) pointed out that the term outcomes is not consistent with the Theory of Human Becoming. Given that quality of life can be described only by each person, "there is no standard against which to measure quality of life, and such measurement is not consistent with this theory" (Young et al., 2001, p. 181). Yet, given that the goal of the human becoming nurse is to be truly present with people as they enhance their quality of life, some standard for enhanced quality of life seems to be required, even if that standard is adjusted for each person or family or community.

 ## CONCLUSION

Parse has made a meaningful contribution to nursing knowledge development by explicating a grand theory that focuses on the human-universe-health process. In addition, she has contributed distinctive methodologies for

basic and applied research and for practice that are consistent with her theory. And, she has begun to extend the theory to community.

The Theory of Human Becoming and the Human Becoming School of Thought have attracted scholars from four continents, with considerable work done by scholars in the United States, Canada, Finland, and Sweden (Parse, 1998, 2001b). The widespread interest in Parse's work is attested to by the establishment of the International Consortium of Parse Scholars. The Consortium began as an interest group in 1988; a few years later, it was officially designated as the Consortium. The purpose of the Consortium is "to contribute to human health and quality of life through practice and research guided by Parse's human becoming theory" (International Consortium of Parse Scholars, 1997, p. 2). The Consortium sponsors annual seminars and conferences and publishes the newsletter *Illuminations*.

Interest in Parse's work also is attested to by the founding of the Institute of Human Becoming. Since 1992, Parse has offered annual summer sessions devoted to the study of the Theory of Human Becoming and its associated research and practice methodologies. In addition, an annual International Colloquium on Human Becoming has been held for more than 10 years. Also, Parse's (1998) book, *The Human Becoming School of Thought: A Perspective for Nurses and Other Health Professionals,* has been translated into Chinese by Wang and published in Taiwan.

In summarizing directions for the future of the Theory of Human Becoming, Parse (2001b) declared:

> Through the efforts of Parse scholars the human becoming school of thought will continue to emerge as a force in the twenty-first century evolution of nursing science. Knowledge gained from the basic research studies will be synthesized to explicate further the meaning of lived experiences. The findings from applied research projects related to evaluation of human becoming practice will be synthesized and conclusions drawn. These syntheses will guide decisions in creating the continuing vision for sciencing and living the art of the human becoming school of thought. (p. 233)

Continued documentation of the use of the Theory of Human Becoming is needed, with special attention given to whether nurses who use the theory contribute to the quality of life of individuals, families, and communities. In addition, the extent to which the Theory of Human Becoming is appropriate for use by health professionals of other disciplines and actually is used by them remains to be determined.

REFERENCES

Bandler, R., & Grinder, J. (1975). The structure of magic I. Palo Alto, CA: Science & Behavior Books.

Barrett, E.A.M. (1998). Unique nursing research methods: The diversity chant of pioneers. Nursing Science Quarterly, 11, 94–96.

Benedict, L.L., Bunkers, S.S., Damgaard, G.A., Duffy, C.E., Hohman, M.L., & Vander Woude, D.L. (2000). The South Dakota Board of Nursing theory-based regulatory decisioning model. Nursing Science Quarterly, 13, 167–171.

Bournes, D. (1997). Interview with Dr. Rosemarie Parse. Illuminations, 6(4), 1–3.

Bournes, D.A. (2000). Concept inventing: A process for creating a unitary definition of having courage. Nursing Science Quarterly, 13, 143–149.

Bournes, D., & Mitchell, G. (Eds.). (1997). Patient focused care: Sailing beyond the boundaries at Sunnybrook Health Science Centre. North York, Ontario, Canada: Nursing Council of Sunnybrook Health Science Centre.

Bruteau, B. (1979). The psychic grid: How we create the world we know. Wheaton, IL: Theosophical Publishing House.

Buber, M. (1965). The knowledge of man (M. Friedman, Ed.). New York: Harper & Row.

Bunkers, S.S. (1998). Considering tomorrow: Parse's theory–guided research. Nursing Science Quarterly, 11, 56–63.

Bunkers, S.S. (1999). Translating nursing conceptual frameworks and theory for nursing practice. In P.A. Solari-Twadell & M.A. McDermott (Eds.), Parish nursing: Promoting whole person health within faith communities (pp. 205–214). Thousand Oaks, CA: Sage.

Bunkers, S.S. (2000). Simple things: Writings of human becoming. Sioux Falls, SD: Health Connections/Simple Things.

Bunkers, S.S. (2003). Community: An emerging mosaic of human becoming. In R.R. Parse, Community: A human becoming perspective (pp. 73–95). Boston: Jones and Bartlett.

Bunkers, S.S., Nelson, M., Leuning, C., Crane, J., & Josephson, D. (1999). The health action model: Academia's partnership with the community. In E. Cohen & V. De Back (Eds.), The outcomes mandate: Case management in health care today (pp. 92–100). St. Louis: Mosby.

Camus, A. (1946). The stranger. New York: Random House.

Camus, A. (1995). The first man (D. Hapgood, Trans.). New York: Knopf.

Cody, W.K. (1995). Of life immense in passion, pulse, and power: Dialoguing with Whitman and Parse—A hermeneutic study. In R.R. Parse (Ed.), Illuminations: The human becoming theory in practice and research (pp. 269–207). New York: National League for Nursing.

Cody, W.K. (2003). Human becoming community change concepts in an academic nursing practice setting. In R.R. Parse, Community: A human becoming perspective (pp. 49–71). Boston: Jones and Bartlett.

Damgaard, G., & Bunkers, S.S. (1998). Nursing science–guided practice and education: A state board of nursing perspective. Nursing Science Quarterly, 11, 142–144.

de Beauvoir, S. (1948). The ethics of ambiguity. Secaucus, NJ: Citadel.

de Beauvoir, S. (1977). A very easy death. New York: Warner.

Dilthey, W. (1961). Pattern and meaning in history: Thoughts on history and society (H.P. Rickman, Ed., Trans.). New York: Harper & Row.

Dilthey, W. (1988). Introduction to the human sciences (R.J. Betanzos, Trans.). Detroit: Wayne State University Press. [Original work published 1883.]

Dossey, L. (1991). Meaning and medicine: A doctor's tales of breakthrough and healing. New York: Bantam.

Edwards, S.D. (2000). Critical review of R.R. Parse's "The Human Becoming School of Thought: A Perspective for Nurses and Other Health Professionals." Journal of Advanced Nursing, 31, 190–196.

Fawcett, J. (2001). The nurse theorists: 21st century updates—Rosemarie Rizzo Parse. Nursing Science Quarterly, 14, 126–131.

Frankl, V.E. (1959). The will to meaning. New York; New American Library.

Gadamer, H.G. (1976). Philosophical hermeneutics (D.E. Linge, Ed., Trans.). Berkeley: University of California Press.

Gadamer, H.G. (1989). Truth and method (2nd rev. ed.). (Translation revised by J. Weinsheimer & D.G. Marshall.) New York: Crossroad. [Original work published 1960.]

Gadamer, H.G. (1993). Truth and method (2nd rev. ed.) (Translation revised by J. Weinsheimer & D.G. Marshall). New York: Continuum.

Gadamer, H.G. (1998). Truth and method (2nd rev. ed.). (Translation revised by J. Weinsheimer & D.G. Marshall.) New York: Continuum. [Original work published 1960.]

Greene, M. (1978). Landscapes of learning. New York: Teachers College Press.

Grinder, J., & Bandler, R. (1976). The structure of magic II. Palo Alto, CA: Science and Behavior Books.

Hall, B.P. (1976). The development of consciousness: A confluent theory of values. New York: Paulist.

Hall, E.T. (1976). Beyond culture. Garden City, NY: Doubleday/Anchor.

Harman, W. (1997). Biology revisioned. Noetic Sciences Review, 41, 12–17, 39–42.

Heidegger, M. (1962). Being and time (J. Macquarrie & E. Robinson, Trans.). New York: Harper & Row.

Hickman, J.S. (2002). Theory of human becoming: Rosemarie Rizzo Parse. In J. B. George (Ed.), Nursing theories: The base for professional nursing practice (5th ed., pp. 427–461). Upper Saddle River, NJ: Prentice Hall.

Holmes, C.A. (1990). Alternatives to natural science foundations for nursing. International Journal of Nursing Studies, 27, 187–198.

International Consortium of Parse Scholars. (1997). Brochure. Toronto, Ontario, Canada: International Consortium of Parse Scholars.

Jacono, B.J., & Jacono, J.J. (1996). The benefits of Newman and Parse in helping nurse teachers determine methods to enhance student creativity. Nurse Education Today, 16, 356–362.

Jourard, S.M. (1971). The transparent self. New York: Van Nostrand Reinhold.

Kelley, L.S. (1999). Hope as lived for native Americans. In R.R. Parse (Ed.), Hope: An international human becoming perspective (pp. 251–272). Boston: Jones and Bartlett.

Kempler, W. (1974). Principles of gestalt family therapy. Costa Mesa, CA: Kempler Institute.

Laing, R.D., Phillipson, H., & Lee, A.R. (1966). Interpersonal perception: A theory and a method of research. New York: Harper & Row.

Langer, S. (1976). Philosophy in a new key. Cambridge: Harvard University Press.

Leonard, G. (1978). The silent pulse. New York: E.D. Dutton.

Linscott, J., Spée, R., Flint, F., & Fisher, A. (1999). Creating a culture of patient-focused care through a learner-centered philosophy. Canadian Journal of Nursing Leadership, 12(4), 5–10.

Marcel, G. (1978). Mystery of being: reflection and mystery (Vol. 1). South Bend, IN: Gateway Editions.

McLeod, E., & Spée, R.T. (2003). Uncovering meaning: How nursing knowledge changes policy in practice. Nursing Science Quarterly, 16, 115–119.

Merleau-Ponty, M. (1974). Phenomenology of perception (C. Smith, Trans.). New York: Humanities Press.

Milton, C.L. (2003). A graduate curriculum guided by human becoming: Journeying with the possible. Nursing Science Quarterly, 16, 214–281.

Mitchell, G.J. (1998). Standards of nursing and the winds of change. Nursing Science Quarterly, 11, 97–98.

Mitchell, G.J. (2002). Rosemarie Rizzo Parse: Human becoming. In A. Marriner Tomey & M.R. Alligood (Eds.), Nursing theorists and their work (5th ed., pp. 527–559). St. Louis: Mosby.

Mitchell, G.J., & Cody, W.K. (1992). Nursing knowledge and human science: Ontological and epistemological considerations. Nursing Science Quarterly, 5, 54–61.

Mitchell, M.G. (2002). Patient-focused care on a complex continuing care dialysis unit: Rose's story. Journal of the Canadian Association of Nephrology Nurses and Technicians, 12(3), 48–49.

Nietzsche, F. (1968). The will to power (W. Kaufmann, Ed., Trans.). New York: Vintage.

Northrup, D.T., & Cody, W.K. (1998). Evaluation of the human becoming theory in practice in an acute care psychiatric hospital. Nursing Science Quarterly, 11, 23–30.

Parse, R.R. (1981). Man-Living-Health: A theory of nursing. New York: Wiley.

Parse, R.R. (1987). Man-Living-Health theory of nursing. In R.R. Parse (Ed.), Nursing Science. Major paradigms, theories, and critiques (pp. 159–180). Philadelphia: Saunders.

Parse, R.R. (1990a). Health: A personal commitment. Nursing Science Quarterly, 3, 136–140.

Parse, R.R. (1990b). Parse's research methodology with an illustration of the lived experience of hope. Nursing Science Quarterly, 3, 9–17.

Parse, R.R. (1992). Human becoming: Parse's theory of nursing. Nursing Science Quarterly, 5, 35–42.

Parse, R.R. (1995). The human becoming theory. In R.R. Parse (Ed.), Illuminations: The human becoming theory in practice and research (pp. 5–8). New York: National League for Nursing.

Parse, R.R. (1997a). Concept inventing: Unitary creations. Nursing Science Quarterly, 13, 63–64.

Parse, R.R. (1997b). The human becoming theory: The was, is, and will be. Nursing Science Quarterly, 10, 32–38.

Parse, R.R. (1997c). The language of nursing knowledge: Saying what we mean. In I.M. King & J. Fawcett (Eds.), The language of nursing theory and metatheory (pp. 73–77). Indianapolis: Sigma Theta Tau International Center Nursing Press.

Parse, R.R. (1998). The human becoming school of thought: A perspective for nurses and other health professionals. Thousand Oaks, CA: Sage.

Parse, R.R. (2001a). Qualitative inquiry: The path of sciencing. Boston: Jones and Bartlett.

Parse, R.R. (2001b). Rosemarie Rizzo Parse: The human becoming school of thought. In M.E. Parker (Ed.), Nursing theories and nursing practice (pp. 227–238). Philadelphia: F.A. Davis.

Parse, R.R. (2003a). Community change concepts. In R.R. Parse, Community: A human becoming perspective (pp. 23–47). Boston: Jones and Bartlett.

Parse, R.R. (2003b). Human becoming research on hope: An interpretation with the community change concepts. In R.R. Parse,

Community: A human becoming perspective (pp. 106–130). Boston: Jones and Bartlett.

Parse, R.R. (2004). The ubiquitous nature of unitary: Major change in human becoming language. Illuminations, 13(1), 1.

Phillips, J.R. (1987). A critique of Parse's man-living-health theory. In R.R. Parse (Ed.), Nursing Science. Major paradigms, theories, and critiques (pp. 181–204). Philadelphia: Saunders.

Pilkington, F.B. (1999). Editor's reply. Illuminations, 8(3), 5–6.

Polanyi, M. (1959). The study of man. Chicago: University of Chicago Press.

Polanyi, M. (1969). Knowing and being. Chicago: University of Chicago Press.

Raths, L.E., Harmin, M., & Simon, S.B. (1978). Values and teaching. Columbus, OH: Merrill.

Ricoeur, P. (1984). Time and narrative: Vol. 1 (K. McLaughlin & D. Pellauer, Trans.). Chicago: University of Chicago Press.

Ricoeur, P. (1987). The rule of metaphor: Multidisciplinary studies of the creation of meaning in language (R. Czerny et al., Trans.). Toronto: University of Toronto Press.

Ricoeur, P. (1988). Time and narrative: Vol. 3 (K. Blamey & D. Pellauer, Trans.). Chicago: University of Chicago Press.

Ricoeur, P. (1992). History and truth (C.A. Kelbley, Trans.). Evanston, IL: Northwestern University Press.

Rogers, M.E. (1970). An introduction to the theoretical basis of nursing. Philadelphia: F.A. Davis.

Rogers, M.E. (1992). Nursing science and the space age. Nursing Science Quarterly, 5, 27–34.

Saltmarche, A., Kolodny, V., & Mitchell, G.J. (1998). An educational approach for patient-focused care: Shifting attitudes and practice. Journal of Nursing Staff Development, 14, 81–86.

Sapir, E. (1966). Culture, language and personality. Berkeley: University of California Press.

Sarter, B. (1988). Philosophical sources of nursing theory. Nursing Science Quarterly, 1, 52–59.

Sartre, J.P. (1966). Being and nothingness. New York: Washington Square.

Schutz, A. (1967). On multiple realities. In M. Natanson (Ed.), The problem of social reality: Collected papers (Vol. 1, pp. 209–212). The Hague: Martinus Nijhoff.

Spée, R. (2000). Shaking shift report: Is it possible? Perspectives, 24(3), 2–8.

Straus, E.W. (1974). Sounds, words, sentences. In E.W. Straus (Ed.), Language and language disturbances (pp. 81–105). New York: Humanities Press.

Takahashi, T. (1992). Perspectives on nursing knowledge. Nursing Science Quarterly, 5, 86–91.

Tillich, P. (1952). The courage to be. New Haven: Yale University Press.

Tillich, P. (1954). Love, power and justice. New York: Oxford University Press.

Toben, B. (1975). Space-time and beyond. New York: E.P. Dutton.

van den Berg, J.H. (1971). Phenomenology and metabletics. Humanitas, 7, 285.

van Kaam, A. (1974). Existential crisis and human development. Humanitas, 10, 109–126.

van Kaam, A., van Croonenburg, B., & Muto, S. (1969). The participant self (Vol. 2). Pittsburgh: Duquesne University Press.

Vander Woude, D. (1998). Nursing theory-based regulatory decisioning model in South Dakota. Issues, 19(3), 14.

Vander Woude, D., & Hutcherson, C. (1999). Health policy and regulatory decisioning based on nursing theory. Nursing Science Quarterly, 12, 209–213.

von Bertalanffy, L. (1959). Human values in a changing world. In A.H. Maslow (Ed.), New knowledge in human values. New York: Harper.

Wang, C-e H. (2000). Developing a concept of hope from a human science perspective. Nursing Science Quarterly, 13, 248–251.

Watzlawick, P. (1978). The language of change. New York: Basic Books.

Watzlawkick, P., Weakland, J., & Fisch, R. (1974). Change: Principles of problem formation and problem resolution. New York: Norton.

Weisskopf, W.A. (1959). Existence and values. In A.H. Maslow (Ed.), New knowledge in human values. New York: Harper.

Whorf, B.E. (1956). Language, thought and reality. Cambridge: Technology.

Wimpenny, P. (1993). The paradox of Parse's theory. Senior Nurse, 13(5), 10–13.

Young, A., Taylor, S.G., & McLaughlin-Renpenning, K. (2001). Connections: Nursing research, theory, and practice. St. Louis: Mosby.

RESEARCH

Allchin-Petardi, L. (1998). Weathering the storm: Persevering through a difficult time. Nursing Science Quarterly, 11, 172–177.

Allchin-Petardi, L. (1999). Hope for American women with children. In R.R. Parse (Ed.), Hope: An international human becoming perspective (pp. 273–285). Boston: Jones and Bartlett.

Banonis, B.C. (1989). The lived experience of recovering from addiction: A phenomenological study. Nursing Science Quarterly, 2, 37–43.

Baumann, S.L. (1994). No place of their own: An exploratory study. Nursing Science Quarterly, 7, 162–169.

Baumann, S.L. (1996). Feeling uncomfortable: Children in families with no place of their own. Nursing Science Quarterly, 9, 152–159.

Baumann, S.L. (1999). The lived experience of hope: Children in families struggling to make a home. In R.R. Parse (Ed.), Hope: An international human becoming perspective (pp. 191–210). Boston: Jones and Bartlett.

Baumann, S.L. (2000). The lived experience of feeling loved: A study of mothers in a parolee program. Nursing Science Quarterly, 13, 332–338.

Baumann, S.L. (2003). The lived experience of feeling very tired: A study of adolescent girls. Nursing Science Quarterly, 16, 326–333.

Baumann, S.L., & Braddick, M. (1999). Out of their element: Fathers of children who are "not the same." Journal of Pediatric Nursing, 14, 369–378.

Baumann, S.L., Carroll, K.A., Damgaard, G.A., Millar, B., & Welch, A.J. (2001). An international human becoming hermeneutic study of Tom Hegg's A Cup of Christmas Tea. Nursing Science Quarterly, 14, 316–321.

Bournes, D.A. (2000). Concept inventing: A process for creating a unitary definition of having courage. Nursing Science Quarterly, 13, 143–149.

Bournes, D.A. (2002a). Having courage: A lived experience of human becoming. Nursing Science Quarterly, 15, 220–229.

Bournes, D.A. (2002b). Research evaluating human becoming in practice. Nursing Science Quarterly, 15, 190–195.

Bournes, D.A. (2003). Stories of courage and confidence: An interpretation within the human becoming community change concepts. In Parse, R.R. (2000) Community: A human becoming perspective (pp. 131–145). Boston: Jones and Bartlett.

Bournes, D.A., & Mitchell, G.J. (2002). Waiting: The experience of persons in a critical care waiting room. Research in Nursing and Health, 25, 58–67.

Bunkers, S.S. (1998). Considering tomorrow: Parse's theory–guided research. Nursing Science Quarterly, 11, 56–63. Reprinted in Parse, R.R. (2001). Qualitative inquiry: The path of sciencing. Boston: Jones and Bartlett. Parse, R.R. (2001). Critical appraisal of "Considering tomorrow: Parse's theory-guided research." In R.R. Parse, Qualitative inquiry: The path of sciencing (pp. 265–270). Boston: Jones and Bartlett.

Bunkers, S.S. (1999). The lived experience of hope for those working with homeless persons. In R.R. Parse (Ed.), Hope: An international human becoming perspective (pp. 227–250). Boston: Jones and Bartlett.

Bunkers, S.S. (2003). Comparison of three Parse method studies on feeling very tired. The lived experience of feeling very tired: A study using the Parse research method. Nursing Science Quarterly, 16, 340–344.

Bunkers, S.S., & Daly, J. (1999). The lived experience of hope for Australian families living with coronary disease. In R.R. Parse (Ed.), Hope: An international human becoming perspective (pp. 45–61). Boston: Jones and Bartlett.

Carson, M.G., & Mitchell, G.J. (1998). The experience of living with persistent pain. Journal of Advanced Nursing, 28, 1242, 1248.

Cody, W.K. (1991). Grieving a personal loss. Nursing Science Quarterly, 4, 61–68.

Cody, W.K. (1995a). Of life immense in passion, pulse, and power: Dialoguing with Whitman and Parse—A hermeneutic study. In R.R. Parse (Ed.), Illuminations: The human becoming theory in practice and research (pp. 269–207). New York: National League for Nursing.

Cody, W.K. (1995b). The lived experience of grieving for families living with AIDS. In R.R. Parse (Ed.), Illuminations: The human becoming theory in practice and research (pp. 197–242). New York: National League for Nursing.

Cody, W.K. (1995c). The meaning of grieving for families living with AIDS. Nursing Science Quarterly, 8, 104–114.

Cody, W.K. (2001). "Mendacity" as the refusal to bear witness: A human becoming hermeneutic study of a theme from Tennessee Williams' "Cat on a Hot Tin Roof." In R.R. Parse, Qualitative inquiry: The path of sciencing (pp. 205–220). Boston: Jones and Bartlett.

Cody, W.K., & Filler, J.E. (1999). The lived experience of hope for women residing in a shelter. In R.R. Parse (Ed.), Hope: An international human becoming perspective (pp. 211–225). Boston: Jones and Bartlett.

Costello-Nickitas, D.M. (1994). Choosing life goals: A phenomenological study. Nursing Science Quarterly, 7, 87–92.

Curley, M.A.Q. (1997). Mutuality—An expression of nursing practice. Journal of Pediatric Nursing, 12, 208–213.

Daly, J. (1995). The lived experience of suffering. In R.R. Parse (Ed.), Illuminations: The human becoming theory in practice and research (pp. 243–268). New York: National League for Nursing.

Davis, D.K., & Cannava, E. (1995). The meaning of retirement for communally-living retired performing artists. Nursing Science Quarterly, 8, 8–16.

Dawson, P. (2000). Exploring the paradoxes and possibilities in life after stroke. Perspectives, 24(4), 30–31.

Fisher, M.A., & Mitchell, G.J. (1998). Patients' views of quality of life: Transforming the knowledge base of nursing. Clinical Nurse Specialist, 12, 99–105.

Fite, S., & Frank, D.I. (1996). Women's perception of social support and obtaining mammography screening. Florida Nurse, 44(2), 18.

Fite, S., Frank, D.I., & Curtin, J. (1996). The relationship of social support to women's obtaining mammography screening. Journal of the American Academy of Nurse Practitioners, 8, 565–569.

Futrell, M., Wondolowski, C., & Mitchell, G.J. (1993). Aging in the oldest old living in Scotland: A phenomenological study. Nursing Science Quarterly, 6, 189–194.

Gates, K.M. (2000). The experience of caring for a loved one: A phenomenological study. Nursing Science Quarterly, 13, 54–59.

Gwilliam, B., & Bailey, C. (2001). The nature of terminal malignant bowel obstruction and its impact on patients with advanced cancer. International Journal of Palliative Nursing, 7, 474–476, 478–481.

Heine, C. (1991). Development of gerontological nursing theory. Applying the man-living-health theory of nursing. Nursing and Health Care, 12, 184–188.

Hellwig, S.D., Yam, M., & DiGiulio, M. (2003). Nurse care managers' perceptions of advocacy: A phenomenological study. Lippincott's Case Mangement, 8(2), 53–65.

Hodges, H.F., Keeley, A.C., & Grier, E.C. (2001). Masterworks of art and chronic illness experiences in the elderly. Journal of Advanced Nursing, 36, 389–398.

Huch, M.H., & Bournes, D.A. (2003). Community dwellers' perspectives on the experience of feeling very tired. Nursing Science Quarterly, 16, 334–339.

Hutchinson, M.K. (1999). Individual, family, relationship predictors of young women's sexual risk perceptions. Journal of Obstetric, Gynecologic, and Neonatal Nursing, 28, 60–67.

Janes, N.M., & Wells, D.L. (1997). Elderly patients' experiences with nurses guided by Parse's theory of human becoming.

Clinical Nursing Research, 6, 205–222. Daley, J. (1997). Commentary. Clinical Nursing Research, 6, 222–224.

Jonas, C.M. (1992). The meaning of being an elder in Nepal. Nursing Science Quarterly, 5, 171–175.

Jonas, C.M. (1995). Evaluation of the human becoming theory in family practice. In R.R. Parse (Ed.), Illuminations: The human becoming theory in practice and research (pp. 347–366). New York: National League for Nursing.

Jonas-Simpson, C. (1997). The Parse research method through music. Nursing Science Quarterly, 10, 112–114.

Jonas-Simpson, C.M. (2001). Feeling understood: A melody of human becoming. Nursing Science Quarterly, 14, 222–230.

Jonas-Simpson, C.M. (2003). The experience of being listened to: A human becoming study with music. Nursing Science Quarterly, 16, 232–238.

Kelley, L.S. (1991). Struggling with going along when you do not believe. Nursing Science Quarterly, 4, 123–129.

Kelley, L.S. (1999a). Evaluating change in quality of life from the perspective of the person: Advanced practice nursing and Parse's goal of nursing. Holistic Nursing Practice, 13, 61–70.

Kelley, L.S. (1999b). Hope as lived for native Americans. In R.R. Parse (Ed.), Hope: An international human becoming perspective (pp. 251–272). Boston: Jones and Bartlett.

Kim, M.S., Shin, K.R., & Shin, S.R. (1998). Korean adolescents' experiences of smoking cessation: A prelude to research with the human becoming perspective. Nursing Science Quarterly, 11, 105–109.

Kruse, B.G. (1999). The lived experience of serenity: Using Parse's research method. Nursing Science Quarterly, 12, 143–150.

Legault, F., & Ferguson-Paré, M. (1999). Advancing nursing practice: An evaluation study of Parse's theory of human becoming. Canadian Journal of Nursing Leadership, 12(1), 30–35.

Major, F., & Pepin, J. (2001). The experience of autonomy for elders living with a family member. Recherche En Soins Infirmiers (64), 36–46. [French; English abstract]

Mattice, M. (1991). Parse's theory of nursing in practice: A manager's perspective. Canadian Journal of Nursing Administration, 4(1), 11–13.

Mitchell, G.J. (1990). The lived experience of taking life day-by-day in later life: Research guided by Parse's emergent method. Nursing Science Quarterly, 3, 29–36.

Mitchell, G.J. (1991). Distinguishing practice with Parse's theory. In I.E. Goertzen (Ed.), Differentiating nursing practice: Into the twenty-first century (pp. 55–58). Kansas City, MO: American Academy of Nursing.

Mitchell, G.J. (1993). Time and a waning moon: Seniors describe the meaning of later life. Canadian Journal of Nursing Research, 25(1), 51–66. Joseph, D. (1994). Critique of "Time and the waning moon: Seniors describe the meaning to later life." Nursing Scan in Research, 7(2), 6–7.

Mitchell, G.J. (1994). The meaning of being a senior: Phenomenological research and interpretation with Parse's theory of nursing. Nursing Science Quarterly, 7, 70–79.

Mitchell, G.J. (1995a). Evaluation of the human becoming theory in practice in an acute care setting. In R.R. Parse (Ed.), Illuminations: The human becoming theory in practice and research (pp. 367–399). New York: National League for Nursing.

Mitchell, G.J. (1995b). The lived experience of restriction-freedom in later life. In R.R. Parse (Ed.), Illuminations: The human becoming theory in practice and research (pp. 159–195). New York: National League for Nursing.

Mitchell, G.J. (1998). Living with diabetes: How understanding expands theory for professional practice. Canadian Journal of Diabetes Care, 22, 30–37.

Mitchell, G.J., Bernardo, A., & Bournes, D. (1997). Nursing theory–guided practice: Nursing guided by Parse's theory— Patient views at Sunnybrook. Nursing Science Quarterly, 10, 55–56.

Mitchell, G.J., & Heidt, P. (1994). The lived experience of wanting to help another: Research with Parse's method. Nursing Science Quarterly, 7, 119–127.

Mitchell, G.J., & Lawton, C. (2000). Living with the consequences of personal choices for persons with diabetes: Implications for educators and practitioners. Canadian Journal of Diabetes Care, 24(2), 23–30.

Moore, L.W. (2000). Severe visual impairment in older women. Western Journal of Nursing Research, 22, 571–595.

Nokes, K.M., & Carver, K. (1991). The meaning of living with AIDs: A study using Parse's theory of man-living-health. Nursing Science Quarterly, 4, 175–179.

Northrup, D.T. (2002). Time passing: A Parse research method study. Nursing Science Quarterly, 15, 318–326.

Northrup, D.T., & Cody, W.K. (1998). Evaluation of the human becoming theory in practice in an acute care psychiatric setting. Nursing Science Quarterly, 11, 23–30. Reprinted in R.R. Parse, (2001). Qualitative inquiry: The path of sciencing. Boston: Jones and Bartlett.

Ortiz, M.R. (2003). Lingering presence: A study using the human becoming hermeneutic method. Nursing Science Quarterly, 16, 146–154.

Overgaard, D. (2002). Being obese is paradoxical living—An exploratory study of five persons' lived experiences of being overweight. Theoria: Journal of Nursing Theory, 11(1), 3–12.

Parse, R.R. (1990). Parse's research methodology with an illustration of the lived experience of hope. Nursing Science Quarterly, 3, 9–17.

R.R. Parse, (1993). The experience of laughter: A phenomenological study. Nursing Science Quarterly, 6, 39–43. Reprinted in R.R. Parse, (2001). Qualitative inquiry: The path of sciencing. Boston: Jones and Bartlett.

Parse, R.R. (1994). Laughing and health: A study using Parse's research method. Nursing Science Quarterly, 7, 55–64.

Parse, R.R. (1996). Quality of life for persons living with Alzheimer's disease: The human becoming perspective. Nursing Science Quarterly, 9, 126–133. Reprinted in R.R. Parse, (2001). Qualitative inquiry: The path of sciencing. Boston: Jones and Bartlett.

Parse, R.R. (1997). Joy-sorrow: A study using the Parse research method. Nursing Science Quarterly, 10, 80–87.

Parse, R.R. (1999). The lived experience of hope for family

members of persons living in a Canadian chronic care facility. In R.R. Parse (Ed.), Hope: An international human becoming perspective (pp. 63–77). Boston: Jones and Bartlett.

Parse, R.R. (2001a). The lived experience of contentment: A study using the Parse research method. In R.R. Parse (2001). Qualitative inquiry: The path of sciencing (pp. 183–203). Boston: Jones and Bartlett.

Parse, R.R. (2001b). The lived experience of contentment: A study using the Parse research method. Nursing Science Quarterly, 14, 330–338.

Parse, R.R. (2003a). Human becoming research on hope: An interpretation with the community change concepts. In R.R. Parse, Community: A human becoming perspective (pp. 106–130). Boston: Jones and Bartlett.

Parse, R.R. (2003b). The lived experience of feeling very tired: A study using the Parse research method. Nursing Science Quarterly, 16, 319–325.

Pilkington, F.B. (1993). The lived experience of grieving the loss of another important other. Nursing Science Quarterly, 6, 130–139.

Pilkington, F.B. (2000a). Persisting while wanting to change: Women's lived experiences. Health Care for Women International, 21, 501–516.

Pilkington, F.B. (2000b). A qualitative study of life after stroke. Journal of Neuroscience Nursing, 31, 336–374.

Pilkington, F.B., & Miller, B. (1999). The lived experience of hope with persons from Wales, UK. In R.R. Parse (Ed.), Hope: An international human becoming perspective (pp. 163–189). Boston: Jones and Bartlett.

Pullen, L., Tuck, I., & Mix, K. (1996). Mental health nurses' spiritual perspectives. Journal of Holistic Nursing, 14(2), 85–97.

Quiquero, A., Knights, D., & Meo, C.O. (1991). Theory as a guide to practice: Staff nurses choose Parse's theory. Canadian Journal of Nursing Administration, 4(1), 14–16.

Rendon, D.C., Sales, R., Leal, I., & Pique, J. (1995). The lived experience of aging in community-dwelling elders in Valencia, Spain: A phenomenological study. Nursing Science Quarterly, 8, 152–157.

Santopinto, M.D.A. (1989). The relentless drive to be ever thinner: A study using the phenomenological method. Nursing Science Quarterly, 2, 29–36. Santopinto, M.D.A. (1989). Reprinted in R.R. Parse, (2001). Qualitative inquiry: The path of sciencing. Boston: Jones and Bartlett.

Santopinto, M.D.A., & Smith, M.C. (1995). Evaluation of the human becoming theory in practice with adults and children. In R.R. Parse (Ed.), Illuminations: The human becoming theory in practice and research (pp. 309–346). New York: National League for Nursing.

Scales, B. (2001). CAMPing in the PACU: Using complementary and alternative medical practices in the PACU. Journal of PeriAnesthesia Nursing, 16, 325–334.

Smith, M.C. (1990). Struggling through a difficult time for unemployed persons. Nursing Science Quarterly, 3, 18–28.

Smith, M.J. (1989). Research and practice application related to man-living-health: A theory of nursing. In J.P. Riehl-Sisca (Ed.),

Conceptual models for nursing practice (3rd ed., pp. 267–276). Norwalk, CT: Appleton & Lange.

Stoltz, P., & Willman, A. (2001). The human becoming school of thought as a framework for the hermeneutic interpretation of persons' experiences of coronary angiography. Theoria: Journal of Nursing Theory, 10(4), 20–29.

Takahashi, T. (1999). Kibou: Hope for persons in Japan. In R.R. Parse (Ed.), Hope: An international human becoming perspective (pp. 115–128). Boston: Jones and Bartlett.

Thornburg, P. (2002). "Waiting" as experienced by women hospitalized during the antepartum period. MCN: American Journal of Maternal Child Nursing, 27, 245–248.

Toikkanen, T., & Muurinen, E. (1999). Toivo: Hope for persons in Finland. In R.R. Parse (Ed.), Hope: An international human becoming perspective (pp. 79–96). Boston: Jones and Bartlett.

Wang, C-e H. (1999). He-bung: Hope for persons living with leprosy in Taiwan. In R.R. Parse (Ed.), Hope: An international human becoming perspective (pp. 143–162). Boston: Jones and Bartlett.

Wang, C-e H. (2000). Developing a concept of hope from a human science perspective. Nursing Science Quarterly, 13, 248–251.

Willman, A. (1999). Hopp: The lived experience for Swedish elders. In R.R. Parse (Ed.), Hope: An international human becoming perspective (pp. 129–142). Boston: Jones and Bartlett.

Wondolowski, C., & Davis, D.K. (1988). The lived experience of aging in the oldest old: A phenomenological study. American Journal of Psychoanalysis, 48, 261–270.

Wondolowski, C., & Davis, D.K. (1991). The lived experience of health in the oldest old: A phenomenological study. Nursing Science Quarterly, 4, 113–118.

Zanotti, R., & Bournes, D.A. (1999). Speranza: A study of the lived experience of hope with persons from Italy. In R.R. Parse (Ed.), Hope: An international human becoming perspective (pp. 97–114). Boston: Jones and Bartlett.

PRACTICE

Andrus, K. (1995). Parse's nursing theory and the practice of perioperative nursing. Canadian Operating Room Nursing Journal, 13(3), 19–22.

Arndt, M.J. (1995). Parse's theory of human becoming in practice with hospitalized adolescents. Nursing Science Quarterly, 8, 86–90.

Balcombe, K., Davis, P., & Lim, E. (1991). A nursing model for orthopaedics. Nursing Standard, 5(49), 26–28.

Baumann, S.L. (1997). Contrasting two approaches in a community-based nursing practice with older adults: The medical model and Parse's nursing theory. Nursing Science Quarterly, 10, 124–130.

Bunkers, S.S. (1996a). Tattered and torn. Nursing Science Quarterly, 9, 134–135.

Bunkers, S.S. (1996b). Thank you, Dorothy: Now I know. Nursing Science Quarterly, 9, 79–80.

Bunkers, S.S. (1998). A nursing theory–guided model of health ministry: Human becoming and parish nursing. Nursing Science Quarterly, 11, 7–8.

Butler, M.J. (1988). Family transformation: Parse's theory in practice. Nursing Science Quarterly, 1, 68–74.

Butler, M.J., & Snodgrass, F.G. (1991). Beyond abuse: Parse's theory in practice. Nursing Science Quarterly, 4, 76–82.

Cody, W.K. (1995). True presence with families living with HIV disease. In R.R. Parse (Ed.), Illuminations: The human becoming theory in practice and research (pp. 115–133). New York: National League for Nursing.

Cody, W.K. (2003). Human becoming community change concepts in an academic nursing practice setting. In R.R. Parse, Community: A human becoming perspective (pp. 49–71). Boston: Jones and Bartlett.

Cody, W.K., Hudepohl, J.H., & Brinkman, K.S. (1995). True presence with a child and his family. In R.R. Parse (Ed.), Illuminations: The human becoming theory in practice and research (pp. 135–146). New York: National League for Nursing.

Galligan, A.C. (2000). That place where we live: The discovery of self through the creative play experience. Journal of Child and Adolescent Psychiatric Nursing, 13, 169–176.

Jonas, C.M. (1994). True presence through music. Nursing Science Quarterly, 7, 102–103.

Jonas, C.M. (1995). True presence through music for persons living their dying. In R.R. Parse (Ed.), Illuminations: The human becoming theory in practice and research (pp. 97–104). New York: National League for Nursing.

Jonas-Simpson, C.M. (1996). The patient-focused care journey: Where patients and families guide the way. Nursing Science Quarterly, 9, 145–146.

Jonas-Simpson, C. (2001). From silence to voice: Knowledge, values, and beliefs guiding healthcare practices with persons living with dementia. Nursing Science Quarterly, 14, 304–310.

Josephson, D.K. (2000). Women of hope—Tiospaye. Nursing Science Quarterly, 13, 300–302.

Kelley, L.S. (1995). Parse's theory in practice with a group in the community. Nursing Science Quarterly, 8, 127–132.

Lee, O.J., & Pilkington, F.B. (1999). Practice with persons living their dying: A human becoming perspective. Nursing Science Quarterly, 12, 324–328.

Letcher, D.C. (2000). Buying your life. Nursing Science Quarterly, 13, 303–305.

Liehr, P.R. (1989). The core of true presence: A loving center. Nursing Science Quarterly, 2, 7–8.

Markovic, M. (1997). From theory to perioperative practice with Parse. Canadian Operating Room Nursing Journal, 15, 13–16, 18–19.

Mattice, M., & Mitchell, G.J. (1991). Caring for confused elders. The Canadian Nurse, 86(11), 16–17.

Mavely, R., & Mitchell, G.J. (1994). Consider karaoke: An audiovisual device that encourages client participation with music. Canadian Nurse, 90(1), 22–24.

Melnechenko, K.L. (1995). Parse's theory of human becoming: An alternative guide to nursing practice for pediatric oncol-ogy nurses. Journal of Pediatric Oncology Nursing, 12, 122–127.

Parse, R.R. (1995). Commentary: Parse's theory of human becoming: An alternative guide to nursing practice for pediatric oncology nurses. Journal of Pediatric Oncology Nursing, 12, 128.

Mitchell, G.J. (1986). Utilizing Parse's theory of man-living-health in Mrs. M.'s neighborhood. Perspectives, 10(4), 5–7.

Mitchell, G.J. (1988). Man-living-health. The theory in practice. Nursing Science Quarterly, 1, 120–127.

Mitchell, G.J. (1991). Human subjectivity: The cocreation of self. Nursing Science Quarterly, 4, 144–145.

Mitchell, G.J. (1993). Parse's theory in practice. In M.E. Parker (Ed.), Patterns of nursing theories in practice (pp. 62–80). New York: National League for Nursing.

Mitchell, G.J. (1996a). Pretending: A way to get through the day. Nursing Science Quarterly, 9, 92–93.

Mitchell, G.J. (1996b). A reflective moment with false cheerfulness. Nursing Science Quarterly, 9, 53–54.

Mitchell, G.J. (2002). Parse's theory of human becoming in nursing practice. In M.R. Alligood & A. Marriner Tomey (Eds.), Nursing theory: Utilization and application (2nd ed., pp. 403–428). St. Louis: Mosby.

Mitchell, G.J., & Copplestone, C. (1990). Applying Parse's theory to perioperative nursing. A nontraditional approach. Association of Operating Room Nurses Journal, 51, 787–798.

Mitchell, M.G. (2002). Patient-focused care on a complex continuing care dialysis unit: Rose's story. Journal of the Canadian Association of Nephrology Nurses and Technicians, 12(3), 48–49.

Pilkington, F.B. (1997). An ethical framework for nursing practice: Parse's human becoming theory. Nursing Science Quarterly, 12, 21–25.

Plank, D.M.P. (1994). Framing treatment options: A method to enhance informed consent. Clinical Nurse Specialist, 8, 174–178.

Rasmusson, D.L. (1995). True presence with homeless persons. In R.R. Parse (Ed.), Illuminations: The human becoming theory in practice and research (pp. 105–113). New York: National League for Nursing.

Rasmusson, D.L., Jonas, C.M., & Mitchell, G.J. (1991). The eye of the beholder: Parse's theory with homeless individuals. Clinical Nurse Specialist, 5, 139–143.

Relf, M.V. (1997). Illuminating meaning and transforming issues of spirituality in human immunodeficiency virus disease and acquired immunodeficiency syndrome: An application of Parse's theory of human becoming. Holistic Nursing Practice, 12(1), 1–8.

Smith, M.J. (1989). Research and practice application related to man-living-health: A theory of nursing. In J.P. Riehl-Sisca (Ed.), Conceptual models for nursing practice (3rd ed., pp. 267–276). Norwalk, CT: Appleton & Lange.

Smith, M.K. (2002). Human becoming and women living with violence: The art of practice. Nursing Science Quarterly, 15, 302–307.

Williamson, G.J. (2000). The test of a nursing theory: A personal view. Nursing Science Quarterly, 13, 124–128.

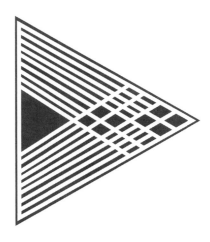

Chapter **14**

Orlando's Theory of the Deliberative Nursing Process

Ida Jean Orlando Pelletier formulated the Theory of the Deliberative Nursing Process after reviewing the data collected for a study of experiences in nursing and teaching that was funded by the National Institute of Mental Health, United States Public Health Service, and was conducted under the auspices of the Yale University School of Nursing. Orlando (1989) explained that as she sorted the data into the categories of good and bad outcomes, she realized that the good outcomes were the result of effective nursing practice in the form of the nurse's nonobservable reaction and observable actions in response to the patient's behavior. She pointed out that the fundamental idea of her work is "directed toward the organization, development and implementation of a system of understanding which makes it possible for nurses to develop and maintain professional responsibility for the patient's care and mutual job responsibility with others who may affect the nurse's care of patients" (Orlando, 1972, p. 3).

Orlando first presented her work in her 1961 book, *The Dynamic Nurse-Patient Relationship: Function, Process and Principles.* In that book, she labeled her work a theory of effective nursing practice but later—in the preface to the 1990 reprint of the 1961 book—referred to the work as the nursing process theory. Explaining the change in label, she stated:

> If I had been more courageous in 1961, when this book was first written, I would have proposed it as "nursing process theory" instead of as a "theory of effective nursing practice." A "deliberative" process was presented as a guide for nurses to practice "effectively." Conversely, an "automatic" process was shown to be "ineffective." "Effectiveness" was conceptualized and illustrated as "improvement" in the patient's behavior. The "improvement" stemmed from the fact that the deliberative process made it possible for the nurse to identify and meet the patient's *need for help.* (Orlando Pelletier, 1990, p. vii)

Orlando presented further development of the Theory of the Deliberative Nursing Process and a research methodology in her 1972 book, *The Discipline and Teaching of Nursing Process (An Evaluative Study).* The 1961 and 1972 books now are regarded as classics.

ANALYSIS OF THE THEORY OF THE DELIBERATIVE NURSING PROCESS

This section presents an analysis of Orlando's theory. The analysis is based on the contents of Orlando's 1961 book, *The Dynamic Nurse-Patient Relationship: Function, Process and Principles*, and her 1972 book, *The Discipline and Teaching of Nursing Process (An Evaluative Study)*.

SCOPE OF THE THEORY

The central thesis of the Theory of the Deliberative Nursing Process is that "(often marvelous) [outcomes are] a result of finding out and meeting the patient's immediate needs for help" (Orlando Pelletier, 1990, p. viii). Inasmuch as the concepts and propositions of the theory are written at a relatively concrete level of discourse, the theory is classified as a middle-range predictive theory that specifies the effects of a particular interpersonal nursing process on identification of the patient's immediate need for help.

CONTEXT OF THE THEORY

Metaparadigm Concepts and Proposition

Even a cursory review of Orlando's books indicates that the Theory of the Deliberative Nursing Process is based on the metaparadigm concepts of *human beings* and *nursing*. Indeed, Orlando (1961) maintained that "learning how to understand what is happening between herself and the patient is the central core of the nurse's practice and comprises the basic framework for the help she gives to patients" (p. 4).

Orlando (1961) focused on a particular nursing process that leads to improvement in the patient's behavior. She stated, "What a nurse says or does is the exclusive mode through which she serves the patient" (p. 6). Hence the metaparadigm proposition that is most relevant is *the nursing actions or processes that are beneficial to human beings*.

Philosophical Claims

Orlando (1961, 1972) made many statements that represent the philosophical basis for the Theory of the Deliberative Nursing Process. Some of those statements re-

507

flect Orlando's philosophical claims about patients, other statements represent philosophical claims about nursing, and still other statements reflect Orlando's philosophical position with regard to interactions between nurses and patients. Two additional statements represent the philosophical basis for Orlando's research methodology. All of those statements are listed here.

Philosophical Claims About Patients

• A patient *may* react with distress to any aspect of an environment which was designed for therapeutic and helpful purposes (Orlando, 1961, p. 17).
• The patient's reactions in the setting which may cause him distress are generally based on an inadequate or incorrect understanding of an experience in the setting (Orlando, 1961, p. 17).
• It is safe to assume that patients become distressed when, without help, they cannot cope with their needs (Orlando, 1961, p. 11).

Philosophical Claims About Nursing

• Nursing is historically rooted in an immediate responsiveness to individuals assumed to be suffering helplessness in immediate situations. Traditionally, the responsiveness has been specific to the individual's cry for help and has provided direct assistance for the purpose of avoiding, relieving or diminishing the helplessness suffered or anticipated (Orlando, 1972, p. 8).
• It may be assumed that [the nurse's] intention is to be of help (Orlando, 1961, p. 70).
• Any nursing, whether one is caring for the self or is being cared for by another, should result in some measure of curative value which is specific to the helplessness suffered or anticipated by individuals in immediate experiences (Orlando, 1972, p. 9).
• The nurse is responsible for helping the patient avoid or alleviate the distress of unmet needs (Orlando, 1961, p. 6).
• It is important for the nurse to concern herself with the patient's distress because the treatment and prevention of disease proceeds best when conditions extraneous to the disease itself and its management do not cause the patient additional suffering (Orlando, 1961, pp. 22–23).
• Nursing in its professional character does not add to the distress of the patient. Instead the nurse assumes the professional responsibility of seeking out and obviating impediments to the patient's mental and physical comfort (Orlando, 1961, p. 9).
• It is the nurse's direct responsibility to see to it that the patient's needs for help are met either by her own activity or by calling in the help of others (Orlando, 1961, p. 22).

• The focus and stimulus of the professional nurse's service is therefore the patient and his needs (Orlando, 1961, p. 8).
• All nursing activities are designed for the benefit of the patient, but sometimes they do not suit the patient because at the same moment he may require something entirely different (Orlando, 1961, p. 8).
• It is reasonable to assume that any activity performed with or for the patient is designed, at least ultimately, for the patient's benefit. But, it sometimes happens that professional and non-professional personnel alike carry out activities which not only do not help the patient but may even hinder his progress (Orlando, 1961, p. 19).

Philosophical Claims About Interactions Between Nurses and Patients

• Since the nurse and patient are both people, they interact, and a process goes on between them (Orlando, 1961, p. 8).
• The nurse-patient situation [is] a dynamic whole—how the patient behaves affects the nurse and the nurse in turn affects the patient (Orlando, 1961, p. 36).
• In order for the nurse to develop and maintain the professional character of her work she must know and be able to validate how her actions and reactions help or do not help the patient or know and be able to validate that the patient does not require her help at a given time (Orlando, 1961, p. 9).
• The nurse … must first realize that the patient cannot clearly state the nature and meaning of his distress or his need without her help or without her first having established a helpful relationship with him (Orlando, 1961, p. 23).

Philosophical Basis for Orlando's Research Methodology

• The [deliberative nursing process] [is] most effective when an explicit verbal form [is] used (Orlando, 1972, p. 51).
• The use of the [deliberative nursing process] would enable the nurse to fulfill her professional and job functions (Orlando, 1972, p. 54).

Forchuk (1991) and Sellers (1991) both noted that some of the philosophical claims on which Orlando's theory is based reflect the totality world view. Sellers (1991) also noted that the theory "illustrates a mechanistic, deterministic, persistence world view. Orlando proposes a reductionistic view of person, in which human behavior is perceived from within a stimulus-response framework and a closed system notion of tension reduction and comfort maintenance. All behavioral activities are considered as purposeful and directed toward the reduction of discomfort from unmet needs" (p. 144).

At the same time, however, the theory "focuses on the reciprocal interaction between the [patient] and the nurse. Both the [patient] and the nurse are affected by the other's behavior" (Sellers, 1991, p. 144). Furthermore, although Orlando's separation of behaviors, perceptions, thoughts, and feelings reflects the totality world view, "she sees each person as unique and as providing her or his own meaning to the situation, as in the simultaneity [world view]" (Forchuk, 1991, p. 41). Thus it can be concluded that Orlando's philosophical claims most closely reflect the *reciprocal interaction* world view.

Conceptual Model

Although Orlando did not explicitly identify the conceptual underpinnings of her theory, she did describe human beings and nursing in some detail. Human beings are described as patients. Human beings become patients when they submit to medical procedures. Orlando (1972) explained:

> Once an individual undergoes medical diagnosis, treatment or supervision, he automatically assumes the status of patient and is vulnerable to the predicament of being a patient. That is, the patient may not be in a position to control all that happens to him and may suffer helplessness as a result. (p. 10)

Professional nurses are needed, according to Orlando (1961; Orlando & Dugan, 1989) when human beings should but do not know why they are helpless, that is, when human beings do not know why they cannot nurse themselves. Professional nurses also are needed when human beings do not know why they are unable to nurse themselves and, therefore, cannot communicate what their immediate need for help is. Moreover, professional nurses are needed when human beings experience distress stemming from physical limitations or adverse reactions to the setting, or when the unique characteristics of the distress cannot be observed directly even if it continues or escalates in intensity. Conversely, nurses are not needed "when the patient is able to meet his own needs and is able to carry out prescribed measures unaided" (Orlando, 1961, p. 5).

Orlando (1961) regarded nursing as distinct from medicine:

> There is a clear distinction between the medical management of a patient and the way the patient would manage his own affairs and his own comforts if he were able to do so. ... The doctor places the patient under the care of the nurse for either or both of the following reasons: (1) the patient cannot deal with what he needs, or (2) he cannot carry out the prescribed treatment or diagnostic plan alone. ... The responsibility of

the nurse is necessarily different [from that of the physician]; it offers whatever help the patient may require for his needs to be met, i.e., for his physical and mental comfort to be assured as far as possible while he is undergoing some form of medical treatment or supervision. (p. 5)

Hence the purpose of nursing "is to supply the help a patient requires in order for his needs to be met" (Orlando, 1961, p. 8). Stated in other words, the nurse's function, which is dictated by patients' predicaments, is "to find out and meet patients' immediate needs for help while undergoing treatment in prescribed settings" (Pelletier, 1967, p. 27). Even more specifically, the function of professional nursing is "attending to individuals when [they are] in distress because they cannot find their own encouragement, look after themselves, nourish, nurture, or protect themselves, nor give themselves curative care when they are ailing" (Orlando & Dugan, 1989, p. 79). The essence of professional nursing, then, is knowing when and validating that the nurse's actions and reactions help or do not help the patient, and knowing when and validating that the patient does *not* need the nurse's help at a particular time (Orlando, 1962).

In a further comparison of nursing and medicine, Orlando (1972) commented:

> Nursing (not necessarily the nurse) is responsive to individuals who suffer or anticipate a sense of helplessness; it is focused on the process of care in an immediate experience; it is concerned with providing direct assistance to individuals in whatever setting they are found for the purpose of avoiding, relieving, diminishing or curing the individual's sense of helplessness. Nursing by another person may take place when an individual is unable to nurse himself and may function independently of whether or not the individual is under medical care. In contrast, medicine is responsive to individuals who suffer or are apt to suffer ill health and commits itself to those who are willing to undergo medical diagnosis, treatment or supervision; it is thus focused on the process of disease; it is concerned with diagnosis and treatment, carried out by advising or directing patients to follow or undergo specific diagnostic, medical, surgical or psychiatric procedures in settings where patients are found or in whatever setting individuals are placed for the purpose of curing, alleviating or preventing disease. Medical practice functions independently of whether or not the patient is able to nurse himself. (p. 12)

The distinction between nursing and medicine also is evident in Orlando's (1961) comment about medically prescribed activities. She stated, "It is important to recognize that the nurse is using a doctor's order for the patient and is not carrying out orders for the doctor" (p. 72). Orlando (1987) also noted that "medical orders are for and directed at patients who are free to comply or not to comply. They may direct a physician's assistant but not a professional nurse. Our commitment is to the individual who may or may not require the nurse's care in response to the doctor's orders or in response to anything else. Helping the patient identify and meet immediate needs for help may result in the patient's more active participation by complying or not complying with the doctor's orders" (p. 411). She went on to point out that her position was logical, because "if the patient were able to carry out the diagnostic or treatment plan alone, in all probability the nurse would not become involved in the first place" (Orlando, 1961, p. 72).

Orlando (1961) provided only a brief description of health, referring to mental health and physical health and to human beings' sense of well-being and adequacy. She did not describe environment, although she implied that the immediate situation is the environment of interest.

Antecedent Knowledge

Orlando did not identify sources of antecedent knowledge. As Forchuk (1991) noted, "Neither book [Orlando, 1961, 1972] contains even a reference list for a hint of other influences" (p. 40). Rather, the Theory of the Deliberative Nursing Process was induced from observations of nurses and patients made as part of a research project. It represents Orlando's (1961) "synthesis of experience in working and learning with teachers, students, nurses, patients, friends and colleagues" (p. ix).

Orlando (1989) recalled that she rejected preexisting frameworks from psychology, social work, and other disciplines for the analysis of the research project data. She explained, "I found what was there [in the data describing nursing outcomes]—I didn't make it up." Elaborating, Schmieding (1990) explained:

> Orlando was one of the first to use field methodology to develop her theoretical perspectives long before it was accepted as appropriate. From participant-observer notes, she devised an ingenious conception of the elements and relationships involved as the nurse determines the meaning of the patient's immediate behavior. (p. xviii)

CONTENT OF THE THEORY

Concepts

Analysis of Orlando's publications revealed that the concepts of the Theory of the Deliberative Nursing Process are **PATIENT'S BEHAVIOR, NURSE'S REACTION,** and **NURSE'S ACTIVITY.** "The interaction of these [concepts] with each other is," according to Orlando (1961), "nursing process" (p. 36).

The concept of **PATIENT'S BEHAVIOR** has two dimensions—**Need for Help** and **Improvement.** The concept

of **NURSE'S REACTION** has three dimensions—**Perception, Thought,** and **Feeling.** The concept of **NURSE'S ACTIVITY** has two dimensions—**Automatic Nursing Process** and **Deliberative Nursing Process.** The dimension of **Deliberative Nursing Process** has three subdimensions—*Activities, Sequence,* and *Requirements.*

Nonrelational Propositions

The definitions for all of the concepts of the Theory of the Deliberative Nursing Process and their dimensions and subdimensions are given here. Those constitutive definitions are the nonrelational propositions of the theory.

PATIENT'S BEHAVIOR

- Behavior [that] is observed by the nurse in an immediate nurse-patient situation (Orlando, 1961, p. 36)

The concept of **Patient's Behavior** encompasses two dimensions—Need for Help and Improvement.

- **Need for Help:** A requirement of the patient which, if supplied, relieves or diminishes his immediate distress or improves his immediate sense of adequacy or well-being (Orlando, 1961, p. 5)
- **Improvement:** To grow better, to turn to profit, to use to advantage (Orlando, 1961, p. 6); an increase in patients' mental and physical health, their well-being, and their sense of adequacy (Orlando, 1961); a change in the behavior of the [patient] indicating either relief from distress or symptoms or that a solution to a living or work problem had been found (Orlando, 1972, p. 61)

The two dimensions of the concept of **Patient's Behavior**—Need for Help and Improvement—can be expressed in both nonverbal and verbal forms (Orlando, 1961). The manifestations of nonverbal behavior encompass several visual and vocal manifestations, which are listed here:

- *Visual Manifestations—Motor Activities:*
  - Eating
  - Walking
  - Twitching
  - Trembling

- *Visual Manifestations—Physiological Activities:*
  - Urinating
  - Defecating
  - Temperature and blood pressure readings
  - Respiratory rate
  - Skin color

• *Vocal Manifestations—Behavior that is heard:*
  • Crying
  • Moaning
  • Laughing
  • Coughing
  • Sneezing
  • Sighing
  • Yelling
  • Screaming
  • Groaning
  • Singing

The manifestations of verbal behavior are:

• *What a patient says:*
  • Complaints
  • Requests
  • Questions
  • Refusals
  • Demands
  • Comments
  • Statements

Orlando (1961) pointed out that "verbal and nonverbal behavior can of course be observed simultaneously" (p. 37). She also pointed out that some patient behaviors, such as refusals or demands, may be regarded as ineffective, that is, "behavior [that] prevents the nurse from carrying out her concerns for the patient's care or from maintaining a satisfactory relationship to the patient" (p. 78). She urged nurses not to dismiss or ignore such behavior, however, because it is "a possible signal of distress or a manifestation of an unmet need" (p. 79). Indeed, "regardless of the form in which it appears, [the patient's behavior] may represent a plea for help" (p. 40).

The dimension of Improvement is, as Orlando (1961) pointed out, "always relative to "what was" when the [nursing process] started, and is concerned with the patient's increased sense of well-being or a change for the better in his condition. The help received by the patient may also have cumulative value as it affects or contributes toward the individual's adequacy in taking better care of himself" (p. 9).

NURSE'S REACTION

• The nurse's nonobservable response to the patient's behavior (Orlando, 1961)

The concept of **Nurse's Reaction** encompasses three dimensions—Perception, Thought, and Feeling.

• **Perception:** A physical stimulation of any one of a person's five senses (Orlando, 1972, p. 59)
• **Thought:** An idea [that] occurs in the mind of a person (Orlando, 1972, p. 59)

• **Feeling:** A state of mind inclining a person toward or against a perception, thought or action (Orlando, 1972, p. 59)

With regard to the **Nurse's Reaction**, Orlando (1961) explained that in the nursing situation, Perception is of the **Patient's Behavior**, and that the nurse's Perception stimulates a Thought. Orlando (1961) went on to explain, "When the nurse perceives a patient, the thoughts which automatically occur to her reflect the meaning or interpretation she attaches to her perception" (p. 40). The nurse's Perception, according to Orlando (1961), "is more often than not correct. [In contrast,] the individual and automatic thought the nurse has about her perception is likely to be inadequate or not completely correct unless it is first investigated with the patient. Indeed, thoughts are sometimes completely incorrect" (p. 43).

Furthermore, in the nursing situation, a Feeling occurs in response to the nurse's Perception and Thought. Orlando (1961) pointed out that the nurse's Feeling must be expressed if it is to benefit the patient:

> Even if feelings are positive but derived from thoughts which are not first checked with the patient, they do not benefit him. ... The patient can make use of the nurse's feeling when she expresses it, provided she explains the basis for it and allows the patient to correct or validate what her feeling is about. (p. 49)

Orlando (1961) acknowledged the difficulty of separating Perception from Thought and Feeling. She maintained, however, that "it is worth trying to do so in order to focus attention on how one aspect of the nurse's reaction may affect the other aspects" (p. 40).

Orlando (1961) noted that "the nurse does not assume that any aspect of her reaction to the patient is correct, helpful or appropriate until she checks the validity of it in exploration with the patient" (p. 56). She also noted, "Reactions [that] the nurse does not resolve may interfere with the interaction between herself and a patient. These reactions may stem from her personal or professional frame of reference, i.e., her personal codes of behavior, her personal value system or her own ideas as to what a nurse should or should not do and say" (p. 56).

NURSE'S ACTIVITY

• The observable action taken by the nurse in response to her reaction (Orlando, 1961)
• Observable behavior, i.e., what the individual says verbally and/or manifests nonverbally (Orlando, 1972, p. 60)
• Only what [the nurse] says or does with or for the benefit of the patient, such as: instructions, suggestions, directions, explanations, information, requests, and

questions directed toward the patient; making decisions for the patient; handling the patient's body; administering medications or treatments; and changing the patient's immediate environment (Orlando, 1961)

The concept of **Nurse's Activity** encompasses two dimensions—Automatic Nursing Process and Deliberative Nursing Process.

• **Automatic Nursing Process:** Actions decided on by the nurse for reasons other than the patient's immediate need (Orlando, 1961, p. 60)

The Automatic Nursing Process dimension of the concept of **Nurse's Activity** is a "nursing process 'without discipline'" (Orlando Pelletier, 1990, p. vii). The Automatic Nursing Process encompasses several activities. "Some automatic activities are ordered by the doctor; others are concerned with routines of caring for patients, and still others are based on principles pertinent to protecting and fostering the health of people in general" (Orlando Pelletier, 1990, p. 60).

• **Deliberative Nursing Process:** A specific set of nurse behaviors or actions directed toward the patient's behavior. Deliberatively decided actions are those [that] ascertain or meet the patient's immediate need (Orlando, 1961, p. 60).

The Deliberative Nursing Process dimension of the concept of **Nurse's Activity** is "nursing process 'with discipline'" (Orlando Pelletier, 1990, p. vii). More specifically, the dimension Deliberative Nursing Process refers to the process of exploration that the nurse initiates "to ascertain how the patient is affected by what she says or does" (Orlando, 1961, p. 67).

The dimension Deliberative Nursing Process has three subdimensions—Activities, Sequence, and Requirements (Orlando, 1961, 1972).

• *Activities*
  1. The nurse initiates a process of helping the patient express the specific meaning of his behavior in order to ascertain his distress.
  2. The nurse helps the patient explore the distress in order to ascertain the help he requires so that the distress may be relieved.

• *Sequence*
  1. The nurse shares with the patient aspects of her perceptions, thoughts, and feelings by expressing in words or nonverbal gestures or tones her wondering, thinking, or questioning in order to learn how accurate or adequate her reaction is.
  2. The response of the patient gives rise to fresh reactions, which the nurse continues to express and explore. The nurse must do this so that both can find out what each is thinking, and why, so that an understanding of the patient's need can be arrived at. When the patient's need is clearly discerned, the nurse can decide on an appropriate course of action.
  3. The nurse then does or says something with or for the patient, or together they decide whether the help of another person is required. Whatever the action, the nurse asks the patient about it in order to find out how her action affects him.

• *Requirements*
  1. What the nurse says to the individual in the contact must match (be consistent with) any or all of the items contained in the immediate reaction and what the nurse does nonverbally must be verbally expressed and the expression must match one or all of the items contained in the immediate reaction.
  2. The nurse must clearly communicate to the individual that the item being expressed belongs to herself.
  3. The nurse must ask the individual about the item expressed in order to obtain correction or verification from that same individual.
  4. The item expressed must be explicitly self-designated by use of a personal pronoun, and a question must be asked about the same item. Examples of this requirement are:
     • I am afraid you will hit me if I ask you a question. Should I be afraid?
     • I don't think you trust anyone. Do you think you do?
     • I think you are very upset today. Are you upset?

The two major Activities of the Deliberative Nursing Process are necessary to meet the patient's needs, and the process follows a definite Sequence. In addition, the Deliberative Nursing Process must meet the four Requirements listed above. The Activities, Sequence, and Requirements clearly demonstrate that the Deliberative Nursing Process "has elements of continuous reflection as the nurse tries to understand the meaning to the patient of the behavior she observes and what he needs from her in order to be helped" (Orlando, 1961, p. 67).

Orlando (1961) pointed out that Deliberative Nursing Activities are effective—that is, they meet the patient's need for help. Deliberative Nursing Activities are effective because:

• The activity comes about after the nurse knows the meaning of the patient's behavior and the specific activity [that] is required to meet his need.
• The activity is carried out in such a way that the patient

is helped to inform the nurse as to how her activity affects him.

- The specific required activity meets the patient's need for help and achieves the nurse's purpose of having helped the patient.
- The nurse is available to respond to the patient's need for help.
- The nurse knows how her activity affects the patient.

In contrast, Automatic Nursing Activities may be "correct" (p. 87), but they are ineffective in meeting the patient's need for help. Thus, although automatic activities may be designed to help the patient, "deliberation is needed to determine whether the activity actually achieves its intended purpose and whether the patient is helped by it" (p. 60). Automatic Nursing Activities are ineffective because:

- The activity is decided on for reasons other than the meaning of the patient's behavior and the unmet need, giving rise to it.
- The activity does not enable the patient to let the nurse know how the activity affects him.
- The activity is unrelated to the patient's immediate need for help.

Relational Propositions

The relational propositions of the Theory of the Deliberative Nursing Process are listed below. The **Patient's Behavior** concept dimension of **Need for Help** and the **Nurse's Reaction** concept dimension of **Perception** are linked in relational proposition A. The concepts of **Nurse's Reaction** and **Nurse's Activity** are linked in relational proposition B. In relational proposition C, the three dimensions of the concept of **Nurse's Reaction** are linked to the concept of **Nurse's Activity**. This sequential proposition describes what Orlando (1972) called the action process. The concepts of **Nurse's Activity** and **Patient's Behavior** are linked in relational propositions D and E. The concept of **Nurse's Activity** is linked with the **Patient's Behavior** concept dimension of **Improvement** in relational propositions F, G, H, and I.

A. The behavior [that] the nurse perceives must be viewed as a possible manifestation of an unmet need [for help] or a signal of distress … unless she has evidence to the contrary (Orlando, 1961, p. 39).

B. What a nurse says or does is necessarily an outcome of her reaction to something in the situation (Orlando, 1961, p. 61).

C. The process of a nurse's activity is based on a specific formulation of the process by which any individual acts. … The process … is comprised of four distinct items. These separate items reside within an individual and at any given moment occur in the following automatic, sometimes instantaneous, sequence: (1) The person perceives with any one of his five sense organs an object or objects; (2) the perceptions stimulate automatic thought; (3) each thought stimulates an automatic feeling; and (4) then the person acts (Orlando, 1972, pp. 24–25).

D. Any observation shared and explored with the nurse is immediately useful in ascertaining and meeting his need [for help] or finding out that he is not in need at that time (Orlando, 1961, p. 36).

E. If the nurse automatically decides on the "right" activity but holds in abeyance what she wants to achieve until she ascertains and meets the patient's need, she helps the patient and achieves her primary objective. If the nurse is not able to carry out what she thinks is indicated, she helps the patient tell her why her judgment is inappropriate or incorrect. She then makes a new decision or continues to explore what is going on so that the patient will understand and accept what the nurse believes is indicated. In either case the purpose is to help the patient. Another way to think of this is that either the patient is willing to go along with the nurse, or the nurse is willing to go along with the patient. They have to move together to achieve a common goal (Orlando, 1961, p. 89).

F. There are … three possible ways for the patient to be affected by nursing activities—the activity may help, may not help, or the result may be unknown (Orlando, 1961, p. 67).

G. The nurse recognizes if she has met the patient's need for help by noting the presence or absence of improvement in his presenting behavior. In the absence of improvement, the nurse knows the patient's need has not yet been met, and, if she remains available, she starts the process all over again with whatever presenting behavior is then observed (Orlando, 1961, p. 68).

H. The product of meeting the patient's immediate need for help is … "improvement" in the immediate verbal and nonverbal behavior of the patient. This observable change allows the nurse to believe or disbelieve that her activity relieved, prevented or diminished the patient's sense of helplessness. In subjective but at least conceptual terms the "improvement" has a measure of curative value to the helplessness suffered by patients in immediate experiences. In this conceptual sense the professional function of nursing is fulfilled and its product is achieved (Orlando, 1972, pp. 21–22).

I. The nurse, in achieving her purpose, contributes simultaneously to the mental and physical health of her patient. This is so because in helping him she affects for the better his sense of adequacy or well-being (Orlando, 1961, p. 9).

EVALUATION OF THE THEORY OF THE DELIBERATIVE NURSING PROCESS

This section presents an evaluation of Orlando's Theory of the Deliberative Nursing Process. The evaluation is based on the results of the analysis of the theory, as well as on publications by others who have used or commented on this nursing theory.

SIGNIFICANCE

The Theory of the Deliberative Nursing Process meets the criterion of significance in part. Orlando did not explicitly identify the metaparadigmatic or paradigmatic origins of the Theory of the Deliberative Nursing Process. The relevant metaparadigm concepts and proposition were, however, extracted from the contents of her books, and a rudimentary conceptual model that describes human beings and nursing, and to a lesser extent, health, was extracted from Orlando's publications. Moreover, although Orlando did not label all of her assumptions as such, the statements that represent the philosophical claims undergirding the Theory of the Deliberative Nursing Process and the associated research methodology were easily extracted from her publications.

Orlando claimed no influences from antecedent knowledge on development of the Theory of the Deliberative Nursing Process. Furthermore, systematic examination of Orlando's publications about the theory revealed no evidence of its derivation from other nursing theories or theories from other disciplines. It is, however, likely that Orlando's implicit conceptual model, which was made explicit here in the analysis section of this chapter, guided here thinking as the theory emerged from the data.

The Theory of the Deliberative Nursing Process is, then, a distinctive nursing theory. As Forchuk (1991) stated, "Orlando's most significant contribution may have been her move away from any existing nursing or nonnursing theory to build her theory entirely on grounded research of actual nursing practice" (p. 43).

The Theory of the Deliberative Nursing Process has definitely enhanced understanding of the nurse-patient relationship, as well as understanding of the nurse's professional role and identity. A particularly noteworthy feature of the theory is the precise specification of the Activities, Sequence, and Requirements making up the Deliberative Nursing Process.

Speaking to the special significance of the theory in a foreword to the 1990 reprint of Orlando's 1961 book, Schmieding (1990) stated:

> Orlando's work was a major force in shifting the nurse's focus from the medical diagnosis to the patient's immediate experience. In her book, Orlando clearly articulates the uniqueness of each patient's immediate need for help as well as the uniqueness of the nurse's deliberative process in determining with the patient his or her specific need. The use of Orlando's theory thus prevents the nurse from acting on invalidated assumptions. … Orlando's theory [emphasizes] the necessity of involving patients in all aspects of their care. Nursing care has become more individualized as a result of this involvement. (p. xvii)

In a more recent explication of the significance of Orlando's theory, Schmieding (2002) stated, "Orlando's theory remains effective and efficient in achieving valued outcome. Identifying the patient's immediate needs for help and the nurse's ability to meet those needs are critically important to patient outcomes and the advancement of nursing practice" (p. 410).

Perhaps the most significant aspect of Orlando's work is the coining of the term "nursing process." Henderson (1978) explained:

> Psychiatric nursing, which was once a stepchild of the nursing profession, came into its own during the 1950s when there was perhaps more money for studies of psychiatric nursing in the USA than for the study of any other branch of clinical nursing. One such study was that of Ida Jean Orlando (1961) at Yale University School of Nursing during which, I believe, she coined the term "nursing process". … The "nursing process" is now a part of the language of nursing in the USA. While Miss Orlando's concept is close kin to the one I had stated in a nursing text in 1955 (Harmer & Henderson), her insistence that the nurse gets the patient to confirm or validate the impression on which the nurse based an assumption of the patient's need was, in my judgment, an important contribution to the concept of nursing. (p. 119)

INTERNAL CONSISTENCY

The Theory of the Deliberative Nursing Process meets the criterion of internal consistency in part. The theory content is congruent with Orlando's philosophical claims, and the theory content is clearly based on her conceptualization of human beings and nursing.

Semantic clarity is evident in the constitutive definitions given for the concepts of the Theory of the Deliberative Nursing Process and their dimensions. As Schmieding (1990) pointed out, "Orlando provided succinct descriptions of the nursing process [which] express elegantly what nurses perceive as the essence of nursing, namely, determining and meeting, directly or indirectly, the patient's need for help in the immediate nurse-patient contact" (p. xvii).

Semantic inconsistency is, however, evident in changes in certain terms, but that appears to be the result of Orlando's (1961, 1972; Orlando Pelletier, 1990) attempt to find terms that would more effectively convey her ideas. Inconsistencies were noted in some terms: help (1961) and need for help (1990); improvement (1961) and helpful outcome (1972); automatic nursing process (1961) and nursing process without discipline (1972); and deliberative nursing process (1961) and process discipline (1972) or nursing process with discipline (1972).

With regard to the inconsistency in the terms help and need for help, Orlando explained in the preface of the 1990 reprint of her 1961 book, "Throughout this text, only the phrase need for help should have been used and not the word need" (Orlando Pelletier, 1990, p. vii). With regard to the inconsistency in the terms deliberative nursing process, process discipline, and nursing process with discipline, Orlando explained, "The deliberative nursing process was renamed nursing process 'with discipline'" (Orlando Pelletier, 1990, p. vii). Orlando did not explain the inconsistency in the terms improvement and helpful outcome.

The analysis of the Theory of the Deliberative Nursing Process revealed structural consistency. The concepts are adequately linked by means of relational propositions, and the progression from **Patient's Behavior** (Need for Help) to **Nurse's Reaction** to **Nurse's Activity** and back to **Patient's Behavior** (Improvement) is clearly specified.

PARSIMONY

The Theory of the Deliberative Nursing Process meets the criterion of parsimony. The theory is elegant in the paucity of words used to convey complex ideas. The theory may, however, be oversimplified. Schmieding (1987) explained:

> A criticism of Orlando's work, despite its elegant specificity, is the lack of repetition and full explanation to accompany important concepts and formulations. The thought may occur to the reader, "if a feature is mentioned, isn't that sufficient?" When learning complex formulations, even if they are clear and precise, and in grasping the meaning and use of abstract concepts, … repetition and more detailed explanations are necessary strategies. (p. 440)

Schmieding (1987) went on to say, "This criticism does not detract from the soundness of Orlando's theory; rather it highlights the fact that practical theories are noted for their simplicity and precision" (p. 440). And, in a later commentary, Schmieding (1990) pointed out that

> the simplicity of [Orlando's] formulations … disguises the complexity of the nurse-patient interaction. The importance

of using perceptions, thoughts, or feelings to understand the meaning of the patient's immediate behavior is not something a person does naturally. It must be developed. (p. xviii)

TESTABILITY

The Theory of the Deliberative Nursing Process meets the criterion of testability for middle-range theories. Orlando (1972) designed a specific **RESEARCH METHODOLOGY** to test the theory. The components of the **RESEARCH METHODOLOGY** are identified and described in Table 14–1.

All components of the **Research Methodology** are completely consistent with and reflect the content of the Theory of the Deliberative Nursing Process. The **Purposes of Research,** the **Phenomena of Interest,** and the **Study Participants** are evident in Orlando's (1961, 1972) books. Furthermore, although Orlando (1961, 1972) labeled some statements as assumptions, they are more appropriately labeled as **Testable Propositions or Hypotheses.** In keeping with the Theory of the Deliberative Nursing Process, Propositions/Hypotheses 1, 2, and 3 refer to the effects of using or not using the **Deliberative Nursing Process;** Propositions/ Hypotheses 4 and 5 refer to the effects of training nurses to use the **Deliberative Nursing Process.** Those propositions indicate that a quasi-experimental or experimental **Study Design** is required. Orlando (1972) advocated nonparticipant observation, tape-recorded person-to-person contacts, and process recordings as the primary **Data Collection Methods.** Other appropriate methods are questionnaires and devices designed to measure particular manifestations of the patient's distress and specific symptoms. For example, Dumas and Leonard (1963) measured the incidence of postoperative vomiting, and Anderson, Mertz, and Leonard (1965) measured blood pressure, pulse rate, and such observable behaviors as sobbing and movements of limbs. Moreover, Williamson (1978) developed an instrument to measure patients' and nurses' awareness of patients' physical and emotional needs, and Potter and Bockenhauer (2000) developed the Bockenhauer/Potter Scale of Immediate Distress to measure nurses' ratings of patient-demonstrated distress (Table 14–2). All of those **Data Collection Methods** are appropriate empirical indicators for the concepts of the Theory of the Deliberative Nursing Process. Orlando (1972) also developed a schema for **Data Analysis,** using precise operational definitions to code the *Characteristics of Verbal Expressions,* the *Outcome,* and the *Consistency of the Nurse's Verbal Expression with the Nurse's Reaction.* The **Data Analysis** schema is in keeping with the Theory of the Deliberative Nursing Process and clearly permits measurement of the relation between the concepts of **Nurse's**

PURPOSES OF THE RESEARCH

To determine the effects of the use of the deliberative nursing process on behavior of patients and other persons (staff and supervisors) in the nursing system.

To test the effects of training in the use of the process discipline on its actual use in practice.

PHENOMENA OF INTEREST

The patient's or other person's behavior, the nurse's reactions, and the nurse's activity.

STUDY PARTICIPANTS

Patients

Staff nurses

Nurse supervisors

TESTABLE PROPOSITIONS/HYPOTHESES

1. Once the patient has been helped, he feels safer to communicate the distress of which he is aware. ... Once he trusts the nurse, his communications are more explicit and he is more likely to spontaneously discuss the experiences which distress him (Orlando, 1961, p. 26).
2. When the reaction of the nurse, in any of its aspects, is not explored with the patient, his condition remains unchanged or becomes worse (Orlando, 1961, p. 45).
3. If a nurse automatically acts on any perception, thought, or feeling without exploring it further with the patient, the activity may very well be ineffective in achieving its purpose or in helping the patient. On the other hand, if the nurse checks her thoughts and explores her reactions with the patient before deciding on which action to follow, what she does is more likely to achieve its purpose and help the patient (Orlando, 1961, p. 61).
4. Training would increase the nurse's use of the [deliberative nursing] process (Orlando, 1972, p. 66).
5. Trained nurses would use the [deliberative nursing] process more than untrained ones (Orlando, 1972, p. 66).

STUDY DESIGN

Quasi-experimental

Experimental

DATA COLLECTION METHODS

Nonparticipant observation

Tape recorded person-to-person contacts

Process recordings

Questionnaires and devices designed to measure particular manifestations of patient distress and specific symptoms

DATA ANALYSIS

Codes for Characteristics of Verbal Expressions

- X   An item is verbally expressed.
- Y   An item is asked about.
- Z   An item that is verbally expressed is designated to the self with a personal pronoun.
- XY   An item is first expressed and the same item is asked about.
- XZ   An item expressed is designated to the self.
- XYZ   An item first expressed is designated to the self and the same item is asked about.

Consistency Between Reactions and Verbal Expressions

- Consistency is defined as whether the verbal behavior matched the reaction.
- Self-designated consistency is defined as whether self-designated verbal expressions were consistent with the reaction.
- No self-designated consistency is defined as whether verbal expressions that were not self-designated were consistent with the reaction.

Codes for Consistency Between Reactions and Verbal Expressions

- Consistent and self-designated
- Consistent and not self-designated
- Inconsistent and self-designated
- Inconsistent and not self-designated

Codes for Outcomes

- High   Verbal and vocal nonverbal indications of improvement
- Medium   Verbal or nonverbal indications of improvement
- Low   No indication of improvement but understanding increased
- Zero   No indications of high, medium, or low improvement; or no indication of distress, symptom, or problem; or no indication of increased distress or symptom or manifestation of a problem

Source: Constructed from Orlando, 1972; data analysis section adapted from Orlando, 1972, pp. 60–61, 63, with permission.

Reaction and **Nurse's Activity**, as well as the relation between the concept of **Nurse's Activity** and the Improvement dimension of the concept of **Patient's Behavior**.

EMPIRICAL ADEQUACY

The Theory of the Deliberative Nursing Process meets the criterion of empirical adequacy for middle-range theories. Published reports of the use of the Theory of the Deliberative Nursing Process as a guide for nursing research are listed in Table 14–3.

A review of those reports, along with the master's theses and doctoral dissertations listed in the chapter bibliography on the CD-ROM, revealed considerable empirical support. In particular, several studies conducted in the early 1960s by faculty and students at the Yale University School of Nursing provided impressive evidence of the beneficial effects of using the Deliberative Nursing Process (see especially Anderson, Mertz, & Leonard, 1965; Barron, 1966; Bochnak, 1963; Cameron, 1963; Dumas, 1963; Dumas & Leonard, 1963; Dye, 1963; Elms & Leonard, 1966; Faulkner, 1963; Fischelis, 1963; Mertz, 1963; Rhymes, 1964; Tryon, 1963, 1966; Tryon & Leonard, 1964).

Although the Yale studies "came to an abrupt halt," Orlando explained that she "continued to develop and refine" her original formulations (Orlando Pelletier, 1990, p. vii). The result of her effort was the publication of the findings of a major National Institute of Mental Health–funded quasi-experimental study that Orlando (1972) conducted at McLean Hospital, a private psychiatric hospital located in Belmont, Massachusetts. The purpose of that study was to test the effectiveness of the use of the deliberative nursing process and the value of its use in patient, staff, and supervisee contacts. Study participants were staff nurses and supervisors, whose contacts with patients, other staff, and supervisees were observed and tape-recorded. Data were obtained from transcribed tape recordings of 144 contacts made by six staff nurses and six supervisors who had been trained in the use of the deliberative nursing process. Other data were obtained from the written records of 280 verbal exchanges submitted by 28 trainees. Analysis of the data revealed that the use of the deliberative nursing process had a significant positive effect on patient and staff behavior, as indicated by a relief from distress or symptoms or the identification of a solution to a living or work problem. Summarizing the results of her research, Orlando (1972) stated:

> The research findings amply document that a verbal form of a [deliberative nursing process] can be isolated, tested and then evaluated in relation to an operational concept of effectiveness in patient, staff and supervisee contacts. Further, the same verbal form is sufficient to measure the use of the [deliberative nursing process] and, therefore, sufficient to measure training results. Still further, findings show that the [deliberative nursing process] and training in its use is effective in achieving helpful outcomes in patient and/or staff and/or supervisee contacts. … These findings, specific to this research, strongly suggest that the [deliberative nursing process] and training in its use is directly relevant to solving the more general problem of inadequate patient care (p. viii).

Instrument or Tool and Citation*	Description
RESEARCH INSTRUMENTS	
Bockenhauer-Potter Scale of Immediate Distress (Potter & Bockenhauer, 2000)	Measures the nurse's rating of the degree of patient-demonstrated distress
Patient's Physical and Emotional Needs Instrument (Williamson, 1978)	Measures patients' and nurses' awareness of patients' physical and emotional needs
PRACTICE TOOLS	
Nursing Process Record (Orlando, 1972, p. 56)	A form that permits recording of perception of or about the patient, thought and/or feeling about the perception, and what the nurse said and/or did to, with, or for the patient
Assessing a Patient by Using Orlando's Theory to Guide the Nurse's Process (Schmieding, 2002)	Contains guidelines for finding out and meeting the patient's immediate need for help

*See the Research Instruments and Practice Tools section of the chapter references for complete citations.

More recently, Potter and Bockenhauer (2000) found evidence of a greater reduction in patients' immediate distress when nurses used the deliberative nursing process than when nurses used a nonspecified nursing intervention. Their sample included 10 registered nurses and 30 patients at a large, university-affiliated state psychiatric hospital, and they used the Bockenhauer/Potter Scale of Immediate Distress to measure patient-demonstrated distress. The investigators explained that the nurses' anecdotal comments indicated that they felt more effective when using the deliberative nursing process as a 'road map' for identifying and meeting the patients' immediate needs for help.

PRAGMATIC ADEQUACY

The Theory of the Deliberative Nursing Process meets the criterion of pragmatic adequacy. Orlando specified the training that is required for use of the theory, and she identified the components of a methodology for applying the theory in the real world of nursing practice.

Nursing Education

Special training is required to learn how to apply the Theory of the Deliberative Nursing Process. Schmieding (2002) contended that every student nurse should receive that special training.

Training in the Deliberative Nursing Process is predicated on Orlando's (1961) claim that "what the individual nurse happens to perceive or think (relevant or otherwise) is not so important as what she does with it. What the nurse automatically perceives or thinks cannot ordinarily be controlled, but she can learn a responsive discipline, the discipline [that] phrases or formulates her perceptions or thoughts by questioning and wondering about the meaning of them to the patient" (p. 41).

Orlando (1972) used the term training to refer to "the process of preparing nurses to impose a specific discipline on the nursing process to fulfill a specific function and achieve a specific product" (p. 2). The purpose of training "is to change the responsiveness of the nurse from the one described as personal and automatic to one [that] is disciplined and professional" (p. 33).

Emphasis in training is, therefore, placed on the **Nurse's Activity** rather than on the dimensions of the **Nurse's Reaction** (Perception, Thought, Feeling). Orlando (1972) found that the Deliberative Nursing Process can be taught successfully to staff nurses in 6 weeks and to supervisors in 3 months. Training is facilitated by use of process recordings of the trainee's reaction and activity. The process recordings are then discussed in individual and group conferences between the trainees and training instructor. The major task, steps, and outcomes of training nurses to use the Deliberative Nursing Process are summarized here.

(Text continues on page 521)

Research Topic	Study Participants	Citation*
DESCRIPTIVE STUDIES		
Effectiveness of student nurses' immediate responses to distressed patients	Senior students in associate degree and baccalaureate degree programs Videotapes of simulated patients' physical and emotional distress	Haggerty, 1987
Effectiveness of nurse managers' responses to problematic situations	Nurse managers Written vignettes about nurse manager–staff nurse situations	Schmieding, 1987
Action processes of nurse administrators in problematic situations	Nurse administrators Written vignettes about patient, nurse, and physician situations	Schmieding, 1988
Types of administrative actions that nurses find helpful	Staff nurses Head nurses Supervisors Written vignettes about patient, nurse, and physician situations	Schmieding, 1990b
Types of head nurse actions that staff nurses find helpful	Staff nurses Head nurses Written vignettes about patient, nurse, and physician situations	Schmieding, 1990a
Immediate responses of staff nurses and head nurses to problematic situations	Staff nurses Head nurses Written vignettes about staff nurse–patient situations	Schmieding, 1991
Nurses' perceptions of the structure of selected nursing care episodes	Master's degree-prepared nurse Adult surgical patients List of 17 nurse-patient situations during postoperative hospitalization	Houfek, 1992
Barriers that prevent effective screening for domestic violence	Registered nurses working in an emergency department	Ellis, 1999
Spouses' identification of their needs	Spouses of dying patients	Hampe, 1975
Patients' satisfaction with nurses' responses to their expressed needs	Adult postoperative patients	Gowen & Morris, 1964
CORRELATIONAL STUDY		
Relation of nurse-expressed empathy to patient-perceived empathy and patient distress	Staff nurses Hospitalized adult medical and surgical patients	Olson & Hanchett, 1997

*See the Research section of the chapter references for complete citations.

(continued)

519

Research Topic	Study Participants	Citation
EXPERIMENTAL STUDIES		
Effect of research-based nursing interventions on spouses' needs	Spouses of patients in a coronary care unit	Dracup & Breu, 1978
Effect of experimental and control educational programs on blood pressure	Patients with hypertension	Powers & Wooldridge, 1982
Effects of an experimental nursing intervention of information-giving and psychological support and a control nursing intervention on spouses' anxiety and attitudes toward hospitalization	Spouses of hospitalized surgical patients	Silva, 1979
Effect of an experimental interpersonal nursing approach and a control nursing approach on patients' hospital-related stress (urine potassium output, anxiety)	Hospitalized medical patients	Pride, 1968
Effect of Orlando's nursing process on exploration of patients' distress	Hospitalized adult medical and surgical patients	Dye, 1963
Effect of Orlando's nursing process on identification of patient concerns	Renal transplant clinic patients 1 year or more after transplant	Nelson, 1978
Effects of an experimental patient-centered admission process and a control admission process on patients' behaviorally displayed distress, systolic blood pressure, and pulse rate	Patients admitted to an emergency department Patients admitted to a mental hospital	Anderson et al., 1965
Effects of an individualized nursing approach and two control nursing approaches on patients' systolic blood pressure, radial pulse rate, respiratory rate, and oral temperature	Patients admitted for elective gynecologic surgery	Elms, 1964 Elms & Leonard, 1966
Effect of psychological preparation for surgery on preoperative patient distress	Gynecologic surgical patients	Dumas, 1963
Effect of experimental and control psychological preparation for surgery on postoperative vomiting	Gynecologic surgical patients	Dumas & Leonard, 1963 Dumas et al., 1965
Effects of an experimental nursing intervention of systematic psychological preparation and continued supportive care and a control intervention on children's distress, cooperation, and posthospital adjustment problems and parents' anxiety and satisfaction with information and nursing care	Hospitalized children and their parents	Wolfer & Visintainer, 1975
Effect of a nondirective, patient-centered nursing approach and a control nursing approach on effectiveness of the predelivery enema	Pregnant women in labor	Tryon, 1962 Tryon & Leonard, 1964

Effects of experimental patient participation in using comfort measures (breathing control, position, back care, elimination, oral care, oral fluids, linen change) and control use of comfort measures on patients' vocal activity, body activity, and control of breathing	Pregnant women in labor	Tryon, 1966
Effect of deliberative and routine nursing approaches on maternal distress associated with breastfeeding	Breastfeeding mothers on a postpartum unit	Princeton, 1986
Effect of deliberative and automatic nursing processes on relief of patients' distress (blood pressure and pulse rate)	Patients in an emergency department	Mertz, 1962
Effect of deliberative and automatic nursing processes on relief of patients' pain	Hospitalized patients	Bochnak et al., 1962 Tarasuk et al., 1965
Effect of deliberative and automatic nursing processes on patients' ability to sleep	Hospitalized medical and surgical patients	Gillis, 1976
Effect of an experimental deliberative nursing process and a control nonspecified nursing intervention on degree of patient-demonstrated distress	Psychiatric patients	Potter & Bockenhauer, 2000 Potter & Tinker, 2000
Effects of experimental nursing care at a local community service center and control emergency department care on children's health and parents' health behaviors	Children with an upper respiratory tract infection and their parents	Thibaudeau & Reidy, 1977
Effects of a high-intensity collaborative practice ambulatory program on patient satisfaction, intensity of medication treatment, and amount and patterns of health services use	Patients with bipolar disorder	Shea et al., 1997

(Text continued from page 518)

- **Major Task**
  - To help the trainee express in full detail (in retrospect) all of the items contained in the immediate reaction in the particular nurse-patient contact being examined. In effect, this helps the trainee experience freedom to acknowledge what the reaction was.

- **Steps of Training**
  - Initially, the training instructor focuses exclusively on eliciting all of the items contained in the trainee's immediate reaction and activity and identifying each item—perception, thought, feeling, action.
  - The trainee records his or her own reaction and activity on a process record that contains parallel columns for "perception of or about the patient," "thought and/or feeling about the perception," and "said and/or did to, with, or for the patient."

- The instructor helps the trainee correct any items of the reaction or activity that were misplaced on the process record form and to add any items that were not included.
- The instructor helps the trainee analyze how the particular reaction and activity affected finding out and meeting the patient's immediate need for help.
- The instructor "literally, but lovingly, coerces the trainee to be herself with the specified discipline" (Orlando, 1972, p. 42) when there are inconsistencies between the trainee's verbal action and the reaction. In that case, the trainee returns to the patient, expresses and explores his or her immediate reaction, and thereby acquires the additional data needed to find out the patient's perception, thought, or feeling and to explain the patient's reaction.

- **Outcomes of Training**
  - To find out what formerly acquired expectation of what origin explains whatever the activity of the trainee was in the same contact being examined; and further, to authoritatively release the trainee from the relevance of the expectation to the same contact being examined. In effect, this helps the trainee not only to experience freedom from expectations of what the trainee "should" perceive, think, feel, say, and do, but to further acknowledge that what he or she "actually" perceived, thought, and felt and what he or she "actually" said and did in the contact being examined.

The need for training is supported by the results of Schmieding's (1988) study of the action process used by nurse administrators in response to hypothetical problematic staff situations. She found that the administrators either did not regard the situations as problematic or responded in an automatic manner. Schmieding indicated that her findings supported Orlando's (1972) contention that special training is required for use of the Deliberative Nursing Process.

The effort expended in training leads to rewards when the Theory of the Deliberative Nursing Process is applied. Orlando (1989) commented, "Nurses who practice their process with discipline will enjoy their practice and can control their practice." Furthermore, Orlando (1972) pointed out that nurses who use the deliberative nursing process express "greater comfort and satisfaction in work situations" (p. 36), and "the trainee's understanding of the process by which she can help a patient in an immediate situation enables her to find her own identity as a professional nurse" (p. 43).

Faust (2002) acknowledged the need for special training to learn the deliberative nursing process but indicated that, after extensive self-directed reading, she was able to apply the process and teach it to nursing staff in an extended care facility. She went on to report that the staff was able to use the deliberative process effectively with two patients who had previously been regarded as creating havoc for both staff and other patients during the night.

Nursing Practice

In keeping with the Theory of the Deliberative Nursing Process, the purpose of nursing practice is "to supply the help a patient requires in order for his needs to be met" (Orlando, 1961, p. 8). More specifically, the function of professional nursing "is conceptualized as finding out and meeting the patient's immediate needs for help" (Orlando, 1972, p. 20). Accordingly, emphasis in nursing practice is placed on the immediate experience of the patient, and the activity performed by a nurse is regarded as professional "only when it deliberatively achieves the purpose of helping the patient" (Orlando, 1961, p. 70).

Orlando (1961, 1972) maintained that the purpose of nursing is achieved when the nurse initiates "a process [that] ascertains the patient's immediate need and helps to meet the need directly or indirectly" (1961, p. 8). The components of that process, which make up Orlando's **PRACTICE METHODOLOGY**, are identified and described in Table 14–4. The central feature of Orlando's **PRACTICE METHODOLOGY** is, of course, the Deliberative Nursing Process. As Orlando (1961) pointed out, although "the natural consequence of observation is a decision to act or not act in relation to what is observed" (p. 7), the direct and indirect observations of the patient "are not adequate for the individual nurse to carry out her responsibility of helping the patient with his needs" (p. 32). Rather, observations must be shared with and validated by the patient. Indeed, "any observation shared and explored with the patient is immediately useful in ascertaining and meeting his need or finding out that he is not in need at that time" (pp. 35–36).

Application of the Theory of the Deliberative Nursing Process by means of the **Practice Methodology** requires that a relationship be established between the nurse and the patient. Orlando (1961) explained:

> Before the nurse establishes her relationship to the patient he does not clearly tell her about his distress or needs; he cannot do so without her help and he does not do so until he is sure she will meet them. Once the relationship is established, his communications to the nurse become clearer and more explicit. When he spontaneously informs the nurse about the specific nature of his distress or what he needs, the nurse can be fairly certain that her professional relationship is established. (p. 28)

A review of published reports of the use of the Theory of the Deliberative Nursing Process in nursing practice (Table 14–5) revealed that the theory is applicable in a wide array of person-to-person encounters in the nursing system and, therefore, in many areas of the real world of nursing practice. As Orlando (1961) pointed out, the theory "has been successfully applied in the nursing of patients with medical, surgical, obstetric and psychiatric conditions and is applicable to the nursing of adults and children whether in the home, hospital or clinic" (p. viii). The theory also has been used in nursing of patients at Brighton Gardens Assisted Living, an extended care facility in Cherry Hill, New Jersey (Faust, 2002).

Orlando (1972) contended that the theory can be applied not only to nurse-patient relationships but also to "contacts with other nurses (line and staff relationships among nurses personnel) and contacts with other professional and nonprofessional people (other staff relationships)" (p., viii). Potter and Bockenhauer (2000) com-

OBSERVATIONS

Observations encompass any and all information pertaining to a patient that the nurse acquires while on duty.

Observations are the raw material with which the nurse makes and implements plans for the patient's care.

Direct observations: The nurse's reaction to the patient's behavior
Direct observations are the nurse's reaction to the patient's behavior.
Direct observations are any perception, thought or feeling the nurse has from his or her own experience of the patient's behavior at any or several moments in time.

Indirect observations: Other information about the patient's behavior
Indirect observations consist of any information that is derived from a source other than the patient. This information pertains to, but is not directly derived from, the patient.

ACTIONS

Actions are carried out with or for the patient.

Nurse's Activity: Deliberative Nursing Process
The process used to share and validate the nurse's direct and indirect observations is the Deliberative Nursing Process.

Clinical Protocols
Clinical protocols contain the specific requirements for the Deliberative Nursing Process
The nurse may express and explore any aspect of his or her reaction to the patient's behavior—perception, thought, or feeling.
If exploration of one aspect of the nurse's reaction does not result in identification of the patient's need for help, another aspect of the reaction can be explored.
If exploration of all aspects of the nurse's reaction does not yield a verbal response from the patient, the nurse may use negative expressions to demonstrate continued interest in the patient behavior and to give the patient permission to respond with his or her own negative reaction.
Examples of negative expressions by the nurse:
* "Is it that you don't think I'll understand?"
* "Am I wrong?"
* "It looked like that procedure was very painful, and you didn't say a word about it."

Direct Help
The nurse meets the patient's need directly when the patient is unable to meet his or her own need and when the activity is confined to the nurse-patient contact.

Indirect Help
The nurse meets the patient's need indirectly when the activity extends to arranging the services of a person, agency, or resource that the patient cannot contact by himself or herself.

REPORTING

The nurse receives reports about the patient's behavior from other nurses and from other health professionals.

The nurse reports his or her observations of the patient's behavior to other nurses and other health professionals.

(continued)

TABLE 14–4
ORLANDO'S PRACTICE METHODOLOGY *(continued)*

RECORDING

The nurse records the nursing process, including:

- The nurse's perception of or about the patient.
- The nurse's thought or feeling about the perception.
- What the nurse said or did to, with, or for the patient.

Constructed from Orlando, 1961, pp. 6–9, 31–36, 42; 1972, p. 56.

mented that nursing administrators at New Hampshire Hospital, a large psychiatric hospital in Concord, New Hampshire, were beginning to plan to use Orlando's theory for clinical supervision. When the theory is extended beyond patients, all references to the patient and patient's behavior are modified to focus on the individual of interest, such as a staff nurse or a supervisee.

The feasibility of implementing practice protocols that reflect the Deliberative Nursing Process is almost self-evident—the recognition, expression, and exploration of Perceptions, Thoughts, and Feelings can occur in any professional nursing situation. The only resources needed are the time and personnel required for proper training. Furthermore, nurses have the legal ability to apply the Theory of the Deliberative Nursing Process in practice and to measure the effectiveness of theory-based nursing actions.

Potter and Tinker (2000) claimed that the use of

TABLE 14–5
PUBLISHED REPORTS OF NURSING PRACTICE GUIDED BY THE THEORY OF THE DELIBERATIVE NURSING PROCESS

Practice Situation	Population	Citation*
Nurse-patient relationships	Surgical patients	Rosenthal, 1996 Schmidt, 1972
	Hospitalized chronically mentally ill patients	Schmieding, 1970
	A man hospitalized for chronic care of pulmonary emphysema	Harrison, 1966
	A pregnant woman who was vomiting	Schmieding, 1986
	A woman diagnosed as having schizophrenia and uterine bleeding	
	A diabetic woman with above-the-knee amputation	
	A man admitted for transurethral resection	
	A man with Raynaud's disease	
	A man with a myocardial infarction	
	A 29-year-old woman with cervical cancer	Schmieding, 2002
	A 57-year-old Vietnamese man with noninfectious tuberculosis	
	Two elderly women residing in an extended care facility	Faust, 2002
Staff-nurse relationships	Staff nurses on two different units	Schmieding, 1986
Supervisor staff-nurse relationships	A head nurse and a senior staff nurse	Schmieding, 1986
Nurse-physician relationships	A staff nurse and a physician A director of nursing and a physician	Schmieding, 1986

*See the Practice section of the chapter references for complete citations.

Orlando's theory at New Hampshire Hospital, "empowers nurses not only to survive, but also to thrive in an unstable [health care] environment" (p. 41). They pointed out that use of the theory is a cost-effective intervention that allows nurses to maximize the time they can spend with patients. They went on to explain, "Because nurses can use the [theory] even with time, energy, and financial constraints, they can reduce frustration associated with 'doing more with less'" (p. 41).

Use of the Theory of the Deliberative Nursing Process is compatible with patients' expectations of nursing practice; there are no reports to date of patients' discomfort or dissatisfaction when the Deliberative Nursing Process has been used. Indeed, a review of the many examples given in Orlando's (1961, 1972) books revealed that patients and staff uniformly reported satisfaction when a nurse used the Deliberative Nursing Process. Potter and Tinker (2000) reported that nurses who use Orlando's theory felt satisfied with their practice.

Many of the studies designed to test the Theory of the Deliberative Nursing Process have included a comparison of outcomes when the Deliberative Nursing Process was used and when it was not used (see Table 14–2). The actual beneficial outcomes of the use of the Deliberative Nursing Process and its problem-solving effectiveness have been documented extensively by Orlando (1972) and other investigators and practitioners (see Tables 14–2 and 14–5). Orlando (1961, 1972) has explained that application of the Theory of the Deliberative Nursing Process yields improvement in the **Patient's Behavior** (or the behavior of a staff nurse or other person) because when one individual in a person-to-person contact expresses and explores his or her own immediate reaction, the other individual in the contact is more able to do the same. Consequently, a more reliable database is available for professional action and decision making, and the person's immediate need for help is more likely to be met. In effect, problems are solved.

 ## CONCLUSION

Continuing interest in the Theory of the Deliberative Nursing Process is attested to by the reprinting of Orlando's 1961 book in 1990. Furthermore, the theory continues to be cited in psychiatric nursing textbooks. For example, Burgess (1997) noted that the Theory of the Deliberative Nursing Process is regarded as an exceptionally influential theory in contemporary psychiatric nursing. International interest in the theory is documented by translations of the 1961 book into Japanese, Hebrew, French, Portuguese, and Dutch (Orlando Pelletier, 1990).

Orlando has made a substantial and significant contribution to nursing knowledge development by explicating a middle-range predictive theory that specifies a nursing process that will meet a person's immediate need for help. "There is no doubt," as Schmieding (1990) pointed out, "that Orlando's formulations ... have had substantial influence on the nursing education, practice, research, and literature that followed [the publication of her theory in 1961]" (p. xviii). Furthermore, use of Orlando's theory helps nurses to "rediscover their unique contribution to patient care—meeting the patient's immediate needs" (Potter & Tinker, 2000, p. 41). Despite the already impressive evidence of the empirical adequacy and pragmatic adequacy of the Theory of the Deliberative Nursing Process, continued study is needed to determine if, as Orlando (1972) predicted, "training in the process discipline is directly relevant to the effectiveness of a nursing system designed to improve the care of patients on a massive scale" (p. 126).

 ## REFERENCES

Anderson, B., Mertz, H., & Leonard, R. (1965). Two experimental tests of a patient-centered admission process. Nursing Research, 14, 151–156.

Barron, M.A. (1966). The effects varied nursing approaches have on patients' complaints of pain [Abstract]. Nursing Research, 15, 90–91.

Bochnak, M.A. (1963). The effect of an automatic and deliberative process of nursing activity on the relief of patients' pain: A clinical experiment [Abstract]. Nursing Research, 12, 191–192.

Burgess, A.W. (1997). Psychiatric nursing. In A.W. Burgess (Ed.), Psychiatric nursing: Promoting mental health (pp. 10–25). Stamford, CT: Appleton & Lange.

Cameron, J. (1963). An exploratory study of the verbal responses of the nurses in 20 nurse-patient interactions [Abstract]. Nursing Research, 12, 192.

Dumas, R., & Leonard, R.C. (1963). The effect of nursing on the incidence of postoperative vomiting. Nursing Research, 12, 12–15.

Dumas, R.G. (1963). Psychological preparation for surgery. American Journal of Nursing, 63(8), 52–55.

Dye, M. (1963). A descriptive study of conditions conducive to an effective process of nursing activity [Abstract]. Nursing Research, 12, 194.

Elms, R.R., & Leonard, R.C. (1966). Effects of nursing approaches during admission. Nursing Research, 15, 39–48.

Faulkner, S. (1963). A descriptive study of needs communicated to the nurse by some mothers on a postpartum service [Abstract]. Nursing Research, 12, 26.

Faust, C. (2002). Clinical outlook. Orlando's deliberative nursing process theory: A practice application in an extended care facility. Journal of Gerontological Nursing, 28(7), 14–18.

Fischelis, M. (1963). An exploratory study of labels nurses attach to patient behavior and their effect on nursing activities [Abstract]. Nursing Research, 12, 195.

Forchuk, C. (1991). A comparison of the works of Peplau and Orlando. Archives of Psychiatric Nursing, 5, 38–45.

Henderson, V. (1978). The concept of nursing. Journal of Advanced Nursing, 3, 113–130.

Mertz, H. (1963). A study of the process of the nurse's activity as it affects the blood pressure readings and pulse ratings of patients admitted to the emergency room [Abstract]. Nursing Research, 12, 197–198.

Orlando, I.J. (1961). The dynamic nurse-patient relationship: Function, process and principles. New York: G.P. Putnam's Sons. [Reprinted 1990. New York: National League for Nursing.]

Orlando, I.J. (1962). Function, process and principles of professional nursing practice. In Integration of mental health concepts with the human relations professions (pp. 87–106). New York: Bank Street College of Education.

Orlando, I.J. (1972). The discipline and teaching of nursing process (an evaluative study). New York: G.P. Putnam's Sons.

Orlando, I.J. (1987). Nursing in the 21st century: Alternate paths. Journal of Advanced Nursing, 12, 405–412.

Orlando, I.J. (1989). The nurse theorists: Portraits of excellence. Athens, OH: Fuld Institute for Technology in Nursing Education. [Videotape.]

Orlando, I.J., & Dugan, A.B. (1989). Independent and dependent paths: The fundamental issue for the nursing profession. Nursing and Health Care, 10, 76–80.

Orlando Pelletier, I.J. (1990). Preface to the NLN edition. In I.J. Orlando, The dynamic nurse-patient relationship: Function, process, and principles (pp. vii–viii). New York: National League for Nursing.

Pelletier, I.O. (1967). The patient's predicament and nursing function. Psychiatric Opinion, 4(1), 25–30.

Potter, M.L., & Bockenhauer, B.J. (2000). Implementing Orlando's nursing theory: A pilot study. Journal of Psychosocial Nursing and Mental Health Services, 38(3), 14–21, 36–37.

Potter, M., & Tinker, S. (2000). Put power in nurses' hands: Orlando's nursing theory supports nurses—simply. Nursing Management, 31(7, Part 1), 40–41.

Rhymes, J. (1964). A description of nurse-patient interaction in effective nursing activity [Abstract]. Nursing Research, 13, 365.

Schmieding, N.J. (1987). Problematic situations in nursing: Analysis of Orlando's theory based on Dewey's theory of inquiry. Journal of Advanced Nursing, 12, 431–440.

Schmieding, N.J. (1988). Action process of nurse administrators to problematic situations based on Orlando's theory. Journal of Advanced Nursing, 13, 99–107.

Schmieding, N.J. (1990). Foreword. In I.J. Orlando, The dynamic nurse-patient relationship: Function, process, and principles (pp. xvii–xix). New York: National League for Nursing.

Schmieding, N.J. (2002). Ida Jean Orlando (Pelletier): Nursing process theory. In A. Marriner Tomey & M.R. Alligood (Eds.), Nursing theorists and their work (5th ed., pp. 399–417). St. Louis: Mosby.

Sellers, S.C. (1991). A philosophical analysis of conceptual models of nursing. Dissertation Abstracts International, 52, 1937B. [University Microfilms No. AAC9126248.]

Tryon, P.A. (1963). An experiment of the effect of patients' participation in planning the administration of a nursing procedure [Abstract]. Nursing Research, 12, 262.

Tryon, P.A. (1966). Use of comfort measures as support during labor. Nursing Research, 15, 109–118.

Tryon, P.A., & Leonard, R.C. (1964). The effect of patients' participation on the outcome of a nursing procedure. Nursing Forum, 3, 79–89.

Williamson, J. (1978). Methodological dilemmas in tapping the concept of patient needs. Nursing Research, 27, 172–177.

RESEARCH

Anderson, B., Mertz, H., & Leonard, R. (1965). Two experimental tests of a patient-centered admission process. Nursing Research, 14, 151–156.

Bochnak, M.A., Rhymes, J.P., & Leonard, R.C. (1962). The comparison of two types of nursing activity on the relief of pain. In Innovations in nurse-patient relationships: Automatic or reasoned nurse action (Clinical papers no. 6, pp. 5–11). New York: American Nurses' Association.

Dracup, K., & Breu, C. (1978). Using nursing research findings to meet the needs of grieving spouses. Nursing Research, 27, 212–216.

Dumas, R.G. (1963). Psychological preparation for surgery. American Journal of Nursing, 63(8), 52–55.

Dumas, R.G., Anderson, B.J., & Leonard, R.C. (1965). The importance of the expressive function in preoperative preparation. In J.K. Skipper & R.C. Leonard (Eds.), Social interaction and patient care (pp. 16–29). Philadelphia: Lippincott.

Dumas, R.G., & Leonard, R.C. (1963). The effect of nursing on the incidence of postoperative vomiting. Nursing Research, 12, 12–15.

Dye, M.C. (1963). Clarifying patients' communications. American Journal of Nursing, 63(8), 56–59.

Ellis, J.M. (1999). Barriers to effective screening for domestic violence by registered nurses in the emergency department. Critical Care Nursing Quarterly, 22, 27–41.

Elms, R.R. (1964). Effects of varied nursing approaches during hospital admission: An exploratory study. Nursing Research, 13, 266–268.

Elms, R.R., & Leonard, R.C. (1966). Effects of nursing approaches during admission. Nursing Research, 15, 39–48.

Gillis, L. (1976). Sleeplessness: Can you help? Canadian Nurse, 72(7), 32–34.

Gowan, N., & Morris, M. (1964). Nurses' responses to expressed patient needs. Nursing Research, 13, 68–71.

Haggerty, L. (1987). An analysis of senior nursing students' immediate response to distressed patients. Journal of Advanced Nursing, 12, 451–461.

Hampe, S. (1975). Needs of the grieving spouse in a hospital setting. Nursing Research, 24, 113–120.

Houfek, J.F. (1992). Nurses' perceptions of the dimensions of nursing care episodes. Nursing Research, 41, 280–285.

Mertz, H. (1962). Nurse actions that reduce stress in patients. In Emergency intervention by the nurse (Clinical papers no. 1, pp. 10–14). New York: American Nurses' Association.

Nelson, B. (1978). A practice application of nursing theory. Nursing Clinics of North America, 13, 157–169.

Olson, J., & Hanchett, E. (1997). Nurse-expressed empathy, patient outcomes, and development of a middle-range theory. Image: Journal of Nursing Scholarship, 29, 71–79.

Potter, M.L., & Bockenhauer, B.J. (2000). Implementing Orlando's nursing theory: A pilot study. Journal of Psychosocial Nursing and Mental Health Services, 38(3), 14–21, 36–37.

Potter, M., & Tinker, S. (2000). Put power in nurses' hands: Orlando's nursing theory supports nurses—simply. Nursing Management, 31(7, Part 1), 40–41.

Powers, M., & Wooldridge, P. (1982). Factors influencing knowledge, research, and compliance of hypertensive patients. Research in Nursing and Health, 5, 171–182.

Pride, L.F. (1968). An adrenal stress index as a criterion measure of nursing. Nursing Research, 17, 292–303.

Princeton, J.C. (1986). Incorporating a deliberative nursing approach with breastfeeding mothers. Health Care for Women International, 7, 277–293.

Schmieding, N.J. (1987). Analyzing managerial responses in face-to-face contacts. Journal of Advanced Nursing, 12, 357–365.

Schmieding, N.J. (1988). Action process of nurse administrators to problematic situations based on Orlando's theory. Journal of Advanced Nursing, 13, 99–107.

Schmieding, N.J. (1990a). Do head nurses include staff nurses in problem-solving? Nursing Management, 21(3), 58–60.

Schmieding, N.J. (1990b). A model of assessing nursing administrators' actions. Western Journal of Nursing Research, 12, 293–306.

Schmieding, N.J. (1991). Relationship between head nurse responses to staff nurses and staff nurse responses to patients. Western Journal of Nursing Research, 13, 746–760.

Shea, N.M., McBride, L., Gavin, C., & Bauer, M.S. (1997). The effects of an ambulatory collaborative practice model on process and outcome of care for bipolar disorder. Journal of the American Psychiatric Nurses Association, 3(2), 49–57.

Silva, M.C. (1979). Effects of orientation information on spouses' anxieties and attitudes toward hospitalization and surgery. Research in Nursing and Health, 2, 127–136.

Tarasuk, M.B., Rhymes, J., & Leonard, R.C. (1965). An experimental test of the importance of communication skills for effective nursing. In J.K. Skipper & R.C. Leonard (Eds.), Social interaction and patient care (pp. 110–120). Philadelphia: Lippincott.

Thibaudeau, M., & Reidy, M. (1977). Nursing makes a difference: A comparative study of the health behavior of mothers in three primary care agencies. International Journal of Nursing Studies, 14, 97–107.

Tryon, P.A. (1962). The effect of patient participation in decision making on the outcome of a nursing procedure. In Nursing and the patients' motivation (Clinical paper no. 19, pp. 14–18). New York: American Nurses' Association.

Tryon, P.A. (1966). Use of comfort measures as support during labor. Nursing Research, 15, 109–118.

Tryon, P.A., & Leonard, R.C. (1964). The effect of the patient's participation on the outcome of a nursing procedure. Nursing Forum, 3, 79–89.

Wolfer, J., & Visintainer, M. (1975). Pediatric surgical patients' and parents' stress responses and adjustment as a function of psychological preparation and stress point nursing care. Nursing Research, 24, 244–255.

RESEARCH INSTRUMENTS AND PRACTICE TOOLS

Orlando, I.J. (1972). The discipline and teaching of nursing process (p. 56). New York: G.P. Putnam's Sons.

Potter, M.L., & Bockenhauer, B.J. (2000). Implementing Orlando's nursing theory: A pilot study. Journal of Psychosocial Nursing and Mental Health Services, 38(3), 14–21, 36–37.

Schmieding, N.J. (2002). Orlando's nursing process theory in nursing practice. In M.R. Alligood & A. Marriner Tomey (Eds.), Nursing theory: Utilization and application (2nd ed., pp. 328). St. Louis: Mosby.

Williamson, J. (1978). Methodological dilemmas in tapping the concept of patient needs. Nursing Research, 27, 172–177.

PRACTICE

Faust, C. (2002). Clinical outlook. Orlando's deliberative nursing process theory: A practice application in an extended care facility. Journal of Gerontological Nursing, 28(7), 14–18.

Harrison, C. (1966). Deliberative nursing process versus automatic nurse action. The care of a chronically ill man. Nursing Clinics of North America, 1, 387–397.

Rosenthal, B.C. (1996). An interactionist's approach to perioperative nursing. Association of Operating Room Nurses Journal, 64, 254–260.

Schmidt, J. (1972). Availability: A concept of nursing practice. American Journal of Nursing, 72, 1986–1089.

Schmieding, N.J. (1970). Relationship of nursing to the process of chronicity. Nursing Outlook, 18, 58–62.

Schmieding, N.J. (1986). Orlando's theory. In P. Winstead-Fry (Ed.), Case studies in nursing theory (pp. 1–36). New York: National League for Nursing.

Schmieding, N.J. (2002). Orlando's nursing process theory in nursing practice. In M.R. Alligood & A. Marriner Tomey (Eds.), Nursing theory: Utilization and application (2nd ed., pp. 315–337). St. Louis: Mosby.

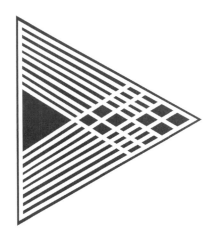

Chapter **15**

Peplau's Theory of Interpersonal Relations

Hildegard Peplau's educational, practice, and teaching experiences "led to an interest in clarifying what happens in a nurse-patient relationship" (Peplau, 1952, p. v). Peplau saw that both the nurse and the patient "participate in and contribute to [a] relationship and, further, that the relationship itself could be therapeutic" (Sills, 1989, p. ix). These notions led to the formulation of what Peplau originally called psychodynamic nursing (Peplau, 1952) and later referred to as a theory of interpersonal relations (Peplau, 1992). The Theory of Interpersonal Relations and a clinical methodology were first taught to nursing students in 1948 and published by Peplau in 1952. Subsequently, Peplau continued to discuss the theory and describe its application to diverse practice problems in a series of papers, many of which are now available in a volume edited by O'Toole and Welt (1989). Peplau presented refinements in her theory in "Interpersonal Constructs for Nursing Practice" (1989 [original work published 1987]) and her 1997 journal article, "Peplau's Theory of Interpersonal Relations." Hildegard Peplau died on March 17, 1999.

Overview

Peplau's work is a middle-range descriptive classification theory that focuses on the phases of the interpersonal process that occur when an ill person and a nurse come together to resolve a health-related difficulty. The one concept of the Theory of Interpersonal Relations and its dimensions are listed here, along with the components of Peplau's clinical methodology. The concept, its dimensions, and the components of the clinical methodology are defined and described later in this chapter.

Key Terms

NURSE-PATIENT RELATIONSHIP
    Orientation Phase

Working Phase
    Identification
    Exploitation
Termination Phase
CLINICAL METHODOLOGY
    Observation
        Participant Observation
        Reframing Empathic Linkages
    Communication
        Interpersonal Techniques
        Principle of Clarity
        Principle of Continuity
    Recording
    Data Analysis
        Phases of the Nurse-Patient Relationship
        Roles
        Relations
        Pattern Integrations

ANALYSIS OF THE THEORY OF INTERPERSONAL RELATIONS

This section presents an analysis of Peplau's Theory of Interpersonal Relations. The analysis is based on Peplau's publications about her theory, drawing primarily from her 1952 book, *Interpersonal Relations in Nursing*, her 1992 journal article, "Interpersonal Relations: A Theoretical Framework for Application in Nursing Practice," and her 1997 journal article, "Peplau's Theory of Interpersonal Relations."

SCOPE OF THE THEORY

The central assertions of the Theory of Interpersonal Relations are that "nursing is a significant, therapeutic, interpersonal process" (Peplau, 1952, p. 16) and that "understanding of the meaning of the experience to the patient is required in order for nursing to function as an educative, therapeutic, maturing force" (Peplau, 1952, p. 41). Although Peplau (1997) commented that "interpersonal relations is a conceptual framework" (p. 162), she labeled her work as a theory and always maintained that it is limited to the phases of interpersonal relations, primarily between the nurse and the patient. These phases represent a relatively concrete and specific taxonomy; therefore, Peplau's work is most accurately categorized as a middle-range theory (O'Toole & Welt, 1989). More specifically, the Theory of Interpersonal Relations is a middle-range descriptive classification theory. The middle-range categorization is further supported by Peplau's own comments regarding the scope of her theory:

> In this inquiry, we are interested in what happens when an ill person and a nurse come together to resolve a difficulty felt in relation to health (Peplau, 1952, p. 18).

> There are, of course, many sources of theory other than interpersonal relations (Peplau, 1997, p. 162).

> The focus of my theory is on interaction phenomena and intrapersonal and interpersonal phenomena and it does not include, for instance, pathophysiology or biological phenomena and other aspects of the human experience. It is focused very specifically on interaction phenomena: person-to-person interaction (Peplau, as cited in Takahashi, 1992, p. 86).

> The theory of interpersonal relations does not provide explanations for [the] medical aspects of the patient's problems.... Concepts contained within interpersonal relations theory are relevant primarily as [descriptions] of the personal behavior of nurse and patient in nursing situations and of psychosocial phenomena. Obviously, then, for the practice of nursing, a

more comprehensive scope of theoretical constructs is needed (Peplau, 1992, p. 13).

CONTEXT OF THE THEORY

Metaparadigm Concepts and Proposition

Peplau (1965) alluded to the metaparadigm of nursing when she stated:

> It seems to me that interpersonal relations is the core of nursing. Basically, nursing practice always involves a relationship between at least two real people—a nurse and a patient. ... The way in which [the nurse] produces the effects of her teaching or of the application of a technical procedure has a good deal to do with the interaction between nurse and patient (p. 274).

That statement indicates that the Theory of Interpersonal Relations is derived from the metaparadigm concepts of *human beings* and *nursing*. Human beings encompass the patient and the nurse, and nursing is the interpersonal process between the nurse and the patient. Moreover, Peplau's statement indicates that the most relevant metaparadigm proposition is *the nursing actions or processes that are beneficial to human beings*.

Philosophical Claims

Peplau made several statements that represent the philosophical claims undergirding the Theory of Interpersonal Relations. These statements focus on human beings and behavior, nurses and nursing, interpersonal relations, and the nurse-patient relationship. Other statements represent the philosophic claims undergirding Peplau's clinical methodology. The philosophical claims are:

Philosophical Claims About Human Beings and Behavior

- The human being is reducible, one way or the other (Peplau, as cited in Takahashi, 1992, p. 88).
- All human behavior is purposeful and goal seeking in terms of feelings of satisfaction and/or security (Peplau, 1952, p. 86).
- Human beings act on the basis of the meaning of events to them, that is, on the basis of their immediate interpretation of the climate and the performances that transpire in a particular relationship (Peplau, 1952, pp. 283–284).
- Each patient will behave, during any crisis, in a way that

has worked in relation to crises faced in the past (Peplau, 1952, p. 255).

- The meaning of behavior of the patient to the patient is the only relevant basis on which nurses can determine needs to be met (Peplau, 1952, pp. 226–227).

Philosophical Claims About Nurses and Nursing

- The kind of person each nurse becomes makes a substantial difference in what each patient will learn as he is nursed throughout his experience with illness (Peplau, 1952, p. xii).
- Fostering personality development in the direction of maturity is a function of nursing and nursing education; it requires the use of principles and methods that permit and guide the process of grappling with everyday interpersonal problems or difficulties (Peplau, 1952, p. xii).
- The professional and personal growth of the nurse requires changes in his or her own behavior (Peplau, 1992, p. 14).
- Nurses do not have the power to change the behavior of patients (Peplau, 1992, p. 14).
- Unwitting "illness-maintenance" by nurses is unacceptable behavior for a professional (Peplau, 1992, p. 14).
- The nursing process is educative and therapeutic when nurse and patient can come to know and to respect each other, as persons who are alike, and yet, different, as persons who share in the solution of problems (Peplau, 1952, p. 9).

Philosophical Claims About Interpersonal Relations

- Interpersonal relationships … are person-to-person interactions that have structure and content and also are situation-dependent (Peplau, 1994, p. 10).
- People need relationships with other persons (Peplau, 1997, p. 166).
- Relationships constitute the social fabric of life (Peplau, 1997, p. 166).
- Interpersonal relationships are the bedrock of quality of life (Peplau, 1994, p. 13).
- Interpersonal relationships are important throughout the entire life span (Peplau, 1994, p. 13).
- Relationship behavior tends to organize around how each person thinks of self (Peplau, 1997, p. 163).
- In an interpersonal relationship there is always interaction between the expectations and perceptions of one person—such as a patient, and the actual behavior of others (Peplau, 1997, p. 166).
- At their best, relationships confirm self worth, provide a sense of connectedness with others, and support self-esteem (Peplau, 1997, p. 166).

- In every contact with another human being there is the possibility for the nurse of working toward common understandings and goals; every contact between two human beings involves the possibility of clash of feelings, beliefs, [and] ways of acting (Peplau, 1952, p. xiii).

Philosophical Claims About the Nurse-Patient Relationship

- The nurse-patient relationship is the primary human contact that is central in a fundamental way to providing nursing care (Peplau, 1997, p. 163).
- The nurse-patient relationship is always unique as to process and outcome (Peplau, 1997, p. 167).
- The nurse-patient relationship is dependent upon both the nurse's style and the theoretical concepts the nurse has, as well as the intellectual and interpersonal competencies which are employed (Peplau, 1997, p. 167).
- Every nurse-patient relationship is an interpersonal situation in which recurring difficulties of everyday living arise (Peplau, 1952, p. xiii).
- The relationship of professional to patient (client) is not the same as more common social relationships (Peplau, 1997, p. 163).
- The nurse needs information about the patient's difficulties for the purpose of providing expert nursing care. Data from the patient about the immediate situation is a major source, superior to case history data, nursing history data, and other sources of information, which the nurse also uses (Peplau, 1992, p. 14).
- The interaction of nurse and patient is fruitful when a method of communication that identifies and uses common meanings is at work in the situation (Peplau, 1952, p. 284).
- To encourage the patient to participate in identifying and assessing his problem is to engage him as an active partner in an enterprise of great concern to him. Democratic method applied to nursing requires patient participation (Peplau, 1952, p. 23).

Philosophical Claims Undergirding Peplau's Clinical Methodology

- What goes on between people can be noticed, studied, explained, understood, and if detrimental changed (Peplau, 1992, p. 14).
- [Three] clearly discernible phases in the [nurse-patient] relationship … are to be thought of as interlocking (Peplau, 1952, p. 17).
- [The phases of the nurse-patient relationship] can be recognized; they enter into every total nursing situation (Peplau, 1952, p. 17).

Sellers (1991) initially maintained that Peplau's theory "espouses the behaviorist philosophy of the medical model. Her [theory] exemplifies a mechanistic, deterministic, persistence ... view" (p. 141). Peplau (1989 [original work presented 1954]), however, rejected that characterization by explicitly stating that her work is dynamic rather than mechanistic. Mechanistic theories, according to Peplau, are "largely partial, one-sided. [They] depend ... on spectator observations made by an individual who presumes detachment from the individual studied" (p. 9). In contrast, as Peplau pointed out, dynamic theories require participant observation and consider data from both the nurse-observer and the patient, which are essential features of the Theory of Interpersonal Relations. These features, along with scrutiny of Peplau's philosophical claims, indicate that the theory is most closely aligned with the *reciprocal interaction* world view, with an emphasis on the elements of totality that are incorporated into that perspective. Indeed, Forchuk (1991a) indicated that Peplau's work reflects the totality world view, and Sellers (1991) ultimately reached the same conclusion.

Conceptual Model

Harry Stack Sullivan's theory of interpersonal relations provided a strong conceptual base for Peplau's theory. She explained that she had studied Sullivan's work during the 1930s and 1940s and used it as a starting point for her theory. Since 1948, however, her work has been "derived from extensive study of data from clinical work primarily with psychiatric patients" (Peplau, 1992, p. 13).

Peplau (1992) regarded the human being as a client or patient who merits "all of the humane considerations: respect, dignity, privacy, confidentiality, and ethical care" (p. 14). She went on to say that "patient-persons ... have problems of one kind or another for which expert nursing services are needed or sought" (p. 14). She regarded the nurse as a professional with particular expertise.

Peplau did not devote much attention to the environment, although she noted the importance of culture on the formation of personality. In particular, she stated that "it is the interaction of cultural forces with the characteristic expression of a particular infant's biological constitution that determines personality" (Peplau, 1952, p. 163). She also commented, "Increasingly, multi-ethnicity is a factor in the contemporary world as well as in health-care systems; therefore, nurses need ... to obtain information from patients about cultures other than their own" (Peplau, 1997, p. 162).

Health, according to Peplau (1952), "has not been clearly defined; it is a word symbol that implies forward movement of personality and other ongoing human processes in the direction of creative, constructive, productive, personal, and community living" (p. 12). Peplau (1952) defined nursing as

a significant, therapeutic, interpersonal process. It functions co-operatively with other human processes that make health possible for individuals in communities. In specific situations in which a professional health team offers health services, nurses participate in the organization of conditions that facilitate natural ongoing tendencies in human organisms. Nursing is an educative instrument, a maturing force, that aims to promote forward movement of personality in the direction of creative, constructive, productive, personal, and community living (p. 16).

Consequently, the aim of professional nursing practice for Peplau (1992) is "to assist patients to become aware of and to solve their problems that interfere with constructive living" (p. 15).

Peplau (1997) identified clear distinctions between nursing and medicine, as well as certain complementary features. She commented:

Physicians are mainly concerned about the incidence, etiology, diagnosis, and treatment of disease. The information which their work requires obtains largely through physical examination and tests which patients undergo.... Much of the medical theoretical framework flows from anatomy, pathology, physiology, biology, chemistry, genetics—the "hard sciences." The relationship (often brief) of physician to patient is largely scripted by the treatment, based on diagnosis and laboratory findings. Nurses collaborate in carrying out orders and in health teaching related to the medical treatment. However, the nurse-patient relationship is unscripted. It is dependent largely upon the conceptual knowledge which each nurse has about the patient's presenting data and the phenomena in the domain of nursing. This knowledge is in the nurse's head, available for recall and application during the interaction. It is this kind of intellectual work by nurses that can transform nurse-patient interactions into a learning event for patients. Much of the current nursing knowledge framework flows from the social sciences—the "soft sciences"—psychology, sociology, and the humanities, with some uses of other basic sciences, such as biology. This may change when *nursing science* is fully developed (pp. 165–166).

Antecedent Knowledge

Peplau explicitly acknowledged the influence of Harry Stack Sullivan and his followers on her ideas. In the preface to her 1952 book, she stated:

The author wishes to express great indebtedness for indirect help gained through the written works of the late Dr. Harry Stack Sullivan and for direct assistance growing out of study with Dr. Erich Fromm, various members of the professional staff of the William Alanson White Institute of Psychiatry and of Chestnut Lodge. The Theory of Interpersonal Relations, as stated by Dr. Sullivan and under further development by these professional workers, is considered by the author to be one of the most useful theories in explaining observations made in nursing. This [book] has drawn heavily upon their contribution in order to make available to nurses in simpler form ideas that are of great value in understanding human behavior (p. v).

Peplau (1989 [original work published 1987]) noted that the term interpersonal relations was coined by Jacob Moreno (1941), the psychiatrist who founded psychodrama, and was later defined and described by Sullivan (1953). She explained that although "Sullivan was a practicing psychoanalyst … his interpersonal constructs were drawn from both his psychiatric clinical work and from the social sciences available in the 1920s to 1950s" (Peplau, 1989 [original work published 1987], p. 58). In a later publication, Peplau (1992) commented that Sullivan's theory of interpersonal relations drew more from theories in the social sciences than from psychoanalytic theories.

Peplau (1989 [original work published 1987]) noted that Sullivan defined interpersonal relations as "the study of what goes on between two or more people, all but one of whom may be completely illusory" (p. 58). She pointed out that the term is interpersonal *relations* rather than interpersonal *relationships*. Relations, Peplau (1989 [original work published 1987]) explained, "refers to connections, linkages, ties and bonds between things and people" (p. 58). She went on to explain that "in a nurse-patient relationship, and most particularly in psychiatric work, the aim of the nurse would be to study the interpersonal relations that go on (or went on) between a client and others, whether family, friends, staff, or the nurse" (p. 59).

Sullivan's work was not, however, the only source of antecedent knowledge for Peplau. Indeed, she explained that she considered other works, rejecting some and keeping others in mind. She stated:

> I hold a BA in interpersonal psychology (1943), studied with Eric Fromm and Frieda Fromm-Reichman, and also in the 1930s was exposed to lectures by top psychiatrists at Bellevue Hospital; and, at the White Institute, I studied with many then well-known interpersonal psychiatrists. And of course, Sullivan's published work greatly illuminated my thinking and my clinical work. I was aware of Helena Render's book, but found it only partially useful in my own early work.… I read extensively on Freud's work under a tutor during my college work, but I never found the theory wholly useful, particularly in clinical work with patients. From the outset, I found such treatments as electroshock and lobotomies outrageous. So Freud and these "therapies" did not appear in my publications (Peplau, 1996, p. 15).

CONTENT OF THE THEORY

Concept

A systematic analysis of Peplau's publications revealed that the Theory of Interpersonal Relations contains one multidimensional concept: NURSE-PATIENT RELATIONSHIP. The phases of the NURSE-PATIENT RELATIONSHIP represent the dimensions of the concept. Initially, Peplau (1952) proposed four phases—orientation, identification, exploitation, and resolution. Later, Peplau (1989 [original work published 1987], 1997) proposed just three phases—the **Orientation Phase**, the **Working Phase**, and the **Termination Phase**. Close examination of Peplau's (1997) discussion of the three phases revealed that the **Working Phase** encompasses the characteristics or processes involved in the original identification and exploitation phases. Consequently, for the purposes of this analysis, the **Working Phase** is divided into an *Identification Subphase* and an *Exploitation Subphase*. The two subphases may be considered subdimensions of the **Working Phase** dimension of the concept of NURSE-PATIENT RELATIONSHIP. Continued examination of Peplau's (1997) discussion indicated that the **Termination Phase** is the term Peplau now uses for the resolution phase.

Nonrelational Propositions

The definition of the concept of NURSE-PATIENT RELATIONSHIP and the definition of each of its dimensions and subdimensions are presented here. All of these constitutive definitions are the nonrelational propositions of the Theory of Interpersonal Relations. Inasmuch as the theory contains just one concept, there are no relational propositions.

NURSE-PATIENT RELATIONSHIP

- An interpersonal process made up of four components—two persons, the professional expertise of the nurse, and the client's problem or need for which expert nursing services are sought (Peplau, 1992)
- An interpersonal process that comprises three sometimes overlapping or interlocking phases (Peplau, 1952, 1997)

The concept of **Nurse-Person Relationship** encompasses three dimensions—the Orientation Phase, the Working Phase, and the Termination Phase. The dimension Working Phase encompasses two subdimensions—the Identification Subphase and the Exploitation Subphase.

- **Orientation Phase:** The phase in which the nurse first identifies herself by name and professional status and states the purpose, nature, and time available for the patient (Peplau, 1997, pp. 163–164). The phase during which the nurse conveys professional interest and receptivity to the patient, begins to know the patient as a person, obtains essential information about the patient's health condition, and sets the tone for further interactions (Peplau, 1997).
- **Working Phase:** The phase in which the major work occurs (Peplau, 1997)
  Identification Subphase: The subphase during which the patient learns how to make use of the nurse-patient relationship (Peplau, 1952)
  Exploitation Subphase: The subphase during which the patient makes full use of available professional services (Peplau, 1952)
- **Termination Phase:** The phase in which the work accomplished is summarized and closure occurs (Peplau, 1997). The phase during which the nurse helps the patient to organize actions so that he or she will want to be free for more productive social activities and relationships (Peplau, 1952).

Peplau (1992) pointed out that the **Nurse-Patient Relationship**

> is a particular kind of interaction. It is not a parent-child relationship. It is not a social relationship of friend-to-friend. It is not a clerk-to-customer relationship. Nor, is it a master-to-servant relationship. Rather, the nurse is a professional, which means a person having a definable expertise. That expert knowledge pertains to the nature of phenomena within the purview of nursing and to the reliable interventions which have been research-tested and therefore have predictable, known outcomes (p. 14).

Furthermore, Peplau (1992) explained that the **Nurse-Patient Relationship** "has a starting point, proceeds through definable phases, and being time-limited, has an end point" (p. 14). Peplau (1952, 1997) regarded the three phases as distinct yet overlapping or interlocking (Fig. 15–1). She explained:

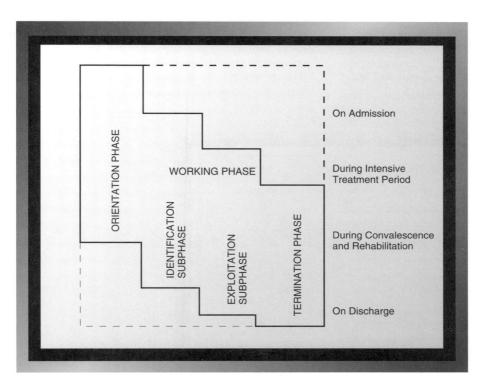

FIGURE 15–1. Overlapping phases of the nurse-patient relationship. (Adapted from Peplau, H.E. (1952). Interpersonal relations in nursing: A conceptual frame of reference for psychodynamic nursing (p. 21). New York: G.P. Putnam's Sons, with permission. Reprinted 1989. London: Macmillan Education. Reprinted 1991. New York: Springer.)

Initially, the patient functions in relation to overlapping situations. That is, he is pulled toward being home where he is sure of familiar responses and he is drawn toward remaining in the hospital and solving the emergent problem (Peplau, 1952, p. 29).

The [working phase subphase] of exploitation overlaps [the subphase of] identification and [the termination phase, which is] the terminal phase of the nurse-patient relationship. Orientation overlapped the previous social or home situation. The phase under discussion represents all prior ones and an extension of the self of the patient into the future. It is characterized by an intermingling of needs and a shuttling back and forth (Peplau, 1952, p. 38).

Peplau's original and continuing discussion of each phase of the **Nurse-Patient Relationship** encompasses a description of the developing interpersonal relationship between the nurse and the patient and the roles each person assumes. As can be seen in Figure 15–2, "each phase is characterized by overlapping roles or functions in relation to health problems as nurse and patient learn to work co-operatively to resolve difficulties" (Peplau, 1952, p. 17).

The **Orientation Phase** occurs as the patient has a felt need signifying a health problem and seeks assistance to clarify the problem. As Peplau (1992) explained, "Seeking assistance on the basis of a need, felt but poorly understood, is often the first step in a dynamic learning experience from which a constructive next step in personal-social growth can occur" (p. 19).

Peplau (1952) further explained that the patient participates in the **Orientation Phase** by asking questions, by trying to find out what needs to be known in order to feel secure, and by observing ways in which professional people respond. The nurse participates in the **Orientation Phase** by helping the patient to recognize and understand the health problem and the extent of need for assistance, to understand what professional services can offer, to plan the use of professional services, and to harness energy from tension and anxiety connected with felt needs (Peplau, 1952).

More specifically, the **Orientation Phase** "sets the stage for the serious work that is to follow. In this phase, for example, the patient begins to know the nurse's name, the nurse's purpose, the time to be made available, and the approach to the work. The nurse begins to know the patient as a person, his/her expectations of the nurse, and the patient's characteristic response patterns. It is the phase in which the nurse makes assessments of the patient's potentials, needs, and interests, and of the patient's inclination to experience fear or anxiety" (Peplau, 1992, p. 14).

Underscoring the importance of the **Orientation Phase**, Peplau (1952) maintained that "orientation is essential to full participation and to full integration of the illness event into the stream of life experiences of the patient. It is the only prevention against repressing or dissociating the event that a nurse can exercise on behalf of the patient" (p. 23). "Orientation to the problem," Peplau (1952) claimed, "leads to expression of needs and feelings, older ones that

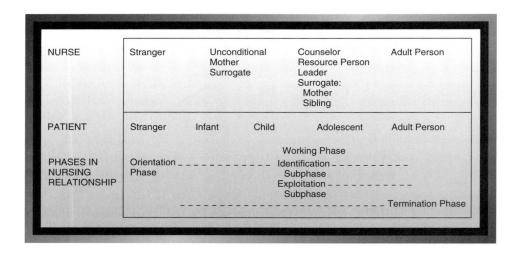

FIGURE 15–2. Phases and changing roles in the nurse-patient relationship. (Adapted from Peplau, H.E. (1952). Interpersonal relations in nursing: A conceptual frame of reference for psychodynamic nursing (p. 54). New York: G.P. Putnam's Sons, with permission. Reprinted 1989. London: Macmillan Education. Reprinted 1991. New York: Springer.)

are reactivated and new ones created by challenges in a new situation" (p. 41).

The nurse's initial role in the **Orientation Phase** is that of stranger, acted out with the patient who is also in the role of stranger (see Fig. 15–2). "A stranger," Peplau (1952) explained, "is an individual with whom another individual is not acquainted" (p. 44). As the **Orientation Phase** progresses, the patient may assume the role of infant and, therefore, cast the nurse into a surrogate role, especially that of unconditional mother. Peplau (1989 [original work presented 1965]) maintained that although the parental role may not be useful in some situations, "this surrogate role may be the logical one for the nurse to fulfill … if the patient is acutely ill and requires continual mothering care" (Peplau, 1952, p. 55).

The **Working Phase** focuses on "patients' reactions to illness and the work to be done by patients toward their development of understanding of themselves, and toward learning what their current health condition requires of them" (Peplau, 1997, p. 164). Overall, "the work of the nurse is broad-based and employs a variety of roles to be taken by the nurse [see Fig. 15–2]" (Peplau, 1997, p. 164). One role is the provider of physical care. "This aspect of interpersonal communication … [which involves] privileged access to the naked body of patients," Peplau (1997) explained, "taps into the needs of patients for respect and dignity and conversely the need to avoid felt shame, embarrassment, and humiliation" (p. 164). Other roles taken by nurses throughout the **Working Phase** include interviewer, health teacher, and counselor. These and other roles are discussed within the context of the subphases of the **Working Phase**.

The **Working Phase** encompasses the *Identification Subphase* and the *Exploitation Subphase*. During the *Identification Subphase,* Peplau (1952) explained, the nurse and the patient come to know and to respect one another, as persons who have like and different opinions about the ways of looking at a situation and in responding to events. At this time, patients may respond "(1) on the basis of participation or interdependent relations with a nurse; (2) on the basis of independence or isolation from a nurse; [or] (3) on the basis of helplessness or dependence upon a nurse" (Peplau, 1952, p. 33). Peplau (1952) went on to say that the nurse-patient relationship may progress from one mode of response to another and that all three modes may be required to achieve goals.

Throughout the *Identification Subphase,* the nurse uses professional education and skill to aid the patient to make full use of the relationship, in order to solve the health problem. Consequently, the nurse may assume several roles, frequently moving from unconditional mother surrogate in response to the patient's roles of infant and child to counselor, resource person, leader, or surrogate in response to the patient's gradual assumption of the role of adolescent (see Fig. 15–2). As a resource person, the nurse gives "specific, needed information that aids the patient to understand [the] health problem and the new situation" (Peplau, 1952, p. 21). As a counselor, the nurse uses investigative inquiry and listens attentively to the patient as he or she narrates and reviews the events that led up to hospitalization and feelings connected with these events. And as a leader, the nurse acts in a democratic, rather than autocratic or laissez-faire, manner. As a surrogate for mother, father, sibling, or other person, the nurse aids the patient by permitting reenactment and examination of older feelings about prior relationships.

Peplau (1952) identified certain benefits of progressing through the *Identification Subphase.* First, "identification with a nurse who consistently symbolizes a helping person, providing abundant and unconditional care, is a way of meeting felt needs and overwhelming problems. When initial needs are met they are outgrown and more mature needs arise" (p. 41). And second, "when a nurse permits patients to express what they feel, and still get all of the nursing that is needed, then patients can undergo illness as an experience that reorients feelings and strengthens positive forces in personality" (p. 31).

During the *Exploitation Subphase,* "the main difficulty seems to be that of trying to strike a balance between a need to be dependent, as during serious illness, and a need to be independent, as following recovery" (Peplau, 1952, p. 38). The nurse's tasks during the *Exploitation Subphase* are to understand what initiates shifts in the patient's behavior from dependence to independence and to guard against excessive exploitation on the patient's part. While in the *Exploitation Subphase,* the nurse initiates discharge planning and continues in the roles of counselor, resource person, leader, or surrogate in response to the patient's role of adolescent (see Fig. 15–2) (Peplau, 1952, 1997).

The benefits of progressing through the *Exploitation Subphase* include "new differentiations of the problem and … the development and improvement of skill in interpersonal relations. [In addition,] new goals to be achieved through personal efforts can be projected" (Peplau, 1952, pp. 41–42).

In the **Termination Phase,** discharge planning is summarized (Peplau, 1997). The patient's wish to terminate the relationship, however, may not coincide with medical recovery (Peplau, 1952). The central task of the **Termination Phase,** then, is the freeing of the patient to move on in life. Both nurse and patient must, of course, participate in the freeing process. As Peplau (1952) explained, "Movement from a hospital situation to participation in community life [requires termination] of nurse-patient relations and the strengthening of personality for new social interdependent relationships. When [termination] occurs on the basis of lacks in a situation, needs are intensified and become longings that, together with unclear meanings of the event itself, limit the possibility of integration of the total experience" (p. 42).

As the **Termination Phase** occurs, both nurse and patient assume the role of adult person (see Fig. 15–2). The benefit of successful progression through the **Termination Phase**, according to Peplau (1952), is enhancement of the patient's ability to be self-reliant. Peplau (1952) explained that this benefit is dependent on successful progression through the other phases of the **Nurse-Patient Relationship:**

> The [termination phase] implies the gradual freeing from identification with helping persons and the generation and strengthening of ability to stand more or less alone. These outcomes can be achieved only when all of the earlier phases are met in terms of "psychological mothering": unconditional acceptance in a sustaining relationship that provides fully for need-satisfaction; recognition of and responses to growth cues, however trivial, as and when they come from the patient; [and] shifting of power from the nurse to the patient as he becomes willing to delay gratification of his wishes and to expend his own efforts in achieving new goals (pp. 40–41).

Peplau (1997) indicated that she expects the nurse to be aware of each role taken and of movement from one role to another. In addition to the roles already discussed in conjunction with each phase of the **Nurse-Patient Relationship,** nurses may assume other roles, including technical expert, consultant, health teacher, tutor, socializing agent, safety agent, manager of the environment, mediator, administrator, recorder, observer, and researcher (Peplau, 1952, 1965). The role of technical expert may be assumed during any or all of the phases of the **Nurse-Patient Relationship.** In this role, the nurse "understands various professional devices and manipulates them with skill and discrimination in the interest of the patient" (Peplau, 1952, p. 22). The role of health teacher also may be assumed at any time. This role is, according to Peplau (1952), "a combination of all [other] roles" (p. 48). In keeping with her focus on the patient, Peplau (1952) advocated a teaching style that "always proceeds from what the patient knows and it develops around his interest in wanting and being able to use additional medical information" (p. 48). Peplau identified the other roles by name, but she did not describe them.

Although nurses assume many different roles during their interactions with patients, they should *not* assume certain roles in which patients may try to cast them. In particular, Peplau (1989 [original work presented 1965]) maintained that the roles of chum, friend, protagonist, and sex object are not useful ones for nurses to take. In essence, then, professional and not social behavior is re-

quired in all nurse-patient relationships. As Peplau (1997) pointed out:

> Some nurses have difficulty making the transition from social to professional modes of behavior in nurse-patient relationships; some even think it is not necessary to do so. As a consequence, those nurses who tell their personal experiences to patients make them into an audience and a sounding board for the nurse's benefit. The nurse's needs, not the patient's, get served (p. 164).

 ## EVALUATION OF THE THEORY OF INTERPERSONAL RELATIONS

This section presents an evaluation of Peplau's Theory of Interpersonal Relations. The evaluation is based on the results of the analysis of the theory, as well as on publications by others who have used or commented on this nursing theory.

SIGNIFICANCE

The Theory of Interpersonal Relations meets the criterion of significance. The metaparadigmatic origin of the theory was easily inferred from Peplau's work, although she never explicitly addressed that underpinning of the theory. Peplau did, however, explicitly identify several philosophical claims undergirding the theory, and others were extracted from her publications.

Peplau has always been especially explicit about the conceptual base for her theory, citing Sullivan's theory of interpersonal relations and the publications of his work as a major source of antecedent knowledge. Indeed, it is difficult to discern exactly where Sullivan's theory leaves off and Peplau's theory begins. Inasmuch as Peplau (1969) regarded nursing as an applied science, the lack of a clear distinction between the theories is not surprising.

Peplau also acknowledged the contributions of Sullivan's followers to her thinking, although she mentioned only Erich Fromm, Frieda Fromm-Reichman, and Helena Render by name and did not provide specific citations to their work. She did, however, provide an extensive bibliography for the many topics she addressed in her 1952 book, including anxiety, child development, communication, conflict, frustration, guilt, illness as an event, leadership, learning, motivation, needs, parental roles, personality, psychopathology, therapeutic methods, and general methods.

Especially noteworthy is the enduring nature of the Theory of Interpersonal Relations. In 1978, Sills pointed out that a literature review spanning the then 25 years since the publication of Peplau's book revealed that the theory, with no revisions, was still useful. The theory continues to be useful more than 50 years later, as documented by the recent literature cited in the chapter bibliography (see CD-ROM), as well as the reprinting of Peplau's 1952 book by Macmillan Education Ltd. in 1989 and by the Springer Publishing Company in 1991. Moreover, Burgess (1997) maintained that the Theory of Interpersonal Relations remains exceptionally influential in contemporary psychiatric nursing. Also, Belcher and Fish (2002) pointed out that the theory has been so fully integrated into nursing practice that it is in the realm of "public domain" (p. 78), as did O' Toole and Welt (1989, p. 365).

Speaking to the significance of her theory, Peplau (1992) stated that the theory is important because "the behavior of the nurse-as-a-person has significant impact on the patient's well-being and the quality and outcome of nursing care" (p. 14). In addition, Peplau (1994) noted that enhancement of interpersonal relations through the use of her theory can enhance a person's quality of life.

The special significance of the Theory of Interpersonal Relations lies in its contributions to understanding the phases of the nurse-patient relationship. "That knowledge," as Sills (1978) explained, "helped give nursing's moral aspirations a concrete basis which narrowed the gap between the ideal and the real" (p. 123).

Furthermore, Peplau (1992; as cited in Takahashi, 1992) pointed out that interpersonal relations theory has led to development of various interviewing techniques and psychotherapeutic modalities, including counseling, psychotherapy, family therapy, and group therapy. In addition, Peplau (1992) claimed that "advanced psychiatric nursing gained considerable impetus from this theory, as did the clinical specialist movement, particularly in psychiatric nursing" (p. 18).

INTERNAL CONSISTENCY

The Theory of Interpersonal Relations meets the criterion of internal consistency in part. The theory clearly reflects Peplau's philosophical claims and is logically derived from the conceptual model, which is based on Sullivan's (1953) theory of interpersonal relations.

The Theory of Interpersonal Relations demonstrates semantic clarity. Peplau provided a clear and concise constitutive definition of the concept of **Nurse-Patient Relationship** and clear constitutive definitions of the phases of the nurse-patient relationship.

However, the theory demonstrates only partial semantic consistency. Peplau's (1952) original work contained four distinct phases of the nurse-patient relationship—orienta-

tion, identification, exploitation, and resolution. Peplau (1989 [original work published 1987]) and later Forchuk (1991b) offered a new term—the working phase—that incorporates the phases of identification and exploitation. Peplau (1989 [original work published 1987], 1997) changed the term for the final phase from resolution to termination without any explanation.

An area of confusion is introduced in Peplau's discussion of nursing roles. In particular, it is unclear whether the various roles assumed by the nurse are associated with particular phases of the nurse-patient relationship, or are taken on during all three phases. The former situation is evident in Figure 15–2, but the latter situation is introduced by the following statement:

> During orientation as well as during the other … phases in the total relationship four interlocking nursing functions may operate: (1) The nurse may function in the role of resource person. … (2) A nurse may function in a counseling relationship. … (3) The patient may cast the nurse into roles, such as surrogate for mother, father, sibling. … (4) The nurse also functions as a technical expert … (Peplau, 1952, pp. 21–22).

The analysis of Peplau's theory revealed structural consistency. The Theory of Interpersonal Relations is a logical product of deduction from Sullivan's interpersonal theory and induction from Peplau's observations of nursing practice. O'Toole and Welt (1989) commented:

> Peplau's method of theory development is both inductive and deductive.… The process of combining induction (observation and classification) with deduction (the application of known concepts and processes to data) provides a creative nonlinear approach to the formation of ideas: one that uses the data of practice, as well as extant theories, as the basis of those formulations (p. 355).

PARSIMONY

The Theory of Interpersonal Relations meets the criterion of parsimony. This middle-range descriptive classification theory consists of one concept with three dimensions (the phases of the **Nurse-Patient Relationship**), two subdimensions (the subphases of the Working Phase of the **Nurse-Patient Relationship**), and the nonrelational propositions that are the constitutive definitions of the concept and its dimensions and subdimensions.

In contrast, Forchuk (1991b) regards the Theory of Interpersonal Relations as "quite complex … due to the many concepts, subconcepts, and … sub-sub-concepts that are interrelated" (pp. 54–55). Indeed, her analysis of Peplau's work yielded a complicated structure that combined what is regarded in this book as the metaparadigm concepts (human beings, environment, health, nursing), the middle-range theory concept of **Nurse-Patient Relationship** and its dimensions (the phases of the **Nurse-Patient Relationship**), and several other concepts and subconcepts (i.e., dimensions). Those concepts and their dimensions are communication, with the dimensions of verbal communication and nonverbal communication; pattern integration; roles; thinking, with the dimensions of preconceptions and self-understanding; learning; competencies; and anxiety.

A middle ground is offered by Howk (2002), who identified four concepts, some of which have dimensions. The concepts and dimensions are: psychodynamic nursing; nurse-patient relationship, with the dimensions orientation, identification, exploitation, and resolution; nursing roles, with the dimensions role of the stranger, role of the resource person, teaching role, leadership role, surrogate role, and counseling role; and psychobiological experiences.

O'Toole and Welt (1989) claimed that loneliness, anxiety, self, hallucinations, thought disorders, focal attention, and learning are "major concepts that form the backbone of Peplau's interpersonal theory" (p. xvi). Repeated readings of Peplau's publications indicated that the additional concepts identified by Forchuk, Howk, and O'Toole and Welt are either an integral part of the description of the phases of the nurse-patient relationship or practice situations for which the Theory of Interpersonal Relations is especially appropriate. Hence, here they are not regarded as concepts of the Theory of Interpersonal Relations.

TESTABILITY

The Theory of Interpersonal Relations meets the criterion of testability for middle-range theories. The theory is testable by means of Peplau's **CLINICAL METHODOLOGY**. The components of the **CLINICAL METHODOLOGY**, which are identified and described in Table 15–1, are

(Text continues on page 540)

TABLE 15–1
PEPLAU'S CLINICAL METHODOLOGY FOR NURSING RESEARCH AND PRACTICE

OBSERVATION

Purpose is the identification, clarification, and verification of impressions about the interactive drama, of the pushes and pulls in the relationship between nurse and patient, as they occur.

Participant Observation
Nurse's Behavior: Observation of the nurse's words, voice tones, body language, and other gestural messages
Patient's Behavior: Observation of the patient's words, voice tones, body language, and other gestural messages
Interpersonal Phenomena: Observation of what goes on between the patient and the nurse
Reframing Empathic Linkages: Occurs when the ability of the nurse, the patient, or both to feel in self the emotions experienced by the other person in the same situation is converted to verbal communications by the nurse asking, "What are you feeling right now?"

COMMUNICATION

Aims are (1) the selection of symbols or concepts that convey both the reference, or meaning, in the mind of the individual, and referent, the object or actions symbolized in the concept; and (2) the wish to struggle toward the development of common understanding for words between two or more people.

Interpersonal Techniques
Verbal interventions used by nurses during nurse-patient relationships aimed at accomplishing problem resolution and competence development in patients.

The nurse uses comments and questions to force the patient to think, to respond, and to use those capacities that will produce the necessary data.

Principle of Clarity
Words and sentences used to communicate are clarifying events when they occur within the frame of reference of common experiences of both or all participants, or when their meaning is established or made understandable as a result of joint and sustained effort of all parties concerned.
Clarity in communication is promoted when the nurse and the patient discuss their preconceptions about the meaning of words and work toward a common understanding.
Clarity is achieved when the meaning of a word to the patient is expressed and talked over and a new view is expanded in awareness.

Principle of Continuity
Continuity in communication occurs when language is used as a tool for the promotion of coherence or connections of ideas expressed and leads to discrimination of relationships or connections among ideas and the feelings, events, or themes conveyed in those ideas.
Continuity is promoted when the nurse is able to pick up threads of conversation that the patient offers in the course of a conversation and over a longer period such as a week, and when he or she aids the patient to focus and to expand these threads.

RECORDING

The written record of the communication between nurse and patient, that is, the data collected through participant observation and reframing of empathic linkages.
Aim is to capture the exact wording of the interaction between the nurse and the patient.
Use a form that permits verbatim recording of the nurse's observations of the patient when initially approached; the nurse's opening remarks, feelings, and thoughts about the patient; the patient's responses; and the nurse's responses (see Table 15–2).
Also can use a tape recorder, or nonparticipant observation by another nurse may be used to record interactions.

DATA ANALYSIS

Focuses on testing the nurse's hypotheses, which are formulated from first impressions or hunches about the patient.

Phases of the Nurse-Patient Relationship
Identify the phase of nurse-patient relationship in which communication occurred:
Orientation Phase
Working Phase
   Identification Subphase
   Exploitation Subphase
Termination Phase

ROLES

Identify the roles taken by the nurse and the patient in each phase of the nurse-patient relationship.

RELATIONS

Identify the connections, linkages, ties, and bonds that go on or went on between a patient and others, including family, friends, staff, or the nurse.
Analyze the relations to identify their nature, origin, function, and mode:
Nature—patterns or themes that represent the patient's characteristic ways of behaving in interpersonal relations, and variations in the patterns or themes.
Origin—the history of the interpersonal relation.
Function—the intent, motive, aim, goal, or purpose of the interpersonal relation.
Mode—the form, style, and method of the interpersonal relation.

(continued)

TABLE 15–1
PEPLAU'S CLINICAL METHODOLOGY FOR NURSING RESEARCH AND PRACTICE *(continued)*

Pattern Integrations
Identify the patterns of the interpersonal relation between two or more people that together link or bind them and
that enable the people to transform energy into patterns of action that bring satisfaction or security in the face of
a recurring problem.
Determine the type of pattern integration:
Complementary—the behavior of one person fits with and thereby complements the behavior of the other
person.
Mutual—the same or similar behaviors are used by both persons.
Alternating—different behaviors used by two persons alternate between the two persons.
Antagonistic—the behaviors of two persons do not fit but the relationship continues.

Source: Constructed from Peplau, 1952, pp. 290–293; 1989 [original work published 1987], pp. 58–59, 61; 1992, pp. 14–15, 18; 1997, pp. 162–163.

(Text continued from page 538)

completely consistent with the content of the Theory of Interpersonal Relations.

The central feature of the **Clinical Methodology** is the nurse's private use of the Theory of Interpersonal Relations "to interpret observations and to guide the patient's work in formulating his or her own interpretations of personal experience" (Peplau, 1992, p. 18). Peplau (1952) explained that "observation, communication, and recording are all interlocking performances in interpersonal relations that make it possible for nurses to study what is happening in their contacts with patients [i.e., analyze the data]" (p. 309).

Communication occurs primarily through interpersonal techniques. These techniques, Peplau (1992) explained, "rest on a one-way focus; the nurse's interests are the concerns and the development of the patient, rather than on having a reciprocal, social relationship. Such techniques are primarily verbal and investigative" (p. 18).

The **Clinical Methodology** is descriptive in nature and yields qualitative data in the form of nurse and patient verbal and nonverbal behaviors. Several alternatives exist for **Recording** the behaviors (Table 15–2). All of these forms and instruments are appropriate empirical indicators of the concept of **Nurse-Patient Relationship** and its dimensions and subdimensions.

The Theory of Interpersonal Relations is tested when the **Data Analysis** focuses on the nurse's hypotheses, which are formulated from first impressions or hunches about the patient. Analysis of the data ultimately yields understanding of the *Phase of the Nurse-Patient Relationship* in which the behaviors occurred; the *Roles* taken by the nurse and the patient in each phase; the nature, origin, function, and mode of *Relations;* and inferences about the *Pattern Integrations* in interpersonal relations.

EMPIRICAL ADEQUACY

The Theory of Interpersonal Relations meets the criterion of empirical adequacy for middle-range theories. A review of the published research designed to test the theory revealed some empirical support. Instrument development research is listed in Table 15–2. Other published research reports are listed in Table 15–3.

Forchuk and Brown's (1989) report of instrument development work provides some of the most direct evidence of the empirical adequacy of the Theory of Interpersonal Relations. Their findings indicated that each phase of the nurse-patient relationship could be documented on the basis of the nurse's and the patient's behaviors. The findings also indicated that "when the nurse can accurately assess the phase of the relationship, appropriate interventions within Peplau's theory are more likely to be selected" (p. 33).

A correlational study of factors that helped and hampered the nature and progression of the nurse-patient relationship provided additional evidence of the empirical adequacy of the Theory of Interpersonal Relations. Forchuk et al. (2000) found that the phases of the nurse-patient relationship observed in a tertiary care psychiatric hospital were consistent with the phases identified in the theory.

Peden's (1992, 1993, 1994, 1996, 1998, 2000; Peden, et al., 2000a, 2000b; Peden et al., 2001) program of research addressing depression in women provides even more evidence of the empirical adequacy of the Theory of Interpersonal Relations. The research program started with the description of a clinical phenomenon—recovering from depression—and has progressed to tests of a nursing intervention designed to reduce negative thinking in depressed women.

▶ TABLE 15–2
INSTRUMENTS TO RECORD THE NURSE-PATIENT RELATIONSHIP

Instrument and Citation*	Description
Nursing Process Study (Peplau, 1952)	A form for recording interpersonal relations in nursing. The form permits recording of the aspects listed here: Initial observation of a patient's behavior. Hypothesis, based on first impressions or hunches about the patient's behavior. Plan to study nurse-patient relationships in order to test the hypothesis. Repeated observations of the patient as the nurse approaches. Nurse's opening remarks, feelings, and thoughts about the patient. Patient's responses to the nurse's remarks and attitudes. Nurse's responses.
Social Interaction Inventory (Methven & Schlotfeldt, 1962; Young et al., 2001)	Measures the nature and type of verbal responses nurses give in emotion-laden practice situations.
Therapeutic Behavior Scale (Spring and Turk, 1962; Young et al., 2001)	Contains categories of verbal behavior evident in psychiatric nurse therapists' communications with their patients and yields a therapeutic behavior score.
Empathy Construct Rating Scale (LaMonica, 1981; Young et al., 2001)	Measures empathy, defined as "a central focus and feeling with and in the client's world. [Empathy] involves accurate perception of the client's world by the helper, communication of this understanding of the client, and the client's perception of the helper's understanding" (LaMonica, 1981, p. 398).
Relationship Form (Forchuk & Brown, 1989; Young et al., 2001)	Measures the progress of the nurse-patient relationship through the orientation, working (identification and exploitation), and resolution (termination) phases.
Stages of Learning Form (Forchuk & Voorberg, 1991)	Measures the eight stages of learning outlined by Peplau (1963)—observe, describe, analyze, formulate, validate, test, integrate, and utilize.

*See the Research Instruments and Practice Tools section of the chapter references for complete citations.

Although the available evidence supporting the empirical adequacy of the Theory of Interpersonal Relations is impressive, and although Peplau's (1952) work "influenced the interpersonal nature and direction of clinical work and studies" (Sills, 1977, p. 203), very few studies that directly tested the Theory of Interpersonal Relations have been conducted in the more than 50 years since the theory was first articulated (see Table 15–3 and the Doctoral Dissertations section of the chapter bibliography on the CD-ROM). That may be due to the tendency to *assume* the empirical adequacy of theories that are an integral part of the history of nursing theory development. As O'Toole and Welt (1989) commented:

Peplau's theoretical ideas … have become a part of the collective culture of the discipline of nursing. Many commonly understood and assumed ideas basic to nursing stem from her work. As we accumulate knowledge, we tend to lose sight of the individual contributions of the originators of that knowledge. In other words, it becomes knowledge in the public domain. For historical and intellectual reasons, it is extremely important to credit and evaluate those early contributions in light of their relevance to our discipline today. It is apparent … that Peplau's [theory] continue[s] to be germane to our research and practice (p. 365).

Clearly, additional systematic research designed to test the empirical adequacy of the phases of the nurse-patient relationship and their generalizability to diverse practice situations is needed to further determine the empirical adequacy of the Theory of Interpersonal Relations.

PRAGMATIC ADEQUACY

The Theory of Interpersonal Relations meets the criterion of pragmatic adequacy. Peplau has identified the educational prerequisites to the use of the theory, and she has explained how the theory can be used as a guide for nursing practice.

(Text continues on page 544)

TABLE 15–3
RESEARCH GUIDED BY THE THEORY OF INTERPERSONAL RELATIONS

Research Topic	Study Participants	Citation*
DESCRIPTIVE STUDIES		
Orientation phase of the nurse-patient relationship	Clients with chronic mental illness	Forchuk, 1992
Orientation phase of the nurse-patient relationship	Newly formed nurse-client dyads	Forchuk, 1994
Case study of a nurse-patient relationship	60-year-old widower living with relatives	Santos, 1998
Development of therapeutic nurse-patient relationships	Nursing home residents with Alzheimer's disease Advanced practice nurses	Williams & Tappen, 1999
Case study of concerns that need to be addressed	A man with AIDS	Gauthier, 2000
Perceptions of the effects of a liver transplant on quality of life	Patients attending an out-patient clinic ≥1 year after liver transplant	Robertson, 1999
Hallucinatory experiences of secluded psychiatric patients	Adult psychiatric inpatients	Kennedy et al., 1994
Teaching psychiatric patients about anxiety	Group of young females with schizophrenia	Hays, 1961
Validation of the nursing diagnosis anxiety	Registered nurses	Whitley, 1988
Pattern integrations	Young depressed women	Beeber, 1996 Beeber & Caldwell, 1996
Assessment of depression	Postpartal women	Almond, 1996
Feasibility of a depressive symptom screening and intervention initiative	Women in a primary care setting	Beeber & Charlie, 1998
Description of negative thoughts experienced by women with major depression	Depressed women	Peden, 2000
Process of recovering from depression	Women recovering from depression	Peden, 1992, 1993, 1996
Strategies used by women recovering from depression	Women recovering from depression	Peden, 1994
Experiences of parenting	Parents of at least one child who had completed high school and who had positive parenting processes	Jacobson, 1999
Patterns that influence adolescent females' nicotine smoking and behavior	Grade 9 Canadian female adolescents	Michael, 1998
Nurses' and patients' perceptions of psychiatric patients' reasons for medication noncompliance	Registered nurses Adult psychiatric patients	Lund & Frank, 1991
Perception of stressful experiences	Student nurses	Garrett et al., 1976

*See the Research section of the chapter references for complete citations.

Nurses' work roles	Psychiatric staff nurses	Morrison et al., 1996
Nurses' knowledge of and misconceptions about suicide	Oncology nurses	Valente et al., 1994
Comparison of perceptions of staff relationships with long-term care facility residents, reports of exposure to disruptive behaviors from residents, and reports of distress related to disruptive behaviors and physical aggression	Staff on special care units and traditional units	Middleton et al., 1999
Nurses' beliefs about the appropriateness of using the technique of therapeutic paradox	Psychiatric–mental health nurses	Hirschmann, 1989

CORRELATIONAL STUDIES

Factors influencing the length of the orientation phase of the nurse-patient relationship	Newly formed nurse-client dyads	Forchuk, 1995a
Factors influencing movement from the orientation to the working phase of the nurse-patient relationship	Nurse-client dyads	Forchuk et al., 1998
Factors influencing the uniqueness of the nurse-client relationship	Nurses and clients	Forchuk, 1995b
Relation of helping and hampering influences to the nature and progression of the nurse-patient relationship	Nurses working in a tertiary care psychiatric hospital	Forchuk et al., 2000
Factors associated with depressive symptoms	Young women	Beeber, 1998
Relation between self-esteem and depressive symptoms, as mediated by negative thinking	Female college students	Peden et al., 2000a
Relation between trait anxiety and anxiety-provoking clinical experiences	Senior year baccalaureate nursing students	Kim,. 2003

EXPERIMENTAL STUDIES

Effects of continued and control type of contact during the perioperative period on patients' readiness to return home and satisfaction with nursing care	Female surgical patients	Vogelsang, 1990
Effects of an individualized nursing approach and two control nursing approaches on patients' systolic blood pressure, radial pulse rate, respiratory rate, and oral temperature	Patients admitted for elective gynecologic surgery	Elms & Leonard, 1966
Effects of a group intervention to reduce negative thinking	Female college students at risk for depression	Peden, 1998 Peden et al., 2000b Peden et al., 2001
Effect of patient education on management of self-care waste	Insulin-dependent diabetic patients	Delpech, 2000

(continued)

Research Topic	Study Participants	Citation
PROGRAM EVALUATION STUDIES		
Evaluation of Theory of Interpersonal Relations–based nursing practice on an affective disorders unit in a large psychiatric hospital in England	Staff nurses Psychiatric patients	Bristow & Callaghan, 1991
Evaluation of a Canadian community mental health program based on the Theory of Interpersonal Relations	Clients in the community mental health program	Forchuk & Voorberg, 1991

(Text continued from page 541)

Nursing Education

The task of nursing education, according to Peplau (1952), "is the gradual development of each nurse as a person who *wants* to nurse patients in a helpful way" (p. xiii). More specifically, the central task of nursing education is "the fullest development of the nurse as a person who is aware of how she functions in a situation" (p. xii). Additional tasks include "release of human interest in others who are in difficulty, liberation of emotional and intellectual capacity for making choices, [and] development of nurses as persons whose enlightened self-interest will lead to no other choice but productive relations with all kinds of patients, students, [and] citizens" (p. xii).

Special education is required for application of the Theory of Interpersonal Relations. In particular, nurses must learn Peplau's **Clinical Methodology** (see Table 15–1). Moreover, nurses must learn to "have control over the signals (stimuli, messages, inputs, cues) that they send to a patient [because the nurse's behaviors] serve as stimuli for evoking behavioral changes by patients" (Peplau, 1992, p. 14). Nurses also must learn "to identify human problems that confront patients, the degrees of skill used to meet situations, and be able to develop with patients the kind of relationships that will be conducive to improvement in skill" (Peplau, 1952, p. xv).

Peplau (1952) maintained that students must engage in productive learning so that they may grow and expand their personalities. She pointed out that as students grow, however, they may experience "frustrations, conflicts, and anxieties as older patterns of behavior are foregone and more productive, new ones are developed" (p. xvi).

Furthermore, nurses must accept responsibility for lifelong learning. Peplau (1952) stated that "although the basic school can do much to foster the development of students as useful, productive persons, each graduate nurse can also take on the responsibility for expanding her own insight into the effects of life experiences on personality functioning and for planning steps that will lead to a mode of life that is more creative and more productive." (p. xvii).

The importance of basic and continuing education is underscored by the comment given here:

> What each nurse becomes—as a functioning personality—determines the manner in which she will perform in each interpersonal contact in every nursing situation. The extent to which each nurse understands her own functioning will determine the extent to which she can come to understand the situation confronting the patient and the way he sees it. Positive, useful nursing actions flow out of understanding of the situation. (Peplau, 1952, p. xii)

Nursing Practice

The purpose of nursing practice "is to promote favorable changes in patients" (Peplau, 1992, p. 13). This purpose is accomplished by application of Peplau's **Clinical Methodology** (see Table 15–1). Indeed, Peplau (1952, 1997) views nursing practice as the study of the **Nurse-Patient Relationship**.

The task of nursing service, according to Peplau (1952), is "concern for the patient" (p. xiii). The operationalization of that task is evident in these characteristics of professional nursing practice (Peplau (1989 [original work presented 1965], 1997):

- The focus is the patient.
- The nurse uses participant observation rather than spectator observation.

- The nurse is aware of the various roles assumed in the nurse-patient relationship.
- Practice is primarily investigative, with emphasis on observation and collection of data that are made available to the patient, rather than task oriented.
- Practice requires major intellectual work, with wide variation in the content of the work.
- Practice is grounded in the application of theory, discretion, and judgment.

The Theory of Interpersonal Relations is widely used in the real world of nursing practice. Martin and Kirkpatrick's (as cited in Forchuk, 1991b) survey, which was conducted at a Canadian tertiary care psychiatric hospital, revealed that Peplau's theory was the most frequently used of 17 different nursing theories to guide staff nurses' practice. In addition, Hirschmann (1989) found that one-half of the 165 psychiatric nurses she surveyed in the United States used Peplau's theory to guide their practice.

Published reports of the application of the Theory of Interpersonal Relations in nursing practice are listed in Table 15–4. Those reports, along with the reports listed in the Commentary: Administration, Commentary: Practice, and Administration sections of the chapter bibliography on the CD-ROM, generally support Peplau's (1992) claim that the theory "is useful in all areas of nursing practice, ... especially in psychiatric nursing, because psychiatric pa-tients, generally, have problems with communication and in relatedness to people" (p. 13).

The Theory of Interpersonal Relations is applicable not only for the study of interpersonal relations between nurses and patients, but also may be applied to relations between the nurse and family members, the nurse and other nurses, the instructor and student, the administrator and staff nurse, and the nurse and other members of the health-care team (Peplau, 1952, 1992). Published reports of such applications could not be located. Systematic examination of the applicability of the theory to other than the nurse-patient relationship is warranted.

There is a question regarding the applicability of the theory with children. As can be seen in Figure 15–2, the **Nurse-Patient Relationship** ends with both nurse and patient assuming the role of adult person. Peplau did not discuss the role that would be assumed by the patient if he or she were a child.

Another question regards the applicability of the theory with patients who have several physiological needs (Belcher & Fish, 2002). The theory has, however, been used successfully with patients who have multiple physiological problems, such as individuals with hemophilia (Hall, 1994) and acquired immunodeficiency syndrome (AIDS) (Hall, 1994; Harding, 1995). Peplau (1992; as cited in Takahashi, 1992) explained that although the theory does not deal with the medical or physiological aspects of the patient's

TABLE 15–4
NURSING PRACTICE GUIDED BY THE THEORY OF INTERPERSONAL RELATIONS

Practice Situation	Population	Citation*
Phases of the nurse-patient relationship	A 23-year-old woman with multiple physical and psychosocial problems	O'Brien & Smith, 1991
	A 32-year-old woman who was admitted to a chemical dependency unit for alcohol abuse	Belcher & Fish, 2002
	A 42-year-old man with shortness of breath—outpatient clinic	Runtz & Urtel, 1983
	A man with acquired AIDS and his fiancée	Harding, 1995
	A man with hemophilia and AIDS and his wife	Hall, 1994
	Patients with depression	Bird, 1992 Stark, 1992
	A 28-year-old man with diabetes	Nordal & Soto, 1980
	A 54-year-old woman with metastatic cancer	
	A 56-year-old man with a stroke	
	An 80-year-old woman who had attempted suicide following the death of a close friend	Doncliff, 1994

*See the Practice section of the chapter references for complete citations.

(continued)

Practice Situation	Population	Citation
Application of the Theory of Interpersonal Relations	New mothers	Normandale, 1995
	Teen-aged boy with emotional and psychological problems	Venn, 1998
	A patient with a serious mental disorder	Thelander, 1997
	A patient with schizophrenia who was not taking prescribed medications	Lan et al., 1997
	Participants in the Bridge to Discharge project— patients with schizophrenia and nurses	Forchuk et al., 1998
	Patients with depression	Beeber, 1989, 1998 Beeber & Bourbonniere, 1998 Feely, 1997a, 1997b Lambert, 1994
	Depressed and self-harming elderly person	Campbell, 2001
	Patients with anxiety	Arnold & Nieswiadomy, 1993 Day, 1990
	Patients who are angry	Thomas et al., 1970
	A patient with a chronic alcohol misuse problem	Buswell, 1997
	Patients with psychosocial problems created by a stroke	Jones, 1995
	A child with cancer	Kelley, 1996
	A 42-year-old man with human immunodeficiency virus (HIV) disease	Beeber et al., 1990
	A man residing in a correctional facility	Schafer, 1999
	A 38-year-old woman with altered body image due to mastectomy	Price, 1998
	A male survivor of sexual abuse	Vardy & Price, 1998
	Adults with multiple sclerosis	McGuinness & Peters, 1999
	A 72-year-old lonely man	Wilford, 1997
	A terminally ill patient in a hospice	Fowler, 1995
	A woman in group psychotherapy	Lego, 1998
	Family caregivers	Yamashita, 1997
	Tense nurse-patient relationships with people living in the community	Edwards, 1996
	A health education group	Jewell & Sullivan, 1996
Nurses' and patients' changing roles	Patients in short-term psychotherapy	Thompson, 1986

problems, it may "be useful when nurses use health teaching to help patients understand [the medical] aspects of their health problem" (Peplau, 1992, p. 13).

Still other questions regard the applicability of the theory when communication between nurses and patients is limited, such as with individuals who are senile, unconscious, or comatose or with newborn infants (Belcher & Fish, 2002; Howk, 2002). Howk (2002) commented, "In such situations, the nurse-patient relationship is often one-sided. The nurse and the patient cannot work together to become more knowledgeable, develop goals, and mature" (p. 388). Williams and Tappen (1999), however, found that 83% of the patients with middle or late stage Alzheimer's disease in their study formed therapeutic relationships with nurses. Therapeutic nurse-patient relationships were not formed primarily when patients had speech difficulties or did not speak at all.

The feasibility of implementing clinical protocols that

reflect the theory is evident in the reports of nursing practice guided by the Theory of Interpersonal Relations (see Table 15–4). The requisite resources typically are limited to the time and personnel required for training in the use of the **Clinical Methodology.**

Peplau (1989 [original work presented 1965]) identified the content and criteria for practice protocols derived from the Theory of Interpersonal Relations that listed here.

Content

- What to observe
- What to do as a consequence of the observation
- A rationale for what is to be done

Criteria

- The situation should be structured so that the patient is clear about the nurse's intentions.
- The nurse should behave like an expert.
- The nurse should show appreciation for what the patient is up against.
- The nurse should provide opportunities for the patient to check the meaning of experiences.

Peplau also developed specific protocols for such practice problems as anxiety, loneliness, and learning (Peplau, 1955, 1962, 1963). Other practice protocols derived from the Theory of Interpersonal Relations include Morrison's (1992) protocol for clinical nurse specialist practice in an inpatient psychiatric unit and Forchuk and co-workers' (1989) protocol for a community mental health promotion program targeted to chronically mentally ill clients who live in boarding homes. An example of a protocol that Peplau (1962, pp. 53–54) designed to abate a patient's severe anxiety is given here.

What to Observe

- Observe the patient's anxiety-related behaviors

What to Do as a Consequence of the Observation

- Encourage the patient to identify the anxiety as such. This is done by having all personnel help the patient to recognize what he or she is experiencing at the point when he or she is actually anxious.
- Encourage the patient to connect the relief-giving patterns that he or she uses to the anxiety that requires such relief.
- Encourage the patient to provide himself or herself and the nurse with data descriptive of situations and interactions that occur immediately before an increase in anxiety is noticed.

- Encourage the patient to formulate from the descriptive data the probable immediate, situational causes for the increase in his or her anxiety.

Rationale

- In keeping with the Theory of Interpersonal Relations, the nursing personnel focus their efforts on maintaining the patient's awareness of the anxiety and connecting it to his or her anxiety-relieving behavior.

Nurses have the legal ability to implement practice protocols derived from the Theory of Interpersonal Relations and to measure the effectiveness of theory-based nursing actions. Indeed, Peplau (1952) maintained that "the nursing profession has legal responsibility for the effective use of nursing and for its consequences to patients" (p. 6). In a later publication, Peplau (1985) commented that "advances in professional practice have, in part, been the result of a sensible balance between self-regulation and external controls" (p. 141). She went on to express her concern that "the privilege of self-regulation is being *given* away or *taken* away" (p. 141) and urged nurses to guard against further erosion of self-regulation.

The extent to which nursing practice based on the Theory of Interpersonal Relations is compatible with expectations for nursing practice is being explored. Bristow and Callaghan (1991) found that the application of Peplau's theory significantly improved nurses' use of the nursing process 3 months after its implementation in a large psychiatric hospital in England. Staff nurse satisfaction, however, changed very little and patient satisfaction decreased. Commenting on their findings, Bristow and Callaghan (1991) stated:

> Patient satisfaction is adversely affected, perhaps because of the increasing administrative tasks of the [theory] which take nurses away from patients. As the [theory] emphasizes the partnership between the nurse and the patient, the added responsibility expected from the patient may invoke an increase in stress. Patients whose very problems may stem from difficulties in assuming responsibilities for their activities of living may see this stress as a deterioration in their health and thus in their satisfaction with nursing care (p. 40).

Conversely, Vogelsang (1990) reported that women who experienced a Theory of Interpersonal Relations–based nursing intervention of continued contact with a familiar nurse from preadmission through postoperative awakening to consciousness reported greater satisfaction with nursing than women who had received a control nursing intervention of contact with various nurses throughout the perioperative period.

Belcher and Fish (2002) maintained that use of the Theory of Interpersonal Relations "directly improves communication" between nurses and patients (p. 76). The reports cited in Table 15–4 indicate that use of the Theory of Interpersonal Relations leads to favorable outcomes for the patient and the nurse and to a solution for the patient's problem. For example, Forchuk and Voorberg's (1991) evaluation of a Theory of Interpersonal Relations–based community mental health program revealed that within the initial 2-year period of the program, the problem identification phase of the nurse-patient relationship was most common, and that just 13% of the 91 clients had not moved beyond the orientation phase. In addition, the clients demonstrated progress in the stages of learning, with 78% at the second (describe) stage, and almost 8% at the fourth stage (formulate) and another 8% at the fifth stage (validate). Furthermore, Forchuk and colleagues (1998) reported that evaluation of the Theory of Interpersonal Relations–based Bridge to Discharge project for schizophrenic patients "improved clients' quality of life and saved taxpayers almost half a million dollars in one year and was supportive of staff's quality of worklife" (p. 197). The project was developed and implemented by the Schizophrenia Intensive Treatment inpatient program of Hamilton Psychiatric Hospital, the Community Mental Health Promotion Program of the Hamilton-Wentworth Department of Public Health Services, and the Mental Health Rights Coalition, all in Hamilton, Ontario, Canada. Also, Middleton, Stewart, and Richardson (1999) found that the Theory of Interpersonal Relations is an appropriate guide for development of strategies for preventing and managing aggressive or aversive behaviors.

None of the reports of application of the Theory of Interpersonal Relations to nursing practice mentioned any comparison of outcomes of use of the theory and outcomes in the same situation when the theory was not used. This work remains to be done (Reynolds, 1997).

 ## CONCLUSION

Peplau proposed her Theory of Interpersonal Relations five decades ago. She has received many accolades for her work. She has been called the psychiatric nurse of the century (Callaway, 2002), the mother of psychiatric nursing (Haber, 2000), and the "inventor of psychiatric–mental health nursing" (Fagin, 1996, p. 11). Fagin explained:

> Peplau's developed ideas went far beyond her predecessors and created a distinct field of study and practice. As a result, she provided the substance for exploration, explanation, and extrapolation, and reached a large and responsive audience of students, scholars, and practitioners. She filled a gap that had begun to hurt nurses practicing in psychiatric settings, who were attempting to become equals with other professionals

but needed a language to describe the uniqueness of nursing's contributions (p. 11).

Adams (1991) credited Peplau with development of the interpersonal paradigm in psychiatric nursing. Furthermore, Peplau was, as Kerr (1990) pointed out, "the first nurse theorist to delineate psychiatric-mental health nursing as an interpersonal process governed by lawful principles" (p. 5). Barker (1998) regards Peplau's work as having the most significant and worldwide influence on the development of psychiatric nursing practice. In a similar vein, Burgess (1997) pointed out that the Theory of Interpersonal Relations has had a greater impact on psychiatric nursing than any other theory. Yet the theory extends beyond psychiatric-mental health nursing and greatly enhances understanding of the nature and substance of interpersonal relations between *all* nurses and patients. Furthermore, the theory is a very useful perspective of the verbal communications between nurses and patients. Most important, as Peplau (1992) pointed out, "the theory assists nurses in their personal growth and in the promotion of growth and understanding in their patients" (p. 18). Peplau's work, then, clearly represents a major contribution to nursing knowledge development. Indeed, as Lethbridge (1997) commented, "Despite its age, Peplau's work remains a part of the contemporary discourse in nursing, as well as an historical treatise that signaled the beginning of a new era in professional nursing" (p. 167). Peden (2001) added,

> Peplau's theory is very timely today, keeping pace with the postmodern influences that have reinformed nurses' awareness of the knowledge-rich context of practice, at the level of the patient. A study of Peplau's work introduces you to a woman whose ideas were ahead of her time. These ideas have arrived (pp. 62–63)!

More evidence of the empirical adequacy of the Theory of Interpersonal Relations is, however, needed. As Kerr (1990) noted, "the task remains for us to develop [and test] theoretical models that define how we are to use acquired interpersonal skills to effect greater degrees of mental health in our clients" (p. 5). Thus, continued documentation of the outcomes of the use of the Theory of Interpersonal Relations is required, with special attention given to the ways in which its utilization promotes favorable changes in patients, as well as the precise nature and stability of those favorable changes.

 ## REFERENCES

Adams, T. (1991). Paradigms in psychiatric nursing. Nursing (London), 4(35), 9–11.

Barker, P. (1998). The future of the theory of interpersonal relations? A personal reflection on Peplau's legacy. Journal of Psychiatric and Mental Health Nursing, 5, 213–220.

Belcher, J.V.R., & Fish, L.J.B. (2002). Interpersonal relations in nursing: Hildegard E. Peplau. In J. B. George (Ed.), Nursing theories: The base for professional nursing practice (5th ed., pp. 61–82). Upper Saddle River, NJ: Prentice Hall.

Bristow, F., & Callaghan, P. (1991). Using Peplau's model in affective disorders. Nursing Times, 87(18), 40–41.

Burgess, A.W. (1997). Psychiatric nursing. In A.W. Burgess (Ed.), Psychiatric nursing: Promoting mental health (pp. 10–25). Stamford, CT: Appleton & Lange.

Callaway, B.J. (2002). Hildegard Peplau: Psychiatric nurse of the century. New York: Springer.

Fagin, C.M. (1996). Commentary. Archives of Psychiatric Nursing, 10, 11–13.

Forchuk, C. (1991a). A comparison of the works of Peplau and Orlando. Archives of Psychiatric Nursing, 5, 38–45.

Forchuk, C. (1991b). Peplau's theory: Concepts and their relations. Nursing Science Quarterly, 4, 54–60.

Forchuk, C., Beaton, S., Crawford, L., Ide, L., Voorberg, N., & Bethune, J. (1989). Incorporating Peplau's theory and case management. Journal of Psychosocial Nursing and Mental Health Services, 27(2), 35–38.

Forchuk, C., & Brown, B. (1989). Establishing a nurse-client relationship. Journal of Psychosocial and Mental Health Services, 27(2), 30–34.

Forchuk, C., Jewell, J., Schofield, R., Sircelj, M., & Velledor, T. (1998). From hospital to community: Bridging therapeutic relationships. Journal of Psychiatric and Mental Health Nursing, 5, 197–202.

Forchuk, C., & Voorberg, N. (1991). Evaluation of a community mental health program. Canadian Journal of Nursing Administration, 4(2), 16–20.

Forchuk, C., Westwell, J., Martin, M., Azzapardi, W.B., Kosterewa-Tolman, D., & Hux, M. (2000). The developing nurse-client relationship: Nurses' perspectives. Journal of the American Psychiatric Nurses' Association, 6, 3–10.

Haber, J. (2000). Hildegard E. Peplau: The psychiatric nursing legacy of a legend. Journal of the American Psychiatric Nurses' Association, 6, 56–62.

Hall, K. (1994). Peplau's model of nursing: Caring for a man with AIDS. British Journal of Nursing, 3, 18–422.

Harding, T. (1995). Exemplar. Professional Leader, 2(1), 20–21.

Howk, C. (2002). Hildegard E. Peplau: Psychodynamic nursing. In A. Marriner Tomey & M.R. Alligood (Eds.), Nursing theorists and their work (5th ed., pp. 379–398). St. Louis: Mosby.

Hirschmann, M. (1989). Psychiatric and mental health nurses' beliefs about therapeutic paradox. Journal of Child Psychiatric Nursing, 2(1), 7–13.

Kerr, N.J. (1990). Editor's corner. Perspectives in Psychiatric Care, 26(4), 5–6.

Lethbridge, D.J. (1997). Book review of Peplau, H.E. (1991). Interpersonal relations in nursing. New York: Springer. Image: Journal of Nursing Scholarship, 29, 197.

Middleton, J.I., Stewart, N.J., & Richardson, J.S. (1999). Caregiver distress related to disruptive behaviors on special care units versus traditional long-term care units. Journal of Gerontological Nursing, 25(3), 11–19.

Moreno, J. (1941). Psychodrama and group psychotherapy. Sociometry, 9, 249–253.

Morrison, E.G. (1992). Inpatient practice: An integrated framework. Journal of Psychosocial Nursing and Mental Health Services, 30(1), 26–29.

O'Toole, A.W., & Welt, S.R. (Eds.) (1989). Interpersonal theory in nursing practice. Selected works of Hildegard E. Peplau. New York: Springer.

Peden, A.R. (1992). The process of recovering in women who have been depressed. Kentucky Nurse, 40(6), 10.

Peden, A.R. (1993). Recovering in depressed women: Research with Peplau's theory. Nursing Science Quarterly, 6, 140–146.

Peden, A.R. (1994). Up from depression: Strategies used by women recovering from depression. Journal of Psychiatric and Mental Health Nursing, 1, 77–83.

Peden, A.R. (1996). Recovering from depression: A one-year follow-up. Journal of Psychiatric and Mental Health Nursing, 3, 289–295.

Peden, A.R. (1998). The evolution of an intervention—The use of Peplau's process of practice-based theory development. Journal of Psychiatric and Mental Health Nursing, 5, 173–178.

Peden, A.R. (2000). Negative thoughts of women with depression. Journal of the American Psychiatric Nurses' Association, 6(2), 41–48.

Peden, A.R. (2001). Hildegard E. Peplau: The process of practice-based theory development. In M.E. Parker (Ed.), Nursing theories and nursing practice (pp. 55–67). Philadelphia: F.A. Davis.

Peden, A.R., Hall, L.A., Reyens, M.K., & Beebe, L. (2000a). Negative thinking mediates the effect of self-esteem on depressive symptoms in college women. Nursing Research, 49, 201–207.

Peden, A.R., Hall, L.A., Reyens, M.K., & Beebe, L. (2000b). Reducing negative thinking and depressive symptoms in college women. Journal of Nursing Scholarship, 32, 145–151.

Peden, A.R., Reyens, M.K., Hall, L.A., & Beebe, L. (2001). Preventing depression in high-risk college women: A report of an 18-month follow-up. Journal of American College Health, 49, 299–306.

Peplau, H.E. (1952). Interpersonal relations in nursing. A conceptual frame of reference for psychodynamic nursing. New York: G.P. Putnam's Sons. [Reprinted 1989. London: Macmillan Education. Reprinted 1991. New York: Springer.]

Peplau, H.E. (1955). Loneliness. American Journal of Nursing, 55, 1476–1481.

Peplau, H.E. (1962). Interpersonal techniques: The crux of psychiatric nursing. American Journal of Nursing, 62, 50–54.

Peplau, H.E. (1963). Process and concept of learning. In S.F. Burd & M.A. Marshall (Eds.), Some clinical approaches to psychiatric nursing (pp. 333–336). New York: Macmillan.

Peplau, H.E. (1965). The heart of nursing: Interpersonal relations. Canadian Nurse, 61, 273–275.

Peplau, H.E. (1969). Theory: The professional dimension. In C.M. Norris (Ed.), Proceedings. First nursing theory conference (pp. 33–46). Kansas City, KS: University of Kansas Medical Center Department of Nursing Education.

Peplau, H.E. (1985). Is nursing's self-regulatory power being eroded? American Journal of Nursing, 85, 140–143.

Peplau, H.E. (1989). Interpersonal constructs for nursing practice. In A.W. O'Toole & S.R. Welt (Eds.), Interpersonal theory in nursing practice. Selected works of Hildegard E. Peplau (pp. 56–70.). New York: Springer. [Original work published 1987.]

Peplau, H.E. (1989). Interpersonal relations in psychiatric nursing. In A.W. O'Toole & S.R. Welt (Eds.), Interpersonal theory in nursing practice: Selected works of Hildegard E. Peplau (pp. 5–20.). New York: Springer. [Original work presented 1954.]

Peplau, H.E. (1989). Interpersonal relationships: The purpose and characteristics of professional nursing. In A.W. O'Toole & S.R. Welt (Eds.), Interpersonal theory in nursing practice: Selected works of Hildegard E. Peplau (pp. 42–55.). New York: Springer. [Original work presented 1965.]

Peplau, H.E. (1992). Interpersonal relations: A theoretical framework for application in nursing practice. Nursing Science Quarterly, 5, 13–18.

Peplau, H.E. (1994). Quality of life: An interpersonal perspective. Nursing Science Quarterly, 7, 10–15.

Peplau, H.E. (1996). Commentary. Archives of Psychiatric Nursing, 10, 14–15.

Peplau, H.E. (1997). Peplau's theory of interpersonal relations. Nursing Science Quarterly, 10, 162–167.

Reynolds, W.J. (1997). Peplau's theory in practice. Nursing Science Quarterly, 10, 168–170.

Sellers, S.C. (1991). A philosophical analysis of conceptual models of nursing. Dissertation Abstracts International, 52, 1937B. [University Microfilms No. AAC9126248.]

Sills, G. (1989). Foreword. In A.W. O'Toole & S.R. Welt (Eds.), Interpersonal theory in nursing practice. Selected works of Hildegard E. Peplau (pp. ix–xi). New York: Springer.

Sills, G.M. (1977). Research in the field of psychiatric nursing 1952–1977. Nursing Research, 26, 201–207.

Sills, G.M. (1978). Hildegard E. Peplau: Leader, practitioner, academician, scholar, and theorist. Perspectives in Psychiatric Care, 16, 122–128.

Sullivan, H.S. (1953). The interpersonal theory of psychiatry [H.S. Perry & M.L. Gawel, Eds.]. New York: Norton.

Takahashi, T. (1992). Perspectives on nursing knowledge. Nursing Science Quarterly, 5, 86–91.

Vogelsang, J. (1990). Continued contact with a familiar nurse affects women's perceptions of the ambulatory surgical experience: A qualitative-quantitative design. Journal of Post Anesthesia Nursing, 5, 315–320.

Williams, C.L., & Tappen, R.M. (1999). Can we create a therapeutic relationship with nursing home residents in the later stages of Alzheimer's disease? Journal of Psychosocial Nursing and Mental Health Services, 37(3), 28–35, 40–41.

RESEARCH

Almond, P. (1996). How health visitors assess the health of postnatal women. Health Visitor, 69, 495–498.

Beeber, L.S. (1996). Pattern integrations in young depressed women: Part I. Archives of Psychiatric Nursing, 10, 151–156.

Beeber, L.S. (1998). Social support, self-esteem, and depressive symptoms in young American women. Image: Journal of Nursing Scholarship, 30, 91.

Beeber, L.S., & Caldwell, C.L. (1996). Pattern integrations in young depressed women: Part II. Archives of Psychiatric Nursing, 10, 157–164.

Beeber, L.S., & Charlie, M.L. (1998). Depressive symptom reversal for women in a primary care setting: A pilot study. Archives of Psychiatric Nursing, 12, 247–254.

Bristow, F., & Callaghan, P. (1991). Using Peplau's model in affective disorders. Nursing Times, 87(18), 40–41.

Delpech, A. (2000). The management of self-care waste: To a hospital training? Recherche en Soins Infirmiers, 60 (March), 67–85. [French; English abstract]

Elms, R.R., & Leonard, R.C. (1966). Effects of nursing approaches during admission. Nursing Research, 15, 39–48.

Forchuk, C. (1992). The orientation phase of the nurse-client relationship: How long does it take? Perspectives in Psychiatric Care, 28, 7–10.

Forchuk, C. (1994). The orientation phase of the nurse-client relationship: Testing Peplau's theory. Journal of Advanced Nursing, 20, 532–537.

Forchuk, C. (1995a). Development of nurse-client relationships: What helps? Journal of the American Psychiatric Nurses Association, 1, 146–153.

Forchuk, C. (1995b). Uniqueness within the nurse-client relationship. Archives of Psychiatric Nursing, 9, 34–39.

Forchuk, C., & Voorberg, N. (1991). Evaluation of a community mental health program. Canadian Journal of Nursing Administration, 4(2), 16–20.

Forchuk, C., Westwell, J., Martin, M., Azzapardi, W.B., Kosterewa-Tolman, D., & Hux, M. (1998). Factors influencing movement of chronic psychiatric patients from the orientation to the working phase of the nurse-client relationship on an inpatient unit. Perspectives in Psychiatric Care, 34, 36–44.

Forchuk, C., Westwell, J., Martin, M., Azzapardi, W.B., Kosterewa-Tolman, D., & Hux, M. (2000). The developing nurse-client relationship: Nurses' perspectives. Journal of the American Psychiatric Nurses' Association, 6, 3–10.

Garrett, A., Manuel, D., & Vincent, C. (1976). Stressful experiences identified by student nurses. Journal of Nursing Education, 15(6), 9–21.

Gauthier, P. (2000). Use of Peplau's interpersonal relations model to counsel people with AIDS. Journal of the American Psychiatric Nurses Association, 6, 119–125.

Hays, D. (1961). Teaching a concept of anxiety. Nursing Research, 10, 108–113.

Hirschmann, M.J. (1989). Psychiatric and mental health nurses' beliefs about therapeutic paradox. Journal of Child and Adolescent Psychiatric Mental Health Nursing, 2(1), 7–13.

Jacobson, G.A. (1999). Parent processes: A descriptive exploratory study using Peplau's theory. Nursing Science Quarterly, 12, 240–244.

Kennedy, B.R., Williams, C.A., & Pesut, D.J. (1994). Hallucinatory experiences of psychiatric patients in seclusion. Archives of Psychiatric Nursing, 8, 169–176.

Kim, K.H. (2003). Baccalaureate nursing students' experiences of anxiety producing situations in the clinical setting. Contemporary Nurse, 14, 145–155.

Lund, V.E., & Frank, D.I. (1991). Helping the medicine go down: Nurses' and patients' perceptions about medication compliance. Journal of Psychosocial Nursing and Mental Health Services, 29(7), 6–9.

Michael, S.B. (1998). A survey of patterns influencing adolescent females' nicotine smoking behaviour. Journal of Substance Misuse for Nursing, Health, and Social Care, 3, 200–205.

Middleton, J.I., Stewart, N.J., & Richardson, J.S. (1999). Caregiver distress related to disruptive behaviors on special care units versus traditional long-term care units. Journal of Gerontological Nursing, 25(3), 11–19.

Morrison, E.G., Shealy, A.H., Kowalski, C., LaMont, J., & Range, B.A. (1996). Work roles of staff nurses in psychiatric settings. Nursing Science Quarterly, 9, 17–21.

Peden, A.R. (1992). The process of recovering in women who have been depressed. Kentucky Nurse, 40(6), 10.

Peden, A.R. (1993). Recovering in depressed women: Research with Peplau's theory. Nursing Science Quarterly, 6, 140–146.
Henderson, D.J. (1994). Commentary on "Recovering in depressed women: Research with Peplau's theory." AWHONN's Women's Health Nursing Scan, 8(2), 19–20.

Peden, A.R. (1994). Up from depression: Strategies used by women recovering from depression. Journal of Psychiatric and Mental Health Nursing, 1, 77–83.

Peden, A.R. (1996). Recovering from depression: A one-year follow-up. Journal of Psychiatric and Mental Health Nursing, 3, 289–295.

Peden, A.R. (1998). The evolution of an intervention—The use of Peplau's process of practice-based theory development. Journal of Psychiatric and Mental Health Nursing, 5, 173–178.

Peden, A.R. (2000). Negative thoughts of women with depression. Journal of the American Psychiatric Nurses Association, 6(2), 41–48.

Peden, A.R., Hall, L.A., Reyens, M.K., & Beebe, L. (2000a). Negative thinking mediates the effect of self-esteem on depressive symptoms in college women. Nursing Research, 49, 201–207.

Peden, A.R., Hall, L.A., Reyens, M.K., & Beebe, L. (2000b). Reducing negative thinking and depressive symptoms in college women. Journal of Nursing Scholarship, 32, 145–151.

Peden, A.R., Reyens, M.K., Hall, L.A., & Beebe, L. (2001). Preventing depression in high-risk college women: A report of an 18-month follow-up. Journal of American College Health, 49, 299–306.

Robertson, G. (1999). Individuals' perception of their quality of life following a liver transplant: An exploratory study. Journal of Advanced Nursing, 30, 497–505.

Santos, S.S.C. (1998). The home health care for elderly person: A help[ing] relationship in nursing. Revista Brasileira de Enfermagem, 51, 665–676. [Portuguese; English abstract]

Valente, S.M., Saunders, J.M., & Grant, M. (1994). Oncology nurses' knowledge and misconceptions about suicide. Cancer Practice, 2, 209–216.

Vogelsang, J. (1990). Continued contact with a familiar nurse affects women's perceptions of the ambulatory surgical experience: A qualitative-quantitative design. Journal of Post Anesthesia Nursing, 5, 315–320.

Whitley, G.G. (1988). A validation study of the nursing diagnosis anxiety. Florida Nursing Review, 3(2), 1–7.

Williams, C.L., & Tappen, R.M. (1999). Can we create a therapeutic relationship with nursing home residents in the later stages of Alzheimer's disease? Journal of Psychosocial Nursing and Mental Health Services, 37(3), 28–35, 40–41.

RESEARCH INSTRUMENTS AND PRACTICE TOOLS

Forchuk, C., & Brown, B. (1989). Establishing a nurse-client relationship. Journal of Psychosocial Nursing and Mental Health Services, 27(2), 30–34.

Forchuk, C., & Voorberg, N. (1991). Evaluation of a community mental health program. Canadian Journal of Nursing Administration, 4(2), 16–20.

LaMonica, E. (1981). Construct validity of an empathy instrument. Research in Nursing and Health, 4, 389–400.

Methven, D., & Schlotfeldt, R.M. (1962). The social interaction inventory. Nursing Research, 11, 83–88.

Peplau, H.E. (1952). Interpersonal relations in nursing. New York: G.P. Putnam's Sons. [Reprinted 1989. London: Macmillan Education Ltd. Reprinted 1991. New York: Springer]

Spring, F.E., & Turk, H. (1962). A therapeutic behavior scale. Nursing Research, 11, 214–218.

Young, A., Taylor, S.G., & McLaughlin-Renpenning, K. (2001). Connections: Nursing research, theory, and practice. St. Louis: Mosby.

PRACTICE

Arnold, W.K., & Nieswiadomy, R. (1993). Peplau's theory with emphasis on anxiety (pp. 153–178). In S.M. Ziegler (Ed.), Theory-directed nursing practice. New York: Springer.

Beeber, L.S. (1989). Enacting corrective interpersonal experiences with the depressed client. An intervention model. Archives of Psychiatric Nursing, 3, 211–217.

Beeber, L.S. (1998). Treating depression through the therapeutic nurse-client relationship. Nursing Clinics of North America, 33, 153–172.

Beeber, L., Anderson, C.A., & Sills, G.M. (1990). Peplau's theory in practice. Nursing Science Quarterly, 3, 6–8.

Beeber, L.S., & Bourbonniere, M. (1998). The concept of interpersonal pattern in Peplau's theory of nursing. Journal of Psychiatric and Mental Health Nursing, 5, 187–192.

Belcher, J.V.R., & Fish, L.J.B. (2002). Interpersonal relations in nursing: Hildegard E. Peplau. In J. B. George (Ed.), Nursing theories: The base for professional nursing practice (5th ed., pp. 61–82). Upper Saddle River, NJ: Prentice Hall.

Bird, J. (1992). Helping Billy move on. Nursing Times, 88(31), 42–44.

Buswell, C. (1997). A model approach to care of a patient with alcohol problems. Nursing Times, 93(3), 34–35.

Campbell, D.M. (2001). Learning to care. Assignment, 7(1), 25–38.

Day, M.W. (1990). Anxiety in the emergency department. Point of View, 27(3), 4–5.

Doncliff, B. (1994). Putting Peplau to work. Nursing New Zealand, 2(1), 20–22.

Edwards, M. (1996). Patient-nurse relationships: Using reflective practice. Nursing Standard, 10(25), 40–43.

Feely, M. (1997a). Using Peplau's theory in nurse-patient relations. International Nursing Review, 44, 115–120.

Feely, M. (1997b). Utilizing Peplau's theory in nurse patient relationship. Professioni Infermieristiche, 50(4), 45–49. [Italian; English abstract]

Forchuk, C., Jewell, J., Schofield, R., Sircelj, M., & Velledor, T. (1998). From hospital to community: Bridging therapeutic relationships. Journal of Psychiatric and Mental Health Nursing, 5, 197–202.

Fowler, J. (1995). Taking theory into practice: Using Peplau's model in the care of patient. Professional Nurse, 10, 226–230.

Hall, K. (1994). Peplau's model of nursing: Caring for a man with AIDS. British Journal of Nursing, 3, 18–422.

Harding, T. (1995). Exemplar. Professional Leader, 2(1), 20–21.

Jewell, J.A., & Sullivan, E.A. (1996). Application of nursing theories in health education. Journal of the American Psychiatric Nurses Association, 2, 79–85.

Jones, A. (1995). Utilizing Peplau's psychodynamic theory for stroke patient care. Journal of Clinical Nursing, 4(1), 49–54.

Kelley, S.J. (1996). "It's just me, my family, my treatments, and my nurse … oh, yeah, and Nintendo": Hildegard Peplau's day with kids with cancer. Journal of the American Psychiatric Nurses Association, 2, 11–14.

Lambert, C. (1994). Depression: Nursing management, part 2. Nursing Standard, 8(48), 57–64.

Lan, C.M., Shiau, S.J., & Huang, R.Y. (1997). Applying Peplau's theory in improving drug compliance of a schizophrenic patient [English abstract]. Journal of Nursing (China), 44, 56–62.

Lego, S. (1998). The application of Peplau's theory to group psychotherapy. Journal of Psychiatric and Mental Health Nursing, 5, 193–196.

McGuinness, S.D., & Peters, S. (1999). The diagnosis of multiple sclerosis: Peplau's interpersonal relations model in practice. Rehabilitation Nursing, 24, 30–33.

Nordal, D., & Soto, A. (1980). Peplau's model applied to primary nursing in clinical practice. In J.P. Riehl & C. Roy (Eds.), Conceptual models for nursing practice (2nd ed., pp. 60–73). New York: Appleton-Century-Crofts.

Normandale, S. (1995). Using a nursing model to structure health visiting practice. Health Visitor, 68, 246–247.

O'Brien, D., & Smith, A. (1991). In search of destiny. Nursing Times, 87(20), 26–28.

Price, B. (1998). Explorations in body image care: Peplau and practice knowledge. Journal of Psychiatric and Mental Health Nursing, 5, 179–186.

Runtz, S.E., & Urtel, J.G. (1983). Evaluating your practice via a nursing model. Nurse Practitioner, 8(3), 30, 32, 37–40.

Schafer, P. (1999). Working with Dave: Application of Peplau's interpersonal nursing theory in the correctional environment. Journal of Psychosocial Nursing and Mental Health Services, 37(9), 18–24, 58–59.

Stark, M. (1992). A system for delivering care. British Journal of Nursing, 1, 85–87.

Thelander, B.L. (1997). The psychotherapy of Hildegard Peplau in the treatment of people with serious mental illness. Perspectives in Psychiatric Care, 33(3), 24–32.

Thomas, M.D., Baker, J.M., & Estes, N.J. (1970). Anger: A tool for developing self-awareness. American Journal of Nursing, 70, 2586–2590.

Thompson, L. (1986). Peplau's theory: An application to short-term individual therapy. Journal of Psychosocial Nursing and Mental Health Services, 24(8), 26–31.

Vardy, C., & Price, V. (1998). The utilization of Peplau's theory of nursing in working with a male survivor of sexual abuse. Journal of Psychiatric and Mental Health Nursing, 5, 149–155.

Venn, R. (1998). Peplau's model in mental health nursing. Paediatric Nursing, 10(6), 18–21.

Wilford, S. (1997). Prisoner of his own fears: Helping John to live again. Mental Health Nursing, 17(3), 22–25.

Yamashita, M. (1997). Family caregiving: Application of Newman's and Peplau's theories. Journal of Psychiatric and Mental Health Nursing, 4, 401–405.

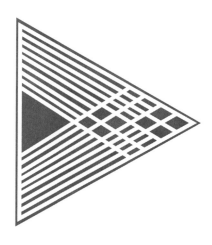

Chapter **16**

Watson's Theory of Human Caring

Jean Watson planned to write a textbook presenting an integrated curriculum for a baccalaureate nursing program. Instead, she developed a novel structure for basic nursing processes. This work, which was published in the book *Nursing: The Philosophy and Science of Caring* (Watson, 1979), solved some of Watson's conceptual and empirical problems about nursing and formed the foundation for the science and art of human caring. Watson (1997) explained that her 1979 book was published

> … before there was any formal movement in nursing related to nursing theory per se. It emerged from my quest to bring new meaning and dignity to the world of nursing and patient care—care that seemed too limited in its scope at the time, largely defined by medicine's [meta]paradigm and traditional biomedical science models. I felt a dissonance between nursing's [meta]paradigm (yet to be defined as such) of caring-healing and health, and medicine's [meta]paradigm of diagnosis and treatment, and concentration on disease and pathology. (p. 49)

As Watson went on to solve other conceptual and philosophical problems about nursing, the Theory of Human Caring was developed, formalized, and presented in her book *Nursing: Human Science and Human Care: A Theory of Nursing* (Watson, 1985). That book also introduced two research methodologies that are consistent with the Theory of Human Caring.

The Theory of Human Caring, which also has been referred to as the Theory of Transpersonal Caring (Watson, 1996), Transpersonal Caring Theory and Transpersonal Caring Science (Watson & Smith, 2002), the Caring Theory (Watson, 2001), and the Caring Model (Watson, 2001), has continued to evolve since the publication of Watson's 1985 book. Indeed, in 1996, Watson noted that she had continued to refine her theory "until this moment in history" (p. 141). In 1997, she commented, "As this work continues to unfold, it is viewed simultaneously as both theory and beyond theory. Both retrospectively and prospectively, it can be read as philosophy, ethic, or even paradigm or worldview" (p. 50). In 2001, Watson noted that the theory "can also be considered a philosophical and moral/ethical foundation for professional nursing and part of the central focus for nursing at the disciplinary level" (p. 349). She went on to point out that the theory can be used as "a theory, model, philosophy, ethic, or ethos for transforming self and practice, or self and system" (p. 349).

Watson (2001) has pointed out that she has "tried to make explicit that nursing's values, knowledge, and practice of human caring were geared toward subjective inner healing processes and the life world of the experiencing person" (p. 345). She went on to explain that in developing the Theory of Human Caring, she "sought to balance the cure orientation of medicine, giving nursing its unique disciplinary, scientific, and professional standing with itself and its public" (p. 345).

Overview

Watson's work is a middle-range explanatory theory that focuses on the human component of caring and the moment-to-moment encounters between the one who is caring and the one who is being cared for, especially the caring activities performed by nurses as they interact with others. The concepts of the Theory of Human Caring and their dimensions are listed here, along with the components of Watson's two research methodologies and her practice methodology. Each concept and its dimensions are defined, and each component of the research and practice methodologies is described later in this chapter.

Key Terms

TRANSPERSONAL CARING RELATIONSHIP
　Self
　Phenomenal Field
　Intersubjectivity
CARING MOMENT/CARING OCCASION
CARING (HEALING) CONSCIOUSNESES
CLINICAL CARITAS PROCESSES
　Practice of Loving Kindness and Equanimity
　　Within the Context of Caring
　　Consciousness
　Being Authentically Present and Enabling
　　and Sustaining the Deep Belief System
　　and Subjective Life World of Self and
　　One-Being-Cared-For
　Cultivation of One's Own Spiritual Practices
　　and Transpersonal Self, Going Beyond Ego
　　Self, Opening to Others with Sensitivity
　　and Compassion
　Developing and Sustaining a Helping-
　　Trusting, Authentic Caring Relationship
　Being Present To, and Supportive Of, the
　　Expression of Positive and Negative
　　Feelings as a Connection With Deeper
　　Spirit of Self and the One-Being-Cared-For

Creative Use of Self and All Ways of Knowing
　as Part of the Caring Process; To Engage in
　Artistry of Caring-Healing Practices
Engaging in Genuine Teaching-Learning
　Experience that Attends to Unity of Being
　and Meaning, Attempting to Stay Within
　Others' Frames of Reference
Creating Healing Environments at All Levels
　(Physical as well as Non-Physical, Subtle
　Environment of Energy and
　Consciousness, Whereby Wholeness,
　Beauty, Comfort, Dignity, and Peace are
　Potentiated)
Assisting with Basic Needs, with an
　Intentional Caring Consciousness,
　Administering "Human Care Essentials,"
　Which Potentiate Alignment of Mind-
　body-spirit, Wholeness, and Unity of
　Being in All Aspects of Care, Tending
　to Both Embodied Spirit and Evolving
　Spiritual Emergence
Opening and Attending to Spiritual-
　Mysterious, and Existential Dimensions
　of One's Own Life-Death; Soul Care for
　Self and the One-Being-Cared-For
RESEARCH METHODOLOGIES
　The Descriptive-Empirical Phenomenological
　　Research Method
　　Phenomenon of Interest
　　Source of Data
　　Guidelines for Data Analysis
　The Transcendental-Poetic Expression of
　　Phenomenology Research Method
　　Phenomenon of Interest
　　Source of Data
　　Guidelines for Data Analysis
PRACTICE METHODOLOGY
　Requirements for a Transpersonal Caring
　　Relationship
　Authentic Presencing

 ## ANALYSIS OF THE THEORY OF HUMAN CARING

This section presents an analysis of Watson's theory. The analysis is based on Watson's publications about her theory, especially *Nursing: The Philosophy and Science of*

Caring (1979), *Nursing: Human Science and Human Care: A Theory of Nursing* (1985), "Watson's Theory of Transpersonal Caring" (1996), "The Theory of Human Caring: Retrospective and Prospective" (1997), *Postmodern Nursing and Beyond* (1999), and "Jean Watson: Theory of Human Caring" (2001).

SCOPE OF THE THEORY

The central thesis of the Theory of Human Caring is that "humans cannot be treated as objects, [and] that humans cannot be separated from self, other, nature, and the larger universe" (Watson, 1997, p. 50). Watson (1989b) claimed that her theory encompasses the whole of nursing; the emphasis, however, is placed on the interpersonal process between the caregiver and the care recipient. In particular, the theory focuses on "the centrality of human caring and on the caring-to-caring transpersonal relationship and its healing potential for both the one who is caring and the one who is being cared for" (Watson, 1996, p. 141). More specifically, the Theory of Human Caring focuses on the relation between use of the clinical caritas processes and the development of a transpersonal caring relationship within the context of the caring occasion/caring moment and caring (healing) consciousness. It is, therefore, appropriately categorized as a middle-range explanatory theory.

CONTEXT OF THE THEORY

Metaparadigm Concepts and Proposition

Watson has begun to identify the influence of the metaparadigm of nursing on her work. In particular, Watson (1996) regards human caring as "an ethic, an ontology, and a critical starting point for nursing's *raison d'être*" (p. 143). A review of her publications led to the conclusion that the Theory of Human Caring, per se, focuses on the metaparadigm concepts of *human beings* and *nursing*. The metaparadigm proposition of interest is *the nursing actions or processes that are beneficial to human beings*.

Philosophical Claims

Analysis of Watson's publications revealed that the Theory of Human Caring is based on a humanitarian, metaphysical, spiritual-existential, and phenomenological orientation that draws from Eastern philosophy. Watson (1989b) regards her theory as metaphysical. She explained that "it goes beyond the rapidly emerging existential-phenomenological approaches in nursing, to perhaps a higher level of abstraction and sense of personhood, incorporating the concept of the soul and transcendence" (p. 221). Accordingly, Watson's evolving ideas and ideals, which are the result of reflective thinking, "are concerned with spirit rather than matter, flux rather than form, inner knowledge and power, rather than circumstance" (p. 219).

Watson's philosophical claims take the form of values about human care and human caring, assumptions about those values, assumptions about caring and about the transpersonal caring relationship, and statements about nursing that can be considered philosophical in nature. Her values about human care and caring are expressed throughout the 1985 book and later in the 1996 book chapter. In addition, Watson (1985, 1996) identified several assumptions about human care and caring values and nursing. More recently, Watson (1999, 2001) identified assumptions about caring and nursing (1999) and about the transpersonal caring relationship (2001). All of those values and assumptions are listed here.

Values About Human Care and Human Caring

- Deep respect is accorded the wonder and mysteries of life (Watson, 1985, pp. 34, 73).
- A spiritual dimension to life and internal power of the human care process are acknowledged (Watson, 1985, pp. 34, 73).
- The power of humans to grow and to change is acknowledged (Watson, 1985, pp. 34, 73).
- Nonpaternalistic values are related to human autonomy and freedom of choice so to preserve personhood, human dignity, and humanity at individual and global levels (Watson, 1985, pp. 34, 73).
- A high regard and reverence is accorded the unfolding subjective-inner-life world of self and other(s) (Watson, 1985, pp. 34, 73).
- A high value is placed on subjectivity-intersubjectivity as evidenced, in a reciprocal relationship between nurse and other(s), by consciousness; intentionality; perceptions and lived experiences related to caring, healing, and health-illness conditions in a given caring moment; and experiences or meanings that transcend the moment and go beyond the actual experience (Watson, 1985, 1996).
- Emphasis is placed on helping other(s), through advanced nursing caring-healing modalities, to gain more self-knowledge, self-control, and even self-healing potential, regardless of the health-illness condition (Watson, 1985, 1996).
- A high value is placed on the relationship between the nurse and other(s), with all parties viewed as coparticipants in the human care process (Watson, 1985).
- Caring is acknowledged as the highest form of commitment to self, to other, to society, to environment, and, at this point in human history, even to the universe (Watson, 1996, p. 146).
- If human caring-healing is not sustained as part of our collective values, knowledge, practices, and global mission, the survival of humankind is threatened (Watson, 1996, p. 147).

Assumptions Related to Human Care and Human Caring Values

- Care and love are the most universal, the most tremendous, and the most mysterious of cosmic forces: they comprise the primal and universal psychic energy (Watson, 1996, p. 149).
- Human needs for care and love are often overlooked; or we know people need each other in loving and caring ways, but often we do not behave well toward each other. If our humanness is to survive, we need to become more caring and loving, thereby nourishing our humanity and evolving as civilized people who can live together (Watson, 1996, pp. 149–150).
- Because nursing is a caring profession, its ability to sustain its caring ideal and ideology (ethic and ethos) in education and practice will affect how humanity develops and evolves toward a moral, caring, peaceful society. In turn, nursing's contribution to society will be determined (Watson, 1996, p. 150).
- To make a beginning, we have to impose our own consciousness, moral ideal, intentionality, and will to care and love on our own behavior and awareness. We must treat ourselves with gentleness and dignity, [and] commit to our own woundedness and healing processes. Only then will we respect and care for others with gentleness, dignity, and caring-healing consciousness (Watson, 1996, p. 150).
- Human care, at the individual, group, community, and societal levels, has received less and less emphasis in the technological systems of medical care in the late 20th century (Watson, 1996, p. 150).

Assumptions About Caring

- Caring is based on an ontology and ethic of relationship and connectedness, and of relationship and consciousness (Watson, 1999, p. 102).
- Caring consciousness, in-relation, becomes primary (Watson, 1999, p. 102).
- Caring can be most effectively demonstrated and practice interpersonally and transpersonally (Watson, 1999, p. 102).
- Caring consists of 'caritas' consciousness, values and motives. It is guided by carative components (Watson, 1999, p. 102).
- A caring relationship and a caring environment attend to 'soul care': the spiritual growth of both the one-caring and the one-being-cared-for (Watson, 1999, p. 103).
- A caring relationship and a caring environment preserve human dignity, wholeness and integrity; they offer an authentic presencing and choice (Watson, 1999, p. 103).
- Caring promotes self-growth, self-knowledge, self-control and self-healing processes and possibilities (Watson, 1999, p. 103).
- Caring accepts and holds safe space (sacred space) for people to seek their own wholeness of being and becoming, not only now but in the future, evolving toward wholeness, greater complexity and connectedness with the deep self, the soul and the higher self (Watson, 1999, p. 103).
- Each caring act seeks to hold an intentional consciousness of caring. This energetic, focused consciousness of caring and authentic presencing has the potential to change the 'field of caring,' thereby potentiating healing and wholeness (Watson, 1999, p. 103).
- Caring, as ontology and consciousness, calls for ontological authenticity and advanced ontological competencies and skills. These, in turn, can be translated into professional ontologically based caring-healing modalities (Watson, 1999, p. 103).

Assumptions About the Transpersonal Caring Relationship

- The nurse's moral commitment, intentionality, and caritas consciousness is to protect, enhance, promote, and potentiate human dignity, wholeness, and healing, wherein a person creates or cocreates his or her own meaning for existence, healing, wholeness, and living and dying (Watson, 2001, p. 348).
- The nurse's will and consciousness affirm the subjective-spiritual significance of the person while seeking to sustain caring in the midst of threat and despair—biological, institutional, or otherwise. This honors the I-Thou relationship versus an I-It relationship (Watson, 2001, p. 348).
- The nurse seeks to recognize, accurately detect and connect with the inner condition of spirit of another through genuine presencing and being centered in the caring moment; actions, words, behaviors, cognition, body language, feelings, intuition, thought, senses, the energy field, and so on. All contribute to transpersonal caring connection (Watson, 2001, p. 348).
- The nurse's ability to connect with another at this transpersonal spirit-to-spirit level is translated via movements, gestures, facial expressions, procedures, information, touch, sound, verbal expressions, and other scientific, technical, aesthetic, and human means of communication into nursing human art/acts or intentional caring-healing modalities (Watson, 2001, p. 348).
- The caring-healing modalities within the context of transpersonal caring/caritas consciousness potentiate harmony, wholeness, and unity of being by releasing some of the disharmony, the blocked energy that interferes with the natural healing processes; thus the nurse

helps another through this process to access the healer within, in the fullest sense of Nightingale's view of nursing (Watson, 2001, p. 348).

- Ongoing personal-professional development and spiritual growth and personal spiritual practice assist the nurse in entering into this deeper level of professional healing practice, allowing the nurse to awaken to the transpersonal condition of the world and to actualize more fully "ontological competencies" necessary for this level of advanced practice of nursing.... Continuous growth is ongoing for developing and maturing within a transpersonal caring model. The notion of health professionals as wounded healers is acknowledged as part of the necessary growth and compassion called forth within this theory/philosophy (Watson, 2001, p. 348).

Assumptions About Nursing

- Human caring is the moral ideal and origin for nursing's professional role and "calling," with the goal of protection, enhancement, and preservation of human dignity (Watson, 1985, p. 74; 1996, pp. 145–146).
- Caring is the essence of nursing and the most central and unifying focus for nursing practice (Watson, 1996, p. 150).
- Caring knowledge and actions [are] a serious ontological, ethical, epistemic, and pragmatic concern for the discipline of nursing (Watson, 1996, p. 146).
- Because nursing phenomena are humans' and life's phenomena, multiple aspects of personal, intuitive, ethical, empirical, aesthetic, and spiritual dimensions are acknowledged as foundational to the ontological and epistemological matrix of the discipline and the profession (Watson, 1996, p. 145).
- As a discipline, nursing has an ethical, social, and scientific responsibility to develop new theories and knowledge about caring, healing, and health practices; to teach them in education and implement them in clinical care; and to promulgate them at the ontological, epistemological, methodological, pedagogical, or praxis level (Watson, 1996, p. 146).
- Nursing, as a profession, exists in order to sustain caring, healing, and health where, and when, they are threatened biologically, institutionally, environmentally, or politically, by local, national, or global influences (Watson, 1996, p. 146).
- Caring and relationships based on caring are being posited as central components that the public is seeking in healing and health outcomes (Watson, 1996, p. 146).
- Nursing has always held a human-care/caring stance in regard to people, society, health-illness, and healing (Watson, 1996, p. 150).

- Human caring can be effectively demonstrated and practiced only interpersonally; however, the process of an interpersonal relationship is defined within a transpersonal context. It transcends each individual and moves in concentric circles from self to other, to environment, to nature, and then to the larger universe (Watson, 1996, pp. 150–151).
- Nursing's social, moral, and scientific contributions to humankind lie in its commitment to a human caring-healing ethic and in consciousness of its knowledge, practices, and paradigmatic matrix in theory, practice, and research endeavors (Watson, 1996, p. 151).
- Caring values of nurses and nursing have been submerged within contemporary medical systems, which are dominated by economics. Nursing and society are, therefore, in crisis as they try to sustain human caring ideals and activities in practice. At the same time, biomedical-technological curing systems proliferate, without regard to costs or to the caring-healing and health needs of the citizenry (Watson, 1996, p. 150).
- Preservation and advancement of caring-healing and health knowledge and practices are ethical, epistemic, and clinical endeavors for all the health sciences. These issues remain particularly significant for further development of nursing science and education, and for advanced clinical care practices today and into the future (Watson, 1996, p. 150).
- The practice of transpersonal caring-healing requires an expanding epistemology and transformative science and art model for further advancement. This practice integrates all ways of knowing. The art and science of a postmodern model of transpersonal caring-healing is complementary to the science of medical curing, modern nursing and medical practices (Watson, 1999, p. 103).

Watson (1985) noted that research methodologies employed to study transpersonal caring "require a nontraditional view of science and reside in methods that are based upon different assumptions about the nature of reality, [the] nature of inquirer-object-subject relationship, [and the] nature of truth statements" (p. 79). She did not, however, explicate any of those assumptions.

Watson's philosophical claims are consistent with humanism (Sellers, 1991). Indeed, Watson (1985) explicitly rejected the mechanistic, reductionistic view of the world in favor of a human science perspective. She declared that "science is emphasized in a human science context" (Watson, 1985, p. 76). Elaborating, Watson (1996), explained that

the context of the [Theory of Human Caring] is both humanitarian and metaphysical. It calls for a return to reverence and a sense of sacredness with regard to life and human experiences, especially those related to caring and healing work with others during their most vulnerable moments of life's journey. Thus, the theory incorporates both the art and science of nursing. (p. 145)

Watson (1997) maintained that some aspects of her theory are dynamic, and that the theory has evolved "toward the simultaneity/unitary-transformative paradigms" (p. 50). She went on to say: "However, some aspects of the [theory] contain components that could be criticized as being located in the totality [paradigm]" (p. 50). Watson later reiterated that the theory is moving toward the unitary transformative paradigm, that is, the simultaneous action world view. She explained, "When you get into transpersonal caring and healing, you are in the unitary-transformative perspective. And that brings in consciousness, intentionality, energy, evolution, transcendence, process, relativity, and things that transcend our conventional medical and modern conventional science models. Although we don't quite have the methodologies, the language, or the tools to be fully into this new paradigm, we are moving in that direction" (Fawcett, 2002a, p. 216). Taken together, Watson's philosophical claims and her discussion of human science, along with her discussion of world views, indicate that the Theory of Human Caring now is most closely aligned with the *simultaneous action* world view.

Conceptual Model

The conceptual model from which the Theory of Human Caring was derived is not yet fully explicit, but it can be inferred from Watson's publications. Statements in her 1996 book chapter suggest that Watson is working on the further development of an explicit conceptual model, referred to as "the caring-healing paradigmatic matrix" (Watson, 1996, p. 142), that will address all four metaparadigm concepts—human beings, environment, health, and nursing. In particular, Watson (1996) commented that her work is evolving "toward a paradigmatic structure for the whole of nursing and its emergence as a distinct caring-healing-health discipline" (p. 142).

Asked whether the content of her book, *Postmodern Nursing and Beyond*, represents a conceptual model, Watson replied, "I see the book entering into caring at the deep ontological level. Though it embraces and is informed by my earlier work, I see it as being beyond theory. I don't know what to call it—a framework, a model, a paradigm, or something else. I was trying to consolidate the components of what a mature structure would look like within the context of a caring and healing framework, in contrast to the dominant medicalized, clinicalized

version of our discipline and our profession" (Fawcett, 2002a, p. 216).

In a recent paper, Watson and Smith (2002) situated the Theory of Human Caring in "the emerging transdisciplinary field of caring science" (p. 458) and outlined the connections between the theory and Rogers' (1992, 1994) Science of Unitary Human Beings. They drew parallels between Rogers' concept of pandimensionality and Watson's notion of transpersonal; Rogers' idea of infinity and Watson's notion of university field of consciousness; Rogers' concept of resonancy and Watson's notion that consciousness is energy; Rogers' notion that the body is an energy field manifestation and Watson's idea of the postmodern body as equivalent to light, energy, and consciousness; Rogers' idea of mutual process and Watson's notion of the mutuality of caring relationships within caring fields; and Rogers' idea of healing modalities and Watson's idea of caring-healing modalities.

Watson and Smith (2002) did not mean to imply that the Theory of Human Caring was derived from Rogers' Science of Unitary Human Beings. Rather, they demonstrated the parallels between the two formulations, which could provide a foundation for continued evolution of the theory.

The evolving conceptual model clearly reflects the metaphysical, spiritual, existential, and phenomenological orientation of Watson's philosophical claims. The conceptual model currently comprises basic descriptions of human beings and human life, environment, health, and nursing.

Watson's (1996) description of human beings indicates that she regards the person as "a unity of mind-body-spirit/nature" (p. 147). Watson's description of human life is based on her definition of the soul. "The concept of the soul," according to Watson (1985) "refers to the *geist*, spirit, inner self, or essence of the person, which is tied to a greater sense of self-awareness, a higher degree of consciousness, an inner strength, and a power that can expand human capacities and allow a person to transcend his or her usual self" (p. 46).

Elaborating on human life, Watson (1985) stated:

My conception of life and personhood is tied to notions that one's soul possesses a body that is not confined by objective space and time. The lived world of the experiencing person is not distinguished by external and internal notions of time and space, but shapes its own time and space, which is unconstrained by linearity. Notions of personhood, then, transcend the here and now, and one has the capacity to coexist with past, present, future, all at once. ... The individual spirit of a person or of collective humanity may continue to exist throughout time, keeping alive a higher sense of humankind. ... [Thus] human life is defined as (spiritual-mental-physical) being-in-the-world, which is continuous in time and space. (pp. 45–47)

Watson (1996) has referred to environment, using such terms as "environments at all levels," "infinity," and "the universal or cosmic level of existence" (p. 147). In keeping with "quantum physics and holographic views of the universe" (p. 149), Watson (1996) views human beings and environment as "a field of connectedness" (p. 147), and she maintains that "everything in the universe is connected" (p. 149).

Watson (1985) has differentiated between health and illness. Her view of health underscores the entire human being in the physical, social, esthetic, and moral realms. Accordingly, "Health refers to unity and harmony within the mind, body, and soul. Health is also associated with the degree of congruence between the self as perceived and the self as experienced". (p. 48)

Illness, according to Watson (1985), is not necessarily disease, although it can lead to disease. She explained, "Illness is subjective turmoil or disharmony with a person's inner self or soul at some level or disharmony within the spheres of the person. ... Illness connotes a felt incongruence within the person such as an incongruence between the self as perceived and the self as experienced. A troubled inner soul can lead to illness, and illness can produce disease" (p. 48).

Watson (1985, 1996) maintained that nursing is a human science discipline and an art, as well as an academic-clinical profession. Human science, which focuses on the whole person, contrasts with natural science, which reduces phenomena to their parts. Watson (1985) explained:

> The mandate for nursing within science as well as within society is a demand for cherishing of the wholeness of human personality. It is thus that I regard nursing as a human science and the human care process in nursing as a significant humanitarian and epistemic act that contributes to the preservation of humanity. (p. 29)

In keeping with her philosophical claim that human caring is the moral ideal of nursing, the ultimate goal of nursing for Watson (1996) is "protection, enhancement, and preservation of human dignity and humanity" (p. 148). Another goal "is to help persons gain a higher degree of harmony within the mind, body, and soul which generates self-knowledge, self-reverence, self-healing, and self-care processes while increasing diversity" (Watson, 1985, p. 49). Watson (1985) went on to say that nursing is directed toward "finding meaning in one's own existence and experiences, discovering inner power and control, and potentiating instances of transcendence and self-healing" (p. 74).

What Watson (1999) called postmodern nursing/beyond nursing "refers to a special way of being-in-relation as a moral starting point for caring for self, for higher/deeper self, other(s), nature and other living things on the plant Earth and in the broader universe. It calls forth a commitment to caring and an intentionality of a caring consciousness" (p. 97).

The process of nursing is human-to-human caring. The individual patient is regarded as the agent of change. The nurse can function as a coparticipant through the human care process, but the "personal, internal mental-spiritual mechanisms of the person [allow] the self to be healed through various internal or external means, or without external agents, [and] through an intersubjective interdependent process wherein both persons may transcend self and usual experiences" (Watson, 1985, p. 74).

Watson (1996, 1999) has distinguished nursing from medicine. She noted that her work is an attempt to articulate a "nursing-qua-nursing" perspective rather than what she regards as the current "nursing-qua-medicine" perspective embraced by so many nurses. She maintained that nursing "needs to emerge as a mature *health* profession capable of interfacing with the *medical* profession" (1996, p. 146). In particular, Watson (1997) associates caring with nursing and curing with medicine, and regards the knowledge contained within the Theory of Human Caring "as a bridge that helps a nurse cross over from a traditional nursing-qua-medicine framework to a more advanced nursing-qua-nursing practice model ... [that is] distinct from, but complementary with curing knowledges and practices associated with modern medicine" (p. 50).

Watson (1985) identified several premises that can be considered propositions of her evolving conceptual model. These propositions are listed here.

- A person's mind and emotions are windows to the soul. Nursing care can be and is physical, procedural, objective, and factual, but at the highest level of nursing the nurses' human care responses, the human care transactions, and the nurses' presence in the relationship transcend the physical and material world, bound in time and space, and make contact with the person's emotional and subjective world as the route to the inner self and the higher sense of self (Watson, 1985, p. 50).
- A person's body is confined in time and space, but the mind and soul are not confined to the physical universe. One's higher sense of mind and soul transcends time and space and helps to account for notions like collective unconscious, causal past, mystical experiences, parapsychological phenomena, [and] a higher sense of power, and may be an indicator of the spiritual evolution of human beings (Watson, 1985, p. 50).

- A nurse may have access to a person's mind, emotions, and inner self indirectly through any sphere—mind, body or soul—provided the physical body is not perceived or treated as separate from the mind and emotions and higher sense of self (soul) (Watson, 1985, p. 50).
- The spirit, inner self, or soul (geist) of a person exists in and for itself. The spiritual essence of the person is related to the human ability to be free, which is an evolving process in the development of humans. The ability to develop and experience one's essence freely is limited by the extent of others' ability to "be." The destiny of one's being (humankind's destiny) is to develop the spiritual essence of the self and in the highest sense, to become more Godlike. However, each person has to question his or her own essence and moral behavior toward others, because if people are dehumanized at a basic level, for example, a human care level, that dehumanizing process is not capable of reflecting humanity back upon itself (Watson, 1985, p. 50).
- People need each other in a caring, loving way. Love and caring are two universal givens. … These needs are often overlooked, or even though we know we need one another in a loving and caring way, we do not behave well toward each other. If our humanness is to survive, we need to become more loving, caring, and moral to nourish our humanity, advance as a civilization, and live together (Watson, 1985, pp. 50–51).
- A person may have an illness that is "completely hidden from our eyes." To find solutions it is necessary to find meanings. A person's human predicament may not be related to the external world as much as to the person's inner world as he or she experiences it (Watson, 1985, p. 50).

Antecedent Knowledge

Watson (1996) credited her experiences in practice and education, along with her philosophical, intellectual, and experiential background as antecedents to the development of the Theory of Human Caring. More specifically, Watson (1985, 1988b, 1989a, 1996, 1997, 2001) noted that her theory developed from her own values and beliefs about human beings and life, which were inspired at least in part by the interpersonal focus of her graduate studies in psychiatric–mental health nursing; her doctoral studies in educational, clinical, and social psychology; and her experiences with other nurses and the indigenous peoples and cultures of New Zealand, Australia, Indonesia, Malaysia, Micronesia, Japan, Korea, the Republic of China, Thailand, India, Egypt, Kuwait, Scandinavia, England, Scotland, Portugal, Brazil, and Canada. She commented:

All of my travels and personal and work experiences have confirmed my sense of witnessing a convergence and expansion of Eastern and Western beliefs, worldviews, and values that affect aspects of humanity, life, death, suffering, caring, healing, and health. Thus, my work seeks to confirm that we are all part of the global human-planet-universe condition and connection—all are part of what I consider both universal and specific nursing phenomena of caring and healing, regardless of setting or country. (Watson, 1997, p. 49)

Watson (1985, 1988b, 1989a, 1996, 1997) also acknowledged and cited the contributions to her thinking made by many noted scholars. She stated that she drew on the work of Carl Rogers (1959) for her definition of the self, and she used Mumford's (1970) notion of the human center as a starting point for the transpersonal process. She also commented that her ideas about transpersonal caring are related to the meaning of that term in transpersonal psychology but were "inspired by Lazarus as a way to expand the field of meaning associated with a human-to-human caring relationship" (Watson, 1997, p. 49). Other ideas were stimulated by the works of Giorgi (1970), Whitehead (1953), de Chardin (1967), Kierkegaard (1941 [original work published 1846]), Taylor (1974), Gadow (1980, 1984), and Zukav (1990). Watson also acknowledged the contributions of Peplau, Marcel, Sartre, and Yalom, although she did not cite any of their works or any of Lazarus' works. Moreover, she acknowledged the tenets of Eastern philosophy but did not cite specific scholars or publications. In addition, Watson (1985) drew from the works of Alexandersson (1981) and Levin (1983) in the development of research methodologies associated with the Theory of Human Caring.

CONTENT OF THE THEORY

Concepts

Analysis of Watson's 1985 book and her 1996 and 2001 book chapters revealed that the concepts of the Theory of Human Caring are **TRANSPERSONAL CARING RELATIONSHIP, CARING MOMENT/CARING OCCASION, CARING (HEALING) CONSCIOUSNESS,** and **CLINICAL CARITAS PROCESSES.** The concept of **TRANSPERSONAL CARING RELATIONSHIP** has three dimensions—**Self, Phenomenal Field,** and **Intersubjectivity.** The concepts of **CARING MOMENT/CARING OCCASION** and **CARING (HEALING) CONSCIOUSNESS** are unidimensional. The concept of **CLINICAL CARITAS PROCESSES** has the 10 dimensions listed here:

> Practice of Loving Kindness and Equanimity Within the Context of Caring Consciousness

Being Authentically Present and Enabling and Sustaining the Deep Belief System and Subjective Life World of Self and One-Being-Cared-For

Cultivation of One's Own Spiritual Practices and Transpersonal Self, Going Beyond Ego Self, Opening to Others with Sensitivity and Compassion

Developing and Sustaining a Helping-Trusting, Authentic Caring Relationship

Being Present To, and Supportive Of, the Expression of Positive and Negative Feelings as a Connection With Deeper Spirit of Self and the One-Being-Cared-For

Creative Use of Self and All Ways of Knowing as Part of the Caring Process; To Engage in Artistry of Caring-Healing Practices

Engaging in Genuine Teaching-Learning Experience that Attends to Unity of Being and Meaning, Attempting to Stay Within Others' Frames of Reference

Creating Healing Environments at All Levels (Physical as well as Non-Physical, Subtle Environment of Energy and Consciousness, Whereby Wholeness, Beauty, Comfort, Dignity, and Peace are Potentiated)

Assisting with Basic Needs, with an Intentional Caring Consciousness, Administering "Human Care Essentials," Which Potentiate Alignment of Mind-body-spirit, Wholeness, and Unity of Being in All Aspects of Care, Tending to Both Embodied Spirit and Evolving Spiritual Emergence

Opening and Attending to Spiritual-Mysterious, and Existential Dimensions of One's Own Life-Death; Soul Care for Self and the One-Being-Cared-For

Nonrelational Propositions

The definitions for all of the concepts of the Theory of Human Caring and their dimensions are presented here. These constitutive definitions are the nonrelational propositions of the theory.

TRANSPERSONAL CARING RELATIONSHIP

- Human-to-human connectedness ... [whereby] each is touched by the human center of the other (Watson, 1989a, p. 131).
- A special kind of relationship [involving] a high regard for the whole person and his or her being-in-the-world (Watson, 1996, p. 151).
- Moves beyond ego self and radiates to spiritual, even cosmic, concerns and connections that tap into healing possibilities and potentials (Watson, 2001, p. 347).

The concept of **Transpersonal Caring Relationship** is further described in terms of transactions, which Watson (1985) views as both science and art. She explained that

transpersonal ... caring transactions are those scientific, professional, ethical, yet esthetic, creative and personalized giving-receiving behaviors and responses between two people (nurse and other) that allow for contact between the subjective world of the experiencing persons (through physical, mental, or spiritual routes or some combination thereof). (p. 58)

Watson's emphasis on the art of the **Transpersonal Caring Relationship** is underscored in four statements:

- The art of transpersonal caring in nursing as a moral ideal is a means of communication and release of human feelings through the coparticipation of one's entire self in nursing (Watson, 1985, p. 70).
- Collectively, the art of transpersonal caring allows humanity to move towards greater harmony, spiritual evolution and perfection (Watson, 1985, p. 70).
- The more the art of transpersonal caring in nursing advances the kinder and more helpful feelings for the human, the more we can define ideal caring with reference to its content and subject matter of nursing (Watson, 1985, p. 70).
- The transpersonal caring process is largely art because of the way it touches another person's soul and feels the emotion and union with another, the goal being the movement of the person toward a higher sense of self and a greater sense of harmony within the mind, body, and soul (Watson, 1985, p. 71).

The concept of **Transpersonal Caring Relationship** encompasses three dimensions—Self, Phenomenal Field, and Intersubjectivity.

- **Self:** The self is transpersonal-mind-body-spirit oneness, an embodied self, and an embodied spirit (Watson, 1996). The self is the organized consistent conceptual gestalt composed of perceptions of the characteristics of the "I" or "me" and the perceptions of the relationships of the "I" or "me" to others and to various aspects of life, together with the values attached to those perceptions. It is a fluid and changing gestalt, a process, but at any moment a specific entity (Rogers, 1959, p. 200, as cited by Watson, 1985, p. 55). The self encompasses the self as it is, the ideal self that the person would like to be, the ego-self, and the spiritual self, which is synonymous with the geist or soul or essence of the person, and which is the highest sense of self (Watson, 1985, 1996).
- **Phenomenal Field:** The totality of human experience (one's being-in-the-world). ... The individual's frame of

reference that can be known only to the person (Watson, 1985, p. 55). The person's subjective reality, which determines perceptions and responses in given situations in conjunction with the objective conditions or external reality (Watson, 1985). The transpersonal caring field resides within a unitary field of consciousness and energy that transcends time, space and physicality (unity of mind-body-spirit nature universe. [Watson & Smith, 2002, p. 458]). Phenomenal field/unitary consciousness [is] unbroken wholeness and connectedness of all (Watson, 2001, p. 345).

- **Intersubjectivity:** Transpersonal refers to an intersubjective human-to-human relationship in which the person of the nurse affects and is affected by the person of the other. Both are fully present in the moment and feel a union with the other. They share a phenomenal field which becomes part of the life history of both and are coparticipants in becoming in the now and the future. Such an ideal of caring entails an ideal of intersubjectivity, in which both persons are involved (Watson, 1985, p. 58). The intersubjective human flow from one to the other [is such that it] has the potential to allow the care giver to become the care receiver (Watson, 1989a, p. 128). Transpersonal conveys a concern for the inner life world and subjective meaning of another who is fully embodied (Watson, 2001, p. 347).

The three dimensions of the concept of **Transpersonal Caring Relationship**—Self, Phenomenal Field, and Intersubjectivity—are regarded as integral. Watson (1985) explained:

> Human care can begin when the nurse enters into the life space or phenomenal field of another person, is able to detect the other person's condition of being (spirit, soul), feels this condition within him- or herself, and responds to the condition in such a way that the recipient has a release of subjective feelings and thoughts he or she had been longing to release. As such, there is an intersubjective flow between the nurse and patient. (p. 63)

CARING MOMENT/CARING OCCASION

- [The coming together of nurse and other(s), which] involves action and choice both by the nurse and the other. The moment of coming together in a caring occasion presents them with the opportunity to decide how to be in the relationship—what to do with the moment (Watson, 1996, p. 157).
- Occurs whenever the nurse and another come together with their unique life histories and phenomenal fields in a human-to-human transaction. The coming together in a given moment becomes a focal point in space and time. It becomes transcendent, whereby experience and perception take place, but the actual caring occasion has a greater field of its own, in a given moment (Watson, 2001, p. 349).
- A caring moment involves an action and a choice by both the nurse and other. The moment of coming together presents the two with the opportunity to decide how to *be in the moment*, in the relationship—what to do with and in the moment (Watson, 2001, p. 349).

Watson (1996) explained that the concept of **Caring Moment/Caring** represents "a focal point in space and time [during which] experience and perception take place" (p. 157). She went on to explain that the moment "goes beyond itself, yet arises from aspects of itself that become part of the life history of each person, as well as part of some larger, deeper, more complex pattern of life" (p. 157).

CARING (HEALING) CONSCIOUSNESS

- A holographic dynamic ... [that] is manifest within a field of consciousness (Watson, 1996, p. 158), [which] exists through time and space and is dominant over physical illness (Watson, 1992, p. 1481).
- Consciousness is energy (Watson, 1996).
- Caring-healing-loving consciousness exists through and transcends time and space and can be dominant over physical dimensions (Watson, 2001, p. 349).
- A nurse's authentic intentionality and consciousness of caring has a higher frequency of energy than noncaring consciousness, opening up connections to the universal field of consciousness and a greater access to one's inner healer (Watson & Smith, 2002, p. 458).

Although Watson (2001) labeled this concept of **Caring (Healing) Consciousness**, when defining and describing the concept, she used the term "caring-healing-loving consciousness" (p. 349). The concept of **Caring (Healing) Consciousness**, Watson (1992, 2001) explained, connects the one caring, the one-being-cared-for, other humans, and the higher energy of the universe. Moreover, the nurse's **Caring (Healing) Consciousness** is communicated to the one-being-cared-for.

CLINICAL CARITAS PROCESSES

- Refers to those aspects of nursing that actually potentiate therapeutic healing processes for both the one caring and the one being cared for (Watson, 1996, pp. 154–155).
- Caritas means to cherish, to appreciate, to give special attention. ... It connotes something that is very fine, that

indeed is precious. … Caritas conveys … love. (Watson, 2001, p. 345).

In her 2001 book chapter, Watson renamed and translated what she had previously called carative factors into the **Clinical Caritas Processes.** She explained, "As carative factors evolve within an expanding perspective, and as my ideas and values evolve, I now offer [a] translation of the original carative factors into clinical caritas processes, suggesting more open ways in which they can be considered" (pp. 346–347). She went on to explain, "What differs in the clinical caritas framework [from the carative factors] is that a decidedly spiritual dimension and an overt evocation of love and caring are merged" (p. 347).

The concept of **Clinical Caritas Processes** refers to nursing interventions, or more precisely, caring processes or caritas processes (Watson, 1985, 2001). Watson (1985) noted that she found the term, intervention, harsh, mechanical, and inconsistent with her ideas and ideals, but had used the term for pedagogical purposes.

Watson (1996, 2001) claimed that the **Clinical Caritas Processes** represent the "core" of nursing, which "is grounded in the philosophy, science, and art of caring" (1996, p. 155). She has contrasted the "core" of nursing with the "trim," a term she uses to refer to "the practice setting, the procedures, the functional tasks, the specialized clinical focus of disease, technology, and [the] techniques surrounding the diverse orientations and preoccupations of nursing" (Watson, 1997, p. 50). The "trim," Watson (1997) went on to explain, is in no way expendable; it is just that it cannot be the center of a professional model of nursing. Trim exists in relation to something larger and deeper. That something deeper is the caring relationship, the health and healing processes that nurses attend to within a larger professional ethic (p. 50).

Watson (1996) maintained that "nurses throughout time have practiced [the clinical caritas processes] in conjunction with the trim activities without naming [the clinical caritas processes] as such" (p. 155). Moreover, Watson (1996, 2001) regards the clinical caritas processes as the foundation for "advanced practices and caring modalities for healing and health processes and outcomes" (1996, p. 157).

The concept of **Clinical Caritas Processes** encompasses ten dimensions (see pages 560 and 561). They are explained here.

- **Practice of Loving Kindness and Equanimity Within the Context of Caring Consciousness:** Translation of the carative factor, Forming a Humanistic-Altruistic System of Values. Focuses on the development of a [humanistic and altruistic] value system over the period of one's life-

time (Watson, 1979, 1996); a qualitative philosophy that guides one's mature life. It is the commitment to and satisfaction of receiving through giving. It involves the capacity to view humanity with love and to appreciate diversity and individuality (Watson, 1979, p. 11; 1996). Human caring is grounded on universal humanistic and altruistic values, and the best professional care is promoted when the nurse subscribes to such a value system (Watson, 1989b).

- **Being Authentically Present and Enabling and Sustaining the Deep Belief System and Subjective Life World of Self and One-Being-Cared-For:** Translation of the carative factor, Enabling and Sustaining Faith-Hope. Refers to the therapeutic effects of faith and hope in both the carative and the curative process (Watson, 1979, 1996). The nurse must instill in the other a sense of faith and hope about the treatment and the nurse's competence (Watson, 1979).

- **Cultivation of One's Own Spiritual Practices and Transpersonal Self, Going Beyond Ego Self, Opening to Others with Sensitivity and Compassion:** Translation of the carative factor, Being Sensitive to Self and Others. Emphasizes the need to recognize one's feelings and to experience those feelings as a foundation for empathy with others (Watson, 1979, 1996). The development of sensitivity to self and others plays a part in the nurse's development of self, the ability to utilize the self with others, and the ability to give holistic care (Watson, 1979).

- **Developing and Sustaining a Helping-Trusting, Authentic Caring Relationship:** Translation of the carative factor, Developing a Helping-Trusting, Caring Relationship. Focuses on the need to develop an effective interpersonal relationship with the one cared for (Watson, 1979, 1996). This process accomplished when the nurse views the other as a separate thinking and feeling being. The attitudinal processes of congruence, or genuineness, empathy, and nonpossessive warmth are essential elements of the helping-trusting, authentic caring relationship, which is a basic element of high-quality nursing care (Watson, 1979).

- **Being Present To, and Supportive Of, the Expression of Positive and Negative Feelings as a Connection With Deeper Spirit of Self and the One-Being-Cared-For:** Translation of the carative factor, Promoting and Accepting the Expression of Positive and Negative Feelings and Emotions. Emphasizes the importance of the expression of both positive and negative feelings and the nurse's acknowledgment and acceptance of those feelings in the self and in others (Watson, 1979, 1996); points to the range of feelings and emotions experienced by both nurse and other(s) and the need to facilitate the expression of such feelings and emotions.

- **Creative Use of Self and All Ways of Knowing as Part of the Caring Process; To Engage in Artistry of Caring-Healing Practices:** Translation of the carative factor, Engaging in Creative, Individualized Problem-Solving Caring Processes. Focuses attention on the creative and individualized aspects of the nursing process, which encompasses assessing, planning, intervening, and evaluating (Watson, 1979, 1989b, 1996). Also focuses attention on the "full use of self and all domains of knowledge, including empirical, aesthetic, intuitive, affective, and ethical knowledge" (Watson, 1989b, p. 230).

- **Engaging in Genuine Teaching-Learning Experience that Attends to Unity of Being and Meaning, Attempting to Stay Within Others' Frames of Reference:** Translation of the carative factor, Promoting Transpersonal Teaching-Learning. Highlights the processes used by both the nurse and the one cared for in the situation of health teaching, including scanning, formulating, appraising, planning, implementing, and evaluating, to facilitate data gathering, decision making, and feedback (Watson, 1979, 1996); emphasizes that nurses and patients are coparticipants in the process of learning.

- **Creating Healing Environments at All Levels (Physical as well as Non-Physical, Subtle Environment of Energy and Consciousness, Whereby Wholeness, Beauty, Comfort, Dignity, and Peace are Potentiated):** Translation of the carative factor, Attending to Supportive, Protective, or Corrective Mental, Physical, Societal, and Spiritual Environments. Focuses attention on the external conditions or factors undergirding a supportive, protective, or corrective environment, including provision of comfort, privacy, safety, and clean aesthetic surroundings (Watson, 1979, 1996); this process is linked with the quality of holistic health care (Watson, 1979).

- **Assisting with Basic Needs, with an Intentional Caring Consciousness, Administering "Human Care Essentials," Which Potentiate Alignment of Mind-body-spirit, Wholeness, and Unity of Being in All Aspects of Care, Tending to Both Embodied Spirit and Evolving Spiritual Emergence:** Translation of the carative factor, Assisting with Gratification of Basic Human Needs While Preserving Human Dignity and Wholeness. Emphasizes the nurse's role in helping others in their activities of daily living, as well as in fostering growth and development. Basic human needs are the need for survival, including needs for food and fluid, elimination, and ventilation; a functional need, including activity-inactivity and sexuality; an integrative need, made up of achievement and affiliation needs; and a need for growth-seeking, which encompasses intrapersonal and interpersonal needs, spiritual development, and self-actualization (Watson, 1979, 1989b, 1996). These are the needs that are most relevant to nursing as human caring (Watson, 1979, 1989b).

- **Opening and Attending to Spiritual-Mysterious, and Existential Dimensions of One's Own Life-Death; Soul Care for Self and the One-Being-Cared-For:** Translation of the carative factor, Allowing For, and Being Open To, Existential-Phenomenological-Spiritual Dimensions of Caring and Healing That Cannot Be Fully Explained Scientifically Through Modern Western Medicine. Underscores the separateness and identity of each person and the personal, subjective experience of each (Watson, 1979, 1996). This process emphasizes the importance of appreciating and understanding the inner world of each person and the meaning each one finds in life, as well as helping others to find meaning in life. "Dealing with another person as he or she *is* and in relation to what he or she would *like* to be or could be is," according to Watson (1979), "a matter of existential-phenomenological [and spiritual] concern for the nurse who practices the science of [human] caring" (p. 205).

The **Clinical Caritas Processes** build on one another, such that being authentically present builds on and draws from the practice of loving kindness to promote holistic professional care and produce positive health. The practice of loving kindness and being authentically present complement each other and further contribute to the cultivation of one's own spiritual self and transpersonal self (Watson, 1979, 2001). Moreover, developing and sustaining a helping-trusting, authentic caring relationship, as well as being present to and supportive of the expression of positive and negative feelings depends on the practice of loving kindness, being authentically present, and cultivation of one's own spiritual self and transpersonal self (Watson, 1979, 2001).

The **Clinical Caritas Processes** are interactive in that all the processes interact for a holistic approach to understanding and studying nursing care (Watson, 1979, 2001). Furthermore, engaging in genuine teaching-learning experience interacts with other clinical caritas processes to promote holistic health care (Watson, 1979, 2001). And, the practice of the clinical caritas process, assisting with basic needs, combined with the other clinical caritas processes, helps gratify higher order needs and provides the essence of what nursing ultimately seeks for high-quality health care (Watson, 1979, 2001).

Relational Propositions

The relational propositions of the Theory of Human Caring are listed below. Relational proposition A links the concept of **Transpersonal Caring Relationship** with the concept of **Caring Moment/Caring Occasion**. Relational propositions B and C link the **Phenomenal Field** dimension of the concept of **Transpersonal Caring Relationship** with the concept of **Caring Moment/Caring Occasion;** and relational proposition D links the **Intersubjectivity** dimension of the concept of **Transpersonal Caring Relationship** with the concept of **Caring Moment/Caring Occasion**. The concepts of **Transpersonal Caring Relationship** and **Caring (healing) Consciousness** are linked in relational proposition E. The **Self** and **Phenomenal Field** dimensions of the concept of **Transpersonal Caring Relationship** are linked with the concept of **Caring (healing) Consciousness** in relational proposition F. The concepts of **Transpersonal Caring Relationship, Caring Moment/Caring Occasion,** And **Caring (healing) Consciousness** are linked in relational propositions G and H and I The **Self** dimension of the concept of **Transpersonal Caring Relationship** is linked with the concepts of **Caring Moment/Caring Occasion** and **Caring (healing) Consciousness** in relational proposition J. Relational proposition K links the **Phenomenal Field** and **Intersubjectivity** dimensions of the concept of **Transpersonal Caring Relationship** with the concepts of **Caring Moment/Caring Occasion** and **Caring (healing) Consciousness.** Relational proposition L links the concepts of **Caring Moment/Caring Occasion** and **Caring (healing) Consciousness.** Relational proposition M links the concepts of **Transpersonal Caring Relationship** and **CLinical Caritas Processes.** The concepts of **Transpersonal Caring Relationship, Caring Moment/Caring Occasion,** And **Clinical Caritas Processes** are linked in relational proposition N.

A. If the caring moment is *transpersonal*, each feels a connection with the other at the spirit level; thus, the moment transcends time and space, opening up new possibilities for healing and human connection at a deeper level than that of physical interaction (Watson, 2001, p. 349).

B. A caring occasion occurs whenever the nurse and other(s) come together with their unique life histories and phenomenal field in a human-to-human transaction (Watson, 1996, p. 157).

C. A transpersonal caring moment transcends the ego level of both nurse and patient, creating a caring field with new possibilities for how to be in the moment (Watson & Smith, 2002, p. 458).

D. Transpersonal ... conveys a concern for the subjective and intersubjective meaning that is fully embodied in a uniquely personal caring moment (Watson, 1996, p. 152).

E. The term transpersonal conveys that the connection has a spiritual dimension that is influenced by the caring consciousness of the nurse (Watson, 1996, p. 152).

F. When [the transpersonal caring] relationship occurs within a caring consciousness, a nurse entering into the life space or phenomenal field of another person is able to detect the other person's condition of being (spirit, or soul level), feels this condition within self, and responds in such a way that the person being cared for has a release of feelings, thoughts, and tension (Watson, 1996, p. 152).

G. Transpersonal caring has the capacity to expand human consciousness, transcend the moment, and potentiate healing and a sense of well-being—a sense of being reintegrated, more connected, more whole (Watson, 1996, p. 160).

H. The transpersonal dimensions of a caring occasion are affected by the nurse's consciousness in the caring moment, which in turn affects the field dynamic of the transaction (Watson, 1996, p. 158).

I. A transpersonal caring relationship connotes a spirit to spirit unitary connection within a caring moment, honouring embodied spirit of both nurse and patient, within the unitary field of consciousness (Watson & Smith, 2002, p. 458).

J. The caring-healing consciousness of a caring moment opens up a higher, deeper energy field of consciousness that has metaphysical and spiritual potentialities for healing and goes beyond the separate ego self and separate body (physical) self (Watson, 1996, pp. 159–160).

K. Transpersonal caring can transpire in a spontaneous "caring moment" or in a caring occasion where two people have arranged to come together. Both meetings are influenced through the intersubjective nature of coming together and the phenomenal field and consciousness energy of the moment (Watson, 1996, p. 152).

L. The whole caring-healing-loving consciousness is contained within a single caring moment (Watson, 2001, p. 349).

M. Transpersonal caring is the full actualization of the [clinical caritas processes] in a human-to-human transaction (Watson, 1989b, p. 232).

N. Transpersonal caring is actualized and "grounded" through ten [clinical caritas processes] that characterize a human-to-human nursing caring transaction within a given caring occasion (Watson, 1996, p. 154).

EVALUATION OF THE THEORY OF HUMAN CARING

This section presents an evaluation of Watson's Theory of Human Caring. The evaluation is based on the results of the analysis of the theory, as well as on publications by others who have used or commented on this nursing theory.

SIGNIFICANCE

The Theory of Human Caring meets the criterion of significance. Watson has begun to focus more explicitly on the metaparadigmatic origins of the Theory of Human Caring, and the metaparadigm concepts and proposition addressed by the theory can be inferred from Watson's publications. Watson clearly explicated the philosophical claims and conceptual orientation for the theory. Although she has only begun to label the conceptual model content presented in the analysis section of this chapter as such, it was possible to extract components of a conceptual model from her writings. It must be noted, however, that the division of statements into philosophical claims and conceptual model seen in the analysis section required certain arbitrary decisions. But the need for those decisions did not come as a surprise inasmuch as Watson (1996) explicitly stated that her work can be read as "a philosophy, an ethic, a conceptual model, or a specific theory" (p. 142).

Watson explicitly acknowledged the importance of her own educational experiences and her immersion in other cultures, and she cited much of the adjunctive knowledge she drew on from other disciplines. She did not, however, provide citations for works by Lazarus, Peplau, Marcel, Sartre, and Yalom, nor did she cite specific sources of adjunctive knowledge from Eastern philosophy. Sarter's (1988) philosophical analysis of Watson's theory revealed influences from Vedic, Hindu, and Buddhist philosophies. In addition, Sarter noted that Watson's portrayal of harmony among body, mind, and soul "may have been indirectly derived from some Eastern source such as Taoism" (p. 57).

A noteworthy feature of the Theory of Human Caring is the attention given to the spiritual aspects of human existence and the soul. Watson's recent writings place even greater emphasis on spirituality (Watson, 1999, 2001; Watson & Smith, 2002). Another noteworthy feature of the theory is the potential for personal growth by nurses as they engage in transpersonal caring relationships. Furthermore, through establishment of intersubjectivity,

the caregiver can become the care receiver. Watson (1989a) explained:

> The one who is cared for (with expanded aesthetic caring processes) can experience a release of subjective feelings and thoughts that had been longing and wishing to be released or expressed. ... Thus, both care provider and care receiver are coparticipants in caring; the release can potentiate self-healing and harmony in both. The release can also allow the one who is cared for to be the one who cares, through the reflection of the human condition that in turn nourishes the humanness of the care provider. (pp. 131–132)

The special significance of the Theory of Human Caring lies in the theory's contributions to understanding a process that nurses can use to effect positive changes in patients' health states. The theory is a comprehensive description of a form of caring that can be used by nurses as they interact with patients, or in Watson's terminology, the other, the ones cared for, the care receivers.

The special significance of the Theory of Human Caring also lies in Watson's rejection of people as objects. Instead, she embraces an orientation that emphasizes "new caring-healing possibilities associated with both the art and science of transpersonal caring-healing and transcendent views of persons in health and illness" (Watson, 1988b, p. 176). Watson's (1988b) orientation leads to a form of nursing that "attends to the human center of both the one caring and the one being cared for" (p. 177).

The Theory of Human Caring reflects a relatively new way for Western society to think about the world. That way of thinking is, however, in keeping with ongoing efforts of several nurses to advance a science that reflects the complexities of human life (see, for example, Fawcett, 2002b). It is likely that not all members of nursing's scientific and practice communities will agree with the orientation that has guided Watson's work, but she should not be faulted for her ongoing efforts.

INTERNAL CONSISTENCY

The Theory of Human Caring meets the criterion of internal consistency in part. Sarter's (1988) philosophical analysis of the Theory of Human Caring raised a question regarding internal consistency. She pointed out that although Watson would undoubtedly describe her work as congruent with a holistic perspective, elements of dualism are evident. She identified dualism in Watson's distinctions between body, mind, and soul; objective and subjective experience; and health and illness. According to Sarter, "whenever Watson speaks of harmony among various aspects of human life, there is an implicit dualism" (p. 56). Similarly, Mitchell and Cody (1992) noted that Watson presented inconsistent views of human beings. They pointed out that, although Watson claimed that people are irreducible wholes, she also referred to several selves (real, inner, ideal) as distinct entities; to the mind, body, spirit, and soul; to physical, emotional, and spiritual spheres; and to the "I" and the "me."

Watson (1992, 1996, 2001) apparently has attempted to overcome the charge of dualism and more effectively convey her idea of a holistic being by using the terms "mind-body-spirit" (1992, 1996) and "mind-body-spirit unity of being" (2001) in her more recent publications. Furthermore, Watson (1997) explicitly acknowledged that some aspects of her work reflect the totality world view, whereas other aspects reflect the simultaneity world view. As her work progresses, it is clear that Watson embraces the simultaneity world view and is attempting to revise the concepts and propositions of the Theory of Human Caring to be in keeping with that world view. One particularly noteworthy example is the change from carative factors to clinical caritas processes, with concomitant changes in wording of the dimensions of the clinical caritas processes (Watson, 2001).

Mitchell and Cody (1992) also pointed out that Watson violated her claim that human beings are free to self-determine and choose. They explained:

First, there are references to the nurse's helping, integrating, and "correcting" the patient's condition to increase harmony and to try to find meaning in the situation. Second, Watson maintains that "*ideally* [italics added], a person should have the opportunity for self-determination of the meaning of a health-illness experience *before professionals make decisions* [italics added] about treatments and interventions" ([Watson], 1985, p. 66).

Furthermore, although Watson claimed allegiance to the human science perspective, her distinction between the person's experience of the world and the world as it actually is, as well as her suggestion of incongruities between the person and nature, are inconsistent with the human science view that humans cannot be separated from their experienced worlds (Mitchell & Cody, 1992). In addition, Watson emphasized the metaphysical, spiritual realm, which Mitchell and Cody (1992) noted is inconsistent with the human science view that the lived experience is the "primal foundation of human knowledge" (p. 58).

Semantic clarity is evident in the constitutive definitions and more elaborate descriptions Watson provided for the concepts of the Theory of Human Caring and most of their dimensions. There is, however, some confusion about the precise definition of intersubjectivity because that term is defined only in conjunction with transpersonal caring.

Although the language Watson uses may not be clear to all readers, she regards the language of her theory as the language of nursing, rather than the language of medicine. She maintained that

for this postmodern era, the [clinical caritas processes] provide a language for caring that is linked to nursing and core processes of professional practice. The language of the [dimensions of the clinical caritas processes] and general caring language help to release nursing from its political and practice history of medical language dominance and orientation. The attention to language is especially critical to an evolving discipline in that during this postmodern era, one's survival depends upon having language; writers in this area remind us "if you do not have your own language you don't exist". (Watson, 1997, p. 50)

Semantic consistency is evident in the consistent use of most terms. One area of potential confusion, however, is evident in the interchangeable use of the terms transpersonal caring and human care relationship throughout Watson's (1985) book and the subsequent discussion of the *components* of transpersonal caring as self, phenomenal field, actual caring occasion, and intersubjectivity (pp. 60–61) and the *concepts* of the human care relationship as phenomenal field, actual caring occasion, and transpersonal caring (p. 73). Watson apparently attempted to overcome confusion in her 2001 book chapter by explicitly listing the concepts of the Theory of Human Caring as **Transpersonal Caring Relationship, Clinical Caritas Processes, Caring Occasion/Caring Moment.** She added the concept of **Caring (Healing) Consciousness** in a separate section of the chapter. Still another area of potential confusion is Watson's use of the terms phenomenal field (1985) and phenomenal field/unitary consciousness (2001); caring-healing (1988b), human caring-healing (1992), and transpersonal caring-healing (1988b); caring-healing consciousness (1988b), caring (healing) consciousness (1996), caring-healing consciousness (2001), caring-healing-loving consciousness (2001), and transpersonal caring-healing human field-consciousness (1992); and actual caring occasion (1985) caring occasion/caring moment (1996), and caring moment/caring occasion (2001).

Evaluation of the structural consistency of the Theory of Human Caring revealed no evidence of contradictions in propositions. The relational propositions adequately link the concepts that make up the theory. Absent, however, is a proposition that links all four concepts of the theory.

PARSIMONY

The Theory of Human Caring meets the criterion of parsimony, although analysis of the evolution of the Theory of Human Caring revealed that the theory has progressed from elegance in its simplicity and relative economy of words to a more complex and verbose work. Indeed, several readings of Watson's various older and more recent publications were required to identify the concepts, their dimensions, and the nonrelational and relational propositions. Although Watson provided what she called a structural overview of the theory in her 1985 book, she did not distinguish between the conceptual and theoretical elements of her work when she identified the subject matter, values, goals, agent of change, interventions, perspective, context, approach, and method. Moreover, the concepts and propositions of the theory were not listed explicitly in the subject matter section of the overview. Rather, Watson stated that the primary subject matter of the theory includes nursing, mutuality of person/self within a context of intersubjectivity, the human care relationship, health-illness, environment, and the universe. Furthermore, Watson's 1996 and 2001 presentations of the content of the theory were not particularly helpful in sorting out concepts, dimensions of concepts, and propositions.

TESTABILITY

The Theory of Human Caring meets the criterion of testability for middle-range theories in part. Watson (1985) noted that "qualitative-naturalistic-phenomenological field methods of inquiry or a combined qualitative-quantitative inquiry" are in keeping with the Theory of Human Caring (p. 79). More specifically, she maintained that the "optimal method for studying the theory is ... through field study that is qualitative in design ... a phenomenological-existential methodology" (p. 76). She went on to present two **RESEARCH METHODOLOGIES** for studying the theory—**The Descriptive-Empirical Phenomenological Research Method** (Table 16–1) and **The Transcendental-Poetic Expression of Phenomenology**

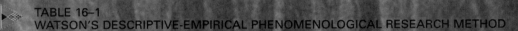

TABLE 16–1
WATSON'S DESCRIPTIVE-EMPIRICAL PHENOMENOLOGICAL RESEARCH METHOD

PHENOMENON OF INTEREST

The notion of essence, that is, the common intersubjective meaning of the human experience of a certain aspect of reality.

Anything that can be said about how people perceive, experience, and conceptualize a given human phenomenon.

SOURCE OF DATA

The researcher obtains naive descriptions from people about their experience of a phenomenon.

GUIDELINES FOR DATA ANALYSIS

The researcher derives essences using descriptive and reduction methods.

The researcher reads a written transcript of each description to get a sense of the whole.

The researcher divides each transcript into "meaning units" or constituents as expressed by the person, marking the transcript each time a transition in meaning is perceived. This is facilitated by asking, "Does this say something different from the previous one with respect to the theme?"

The researcher interrogates each meaning unit for its psychological-nursing-human care relevance.

The researcher reduces the meaning units to those that characterize the person's experience by carrying out a "free-imaginative variation" on each meaning unit to check that these statements capture the essence of the experience.

The researcher integrates the statements into a structure, synthesizing the statements into an integrated whole that embodies the structure of the experience in such a way that it could be compared with structures derived from other experiences.

Constructed from Watson, 1985, pp. 83–84.

Research Method (Table 16–2). These two **RESEARCH METHODOLOGIES** are completely consistent with the philosophical foundation of the Theory of Human Caring.

Watson (1990b) also indicated that the Theory of Human Caring can be tested by means of illustrations of human care and caring as expressed in art and metaphor. Such methods also are consistent with the philosophical foundation of the theory. None of the methodologies, however, is directed toward measurement of the relation between the **Clinical Caritas Processes** and the **Transpersonal Caring Relationship**, which is a central focus of the Theory of Human Caring.

Watson (1985) advocated the use of the **RESEARCH METHODOLOGIES,** but she also cautioned that any one method should not supersede the research question. Thus, although she encouraged investigators to consider "creative-paradigm transcending" (p. 76) methods that are consistent with human science, rather than quantitative rationalistic methods that are more consistent with natural and medical sciences, she was not dogmatic about a particular method. This is an especially important point to consider as investigators struggle to identify the best ways not only to describe human life and human conditions from a human science perspective but also to further develop theories so that predictions may be made with some degree of certainty about the effects of nursing interventions on human life and human conditions from a human science perspective.

Holmes (1990) questioned the generalizability of Watson's research methodologies:

> Unfortunately, Watson adumbrates only one case [in her 1985 book], which concerns experiences of grief and loss among Aboriginal people in Western Australia, and it requires a considerable leap of imagination to transpose the technique into other settings, particularly complex, urbanized ones. Nevertheless, it must be regarded as a courageous attempt to explore the phenomenological epoche as a practical tool for health care purposes, and is a powerful stimulus to innovation. (pp. 192–193)

Empirical indicators designed to measure the concepts of the Theory of Human Caring have begun to be developed (Table 16–3). Some instruments have been developed to measure the concept of carative factors (now known as the **Clinical Caritas Processes**) and the related idea of caring activities. And, the Caring Efficacy Scale represents a step toward measurement of the concept of **Transpersonal Caring Relationship**.

It is not appropriate to assume that instruments designed to measure the carative factors also measure those factors as translated into the **Clinical Caritas Processes**, especially given the "decidedly spiritual" emphasis of those processes (Watson, 2001, p. 347). Consequently, psychometric testing is needed to determine whether instruments designed to measure the carative factors are valid measures of the **Clinical Caritas Processes**. Noteworthy in this regard

---

TABLE 16–2
WATSON'S TRANSCENDENTAL-POETIC EXPRESSION OF PHENOMENOLOGY RESEARCH METHOD

PHENOMENON OF INTEREST

The depth of one's experience, an openness to one's nature, one's potential for being.

SOURCE OF DATA

Articulations of experience as felt and lived, which transcend the facts and pure description of the experience.

GUIDELINES FOR DATA ANALYSIS

The researcher allows for the level of depth or transcendence of the description of the experience, to contact another dimension of his or her being.

The researcher is true to his or her self and acknowledges the openness of the process.

The researcher uses a language that has a transcendental and no longer mundane relationship to the experience, and that encourages existential authenticity. The transcendental reduction changes how words relate to the experience, rather than the meaning of the words per se.

The researcher expresses the data analysis through poetic language.

Source: Constructed from Watson, 1985, pp. 89–93.

Instrument or Tool and Citation*	Description
RESEARCH INSTRUMENTS	
Caring Behaviors Assessment Tool (Cronin & Harrison, 1988; Harrison, 1988; Stanfield, 1992; Watson, 2002; Young et al., 2001)	Measures nurse caring behaviors in terms of the carative factors (now known as the clinical caritas processes)
Caring Assessment Tool (Duffy, 1991, 1992; Watson, 2002)	Measures nurses' caring activities, in terms of the carative factors (now known as the clinical caritas processes)
Caring Assessment Tool-Admin (Duffy, 1993; Watson, 2002)	Measures staff nurses' perceptions of their managers in terms of the carative factors (now known as the clinical caritas processes)
Caring Assessment Tool-Edu (Watson, 2002)	Measures students' perceptions of faculty caring behaviors in terms of the carative factors (now known as the clinical caritas processes)
Caring Behaviors Inventory (Watson, 2002; Wolf, 1986; Wolf et al., 1994, 1998; Young et al., 2001)	Measures nurses' caring behaviors within the context of the carative factors
Caring Efficacy Scale (Coates, 1997; Watson, 2002)	Assesses the nurse's belief in his or her ability to express a caring orientation and to develop caring relationships with patients
Nyberg Caring Assessment (Attributes) Scale (Nyberg, 1989, 1990; Watson, 2002)	Measures caring attributes, the subjective aspect of caring
Conversation Guide (Nyman & Lützen, 1999	Assessment of needs of women with rheumatoid arthritis, using open-ended questions for each of the 10 carative factors
PRACTICE TOOLS	
Caring Documentation Instrument (Ekebergh & Dahlberg, as cited in Watson, 1996)	Permits recording of nurse caring activities
Watson's Carative Factors Redefined, Patients' Subjective Worlds, and Nurses' Reflections Tool (McGraw, (2002)	Provides a list of each Clinical Caritas Process, along with aspects of the patient's subjective world and questions to guide the nurse's reflections about the patient.
Community Assessment Guided by Watson's Theory (Rafael, 2000)	A tool to assess community identity, community spirit, internal and external environments, community capacity to meet basic needs of members, community capacity to care for its most vulnerable members, community capacity to meet social needs of members, community capacity to promote growth and development of its members

*See the Research Instruments/Practice Tools section of the chapter references for complete citations.

is McGraw's (2002) development of a practice tool to guide application of the **Clinical Caritas Processes** as defined and described by Watson (2001) (see Table 16–3).

Recently, Watson (2002a) published a compendium of 21 instruments designed to "assess and measure caring ... that have relevance in assessing caring among students as well as patients and nurses" (p. xiii). The instruments are:

• Caring Assessment Report Evaluation Q-sort (CARE-Q)
• Caring Satisfaction (CARE/SAT)
• Caring Behaviors Inventory

- Caring Behaviors Assessment Tool
- Caring Behaviors of Nurses Scale
- Professional Caring Behaviors
- Nyberg Caring Assessment (Attributes) Scale
- Caring Ability Inventory
- Caring Behavior Checklist
- Client Perception of Caring
- Caring Assessment Tool
- Caring Assessment Tool-Admin
- Caring Assessment Tool-Edu
- Peer Group Caring Interaction Scale
- Organizational Climate for Caring Questionnaire
- Caring Efficacy Scale
- Holistic Caring Inventory
- Caring Dimensions Inventory
- Caring Attributes, Professional Self-Concept Technological Influences Scale
- Caring Professional Scale
- Methodist Health Care System Nurse Caring Instrument

Some of those instruments were derived directly from the Theory of Human Caring (see Table 16–3); others are more generic measures of caring whose theoretical origins were not always made explicit by the nurses who developed them or were based on other theories of caring. Acknowledging the need for further instrument development work, Watson (1989b) stated, "The [carative] factors and the human process of caring need to be further delineated, expanded, and researched" (p. 227). In particular, empirical indicators must be developed to measure the complexity of the concepts of **Transpersonal Caring Relationship, Caring Moment/Caring Occasion,** and **Caring (Healing) Consciousness** in the real world of nursing practice. In addition, data analysis techniques must be developed to measure the relation between the concepts of **Clinical Caritas Processes** and **Transpersonal Caring Relationship.**

EMPIRICAL ADEQUACY

The Theory of Human Caring has begun to meet the criterion of empirical adequacy for middle-range theories. Investigators have employed a variety of methodologies, including various forms of phenomenology and grounded theory, as well as the Theory of Human Caring–based **Descriptive-Empirical Phenomenological Research Method** and the **Transcendental-Poetic Expression of Phenomenology Research Method.** Published research reports have begun to provide evidence regarding the empirical adequacy of the Theory of Human Caring (Table 16–4). For example, Mullaney (2000) reported that de-

pressed woman who experienced the actual caring occasion during therapy persisted in treatment. Bollinger (2001) found that use of the theory contributed to change of affect and commitment to take positive action in an 11-year-old boy and his mother. Bollinger also found that the nurse practitioner who cared for the boy and his mother experienced a renewal of spirit and sense of gratitude, which supports Watson's (1988b) assertion that use of the theory can have benefits not only for the one-cared-for but also for the one who is caring. In addition, the findings of one experimental study suggest that use of the carative factors (now known as the **Clinical Caritas Processes**) resulted in increased quality of life and decreased systolic and diastolic blood pressure for patients with hypertension (Erci et al., 2003). The findings of another experimental study revealed that hospitalized adults who were fed by college students trained to feed people in a caring manner ate twice as much as their counterparts who were fed by the nursing staff (Robinson et al., 2002).

Despite the growing number of published reports of Theory of Human Caring–based research (see Table 16–4), as well as the doctoral dissertations and master's theses listed in the chapter bibliography on the CD-ROM, the outcomes of a **Transpersonal Caring Relationship** and the effects of the **Clinical Caritas Processes** have not yet been fully documented empirically. Additional research is needed to further establish or refute the empirical adequacy of the Theory of Human Caring. In particular, Watson's (1979, 1996) claims that the use of the carative factors (now known as the **Clinical Caritas Processes**) represents a high quality of holistic nursing care (1979) and that the carative factors are "the primary ingredients for effective nursing practice" (1996, p. 155) have not yet been substantiated empirically. Inasmuch as all research to date, including instrument development work (see Table 16–3) has focused on an earlier version of the Theory of Human Caring, especially with regard to the carative factors, future studies should address the empirical adequacy of the **Clinical Caritas Processes** per se, as well as the relation between the **Clinical Caritas Processes** and the **Transpersonal Caring Relationship.**

PRAGMATIC ADEQUACY

The Theory of Human Caring meets the criterion of pragmatic adequacy. Watson has identified the special educational requirements for application of the theory, and she has outlined a particular approach to nursing practice.

(Text continues on page 574)

Research Topic	Study Participants	Citation*
DESCRIPTIVE STUDIES		
Transpersonal caring interactions	Nurse-elderly person dyads	Clayton, 1989
Essential elements of spirituality	Well adults	Burns, 1991
Components of spiritual nursing care	Registered nurses	Dennis, 1991
Definition of hope	Well and hospitalized adolescents	Hinds, 1984
What homeless children regard as special	Photographs taken by children living in a public shelter	Percy, 1995
Educational needs of prospective family caregivers	Prospective family caregivers of newly disabled adults	Weeks, 1995
Categories of family members' involvement in the care of a dying relative	Spouses of persons with grave, incurable cancer of the colon, liver, or bile duct being cared for at a medical center in Sweden	Andershed, & Ternestedt, 1999
Perceptions of nurse caring behaviors	Childbearing women	Manogin, Bechtel, & Rami, 2000
Description of nurse caring behaviors as important indicators of caring	Emergency department patients	Baldursdottir & Jonsdottir, 2002
Differences in perceptions of nurses' caring behaviors	Adults with sickle cell disease and adults with general medical conditions	Dorsey et al., 2001
Identification of nurse caring behaviors	Older adults residing in institutions	Marini, 1999
Parents' perceptions of nurses' and physicians' expressions of caring	Bereaved parents who experienced a perinatal loss	Lemmer, 1991
Patients' perceptions of perioperative nurses' use of the carative factors	Adult surgical patients	Parsons et al., 1993
Perioperative nurses' perceptions of their use of the carative factors	Registered nurses	McNamara, 1995
Student nurses' perceptions of the meaning and value of caring	Second-year diploma nursing students	Chipman, 1991
Nurses' and patients' perceptions of the experience of caring in the acute care setting	Nurses Adult medical-surgical patients	Miller et al., 1992
Nurses', educators', and patients' perceptions of caring needs and experiences	Staff nurses Nurse educators Kidney transplant patients	Watson, 1996
Nurses' and caregivers' perceptions of helpful nursing behaviors	Primary caregivers Hospice nurses	Ryan, 1992

*See the Research section of the chapter references for complete citations.

Generation of a theory of caring	Women who had miscarried Parents and health professionals (nurses, physicians, social worker, biomedical ethicist) in a newborn intensive care unit Socially at-risk young mothers	Swanson, 1991
Essential structure of the lived experience of depressed women who enter therapy and experience Watson's actual caring occasion with the transpersonal caring relationship	Women who were depressed	Mullaney, 2000
Experience of living in a nursing home	Nursing home residents age 80 years and older	Running, 1997
Experience of growing up with a chronic illness	Adults with cystic fibrosis	Tracy, 1997
Caring needs specific to the human experience of having rheumatoid arthritis and undergoing acupuncture treatment within the context of the 10 carative factors	Swedish women with rheumatoid arthritis who sought acupuncture treatment	Nyman & Lützen, 1999
Knowledge, attitudes, and family planning decisions[†]	Persons with adult polycystic kidney disease and their at-risk family members	Shindel-Martin, 1991
Stories of living with HIV disease/AIDS	Clients at a nurse-directed HIV/AIDS facility	Schroeder & Neil, 1992
Description of difficulties, wishes, anxieties, frustrations, emotions, expectations, fears, doubts, preconceptions and feelings of insecurity, discouragement, satisfaction, and apathy	Breastfeeding mothers	Rozario & Zongonel, 2000
Descriptions of the use of humor as a coping skill and the association of humor with nursing and spirituality	Women in breast cancer support groups	Johnson, 2002
Meaning of caring	A 30-year-old man with HIV disease receiving home care, his life-partner, and his parents	Beauchamp, 1993
[†]Description of caring and loss	Tribal Aboriginal men in Cundeelee, Western Australia	Watson, 1985a
[‡]Poetic expression of the researcher's subjective experiences of patients' and nurses' day-to-day lives	Researcher	Krysl & Watson, 1988
[‡]Poetic expression of the researcher's experience and Aborigines' loss-caring experiences	Researcher Tribal Aboriginal men in Cundeelee, Western Australia	Watson, 1985b
Application of transpersonal caring	Cancer patients and their families	Souza & Lacerda, 2000
Nurses' knowledge of and attitudes toward organ donation	Registered nurses	Bishop, 1996

[†]Used the Descriptive-Empirical Phenomenological Research Method.
[‡]Used the Transcendental-Poetic Expression of Phenomenology Research Method.

(continued)

TABLE 16–4
PUBLISHED REPORTS OF RESEARCH GUIDED BY THE THEORY OF HUMAN CARING *(continued)*

Research Topic	Study Participants	Citation
Nurses' views of key elements of nursing practice	Oncology nurses	Perry, 1998
Characteristics of Swedish nurses considered to have a "green thumb" for nursing and description of caring moments	Swedish staff nurses	Jensen et al., 1993
Description of how and why nurses provide for patients' aesthetic needs	Registered nurses working in hospitals in Sweden	Wikström, 2002
Exploration of the practice of caring for caregivers [nurses]	Nurses and nurse managers working in hospitals in KwaZulu-Natal, South Africa	Minnaar, 2001
Characteristics of excellent nurses	Danish women with breast cancer	Jensen et al., 1996
Personal and professional impact of a 15-week degree level module on nursing as human caring	Students in a 4-year, post-registration nursing degree course in Wales, United Kingdom	Hoover, 2002
CORRELATIONAL STUDY		
Relation of nurse caring behaviors to patient satisfaction, health status, length of stay, and nursing care costs	Patients with a medical or surgical diagnosis	Duffy, 1992
EXPERIMENTAL STUDIES		
Effect of use of Watson's theory of human caring on blood pressure and quality of life	Adult patients with hypertension attending health clinics in Turkey	Erci et al., 2003
Effects of feeding hospitalized patients >65 years of age who required assistance with feeding	College-aged volunteers Nursing staff	Robinson et al., 2002
Effects of experimental therapeutic massage and control nurse interaction on pain intensity, pain distress, sleep quality, symptom distress, and anxiety	Hospitalized male and female cancer patients receiving chemotherapy or radiation treatment	Smith et al., 2002

(Text continued from page 571)

Nursing Education

A commitment to transpersonal caring, according to Watson (1988b), is a moral ideal and a standard for nursing care. Furthermore, as Watson (1999) explained, a transpersonal caring relationship depends upon:

1. A moral commitment to protect and enhance human dignity and the deeper/higher self; the soul of the person honored.

2. The caring consciousness of the nurse is communicated with the other on a level that both embodies and honors the other's physicality, but transcends the physical by preserving and honoring the embodied spirit; the person is not therefore reduced to the moral status of 'object.' There is then a connection between the persons, but also a new energy field is created by the consciousness and intentionality held in the moment.

3. A transpersonal caring connection is a focal point in time and space from which experience, perception and

intentional connection are taking place. Such a caring consciousness and connection, one to another, has a healing potential. It is grounded in the individual experiences of the two separate persons, but goes beyond the two; the self connection is every self—the universal self. We learn to recognize ourselves in others by engaging in a transpersonal caring moment (pp. 154–155).

The delivery of nursing care based on the Theory of Human Caring requires considerable education to better understand the expanded view of nursing, science, person, and health-illness that is reflected in the theory (Watson, 1990b, 1996). Some of the education required for use of the Theory of Human Caring comes from nurses themselves. "Valuable teachers for this work," Watson (2001) declared, "include the nurse's own life history and previous experiences, which provide opportunities for focused studies, the nurse having lived through or experienced various human conditions and having imagined others' feelings in various circumstances" (p. 348).

Watson (2001) identified several facilitators of the understanding required for use of the Theory of Human Caring. The facilitators include the nurse's work with peoples of diverse cultures; the study of the humanities, including art, drama, literature, and personal story narratives of illness; the nurse's exploration of his or her own values, beliefs, relationship with self and others, and his or her own world; and such personal growth experiences as psychotherapy, transpersonal psychology, meditation, bioenergetics work, and other methods of spiritual awakening. Watson (2001) went on to point out that "to truly 'get it,' one has to experience it personally; thus, the [theory] is both an invitation and an opportunity to interact with the ideas, experiment with and grow within the philosophy, and to live it out in one's personal/professional life" (p. 349).

Watson (1988a, 1996; Fawcett, 2002) proposed that professional nursing education be at the postbaccalaureate level of the Doctorate of Nursing (ND); such a program is offered at the University of Colorado Health Sciences Center School of Nursing (Watson & Phillips, 1992; Nursing Doctorate, retrieved July 15, 2003 from http://www2.uchsc.edu/son). Watson presented a clear rationale for her position when she declared:

Although the bachelor's degree is considered still the [unresolved and impossible to implement] minimal entry into the professional practice of nursing, the mature practice of nursing, as a career health professional, ideally should be at the professional doctoral level, or at least the graduate level. Why should nursing differ from every other practicing discipline (e.g., dentistry, medicine, pharmacy, psychology, law). It is so ironic and amazing to me that, even as we enter the 21st century, we who are the oldest of the caring/health/healing professions, and we, who deal with the most complex human experiences and health-related phenomena, have never made the connection for the need for additional education to deal with these complex, technological, and evolving human phenomena. Instead, we talk about less education or the same education, resist upping the ante for required higher education for entry. … I think every major academic health science center nursing program should convert its baccalaureate nursing programs into non-practice degrees in caring science and health, or at least make that degree a major in the field. Such a framework for a general undergraduate degree could be preparatory as pre-med, pre-nursing, etc. But this hard transition into professionalism would entail letting go of the baccalaureate degree as entry level into nursing, moving quickly to graduate-doctoral level, parallel with all other health professionals. Almost all other practicing professions have made this turn—witness pharmacy's quick shift in the last decade, from baccalaureate degree to Pharm. D. [Doctorate of Pharmacy]; similar shifts have occurred in physiotherapy, psychology, law, and so on (Fawcett, 2002, p. 217).

In keeping with academic preparation at the ND level, Watson (1996) proposed that professional practice should be advanced practice in nursing, with expertise in caring-healing and health and "attending nurse" status in healthcare organizations, "working alongside other members of the health team, while assuming responsibility for the caring-healing focus of care" (p. 163). Watson and Foster (2003) then described a professional practice model for the attending nurse, which they called the Attending Nursing Caring Model®. The proposed model for professional practice within the context of Watson's Theory of Human Caring is evidence-based and reflective.

The nature of human life, according to Watson (1988a), is the subject matter of nursing. Hence, nursing education focuses on clarification of the values and views regarding human life. A moral context for nursing education that emphasizes a way of being as a caring professional is required. In particular, a curriculum based on the Theory of Human Caring acknowledges caring as a moral ideal and incorporates philosophical theories of human caring, health, and healing. The special education requirements for learning and applying the Theory of Human Caring are listed here (Watson, 1989b, 1996, 1997).

- Continual study, development, and research are required to understand the content of the theory and its implications for nursing practice.
- Core areas of content include the arts and humanities, social-biomedical sciences, emerging sciences, and human caring content and process.
- Additional content includes knowledge of human behavior and human responses to actual or potential health problems; knowledge and understanding of individual

needs; knowledge of how to respond to others' needs; knowledge of own and others' strengths and limitations; knowledge of the meaning of the situation for the person; and knowledge of how to provide comfort, offer compassion, and express empathy.

- Reflection on and critique of one's own values, beliefs, and practices with regard to their congruence with the values, beliefs, and practices associated with the Theory of Human Caring are essential.
- Personal experience with the Theory of Human Caring in the form of opportunities to interact and grow within the philosophical claims and content of the theory also is essential.
- A personal, social, moral, and spiritual engagement of self is required, which may necessitate a radical transformation of traditional ways of thinking about nursing.
- Each person working within the Theory of Human Caring should cultivate a time for daily contemplation, that is, for soul care, by engaging in such practices as centering, meditation, breath work, yoga, prayer, and connections with nature.
- Learn the Practice Methodology for the Theory of Human Caring (Table 16–5).

Watson (1988a) claimed that new approaches to studying the concepts of caring are needed, such as courses using art, music, literature, poetry, drama, and movement to facilitate understanding of responses to health and illness, and new caring-healing modalities. Thus, considerable change in the typical curriculum of most schools of nursing is required.

The curriculum of the ND program at the University of Colorado Health Sciences Center School of Nursing serves as an exemplar. The 4-year curriculum of that program is made up of a clinical sciences core, a clinical arts and humanities caring core, a discipline-specific human caring nursing core, a health professional and ethical foundation core, and a professional practice residency (Watson & Phillips, 1992; Doctor of Nursing, retrieved July 15, 2003 from http://www2.uchsc.edu/son).

Nurses who are not prepared at the ND level require additional professional development and continuing education to learn the Theory of Human Caring and its associated advanced caring-healing modalities. The University of Colorado Health Sciences Center School of Nursing in Denver, and Naropa University in Boulder, Colorado, offer on-site course modules as part of an International Certificate Program in Caring and Healing; other courses are available online. The School of Nursing also can accommodate visiting scholars from throughout the world who would like to study Watson's work. In addition, information about Watson's work is available online (see http://www2.uchsc.edu/son).

As part of the education needed to use the Theory of Human Caring, each nurse should consider "What is one's view of 'human'? And what does it mean to be human, caring, healing, becoming, growing, transforming, and so on?" (Watson, 2001, p. 350). The decision to proceed with use of the theory should be based on affirmative answers to several questions (Watson, 2001, pp. 349–350). The questions are:

- Is there congruence between the values and major concepts and beliefs in the [theory] and the given nurse, group, system, organization, curriculum, population needs, clinical administrative setting, or other entity that is considering interactions with the caring [theory] to transform and/or improve practice?
- Are those interacting and engaging in the [theory] interested in their own personal evolution: Are they committed to seeking authentic connections and caring-healing relationships with self and others?
- Are those involved "conscious" of their caring caritas or noncaring consciousness and intentionally in a given moment, at individual and system level? Are they interested and committed to expanding their caring consciousness and actions to self, other, environment, nature, and wider universe?
- Are those working within the [theory] interested in shifting their focus from a modern medical science-technocure orientation to a true caring-healing-loving [theory]?

Nursing Practice

Human caring, according to Watson (1990b), is required when curing is possible, but especially when curing has failed. Drawing on Gaut's (1983) philosophical analysis of caring, Watson (1989b) noted that the provision of human care through application of the carative factors (now known as the **Clinical Caritas Processes**) requires "an intention, caring values, knowledge, a will, a relationship, and actions" (p. 227). Elaborating on actions, Watson (1989b) explained that the provision of human care "requires enabling actions—that is, actions that allow another to solve problems, grow, and transcend the here and now, actions that are related to general and specific knowledge of caring and human responses" (p. 227).

Holistic nursing practice based on the Theory of Human Caring requires the integration of all 10 **Clinical Caritas Processes**. Watson (1979) explained, "No one [process] can be effective alone. The student nurse and the practicing nurse must continue to integrate the [processes] that effect positive health care" (p. 214).

Nursing practice based on the Theory of Human Caring is not necessarily easy. Indeed, Watson (1989a) pointed out that human caring, "with its need for ethics, emotions, compassion, knowledge, wisdom, intentions, and so on, is always fragile and threatened because it requires a personal, social, moral, and spiritual engagement of self and a commitment to one*self* and to others' *self* and dignity" (p. 129). Thus "a radical transformation of traditional professional relationships" is required (p. 132). Furthermore,

nurses must continuously "question and be open to new possibilities" (Watson, 1992, p. 1481). A **PRACTICE METHODOLOGY** for the Theory of Human Caring, which was extracted from Watson's publications, guides the application of the theory in practice situations (see Table 16–5).

The **Practice Methodology** incorporates what Watson (1999; Watson & Smith, 2002) calls transpersonal caring-healing modalities or advanced transpersonal caring modalities. Those caring modalities "draw upon multiple ways of knowing and being; then encompass ethical, and

---

▶ TABLE 16–5
PRACTICE METHODOLOGY FOR THE THEORY OF HUMAN CARING

REQUIREMENTS FOR A TRANSPERSONAL CARING RELATIONSHIP

The nurse considers the person to be valid and whole, regardless of illness or disease.

The nurse makes a moral commitment and directs intentionality and consciousness to the protection, enhancement, and potentiation of human dignity, wholeness, and healing, such that a person creates or co-creates his or her own meaning for existence, healing, wholeness, and caring.

The nurse orients intent, will, and consciousness toward affirming the subjective/intersubjective significance of the person; a search to sustain mind-body-spirit unity and I-Thou versus I-It relationships.

The nurse has the ability to realize, accurately detect, and connect with the inner condition (spirit) of another. The nurse recognizes that actions, words, behaviors, cognition, body language, feelings, intuition, thought, senses, and the energy field gestalt all contribute to the interconnection.

The nurse has the ability to assess and realize another's condition of being-in-the-world and to feel a union with the other. This ability is translated via movements, gestures, facial expressions, procedures, information, touch, sound, verbal expressions, and other scientific, aesthetic, and human means of communication into nursing-art acts wherein the nurse responds to, attends to, or reflects the condition of the other. Drawn from the ontological caring-consciousness stance and basic competencies of the nurse, this ability expands and translates into advanced caring-healing modalities, nursing arts, advanced nursing therapeutics, and healing arts.

The nurse understands that the caring-healing modalities potentiate harmony, wholeness, and comfort and produce inner healing by releasing some of the disharmony and blocked energy that interfere with the natural healing processes.

Transpersonal caring-healing modalities include:

- Intentional conscious use of auditory modalities, such as music; sounds of nature, wind, sea, chimes, and chants; and familiar sounds
- Intentional conscious use of visual modalities, such as light, color, form, texture, and works of art
- Intentional conscious use of olfactory modalities, such as aromatherapy, breathwork, breathing fresh air, and inhalation-exhalation.
- Intentional conscious use of the tactile modality, including such body touch therapies as acupressure, body therapy, caring touch, foot reflexology, shiatsu, and therapeutic massage.
- Intentional conscious use of gustatory modalities, with a focus on particular foods in one's diet.
- Intentional conscious use of mental-cognitive modalities, with a focus on the importance of the mind and the imagination through story.
- Intentional conscious use of kinesthetic modalities, such as basic skin care, deep massage and deep cellular tissue work (e.g., Rolfing), movement, dance, yoga, Tai Chi, applied kinesiology, chiropractic, Feldendrais work, Jin shin jyutsu, polarity work, Reiki, and Trager work.
- Intentional conscious use of 'caring consciousness' as modality, with a focus on physical presence, psychological presence, and therapeutic presence.

The nurse understands that his or her own life history and previous experiences, including opportunities, studies, consciousness of having lived through or experienced human feelings and various human conditions, or of having imagined others' feelings in various circumstances, are valuable contributors to the transpersonal caring relationship.

▶ ◄ **TABLE 16–5**
PRACTICE METHODOLOGY FOR THE THEORY OF HUMAN CARING *(continued)*

AUTHENTIC PRESENCING

The nurse is authentically present as self and other in a reflective mutuality of being and becoming.

The nurse centers consciousness and intentionality on caring, healing, and wholeness, rather than on disease, problems, illness, complications, and technocures.

The nurse attempts to:

- Stay within the other's frame of reference.
- Join in a mutual search for meaning and wholeness of being.
- Potentiate comfort measures, pain control, a sense of well-being, or spiritual transcendence of suffering.

Source: Constructed from Watson, 1996, pp. 152–154; 1997, pp. 50–51; 1999, pp. 206–227.

relational caring along with those intentional consciousness modalities that are energetic in nature, e.g., form, colour, light, sound, touch, visual, olfactory, etc. that potentiate wholeness, healing, comfort, and well-being" (Watson & Smith, 2002, p. 458). The caring-healing modalities, which emerge from the **Clinical Caritas Processes,** can be traced to Nightingale's (1859/1946) writings (Watson, 1999).

Despite the potential difficulty of using the Theory of Human Caring, evidence of its utility is beginning to emerge in the form of several published reports of nursing practice and implementation projects with a variety of persons in diverse settings (Table 16–6).

The reports listed in Table 16–6, along with the reports listed in the Commentary: Administration and Commentary: Practice sections of the chapter bibliography on the CD-ROM, document the use of the Theory of Human Caring in the real world of nursing practice with various populations. The reports lend support to Watson's (1996) claim that nurses who use the Theory of Human Care practice "wherever the patients/clients are located: in and outside of institutions, schools, homes, clinics, and community settings" (p. 163). Kelley and Johnson (2002) added that the literature indicates that the theory "has the potential to apply to any situation in which nursing occurs" (p. 419).

Moreover, various projects designed to implement Watson's Theory of Human Caring document the feasibility of implementing practice protocols and practitioners' legal ability to implement nursing actions based on the **Clinical Caritas Processes** and to measure the effectiveness of those actions. The sites of the implementation projects are listed here. The complete citations to the published reports of the projects are given in the Administration section of the chapter references.

- Denver Nursing Project in Human Caring in Denver, Colorado (Astorino et al., 1994; Leenerts et al., 1996; Lyne & Waller, 1990; Neil, 1995, 2001; Nyberg, 1994; Quinn, 1994; Schroeder, 1993a, 1993b; Schroeder & Astorino, 1996; Schroeder & Maeve, 1992; Schroeder & Neil, 1992; Smith, 1994, 1997; Watson, 1996)
- Dementia Unit in a Nursing Home (Residents with dementia) (Marckx, 1995)
- Baycrest Centre for Geriatric Care in Toronto, Ontario, Canada (Cappell & Leggat, 1993; Watson, 1996)
- Nursing Partners at Providence Hospital in Sandusky, Ohio (Sanford & Lamb, 1997)
- Our Lady of the Resurrection Medical Center in Chicago, Illinois (Brooks & Rosenberg, 1995)
- Rockford Health System, University of Illinois at Chicago, College of Nursing Rockford Program (Watson, 1996)
- University of Natal School of Nursing Decentralised Programmes, South Africa (Minnaar, 2002)
- Kent State University, Kent, Ohio (A faculty mentoring program based on a caring theoretical perspective) (Snelson et al., 2002)

Evidence of the extent to which **Clinical Caritas Processes**–based actions are compatible with expectations for nursing practice and the effects of those actions on both the one-cared-for and the one caring is mounting. The outcomes achieved by the Denver Nursing Project in Human Caring (DNPHC) during its existence serve as an exemplar. The DNPHC, a nurse-managed center devoted to the care of persons living with human immunodeficiency virus (HIV) and acquired immunodeficiency syndrome (AIDS), was established in 1988 as a clinical demonstration project of the University of Colorado School of Nursing and the Center for Human Caring; the

► ▸ **TABLE 16–6**
PUBLISHED REPORTS OF NURSING PRACTICE GUIDED BY THE THEORY OF HUMAN CARING

Practice Situation	Population	Citation*
Use of the carative factors (now know as the clinical caritas processes)	Premature infants and their parents	Sithichoke-Rattan, 1989
	A young woman with life-threatening postpartal complications	Saxton, 1994
	A patient with HIV	Nelson-Marten et al., 1998
	A patient with AIDS	
	A group of elderly residents of a nursing home	Carson, 1992
Application of the Theory of Human Caring	An 11-year-old boy and his mother	Bollinger, 2001
	A 29-year-old woman with cervical cancer	McGraw, 2002
	A 35-year-old man dying of AIDS	
	Patients with Alzheimer's disease and their families	Wykle & Morris, 1994
	A dying patient in the intensive care unit and family members	Mendyka, 1993
	Bereaved persons	Hubner, 1999
Application of the Theory of Human Caring—use of art	Patients with Alzheimer's disease and other dementias	Sterritt & Pokorny, 1994
	Patients with cancer	Gullo, 1997
Application of the Theory of Human Caring—psychiatric consultation liaison nursing	A support group of nurses working in a neurological intensive care unit	Brandman, 1996
Theory of Human Caring–based teaching program about AIDS	Preadolescents	Jones, 1991
Ethical aspects of caring	A 12-year-old boy with AIDS	Weiser, 1992
Maintenance of authentic caring	Nurses caring for patients with HIV/AIDS	Montgomery, 1994 Neil, 1994
Nursing strategies to increase hope and facilitate spirituality	People with HIV	Harrison, 1997

*See the Practice section of the chapter references for complete citations.

project ended in 1996 (Smith, 1997; Watson, 1996). The DNPHC, where nursing practice was based on Watson's philosophy and science of human caring, and care was delivered through the carative factors (now known as the **Clinical Caritas Processes**), became an international prototype for caring-based practice. Smith (1997) reported that DNPHC clients stated that each one was "seen as a whole person with a life and a family," that nursing care was "coming home," that they were helped to discover "a personal path for healing," and that they felt "the energy of love and compassion" (pp. 57–58). In addition, Watson (1996) noted that caring extended beyond the nurse-client relationship to staff-staff, client-client, and staff-client-community relationships.

The reports of implementation projects indicate that some comparisons have been made between outcomes before and after implementation of the Theory of Human Caring. The results of the various projects revealed that staff job satisfaction increased, hospital length of stay decreased, and health-care costs decreased when the theory was used to guide nursing practice. Furthermore, the reports of the implementation projects, as well as the reports of nursing practice applications (see Table 16–6), indicate that use of the Theory of Human Caring helps people solve their health-related problems.

 ## CONCLUSION

Watson has made a substantial contribution to nursing by explicating a new way of thinking about nursing. Her theory clearly reflects her commitment "to preserve and restore the human mind-body-spirit in theory and practice" (Watson, 1992, p. 1481). Yet Watson (1996) is not content with the current status of her work. Indeed, she explained that her work is evolving "toward a paradigmatic structure for the whole of nursing and its emergence as a distinct caring-healing-health discipline and profession for the next century" (p. 142). Later, Watson explained, "I seek to bring my work into a more meaningful level for how we live our lives and how we bring this caring-healing to our day-to-day existence" (Fawcett, 2002, p. 218). Watson's 1999 book and 2001 book chapter, as well as her 2002 journal article co-authored with Smith clearly reflect her evolution in thinking.

In summarizing Watson's contributions to nursing, Kelley and Johnson (2002) stated:

> Watson's work is transformative at all levels and realms of nursing. The theory directs the focus back onto the person and mandates that technology be used selectively for the betterment of humankind rather than as the sole guiding factor in health care. Watson attempts to rekindle the passion of nursing for the sacredness of being human and the sacred traditions of health and healing (p. 421).

Evidence of the empirical and pragmatic adequacy of the Theory of Human Caring is increasing. Watson's 1985 book has been translated into Chinese, German, Japanese, Korean, and Swedish (Watson, 1997). Moreover, during its existence, the Center for Human Caring, which fostered "the study, teaching, and practice of human caring" (Watson, 1990a, p. 47), established the formal mechanism of International Affiliates for shared activities throughout the world. Watson (1996) reported that International Affiliates include the Scottish Highlands Center in the United Kingdom; Baycrest Centre for Geriatric Care in Toronto, Ontario, Canada; the Collaborative Nursing Education Project in Victoria, British Columbia, Canada; and Victoria University Department of Graduate Nursing and Midwifery in Wellington, New Zealand. Investigators

and practitioners throughout the world, then, should continue to compile evidence so that the efficacy of Watson's ideas and the generalizability of the theory and its associated research and practice methodologies can be fully determined. With its closing, most Center for Human Caring activities were reorganized into a larger nursing research center at the University of Colorado Health Sciences Center School of Nursing (see *www2.uchsc.edu/son*).

Walker (1989) raised a particularly intriguing issue regarding Watson's notion of caring: "That is whether caring is equally the moral ideal for all helping relationships: minister-sinner, doctor-patient, therapist-client. If so, then Watson's work is relevant to all these relationships not just nurse-patient ones" (p. 154). Watson (2001) declared,

> This work, in both its original and evolving forms, seeks to develop caring as an ontological and theoretical-philosophical-ethical framework for the profession and discipline of nursing and to clarify its mature relationship and distinct intersection with other health sciences.... The future already revels that all health-care practitioners will need to work within a shared framework of caring relationships, mind-body-spirit medicine, embracing the healing arts and caring practices and processes and the spiritual dimensions of care much more completely. (p. 350)

Later, Watson added,

> I see the value of human caring theory as a foundational ethic and philosophy for any health professional. Though my work comes from nursing, the current momentum for a focus on caring in several health disciplines is congruent with the caring stance that nursing has had across time. The core of the human caring theory is about human caring relationships and the deeply human experiences of life itself, not just health-illness phenomena, as traditionally defined within medicine [Watson, 2002b, 2002c]. The theory is about a different way of being human, a different way of being present, attentive, conscious, and intentional as the nurse works with another person. All of this perspective has relevance for medicine as well as for nursing or other health professions. The mature practice of human caring theory is most fully actualized in a nursing model because nursing allows for the continuous caring component that medicine does not have; nurses and nursing working from a human caring philosophy bring a different consciousness and energy of wholeness to any setting, offering a counterpoint to the medicalizing-clinicalizing of human experiences in the conventional institutional industrial models of practice.... I see [my work] as *transdisciplinary*, in that the future calls for all of health care to enter into an expanded model of wholeness and healing, beyond conventional medicine. Thus, as I see it, eventually all health practitioners will need to be in an expanded model of caring and healing to serve the changing needs and expectations of the public. The shared caring healing work from this expanded consciousness transcends any one discipline or profession. Inasmuch as it is

beyond cross-disciplinary, it is transdisciplinary (Fawcett, 2002a, pp. 215–216).

Clearly, the issue of whether and how the theory is relevant to all helping relationships requires continued discussion so that the distinctive contribution of Watson's work to nursing knowledge and the contributions of that work to the knowledge base of other disciplines can be determined. Indeed, as Watson (1995) has begun to locate her work within the broader area of alternative caring-healing practices, and as she raises the question of the continued existence of the discipline of nursing (Watson, 1996, 1997), continued discussion of that issue is even more crucial.

REFERENCES

Alexandersson, C. (1981). Amedeo Giorgi's empirical phenomenology. Publication no. 3. Goteborg, Sweden: Swedish Council for Research in Humanities and Social Sciences, Department of Education, University of Goteborg.

Bollinger, E. (2001). Applied concepts of holistic nursing. Journal of Holistic Nursing, 19, 212–214.

de Chardin, T. (1967). On love. New York: Harper & Row.

Erci, B., Sayan, A., Tortumluoglu, G., Kikiç, D., Sahin, O, & Güngörmüs, Z. (2003). The effectiveness of Watson's caring model on the quality of life and blood pressure of patients with hypertension. Journal of Advanced Nursing, 41, 130–139.

Fawcett, J. (2002a). The nurse theorists: 21st century updates—Jean Watson. Nursing Science Quarterly, 15, 214–219.

Fawcett, J. (2002b). On science and human science: A conversation with Marilyn M. Rawnsley. Nursing Science Quarterly, 15, 41–45.

Gadow, S. (1980). Existential advocacy: Philosophical foundation of nursing. In S. Spicker & S. Gadow (Eds), Nursing: Images and ideals: Opening dialogue with the humanities (pp. 79–101). New York: Springer.

Gadow, S. (1984, March). Existential advocacy as a form of caring: Technology, truth, and touch. Paper presented to the Research Seminar Series: The Development of Nursing as a Human Science. University of Colorado School of Nursing, Denver.

Gaut, D.A. (1983). Development of a theoretically adequate description of caring. Western Journal of Nursing Research, 5, 313–324.

Giorgi, A. (1970). Psychology as a human science. New York: Harper & Row.

Holmes, C.A. (1990). Alternatives to natural science foundations for nursing. International Journal of Nursing Studies, 27, 187–198.

Kelley, J.H., & Johnson, B. (2002). Theory of transpersonal caring: Jean Watson. In J. B. George (Ed.), Nursing theories: The base for professional nursing practice (5th ed., pp. 427–461). Upper Saddle River, NJ: Prentice Hall.

Kierkegaard, S. (1941). Concluding unscientific postscript (New ed., H.J. Patton, Trans.). Princeton, NJ: Princeton University Press. [Original work published 1846.]

Levin, D. (1983). The poetic function in phenomenological discourse. In W. McBride & C. Schrag (Eds.), Phenomenology in a pluralistic context (pp. 216–234). Albany, NY: State University of New York Press.

McGraw, M-J. (2002). Watson's philosophy in nursing practice. In M.R. Alligood & A. Marriner Tomey (Eds.), Nursing theory: Utilization and application (2nd ed., pp. 97–121). St. Louis: Mosby.

Mitchell, G.J., & Cody, W.K. (1992). Nursing knowledge and human science: Ontological and epistemological considerations. Nursing Science Quarterly, 5, 54–61.

Mullaney, J.A.B. (2000). The lived experience of using Watson's actual caring occasion to treat depressed women. Journal of Holistic Nursing, 18, 129–142.

Mumford, L. (1970). The myth of the machine: The pentagon of power. New York: Harcourt Brace Jovanovich.

Nightingale, F. (1859). Notes on nursing: What it is, and what it is not. London: Harrison. [Reprinted 1946. Philadelphia: Lippincott.]

Robinson, S., Clump, D., Weitzel, T., Henderson, L., Lee, K., Schwartz, C., Egizii, P., & Metz, L. (2002). The Memorial Meals Mates: A program to improve nutrition in hospitalized older adults. Geriatric Nursing, 23, 332–335.

Rogers, C.R. (1959). A theory of therapy, personality, and interpersonal relationships, as developed in the client-centered framework. In S. Koch (Ed.), Psychology: A study of a science (Vol. 3, pp. 184–256). New York: McGraw-Hill.

Rogers, M.E. (1992). Nursing science and the space age. Nursing Science Quarterly, 5, 27–34.

Rogers, M.E. (1994). The science of unitary human beings: Current perspectives. Nursing Science Quarterly, 7, 33–35.

Sarter, B. (1988). Philosophical sources of nursing theory. Nursing Science Quarterly, 1, 52–59.

Sellers, S.C. (1991). A philosophical analysis of conceptual models of nursing. Dissertation Abstracts International, 52, 1937B. [University Microfilms No. AAC9126248.]

Smith, M.C. (1997). Nursing theory–guided practice: Practice guided by Watson's theory—The Denver Nursing Project in Human Caring. Nursing Science Quarterly, 10, 56–58.

Taylor, R. (1974). Metaphysics. Englewood Cliffs, NJ: Prentice-Hall.

Walker, L.O. (1989). Book review of Wastson, J. (1985). Nursing: Human science and human care. A theory of nursing. Nursing Science Quarterly, 2, 153–154.

Watson, J. (1979). Nursing: The philosophy and science of caring. Boston: Little, Brown.

Watson, J. (1985). Nursing: Human science and human care: A theory of nursing. Norwalk, CT: Appleton-Century-Crofts. [Reprinted 1988. New York: National League for Nursing.]

Watson, J. (1988a). Human caring as moral context for nursing education. Nursing and Health Care, 9, 422–425.

Watson, J. (1988b). New dimensions of human caring theory. Nursing Science Quarterly, 1, 175–181.

Watson, J. (1989a). Human caring and suffering: A subjective model for health sciences. In R.L. Taylor & J. Watson (Eds.), They shall not hurt: Human suffering and human caring (pp. 125–135). Boulder, CO: Colorado Associated University Press.

Watson, J. (1989b). Watson's philosophy and theory of human caring in nursing. In J.P. Riehl-Sisca (Ed.), Conceptual models for nursing practice (3rd ed., pp. 219–236). Norwalk, CT: Appleton & Lange.

Watson, J. (1990a). Human caring: A public agenda. In J.S. Stevenson & T. Tripp-Reimer (Eds.), Knowledge about care and caring. State of the art and future developments (pp. 41–48). Kansas City, MO: American Academy of Nursing.

Watson, J. (1990b). Transpersonal caring: A transcendent view of person, health, and nursing. In M.E. Parker (Ed.), Nursing theories in practice (pp. 277–288). New York: National League for Nursing.

Watson, J. (1992). Window on theory of human caring. In M. O'Toole (Ed.), Miller-Keane encyclopedia and dictionary of medicine, nursing, and allied health (5th ed., p. 1481). Philadelphia: Saunders.

Watson, J. (1995). Nursing's caring-healing paradigm as exemplar for alternative medicine? Alternative Therapies in Health and Medicine, 1(3), 64–69.

Watson, M.J. (1996). Watson's theory of transpersonal caring. In P. Hinton Walker & B. Neuman (Eds.), Blueprint for use of nursing models (pp. 141–184). New York: NLN Press.

Watson, J. (1997). The theory of human caring: Retrospective and prospective. Nursing Science Quarterly, 10, 49–52.

Watson, J. (1999). Postmodern nursing and beyond. New York: Churchill Livingstone.

Watson, J. (2001). Jean Watson: Theory of human caring. In M.E. Parker (Ed.), Nursing theories and nursing practice (pp. 343–354). Philadelphia: F.A. Davis.

Watson, J. (2002a). Assessing and measuring caring in nursing and health science. New York: Springer.

Watson, J. (2002b). Caring and healing our living and dying. The International Nurse, 15(2), 4–5.

Watson, J. (2002c). Nursing: Seeking its source and survival. [Guest Editorial.] ICUs and Nursing Web Journal, 9, 1–7. Available at: www. nursing.gr/(Click on Issue 9)

Watson, J. & Foster, R. (2003). The Attending Nurse Caring Model®: Integrating theory, evidence and advanced caring-healing therapeutics for transforming professional practice. Journal of Clinical Nursing, 12, 360–365.

Watson, J., & Phillips, S. (1992). A call for educational reform: Colorado nursing doctorate model as exemplar. Nursing Outlook, 40, 20–26.

Watson, J., & Smith, M.C. (2002). Caring science and the science of unitary human beings: A trans-theoretical discourse for nursing knowledge development. Journal of Advanced Nursing, 37, 452–461.

Whitehead, A.N. (1953). Science and the modern world. Cambridge: Cambridge University Press.

Zukav, G. (1990). The seat of the soul. New York: Fireside Books.

RESEARCH

Andershed, B., & Ternestedt, B-M. (1999). Involvement of relatives in care of the dying in different care cultures: Development of a theoretical understanding. Nursing Science Quarterly, 12, 45–51.

Baldursdottir, G., & Jonsdottir, H. (2002). The importance of nurse caring behaviors as perceived by patients receiving care at an emergency department. Heart and Lung, 31, 67–75.

Beauchamp, C.J. (1993). The centrality of caring: A case study. In P.L. Munhall & C.O. Boyd (Eds.), Nursing research: A qualitative perspective (2nd ed., pp. 338–358). New York: National League for Nursing.

Bishop, M.E. (1996). Nurses' knowledge, attitude may influence organ donation. Michigan Nurse, 69(5), 14.

Burns, P. (1991). Elements of spirituality and Watson's theory of transpersonal caring: Expansion of focus. In P.L. Chinn (Ed.), Anthology on caring (pp. 141–153). New York: National League for Nursing.

Chipman, Y. (1991). Caring: Its meaning and place in the practice of nursing. Journal of Nursing Education, 30, 171–175.

Clayton, G.M. (1989). Research testing Watson's theory: The phenomena of caring in an elderly population. In J.P. Riehl-Sisca (Ed.), Conceptual models for nursing practice (3rd ed., pp. 245–252). Norwalk, CT: Appleton & Lange.

Dennis, P.M. (1991). Components of spiritual nursing care from the nurse's perspective. Journal of Holistic Nursing, 9, 27–42.

Dorsey, C., Phillips, K.D., & Williams, C. (2001). Adult sickle cell patients' perceptions of nurses' caring behaviors. Association of Black Nursing Faculty Journal, 12, 95–100.

Duffy, J.R. (1992). The impact of nursing caring on patient outcomes. In D. Gaut (Ed.). The presence of caring in nursing (pp. 113–136). New York: National League for Nursing.

The findings of experimental studies suggest that use of the carative factors (now known as the CLINICAL CARITAS PROCESSES) resulted in increased quality of life and decreased systolic and diastolic blood pressure for patients with hypertension Erci, Sayan, Tortumluoglu, Kikiç, Sahin, & Güngörmüs, 2003)

Erci, B., Sayan, A., Tortumluoglu, G., Kikiç, D., Sahin, O, & Güngörmüs, Z. (2003). The effectiveness of Watson's caring model on the quality of life and blood pressure of patients with hypertension. Journal of Advanced Nursing, 41, 130–139.

Hinds, P.S. (1984). Inducing a definition of hope through the use of grounded theory methodology. Journal of Advanced Nursing, 9, 357–362.

Hoover, J. (2002). The personal and professional impact of undertaking an educational module on human caring. Journal of Advanced Nursing, 37, 79–86.

Jensen, K.P., Back-Pettersson, S.R., & Segesten, K.M. (1993). The caring moment and the green-thumb phenomenon among Swedish nurses. Nursing Science Quarterly, 6, 98–104.

Jensen, K.P., Back-Pettersson, S.R., & Segesten, K.M. (1996). "Catching my wavelength": Perceptions of the excellent nurse. Nursing Science Quarterly, 9, 115–120.

Johnson, P. (2002). The use of humor and its influences on spirituality and coping in breast cancer survivors. Oncology Nursing Forum, 29, 691–695.

Krysl, M., & Watson, J. (1988). Existential moments of caring: Facets of nursing and social support. Advances in Nursing Science, 10(2), 12–17.

Lemmer, C.M. (1991). Parental perceptions of caring following perinatal bereavement. Western Journal of Nursing Research, 13, 475–494.

Manogin, T.W., Bechtel, G.A., & Rami, J.S. (2000). Caring behaviors by nurses: Women's perceptions during childbirth. Journal of Obstetric, Gynecologic, and Neonatal Nursing, 29, 153–157.

Marini, B. (1999). Institutionalized older adults' perceptions of nurse caring behaviors: A pilot study. Journal of Gerontological Nursing, 25(5), 10–16.

McNamara, S.A. (1995). Perioperative nurses' perceptions of caring practices. Association of Operating Room Nurses Journal, 61, 377, 380–382, 384–385, 387–388. Hinojosa, R.J. (1996). Perioperative nurses' perceptions of caring practices: A research critique. Plastic Surgical Nursing, 16, 259–262.

Miller, B.K., Haber, J., & Byrne, M.W. (1992). The experience of caring in the acute care setting: Patient and nurse perspectives. In D. Gaut (Ed.), The presence of caring in nursing (pp. 137–155). New York: National League for Nursing.

Minnaar, A. (2001). Caring for the caregivers: A nursing management perspective. Curationis, 24(3), 19–26.

Mullaney, J.A.B. (2000). The lived experience of using Watson's actual caring occasion to treat depressed women. Journal of Holistic Nursing, 18, 129–142.

Nyman, C.S., & Lützen, K. (1999). Caring needs of patients with rheumatoid arthritis. Nursing Science Quarterly, 12, 14–169.

Parsons, E.C., Kee, C.C., & Gray, D.P. (1993). Perioperative nurse caring behaviors: Perceptions of surgical patients. Association of Operating Room Nurses Journal, 57, 1106–1107, 1110–1114.

Percy, M.S. (1995). Children from homeless families describe what is special in their lives. Holistic Nursing Practice, 9(4), 24–33.

Perry, B. (1998). Beliefs of eight exemplary oncology nurses related to Watson's nursing theory. Canadian Oncology Nursing Journal, 8, 97–101.

Robinson, S., Clump, D., Weitzel, T., et al. (2002). The Memorial Meals Mates: A program to improve nutrition in hospitalized older adults. Geriatric Nursing, 23, 332–335.

Rozario, P.S., & Zongonel, I.P.S. (2000). A proposal of nursing care with an educational focus for breasfeeding mothers. Revista Brasilerira De Enfermagem, 53, 401–409. [Portuguese; English abstract]

Running, A. (1997). Snapshots of experience: Vignettes from a nursing home. Journal of Advanced Nursing, 25, 117–122.

Ryan, P.Y. (1992). Perceptions of the most helpful nursing behaviors in a home-care hospice setting: Caregivers and nurses. American Journal of Hospice and Palliative Care, 9(5), 22–31.

Schindel-Martin, L. (1991). Using Watson's theory to explore the dimensions of adult polycystic kidney disease. American Nephrology Nurses' Association Journal, 18, 493–496.

Schroeder, C., & Neil, R.M. (1992). Focus groups: A humanistic means of evaluating an HIV/AIDS programme based on caring theory. Journal of Clinical Nursing, 1, 265–274.

Souza, S.M., & Lacerda, M.R. (2000). Home nursing transpersonal care to neoplastic patients and their families. Texto and Contexto Enfermagem, 9(2 Part 2), 726–736. [Portuguese; English abstract]

Smith, M.C., Kemp, J., Hemphill, L., & Vojir, C.P. (2002). Outcomes of therapeutic massage for hospitalized cancer patients. Journal of Nursing Scholarship, 34, 257–262.

Swanson, K.M. (1991). Empirical development of a middle range theory of caring. Nursing Research, 40, 161–166.

Tracy, J.P. (1997). Growing up with chronic illness: The experience of growing up with cystic fibrosis. Holistic Nursing Practice, 12(1), 27–35.

Watson, J. (1985a). Nursing: Human science and human care (pp. 84–89). Norwalk, CT: Appleton-Century-Crofts. [Second printing, 1988. Boulder, CO: Colorado Associated University Press. Third printing, 1988. New York: National League for Nursing.]

Watson, J. (1985b). Nursing: Human science and human care (pp. 89–100). Norwalk, CT: Appleton-Century-Crofts. [Second printing, 1988. Boulder, CO: Colorado Associated University Press. Third printing, 1988. New York: National League for Nursing.]

Watson, J. (1996). The wait, the wonder, the watch: Caring in a transplant unit. Journal of Clinical Nursing, 5, 199–200.

Weeks, S.K. (1995). What are the educational needs of prospective family caregivers of newly disabled adults? Rehabilitation Nursing, 20, 256–260, 272, 298.

Wikström, B.M. (2002). Nurses' strategies when providing for patients' aesthetic needs: Personal experiences of aesthetic means of expression. Clinical Nursing Research, 11, 22–33.

RESEARCH INSTRUMENTS AND PRACTICE TOOLS

Coates, C.J. (1997). The Caring Efficacy Scale: Nurses' self-reports of caring in practice settings. Advanced Practice Nursing Quarterly, 3(1), 53–59.

Cronin, S.N., & Harrison, B. (1988). Importance of nurse caring behaviors as perceived by patients after myocardial infarction. Heart and Lung, 17, 374–380.

Duffy, J.R. (1991). An analysis of the relationships among nurse caring behaviors and selected outcomes of care in hospitalized medical and/or surgical patients. Dissertation Abstracts International, 51, 3777B.

Duffy, J.R. (1992). The impact of nursing caring on patient outcomes. In D. Gaut (Ed.), The presence of caring in nursing (pp. 113–136). New York: National League for Nursing.

Duffy, J. (1993). Caring behaviors of nurse managers: Relationship to staff nurse satisfaction and retention. In D. Gaut (Ed.), A global agenda for caring (pp. 365–378). New York: National League for Nursing.

Harrison, B.P. (1988). Development of the caring behaviors assessment based on Watson's theory of caring. Master's Abstracts International, 27, 95.

McGraw, M-J. (2002). Watson's philosophy in nursing practice. In M.R. Alligood & A. Marriner Tomey (Eds.), Nursing theory: Utilization and application (2nd ed., pp. 97–121). St. Louis: Mosby.

Nyberg, J. (1989). Human care and economics: A nursing study. Dissertation Abstracts International, 50, 5549B.

Nyberg, J. (1990). The effects of care and economics on nursing practice. Journal of Nursing Administration, 20(5), 13–18.

Nyman, C.S., & Lützen, K. (1999). Caring needs of patients with rheumatoid arthritis. Nursing Science Quarterly, 12, 14–169.

Rafael, A.R.F. (2000). Watson's philosophy, science, and theory of human caring as a conceptual framework for guiding community health nursing practice. Advances in Nursing Science, 23(2), 34–49.

Stanfield, M.H. (1992). Watson's caring theory and instrument development. Dissertation Abstracts International, 52, 4128B.

Watson, M.J. (1996). Watson's theory of transpersonal caring. In P. Hinton Walker & B. Neuman (Eds.), Blueprint for use of nursing models [Ekebergh & Dahlberg cited, pp. 178–179]. New York: NLN Press.

Watson, J. (2002). Assessing and measuring caring in nursing and health science. New York: Springer.

Wolf, Z.R. (1986). The caring concept and nurse identified caring behaviors. Topics in Clinical Nursing, 8, 84–93.

Wolf, Z.R., Colahan, M., Costello, A., Warwick, F., Ambrose, M.S., & Giardino, E.R. (1998). Research utilization: Relationship between nurse caring and patient satisfaction. MEDSURG Nursing, 7, 99–105.

Wolf, Z.R., Giardino, E.R., Osborne, P.A., & Ambrose, M.S. (1994). Dimensions of nurse caring. Image: Journal of Nursing Scholarship, 26, 107–111.

Young, A., Taylor, S.G., & McLaughlin-Renpenning, K. (2001). Connections: Nursing research, theory, and practice. St. Louis: Mosby.

ADMINISTRATION

Astorino, G., Hecomovich, K., Jacobs, T., Laxson, L., Mauro, P., Neil, R.M., & Talley, S. (1994). The Denver Nursing Project in Human Caring. In J. Watson (Ed.), Applying the art and science of human caring (pp. 19–39). New York: National League for Nursing.

Brooks, B.A., & Rosenberg, S. (1995). Incorporating nursing theory into a nursing department strategic plan. Nursing Administration Quarterly, 20(1), 81–86.

Cappell, E., & Leggat, S. (1993). Implementation of theory-based nursing practice: Laying the groundwork for total quality management within a nursing department. Canadian Journal of Nursing Administration, 7, 31–41.

Leenerts, M.H., Koehler, J.A., & Neil, R.M. (1996). Nursing care models increase care quality while reducing costs. Journal of the Association of Nursing in AIDS Care, 7(4), 37–49.

Lyne, B.A., & Waller, P.R. (1990). The Denver Nursing Project in Human Caring: A model for AIDS nursing and professional education. Family and Community Health, 13, 78–84.

Marckx, B.B. (1995). Watson's theory of caring: A model for implementation in practice. Journal of Nursing Care Quality, 9(4), 43–54.

Minnaar, A. (2002). A framework for caring in the human resource management process of nurses. Curationis; South African Journal of Nursing, 25, 35–40.

Neil, R.M. (1995). Evidence in support of basing a nursing center on nursing theory: The Denver Nursing Project in Human Caring. In B. Murphy (Ed.), Nursing centers: The time is now (pp. 33–46). New York: National League for Nursing.

Neil, R.M. (2001). Caring for the human spirit in the workplace. In M.E. Parker (Ed.), Nursing theories and nursing practice (pp. 355–360). Philadelphia: F.A. Davis.

Nyberg, J. (1994). Implementing Watson's theory of caring. In J. Watson (Ed.), Applying the art and science of human caring (pp. 53–61). New York: National League for Nursing.

Quinn, J.F. (1994). Caring for the caregiver. In J. Watson (Ed.), Applying the art and science of human caring (pp. 63–71). New York: National League for Nursing.

Sanford, S., & Lamb, C.R. (1997). Nurse partners: Going beyond the delivery room. Mother Baby Journal, 2(6), 8–12.

Schroeder, C. (1993a). Cost effectiveness of a theory-based nurse-managed center for persons living with HIV/AIDS. In M.E. Parker (Ed.), Patterns of nursing theories in practice (pp. 159–179). New York: National League for Nursing.

Schroeder, C. (1993b). Nursing's response to the crisis of access, costs, and quality in health care. Advances in Nursing Science, 16(1), 1–20.

Schroeder, C., & Astorino, G. (1996). The Denver Nursing Education Project: Promoting the health of persons living with HIV/AIDS. In E.L. Cohen (Ed.), Nurse case management in the 21st century (pp. 63–67). St. Louis: Mosby.

Schroeder, C., & Maeve, M.K. (1992). Nursing care partnerships at the Denver Nursing Project in Human Caring: An application and extension of caring theory in practice. Advances in Nursing Science, 15(2), 25–38.

Schroeder, C., & Neil, R.M. (1992). Focus groups: A humanistic means of evaluating an HIV/AIDS programme based on caring theory. Journal of Clinical Nursing, 1, 265–274.

Smith, M.C. (1994). Case management in the caring-healing paradigm. In J. Watson (Ed.), Applying the art and science of human caring (pp. 47–52). New York: National League for Nursing.

Smith, M.C. (1997). Nursing theory–guided practice: Practice guided by Watson's theory—The Denver Nursing Project in Human Caring. Nursing Science Quarterly, 10, 56–58.

Snelson, C.M., Martsolf, D.S., Dieckman, B.C., Anaya, E.R.,

Cartechine, K.A., Miller, B., Roche, M., & Shaffer, J. (2002). Caring as a theoretical perspective for a nursing faculty mentoring program. Nurse Education Today, 22, 654–660.

Watson, M.J. (1996). Watson's theory of transpersonal caring. In P. Hinton Walker & B. Neuman (Eds.), Blueprint for use of nursing models (pp. 166–173). New York: NLN Press.

PRACTICE

Brandman, W. (1996). Intersubjectivity, social microcosm, and the here-and-now in a support group for nurses. Archives of Psychiatric Nursing, 10, 374–378.

Bollinger, E. (2001). Applied concepts of holistic nursing. Journal of Holistic Nursing, 19, 212–214.

Carson, M.G. (1992). An application of Watson's theory to group work with the elderly. Perspectives, 16(4), 7–13.

Gullo, S. (1997). Oncology nurses: Masters in the art of caring. Oncology Nursing Forum, 24, 971–978.

Harrison, R.L. (1997). Spirituality and hope: Nursing implications for people with human immunodeficiency virus disease. Holistic Nursing Practice, 12(1), 9–16.

Hubner, L.L. (1999). Nurses as caregivers of bereaved individuals: Applying Watson's theory. DNA Reporter, 24(3), 8–9.

Jones, S.B. (1991). A caring-based AIDS educational model for pre-adolescents: Global health human caring perspective. Journal of Advanced Nursing, 16, 591–596.

McGraw, M-J. (2002). Watson's philosophy in nursing practice. In M.R. Alligood & A. Marriner Tomey (Eds.), Nursing theory: Utilization and application (2nd ed., pp. 97–121). St. Louis: Mosby.

Mendyka, B.E. (1993). The dying patient in the intensive care unit: Assisting the family in crisis. AACN Clinical Issues in Critical Care Nursing, 4, 550–557.

Montgomery, C. (1994). The caring/healing relationship of "maintaining authentic caring." In J. Watson (Ed.), Applying the art and science of human caring (pp. 39–45). New York: National League for Nursing.

Neil, R.M. (1994). Authentic caring: The sensible answer for clients and staff dealing with HIV/AIDS. Nursing Administration Quarterly, 18(2), 36–40.

Nelson-Marten, P., Hecomovich, K., & Prangle, M. (1998). Caring theory: A framework for advanced practice nursing. Advanced Practice Nursing Quarterly, 4(1), 70–71.

Saxton, M. (1994). How could theory affect practice? Nursing Praxis in New Zealand, 9(1), 13–17.

Sithichoke-Rattan, N. (1989). A clinical application of Watson's theory. Pediatric Nursing, 15, 458–462.

Sterritt, P.F., & Pokorney, M.E. (1994). Art activities for patients with Alzheimer's and related disorders. Geriatric Nursing, 15, 155–159.

Weiser, M.L. (1992). Caring and hope for Jon. Imprint, 39, 120, 19.

Wykle, M.L, & Morris, D.L. (1994). Nursing care in Alzheimer's disease. Clinics in Geriatric Medicine, 10, 351–365.

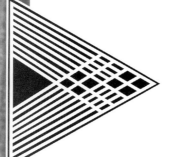

Part Four

NURSING KNOWLEDGE IN THE 21st CENTURY

Part Four introduces the reader to the possibilities of nursing knowledge now and in the future.

Chapter 17, the last chapter in this book, offers the reader an opportunity to consider a strategy to promote the integration of nursing knowledge with nursing research and nursing practice and to explore the future of the discipline of nursing.

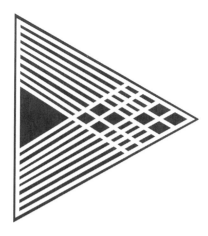

Chapter **17**

Integrating Nursing Models, Theories, Research, and Practice

The use of explicit conceptual models of nursing and nursing theories fosters a systematic approach to nurses' activities. The use of any one nursing model or theory—or of a comprehensive conceptual-theoretical-empirical system (C-T-E system) of nursing knowledge (see Chapter 2)—can easily close the theory-practice and research-practice gaps. This final chapter begins with a discussion of nursing as a professional discipline. Next, the value of nursing discipline-specific C-T-E systems is discussed. The chapter continues with presentation of a strategy for the integration of C-T-E systems, nursing research, and nursing practice. The chapter concludes with a proposal that will enhance the probability of the survival of the discipline of nursing.

Overview

The professional discipline of nursing is mandated by society not only to develop and disseminate nursing knowledge but also to use that knowledge to improve the well-being of human beings. Nursing knowledge is formalized in conceptual models of nursing and nursing theories. Chapters 4 through 10 and 12 through 17 of this book present discussions of the development of the most widely recognized conceptual models of nursing and nursing theories and bibliographies that document the dissemination of those nursing models and theories. Those chapters also document the utilization of each nursing model or theory as a guide to the separate activities of nursing research, education, administration, and practice. The major components of this chapter, which emphasizes the integration of nursing research and nursing practice within the content of ex-

plicit nursing discipline-specific C-T-E systems, are listed here. Each component is described in detail in the chapter.

Key Terms

THE DISCIPLINE OF NURSING
    Professional Discipline
    Academic Discipline
    Nursing Science and the Nursing Profession
    Nursing Research and Nursing Practice
        C-T-E System Development and
            Dissemination
        C-T-E System Utilization and Evaluation
            in Practice
    Discipline-Specific Research
    Discipline-Specific Methodologies
    Discipline-Specific Practice

THE DISCIPLINE OF NURSING

The term discipline comes from the Latin *disciplina,* meaning a branch of instruction or learning (Simpson & Weiner, 1989). Some scholars maintain that disciplines exist and are distinguished by the subject matter of interest to their members (e.g., Schwab, 1962; Walton, 1963). The subject matter of a discipline, according to Walton (1963), encompasses "concepts, facts, and theories, so ordered that it can be deliberately and systematically taught" (p. 5). Elaborating, Scheffler (1963) maintained that disciplines are "branches of knowledge or bodies of science ... [that strive] to offer a complete, systematic account of some realm of things in the world. [Each discipline] seeks a comprehensive body of true principles describing and explaining the realm it takes as its proper object" (p. 49). Meleis (1997) stated that a discipline "provides a unique way of considering the phenomena that are of interest to its members" (p. 42). Shermis (1962) added that what he called intellectual disciplines are characterized by "(1) a rather impressive body of time-tested works, (2) a technique suitable for dealing with their concepts, (3) a defensible claim to being an intimate link with basic human activities and aspirations, (4) a tradition that both links the present with the past and provides inspiration and sustenance for the future, [and] (5) a considerable achievement in both eminent men [sic] and significant ideas" (p. 84). According to those scholars, each discipline claims a distinctive body of knowledge and specifies the ways in which that knowledge is generated and tested, that is, the way in which knowledge is developed.

Peters (1963), in contrast, regards the idea of disciplines having subject matter as "an archaic relic of the old Baconian myth about scientific method" (p. 17). He went on to say that "A discipline develops when there are some reasonably well-worked out and structured answers to such questions which come to form a body of knowledge, together with techniques and procedures for developing better answers or for dealing with new problems which these answers give rise to" (pp. 17–18). Peters' point is that disciplines exist but are not distinguished by what he understands to be subject matter. Instead, for Peters, disciplines are distinguished by the questions asked, the answers to those questions, and the methods used to obtain the answers, all of which constitute a body of knowledge that can be taught and learned. Kuethe (1963) argued that disciplines are not distinguished by unique bodies of knowledge nor can they be identified by unique methods of inquiry. He maintained that a discipline is distinguished by its unique concern with "certain relations between facts" (p. 76).

Regardless of one's position, the designation of discipline has come to be a way of organizing knowledge. The designation of discipline also has some utility as an administrative structure for education. Within colleges and universities, for example, disciplines frequently are divided into separate schools and departments, such as nursing, psychology, sociology, education, and physics. Within health-care institutions, disciplines frequently are divided into departments, such as nursing and physical therapy.

Nursing, according to Donaldson and Crowley (1978), is a **Professional Discipline**. The term, profession, refers to a vocation requiring knowledge of some branch of learning (Simpson & Weiner, 1989). Professions are constrained by certain standards, policies, and regulations imposed by society.

Donaldson and Crowley (1978) explained that a professional discipline has a societal mandate to conduct what they labeled basic research, applied research, and clinical research. Thus, the professional discipline of nursing is responsible not only for the generation and dissemination of new knowledge (basic research) and the determination of the limits of that knowledge in various situations (applied research) but also for the determination of the effects of nursing practices (clinical research). Education, engineering, and physical therapy are examples of other professional disciplines. **Academic Disciplines**, in contrast, are responsible only for basic and applied research. Physics, chemistry, biology, psychology, and sociology are examples of academic disciplines.

Donaldson and Crowley's (1978) assertion that nursing is a professional discipline remained unchallenged for more than 20 years. Recently, however, Parse (Fawcett, 2001) stated that she disagrees with Donaldson and Crowley's assertion. She prefers to separate the discipline from the profession. In particular, she maintained that the discipline is a basic science and the knowledge base of nursing, and that the goal of the discipline is to "expand knowledge about human experiences through research and creative conceptualization" (Fawcett, 2001, p. 127). Parse maintained that the profession of nursing, in contrast, "consists of persons educated in the discipline according to nationally defined, regulated, and monitored standards. People join the profession and practice the performing art" (Fawcett, 2001, p. 127). Although Parse's position certainly has merit, the notion of a professional discipline as one entity, albeit with two dimensions, is used in this book.

The two dimensions of the professional discipline of nursing are nursing science and the nursing profession (Fig. 17–1). **Nursing Science** is accomplished by means of **Nursing Research**. The product of nursing research is *C-T-E System Development and Dissemination*. **The Nursing Profession** is actualized through **Nursing Practice**. The major activity of nursing practice is *C-T-E System Utilization and Evaluation in Practice*.

As depicted in Figure 17–1, the relation between **Nursing Science** and the **Nursing Profession** is reciprocal, as is the relation between **Nursing Research** and **Nursing Practice** and the relation between C-T-E system development and dissemination and C-T-E system utilization and evaluation in practice. The reciprocal relation means that although the knowledge contained in a C-T-E system is "the most important source of influence on practice" (Kerlinger, 1979, p. 296) and "practice is the medium for transforming nursing science knowledge from the world of ideas into the world of events" (Rawnsley, 2003, p. 11), the

results of utilizing knowledge in practice are used to refine the C-T-E knowledge system. In other words, the reciprocal relation means that the C-T-E systems developed through research are used in practice, and the outcomes of utilization of the C-T-E systems are used to refine those C-T-E systems. The reciprocal relation also can be seen when practical problems act as a catalyst for C-T-E-based research, the results of research suggest solutions for the problems, and the results of tests of those solutions in practice influence the further development of the C-T-E knowledge system.

Recognition of a reciprocal relation between the development and utilization of C-T-E systems underscores that C-T-E systems are *not* "engraved in tablets of stone" (Kalideen, 1993, p. 5). Indeed, the development and dissemination of a C-T-E system informs and transforms the ways in which practice is understood and experienced, and the utilization and evaluation of that C-T-E system informs and transforms the C-T-E system by informing and transforming its further development (Speedy, 1989).

Recognition of nursing as a distinct discipline confers a certain status on nurses. The status conferred by being a member of the professional discipline of nursing, rather than of an occupation or a trade, carries with it the responsibility to develop, disseminate, use, and evaluate explicit nursing discipline-specific C-T-E systems. In particular, the responsibility and goal of the professional discipline of nursing is to conduct **Discipline-Specific Research** (Mitchell, 1994), using **Discipline-Specific Methodologies** (Thorne, Kirkham, & MacDonald-Emes, 1997) and to engage in **Discipline-Specific Practice** (Smith, 1995).

Anderson (1995) explained that as members of a professional discipline, nurses "must ensure that we have a solid scholarly and scientific foundation upon which to base our practice" (p. 247). The development and dissemination of explicit C-T-E systems already is a hallmark of success in nursing theory development (Fawcett, 1983). But nurses must continue the development of existing nursing discipline-specific C-T-E systems and must develop new ones if the discipline is to thrive.

The use of nursing discipline-specific C-T-E systems "distinguishes nursing as an autonomous health profession" and represents "nursing's unique contribution to the health care system" (Parse, 1995, p. 128). The use of explicit C-T-E systems as guides for nursing practice already is a hallmark of professional nursing practice (Fawcett & Carino, 1989). But it is incumbent on *all* nurses to continue to use and to evaluate explicit nursing discipline-specific C-T-E systems if the professional discipline of nursing is to retain its rightful place in the multidisciplinary health-care arena.

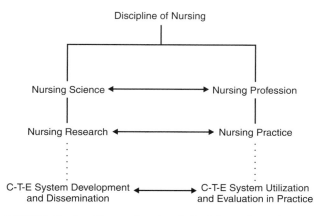

FIGURE 17–1. The professional discipline of nursing: reciprocal relations between nursing science and the nursing profession, nursing research and nursing practice, and C-T-E system development/dissemination and C-T-E system utilization/evaluation.

THE VALUE OF NURSING DISCIPLINE-SPECIFIC C-T-E SYSTEMS

The rapid growth of advanced practice nursing programs, especially nurse practitioner programs, during the last decade of the 20th century and continuing into the early years of the 21st century, has diverted attention away from nursing discipline-specific C-T-E systems and toward a medical perspective as the base for research and practice. Consequently, nursing, along with human experiences of health, have been medicalized (Chinn, 1999), and nursing practice tends to be evaluated within the context of medical outcomes rather than outcomes identified by *nursing* conceptual models and theories. Furthermore, independent functioning as a nurse has been equated with performing skills that physicians perform (McBride, 1999). Indeed, some nurse practitioners, clinical specialists, nurse midwives, and nurse anesthetists strive to become "quasi practitioners of medicine" (Orlando, 1987, p. 412), physician's assistants (Martha Rogers, as cited in Huch, 1995), physician substitutes (McBride, 1999), physician extenders (Sandelowski, 1999), junior doctors (Meleis, 1993), mini-doctors (Barnum, 1998), or pseudo doctors (Kendrick, 1997), engaged in nursing-qua-medicine (Watson, 1996) and primary care medicine, rather than primary care nursing (Barrett, 1993). Those nurses who emulate physicians most likely do so because "the lure of following the medical model is sanctioned and well rewarded in some settings" (Hawkins & Thibodeau, 1996, p. 11). In essence, then, so-called advanced nursing practice may represent limited medical practice rather than full nursing practice, and many nurses, as Sandelowski (1999) pointed out, continue to perform work that relieves deliberately controlled shortages of physicians, which preserves their market value but has lead to an oversupply of nurse practitioners (Anderson, 1999; Barnum, 1998).

Clearly, it is mandatory that the value of using nursing discipline-specific C-T-E systems to guide nursing practice is underscored, so that all nurses can become *nursing* practitioners (Orem, 2001), senior nurses (Meleis, 1993), and maximally functioning nurses (Barnum, 1998) who have the freedom and autonomy (Hawkins & Thibodeau, 1996) that comes from engaging in nursing-qua-nursing (Watson, 1997). Fortunately, the number of nurses throughout the world who recognize **THE VALUE OF NURSING DISCIPLINE-SPECIFIC C-T-E SYSTEMS** is rapidly increasing. Indeed, Cash's (1990) claim that "there is no central core that can distinguish nursing theoretically from a number of other occupational activities" (p. 255) has been readily offset by many claims to the contrary, including the numerous publications cited in the references and bibliography for each chapter of this book.

Furthermore, as Chalmers (as cited in Chalmers et al., 1990) pointed out, "Nursing models [and theories] have provided what many would argue is a much needed alternative knowledge base from which nurses can practice in an informed way. An alternative, that is, to the medical [perspective] which for so many years has dominated many aspects of health care" (p. 34). Nursing discipline-specific C-T-E systems also provide an alternative to the institutional model of practice, in which "the most salient values [are] efficiency, standardized care, rules, and regulations" (Rogers, 1989, p. 113). The institutional model, moreover, typically upholds, reinforces, and supports a medical perspective (Grossman & Hooton, 1993).

Nursing discipline-specific C-T-E systems collectively identify the distinctive nursing territory within the vast arena of health care (Feeg, 1989). Each nursing model and theory provides a holistic orientation that reminds nurses of the concepts and propositions of the metaparadigm of nursing (see Chapter 1) and reinforces the view that nursing practice ultimately is "for our patients' sake" (Dabbs, 1994, p. 220). Admittedly, some nurses believe that nursing conceptual models are "dinosaurs that are irrelevant for contemporary research and practice" (Fawcett, 2003, p. 229), or hold the "unfortunate view [that nursing models and theories] are the inventions and predictions only of scholars and academics [and have] little significance for their own practice environments" (Hayne, 1992, p. 105). Many other nurses, however, recognize the beneficial effects of nursing models and theories on practice. Indeed, nursing discipline-specific C-T-E system-based nursing practice "help[s] nurses better communicate what they do" (Neff, 1991, p. 534) and why they do it.

In particular, nursing discipline-specific C-T-E systems provide a nursing knowledge base that has a positive effect on practice "by enabling well-coordinated [nursing] to take place, by providing a basis for the justification of [nursing] actions and by enabling [all] nurses to *talk nursing*" (Chalmers, as cited in Chalmers et al., 1990, p. 34), to *think nursing* (Nightingale, 1993; Perry, 1985), and to engage in *thinking nursing* (Allison & Renpenning, 1999) rather than just doing tasks and carrying out physicians' orders (Le Storti et al., 1999). Nurses are able to talk nursing and think nursing because the nursing models and theories and methodologies that make up C-T-E systems provide a distinctive nursing language. The lack of a nursing language in the past, and in the present when nursing models and theories are not used "has been a handicap in nurses' communications about nursing to the public as well as to persons with whom they work in the health field" (Orem, 1997, p. 29).

Thinking nursing within the context of nursing discipline-specific C-T-E systems helps nurses in various specialties to "clarify their thinking on their role, especially at a time when the roles of many health professionals are becoming blurred" (Nightingale, 1993, p. 2). Moreover, thinking nursing within the context of nursing discipline-specific C-T-E systems may shape the way in which specialized nursing practice is viewed. Nurses may elect to specialize in the use of a particular nursing model or theory as the starting point for construction of C-T-E systems; or nurses may elect to specialize in a particular concept of a particular nursing model or theory. A nurse could, for example, specialize in one behavioral subsystem of Johnson's Behavioral System Model (Rogers, 1973).

Research findings indicate that nurses feel vulnerable and experience a great deal of stress as they attempt to achieve professional aspirations within a constantly changing, medically-dominated, bureaucratic health-care delivery system (Graham, 1994; Mark, 2002). As structures for critical thinking within a distinctively nursing context, nursing discipline-specific C-T-E systems provide the intellectual and organizational skills that nurses need to survive during times when cost containment through reduction of professional nursing staff is the *modus operandi* of managed care and the administrators of health-care delivery systems, including hospitals, home health-care agencies, and health maintenance organizations. Nursing discipline-specific C-T-E systems also provide the intellectual and organizational skills that nurses need to survive during times of nursing shortages (Mitchell, 2003). That is because C-T-E systems represent structures for thinking coherently and organizing practice consistently and efficiently, which allows the required time for direct care of those who need nursing.

Johnson (1990) noted that, although individual nurses and nursing departments take risks when the decision is made to use an explicit nursing discipline-specific C-T-E system to guide nursing practice, the rewards far outweigh the risks. She stated:

> To openly use a nursing model is risk-taking behavior for the individual nurse. For a nursing department to adopt one of these models for unit or institution use is risk-taking behavior of an even higher order. The reward for such risk-taking for the individual practitioner lies in the great satisfaction gained from being able to specify explicit concrete *nursing goals* in the care of patients and from documenting the actual achievement of the desired outcomes. The reward for the nursing department is having a rational, cohesive, and comprehensive basis for the development of standards of nursing practice, for the evaluation of practitioners, and for the documentation of the contribution of nursing to patient welfare. (p. 32)

The continually accumulating anecdotal and empirical evidence cited in Chapters 4 through 10 and 12 through 16 indicates that additional rewards of using explicit nursing discipline-specific C-T-E systems to guide nursing practice include reduced staff nurse turnover, more rapid movement from novice to expert nurse, increased patient and family satisfaction with nursing, increased nurse job satisfaction, and considerable cost savings. Furthermore, as the use of C-T-E systems moves nursing practice from a base of implicit knowledge to explicit nursing knowledge, both nurses and participants in nursing are empowered. Indeed, "[nursing] knowledge is power" (Orr, 1991, p. 218), and the power of nursing knowledge can be used to empower individuals, families, and communities to fully participate in decisions about their health care (Lister, 1991; Malin & Teasdale, 1991). The challenge, then, is to use the strategies identified in Chapter 2 to help each nurse to adopt an explicit nursing discipline-specific C-T-E system and each health-care organization to implement nursing discipline-specific C-T-E systems.

 ## INTEGRATING C-T-E SYSTEMS, RESEARCH, AND PRACTICE

Earlier in this chapter, the relation between C-T-E system development and dissemination and C-T-E system utilization and evaluation in practice was described as reciprocal. A reciprocal relation means that two discrete entities interact with one another. Viewing C-T-E system development and dissemination and C-T-E system utilization and evaluation in practice as discrete yet interacting entities certainly has merit. But how much more might be accomplished if the two entities were viewed as one integrated process? It is proposed that the development, dissemination, utilization, and evaluation of nursing knowledge in the form of explicit nursing discipline-specific C-T-E systems can best be advanced through the integration of nursing research and nursing practice, which can best be advanced through the integration of nursing science and the nursing profession. Figure 17–2, which is an alternative to Figure 17–1, presents an integrated view of the dimensions of the professional discipline of nursing and the activities associated with the dimensions. Here, the dimensions of nursing science and the nursing profession are regarded as integrated, as are the research and practice activities that flow from those integrated dimensions and the C-T-E system activities that flow from the integration of research and practice. Note that the integration of nursing research and practice means that research is practice and practice is research.

Integrating C-T-E systems, research, and practice is a seemingly complex activity that has, to date, eluded most nurses, as the integration of research and practice has eluded most members of other professional disciplines. Integration, however, can be straightforward. **A STRATEGY TO INTEGRATE C-T-E SYSTEMS, RESEARCH, AND PRACTICE** is to use an explicit nursing discipline-specific C-T-E system to guide nursing practice and to use

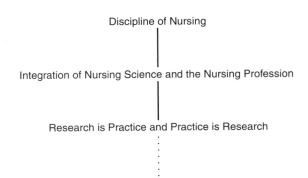

FIGURE 17–2. The professional discipline of nursing—an alternative view: integration of nursing science and the nursing profession, nursing research and nursing practice, and C-T-E system development/dissemination and C-T-E system utilization/evaluation.

practice information gained from the implementation of that C-T-E system as research data for **Single-Case Studies.** In other words, every nursing situation for the purpose of the delivery of nursing services also is for the purpose of research. Every nursing situation, then, is a single-case study of an experiment in which the intervention is hypothesized to have a certain outcome (Feinstein, 1967; Wood, 1978). Thus, the data available in every nursing practice situation are used to refine or reject existing C-T-E systems and to develop new C-T-E systems. The steps of the single-case study approach are listed here.

- Develop a prototype conceptual-theoretical-empirical system of nursing knowledge (C-T-E system) for a population of nursing participants.
- Develop an individualized C-T-E system for a particular nursing participant.
- Provide nursing in accordance with the practice methodology of the C-T-E system.
- Document all aspects of the application of the practice methodology.
- Use the documented information about C-T-E system-based nursing actions and the outcome for the nursing participant as single-case study research data.

The key to the integration of research and practice is recognition and acceptance of the similarity between the process of research and the process of practice, and recognition and acceptance that both research and practice are guided by the same C-T-E system. Drawing from discussions of nursing practice and nursing research

(Whitney & Roncoli, 1986), social work research and casework processes (Wood, 1978), the science and art of medicine (Feinstein, 1967), the interests of industrial management theorists-researchers and practitioners (Dubin, 1976), and the purposes of documentation (Johnson, Ludwig-Beymer, & Micek, 1999), the steps of the nursing process, or the components of a practice methodology, can be viewed as the steps of the nursing research process. That is, "The processes of [practice] … are exactly the same processes as those of research" (Wood, 1978, p. 454). Even more to the point, "A clinician performs an experiment every time he [or she] treats a patient. … [Thus,] every aspect of clinical management can be designed, executed, and appraised with intellectual procedures identical to those used in any experimental situation" (Feinstein, 1967, pp. 14, 21).

Nurses who are engaged in nursing practice, then, are researchers (Fawcett, Aber, & Weiss, 2003; Rolfe, 1993; Whitney & Roncoli, 1986), and nursing participants are their own controls in quasi-experimental single-case studies guided by explicit nursing discipline-specific C-T-E systems. Within the context of a particular C-T-E system, the **Nursing Practice Process** is the same as the **Nursing Research Process** (Table 17–1). Thus, the results of *Assessment* comprise the *Baseline Data*. The *Labeling* used to summarize the nursing participant's health condition represents the *Statement of the Problem* to be studied. *Goal Setting* represents the *Hypothesis* that specifies the desired nurse-sensitive outcome and the means to achieve that outcome. The desired outcome is the dependent variable, and the means to achieve that outcome is the independent variable. *Implementation* is the means to achieve the outcome, that is, the intervention or the *Experimental Treatment*, which is the independent variable. *Evaluation* is analysis of the desired *Nurse-Sensitive Outcome*, that is, the dependent variable. Written or computerized documentation of each step of the nursing practice process provides the actual data from which a conclusion regarding the hypothesis may be drawn.

The generic nursing practice process listed in Table 17–1 is replaced by the components of the particular practice methodology associated with the nursing model or theory of the C-T-E system. The practice methodologies associated with the nursing models and theories included in this book are presented in Chapters 4 through 10 and 12 through 16. The practice tools and research instruments derived from each nursing model and nursing theory, also presented in Chapters 4 through 10 and 12 through 16, should be used to collect and record information for the assessment, labeling, goal-setting, and evaluation steps of the nursing practice process that will then be used for the single-case study. Thus, practice tools are useful for re-

TABLE 17–1
THE PARALLEL BETWEEN THE NURSING PRACTICE PROCESS AND THE NURSING RESEARCH PROCESS

Nursing Practice Process*	Nursing Research Process
Assessment	Baseline data
Labeling	Statement of the problem
Goal setting	Hypothesis
Desired nurse-sensitive outcome	Dependent variable
Means to achieve outcome	Independent variable
Implementation of intervention	Experimental treatment Independent variable
Evaluation	Nurse-sensitive outcome
Outcome actually achieved	Dependent variable
Documentation of practice information	Record of data to be analyzed Conclusion regarding hypothesis

*See Chapters 4 through 10 and 12 through 16 for the practice methodologies associated with particular nursing models and theories.

search purposes, and research instruments can be examined for their utility in practice situations.

Here it is important to emphasize that practice tools and research instruments derived from *nursing* conceptual models and theories be used. Using tools and instruments from other disciplines, which Jukes (1988) found to be favored by some nurses, does not allow the nurse to collect and record the information needed for *nursing* practice processes.

The experimental treatment, that is, the intervention, should be written in the form of a script that specifies exactly how the goal will be achieved for the particular nursing participant. The script then is viewed as a research protocol. Any necessary deviations from the *a priori* script for the intervention should be recorded, so that it is possible to link what was to be done with what actually was done and with what outcome occurred.

Single-case studies can be aggregated for the purposes of quality assurance or quality improvement programs. The use of an explicit nursing discipline-specific C-T-E system to guide each case study ensures that the outcome is a nurse-sensitive outcome. That is, the outcome is directly associated with a nursing assessment, a nursing label, and a nursing intervention. Thus, quality assurance and quality improvement programs dealing with nursing yield data that are relevant to nursing. The long–sought-after and

much-desired **Evidence-Based Best Practices** (Anderson, 1998a; Fagin, 1998) are the collective result of both single-case studies and quality assurance or quality improvement programs.

A PROPOSAL TO ENHANCE SURVIVAL OF THE DISCIPLINE OF NURSING

The discipline of nursing may be on the brink of extinction (Fawcett, 2000; Nagle, 1999; Mitchell, 1994; Watson & Foster, 2003). If the discipline is to survive, nurses cannot take pride in or be satisfied with practicing "atheoretically" or apply nursing knowledge "without conscious recognition" (Lenz, 1998, p. 63). They cannot continue to condone the disparagement of nursing knowledge that occurs all too frequently in practice settings (Lenz, 1998). Instead, nurses must be proactive in convincing themselves and their colleagues that utilization of explicit nursing discipline-specific C-T-E systems of nursing knowledge is *not* "difficult, boring, [or] esoteric" (Lenz, 1998, p. 64) but rather easy, stimulating, and understood by all nurses. The discipline of nursing will continue to exist and thrive in the 21st century *only* if nurses use explicit nursing discipline-specific C-T-E systems to guide practice and conduct research to determine the effectiveness of those C-T-E systems in achieving specified goals. **A PROPOSAL TO ENHANCE SURVIVAL OF THE DISCIPLINE OF NURSING** is offered. The components of the proposal are **Nurse Scholars, Nurse Corporations,** and **Nurse Entrepreneurs.**

NURSE SCHOLARS

It is proposed that nursing is more likely to continue to exist and thrive as a discipline if nursing research and nursing practice are integrated within the context of nursing discipline-specific C-T-E systems. It is further proposed that the integration of nursing research and nursing practice within the context of C-T-E systems is more likely to occur if the roles of researcher and practitioner are integrated into the single role of **Nurse Scholar.** The essential characteristics of **Nurse Scholars** are given here.

- Nurse Scholars are first and foremost nurses who *think nursing,* "because nursing first and foremost is a *thinking* [discipline]" (Anderson, 1998b, p. 198).
- Nurse Scholars "have the courage to take a position about why people need nursing and about what nursing can and should be" (Orem, 2001, p. 470).
- Nurse Scholars are knowledge workers (Cappell, & Leggat, 1994) who understand that an explicit nursing discipline-specific C-T-E system is an intellectual and practical framework that fosters talking nursing and thinking nursing.
- Nurse Scholars understand that talking nursing and thinking nursing are the keys to integrating nursing research and nursing practice, which, in turn, is the key to evidence-based best practices that will improve the well-being of human beings.
- Nurse Scholars understand that development, dissemination, utilization, and evaluation of explicit nursing discipline-specific C-T-E systems is the only way in which the discipline of nursing can demonstrate its distinctive contributions to the well-being of human beings.
- Nurse Scholars understand that development, dissemination, utilization, and evaluation of explicit nursing discipline-specific C-T-E systems is the only way that nursing can move from a "silent service" recognized primarily by its absence (Allison & Renpenning, 1999, p. 26) to a very visible and vocal public service, the need for which is widely recognized.
- Nurse Scholars understand that nursing has "no dependent functions … [but rather] like all other professions, nursing has many collaborative functions, which are indispensable to providing society with a higher order of service than any one profession can offer" (Rogers, 1985, p. 381).

- Nurse Scholars understand that "each profession has the knowledge, competence, or prerogative to delegate anything to another profession. Each profession is responsible for determining its own boundaries within the context of social need" (Rogers, 1985, p. 381).
- Nurse Scholars understand that, collectively, the development, dissemination, utilization, and evaluation of explicit nursing discipline-specific C-T-E systems is the way in which nursing is explained and the distinctive contributions nurses make to collaborative practice and multidisciplinary research are demonstrated and documented. Thus, the development, dissemination, utilization, and evaluation of explicit nursing discipline-specific C-T-E systems will end the journey on the dependent path that has led to nurses functioning primarily as handmaidens to physicians and will facilitate the journey along the independent path of professional nursing (Orlando, 1987).
- Nurse Scholars function as attending nurses, that is, nurses who are with people continuously wherever they are—"in and outside of institutions, schools, homes, clinics, and community settings" (Watson, 1996, p. 163). Thus, each participant in nursing always has his or her own Nurse Scholar, who collaborates with other health professionals when the participant requires services from others. Attending nurses, of course, integrate research and practice within the context of explicit nursing discipline-specific C-T-E systems. The Attending Nurse Caring Model®, which is based on Watson's Theory of Human Caring (see Chapter 16), is just one example of how attending nurses might function and enhance nursing practice in service to human beings (Watson & Foster, 2003).

The depth and breath of knowledge needed by Nurse Scholars mandate post-baccalaureate education. In other words, the education required for entry into professional nursing should be the doctorate of nursing (ND) (Fawcett, 1999; Fawcett & Bourbonniere, 2001; Rawnsley, 2003).

NURSE CORPORATIONS AND NURSE ENTREPRENEURS

Nurse Scholars may work in **Nurse Corporations,** which are made up of Nurse Scholars in equal partnership with one another, or they may elect to be self-employed **Nurse Entrepreneurs.** Nurse corporations and self-employed nurse entrepreneurs contract with individuals, families, communities, medical centers, community and specialty hospitals, home care agencies, hospices, and other agencies and institutions for the provision of distinctively nursing services guided by explicit nursing discipline--ecific C-T-E systems. The idea of nurse corporations is not new. Indeed, Sills (1983) initially proposed that idea more than 20 years ago:

> The conceptual key to the corporation proposal is that it changes the fundamental nature of the social contract. The professional nurse would no longer be an employee of the hospital or agency, but rather a member of a professional corporation which provides nursing services to patients and clients on a fee-for-service basis. ... Such a change in the nature of the social contract is, it seems to me, fundamentally necessary for the survival of nursing as a profession rather than an occupational group of workers employed by other organizations (Sills, 1983, p. 573).

Nurse corporations are a solution to the problem of collective bargaining by nurses (Sills, 1983). Contracts are between the nurse corporation, which is a professional entity rather than a union, and individuals or organizations. Nurse corporations also are an organizational way to address the economics of nursing practice (Sills, 1983), because nurse corporations operate on a fee-for-(nursing) service basis. Thus, nurses determine the cost for their distinctive services and charge individuals and organizations directly for those services.

Nurse Scholars, whether in nurse corporations or self-employed entrepreneurs, also act as mentors for students. Indeed, the integration of research and practice within the context of nursing discipline-specific C-T-E systems most likely would be greatly facilitated and the emotional and cognitive difficulties inherent in perspective transformation (see Chapter 2) might be reduced or eliminated if the process of learning and applying explicit nursing discipline-specific C-T-E systems were taught in an explicit manner in nursing education programs by Nurse Scholars who serve as role models for students. The curricula of some schools of nursing in the United States and other countries already are based on one or more nursing models or theories (see Chapters 4 through 10 and 12 through 16, and many schools offer at least one required or elective course dealing with nursing models and theories. Yet little attention is paid to the process underlying learning the content of any nursing model or theory and the process of using an explicit nursing discipline-specific C-T-E system to guide nursing practice and nursing research (McEwen, 2000). Even less attention is given to the integration of nursing practice and research (McEwen, 2000). It is, therefore, recommended that relevant courses include content on the substantive and process elements of implementing C-T-E system-based nursing practice (see Chapter 2), as well as content on strategies to integrate nursing practice and nursing research, such as the single-case study method described in this chapter.

 ## CONCLUSION

In conclusion, as Parse (1999) so eloquently declared, "Nursing knowledge-based practice is not something 'I put on.' It shows itself in 'what I am' to the other" (p. 1385). Nursing knowledge-based practice (that is, practice based on explicit nursing discipline-specific C-T-E systems) not only shows the "What I am" of each nurse to the public and other health professionals but also shows potential applicants to nursing education programs what nursing is—an intellectual as well as a practical enterprise, a science and an art, focused on development and use distinctive of knowledge that "brings with it increased capacity for meaningful service" to human beings (Rogers, 1970, p. xi).

The belief that conceptual models of nursing and nursing theories—rather than a medical point of view, an institutional model, or theories from other disciplines—are the proper starting points for nursing practice, and the belief that nursing research and nursing practice should be guided by explicit nursing discipline-specific C-T-E systems—rather than implicit private images—have permeated the discussion throughout this book. This author is convinced that the discipline of nursing can survive and thrive *only* if nurses celebrate their own heritage and acknowledge their own knowledge base by adopting explicit nursing discipline-specific C-T-E systems to guide their activities. Whether the conceptual model and theories selected by each nurse are among the existing public nursing models or theories or are of his or her own design does not matter; what does matter is that the C-T-E system chosen be explicit and open to public scrutiny. But it is imperative that conceptual models of nursing and nursing theories not be treated as ideologies that cannot be refined, modified, or rejected. Thus the information collected when explicit nursing discipline-specific C-T-E systems are implemented in nursing practice must be used as research data to determine the extent to which the conceptual models are credible and the theories are empirically adequate. Such data will provide the much-needed definitive evidence of best nursing practices within the context of explicit *nursing* knowledge.

 ## REFERENCES

Allison, S.E., & Renpenning, K. (1999). Nursing administration in the 21st century. Thousand Oaks, CA: Sage.

Anderson, C.A. (1995). Scholarship: How important is it? Nursing Outlook, 43, 247–248.

Anderson, C.A. (1998a). Does evidence-based practice equal quality nursing care? Nursing Outlook, 46, 257–258.

Anderson, C.A. (1998b). Nursing: A thinking profession. Nursing Outlook, 46, 197–198.

Anderson, C.A. (1999). Hitting the wall. Nursing Outlook, 47, 153–154.

Barnum, B.S. (1998). The advanced nurse practitioner: Struggling toward a conceptual framework. Nursing Leadership Forum, 3, 14–17.

Barrett, E.A.M. (1993). Nursing centers without nursing frameworks: What's wrong with this picture? Nursing Science Quarterly, 6, 115–117.

Cappell, E., & Leggat, S. (1994). The implementation of theory-based nursing practice: Laying the groundwork for total quality management within a nursing department. Canadian Journal of Nursing Administration, 7, 31–41.

Cash, K. (1990). Nursing models and the idea of nursing. International Journal of Nursing Studies, 27, 249–256.

Chalmers, H., Kershaw, B., Melia, K., & Kendrich, M. (1990). Nursing models: Enhancing or inhibiting practice? Nursing Standard, 5(11), 34–40.

Chinn, P.L. (1999). From the Editor. Advances in Nursing Science, 21(4), v.

Dabbs, A.D.V. (1994). Theory-based nursing practice: For our patients' sake. Clinical Nurse Specialist, 8, 214, 220.

Donaldson, S.K., & Crowley, D.M. (1978). The discipline of nursing. Nursing Outlook, 26, 113–120.

Dubin, R. (1976). Theory building in applied areas. In M.D. Dunnette (Ed.), Handbook of industrial and organizational psychology (pp. 17–39). Chicago: Rand McNally.

Fagin, C.M. (1998). Nursing research and the erosion of care. Nursing Outlook, 46, 259–260.

Fawcett, J. (1983). Hallmarks of success in nursing theory development. In P.L. Chinn (Ed.), Advances in nursing theory development (pp. 3–17). Rockville, MD: Aspen.

Fawcett, J. (1999). The state of nursing science: Hallmarks of the 20th and 21st centuries. Nursing Science Quarterly, 12, 311–315.

Fawcett, J. (2000). The state of nursing science: Where is the nursing in the science? Theoria: Journal of Nursing Theory, 9(3), 3–10.

Fawcett, J. (2001). The nurse theorists: 21st century updates—Rosemarie Rizzo Parse. Nursing Science Quarterly, 14, 126–131.

Fawcett, J. (2003). Guest editorial: On bed baths and conceptual models of nursing. Journal of Advanced Nursing, 44, 229–230.

Fawcett, J., Aber, C., & Weiss, M. (2003). Teaching, practice, and research: An integrative approach benefiting students and faculty. Journal of Professional Nursing, 19, 17–21.

Fawcett, J., & Bourbonniere, M. (2001). Utilization of nursing knowledge and the future of the discipline. In N.L. Chaska (Ed.), The nursing profession: Tomorrow's vision (pp. 311–320). Thousand Oaks, CA: Sage.

Fawcett, J., & Carino, C. (1989). Hallmarks of success in nursing practice. Advances in Nursing Science, 11(4), 1–8.

Feeg, V. (1989). From the editor: Is theory application merely an intellectual exercise? Pediatric Nursing, 15, 450.

Feinstein, A.R. (1967). Clinical judgment. Baltimore: Williams and Wilkins.

Graham, I. (1994). How do registered nurses think and experience nursing: A phenomenological investigation. Journal of Clinical Nursing, 3, 235–242.

Grossman, M., & Hooton, M. (1993). The significance of the relationship between a discipline and its practice. Journal of Advanced Nursing, 18, 866–872.

Hawkins, J.W., & Thibodeau, J.A. (1996). The advanced practice nurse: Current issues (4th ed.). New York: Tiresias Press.

Hayne, Y. (1992). The current status and future significance of nursing as a discipline. Journal of Advanced Nursing, 17, 104–107.

Huch, M.H. (1995). Nursing and the next millennium. Nursing Science Quarterly, 8, 38–44.

Johnson, B., Ludwig-Beymer, P., & Micek, W.T. (1999). Documenting the practice. In P.A. Solari-Twadell & M.A. McDermott (Eds.), Parish nursing: Promoting whole person health within faith communities (pp. 233–245). Thousand Oaks, CA: Sage.

Johnson, D.E. (1990). The behavioral system model for nursing. In M.E. Parker (Ed.), Nursing theories in practice (pp. 23–32). New York: National League for Nursing.

Jukes, M. (1988). Nursing model or psychological assessment? Senior Nurse, 8(11), 8–10.

Kalideen, D. (1993). Is there a place for nursing models in theatre nursing? British Journal of Theatre Nursing, 3(5), 4–6.

Kendrick, K. (1997). What is advanced nursing? Professional Nurse, 12(10), 689.

Kerlinger, F.N. (1979). Behavioral research: A conceptual approach. New York: Holt, Rinehart & Winston.

Kuethe, J.L. (1963). Education: The discipline that concern built. In J. Walton & J.L. Kuethe (Eds.), The discipline of education (pp. 73–84). Madison: University of Wisconsin Press.

Lenz, E.R. (1998). The role of middle-range theory for nursing research and practice. Part 2. Nursing practice. Nursing Leadership Forum, 3, 62–66.

Le Storti, L.J., Cullen, P.A., Hanzlik, E.M., Michiels, J.M., Piano, L.A., Ryan, P.L., & Johnson, W. (1999). Creative thinking in nursing education: Preparing for tomorrow's challenges. Nursing Outlook, 47, 62–66.

Lister, P. (1991). Approaching models of nursing from a postmodernist perspective. Journal of Advanced Nursing, 16, 206–212.

Malin, N., & Teasdale, K. (1991). Caring versus empowerment: Considerations for nursing practice. Journal of Advanced Nursing, 16, 657–662.

Mark, B.A. (2002). What explains nurses' perceptions of staffing adequacy? Journal of Nursing Administration, 32, 234–241.

McBride, A.B. (1999). Breakthroughs in nursing education: Looking back, looking forward. Nursing Outlook, 47, 114–119.

McEwen, M. (2000). Teaching theory at the master's level: Report of a national survey of theory instructors. Journal of Professional Nursing, 16, 354–361.

Meleis, A.I. (1993, April). Nursing research and the Neuman

model: Directions for the future. Panel discussion at the Fourth Biennial International Neuman Systems Model Symposium (B. Neuman, A.I. Meleis, J. Fawcett, L. Lowry, M.C. Smith, A. Edgil, participants), Rochester, NY.

Meleis, A.I. (1997). Theoretical nursing: Definitions and interpretations. In I.M. King & J. Fawcett (Eds.), The language of nursing theory and metatheory (pp. 41–50). Indianapolis: Sigma Theta Tau International Center Nursing Press.

Mitchell, G. (1994). Discipline-specific inquiry: The hermeneutics of theory-guided nursing research. Nursing Outlook, 42, 224–228.

Mitchell, G.J. (2003). Nursing shortage or nursing famine: Looking beyond numbers? Nursing Science Quarterly, 16, 219–224.

Nagle, L.M. (1999). A matter of extinction or distinction. Western Journal of Nursing Research, 21, 71–82.

Neff, M. (1991). President's message: The future of our profession from the eyes of today. American Nephrology Nurses Association Journal, 18, 534.

Nightingale, K. (1993). Editorial. British Journal of Theatre Nursing, 3(5), 2.

Orem, D.E. (1997). Views of human beings specific to nursing. Nursing Science Quarterly, 10, 26–31.

Orem, D.E. (2001). Nursing: Concepts of practice (6th ed.). St. Louis: Mosby.

Orlando, I.J. (1987). Nursing in the 21st century: Alternate paths. Journal of Advanced Nursing, 12, 405–412.

Orr, J. (1991). Knowledge is power. Health Visitor, 64, 218.

Parse, R.R. (1995). Commentary. Parse's theory of human becoming: An alternative guide to nursing practice for pediatric oncology nurses. Journal of Pediatric Oncology Nursing, 12, 128.

Parse, R.R. (1999). Nursing science: The transformation of practice. Journal of Advanced Nursing, 30, 1383–1387.

Perry, J. (1985). Has the discipline of nursing developed to the stage where nurses do 'think nursing'? Journal of Advanced Nursing, 10, 31–37.

Peters, R.S. (1963). Comments [On "A discipline of education."] In J. Walton & J.L. Kuethe (Eds.), The discipline of education (pp. 17–22). Madison: University of Wisconsin Press.

Rawnsley, M.M. (2003). Dimensions of scholarship and the advancement of nursing science: Articulating a vision. Nursing Science Quarterly, 16, 6–13.

Rogers, C.G. (1973). Conceptual models as guides to clinical nursing specialization. Journal of Nursing Education, 12(4), 2–6.

Rogers, M. E. (1970). An introduction to the theoretical basis of nursing. Philadelphia: F. A. Davis.

Rogers, M.E. (1985). The nature and characteristics of profes-

sional education for nursing. Journal of Professional Nursing, 1, 381–383.

Rogers, M.E. (1989). Creating a climate for the implementation of a nursing conceptual framework. Journal of Continuing Education in Nursing, 20, 112–116.

Rolfe, G. (1993). Closing the theory-practice gap: A model of nursing praxis. Journal of Clinical Nursing, 2, 173–177.

Sandelowski, M. (1999). Venous envy: The post-World War II debate over IV nursing. Advances in Nursing Science, 22(1), 52–62.

Scheffler, I. (1963). Is education a discipline? In J. Walton & J.L. Kuethe (Eds.), The discipline of education (pp. 47–61). Madison: University of Wisconsin Press.

Schwab, J. (162). The concept of the structure of a discipline. Educational Record, 43, 197–204.

Shermis, S.S. (1962, November). On becoming an intellectual discipline. Phi Delta Kappan, 84–86.

Sills, G.M. (1983). The role and function of the clinical nurse specialist. In N.L. Chaska (Ed.), The nursing profession: A time to speak (pp. 563–579). New York: McGraw-Hill.

Simpson, J.A., & Weiner, E.S.C. (1989). The Oxford English dictionary (2nd ed.). New York: Oxford University Press.

Smith, M.C. (1995). The core of advanced practice nursing. Nursing Science Quarterly, 8, 2–3.

Speedy, S. (1989). Theory-practice debate: Setting the scene. Australian Journal of Advanced Nursing, 6(3), 12–20.

Thorne, S., Kirkham, S.R., & MacDonald-Emes, J.(1997). Interpretive description: A noncategorical qualitative alternative for developing nursing knowledge. Research in Nursing and Health, 20, 169–177.

Walton, J. (1963). A discipline of education. In J. Walton & J.L. Kuethe (Eds.), The discipline of education (pp. 3–16). Madison: University of Wisconsin Press.

Watson, J. (1997). The theory of human caring: Retrospective and prospective. Nursing Science Quarterly, 10, 49–52.

Watson, M.J. (1996). Watson's theory of transpersonal caring. In P. Hinton Walker & B. Neuman (Eds.), Blueprint for use of nursing models: Education, research, practice, and administration (pp. 141–184). New York: NLN Press.

Watson, J., & Foster, R. (2003). The Attending Nurse Caring Model®: Integrating theory, evidence and advanced caring-healing therapeutics for transforming professional practice. Journal of Clinical Nursing, 12, 360–365.

Whitney, F.W., & Roncoli, M. (1986). Turning clinical problems into research. Heart and Lung, 15, 57–59.

Wood, K.W. (1978). Casework effectiveness: A new look at the research evidence. Social Work, 23, 437–458.

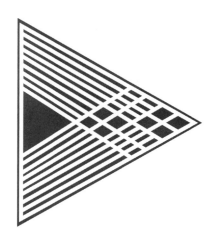

Appendix

Resources for Conceptual Models of Nursing and Nursing Theories*

GENERAL RESOURCES

The initial dates of publication for the major nursing conceptual models, grand theories, and middle-range theories are listed in Table AP–1.

NURSING THEORIES WEBSITES

www.sandiego.edu/nursing/theory/
www.nurses.info/nursing_theory.htm
healthsci.clayton.edu/eichelberger/nursing.htm

Links to websites for Imogene King, Myra Levine, Betty Neuman, Margaret Newman, Dorothea Orem, Rosemarie Parse, Hildegard Peplau, Martha Rogers, Callista Roy, Jean Watson, Virginia Henderson, Florence Nightingale, and other theorists. Links also to websites for nursing conceptual model and theory-related teaching tools and study guides, discussion forums and networking, scholars and experts, books, journals, and conferences and events.

INTERNATIONAL PHILOSOPHY OF NURSING SOCIETY (IPONS)

The purpose of IPONS, which was founded in September 2003, is to form an international network to promote and support the philosophy of nursing. IPONS publishes a

*NOTE: Some audio and video productions may no longer be available directly from the producer/distributor. Internet addresses may change.

journal, *Nursing Philosophy,* and sponsors an annual conference. Website: *www.ipons.dundee.ac.uk*

AUDIO PRODUCTIONS
The Second Annual Nurse Educator Conference

Audiotapes originally available from Teach 'em, Inc., 160 E. Illinois Street, Chicago, IL 60611. (Tapes are no longer available from the distributor.)

Audiotapes of the papers presented at the Nurse Educator Conference held in New York, New York, in December 1978. Presentations are by Johnson, King, Levine, Orem, Rogers, Roy, Newman, and Paterson and Zderad. A presentation by Dickoff and James was also taped.

Nurse Theorist Conference

Audiotapes available from Kennedy Recordings, RR5, Edmonton, Alberta, Canada T5P 4B7.

Audiotapes of the papers presented at the Nurse Theorist Conference held in Edmonton, Alberta, Canada, in August 1984. Presenters include King, Levine, Rogers, Roy, and Newman.

Nursing Theory in Action

Audiotapes available from Kennedy Recordings, RR5, Edmonton, Alberta, Canada T5P 4B7.

Audiotapes of the papers and concurrent sessions on applications to practice, research, and education presented

Publication Date	Nursing Conceptual Model Or Theory
1952	Hildegard Peplau: Theory of Interpersonal Relations (Middle-range theory)
1961	Ida Jean Orlando: Theory of the Deliberative Nursing Process (Middle-range theory)
1969	Myra Levine: Levine's Conservation Model (Conceptual model)
1970	Martha Rogers: Science of Unitary Human Beings (Conceptual model)
1971	Dorothea Orem: Orem's Self-Care Framework (Conceptual model)
1972	Betty Neuman: Neuman's Systems Model (Conceptual model)
1974	Callista Roy: Roy's Adaptation Model (Conceptual model)
1980	Dorothy Johnson: Johnson's Behavioral System Model (Conceptual model)
1981	Imogene King: King's General Systems Framework (Conceptual model)
1981	Rosemarie Parse: Theory of Human Becoming (Grand theory)
1985	Jean Watson: Theory of Human Caring (Middle-range theory)
1986	Margaret Newman: Newman's Theory of Health as Expanding Consciousness (Grand theory)

at the Nursing Theory in Action Conference held in Edmonton, Alberta, Canada, in August 1985. Presenters include King, Levine, Neuman, Orem (presented by S. Taylor), Rogers, Roy, Newman, and Parse. In addition, a presentation on the Roper/Logan/Tierney Framework also is available.

Nursing Theory Congress, 1986
Audiotapes available from Audio Archives International, 100 West Beaver Creek, Unit 18, Richmond Hill, Ontario, Canada L4B 1H4.

Audiotapes of the papers and concurrent sessions on applications to practice, research, and education presented at the Nursing Theory Congress, "Theoretical Pluralism: Direction for a Practice Discipline," held in Toronto, Ontario, Canada in August 1986. Presentations are by

King, Levine, Neuman, Rogers, Roy, Holaday (Johnson's model), Taylor (Orem's framework), Parse, Allen (a developmental health model), Kritek (nursing diagnosis), Dickoff and James (theoretical pluralism), and McGee (criteria for selection and use of a nursing model for practice).

Nursing Theory Congress, 1988
Audiotapes available from Audio Archives International, 100 West Beaver Creek, Unit 18, Richmond Hill, Ontario, Canada L4B 1H4.

Audiotapes of the papers presented at the Nursing Theory Congress, "From Theory to Practice," held in Toronto, Ontario, Canada in August 1988. Presentations are by Parse (nursing science as a basis for research and practice), Watson (one or many models), Henderson

602

(historical perspective), Lindeman (elitism or realism of nursing theory), Moccia (emerging world views), Gordon (nursing diagnosis), and Kritek (agendas for the future). In addition, a panel presentation on the impact of nursing theory on the profession is moderated by Kritek. Concurrent sessions focus on the application of nursing models and theories to practice, education, research, and quality assurance and administration.

VIDEO PRODUCTIONS

The Nurse Theorists: Portraits of Excellence

Videotapes and CD-ROMs available from Fuld Institute for Technology in Nursing Education (FITNE), 5 Depot Street, Athens, OH 45701 (1-800-691-8480; 740-592-2511; E-mail: *info@fitne.net*; Website: *www.fitne.net*).

A series of videotapes, now available as interactive CD-ROMs, funded by the Helene Fuld Health Trust and produced by Studio Three of Samuel Merritt College of Nursing in Oakland, California, depicting the major events and incidents in the lives of 16 nurse theorists. Interviews were conducted by Jacqueline Fawcett. The series includes separate videotapes of Johnson, King, Levine, Neuman, Orem, Rogers, Roy, Leininger, Newman, Orlando, Parse, Peplau, Watson, Rubin, Henderson, and Nightingale.

The Nurse Theorists: Excellence in Action

Videotapes available from Fuld Institute for Technology in Nursing Education (FITNE), 5 Depot Street, Athens, OH 45701 (1-800-691-8480; 740-592-2511; E-mail: info@fitne. net; Website: *www.fitne.net*).

Two videotapes, funded by the Helene Fuld Health Trust and produced by Studio Three of Samuel Merritt College of Nursing in Oakland, California, depicting the implementation of the works of nurse theorists in nursing practice. The series includes separate videotapes of the application of Orem's Self-Care Framework and Roy's Adaptation Model.

Nursing Theory: A Circle of Knowledge

Videotape available from National League for Nursing, 61 Broadway, New York, NY 10006.

Patricia Moccia interviews several nurse theorists, including Orem, Rogers, Roy, Watson, Henderson, and Benner. The discussion emphasizes philosophy of science.

AUDIO AND VIDEO PRODUCTIONS

Nurse Theorist Conference, 1985

Audiotapes and videotapes available from Veranda Communications, Inc., 1200 Delor Avenue, Louisville, KY 40217.

Audiotapes and videotapes from the 1985 Nurse Theorist Conference sponsored by Discovery International, Inc. Audiotaped presentations are by King, Orem, Rogers, Roy, and Parse, followed by critiques of each model or theory. In addition, Peplau presents a historical overview of nursing science, and a panel presentation features all conference speakers. Videotapes are available for the presentations by Orem and Peplau, as well as for the panel presentation.

Nurse Theorist Conference, 1987

Audiotapes and videotapes available from Veranda Communications, Inc., 1200 Delor Avenue, Louisville, KY 40217.

Audiotapes and videotapes from the 1987 Nurse Theorist Conference sponsored by Discovery International, Inc. Presentations are by King, Rogers, Roy, Parse, and Watson. In addition, Peplau presents a paper on the art and science of nursing, Schlotfeldt presents a paper on nursing science in the twenty-first century, and a panel presentation features all conference speakers. Audiotapes are also available of the small group sessions led by King, Rogers, Roy, Parse, and Watson.

Nurse Theorist Conference, 1989

Audiotapes and videotapes available from Veranda Communications, Inc., 1200 Delor Avenue, Louisville, KY 40217.

Audiotapes and videotapes from the 1989 Nurse Theorist Conference sponsored by Discovery International, Inc. Presentations are by King, Neuman, Rogers, and Parse. In addition, Meleis presents a paper on being and becoming healthy, Pender presents a paper on expression of health through beliefs and actions, and a panel presentation features all conference speakers.

Nurse Theorist Conference, 1993

Audiotapes and videotapes available from Veranda Communications, Inc., 1200 Delor Avenue, Louisville, KY 40217.

Audiotapes and videotapes from the 1993 Nurse Theorist Conference sponsored by Discovery International, Inc. Presentations are by King, Parse, Peplau, and Rogers. In addition, M.C. Smith, C. Forchuk, G.J. Mitchell, and J. Chapman present a session on nursing theory–based research and practice in Canada, and a panel presentation features all conference speakers.

National Nursing Theory Conference, 1990

Audiotapes available from Convention Recorders, 5401 Linda Vista Road, Suite C, San Diego, CA 92110.

Videotape available from UCLA Neuropsychiatric Institute and Hospital, Nursing Department, 760 Westwood Plaza, Room 17–364, Los Angeles, CA 90024–1759.

Audiotapes of the papers presented at the National Nursing Theory Conference held at the University of California-Los Angeles Neuropsychiatric Institute and Hospital in September 1990. Presentations are by Flaskerud, Fawcett, and Meleis, as well as by numerous nurses who report the results of their use of the works of Johnson, Neuman, Orem, Rogers, Roy, and Parse. In addition, both audiotapes and videotapes of a panel presentation featuring the nurse theorists, which is moderated by Randell, are available.

SPECIFIC RESOURCES

KING'S CONCEPTUAL SYSTEM AND THEORY OF GOAL ATTAINMENT
Contact Imogene King directly via e-mail at *imkn@earthlink.net*

LEVINE'S CONSERVATION MODEL
Website:*www2.oakland.edu/nursing/levinebib.cfm*
Or link to this home page through *www.sandiego.edu/nursing/theory/*

NEUMAN'S SYSTEMS MODEL
Neuman Systems Model Archives
    Neumann College Library
    One Neumann Drive
    Aston, PA 19014–1298
    610-361-5206; 610-558-5545
    Websites:*www.neumansystemsmodel.com*
Or link to this home page through: *www.sandiego.edu/nursing/theory/*
Neuman News is available on the Neuman Systems Model Website.

OREM'S SELF-CARE FRAMEWORK
International Orem Society for Nursing Science and Scholarship
    Sinclair School of Nursing
    University of Missouri–Columbia
    Columbia, MO 65211
Websites:*www.muhealth.org/%7Enursing/scdnt/scdnt.html*
Link to other Orem Self-Care Framework websites through *www.sandiego.edu/nursing/theory/*

Video Productions
Teaching the Self-Care Deficit Nursing Theory
Videotapes available from Media Sales, Biomedical Communications, University of British Columbia, 2194 Health Sciences Mall, Room B-32, Vancouver, British Columbia, Canada V6T 1Z3.

Eight videotapes, which were produced by the Vancouver Health Department, explain the content and use of Orem's Self-Care Framework in nursing practice. A teaching manual and a facilitator's manual are included with the package of videotapes. The package is designed for use by individuals or groups.

Care with a Concept
Videotape available from Health Sciences Consortium, 201 Cedar Court, Chapel Hill, NC 27514.

Mary Hale and Gates Rhodes of the University of Pennsylvania School of Nursing produced this videotape documenting the use of Orem's Self-Care Framework at Children's Seashore House, when it was located in Atlantic City, New Jersey.

Care Plans That Work
Videotape available from St. Clare Hospital Video Productions, Dept. No. BB, 515 22nd Avenue, Monroe, WI 53566.

An instructional video that demonstrates the use of Orem's Self-Care Framework and Roy's Adaptation Model to guide nursing care planning.

ROGERS' SCIENCE OF UNITARY HUMAN BEINGS
Website:*medweb.uwcm.ac.uk/martha*
Or link to this home page through *www.sandiego.edu/nursing/theory/*
The Martha E. Rogers Center
    Dr. Joanne Griffin, Director
    New York University
    Steinhardt School of Education
    Division of Nursing
    246 Greene Street
    New York, NY 10003–5300
    212-998-5324
    Society of Rogerian Scholars, Inc.
    Canal Street Station
    P.O. Box 1195
    New York, NY 10013
Instructions for subscribing to the Rogers listserv are available at: *http://groups.yahoo.com/group/Martha_E.Rogers*
The Martha E. Rogers Collection
    Boston University
    Mugar Library Department of Special Collections
    History of Nursing Archives
    Boston, MA
    617-353-3696
    e-mail: *speccol@bu.edu*
    See *Visions: The Journal of Rogerian Nursing Science, 8,* 74, 2000, for a discussion about the archives.

Video Production
The Art of Nursing
Videotape and workbook available from Personalized Nursing Corporation, P.C.,

575 S. Main Street, Plymouth, MI 48170.

Interactive videotape featuring Marcia Anderson, who explains her Personalized LIGHT Model, which is derived from Rogers' Science of Unitary Human Beings, and applies the model with her own patients.

ROY'S ADAPTATION MODEL
Roy Adaptation Association
Sister Callista Roy
William F. Connell School of Nursing
Boston College
140 Commonwealth Avenue
Chestnut Hill, MA 02467
617-552-8862
e-mail: *callista.roy@bc.edu*
Website:*www2.bc.edu/~royca/htm/ram.htm*
Or link to this home page through*www.sandiego.edu/nursing/theory/*

NEWMAN'S THEORY OF HEALTH AS EXPANDING CONSCIOUSNESS
Website:*www.healthasexpandingconsciousness.org/*
Or link to this website through *www.sandiego.edu/nursing/theory/*

Margaret Newman's professional papers are stored in the Health Sciences Historical Collections in the University of Tennessee Health Sciences Library. Contact:
Richard Nollan
Assistant Professor and Curator
Health Sciences Historical Collections
University of Tennessee Health Sciences Center
877 Madison Avenue
Memphis, TN 38163
901-338-6053
rnollan@utmem.edu
http://library.utmem.edu/HSLBC/history
See Nursing Science Quarterly, 14, 254, July 2001.

ORLANDO'S THEORY OF THE DELIBERATIVE NURSING PROCESS
Website:*www.uri.edu/nursing/schmieding/orlando/*
Or link to this website through *www.sandiego.edu/nursing/theory/*

PARSE'S THEORY OF HUMAN BECOMING
International Consortium of Parse Scholars
P.O. Box 94058
3332 Yonge Street
Toronto, Ontario, Canada M4N 3R1
Website:*www.humanbecoming.org/*
Or link to this website through *www.sandiego.edu/nursing/theory/*
Listserv: PARSE-L

To Subscribe to Parse-L, send an e-mail to: *listserv@listserv.utoronto.ca*

In the body of the note say ONLY: sub parse-L yourfirstname yourlastname

For further information contact Pat Lyon *pat.lyon@sympatico.ca*

Institute of Human Becoming
Discovery International, Inc.
P.O. Box 22034
Pittsburgh, PA 15222
412-391-8471 (office)
412-391-8458 (fax)
Website: *www.discoveryinternationalonline.com*

Audio Productions
Research Seminar: Research Related to Man-Living-Health: An Emerging Methodology
Audiotapes available from Meetings Internationale, Ltd., 1200 Delor Avenue, Louisville, KY 40217.

Audiotapes from a research seminar sponsored by Discovery International, Inc., with a paper by Parse describing her research methodology, papers by Sklar and M.J. Smith reporting research results, and a panel discussion moderated by M. Smith.

Research Seminar: Research and Practice Related to Parse's Theory of Nursing
Audiotapes available from Meetings Internationale, Ltd., 1200 Delor Avenue, Louisville, KY 40217.

Audiotapes from a research seminar sponsored by Discovery International, Inc. Parse describes her research and practice methodologies; Cody, Beauchamp, and M. Smith report results of their research; and Menke critiques the research reports. In addition, Mitchell and Santopinto discuss their experiences using Parse's theory in practice, and Menke moderates a panel discussion.

Research Seminar: Guided Practice in Qualitative Research
Audiotapes available from Meetings Internationale, Ltd., 1200 Delor Avenue, Louisville, KY 40217.

Audiotapes from a research seminar sponsored by Discovery International, Inc., with four papers by Parse describing qualitative and quantitative research methodology, the phenomenological method (two parts), and the ethnographic method; and two papers by

M.J. Smith describing the descriptive method and other qualitative methods.

Research Seminar: General Topics
Audiotape available from Meetings Internationale, Ltd., 1200 Delor Avenue, Louisville, KY 40217.

Audiotape of a paper by Parse discussing nursing education in the twenty-first century.

Video Productions
The Theory of Human Becoming: Living
True Presence in Nursing Practice
The Lived Experience of Serenity
Available from Pat Lyon, 1 Meredith Avenue, Cobourg, Ontario, Canada K9A 4G6; 905-377-1665 (phone), 905-377-1533 (fax); e-mail: *pat.lyon@sympatico.ca*

Order form available at *www.humanbecoming.org/*

Print Resources
The Theory of Human Becoming:
A Learning Guide (2nd ed.)
Available from Pat Lyon, 1 Meredith Avenue, Cobourg, Ontario, Canada K9A 4G6; 905-377-1665 (phone), 905-377-1533 (fax); e-mail: *pat.lyon@sympatico.ca*

Order form available at *www.humanbecoming.org/*

Patient Focused Care: Sailing Beyond the Boundaries at Sunnybrook Health Science Centre
Available from Donna Empacher, Sunnybrook Health Science Centre, D404A-2075 Bayview Avenue, North York, Ontario, Canada M4N, 3M5; 416-480-5207 (fax)

Simple Things: Writings of Human Becoming by Sandra Schmidt Bunkers
Available from Health Connections/Simple Things, 1119 Plum Creed Road, Sioux Falls, SD 57105

Order form available at *www.humanbecoming.org/*

Mitchell, G.J., & Bournes, D.A. (1998). *Finding the way: A guide to patient focused care.* Toronto: Sunnybrook and Women's College Health Sciences Centre.

PEPLAU'S THEORY OF INTERPERSONAL RELATIONS
Website:*publish.uwo.ce/%7Ecforchuck/peplau/hpcb. html/*
Or link to this website through *www.sandiego.edu/ nursing/theory/*

Audio Production
Life of an Angel: An Interview with Hildegard Peplau
Audiotape available from American Psychiatric Nurses Association, 1200 19th St. NW, Suite 300, Washington DC 20036–2422, 202-857-1133, 202-223-4579 (fax). An interview with Hildegard Peplau conducted by Dr. Frederic Flach in 1998.

WATSON'S THEORY OF HUMAN CARING
Website: *www2.uchsc.edu/son/caring/content/*Or link to this website through *www.sandiego.edu/nursing/theory/*
Listserv: Carenet
To subscribe, send mail to *LISTSERV@ADMIN. HUMBERC.ON.CA* with the command: *SUBSCRIBE CARENETL*
International Association for Human Caring
2090 Linglestown Road
Suite 107
Harrisburg, PA 17110
Phone: 717-703-0033; Fax: 717- 234-6798
Website:*www.humancaring.org/*
Or link to this website through *www.sandiego.edu/nursing/ theory/*

Video Productions
A Guide to Applying the Art and Science of Human Caring: A Consultation with Jean Watson and Colleagues
Videotapes available from National League for Nursing, 61 Broadway, New York, NY 10006. Telephone: 800-669-1656; 212-363-5555

Two videotapes demonstrate the use of Watson's Theory of Human Caring in nursing practice. The first tape is an interview with Jean Watson and includes a concise overview of the theory. The second tape is a panel discussion with Watson and her colleagues, including Peggy Chinn, Ruth Neill, Jan Nyberg, and Carol Montgomery, that focuses on strategies used to implement the Theory of Human Caring in diverse practice settings.

Theories at Work
Videotape available from National League for Nursing, 61 Broadway, New York, NY 10006. Telephone: 800-669-1656; 212-363-5555.

Videotape of innovative applications of nursing theory in actual practice settings. Patricia Moccia interviews Jean Watson, Janet Quinn, Dorothy Powell, Bernadine Lacey, Sunny Sutton, and Maria Mitchell. Coverage includes the work with the homeless spearheaded by Powell and Lacey at Howard University College of Nursing, and the Center for Human Caring (Watson and Quinn). Sutton and Mitchell discuss the importance of home care, which they contend will be the major health care delivery system of the future.

A Conversation on Caring with Jean Watson and Janet Quinn
Videotape available from National League for Nursing, 61 Broadway, New York, NY 10006.Telephone: 800-669-1656; 212-363-5555.

Videotape of Patricia Moccia's interviews with Jean Watson and Janet Quinn. Watson and Quinn discuss their views of human caring and health. Coverage includes the Denver Nursing Project in Human Caring, which focuses on individuals with acquired immunodeficiency syndrome (AIDS), and Quinn's Senior Citizen's Therapeutic Touch Education Program.

COMPUTER SEARCH STRATEGIES

NOTE: The search strategies given here yielded the most targeted searches in 2003. Inasmuch as different vendors may use different keywords, readers are advised to seek help from a librarian if the strategies given here are not effective at a later time. Readers also are advised to read abstracts and articles carefully to determine if the indexing is accurate.

Cumulative Index to Nursing and Allied Health Literature

The Cumulative Index to Nursing and Allied Health Literature (CINAHL) may be accessed via various on-line vendors (e.g., OVID, First Search), CD-ROMs available at libraries, and other databases. The headings listed below yield the most relevant citations for specific conceptual models of nursing and nursing theories when searching CINAHL:

> Johnson-Behavioral-System-Model
> King-Open-Systems-Model
> Kings-Theory-of-Goal-Attainment
> Levine-Conservation-Model
> Neuman-Systems-Model
> Orem-Self-Care-Model
> Rogers-Science-of-Unitary-Human-Beings
> Roy-Adaptation-Model
> Newman-Health-Model
> Orlandos-Nursing-Theory
> Parses-Theory-of-Human-Becoming
> Peplau-Interpersonal-Relations-Model
> Watsons-Theory-of-Caring

Citations for general literature about conceptual models and theories can be obtained using the following headings:

> Nursing-Models-Theoretical
> Conceptual-Framework
> Nursing-Theory

Before 1988, the most relevant citations for specific conceptual models of nursing and nursing theories in the CINAHL database can be located by using the following subject headings. The same subject headings can be used to locate citations for general materials about nursing models and theories.

> Models-Theoretical
> Nursing-Theory

Medline

Medline may be accessed via on-line PubMed, various on-line vendors (e.g., OVID, First Search), and other data-

bases. The following subject headings yield the most relevant citations for *conceptual models of nursing* when searching Medline:

> Nursing Models
> Nursing Theories

Dissertation Abstracts International

Dissertation Abstracts International (DAI), which also includes Master's Abstracts, may be accessed via various on-line vendors (e.g., First Search) and other databases, including ProQuest (*wwwlib.umi.com/dissertations/*). The search strategies listed below yield the most relevant citations for conceptual models of nursing and nursing theories when searching DAI:

> behavioral system (keyword) AND nursing (subject)
> King (keyword) AND nursing (subject)
> King's (keyword) AND nursing (subject)
> goal attainment (keyword) AND nursing (subject)
> Levine (keyword) AND nursing (subject)
> Levine's (keyword) AND nursing (subject)
> conservation (keyword) AND nursing (subject)
> Neuman (keyword) AND nursing (subject)
> Neuman's (keyword) AND nursing (subject)
> Orem's (keyword) AND nursing (subject)
> science of unitary human beings (keyword) AND nursing (subject)
> Roy's (keyword) AND nursing (subject)
> adaptation model (keyword) AND nursing (subject)
> Newman's (keyword) AND nursing (subject)
> expanded consciousness (keyword) AND nursing (subject)
> Orlando's (keyword) AND nursing (subject)
> Parse's (keyword) AND nursing (subject)
> human becoming (keyword) AND nursing (subject)
> Peplau's (keyword) AND nursing (subject)
> Watson's (keyword) AND nursing (subject)

Sigma Theta Tau International Registry of Nursing Research

The Sigma Theta Tau International Registry of Nursing Research is available on-line via the Virginia Henderson International Nursing Library. The Registry and other research-oriented databases provided by the Virginia Henderson International Nursing Library contain information on both completed and ongoing research. Contact Sigma Theta Tau International, 550 W. North Street, Indianapolis, IN 46209–0209, 1-888-634-7575, 317-634-8171, for instructions on access to the on-line databases.

Websites: *www.nursingsociety.org* and *www.stti.iupui.edu/library/*

The subject headings for conceptual models of nursing and nursing theories are as follows:

> Johnson Behavioral System

King Interacting System
Levine Conservation
Neuman Systems
Orem Self Care
Rogers' Science of Unitary Human Beings
Roy Adaptation
Newman Health
Orlando
Parse Man-Living-Health

Peplau Interpersonal Relations
Watson Human Caring

A discussion of computer and hand searches is given in Johnson, E.D. (1989). In search of applications of nursing theories: The Nursing Citation Index. Bulletin of the Medical Library Association, 77, 176–184. See also Allen, M. Searching bibliographic databases for nursing theory. On-line at *www.sandiego.edu/nursing/theory/student.htm*

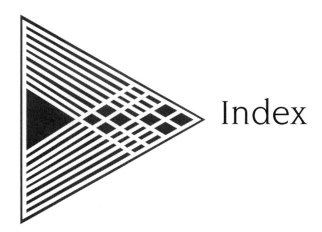

Index

Page numbers followed by f indicate figures; page numbers followed by t indicate tables.

ISBN 13: 978-0-8036-1194-8
ISBN 10: 0-8036-1194-3

9 780803 611948